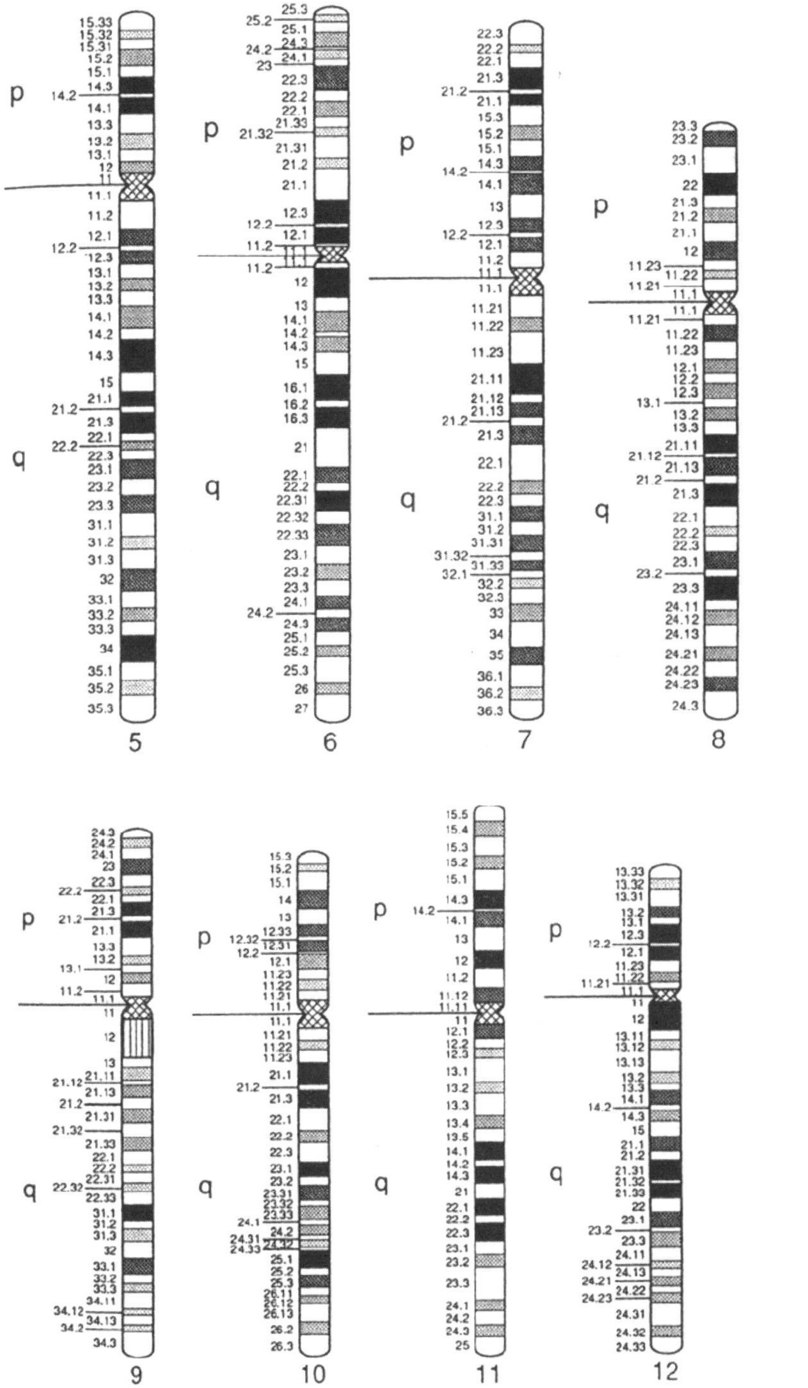

Figure Continued

OXFORD MEDICAL PUBLICATIONS

Oxford Desk Reference
Clinical genetics

Cover image: The polydactyl hands image is reproduced here from Winship, W.S. (2003). *Handbook of Genetics and Congenital Syndromes for Southern Africa*, Oxford University Press Southern Africa, with permission from Oxford University Press Southern Africa.

Oxford Desk Reference
Clinical genetics

Helen V. Firth

Consultant Clinical Geneticist, Addenbrooke's
Hospital, Cambridge, UK

Jane A. Hurst

Consultant in Clinical Genetics, Oxford Radcliffe
Hospitals, Oxford, UK

with

Judith G. Hall (Consulting Editor)

Emeritus Professor of Pediatrics and Medical
Genetics, University of British Columbia,
Vancouver, Canada

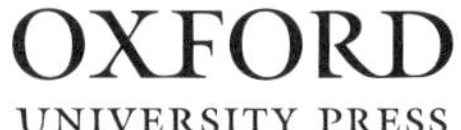

OXFORD

UNIVERSITY PRESS

OXFORD
UNIVERSITY PRESS

Great Clarendon Street, Oxford OX2 6DP

Oxford University Press is a department of the University of Oxford.
It furthers the University's objective of excellence in research, scholarship,
and education by publishing worldwide in

Oxford New York

Auckland Cape Town Dar es Salaam Hong Kong Karachi
Kuala Lumpur Madrid Melbourne Mexico City Nairobi
New Delhi Shanghai Taipei Toronto

With offices in

Argentina Austria Brazil Chile Czech Republic France Greece
Guatemala Hungary Italy Japan Poland Portugal Singapore
South Korea Switzerland Thailand Turkey Ukraine Vietnam

Oxford is a registered trade mark of Oxford University Press
in the UK and in certain other countries

Published in the United States
by Oxford University Press Inc., New York

© Oxford University Press, 2005

The moral rights of the authors have been asserted
Database right Oxford University Press (maker)

First published 2005
Reprinted 2005, 2006 (twice), 2007 (with correction), 2008

All rights reserved. No part of this publication may be reproduced,
stored in a retrieval system, or transmitted, in any form or by any means,
without the prior permission in writing of Oxford University Press,
or as expressly permitted by law, or under terms agreed with the appropriate
reprographics rights organization. Enquiries concerning reproduction
outside the scope of the above should be sent to the Rights Department,
Oxford University Press, at the address above

You must not circulate this book in any other binding or cover
and you must impose the same condition on any acquirer

British Library Cataloguing in Publication Data
Data available

Library of Congress Cataloging in Publication Data
Oxford desk reference : clinical genetics / Helen V. Firth,
Jane A. Hurst, with Judith G. Hall (consulting editor).

Includes bibliographical references and index.
1. Medical genetics—Handbooks, Manuals, etc.
[DNLM: 1. Genetics, Medical—Handbooks. 2. Chromosome Aberrations—Handbooks.
3. Genetic Diseases, Inborn—Handbooks. 4. Genetic Predisposition to
Disease—Handbooks. QZ 39 FS270 2005]
I. Title: Desk reference: clinical genetics. II. Hurst, Jane A.
III. Hall, Judith G. IV. Title.
RB155.F55 2005 616'.042—dc22 2004029397

Typeset by Newgen Imaging Systems (P) Ltd., Chennai, India
Printed in Great Britain
on acid-free paper by
Biddles Ltd, King's Lynn

ISBN 978-0-19-262896-1 (Hbk.)

10 9 8 7 6

Preface

When Helen and Jane asked me whether a desk reference in clinical genetics would be useful, I, enthusiastically replied 'yes'. Who has not been asked to see a child on the ward and not been able to remember the approach to a relatively common, but recently forgotten disorder? During an outreach clinic, you are scheduled to see a family with a common disorder and they turn out to have two or three rare complications, and you do not have access to 'real' textbooks. You get a call from a good colleague who asks you 'simple' questions about the workings of a well-known syndrome and you do not want to appear stupid to your friend. This book can be your 'lifesaver' in many situations.

The book includes many common sense approaches, useful standards and definitions, suggestions for appropriate testing, and excellent references. It is meant to be 'first line' and a way to jog your memory. Certainly, you will need to consult other texts and data sources. However, this book can be carried around in your briefcase or handbag—so to speak a peripheral brain. Blank pages are distributed throughout the book to enable you to update and personalize your copy with notes from current journals, guidelines, seminars, and lectures.

If it turns out to be useful, and I certainly expect that it will, there will surely be additional editions. The authors would therefore like feedback and suggestions. Genetic information is changing so quickly that a 2-year half-life can be expected.

Medical genetics registrars, residents, and fellows should particularly find this book useful, but I would anticipate that the mature and experienced clinical geneticist would also find it useful and thoughtfully constructed.

If you are the lucky new purchaser of *Oxford Desk Reference*: Clinical Genetics, 'Congratulations'. If you are considering buying it—'do it'. If you need an easy to use, handy reference that can be carried around so you appear more competent and well informed—'don't hesitate'.

Enjoy this new approach.

Judith G Hall, OC, MD, FRCP(C), FAAP, FCCMG, FABMG
Emeritus Professor of Pediatrics and Medical Genetics, University of British Columbia,
Vancouver, Canada

Companion web site: www.oup.com/uk/booksites/content/0192628968

Acknowledgements

In writing this book we are indebted to the many colleagues and friends who have kindly given of their time and expertise to review each section of the book. Their wide experience of particular clinical areas has enhanced the book in many ways, improving accuracy and clarity and ensuring that the entries are as up to date as we can make them. We owe special thanks to Martin Bobrow, Katie Bushby, Lyn Chitty, Angus Clarke, Jill Clayton-Smith, Dian Donnai, Ian Frayling, Tony Moore, Danielle Pilz, Jo Poulton, Virginia Sybert, Andrew Wilkie, and Ian Young who each advised on several sections, to Rachel Firth for her help with some of the illustrations to Sandra Wombwell for secretarial assistance, and to Mark Bateman for his help in preparing the karyotypes. Thanks also to Catherine Barnes at Oxford University Press for her commitment to this project over several years and to Laura Johnstone for overseeing the production of the book.

We also owe a debt of gratitude to Judy for her sustained encouragement and enthusiasm and especially to our husbands and children for their love and forbearance.

Reviews

'It is very refreshing to review a book written for clinicians by clinicians, which is in a format that reflects situations actually encountered in practice. Information provided by the referring doctor to a clinical geneticist or other specialist before a clinic or ward consultation is usually limited. This new text takes common referral indications and, in a standardized format that manages to be brief and clear without skimping on detail, reminds the clinician of diagnostic possibilities and strategies for investigation and management. This will allow the best possible use to be made of an individual consultation by both the patient and the doctor.'

Dian Donnai, Professor of Medical Genetics, University of Manchester, Consultant Clinical Geneticist, Regional Genetics Service, St Mary's Hospital, Manchester, UK.

'I have been impressed with the thoughtfulness of the topics. This should be a great help to many people who are part of the clinical genetics team....There are up-to-date summaries for the staff member who needs a refresher, as well as the glossary and the headings on fundamental topics, like AD inheritance, for those just starting out.'

Lewis B. Holmes, Professor of Pediatrics, Harvard Medical School and Chief, Genetics and Teratology Unit, Massachusetts General Hospital for Children, Boston, Massachusetts, USA.

'This is going to be an extremely useful reference source. The authors have done an outstanding job of summarizing, in one or two pages, pertinent recommendations regarding diagnoses and management of specific disorders as well as practical approaches to a variety of problems that commonly present in real life.'

Marilyn Jones, Adjunct Professor of Pediatrics, University of California, San Diego and Director, Dysmorphology and Genetics, Children's Hospital San Diego, San Diego, California, USA.

Brief contents

Detailed contents *xi*
System-based contents *xv*
Glossary of terms used in dysmorphology *xix*
Glossary of terms used in genetics *xxiv*
Abbreviations *xxxiii*
Expert advisers *xli*

1 **Introduction** — 1

2 **Clinical approach** — 37

3 **Common consultations** — 259

4 **Cancer** — 425

5 **Chromosomes** — 489

6 **Pregnancy and fertility** — 565

Appendix — 645

Index *701*

Detailed contents

System-based contents *xv*
Glossary of terms used in dysmorphology *xix*
Glossary of terms used in genetics *xxiv*
Abbreviations *xxxiii*
Expert advisers *xli*

1 Introduction *1*

Adoption *2*
Approach to the consultation with a child with dysmorphism, congenital malformation, or developmental delay *4*
Autosomal dominant (AD) inheritance *6*
Autosomal recessive (AR) inheritance *8*
Communication skills *10*
Confidentiality *12*
Confirmation of diagnosis *14*
Consent for genetic testing *16*
The genetic code and mutations *18*
Genomic imprinting *20*
Mitochondrial inheritance *22*
Multifactorial inheritance *24*
Reproductive options *26*
Testing for genetic status *28*
Useful resources *30*
X-linked dominant (XLD) inheritance *32*
X-linked recessive (XLR) inheritance *34*

2 Clinical approach *37*

Ambiguous genitalia (including sex reversal) *38*
Anal anomalies (atresia, stenosis) *42*
Anterior segment eye malformations *46*
Arthrogryposis (arthrogryposis multiplex congenita) *48*
Ataxic adult *50*
Ataxic child *52*
Brachydactyly *56*
Broad thumbs *58*
Cardiomyopathy in children under 10 years *60*
Cataract *64*
Cerebellar anomalies *66*
Cerebral palsy *70*
Chondrodysplasia punctata *72*
Cleft lip and palate *74*
Coarse facial features *78*
Coloboma *82*
Congenital heart disease *84*
Corneal clouding *88*

Severe deafness in early childhood *90*
Developmental delay in the child with consanguineous parents *94*
Developmental regression *96*
Duane retraction syndrome *100*
Dysmorphic child *102*
Dystonia *106*
Ear anomalies *108*
Facial asymmetry *112*
Failure to thrive *116*
Floppy infant *118*
Fractures *122*
Generalized disorders of skin pigmentation (including albinism) *126*
Hemihypertrophy and limb asymmetry *128*
Holoprosencephaly (HPE) *130*
Hydrocephalus *134*
Hypermobile joints *138*
Hypoglycaemia in the neonate and infant *140*
Hypospadias *142*
Increased bone density *144*
Large fontanelle *146*
Laterality disorders including heterotaxy and isomerism *148*
Leukodystrophy/leukoencephalopathy *150*
Limb reduction defects *152*
Lissencephaly and neuronal migration disorders *156*
Lumps and bumps *160*
Macrocephaly *162*
Mental retardation with apparent X-linked inheritance *164*
Mental retardation *168*
Microcephaly *172*
Micrognathia and Robin sequence *174*
Microphthalmia and anophthalmia *176*
Minor congenital anomalies *180*
Nasal anomalies *182*
Neonatal encephalopathy and intractable seizures in the neonate *186*
Nystagmus *190*
Obesity with and without developmental delay *192*
Ocular hypertelorism *196*
Oedema—generalized or puffy extremities *198*
Oesophageal and intestinal atresia (including tracheo-oesophageal fistula) *200*

Optic nerve hypoplasia 204
Overgrowth 206
Patchy hypomelanotic skin lesions 208
Patchy pigmented skin lesions
(including café-au-lait spots) 210
Plagiocephaly and abnormalities of
skull shape 212
Postaxial polydactyly 214
Preaxial polydactyly 218
Prolonged neonatal jaundice and jaundice in
infants below 6 months 220
Ptosis, blepharophimosis, and other eyelid
anomalies 224
Radial ray defects and thumb hypoplasia 228
Retinal dysplasia 230
Retinal receptor dystrophies 232
Scalp defects 236
Seizures with developmental delay/mental
retardation 238
Short stature 242
Skeletal dysplasia 246
Structural intracranial anomalies (agenesis
of the corpus callosum, septo-optic dysplasia,
and arachnoid cysts) 248
Suspected non-accidental injury 252
Syndactyly (other than 2, 3 toe syndactyly) 254
Unusual hair, teeth, nails, and skin 256

3 **Common consultations** 259

Achondroplasia 260
Autosomal dominant polycystic kidney
disease (ADPKD) 262
X-linked adrenoleukodystrophy (X-ALD) 264
Alpha₁-antitrypsin deficiency 266
Alport syndrome 268
Androgen insensitivity syndrome (AIS) 270
Angelman syndrome 272
Autism and austism spectrum disorders 274
Beckwith–Wiedemann syndrome (BWS) 278
Congenital adrenal hyperplasia (CAH) 282
Consanguinity 284
Craniosynostosis 288
Cystic fibrosis (CF) 292
Dementia 296
Diabetes mellitus 298
Dilated cardiomyopathy (DCM) 302
DNA repair defects 304
Duchenne and Becker muscular dystrophy
(DMD and BMD) 308
Ehlers–Danlos syndrome (EDS) 312
Epilepsy in infants and children 314
Epilepsy 318

Facioscapulohumeral muscular dystrophy
(FSHD) 322
Fragile X syndrome (FRAX) 324
Glaucoma 328
Haemochromatosis 330
Haemoglobinopathies 334
Haemophilia and other inherited coagulation
disorders 338
Hereditary haemorrhagic
telangiectasia (HHT) 342
Hereditary motor and sensory neuropathy
(HMSN) 344
Hereditary spastic paraplegias (HSP) 348
Hirschsprung disease 352
Huntington disease (HD) 354
Hyperlipidaemia 358
Hypertrophic cardiomyopathy (HCM) 360
Immunodeficiency and recurrent
infection 364
Incest 370
Leigh encephalopathy 372
Limb girdle muscular dystrophies 374
Long QT and Brugada syndromes 378
Marfan syndrome 380
Mitochondrial DNA diseases 384
Myotonic dystrophy (DM) 388
Neural tube defects 392
Neurofibromatosis type 1 (NF1) 396
Noonan syndrome (NS) 402
Parkinson disease 404
Retinitis pigmentosa (RP) 406
Rett syndrome 408
Sensitivity to anaesthetic agents 410
Spinal muscular atrophy (SMA) 412
Stickler syndrome 414
Thrombophilia 416
Tuberous sclerosis (TSC) 420

4 **Cancer** 425

BRCA1 and BRCA2 426
Breast cancer 430
Cancer surveillance methods 434
Colorectal cancer (CRC) 436
Confirmation of diagnosis of cancer 440
Cowden syndrome (CS) 442
Familial adenomatous polyposis (FAP) 444
Gastric cancer 450
Gorlin syndrome 452
Hereditary nonpolyposis colorectal cancer
(HNPCC) 454
Juvenile polyposis syndrome (JPS) 460

Lifestyle factors in cancer: smoking, alcohol, obesity, diet, and exercise 462
Li–Fraumeni syndrome (LFS) 464
Multiple endocrine neoplasia (MEN) 466
Neurofibromatosis type 2 (NF2) 470
Ovarian cancer 472
Peutz–Jeghers syndrome (PJS) 474
Phaeochromocytoma 478
Retinoblastoma 480
von Hippel–Lindau (VHL) disease 484
Wilms tumour 486

5 **Chromosomes** 489

22q11 deletion syndrome 490
47,XXX 494
47,XXY 496
47,XYY 498
Autosomal reciprocal translocations—background 500
Autosomal reciprocal translocations—familial 504
Autosomal reciprocal translocations—postnatal 506
Autosomal reciprocal translocations—prenatal 508
Cell division—mitosis, meiosis, and non-disjunction 510
Chromosomal mosaicism—postnatal 514
Chromosomal mosaicism—prenatal 516
Deletions and duplications 520
Down syndrome (trisomy 21) 524
Edwards' syndrome (trisomy 18) 526
Inversions 528
Mosaic trisomy 8 530
Mosaic trisomy 16 532
Patau syndrome (trisomy 13) 534
Prenatal diagnosis of sex chromosome aneuploidy 536
Ring chromosomes 538
Robertsonian translocations 540
Sex chromosome mosaicism 544
Submicroscopic chromosomal abnormalities and the chromosomal phenotype 546
Supernumerary marker chromosomes (SMCs)—postnatal 552
Supernumerary marker chromosomes (SMCs)—prenatal 554
Triploidy (69,XXX, 69,XXY, or 69,XYY) 556
Turner syndrome, 45,X and variants 558
X-autosome translocations 562

6 **Pregnancy and fertility** 565

Anterior abdominal wall defects 566
Assisted reproductive technology: *in vitro* fertilization (IVF), intracytoplasmic sperm injection (ICSI), and pre-implantation genetic diagnosis (PGD) 568
Bowed limbs 572
Club-foot (talipes) 574
Congenital cystic lung lesions, Currarino syndrome, and sacrococcygeal teratoma 576
Congenital diaphragmatic hernia 578
Cytomegalovirus (CMV) 580
Dandy–Walker malformation 582
Drugs in pregnancy 584
Female infertility and amenorrhoea: genetic aspects 586
Fetal alcohol syndrome (FAS) 588
Fetal anticonvulsant syndrome (FACS) 590
Fetomaternal alloimmunization (rhesus D and thrombocytopenia) 592
Hyperechogenic bowel 594
Hypoplastic left heart 596
Imaging in prenatal diagnosis 598
Invasive techniques and genetic tests in prenatal diagnosis 600
Low maternal serum oestriol 604
Male infertility: genetic aspects 606
Maternal age 610
Maternal diabetes mellitus and diabetic embryopathy 612
Maternal phenylketonuria (PKU) 614
Miscarriage and recurrent miscarriage 616
Oedema—increased nuchal translucency, cystic hygroma, and hydrops 618
Premature ovarian failure (POF) 620
Radiation exposure chemotherapy and landfill sites 622
Renal tract anomalies 624
Rubella 628
Short limbs 630
Toxoplasmosis 634
Twins and twinning 636
Varicella 640
Ventriculomegaly 642

Appendix 645

Bayes' theorem 646
Behavioural pattern profile (Shalev and Hall 2004) 648
Carrier frequency and carrier testing for autosomal recessive disorders 650

Centile charts for boys height and weight *652*
Centile charts for girls height and weight *656*
Centile charts for occipital-frontal circumference (OFC) *660*
CK (Creatine kinase) levels in carriers of Duchenne muscular dystrophy (DMD) *662*
Conversion charts from English to metric units for height and weight *664*
Denver Developmental Screening Test *666*
Distribution of muscle weakness in different types of muscular dystrophy *668*
Dysmorphology examination checklist *670*
Embryonic fetal development (overview) *672*
Family tree sheet and symbols *674*
Haploid autosomal lengths of human chromosomes *676*

Investigation of lethal metabolic disorder or skeletal dysplasia *678*
ISCN Nomenclature *680*
Karyotypes *682*
Normal range of aortic root dimensions *684*
Paternity testing *688*
Patterns of cancer *690*
Radiological investigations including magnetic resonance imaging (MRI) *694*
Skeletal dysplasia charts *696*
Staging of puberty *700*

Index *701*
Human chromosome ideograms *inside front and back covers*

System-based contents

Cardiac disorders

22q deletion syndrome
in **Chromosomes** 490

Cardiomyopathy in children under 10 years
in **Clinical approach** 60

Congenital heart disease
in **Clinical approach** 84

Dilated cardiomyopathy
in **Common consultations** 302

Hypertrophic cardiomyopathy
in **Common consultations** 360

Hypoplastic left heart
in **Pregnancy and fertility** 596

Laterality disorders including heterotaxy
and isomerism
in **Clinical approach** 148

Long QT syndrome
in **Common consultations** 378

Marfan syndrome
in **Common consultations** 380

Normal range of aortic root dimensions in
Appendix 684

Cranial imaging abnormalities

Cerebellar anomalies
in **Clinical approach** 66

Cerebral palsy
in **Clinical approach** 70

Dandy–Walker malformation
in **Pregnancy and fertility** 582

Holoprosencephaly
in **Clinical approach** 130

Hydrocephalus
in **Clinical approach** 134

Lissencephaly and neuronal migration disorders
in **Clinical approach** 156

Leukodystrophy
in **Clinical approach** 150

Neural tube defects
in **Common consultations** 392

Structural intracranial anomalies
in **Clinical approach** 248

Ventriculomegaly
in **Pregnancy and fertility** 642

Cranial size and shape abnormal

Craniosynostosis
in **Common consultations** 288

Head circumference charts
in **Appendix** 660

Large fontanelle
in **Clinical approach** 146

Macrocephaly
in **Clinical approach** 162

Microcephaly
in **Clinical approach** 172

Plagiocephaly and abnormalities of skull shape
in **Clinical approach** 212

Developmental delay/ learning disability and neurodevelopmental disorders

Approach to the child with dysmorphism or
developmental delay
in **Introduction** 4

Autism and austism spectrum disorders
in **Common consultations** 274

Cerebral palsy
in **Clinical approach** 70

Denver Developmental Screening Test
in **Appendix** 666

Developmental delay in the child with
consanguineous parents
in **Clinical approach** 94

Developmental regression
in **Clinical approach** 96

Fragile X syndrome
in **Common consultations** 324

Mental retardation
in **Clinical approach** 168

Mental retardation with apparent
X-linked inheritance
in **Clinical approach** 164

Rett syndrome
in **Common consultations** 408

Seizures with developmental delay
in **Clinical approach** 238

Dysmorphology

Approach to the child with dysmorphism or developmental delay
in **Introduction** 4

Coarse facial features
in **Clinical approach** 78

Cleft lip/palate
in **Clinical approach** 74

Dysmorphic child
in **Clinical approach** 102

Dysmorphology examination checklist
in **Appendix** 670

Ear anomalies
in **Clinical approach** 108

Facial asymmetry
in **Clinical approach** 112

Micrognathia and Robin sequence
in **Clinical approach** 174

Nasal anomalies
in **Clinical approach** 182

Ocular hypertelorism
in **Clinical approach** 196

Eye disorders

Anterior segment eye malformations
in **Clinical approach** 46

Coloboma
in **Clinical approach** 82

Corneal clouding
in **Clinical approach** 88

Duane retraction syndrome
in **Clinical approach** 100

Glaucoma
in **Common consultations** 328

Microphthalmia and anophthalmia
in **Clinical approach** 176

Nystagmus
in **Clinical approach** 190

Ocular hypertelorism
in **Clinical approach** 196

Optic nerve hypoplasia
in **Clinical approach** 204

Ptosis, blepharophimosis, and other eyelid anomalies
in **Clinical approach** 224

Retinal dysplasia
in **Clinical approach** 230

Retinitis pigmentosa
in **Common consultations** 406

Retinal receptor dystrophies
in **Clinical approach** 232

Growth

Centile charts for boys' height and weight
in **Appendix** 652

Centile charts for girls' height and weight 656
in **Appendix** 656

Centile charts for occipital-frontal circumference (OFC) in **Appendix** 660

Failure to thrive
in **Clinical approach** 116

Hemihypertrophy and limb asymmetry
in **Clinical approach** 128

Obesity with and without developmental delay
in **Clinical approach** 192

Overgrowth
in **Clinical approach** 206

Short limbs
in **Pregnancy and fertility** 630

Short stature
in **Clinical approach** 242

Skeletal dysplasia
in **Clinical approach** 246

Staging of puberty
in **Appendix** 700

Haematological disorders

Haemochromatosis
in **Common consultations** 330

Haemoglobinopathies
in **Common consultations** 334

Haemophilia
in **Common consultations** 338

Thrombophilia
in **Common consultations** 416

Limb anomalies

Brachydactyly
in **Clinical approach** 56

Broad thumbs
in **Clinical approach** 58

Club-foot (talipes)
in **Pregnancy and fertility** 574

Limb reduction defects
in **Clinical approach** 152

Postaxial polydactyly
in **Clinical approach** 214

Preaxial polydactyly
in **Clinical approach** 218

Radial ray and thumb hypoplasia
in **Clinical approach** 228

Syndactyly
in **Clinical approach** 254

Muscle disorders

Arthrogryposis
in **Clinical approach** 48

Creatine kinase (CK) levels in carriers of
Duchenne muscular dystrophy
in **Appendix** 662

Distribution of muscle weakness in different
types of muscle dystrophy
in **Appendix** 668

Duchenne and Becker muscular dystrophies
in **Common consultations** 308

Facioscapulohumeral muscular dystrophy
in **Common consultations** 322

Floppy infant
in **Clinical approach** 118

Limb girdle dystrophy
in **Common consultations** 374

Myotonic dystrophy
in **Common consultations** 388

Neonatal disorders

Floppy infant
in **Clinical approach** 118

Hypoglycaemia in neonate and infant
in **Clinical approach** 140

Minor congenital anomalies
in **Clinical approach** 180

Neonatal encephalopathy and intractable seizures
in **Clinical approach** 186

Prolonged neonatal jaundice and jaundice
in infants under 6 months
in **Clinical approach** 220

Neurological disorders

Adrenoleukodystrophy (X-linked)
in **Common consultations** 264

Arthrogryposis
in **Clinical approach** 48

Ataxic adult
in **Clinical approach** 50

Dementia
in **Common consultations** 296

Dystonia
in **Clinical approach** 106

Floppy infant
in **Clinical approach** 118

Hereditary spastic paraparesis
in **Common consultations** 348

Huntington disease
in **Common consultations** 354

Parkinson disease
in **Common consultations** 404

Spinal muscular atrophy
in **Common consultations** 412

Seizures

Epilepsy
in **Common consultations** 318

Epilepsy in infants and children
in **Common consultations** 314

Fetal anticonvulsant syndrome
in **Pregnancy and fertility** 590

Neonatal encephalopathy and intractable seizures
in **Clinical approach** 186

Seizures with developmental delay
in **Clinical approach** 238

Skeletal disorders

Achondroplasia
in **Common consultations** 260

Bowed limbs
in **Pregnancy and fertility** 572

Centile charts for height/weight in boys
in **Appendix** 652

Centile charts for height/weight in girls
in **Appendix** 656

Chrondrodysplasia punctata
in **Clinical approach** 72

Fractures
in **Clinical approach** 122

Increased bone density
in **Clinical approach** 144

Radiological investigations including magnetic
resonance imaging (MRI)
in **Appendix** 694

Short limbs
in **Pregnancy and fertility** 630

Skeletal dysplasia
in **Clinical approach** 246

Skeletal dysplasias presenting at birth
in **Appendix** 696

The non-lethal skeletal dysplasias
in **Appendix** 698

Skin disorders

Generalized disorders of skin pigmentation
(including albinism)
in **Clinical approach** 126

Patchy hypomelanotic skin lesions
in **Clinical approach** 208

Patchy pigmented skin lesions (including
café-au-lait patches)
in **Clinical approach** 210

Unusual hair, teeth, nails, and skin
in **Clinical approach** 256

Teratogens

Cytomegalovirus
   in **Pregnancy and fertility** *580*

Drugs in pregnancy
   in **Pregnancy and fertility** *584*

Fetal alcohol syndrome
   in **Pregnancy and fertility** *588*

Fetal anticonvulsant syndrome
   in **Pregnancy and fertility** *590*

Maternal diabetes and diabetic embryopathy
   in **Pregnancy and fertility** *612*

Maternal phenylketonuria (PKU)
   in **Pregnancy and fertility** *614*

Radiation chemotherapy and landfill sites
   in **Pregnancy and fertility** *622*

Rubella
   in **Pregnancy and fertility** *628*

Toxoplasmosis
   in **Pregnancy and fertility** *634*

Varicella
   in **Pregnancy and fertility** *640*

Glossary of terms used in dysmorphology

Accessory nipple Additional nipple arising on the 'milk line' that runs caudally from the normally sited nipple and cranially towards the axilla

Agenesis A condition in which a body part is absent or does not develop completely

Ala nasi The flaring cartilaginous area forming the outer side of each nostril

Alopecia Absence, loss, or deficiency of hair; may be patchy or total

Amelia Complete absence of one or more limbs from the shoulder or pelvic girdle

Ankyloglossia A short or tight lingual frenulum attaching the anterior half of the inferior aspect of the tongue to the floor of the mouth, just beneath or directly onto the posterior alveolar ridge, which restricts tongue movement

Aniridia Absence of the iris

Anisocoria Unequal pupil size

Ankyloblepharon Adhesion of the eyelids by synechiae or fibrous bands

Anodontia Absence of teeth

Anonychia Absence of nails

Anophthalmia Congenital absence of one or both eyes. Genetically, anopthalmia may represent an extreme form of microphthalmia and both forms may coexist in the same patient or in different family members

Antimongoloid slant Downward slant of the palpebral fissure of the eye, with the outer canthus (outer corner) lying below the level of the inner canthus

Aphakia Absence of the ocular lens

Arachnodactyly Long slender hands, feet, fingers, and toes. Literally 'spider digits'

Areola Pigmented skin surrounding the nipple

Arrhinia Congenital absence of the nose

Atresia A condition in which an opening or passage for the tracts of the body is absent or closed, e.g. anal atresia, duodenal atresia

Bathing trunk naevus A congenital giant pigmented naevus over the area of the body covered by swimming trunks. The naevus can be hairy, deeply pigmented, and very large. It may undergo malignant transformation, so expert advice from a paediatric dermatologist is essential

Birthmark An area of altered skin colour present from birth or arising in early infancy and caused by vascular or pigment-distribution anomalies

Blaschko line Streak of abnormally pigmented skin following the line of a dermatome. Linear distribution along limbs; hemicircumferential on trunk

Body mass index (BMI) BMI = weight (kg)/height^2 (m^2). See section on Obesity in *Clinical approach* for table

Bone age Radiological assessment of skeletal maturity based on ossification of the carpal and hand bone epiphyses. By convention a radiograph of the left wrist is taken. The skeletal age is compared with the chronological age. Normal values and standard deviations are defined and thus an assessment can be made as to whether skeletal maturation is delayed, normal, or advanced. A more accurate assessment can be made under the age of two years by evaluation of the epiphyses at the knees by comparison with an atlas of normal knees at different ages

Blepharophimosis Decrease in palpebral fissure aperture; the distance between the inner and outer canthi of each eye is reduced

Brachycephaly Flattening of the back of the head

Brachydactyly Short fingers

Brushfield spot Mottle, marbled, or speckled elevation of the iris due to increased density of the anterior border layer of the iris. Present in 85% of individuals with Down syndrome—similar appearances may also be seen in nomal individuals

Buphthalmos Congenital enlargement of the eye, usually secondary to congenital glaucoma

Café au lait spot Macular area of coffee-coloured pigmentation >0.5 cm in diameter

Calvarium Upper, dome-like portion of the skull

Camptodactyly Literally 'bent fingers'; usually involving contractures of the fingers

Campomelia Literally 'bent limb' as seen in campomelic dysplasia or oto-palato-digital syndrome type II

Canthal distance, inner Distance between the inner canthi (inner corners) of the two eyes

Canthal distance, outer Distance between the outer canthi (outer corners) of the two eyes

Carrying angle With the arms hanging by the sides and palms facing forwards, the deviation of the forearm relative to the humerus

Cavernous haemangioma Elevated vascular naevus or 'strawberry mark'; usually a dense red colour. Often not apparent or minimal at birth and growing rapidly during infancy; usually involuting spontaneously from the first birthday

Cebocephaly Severe form of holoprosencephaly with ocular hypotelorism and a centrally placed nose with a single blind-ended nostril

Cheilion Most lateral point of the corner of the mouth

Chordee Abnormal postion of the penis caused by a band of tissue that holds the penis in a ventral or lateral curve

Clinodactyly Lateral or medial curve of one or more fingers or toes away from the third finger. Mild fifth finger clinodactyly is a common autosomal dominant (AD) trait

Club-foot Abnormal resting position of the foot. May be positional or structural. The two most common types are talipes equinovarus (forefoot is plantar-flexed and medially rotated) and talipes calcaneovalgus (forefoot is dorsiflexed and everted)

Coloboma Congenital fissure of the eye. May involve iris and/or retina or eyelid. Inferior colobomas arise early in embryonic life due to incomplete fusion of the optic cup. Colobomas of the lower eyelid may be found in Treacher–Collins syndrome

Columella nasi Fleshy inferior border of the nasal septum, between the nostrils

Craniorachischisis Congenital failure of closure of the skull and spinal column

Crown–rump length (CRL) Distance from the top of the head to the bottom of the buttock. The most accurate measure of gestational age in the embryo between 6 and 11+ weeks gestation

Cubitus valgus Increased carrying angle at the elbow

Cupid's bow The upper edge of the upper lip; shaped like the double-curved bow carried by Cupid

Cutis aplasia Absence of skin in specific area—commonly on scalp over vertex

Cryptophthalmos Complete congenital adhesion of the eyelids; fused eyelid

Cryptorchidism Failure of the testis to descend into the scrotum; undescended testes

Cystic hygroma Accumulation of lymphatic fluid found usually at the back of the neck

Depigmentation Area of absent or reduced pigment due to lack of functional melanocytes

Dermatoglyphics Pattern of ridges and grooves over the fingertips, palms, and soles

Dermatome Segmental area of skin supplied by nerves from a single spinal nerve root

Dermis Inner layer of the skin; outer layer is the epidermis. Thickness of the dermis varies from <0.5 mm over eyelid to 2–3 mm over back

Developmental delay Delayed acquisition of developmental milestones (e.g. smiling, sitting independently, walking, first words) in comparison with normal range for chronological age

Developmental quotient Ratio of developmental age/chronological age

Dimple Indentation or depression of the skin where the subcutaneous tissues are deficient and the skin may be tethered to underlying structures, e.g. bone

Distichiasis A second row of eyelashes arising from the meiobian glands as seen in the lymphoedema–distichiasis syndrome caused by mutations in *FOXC2*

Dolicocephaly Elongation of the skull. The skull is long in its anteroposterior dimension and narrow in its bitemporal dimension

Drusen Drusen are deposits on the optic nerve head present in 0.3% of the population, of which 70% occur bilaterally. An irregular knobbly disc margin, anomalous branching of the vessels, and autofluorescence help the differentiation from papilloedema

Dystopia canthorum Lateral displacement of the innner canthi of the eye (e.g. Waardenburg type 1)

Eclabion Eversion of the lips, as seen in congenital Harlequin ichthyosis

Ectrodactyly Commonly used to describe a 'split hand' or 'split foot' where there is deficiency of the middle ray(s) of the hand/foot.

Ectopia lentis Displacement of the ocular lens as seen in Marfan syndrome, and homocysteinuria

Ectopic Abnormally sited

Ectropion Eversion of the eyelid

Encephalocele Congenital herniation of the brain through a bony deficiency of the skull. May be frontal or occipital (e.g. Meckel syndrome)

Enophthalmos Abnormal retraction of the eye into the orbit, producing deeply set eyes

Entropion Inversion of the eyelid

Epicanthic fold Congenital fold of skin medial to the eye, sometimes covering the inner canthus. It is commonly seen in association with a hypoplastic nasal bridge

Epicanthus inversus Congenital fold of skin medial to the eye, sometimes covering the inner canthus, with the fold broader inferiorly than superiorly. May occur in association with blepharophimosis and ptosis in BPES (blepharophimosis–ptosis–epicanthus inversus) syndrome due to mutations in *FOXL2*

Epidermis Superficial keratinized layer of the skin

Epiphora Flow of tears down the cheek due to blockage or stenosis of the nasolacrimal duct

Epispadias Abnormal location of the urethral meatus on the dorsal surface of the penis

Esotropia Inward deviation of an eye when both eyes are open and uncovered; convergent strabismus (squint)

Exophthalmos Abnormal protrusion of the eyes (as seen in Crouzon or Apert syndromes)

Exotropia Outward deviation of an eye when both eyes are opened and uncovered; divergent strabismus (squint)

Flexion crease Crease in skin on the ventral surface of a joint, secondary to movement at that joint

Fontanelle Membrane-covered space remaining in the incompletely ossified skull of a fetus or infant in the line of the sutures. Anterior fontanelle at the junction of the saggital, coronal, and metopic sutures is patent in the first 6–12 months of life and usually closes by the end of the first year

Frenulum Small fold of mucous membrane, e.g. arising between the upper central incisors and extending to the upper lip, or beneath the tongue. Additional frenulae may be found in oral–facial–digital (OFD) syndrome

Frontal bossing Prominence of the anterior portion of the frontal bone of the skull

Gastroschisis Congenital fissure of the anterior abdominal wall, adjacent to but not involving the insertion of the umbilical cord. Part of the intestine may herniate through the defect

Genu valgum Outward bowing of the knee; bow-leg

Genu varum Inward deviation of the knee; knock-knee

Gibbus Extreme kyphosis or hump: deformity of the spine in which there is a sharply angulated segment, the apex of the angle being posterior

Glabella The most prominent midline point between the eyebrows

Glossoptosis Downward displacement or retraction of the tongue; sometimes held by a frenulum (tongue-tie)

Gnathion The lowest median point on the inferior border of the mandible

Gonion The most lateral point of the posteroinferior angle of the mandible

Height Distance from the top of the head to the sole of the foot in a standing position

Heterochromia iridis Unequal colour of the irises, where the entire iris of one eye is of a distinctly different colour as seen in Waardenburg syndrome. A wedge-shaped segment of anomalous eye colour is called heterochromia iridum

Hirsutism Excessive body and facial hair

Holoprosencephaly Failure of midline cleavage of the embryonic forebrain

Hydrocephalus Abnormal increase in the amount of cerebrospinal fluid accompanied by dilatation of the cerebral ventricles

Hyperextensibility Excessive stretch of the skin or excessive range of movement of a joint

Hypertelorism Increased distance between two paired structures such as the nipples or eyes. Ocular hypertelorism is used to describe the appearance of wide-set eyes due to an increased interpupillary distance

Hypertrichosis Excessive body hair that is long and often involves the face

Hypodontia Reduced number and/or size of teeth due to disturbance of tooth bud development/patterning

Hyponychia Small dysplastic nails

Hypospadias Abnormal location of the urethral meatus on the ventral surface of the penis: may be glandular (1°), penile (2°), scrotal (3°), or perineal (4°)

Hypotelorism Decreased interpupillary distance; eyes unusually close together

Imperforate anus Absence of the normal anal opening. Usually results from abnormal development of the urorectal septum resulting in incomplete separation of the cloaca into urogenital and anorectal portions

Intelligence quotient (IQ) Measure of intellectual funtioning as assessed by standardized tests: usually measures verbal and nonverbal reasoning and expresses results as a quotient standardized for age, with 100 being the mean

Interpupillary distance Distance between the centres of the pupils of the eyes

Iridodonesis Tremor of the iris on movement, usually secondary to dislocation of the lens

Keratoconus Conical protrusion of the cornea usually associated with thinning of the cornea

Koilonychia Spoon-shaped nails

Kyphoscoliosis Abnormal curvature of the spinal column, both anteroposteriorly and laterally

Kyphosis Curvature of the spine in the anteroposterior plane. A normal kyphosis exists in the shoulder area

Lagophthalmos Condition in which the eyelid cannot be completely closed

Lanugo Embryonic or fetal hair: fine, soft, unmedullated

Length Distance between the top of the head and the sole of the foot when the individual is lying down—used as a surrogate for height in the first year of life

Lentigo Round or oval, flat, brown, pigmented skin spot due to deposition of melanin by an increased number of melanocytes at the epidermodermal junction

Leukocoria White pupillary reflex. The pupillary reflex is usually red

Leukonychia White spots or stripes on the nails; may involve the whole nail

Lingua plicata Fissured tongue

Lisch nodule Hamartomatous iris structure seen in neurofibromatosis type 1 (NF1). Lisch nodules are iris freckles that project above the surface of the iris (unlike normal iris pigmentation) and thus are detectable by slit-lamp examination

Lordosis Curvature of the spinal column with a forward (ventral) convexity. A normal lordosis exists in the lumbar area

Lower segment Distance from the top of the pubic bone to the sole of the foot

Macrocephaly Abnormally large skull. Occipital-frontal circumference >3 standard deviations

Macrodactyly Abnormally large digit

Macroglossia Abnormally large or hypertrophic tongue (as seen in Beckwith–Wiedemann syndrome)

Madelung deformity A developmental abnormality of the wrist characterized by anatomical changes in the radius, ulna, and carpal bones, leading to palmar and ulnar wrist subluxation ('dinner-fork deformity'). It is seen in individuals with deletions or mutations of the *SHOX* gene on Xp22.3 (e.g. Leri–Weill syndrome) and sometimes in Turner syndrome. The deformity usually becomes evident clinically between the ages of 6 and 13 years. Madelung deformity can result in wrist pain and restriction of forearm rotation (pronation/supination)

Male pattern baldness Loss of hair at the temples and on the top of the head

Manubrium Cranial portion of the sternum that articulates with the clavicles and the first two pairs of ribs

Melanocyte Pigment cell in the skin

Meromelia Partial absence of a limb

Mesomelic Referring to the middle segment of the limb

Microcephaly Abnormally small head. Occipital-frontal circumference <3 standard deviations

Micrognathia Abnormally small mandible giving a small chin

Microphthalmia Abnormally small eye

Microstomia Abnormally small opening of the mouth

Microphallus Abnormally small penis: micropenis. If the genitalia are ambiguous it may be difficult to distinguish a micropenis from an enlarged clitoris

Mid-parental height Sum of parents' heights divided by two

Miosis Small contracted pupil

Mole Circumscribed area of darkly pigmented skin, which is often raised

Mongolian blue spot Bluish area of skin, mostly over the sacrum. The discoloured area of skin is not raised. More frequent in Black, Hispanic, and Asian people

Müllerian duct Embryonic precursor of the female reproductive tract (Fallopian tubes, uterus, and upper one-third of vagina)

Mydriasis Large, dilated pupil. Mydriatics are used to facilitate fundoscopy

Naevus sebaceous Raised waxy patch with a mostly linear distribution

Nyctalopia Poor night vision due to loss or dysfunction of rod photoreceptors in the retina, e.g. in retinitis pigmentosa

Nystagmus Involuntary rapid movement of the eyeball that may be horizontal, vertical, rotatory, or mixed

Occipital-frontal circumference (OFC) Distance around the head. The largest measurement with the tape measure passing across the forehead, over the ears, and over the occiput

Oligodontia Less than the normal number of teeth (see also hypodontia)

Omphalocele Failure of embryonic herniation of the intestines to return inside the abdominal cavity. The intestines (and sometimes parts of the liver) protrude through a defect in the abdominal wall at the umbilicus and are covered by a thin membrane composed of amnion and peritoneum

Ophthalmoplegia Paralysis of the eye muscles (may occur in some mitochondrial disorders)

Pachyonychia Thickened nails

Palpebral fissure length Distance between the inner and outer canthus of one eye

Patterning Process whereby embryonic cells acquire their spatial identities

Pectus carinatum Undue prominence of the sternum, often referred to as a pigeon chest

Pectus excavatum Undue depression of the sternum, often referred to as a funnel chest

Pes cavus High arched foot

Philtrum Vertical groove in the midline extending from beneath the nose to the cupid's bow in the vermilion border of the upper lip

Pili torti Hair twisted by 180° angle

Plagiocephaly Asymmetric head shape

Poland anomaly Hypoplastic pectoral muscle often found in association with ipsilateral breast hypoplasia. Often found in association with a terminal transverse limb defect

Polydactyly Extra digit(s)—may be preaxial or postaxial or insertional

Polysyndactyly Extra digit(s) with fused digit(s)

Polythelia Occurrence of an extra nipple(s)—usually found in the milk line that runs caudally from the normal position of the nipples and cranially towards the axilla

Postaxial Posterior or lateral to the axis (e.g. postaxial polydactyly where the extra digit is lateral to the fifth finger or fifth toe)

Portwine naevus Dark angioma that can be purple in colour (as seen in Sturge–Weber syndrome)

Preaxial Anterior or medial to the axis (e.g. preaxial polydactyly where the extra digit is medial to the thumb or hallux)

Prognathism Prominence of the jaw leading to an unusually prominent chin

Pterygium A wing-shaped web, e.g. a skin web across a joint

Ptosis Drooping of the upper eyelid

Range of movement Range of place or position through which a particular joint can move

Rhizomelic Referring to the proximal portion of the limb

Scaphocephaly Abnormally long and narrow skull as a result of premature closure of the sagittal suture

Scoliosis Appreciable lateral deviation from the normally straight vertical line of the spine

Shawl scrotum Congenital ventral insertion of the scrotum

Sidney crease Proximal flexion crease of the palm that extends all the way across the palm; the distal flexion crease is still present

Simian crease Single palmar crease

Sitting height Distance from the top of the head to the buttocks when in sitting position

Skin-fold thickness Thickness of skin in designated areas (e.g. triceps, subscapular, suprailiac) used to assess subcutaneous fat and nutrition

Span Distance between the tips of the middle fingers of each hand when the arms are stretched out horizontally from the body with the palms facing forwards

Sprengel deformity Congenital upward displacement of the scapula

Stadiometer Upright measuring device for accurate assessment of height

Stellate iris A lacy 'star-like' reticulate pattern radiating out from the pupil

Strabismus Deviation of the eye (squint); the visual axes assume a position relative to each other different from that required by physiological conditions

Stork mark Pink vascular mark localized over the middle of the forehead, or nape of the neck in the newborn. It represents the fetal circulatory pattern in the skin and those on the face resolve spontaneously

Symblepharon Adhesion of the eyelid to the eyeball

Symphalangism Bony fusion of interdigital spaces resulting in fixed extension of joints

Syndactyly Webbing or fusion of fingers or toes

Synechia Adhesion of parts; especially adhesion of the iris to the cornea or to the lens

Syngnathia Intraoral bands, possibly remnants of the buccopharyngeal membrane extending between the jaws

Synophyrys Confluent eyebrow growth across the glabella

Tanner stages Grading system to establish standards for the stages of puberty

Telangiectasis Prominence of blood vessels on the surface of the skin

Telecanthus Increased distance between the inner canthi of the eyes

Teratogenic effect Any harmful fetal effect arising from an exposure during pregnancy

Torticollis 'Wry neck'—contracted state of the cervical muscles resulting in twisting of the neck and restriction of movement, especially rotation. The most common causes are trauma, inflammation, or a congenital malformation involving the cervical vertebrae and or the sternocleido-mastoid muscle on one side

Trichorrhexis Nodular swelling of the hair. The hair is light-coloured and breaks easily

Trigonocephaly Triangular-shaped head and skull resulting from premature synostosis of the portions of the frontal bone with prominence of the metopic suture

Triphalangeal thumb Thumb with three phalanges (as in the fingers)

Triradii Dermatoglyphic pattern where three sets of ridges converge

Turricephaly Tall or high skull; the top of the head is pointed—may be caused by premature closure of the lamboid and coronal sutures

Vermilion border Red-coloured edge to the lip where it meets the normal skin of the face

Vertex Highest point of the head in the midsagittal plane, when the head is held erect

Widow's peak Pointed frontal hairline in the midline

Wolffian duct Embryonic precursor of the male reproductive tract (vas deferens, seminal vesicles, and prostate)

Woolly hair Tightly curled kinky hair with a reduced shaft diameter

Wormian bone Small irregular bone in the suture between the bones of the skull

Expert adviser: Judith G. Hall, Emeritus Professor of Pediatrics and Medical Genetics, University of British Columbia, Vancouver, Canada

Reference

Hall JG, Froster-Iskenius UG, Allanson JE. *Handbook of normal physical measurements.* Oxford University Press, Oxford, 1995.

Glossary of terms used in genetics

Acrocentric A chromosome where the centromere is near one end. The gene coding material is usually located only on the long arm. The human acrocentric chromosomes are 13, 14, 15, 21, and 22

Allele One of several alternative forms of a gene occupying a given locus on a chromosome

Allele drop-out (ADO) The failure, for technical reasons, to detect an allele that is present in a sample; the failure to amplify an allele during a polymerase chain reaction

Allele frequency The frequency in a population of each allele at a polymorphic locus

Alternative splicing A mechanism by which different forms of mature mRNAs are generated from the same gene. Different exons from a single gene are used to produce isoforms of a protein

Aneuploidy In *full aneuploidy* there is an abnormal chromosome number differing from the usual diploid or haploid set by loss or addition of one or a small number of chromosomes, e.g. 45,X or 47,XY + 21. It can be the result of non-disjunction in (i) a premeiotic mitotic division in the germline of either parent, (ii) a first or second meiotic division in either parent, or (iii) an early embryonic mitotic (postzygotic) division in an affected individual. In *partial aneuploidy*, the imbalance involves the gain or loss of part of a chromosome.

Anticipation Worsening of disease severity in successive generations. Characteristically occurs in triplet repeat disorders where there is expansion of the triplet repeat in the maternal or paternal line, e.g. myotonic dystrophy

Antisense mRNA mRNA transcript that is complementary to endogenous mRNA. Introducing a transgene coding for antisense mRNA is a strategy used experimentally, but not currently in clinical practice, to block expression of an endogenous gene of interest

Apoptosis Programmed cell death

Array-CGH Microarray based comparative genomic hybridisation (see 'microarray' and 'CGH')

ARMS (amplification refractory mutation system) A specific robust polymerase chain reaction system for routine genetic testing that can be readily multiplexed, e.g. 29-mutation kit for cystic fibrosis (CF) testing

ART (assisted reproductive technologies) Assisted reproductive technology, e.g. *in vitro* fertilization (IVF) and intracytoplasmic sperm injection (ICSI), has revolutionized the treatment of infertility. In conjunction with single-cell genetic analysis based on polymerase chain reaction (PCR) or fluorescent *in situ* hybridization (FISH) it has also made pre-implantation genetic diagnosis (PGD) possible for some genetic disorders. See 'Assisted reproductive technologies: *in vitro* fertilization (IVF), intracytoplasmic sperm injection (ICSI), and pre-implantation genetic diagnosis (PGD)' page 568

Ascertainment bias A tendency for a study to be non-representative of the true population, because individuals of a particular type are more likely to be sampled

Autosome A chromosome that is not an X or Y chromosome. There are 22 pairs of autosomes in the human chromosome complement

BAC (bacteria artificial chromosome) A cloning vector derived from an E. coli plasmid. BACs can be used in the cloning of large DNA fragments, on average approximately 200kb long, and are ideal as cloning vectors for the sequencing of whole genomes. BACs are convenient for use as FISH probes

Band/banding Differential staining of a chromosome leading to distinction of chromosomal segments. A Giemsa-stained (G-banded) karyotype has 850 bands visible at prometaphase (Mitelman 1995)

Birth prevalence The number of cases of disorder/condition per number of live births (usually per 1000)

Bivalent Describes a pair of homologous chromosomes that align and undergo synapsis and recombination. The double structure is termed a bivalent

bp (base pair) In DNA a purine and pyrimidine base on each strand that interact with each other through hydrogen bonding

cDNA DNA complimentary to, and copied from an RNA molecule. cDNA libraries of living cells therefore represent the RNA content of those cells, and thereby represent expressed gene sequences.

Centimorgan (cM) Unit of genetic map distance corresponding to a recombination fraction of 0.01.

Centromere The constricted region of a chromosome that includes the site of attachment to the mitotic or meiotic spindle

Chimerism The presence in an organism of two or more cell lines that are derived from different zygotes. Such an organism is termed a chimera. Chimerism is extremely rare in humans

Chip (see microarray)

Chromatid A chromosome that has undergone replication has two identical sister chromatids that are joined at the centromere before they separate into two distinct chromosomes during cell division

Chromatin The DNA helix is wrapped around core histones to form a simple 'beads on a string' configuration, where the beads represent nucleosomes. This is then folded into higher-order chromatin. Chromatin can be modified by processes such as DNA methylation and histone modification (acetylation, phosphorylation, methylation, and ubiquitylation). The regulation of higher-order chromatin structures is crucial for genome reprogramming during early embryogenesis and gametogenesis and for tissue-specific gene expression and global gene silencing

Chromosome A thread-like structure composed mainly of chromatin that carries a highly ordered sequence of linked genes and resides in the nucleus of eukaryotic cells

Chromosome walking The method of moving from a linked marker to a gene

Cloning Production of genetically identical cells (or organisms from a single ancestral cell (or nucleus)). Also a technique used in molecular biology to propagate single or discrete DNA fragments of interest. See also 'Reproductive cloning', this glossary

Coding strand The coding strand of DNA has a complementary sequence to mRNA since it serves as the template for mRNA synthesis

Comparative genomic hybridization (CGH) Reference and test DNA samples are fluorescently labelled, e.g. one with green probes, the other with red probes. After hybridization of labelled probe mixes to metaphase chromosome spreads, the ratio of green to red fluorescence along each chromosome is compared in an attempt to identify genomic imbalance in the test DNA

Compound heterozygote An individual that has altered gene function because each copy of the gene is altered by different mutations, e.g. an individual with cystic fibrosis may have the *CFTR* genotype deltaF508/G542X, i.e. there are two mutations in both alleles at the *same* locus. (NB. A double heterozygote is an individual who is heterozygous at two different loci)

Concordance Presence of the same trait in both members of a pair (as in twins) or in all members of a set of similar individuals.

Confidence interval (CI) The CI provides a means of quantifying the range of uncertainty around a result (e.g. for a relative risk (RR) = 0.7 with a 95% CI, the range is 0.5–0.8). The smaller the range of the CI, the more precise the estimate is likely to be. Where a CI spans 1.0, this indicates no significant observed effect

Consanguinity Parents are related (i.e. have a recent common ancestor) and share a proportion of their genetic material. In practice, a consanguineous relationship is often considered as one between individuals who are second cousins or closer

Consultand An individual seeking advice about a genetic disorder

Contig A set of overlapping sequences or clones from which a sequence can be obtained

Copy Number The number of copies of a given chromosomal locus which are present. For an autosomal locus with a heterozygous deletion eg. Smith-Magenis syndrome on 17p11.2, the copy number for the deleted region is 1, compared with 2 for normal individuals and 3 for individuals carrying a 17p11.2 duplication. For a male with an AZFa deletion on his Y chromosome, the copy number will be 0, compared with 1 for a normal male.

Cumulative risk Cumulative risk of a disease by age *n* is the probability of an individual being diagnosed with that disease by their *n*th birthday

Deletion Loss of part of a chromosome, or part or all of a gene or DNA sequence

dHPLC (denaturing high-performance liquid chromatography) A high-resolution method for separating large molecules that is often used as an automated method for the detection of DNA sequence variants. dHPLC-based mutation or single nucleotide polymorphism (SNP) screening relies on different DNA thermodynamic properties between perfectly matched base pairs in homoduplex molecules and mismatches in heteroduplex DNAs. dHPLC analysis is conducted on a WAVE machine

Differentially methylated region (DMR) DNA segments in imprinted genes that show different methylation patterns between paternal and maternal alleles, e.g. SNRP (small nuclear ribonuclear protein). Some DMRs

acquire DNA methylation in the germ cells, whereas others acquire DNA methylation during embryogenesis

Digenic inheritance Two genes are involved, with at least one mutation at both loci needed, in order to produce the phenotype e.g. Connexin 26 and 30 in sensorineural deafness, and *HFE* and *HAMP* in juvenile haemochromatosis and BBS2 and BBS4 in Bardet-Biedl syndrome.

Diploid (2*n*) A paired set of chromosomes comprising two of each autosome and two sex chromosomes. Diploid chromosome sets occur in somatic cells, e.g. 46,XX and 46,XY. Often used as diploid cell or diploid organism

Discordance A twin pair or set of individuals in which the members differ in whether they exhibit a certain trait.

Dizygotic twins (DZ) Two individuals born together derived from two separate eggs fertilized by two separate sperm

Domain A discrete portion of a gene or protein with its own function

Dominant A trait in which the mutant allele is dominant to the wild-type allele, i.e. the disease or disorder is manifest when one copy of the mutant allele is inherited, e.g. achondroplasia

Dominant negative mutation A mutation in one copy of a gene resulting in a mutant protein that has not only lost its own function, but also prevents the wild-type protein of the same gene from functioning normally. Commonly acts by producing an altered polypeptide (subunit) that prevents the assembly of a multimeric protein

Double heterozygote An individual who is heterozygous at two *different* loci. (NB. An individual who is a compound heterozygote has two different mutations at the same locus)

Downstream A region of DNA that lies 3′ to the point of reference

Duplicon A duplicated segment of the genome. Pericentromeric regions of human chromosomes are preferential sites for the integration of duplicated DNA, or 'duplicons', which often contain gene fragments. Duplicons appear to mediate genomic fluidity in both disease and evolutionary processes. Duplicons are implicated in the recurring 15q11–q13 deletion seen in PWS/AS (Prader–Willi syndrome/Angelman syndrome) and also in 22q11 deletion syndrome

Dynamic mutation A trinucleotide repeat expansion that can change in size during meiosis or, in some instances, mitosis

Embryonic stem cell Cell derived from the inner cell mass of an early embryo that can replicate indefinitely and differentiate into many cell types

Empiric risk Risk of recurrence that has been observed based on family studies—often used for complex multifactorial disorders

Epigenetic Any heritable influence (in the progeny of cells or of individuals) on chromosome or gene function that is not acompanied by a change in DNA sequence, e.g. X-chromosome inactivation, imprinting, centromere inactivation, and position effect variegation

ESAC (extra structurally abnormal chromosome) Term synonymous with 'marker chromosome'. Some are composed entirely of heterochromatin and do not influence phenotype, others contain euchromatin and may adversely affect phenotype

EST (expressed sequence tag) A small segment of DNA with a characteristic (or perhaps unique) sequence derived from a cDNA clone. Used to map the positions of expressed sequences

Euchromatin The lightly staining regions of the nucleus that generally contain decondensed, transcriptionally active regions of the genome; gene-rich areas of chromatin that are typically decondensed and therefore light-staining in nuclei and chromosomes

Exon A segment of an interrupted gene that is represented in the mature RNA product

Expressivity Variation in the severity of a disorder in individuals who have inherited the same disease alleles. Note the difference from *penetrance*, which is the percentage of individuals expressing the disorder to any degree, from the most trivial to the most severe

FISH (fluorescence *in situ* hybridization) *In situ* hybridization in which the DNA-probe is labelled with a fluorophore. Using fluorescence microscopy, the probe can be visualized binding to a specific chromosomal region. The efficacy of FISH is limited in some applications by low-resolution sensitivity

Founder effect A high prevalence of a genetic disorder in an isolated or inbred population due to the fact that many members of the population are derived from a common ancestor who harboured a disease-causing mutation. Founder effects are seen both for dominant and recessive disorders and, if the disorder is due to a founder effect, the affected individuals in a given population carry the same mutation (founder mutation). Examples include the recessive disorders Meckel syndrome, hydrolethalus syndrome, Cohen syndrome, and congenital Finnish nephropathy, which all occur with disproportionately high incidence in Finland compared with other European populations

Founder mutation A disease-causing mutation that is found repeatedly in a given population and is derived from a common ancestor who harboured that mutation

Frameshift mutation Deletion or insertion of a number of bases, that is not a multiple of three, leading to alteration of the reading frame

Gene The fundamental unit of heredity. A sequence of DNA involved in producing a polypeptide chain—it includes coding segments (exons) and intervening sequences (introns) together with regulatory elements, e.g. promoter. A gene is functionally defined by its product

Gene conversion A non-reciprocal recombination process between alleles or loci that results in an alteration of the sequence of a gene to that of its homologue. Gene conversion occurs as a consequence of mismatch repair after heteroduplex formation. Gene conversion events are common between the telomeric and centromeric SMN genes (spinal muscular atrophy (SMA)) and between the NEMO gene and its pseudogene in incontinentia pigmenti (IP).

Genetic counselling The process by which individuals or relatives at risk of a disorder that may be hereditary are advised of the consequences of the disorder, the probability of developing or transmitting it and the ways in which this may be prevented, avoided or ameliorated.' (Harper 1998)

Genome The entire genetic complement of a prokaryote, virus, mitochondria or chloroplast or the haploid nuclear genetic complement of a eukaryotic species. The human genome contains ^32,000 genes

Genome architecture The structure, content, and organization of a genome, including the location and order of genes

Genome-wide scan A systematic survey to discover if a phenotypic trait or genetic disease is linked to a genetic mapping marker(s) used to try and identify the gene(s) responsible for a given disease

Genotype The genetic constitution of an individual, at one or more gene loci

Germline mosaicism The presence in a gonad of genetically distinct populations of cells, usually implying that the mosaicism is confined to the ovary/testis. If both parents appear unaffected, but one parent is a germline mosaic, this can result in recurrence of affected children eg. TSC.

Haploid (*n*) A set of chromosomes comprising one of each autosome and one sex chromosome. Haploid chromosome sets (*n*) occur in the gametes, e.g. 23,X and 23,Y

Haploinsufficiency Situation in which the product of only one allele is produced and is insufficient for normal function. It arises when the normal phenotype requires the protein product of two alleles, and reduction of 50% of gene product results in an abnormal phenotype

Haplotype A set of closely linked alleles on a single chromosome that tend to be inherited *en bloc*, i.e. not separated by recombination at meiosis

Hedgehog genes A highly conserved family of genes that encode signalling molecules. Sonic hedgehog (SHH) plays a major part in the growth and patterning of many tissues and organ systems, Indian hedgehog (IHH) is important in endochondral bone formation, and desert hedgehog (DHH) regulates male germline development

Helicases Enzymes that unwind double-stranded DNA into two single strands

Hemizygous The presence of only one copy of a gene. Males are hemizygous for most genes on the X chromosome (with the exception of the pseudoautosomal regions, which are also represented on Y)

Heritability The proportion of the variation in a given characteristic or state within a particular population that can be attributed to genetic factors

Heterochromatin Regions of the genome that are permanently in a highly condensed condition, are not transcribed, and are late-replicating. Heterochromatin includes both repetitive DNA (e.g. highly repetitive satellite DNA and ribosomal DNA gene clusters) and some protein-coding genes

Heterodisomy See 'uniparental disomy (UPD)', this glossary

Heteroduplex Double-stranded DNA fragment that has a mismatch between the two strands due to a mutation. The mismatched bases cannot pair as normal and so destabilize the DNA molecule

Heteroplasmy The existence of more than one mitochondrial DNA (mtDNA) type in the same cell, tissue, or individual, e.g. mitochondria containing a mixture of mtDNA carrying the MELAS 3243 point mutation and mtDNA with the wild-type sequence. In mitochondrial disorders because of the thousands of mitochondria in each cell there are often a variable percentage of mutant and wild-type mtDNAs between different cells and especially between different tissues. See 'homoplasmy', this glossary

Heterozygous The presence of two different alleles at a specified locus

Histones Small, highly conserved basic proteins that associate with DNA to form a nucleosome (the basic structural subunit of chromatin)

Homeobox The conserved 60 amino acid DNA-binding homeodomain in a HOX gene

Homeobox (HOX) genes A family of genes that encode proteins with a conserved DNA-binding homeobox domain that are involved in regulating patterning events of early embryonic development. The HOX genes provide a remarkably conserved system for providing regional identity to the primary body axis of developing embryos. They encode transcription factors with a conserved 60 amino acid DNA-binding homeodomain (homeobox) and are organized in four clusters on the chromosomes (*HOXA*, *HOXB*, *HOXC*, and *HOXD*). In *Drosophila* they specify segment identity along the rostrocaudal axis. To date, only two HOX genes, *HOXD13* (synpolydactyly) and *HOXA13* (hand–foot–genital syndrome), have been found to be mutated in human malformation syndromes. Both genes are located at the 5' end of their respective clusters and play a role in the specification of the most caudal structures, i.e. the most distal parts of the limb and the genital tubercle

Homeotic genes A class of genes that are crucial for controlling the early development and differentiation of embryonic tissues, e.g. homeobox (HOX) genes and paired box (PAX) genes

Homoplasmy The existence of only one mitochondrial DNA (mtDNA) type in the same cell, tissue, or individual, e.g. mitochondria containing only mtDNA carrying the A1555G sensorineural deafness sequence. See 'heteroplasmy', this glossary

Homozygosity by descent Seen in consanguineous families where both copies of an allele or haplotype arise from a common ancestor. Can be a useful mapping steategy for autosomal recessive (AR) disorders

Homozygous The presence of two identical alleles at a specified locus

Housekeeping gene A gene that is ubiquitously expressed and encodes a protein performing a basic function common to most cells

HOX genes See 'homeobox (HOX) genes', this glossary

Hybridization The artificial pairing of two complementary strands of DNA (or one strand of DNA and one of RNA) to form a double-stranded molecule. One strand is often labelled and used as a probe to detect the presence of the other

Hypomorphic mutation/allele A mutation which leads to impaired function of the gene product, in contrast to a null mutation which leads to absence or complete loss of function of the gene product

ICSI (intracytoplasmic sperm injection) Used as an adjunct to IVF to overcome infertility due to oligospermia and/or immotile sperm and for polymerase chain reaction - (PCR)-based pre-implantation genetic diagnosis (PGD) techniques, to avoid the risk of extra sperm buried in the zona pellucida contaminating the assay

Incidence The number of new cases arising in a specified population over a given period of time

Imprinting A genetic mechanism by which genes are selectively expressed from the maternal or paternal homologue of a chromosome. This expression may be time specific and even tissue specific. For a small number of genes, epigenetic mechanisms can determine expression from one generation of the organism to the next. Imprinting invokes a variety of mechanisms that distinguish the maternal and paternal homologue and affect the chromatin structures that determine transcriptionally silent and active states. The inactive allele is epigenetically marked by histone modification, cytosine methylation, or both. Imprints once established are erased during the early development of the male and female germ cells and then reset prior to germ cell maturation. In humans about 50 genes are imprinted, i.e. differentially expressed according to their origin in either the oocyte or spermatozoa. These imprinted genes have roles in growth and development as well as in tumour suppression.

Imprinting centre Controls resetting of a cluster of closely linked imprinted genes during transmission through the opposite sex, e.g. UBE3A in Angelman syndrome

Incest Incest is defined as sexual intercourse between close relatives. In English law it is the crime of sexual intercourse between parent and child or grandchild, or between siblings or half-siblings (*Shorter Oxford English Dictionary*)

Informed choice 'An informed choice is one that is based on relevant knowledge consistent with the decision maker's values and behaviourally implemented' (Marteau 2001)

In-frame mutation Deletion or insertion of multiples of three bases that lead to a deletion or insertion to the encoded protein, but not to early termination

In situ Refers to carrying out experiments with intact tissue

Interphase The period between mitotic cell divisions; divided into G1, S, and G2

Intron A segment of DNA that is transcribed, but removed from within the transcript by splicing together the coding sequences (exons) on either side of it

Inverse PCR (iPCR) iPCR is a technique to amplify genomic DNA flanking the insertion site of a tranposon. The flanking genomic DNA obtained can be sequenced to determine the position of insertion of the transposon.

Isodisomy See 'uniparental disomy (UPD)', this glossary

Isoelectric focusing gels Thin-layer acrylamide gels that separate proteins by mass and charge, e.g. the different mutants of alpha₁-antitrypsin have characteristic migration profiles

IVF (*in vitro* fertilization) An assisted reproductive technology (ART) procedure that involves collecting eggs from a woman's ovaries (egg retrieval) and fertilizing them in the laboratory. The resulting embryos are then transferred back into the uterus through the cervix. Hormone therapy is administered to stimulate ovulation prior to egg collection, and to prepare the endometrium to facilitate implantation of the embryo(s). Usually a maximum of two embryos is implanted to minimize the risk of triplets and higher-order multiple births

kb (kilobase) 10^3 base pairs of DNA

Karyotype The chromosome complement of a cell or species. In humans, the karyotype of a normal male is 46,XY and that of a normal female is 46,XX

Knock-out Usually refers to a genetically engineered organism (e.g. a mouse) carrying a targeted mutation (in all of their somatic and germline cells) that inactivates the gene of interest. Interbreeding of heterozygous knock-out mice can generate homozygous knock-outs

Lambda (λ) The ratio of the frequency of a multifactorial disease in the relative of an affected person compared with its rate in the general population, e.g. in sib pair studies lambda$_s$ is the ratio of the frequency of the disease in siblings compared with the general population. Lambda$_s$ is a measure of relative risk and hence disease heritability

LCR (low-copy repeat element) LCRs have been found to mediate the recurrent interstitial deletions on 7q (Williams), 15q11–q13 (PWS/AS (Prader–Willi syndrome/Angelman syndrome)), and 22q11. LCRs are either chromosome-specific, e.g. LCR-22 or specific to a particular chromosomal region(s). Three large region-specific LCRs, composed of different blocks (A, B, and C), flank the Williams syndrome deletion interval and are thought to predispose to misalignment and unequal crossing-over, causing the deletions

Linkage disequilibrium Linkage disequilibrium occurs when the probability of the occurrence of particular DNA variants at two sites physically close to one another on the chromosome is significantly greater than that expected from the product of the observed allelic frequencies at each site independently, i.e. the DNA variants occur together more frequently on individual chromosomes in the population than expected by chance

Locus A unique chromosomal region that corresponds to a gene or some other DNA sequence

Locus heterogeneity The disease phenotype caused by mutation in one gene can also be caused by mutations in another gene at a different location in the genome, e.g. tuberous sclerosis can be caused by a mutation in *TSC1* on 9q or by a mutation in *TSC2* on 16p

LOD (logarithm of the odds ratio) score A measure of genetic linkage, defined as the $\log_{10}$ ratio of the probability that the data would have arisen if the loci are linked, to the probability that the data could have arisen from unlinked loci. The conventional threshold for declaring linkage is a LOD score of 3.0, i.e. a 1000:1 ratio (which must be compared with the 50:1 probability that any random pair of loci will be linked)

LOF (loss of function) Referring to a type of mutation resulting in inactivation of the gene product

LOH (loss of heterozygosity) When a region of a chromosome becomes homozygous for alleles that were expected to be heterozygous (usually due to a deletional event or loss of chromosomal material, often seen in the evolution of tumours)

LOI (loss of imprinting) Loss of imprinting is a phenomenon seen in many cancers

Marker chromosome Term synonymous with ESAC (extra structurally abnormal chromosome)

Mb (megabase) 10^6 base pairs of DNA

Meiosis The process by which haploid (*n*) germ cells are produced by two successive cell divisions without an intervening round of DNA replication. The first meiotic division (MI) is called the reduction division because it reduces the chromosome number from 2*n* to *n*. Sister chromatids separate from each other only at the second meiotic division (MII). This yields haploid cells that differentiate into ova or sperm. Recombination occurs in the prophase of MI

Microarray (Chip) A high-density miniaturized array of oligonucleotides spotted onto a glass slide. Expression arrays hybridise mRNA to quantify gene expression Genomic arrays hybridise DNA to identify cryptic deletions and duplications

Microsatellite A stretch of DNA in which a short motif (usually one to 5 nucleotides long) is repeated several times, e.g. a poly A tract (A)$_{13}$. The most common microsatellite in humans is a (CA)$_n$ repeat which occurs in tens of thousands of places in the genome. Microsatellites are often polymorphic, e.g. (CA)$_{11}$, (CA)$_{14}$, (CA)$_{15}$, and (CA)$_{20}$

Microsatellite instability (MSI) The situation in which germline microsatellite alleles (see above) gain or lose repeat units during mitosis. This generates a variety of repeat lengths for specific microsatellites in different somatic cells of the same individual. Microsatellite instability is a feature of Hereditary Nonpolyposis Colorectal Cancer (HNPCC)

Minisatellite see 'VNTR (variable number tandem repeat)', this glossary

Missense mutation Nucleotide substitution that results in an altered amino acid residue in the encoded protein

Mismatch repair Nucleotide mismatches occur normally when two strands of DNA replicate, but almost all such errors are quickly corrected by a molecular proofreading mechanism (encoded by the mismatch repair genes, e.g. *MSH2* and *MLH1*). Defective mismatch repair facilitates malignant transformation by allowing the rapid accumulation of mutations that inactivate genes that ordinarily have key functions in the cell

Mitosis The process by which the genetic material in a cell is duplicated and divided equally between two daughter cells. Each chromosome undergoes duplication to produce two closely adjacent sister chromatids that separate from each other to become two daughter chromosomes

Modifier gene A gene whose expression can influence a phenotype resulting from mutation at another locus

Monogenic A trait or disease governed by the individual action of a single gene (as in classical Mendelian disorders)

Monosomy One copy of a chromosome. Usually two copies are present in a somatic cell (2*n*). Autosomal monosomy is invariably lethal in early pregnancy. Females with Turner syndrome are typically monosomic for X, i.e. 45,X

Monozygotic twins (MZ) Two individuals born together derived from one sperm and one egg

Mosaicism The presence of two or more cell populations derived from the same conceptus, but in which one has subsequently acquired a genetic difference, either by mitotic non-disjunction, trisomy rescue, or occurrence of a somatic new mutation. Examples include trisomy 21 mosaicism arising either from a normal conceptus with mitotic non-disjunction in the early zygote or from a trisomy 21 conceptus with subsequent trisomy rescue establishing a euploid cell line 47XY + 21/46XY, or segmental neurofibromatosis type 1 (NF1) in which cells in just a few dermatomes have acquired a neurofibromin mutation

Multifactorial disease A disease caused by the interaction of several genes and the environment

Multiplex ligation-dependent probe amplification (MLPA) A new method for the relative quantification of up to 40 different DNA sequences. Each MLPA probe consists of two oligonucleotides that are ligated by a thermostable ligase if they bind to the target sequence. Target sequences are small (50–70 nucleotides). The ligated probe is then amplified by polymerase chain reaction (PCR) rather than the target sequence as in conventional assays). Each MLPA probe is designed to have a specific size so that, when the amplification products of the PCR are run on a gel, the product of each probe can be identified by its size. This technique can be used to identify exon deleletions and duplications and, potentially, the copy number of any unique sequence

Multiplex polymerase chain reaction (PCR) In this test PCR is used with a mixture of different primer pairs. Each primer pair is designed to amplify a single region of interest (e.g. an exon of dystrophin) using genomic DNA as a template

Mutation A permanent change in the genetic material that can be transmitted to offspring. A pathogenic mutation results in an alteration in the function of the gene product

Nested polymerase chain reaction (PCR) A technique for improving the sensitivity and specificity of PCR by the sequential use of two sets of oligonucleotide primers in two rounds of PCR. The second pair (known as 'nested primers') are located within the segment of DNA that is amplified by the first pair

Non-disjunction The failure of homologous chromosomes to segregate at meiosis, resulting in one daughter cell with two copies, and one daughter cell with no copies of the chromosome in question. Trisomy 21 usually arises by non-disjunction in maternal meiosis

Nonsense-mediated decay (NMD) A pathway ensuring that mRNAs that bear premature stop codons are eliminated as templates for translation

Nonsense mutation A mutation resulting in the introduction of a stop codon that causes the premature truncation of a protein

Northern blotting Technique for transferring RNA from an agarose gel to a nitrocellulose filter on which it can be hybridized to complementary DNA

Nucleosome The basic structural subunit of chromatin consisting of 200 bp of double-helical DNA and an octamer of histone proteins, comprising two of each core histone (H2A, H2B, H3, and H4)

Nucleotide A purine or pyrimidine base to which a sugar and phosphate groups are attached

Null mutation/allele A mutation which leads to absence or complete loss of function of the gene product in contrast to a hypomorphic mutation which leads to impaired function of the gene product

Odds ratio (OR) The association of an exposure and an outcome measure can be estimated by the calculation of an odds ratio, which is the ratio of the odds of exposure among cases to the odds of exposure among controls. An OR greater than one (>1) means the exposure is estimated to increase the odds of an event, conversely, an OR < 1 will decrease the odds. If the OR = 1 then the exposure is estimated to have no effect on the outcome

Offspring risk The risk that an affected parent will have an offspring with the same genetic condition. For a fully penetrant autosomal dominant condition, this risk will be 50%. See relevant sections of Chapter 1, 'Introduction'

Oligogenic A trait or disease governed by the simultaneous action of a few (2–3) gene loci

Oligonucleotide (oligo) A short fragment of single-stranded DNA that is typically 5–50 nucleotides long

Oncogene A gene normally involved in promoting cell proliferation or differentiation, whose overactivity contributes to carcinogenesis. Oncogenes usually act dominantly at the cellular level, i.e. an activating mutation in just one copy of the gene is sufficient to drive carcinogenesis

Open reading frame (ORF) A sequence of DNA following an initiation codon that does not contain a stop codon. Implies the presence of a gene that codes for a protein or functional RNA

Paracentric inversion A structural alteration to a chromosome that results from breakage, inversion, and reinsertion at the sites of breakage of the fragment at the same breakpoints, where both breakpoints lie on the same arm of the chromosome, i.e. the inversion does not span the centromere

Paralogues Homologous genes that are related by a duplication event

Parent of origin (PoO) When inheritance expression differs depending on which parent (mother or father) a gene or trait is inherited from (see 'imprinting') and allelic expansion

PAX (paired box) genes Genes that encode transcription factors involved in early embryological development of many tissues. Their DNA-binding domain resembles that of paired genes of *Drosophila*

PCR (polymerase chain reaction) A technique in which cycles of denaturation, annealing with primer, and extension with DNA polymerase are used to amplify the number of copies of a target DNA sequence by >10^6 times (Lewin 2000)

Penetrance The probability of the carrier of a germline mutation showing signs of the disease, from the most trivial to the most severe. If all individuals who have a disease genotype show the disease phenotype, then the disease is said to be 'fully penetrant' or to have a penetrance of 100%

Pericentric inversion A structural alteration to a chromosome that results from breakage, inversion and reinsertion of the fragment at the same breakpoints, where one breakpoint lies on the p arm and the other on the q arm, i.e. the inversion spans the centromere

PGD (pre-implantation genetic diagnosis) IVF (*in vitro* fertilization) techniques are used (ovarian hyperstimulation, oocyte retrieval, and *in vitro* fertilization) to obtain fertilized embryos. 1–2 cells are removed for genetic analysis from several cleavage stage embryos at the 8–16 cell stage (day 3). Only embryos in which genetic testing predicts that the developing embryo will not develop the genetic disorder under test are then implanted in the mother

Phase Describes whether particular alleles at adjacent loci are on the same (*cis*) or different (*trans*) chromosomes

Phenocopy The mimicking of a disorder usually caused by mutations in a given gene, by mutations in a different gene, or by environmental factors

Phenotype The appearance or other characteristics of the organism, resulting from the interaction of its genetic constitution with the environment

Pleiotropy The production by a single gene of two or more apparently unrelated diseases, e.g. limb-girdle dystrophy, partial lipodystrophy, and Charcot–Marie–Tooth disease can all be caused by different mutations in the lamin A/C (*LMNA*) gene on 1q21. Conversely, the term may refer to the pleiotropic effects (e.g. multiple system involvement) of a single gene, (e.g. eye, bone and heart involvement in Marfan syndrome due to mutations in *FBN1*)

Polygenic A trait or disease governed by the simultaneous action of many (>3) gene loci

Polyploid (3*n* or 4*n*) Multiple sets of chromosomes, e.g. triploid 69,XXX or 69,XXY, or 69,XYY or tetraploid 92,XXXX or 92,XXYY sometimes found in spontaneous abortions

Polymorphism The existence of two or more variants (alleles, sequence variants, chromosomal variants) that are nonpathogenic, the less common occurring at a frequency of >1% in a normal population.

Predictive testing Determining the genotype of an individual at risk for an inherited disorder who at the time of testing has no symptoms or features of the disorder. Usually contemplated in the context of adult onset degenerative disorders, e.g. Huntington disease or disorders for which burdensome screening will be undertaken in at-risk individuals, e.g. familial amyloid polyneuropathy, retinoblastoma

Premutation A mutation that has no phenotypic effect, but that predisposes to a pathogenic mutation in subsequent generations, e.g. triplet repeat expansions in fragile X syndrome

Primers Oligonucleotides that anneal to template DNA to prime synthesis mediated by DNA polymerase

PRINS (primed *in situ* labelling) PRINS is based on specific hybridization of an unlabelled oligonucleotide with a denatured template and synthesis of a single-strand DNA *in situ*. This method may represent a powerful alternative to fluorescent *in situ* hybridization (FISH) for gene mapping and the detection of small deletions because of its ability to generate multiple independent signals within the same gene segment

Private mutation A mutation unique to a given individual or family

Proband The first person in a pedigree to be identified clinically as being affected by a genetic disorder

Promotor A region of DNA involved in the binding of RNA polymerase to initiate transcription of a gene

Proteome The set of all expressed proteins for a given organism

Proto-oncogene A normal cellular gene that, by activating mutations, can be converted into an oncogene

Pseudogene A DNA sequence that was derived originally from a functional protein-coding gene that has lost its function, owing to the presence of one or more inactivating mutations

PSV (paralogous sequence variant) Sequence variants observed between duplicated segments of the genome

Quantitative real-time polymerase chain reaction (PCR) A procedure in which the PCR reaction is tracked as it progresses, by monitoring the accumulating signal that is provided by a fluorescent dye released during each PCR cycle

QTL (quantitative trait locus) A genetic locus or chromosomal region that contributes to variability in complex quantitative traits (e.g. height, weight, IQ). Quantitative traits are typically affected by several genes and by the environment

Recessive A trait in which the mutant allele is recessive to the wild-type allele, i.e. the disease is manifest only when two mutant alleles are inherited, e.g. cystic fibrosis

Recurrence risk The chance of an event happening again. In genetic counselling this term is usually used when advising parents who have experienced the birth of a child with a specific problem about the chance of that problem occurring again in a subsequent pregnancy. For a Mendelian condition following autosomal recessive inheritance, the recurrence risk will be 25% for each pregnancy (see relevant sections in Chapter 1, 'Introduction')

Relative risk (RR; or risk ratio) The ratio of the risk of developing a disease in individuals who have been exposed to (or inherited) a risk factor to that in individuals who have not been exposed (or not inherited) the risk factor. An RR > 1 means a person is estimated to be at an increased risk, while an RR < 1 represents a decrease in risk. An RR of 1.0 means there is no apparent effect on risk

Repeat sequences Roughly half of the human genome is composed of repeat sequences. The majority of repeated sequences are transposable 'parasitic' elements such as long interspersed elements (LINEs) and short interspersed elements (SINEs) (e.g. Alu elements). Together LINE1 and Alu account for >60% of all repeated sequences in our genome. About 5% of the genome is made up of large duplicated regions e.g. chromosome specific low-copy repeats (LCRs)

Reporter gene Easily detected gene/gene product used to report expression of gene of interest, e.g. β-galactosidase (enzyme encoded by bacterial *LacZ* gene that converts substrate to fluorescent compounds), green fluorescent protein (protein derived from jellyfish that fluoresces spontaneously when excited by light of an appropriate wavelength)

Reproductive cloning The use of cloning technology to create a new organism. A reproductive clone is an organism that develops from the genetic information contained in one somatic cell of its parent and is genetically identical to that parent

Restriction fragment length polymorphism (RFLP) A genetic marker based on presence or absence of a target for a restriction enzyme due to a polymorphism at a single base pair

RNA interference (RNAi) RNA interference is a natural process through which small interfering RNAs (siRNAs)—small stretches of double-stranded RNA—act as guides for an enzyme complex that uses the sequence of the siRNAs to identify and destroy complementary messenger RNA, thus silencing gene expression in a sequence-specific manner

RT-PCR (reverse transcriptase polymerase chain reaction) A form of PCR that amplifies RNA by first converting it to cDNA using reverse transcriptase

SAGE (serial analysis of gene expression) SAGE can be used to profile genome-wide transcript levels

Satellite DNA Consists of many tandem repeats (identical or related) of a short basic repeating unit

Screening The systematic application of a test or enquiry in order to identify individuals at sufficient risk of a specific disorder to warrant further investigation or direct preventive action among persons who have not sought medical attention on account of symptoms of that disorder. (UK National Screening Committee)

Segmental aneusomy An unbalanced karyotype arising from a deletion or duplication, such that a segment of the genome is represented in additional or fewer copies than normal, e.g. 46,XY del 7q11.2 (Williams syndrome)

Segregation analysis A means to trace a DNA change through a family to test whether the change is co-inherited with the disease state

Sensitivity The frequency with which a test result is positive when the disorder/disease is present

Silent substitution (synonymous change) A nucleotide substitution that does not result in an amino acid substitution in the encoded protein because of the redundancy of the genetic code

Small interfering RNAs (siRNAs) See 'RNA interference', this glossary

SNP (single nucleotide polymorphism, 'Snip') The occurrence in a population of different nucleotides at particular sites in the genome. SNPs are not disease-causing and are present at an appreciable frequency. They can be used in association studies and several adjacent SNPs can be combined into a haplotype

Somatic mosaicism The presence in a given individual of genetically distinct populations of somatic cells that have derived from one zygote, usually implying the germline is not affected by the genetic change

Somatic recombination Pairing of homologous chromosomes, followed by recombination (crossing-over) is a central feature of meiosis. In contrast, chromosomes do not generally pair during mitotic cell division and recombination (homologous or heterologous) is a rare event. Occasional cells do, however, undergo recombination events and this can be an important mechanism in disease. For example, mosaicism for paternal uniparental isodisomy (UPD) occurring as a result of somatic recombination may underly some cases of Beckwith–Wiedemann syndrome (BWS). Somatic recombination can cause loss of heterozygosity (LOH), which is often an important step in tumour development

Southern blotting Procedure for transferring denatured DNA that has been cut with restriction enzymes from an agarose gel to a nitrocellulose filter where it can be hybridized with a radioactively labelled probe (complementary nucleic acid sequence). Used to size high-copy repeats, e.g. in Huntington disease, myotonic dystrophy, fragile X

SOX genes Group of genes that encode transcription factors which influence embryonic development of many tissues. Sox refers to Sry-like high mobility group box transcription factor

Specificity The frequency with which a test result is negative when the disorder/disease is absent

Splice acceptor site Junction between the dinucleotide AG at the end of an intron and the start of the next exon

Splice donor site Junction between the end of an exon and the dinucleotide GT at the start of the next intron

Splicing The process by which introns are removed from the primary transcript, and the exons are joined together. Some genes have alternative splice variants, where a single gene gives rise to more than one mRNA sequence which may have different tissue distributions

SSCP (single-strand conformational polymorphisms) A mutation detection technique in which reference wild-type and test DNA samples are cleaved into short sections of <200 bp and amplified by polymerase chain reaction (PCR). The PCR reaction is stopped at the denaturation stage of the cycle. The products are loaded on to a native poly-acrylamide gel that allows the single-stranded DNA molecules to form a secondary structure that affects their rate of migration. Since each strand takes up a different structure, two bands are seen in wild-type DNA. A mutation affecting the secondary structure produces two novel bands

Stem cell A cell of a multicellular organism that is pluripotent and capable of giving rise to indefinitely more cells of the same type, and that retains the potential to undergo terminal differentiation, e.g. into a neuron or an oligodendrocyte or into a red blood cell or a white blood cell

Stutter bands The signals that indicate the presence of DNA fragments that are one or two repeats shorter than the true allele, owing to a 'slippage' artefact that arises from the polymerase chain reaction (PCR)

STR (short tandem repeat) An array of short sequences each normally 2–4 bp nucleotides in length. Often used in DNA profiling

STS (sequence-tagged-sites) Short segments of genomic DNA for which the base sequence is known; they serve as physical landmarks for mapping

Synapsis Side-by-side pairing and union of homologous chromosomes

Taqman A propietary system that allows the progression of a polymerase chain reaction (PCR) to be monitored in real time

Targeting vector DNA fragment usually derived from a virus or plasmid that carries the mutation to be introduced during gene targeting (genetic engineering). It contains the mutation and is flanked by long stretches of homologous DNA sequences to ensure proper exchange with the targeted endogenous gene

T-box genes A highly conserved family of genes, found in vertebrates and invertebrates, encoding transcription factors that bind DNA through a motif called the T-box and are important in the development of many organ systems

Telomere The tip of a chromosome: in humans it consists of a tandem repeat of the sequence TTAGGG and ends in a 3′ extension that may be bent over like a hairpin. All ends of human chromosomes must have a telomeric cap to be stable. If a telomere is lost in a terminal deletion, at least three mechanisms exist to maintain the chromosome end: stabilization of a terminal deletion through a process of telomere regeneration ('telomere healing'); retention of the original telomere producing an interstitial deletion; and formation of a derivative chromosome by obtaining a different telomeric sequence through cytogenetic rearrangement ('telomere capture')

Tiling path The set of clones that represents the sequence of a region or entire chromosome with the minimum overlap

Transcription factor A protein that regulates expression of one or more genes (its target genes). To do so, it must enter the nucleus and bind to a specific sequence in its target gene's DNA

Transgenerational When effects occur across more than one generation, e.g. from grandparent to grandchild

Transgene A foreign gene, typically a gene produced by recombinant DNA techniques. In reference to mice, transgenic refers to mice whose genetic make-up has been changed by introduction of a transgene (see next entry)

Transgenic An organism (often a mouse) whose genome has been modified by introducing a new DNA sequence (e.g. a human gene) into the germline (by manipulation of the egg)

Transposons (Transposable element) A DNA sequence that can move from one chromosomal location to another

Trisomy Three copies of a chromosome. Usually two copies are present in a somatic cell (2*n*). The most common human trisomy surviving to livebirth is Down syndrome, e.g. 47,XY + 21

Truncating mutation A deletion or insertion of one or more bases (but not multiples of three) that disrupt the open reading frame, or a substitution leading to the creation of a stop codon. All result in premature termination of translation

Tumour suppressor gene A gene normally involved in inhibition of cell proliferation or differentiation, whose inactivation contributes to carcinogenesis. Tumour suppressor genes usually act recessively at the cellular level, i.e. inactivating mutations in both copies of the gene are necessary to drive carcinogenesis

Two-dimensional gel electrophoresis A method by which proteins are separated by charge in the first dimension and by size in the second

Uniparental disomy (UPD) A euploid cell in which one of the chromosome pairs has been inherited exclusively from one parent. If two identical homologues are inherited this is called *isodisomy*; if non-identical homologues are inherited the term *heterodisomy* is used. This occurs when non-disjunction during meiosis in one parent leads to formation of a disomic gamete. A trisomic zygote is formed and trisomic rescue with loss of the chromosome from the other parent occurs. UPD is of particular importance in imprinted regions of the genome

Upstream A region of DNA that lies 5′ to the point of reference

VNTR (variable number tandem repeat) Also known as minisatellites these are a class of highly repetitive sequences that consist of a sequence 10–100 bp long repeated in tandem arrays which vary in size from 0.5 to 40 kb. They tend to occur near telomeres

Wave machine Automated method for the detection of DNA sequence variants using denaturing high-performance liquid chromatography (dHPLC)

Western blot Detection of specific proteins by transfer to a membrane and reaction with labelled antibodies

Wild-type The term used to indicate the normal allele (often symbolized as +) or the normal phenotype

X-inactivation The process by which most of the genes on one of the X chromosomes in female somatic cells are inactivated or turned off during embryonic development. Also termed Lyonization.

YAC (yeast artificial chromosome) Cloning vector system able to accommodate large genomic fragments. YACs are grown in yeast

Zygote A diploid cell resulting from the fusion of two haploid gametes; a fertilized ovum

Expert advisers: Martin Bobrow, Professor of Medical Genetics, University of Cambridge, Cambridge, England and Judith G. Hall, Emeritus Professor of Pediatrics and Medical Genetics, University of British Columbia, Vancouver, Canada

References

Gardner RJM, Sutherland GR. *Chromosome abnormalities and genetic counselling*, Oxford Monographs on Medical Genetics No 31, 3rd edn. Oxford University Press, New York, 2004.

Goodman FR. Congenital abnormalities of body patterning: embryology revisited. *Lancet* 2003; **362**: 651–62.

Harper PS. Practical genetic counselling. 6th edn. 2004.

Lewin B. *Genes VII*. Oxford University Press, Oxford, 2000.

Mitelman F. (ed.). *ISCN (1995): an international system for human cytogenetic nomenclature*. Karger, Basel, 1995.

Strachan T, Read AP. *Human molecular genetics*, 3rd edn. Garland Science, Philadelphia, 2003.

Sudbery P. *Human molecular genetics*. Longman, Essex, 1998.

Abbreviations

11β-OHase	11β-hydroxylase (deficiency)
17β-HSD	17β-hydroxysteroid dehydrogenase
17-OHP	17-OH-progesterone
21-OHase	21-hydroxylase (deficiency)
3C	craniocerebellocardiac (dysplasia)
AAA	achalasia–addisonianism–alacrima (syndrome)
AC	abdominal circumference
ACALD	adult cerebral adrenoleukodystrophy
ACC	agenesis of the corpus callosum
ACE	angiotensin-converting enzyme
ACMG	American College of Medical Genetics
ACS	acrocallosal syndrome
ACTH	adrenocorticotrophic hormone
AD	autosomal dominant
ADA	adenosine deaminase
ADCA	autosomal dominant cerebellar ataxia
ADHD	attention deficit hyperactivity disorder
ADNFLE	autosomal dominant nocturnal frontal lobe epilepsy
ADO	allele drop-out
AdolCALD	adolescent cerebral adrenoleukodystrophy
ADPKD	autosomal dominant polycystic kidney disease (adult PKD)
ADRP	autosomal dominant retinitis pigmentosa
ADULT	acro-dermato-ungual-lacrimal-tooth (syndrome)
AEC	ankyloblepharon–ectodermal dysplasia–clefting (syndrome)
AEG	anophthalmia–(o)esophageal atresia–genital anomalies (syndrome)
AF	amniotic fluid
AFAP	attenuated familial adenomatous polyposis
AFP	alpha-fetoprotein
AFO	ankle–foot orthosis
AHO	Albright hereditary osteodystrophy
AID	artificial insemination by donor
AIS	androgen insensitivity syndrome
ALD	adrenoleukodystrophy
ALK	activin-like receptor kinase
ALL	acute lymphocytic leukaemia
AMH	anti-Müllerian hormone
AML	acute myeloid leukaemia
AML	angiomyolipoma
AMN	adrenomyeloneuropathy
ANCL	adult neuronal ceroid lipofuscinosis
ANF	antinuclear factor
AOA	ataxia with oculomotor apraxia
AP	anteroposterior
APC	activated protein C
APECED	autoimmune polyendocrinopathy–candidiasis–ectodermal dystrophy
APOE	apolipoprotein E
APTT	activated partial thromboplastin time
AR	autosomal recessive
ARAD	autosomal recessive Alport syndrome
ARH	autosomal recessive hypercholesterolaemia
ARMS	amplification refractory mutation system
ARND	alcohol-related neurodevelopmental disorder
ARPKD	autosomal recessive polycystic kidney disease (infantile PKD)
ART	assisted reproductive technology
ARVC	arrythmogenic right ventricular cardiomyopathy
ARVD	arrythmogenic right ventricular dysplasia
ARX	Aristaless related homeobox (gene)
AS	Alport syndrome
AS	Angelman syndrome
ASD	atrial septal defect
ASH	asymmetric septal hypertrophy
ASHG	American Society of Human Genetics
ASPA	aspartoacylase
ASSA	aminopterin syndrome sine amniopterin
AST	aspartate transaminase
AT	ataxia telangiectasia
ATLD	ataxia telangiectasia-like disorder
ATP	adenosine triphosphate
ATR-X	X-linked alpha-thalassaemia/mental retardation syndrome
AVM	arteriovenous malformation
AVR	aortic valve replacement
AVSD	atrioventricular septal defect
AZF	azoospermia factor (e.g. AZFa, AZFb)
BAC	bacteria artificial chromosome
BAER	brainstem auditory evoked response
BAV	bicuspid aortic valve
BBS	Bardet–Biedl syndrome
BCC	basal cell carcinoma
BCECTS	benign childhood epilepsy with centrotemporal spikes
BCG	bacille Calmette–Guérin (immunization)
BMD	Becker muscular dystrophy
BMI	body mass index
BMPR2	bone morphogenetic protein receptor II

BMT	bone marrow transplantation
BOCA	brown oculocutaneous albinism
BOF	branchio-oculo-facial (syndrome)
BOR	branchio-oto-renal (syndrome)
bp	base pair
BP	blood pressure
BPD	biparietal diameter
BPES	blepharophimosis–ptosis–epicanthus inversus syndrome
BPNH	bilateral periventricular nodular heterotopia
BRR	Banayan–Riley–Ruvalcaba (syndrome)
BRR–CS	Banayan–Riley–Ruvalcaba/Cowden syndrome
BSA	body surface area
BSO	bilateral salpingo-oophorectomy
BWS	Beckwith–Wiedemann syndrome
CA	chronological age
CA125	cancer antigen 125
CADASIL	cerebral autosomal dominant arteriopathy with subcortical infarcts and leukoencephalopathy
CAH	congenital adrenal hyperplasia
CAIS	complete androgen insensitivity syndrome
CAL	café au lait (spot)
CAUV	congenital absence of the uterus and vagina
CAVM	cerebral arteriovenous malformation
CBAVD	congenital bilateral absence of the vas deferens
CCA	congenital contractural arachnodactyly
CCALD	childhood cerebral adrenoleukodystrophy
CCAM	congenital cystic adenomatoid malformation
CCD	central-core disease
CCMS	cerebrocostomandibular syndrome
CDG	congenital disorders of glycosylation
CDH	congenital dislocation of the hip
CDP	chondrodysplasia punctata
CES	cat-eye syndrome
CF	cystic fibrosis
CFC	cardiofaciocutaneous (syndrome)
CFNS	craniofrontonasal dysplasia
CFTR	cystic fibrosis transmembrane conductance regulator (gene)
CGD	chronic granulomatous disease
CGH	comparative genomic hybridization
CGRP	calcitonin-gene related peptide
CHARGE	coloboma–heart defects–atresia choanae–retardation of growth and/or development–genital defect–ear anomalies and/or deafness
CHD	congenital heart disease
CHILD	congenital hemidysplasia–ichythiosiform erythroderma–limb defects (syndrome)
CHRPE	congenital hypertrophy of the retinal pigment epithelium
CHS	Chediak–Higashi syndrome
CHSPs	complex hereditary spastic paraplegias
CI	confidence interval
CIPA	congenital insensitivity to pain with anhidrosis
CJD	Creutzfeld–Jakob disease
CK	creatine kinase
CLE	congenital lobar emphysema
CL/P	cleft lip and palate
CLS	Coffin–Lowry syndrome
CLS	cholestasis–lymphoedema syndrome
cM	centimorgan
CM	complete hydatidiform mole
CMD	congenital muscular dystrophy
CMG2	capillary morphogenesis protein 2
CML	chronic myelogenous leukaemia
CMT	Charcot–Marie–Tooth (disease)
CMV	cytomegalovirus
CNC	Carney complex
CNS	central nervous system
COACH	cerebellar vermian hypoplasia–oligophrenia–ataxia–coloboma–hepatic fibrosis (syndrome)
COD–MD	cerebroocular dysplasia–muscular dystrophy
COFS	cerebro-oculo-facial-skeletal (syndrome)
CORS	cerebello-oculo-renal syndrome
COX	cytochrome oxidase
CP	cerebral palsy
CP	cleft palate
CPAP	continuous positive airway pressure
CPEO	chronic progressive external ophthalmoplegia
CPHD	combined pituitary hormone deficiency
CPK	creatine phosphokinase
CPM	confined placental mosaicism
CRC	colorectal cancer
CRF	chronic renal failure
CRL	crown–rump length
CRS	congenital rubella syndrome
CS	Cockayne syndrome
CS	Cowden syndrome
CSF	cerebrospinal fluid
CT	computerized tomography
CVID	common variable immunodeficiency
CVS	chorionic villus sampling
D	diversity (region of an immunoglobulin chain)
D & C	dilatation and curettage
DCIS	ductal carcinoma *in situ*
DCM	dilated cardiomyopathy
DDAVP	1-deamino-8-D-arginine vasopressin

DDS	Denys–Drash syndrome
DEB	diepoxybutane
DGS	DiGeorge syndrome
DHA	dehydroepiandosterone
DHH	desert hedgehog (gene)
dHPLC	denaturing high-performance liquid chromatography
DHT	dihydrotestosterone
DI	dentinogenesis imperfecta
DIDMOAD	diabetes insipidus–diabetes mellitus–optic atrophy–deafness (syndrome)
DM	myotonic dystrophy
DMD	Duchenne muscular dystrophy
DMR	differentially methylated region
DNA	deoxyribonucleic acid
DOOR	deafness–onychodystrophy–onycholysis–retardation (syndrome)
DORV	double-outlet right ventricle
DPNH	dinitrophenylhydrazine
DR	MHC class 2
DRD	dopa-responsive dystonia
DRPLA	dentatorubropallidoluysian atrophy
DSA	digital subtraction angiography
DSP	desmoplakin
DTPA	diethyltriaminepentaacetic acid
DTR	deep tendon reflex
DVLA	Driver and Vehicle Licensing Agency (UK)
DWM	Dandy–Walker malformation
DZ	dizygotic (twin)
EBD	epidermylosis bullosa dystrophica
EBP	emopamil binding protein
EBV	Epstein–Barr virus
ECG	electrocardiogram
ED	ectodermal dysplasia
EDD	estimated date of delivery
EDS	Ehlers–Danlos syndrome
EDTA	ethylenedinitrilotetraacetate
EEC	ectrodactyly–ectodermal dysplasia–clefting (syndrome)
ESHRE	European Society of Human Reproduction and Embryology
EM	electron microscopy
EMG	electromyography
EMG	exomphalos–macroglossia–gigantism (syndrome)
ENaC	epithelial sodium channel
ENG	endoglin
ENT	ear, nose, and throat
EPL	early pregnancy loss
ERG	electroretinography
ERT	enzymatic replacement therapy
ESAC	extrastructurally abnormal chromosome
ESR	erythrocyte sedimentation rate
ESRF	end-stage renal failure
EST	expressed sequence tag
EVC	Ellis–van Creveld (syndrome)
FA	Fanconi anaemia
FACS	fetal anticonvulsant syndrome
FAO	fatty acid oxidation (disorders)
FAP	familal adenomatous polyposis
FAS	fetal alcohol syndrome
FBC	full blood count
FBS	fetal blood sampling
FCMD	Fukayama congenital muscular dystrophy
FDB	familial defective apoB-100
FE1	faecal elastase 1
FEV$_1$	forced expiratory volume in 1 second
FEVR	familial exudative vitreoretinopathy
FFU	femur–fibula–ulna (complex)
FGF	fibroblast growth factor
FH	familial hypercholesterolaemia
FHS	floating harbour syndrome
FIHP	familial isolated hyperparathyroidism
FISH	fluorescent *in situ* hybridization
FKRP	fukutin-related protein
FLAIR	fluid-attenuated inversion recovery (sequence in MRI)
FMTC	familial medullary thyroid cancer
FOP	fibrodysplasia ossificans progressiva
FRAX	fragile X (syndrome)
FRDA	Friedreich's ataxia
FSH	follicle-stimulating hormone
FSHD	facioscapulohumeral muscular dystrophy
FVC	forced vital capacity
FXTAS	fragile X tremor ataxia syndrome
G6PD	glucose-6-phosphate dehydrogenase (deficiency)
GAD	glutamic acid decarboxylase
GAG	glycosaminoglycan
GALT	galactose-1-phosphate uridyl-transferase
GAP	GTPase-activating protein
GBM	glomerular basement membrane
G-CSF	granulocyte colony-stimulating factor
GEFS(+)	generalized epilepsy with febrile seizures
GFAP	glial fibrillary acidic protein
GH	growth hormone
GI	gastrointestinal
GnRH	gonadotrophin-releasing hormone
GSD	Gerstmann–Straussler disease
GSD	glycogen storage disease
GT	glutamyl transpeptidase
GTP	guanosine triphosphate
GTT	gestational trophoblastic tumour
GUCH	grown-up congenital heart disease (clinic)
HADHB	hydroxyacyl-CoA dehydrogenase/3-ketoacyl-coa thiolase/enoyl-CoA hydratase, β-subunit

HAL	haploid autosomal length
HARD ± E	hydrocephalus–agyria–retinal dystrophy ± encephalocele (alternative name for WWS)
Hb	haemoglobin (HbA, HbH, etc.)
HC	head circumference
hCG	human chorionic gonadotrophin
HCM	hypertrophic cardiomyopathy
HD	Huntington disease
HDGC	hereditary diffuse gastric cancer
HDN	haemolytic disease of the newborn
HDR	hypoparathyroidism–sensorineural deafness–renal dysplasia (syndrome)
HED	hypohidrotic ectodermal dysplasia
HEM	hydrops–ectopic calcification–moth-eaten appearance
HFEA	Human Fertilisation and Embryology Authority (UK)
HH	hereditary haemochromatosis
HHS	Hoyerall–Hreidarsson syndrome
HHT	hereditary haemorrhagic telangiectasia
Hib	*Haemophilus influenzae* type b
HIE	hypoxic ischaemic encephalopathy
HIF	hypoxia-inducible factor-1
HIV	human immunodeficiency virus
HLA	human leukocyte antigen
HLCS	holocarboxylase synthetase
HLH	hypoplastic left heart
HLHS	hypoplastic left heart syndrome
HME	hereditary multiple exostoses
HMG-CoA	hydroxymethyl glutaryl coenzyme A
HMPS	hereditary mixed polyposis syndrome
HMSN	hereditary motor and sensory neuropathy
HNF-1β	hepatocyte nuclear factor-1β
HNPCC	hereditary nonpolyposis colorectal cancer
HNPP	hereditary neuropathy with liability to pressure palsies
HOCM	hypertrophic obstructive cardiomyopathy
HOS	Holt–Oram syndrome
HOX	homeobox (gene)
HPA	human platelet antigen
HPE	holoprosencephaly
HPFH	hereditary persistence of fetal haemoglobin
HPS	Hermansky–Pudlak syndrome
HPT-JT	hyperparathyroidism–jaw tumour (syndrome)
HRC	HNPCC-related
HRT	hormone replacement therapy
HSP	hereditary spastic paraplegia
HSS	Hallervorden–Spatz syndrome
IC	imprinting centre
ICA	intracranial aneurysm
ICD	implantable cardioverter defibrillator
ICEGTC	intractable childhood epilepsy with generalized tonic–clonic seizures
ICSI	intracytoplasmic sperm injection
IDDM	insulin-dependent diabetes mellitus
idic	isodicentric marker chromosome
IDMs	infants of diabetic mothers
IFNγ	interferon γ
IGF	insulin-like growth factor
IGFR	insulin-like growth factor receptor
IHC	immunohistochemistry
IHH	Indian hedgehog (gene)
IHH	isolated hemihyperplasia
IHH	isolated hemihypertrophy
ILNR	intralobar nephrogenic rest
IL-7R	interleukin 7 receptor
ILS	isolated lissencephaly sequence
IM	intramuscular
INCL	infantile neuronal ceroid lipofuscinosis
IP	incontinentia pigmenti
IP	interphalangeal (joints)
IPD	interpupillary distance
IPEX	immunodysregulation–polyendocrinopathy–enteropathy, X-linked
IPF1	insulin promoter factor-1 (gene)
IQ	intelligence quotient
IR	insulin receptor
IRT	immunoreactive trypsinogen
ISH	infantile systemic hyalinosis
ITP	idiopathic thrombocytopenia purpura
IUD	intrauterine (fetal) death
IUGR	intrauterine growth retardation
IV	intravenous
IVC	inferior vena cava
IVF	*in vitro* fertilization
IVH	intraventricular haemorrhage
IVU	intravenous urography
J	joining (region of an immunoglobulin chain)
Jak-3	Janus-associated kinase 3
JBS	Johanson–Blizzard syndrome
JHF	juvenile hyaline fibromatosis
JME	juvenile myoclonic epilepsy
JNCL	juvenile neuronal ceroid lipofuscinosis
JPS	juvenile polyposis
JS	Joubert syndrome
JVP	jugular venous pressure
kb	kilobase
KS	Kallmann syndrome
KSS	Kearns–Sayre syndrome
KTS	Klippel–Trenauny syndrome
KTW	Klippel–Trenauney–Weber (syndrome)
LADD	lacrimo-auriculo-dental-digital (syndrome)

LCA	Leber congenital amaurosis
LCH	lissencephaly with cerebellar hypoplasia
LCHAD	long-chain hydroxy acyl-CoA dehydrogenase
LCR	low-copy repeat (LCR22 = LCR on chromosome 22)
LDD	Lhermitte–Duclos disease
LDDB	London Dysmorphology Database
LDH	lactate dehydrogenase
LDL	low-density lipoprotein
LEOPARD	(syndrome comprising) lentigines–ECG abnormalities–ocular hypertelorism–pulmonary stenosis–abnormal genitalia–retardation of growth–deafness
LFS	Li–Fraumeni syndrome
LFT	liver function test
LGA	large for gestational age
LGMD	limb-girdle muscular dystrophy
LH	luteinizing hormone
LHON	Leber hereditary optic neuropathy
LINCL	late infantile neuronal ceroid lipofuscinosis
LMNA	lamin A (gene)
LMPS	lethal multiple pterygium syndrome
LOD	logarithm of the odds ratio (score)
LOF	loss of function
LOH	loss of heterozygosity
LOI	loss of imprinting
LPS	levator palpebrae superioris (muscle)
LSA	learning support assistant
LSCS	lower segment Caesarean section
LTC	long-term culture
LTE	laryngo-tracheo-(o)esophageal (defects)
LV	left ventricle
LVD	left ventricle diameter
LVH	left ventricular hypertrophy
MADD	multiple acyl CoA dehydrogenation deficiency
MAE	myoclonic–astatic epilepsy
MASA	mental retardation–aphasia–shuffling gait–adducted thumbs
MASS	mitral valve prolapse–aortic involvement–skeletal anomalies–skin anomalies
MatUPD7	maternal uniparental disomy 7
Mb	megabase
MCAD	medium-chain acyl-CoA dehydrogenase (deficiency)
MCD	multiple carboxylase deficiency
MCDK	multicystic dysplastic kidney
MCH	mean corpuscular haemoglobin
M-CMTC	macrocephaly–cutis marmorata–telangiectatica congenita
MCP	metacarpophalangeal (joint)
MCUG	micturating cysturethrogram
MCUL	multiple cutaneous and uterine leiomyomatosis
MCV	mean corpuscular volume
MDC1C	congenital muscular dystrophy 1C
MDS	Miller–Dieker syndrome
MEB	muscle–eye–brain (disease)
MED	multiple epiphyseal dysplasia
MELAS	mitochondrial myopathy–encephalopathy–lactic acidosis–stroke-like episodes
MEN	multiple endocrine neoplasia (MEN1 and MEN2)
MERRF	myoclonic epilepsy with ragged red fibres
MFS	Marfan syndrome
MH	malignant hyperthermia
MHC	major histocompatibility complex
MHC	myosin heavy chain
MIM	Mendelian Inheritance in Man (database)
MLC	megalencephalic leukoencephalopathy with subcortical cysts
MLPA	multiplex ligation-dependent probe amplification
MLS	microphthalmia with linear skin defects
MMC	mitomycin C
MMIH	megacystis–microcolon–intestinal hypoperistalsis (syndrome)
MMR	mismatch-repair (genes)
MMR	measles, mumps, rubella (vaccine)
MODED	microcephaly–oculo–digito–(o)esophageal–duodenal (syndrome)
MODY	maturity-onset diabetes of the young
MoM	multiple of the median
MOPDII	Majewski osteodysplastic primordial dwarfism II
MPH	mid-parental height
MPNST	malignant peripheral nerve sheath tumour
MPS	mucopolysaccharide (disorders)
MR	mental retardation
MR/MCA	mental retardation/multiple congenital anomalies (syndrome)
MRA	magnetic resonance angiography
MRC	mitochondrial respiratory chain
MRI	magnetic resonance imaging
MS	multiple sclerosis
MSI	microsatellite instability
MSUD	maple syrup urine disease
mSv	millisievert
MTC	medullary thyroid cancer
mtDNA	mitochondrial DNA
MTHFR	5,10-methylenetetrahydrofolate reductase (gene)
mTOR	mammalian target of rapamycin
MTS	Muir–Torre syndrome

MURCS	Müllerian duct anomalies–renal aplasia–cervicothoracic somite dysplasia (Klippel–Feil anomaly)
MVA	mosaic variegated aneuploidy
MVP	mitral valve prolapse
MVR	mitral valve replacement
MZ	monozygotic (twin)
NAA	*N*-acetylaspartic acid
NAD	nicotinamide–adenine dinucleotide
NADH	reduced nicotinamide–adenine dinucleotide
NADP	nicotinamide–adenine dinucleotide phosphate
NADPH	reduced nicotinamide–adenine dinucleotide phosphate
NAI	non-accidental injury
NAIT	neonatal alloimmune thrombocytopenia
NARP	neuropathy–ataxia–retinitis pigmentosa
NBS	Nijmegen breakage syndrome
NBS	National Blood Service
NBT	nitroblue tetrazolium
NC	non-collagenous (domain)
NCL	neuronal ceroid lipofuscinosis
NCV	nerve conduction velocity (test)
NE	Northern epilepsy
NER	nucleotide excision repair
NF	neurofibromatosis (NF1 and NF2)
NHL	non-Hodgkins lymphoma
NHSBSP	NHS breast screening programme
NICE	National Institute of Clinical Excellence
NICU	neonatal intensive care unit
NIDDM	non-insulin-dependent diabetes mellitus
NK	natural killer (cells)
NKH	non-ketotic hyperglycinaemia
NLGN4	neuroligin 4 (gene)
NMD	nonsense-mediated decay
NOR	nucleolar organizing region
NPS	nail patella syndrome
NPV	negative predictive value
NR	nephrogenic rests
NS	Noonan syndrome
NSAIDs	nonsteroidal anti-inflammatory drugs
NTD	neural tube defect
NTx	*N*-telopeptide of type 1 collagen
OA	oesophageal atresia
OAG	open angle glaucoma
OAVS	oculoauriculovertebral spectrum
OCA	oculocutaneous albinism
ocp	oral contraceptive pill
ODD	oculodentodigital (syndrome)
OEIS	(combination of) omphalocele–exstrophy of the cloaca–imperforate anus–spinal defects
OFC	occipital-frontal circumference
OFD	oral–facial–digital (syndrome; OFD1, OFD2, etc.)
OGD	oesophagogastroduodenoscopy
OHP	OH-progesterone
OHSS	ovarian hyperstimulation syndrome
OI	osteogenesis imperfecta
OMIM	Online Mendelian Inheritance in Man (database)
OMLH	oromandibular–limb–hypogenesis (syndrome)
ONH	optic nerve hypoplasia
OPD	otopalatodigital syndrome (OPD-1 and OPD-2)
OPG	optic pathway glioma
OPG	orthopantogram
OPMD	oculopharyngeal muscular dystrophy
OR	odds ratio
ORF	open reading frame
OSMED	otospondylomegaepiphyseal dysplasia
OTC	ornithine transcarbamylase
OXPHOS	oxidative phosphorylation
PA	posteroanterior
PAIS	partial androgen insensitivity
PA–JEB	pyloric atresia associated with junctional epidermolysis bullosa
PAP	postaxial polydactyly
PAPP-A	pregnancy-associated plasma protein A
PAR	pseudoautosomal region
PAVM	pulmonary arteriovenous malformation
PAX	paired box (gene)
PCP	*Pneumocystis carinii* pneumonia
PCR	polymerase chain reaction
PCS	premature chromatid separation
PDA	patent ductus arteriosus
PDH	pyruvate dehydrogenase
PEHO	progressive encephalopathy–(o)edema–hypsarrthymia–optic atrophy (syndrome)
PESA	percutaneous epididymal sperm aspiration
PET	pre-eclampsia
PFIC	progressive familial intrahepatic cholestasis
PFO	persistent foramen ovale
PGD	pre-implantation genetic diagnosis
PGS	pre-implantation genetic screening
PHHI	persistent hyperinsulinaemic hypoglycaemia of infancy
PHP	pseudohypoparathyroidism
PHPV	persistent hyperplastic primary vitreous
PHSP	pure hereditary spastic paraplegia
PHTS	*PTEN* hamartoma tumour syndrome (also known as Cowden syndrome)
PI3K	phosphoinositide 3-kinase
PIP	proximal interphalangeal (joints)
PJS	Peutz–Jeghers syndrome

PKD	polycystic kidney disease
PKU	phenylketonuria
PLIC	posterior limb of the internal capsule
PLNR	perilobar nephrogenic rest
PM	partial hydatidiform mole
PMD	Pelizaeus–Merzbacher disease
PME	progressive myoclonic epilepsy
PMG	polymicrogyria
PMM	phosphomannomutase
PNET	primitive neuroectodermal tumour
PNP	purine nucleoside phosphorylase
POADS	postaxial acrofacial dysostosis syndrome
POAG	primary open angle glaucoma
POC	product of conception
POF	premature ovarian failure
Poly-T	polythymidine
POMC	pro-opiomelanocortin
PoO	parent of origin
PPD	preaxial polydactyly
PPH	post-partum haemorrhage
PPHP	pseudo-pseudohypoparathyroidism
PPM-X	X-linked psychosis–pyramidal signs–macroorchidism
PPNAD	primary pigmented nodular adrenocortical disease
PPT	palmitoyl-protein thioesterase
PPV	positive predictive value
PRINS	primed *in situ* labelling
PROMM	proximal myotonic myopathy
psudic	pseudo-dicentric (marker chromosome)
PSV	paralogous sequence variant
PT	prothrombin time
PUBS	periumbilical blood sampling
PUJ	pelvi-ureteral junction
PUV	posterior urethral valve
PVNH	periventricular nodular heterotopia
PWACR	Prader–Willi/Angelman syndrome critical region
PWS	Prader–Willi syndrome
QTL	quantitative trait locus
RAG	recombinase-activating gene (*RAG1*, *RAG2*)
RB	retinoblastoma
RCAD	renal cysts and diabetes
RCDP	rhizomelic chondrodysplasia punctata
Rcp	reciprocal translocations
RFLP	restriction fragment length polymorphism
RhD	rhesus D
RNA	ribonucleic acid
RNAi	RNA interference
RP	retinitis pigmentosa
RR	relative risk (or risk ratio)
RTA	renal tubular acidosis
RT-PCR	reverse transcriptase polymerase chain reaction
RTS	Rubinstein–Taybi syndrome
RVOT	right ventricular outflow tract obstruction
RYR	ryanodine receptor
SA	sinoatrial (node)
SACS	Charlevoix–Saguenay syndrome
SAGE	serial analysis of gene expression
SAH	subarachnoid haemorrhage
SAM	systolic anterior motion
SaO_2	arterial oxygen saturation
SB	serum bilirubin (concentration)
SB	stillbirth
SBE	subacute bacterial endocarditis
SBH	subcortical band heterotopia
SCA	spinocerebellar ataxia
SCE	sister chromatid exchange
SCID	severe combined immunodeficiencies
SCS	Saethre–Chotzen syndrome
SCTAT	sex cord tumour with annular tubules
SD	standard deviation
SDH	subdural haemorrhage
SDH	succinate dehydrogenase
SEDC	spondyloepiphyseal dysplasia congenita
SEGA	subependymal giant cell astrocytoma
SEN	subependymal nodule
SGB	Simpson–Golabi–Behmel (syndrome)
SHH	sonic hedgehog (gene)
siRNA	small interfering RNAs
SLE	systemic lupus erythematosus
SLO	Smith–Lemli–Opitz (syndrome)
SMA	spinal muscular atrophy
SMARD	SMA with respiratory distress
SMC	supernumerary marker chromosome
SMEI	severe myoclonic epilepsy in infancy
SMS	Smith–Magenis syndrome
SNP	single nucleotide polymorphism
SNRP	small nuclear ribonuclear protein
SNRPN	small nuclear ribonuclear protein-associated polypeptide N (gene)
SOD	septo-optic dysplasia
SRS	Silver–Russell syndrome
SSCP	single-strand conformational polymorphisms
STC	short-term culture
STR	short tandem repeat
STS	sequence-tagged-sites
STS	steroid sulphatase
SUDEP	sudden unexplained death in epilepsy
SVAS	supravalvular aortic stenosis
SXR	spine X-ray
T1D	type 1 diabetes

T2D	type 2 diabetes
T3	triiodothyronine
T4	thyroxine
TA	transabdominal
TAPVD	total anomalous pulmonary venous drainage
TAR	thrombocytopenia–absent radius (syndrome)
TBS	Townes–Brock syndrome
TC	transcervical
TCC	transitional cell carcinoma
TCS	Treacher–Collins syndrome
TD	thanatophoric dysplasia
tds	*ter die sumendus* = three times a day
TEV	talipes equinovarus
TGA	transposition of the great arteries
TGF-β	transforming growth factor β
TIA	transient ischaemic attack
TND	transient neonatal diabetes
TNSALP	tissue-non-specific alkaline phosphatase
TOC	tylosis oesophageal cancer
TOF	tracheo-oesophageal fistula
TOP	termination of pregnancy
TORCH	(screen for) toxoplasmosis–other (including syphilis, varicella zoster, parvovirus)–rubella–cytomegalovirus–herpes simplex virus
TPP	tripeptidyl-peptidase
TRH	thyroid-releasing hormone
TRPS	trichorhinophalangeal syndrome
TS	Turner syndrome
TSC	tuberous sclerosis
TSH	thyroid-stimulating hormone
TTD	trichothiodystrophy
TYRP1	tyrosinase-related protein 1
U & E	urea and electrolytes
UBOs	unidentified bright objects (in MRI scan)
UDS	unscheduled DNA synthesis (assay)
uE3	unconjugated (o)estriol
UG	urogenital
UKFOCSS	UK Familial Ovarian Cancer Screening Study
UP	urticaria pigmentosa
UPD	uniparental disomy
USS	ultrasound scan
UTI	urinary tract infection
UV	ultraviolet
V	variable (region of an immunoglobulin chain)
VA	visual acuity
VACTERL	(combination of) vertebral defects–anal atresia–cardiac anomalies–tracheo-oesophageal fistula–(o)esophageal atresia–renal anomalies–limb defects
VATER	(combination of) vertebral defects–anal atresia–tracheo-oesophageal fistula–(o)esophageal atresia–renal anomalies
VCFS	velocardiofacial syndrome
VEGF	vascular endothelial growth factor
VEP	visual evoked potential
VER	visual evoked response
VF	ventricular fibrillation
VHL	von Hippel–Lindau (disease)
VIP	vasoactive intestinal peptide
VLCFA	very-long-chain fatty acid
VLNT	venterolateral nucleus of the thalamus
VMA	vanillylmandelic acid
VNTR	variable number tandem repeat
VP	ventriculoperitoneal (shunt)
VPA	valproate
VSD	ventricular septal defect
VTE	venous thromboembolism
VUR	vesicoureteral reflux
VWD	Von Willebrand disease
VWF:Ag	Von Willebrand factor antigen
VWF:RiCof	ristocetin cofactor of Von Willebrand factor
VWS	van der Woude (syndrome)
WAGR	Wilms tumour–aniridia–genitourinary anomalies–mental retardation
WBC	white blood cell
WRS	Wiedemann–Rautenstrauch syndrome
WS	Waardenburg syndrome
WWS	Walker–Warburg syndrome
X-ALD	X-linked adrenoleukodystrophy
X-HMSN	X-linked hereditary motor and sensory neuropathies
Xic	X-chromosome inactivation centre
XL	X-linked
XLA	X-linked agammaglobulinaemia
XLAG	X-linked lissencephaly with abnormal genitalia
XLAS	X-linked Alport syndrome
XLD	X-linked dominant
XLEDMD	X-linked Emery–Dreifuss muscular dystrophy
XLI	X-linked ichthyosis
XLIS	X-linked isolated lissencephaly sequence
XLMR	X-linked mental retardation
XLOA	X-linked ocular albinism
XLP	X-linked lymphoproliferative (syndrome)
XLR	X-linked recessive
XLRP	X-linked retinitis pigmentosa
XP	xeroderma pigmentosum
YAC	yeast artificial chromosome

Expert advisers

Judith Allanson Professor of Pediatrics, University of Ottawa, Ottawa, Ontario, Canada

Derek Applegarth Emeritus Professor of Pediatrics, University of British Columbia, Vancouver, British Columbia, Canada

Trevor Baglin Consultant Haematologist, Addenbrooke's Hospital, Cambridge, England

Michael Baraitser Emeritus Consultant Clinical Geneticist, Great Ormond Street Hospital, London, England

Angela Barnicoat Consultant in Clinical Genetics, Institute of Child Health, London, England

Philip Beales Wellcome Trust Senior Research Fellow and Honorary Consultant, Institute of Child Health, London, England

Di Bilton Consultant Respiratory Physician and Director of the Adult Cystic Fibrosis Unit, Papworth Hospital, Cambridge, England

Nick Bishop Professor of Paediatric Bone Disease, University of Sheffield, Sheffield, England

Maria Bitner-Glindzicz Senior Lecturer and Honorary Consultant Geneticist, Institute of Child Health, London, England

Martin Bobrow Professor of Medical Genetics, University of Cambridge, Cambridge, England

Patrick Bolton Professor of Child and Adolescent Psychiatry, The Institute of Psychiatry, London, England

Paula Bolton-Maggs Consultant Haematologist, Manchester Comprehensive Care Haemophilia Centre, Manchester Royal Infirmary, Manchester, England

Patricia Boyd Associate Specialist in Clinical Genetics for Prenatal Diagnosis, John Radcliffe Hospital, Oxford, England

Garry Brown University Lecturer, Genetics Unit, Department of Biochemistry, University of Oxford, Oxford, England

Han G. Brunner Professor, Department of Human Genetics, University of Nijmegen, Nijmegen, The Netherlands

Nigel Burrows Consultant Dermatologist, Addenbrooke's Hospital, Cambridge, England

Kate Bushby Action Research Professor in Neuromuscular Genetics, Institute of Human Genetics, University of Newcastle, Newcastle-upon-Tyne, England

Carlos Caldas Professor, Cancer Genomics Programme, Department of Oncology, University of Cambridge, Cambridge, England

Hilary Cass Wolfson Centre, Great Ormond Street Children's Hospital NHS Trust, London, England.

Edwin Chilvers Professor of Respiratory Medicine, University of Cambridge, Cambridge, England

Lyn Chitty Consultant in Genetics and Fetal Medicine, University College Hospital, London, England

Angus Clarke Professor in Clinical Genetics, University of Wales College of Medicine, Cardiff, Wales

Jill Clayton-Smith Consultant Clinical Geneticist, St Mary's Hospital, Manchester, England

Trevor Cole Consultant Clinical Geneticist, Birmingham, England

Amanda Collins Consultant Clinical Geneticist, Wessex Regional Genetics Service, Southampton, England

Helen Cox Specialist Registrar in Clinical Genetics, University of Southampton, Southampton, England

T.M. Cox Professor of Clinical Medicine, University of Cambridge, Cambridge, England

John Crolla Clinical Molecular Cytogeneticist, Wessex Regional Genetics Laboratories, Salisbury, England

Melanie Davies Consultant Obstetrician and Gynaecologist (Reproductive Medicine), University College Hospital, London, England

Sally J. Davies Consultant in Medical Genetics, University Hospital of Wales, Cardiff, Wales

Bert B.A. de Vries Clinical Geneticist, University Medical Centre, Nijmegen, The Netherlands

Dian Donnai Professor of Medical Genetics, University of Manchester, Manchester, England

David Dunger Professor of Paediatrics, University of Cambridge, Cambridge, England

Douglas Easton Director Cancer Research UK Genetic Epidemiology Unit, Cambridge, England

Diana Eccles Consultant/Professor of Cancer Genetics, University of Southampton, Southampton, England

John Edwards Emeritus Professor of Genetics, University of Oxford, Oxford, England

Charis Eng Professor and Director, Clinical Cancer Genetics Program, Ohio State University, Columbus, Ohio, USA

Gareth Evans Professor of Cancer Genetics, University of Manchester, Manchester, England

Peter Farndon Professor of Clinical Genetics, University of Birmingham, Birmingham, England

Sadaf Farooqi Wellcome Clinician Scientist Fellow, Department of Clinical Biochemistry, University of Cambridge, Cambridge, England

John Firth Consultant Physician and Nephrologist, Addenbrooke's Hospital, Cambridge, England

David FitzPatrick Senior Clinical Scientist and Hon. Consultant Clinical Geneticist, Western General Hospital, Edinburgh, Scotland

Frances Flinter Consultant Clinical Geneticist, Guy's Hospital, London, England

Charles ffrench-Constant Professor of Neurogenetics, University of Cambridge, Cambridge, England

Ian M. Frayling Consultant in Clinical Genetics and Director of Clinical Genetics Laboratory, University Hospital of Wales, Cardiff, Wales

R.M. Gardiner Professor, Department of Paediatrics and Child Health, Royal Free and University College Medical School, London, England

Paul Giangrande Consultant Haematologist, Oxford Haemophilia Centre and Thrombosis Unit, Churchill Hospital, Oxford, England

Richard Gibbons Lecturer in Clinical Biochemistry and Honorary Consultant in Clinical Genetics, Oxford, England

Karen Goldstone Radiation Protection Advisor, Addenbrooke's Hospital, Cambridge, England

Frances R. Goodman Former Honorary Clinical Lecturer, Molecular Medicine Unit, Institute of Child Health, London, England

Judith Goodship Professor of Medical Genetics, University of Newcastle, Newcastle-upon-Tyne, England

Robert J. Gorlin Professor (retired), Department of Oral Pathology and Genetics, University of Minnesota, Minneapolis, Minnesota, USA

Andrew Grace Consultant Cardiologist, Papworth Hospital, Cambridge, England

Christine Hall Professor of Paediatric Radiology, Institute of Child Health, London, England

Judith G. Hall Emeritus Professor of Pediatrics and Medical Genetics, University of British Columbia, Vancouver, British Columbia, Canada

Ann Harding-Bell Speech Therapist to the Eastern Region Cleft Network, Addenbrooke's Hospital, Cambridge, England

Peter S. Harper Professor of Genetics, University of Wales College of Medicine, Cardiff, Wales

David Hilton-Jones Consultant Neurologist, Oxford Kadcliffe Hospitals NHS Trust, Oxford, England.

Lewis B. Holmes Professor of Pediatrics, Harvard Medical School and Chief, Genetics and Teratology Unit, Massachusetts General Hospital for Children, Boston, Massachusetts, USA

Tony Hope Professor, Director of Ethox, Institute of Health Sciences, University of Oxford, Oxford, England

Ieuan Hughes Professor of Paediatrics, University of Cambridge, Cambridge, England

Steve E. Humphries Professor of Cardiovascular Genetics, British Heart Foundation Laboratories, Royal Free and Universty College Medical School, London, England

Susan M. Huson Hon Consultant in Clinical Genetics, Oxford Regional Genetics Service, Manchester, England

Alison Jones Consultant Paediatric Immunologist/ Honorary Senior Lecturer, Great Ormond Street Hospital/Institute of Child Health, University College, London, England

Alison Kerr Consultant Paediatrician and Senior Lecturer, Department of Psychological Medicine, University of Glasgow, Glasgow, Scotland

Samantha J.L. Knight University Research Lecturer and Wellcome Trust Research Fellow, Wellcome Trust Centre for Human Genetics, Oxford, England

Ian D. Krantz The Children's Hospital of Philadelphia, The University of Pennsylvania School of Medicine, Philadelphia, Pennsylvania, USA

Alison Lashwood Consultant Nurse in Preimplantation Genetic Diagnosis, Guy's Hospital, London, England

Alan Lehmann Professor and Chairman, Genome Damage and Stability Centre, University of Sussex, Brighton, England

Mary Linden Genetic Counsellor, Kimball Genetics Inc., Denver, Colorado, USA

David Lomas Professor, Department of Radiology, University of Cambridge, Cambridge, England

David A. Lomas Professor of Respiratory Medicine, Department of Medicine, University of Cambridge, Cambridge, England

Peter Lunt Consultant Clinical Geneticist, St. Michael's Hospital, Bristol, England

Stanislas Lyonnet Professor of Genetics, Hôpital Necker–Enfants Malades, Paris, France

Eamonn Maher Professor of Medical Genetics, University of Birmingham, Birmingham, England

Kenny McCormick Consultant Neonatologist, John Radcliffe Hospital, Oxford, England

Patricia McElhatton Consultant Teratologist and Head of National Teratology Information Service, Newcastle-upon-Tyne, England

R.J. McKinlay Gardner Medical Geneticist, Genetic Health Services Victoria and Murdoch Children's Research Institute, Melbourne, Australia

Peter Mortimer Professor of Dermatological Medicine, St George's Hospital, London, England

Hugo Moser Professor of Neurology and Pediatrics, Johns Hopkins University, Baltimore, Maryland, USA

Jessica Mozersky Cancer Research UK and UCL Cancer Trials Centre, University College, London, England

Maximilian Muenke Chief, Medical Genetics Branch, National Institutes of Health, Bethesda, Maryland, USA

Andrea Németh Consultant and Lecturer in Clincal Genetics, University of Oxford, Oxford, England

Ruth Newbury-Ecob Consultant in Clinical Genetics, St Michael's Hospital, Bristol, England

John Old National Haemoglobinopathy Reference Laboratory, Churchill Hospital, Oxford, England

John Optiz Professor of Human Genetics, Pediatrics, Obstetrics and Gynaecology, and Pathology, University of Utah, Salt Lake City, Utah, USA

Ingegerd Östman-Smith Professor of Paediatric Cardiology, Gothenburg University, Gothenburg, Sweden

Willem H. Ouwehand Lecturer in Haematology, University of Cambridge, Cambridge, England

Ozkan Ozturk Senior Lecturer in Obstetrics and Gynaecology (Reproductive Medicine), University College Hospital, London, England

Gilbert Park Director of Intensive Care Research, Addenbrooke's Hospital, Cambridge, England

Donald Peebles Consultant in Fetal Medicine, University College Hospital, London, England

Paul Pharaoh Cancer Research UK Senior Clinical Research Fellow, Strangeways Research Laboratory, Cambridge, England

Robin Phillips Professor, St Mark's Hospital, London, England

Daniela Pilz Consultant Clinical Geneticist, Institute of Medical Genetics, University Hospital of Wales, Cardiff, Wales

Bruce Ponder Professor of Oncology, University of Cambridge, Cambridge, England

Mary Porteous Consultant Clinical Geneticist, Edinburgh, Scotland

Joanna Poulton Professor of Mitochondrial Genetics, University of Oxford, Oxford, England

Sue Price Consultant Geneticist, Oxford Regional Genetics Service, Oxford, England

Kathy Pritchard-Jones Senior Lecturer and Honorary Consultant in Paediatric Oncology, Institute of Cancer Research and Royal Marsden Hospital, London, England

Nicola Ragge Consultant Paediatric Opthalmologist, Moorfields Eye Hospital, London, England

Nazneen Rahman Senior Lecturer and Honorary Consultant in Clinical Genetics, Institute of Cancer Research, Sutton, Surrey, England

Uma Ramaswami Consultant Paediatrician (Metabolic Disorders), Addenbrooke's Hospital, Cambridge, England

Evan Reid University Lecturer and Honorary Consultant in Medical Genetics, University of Cambridge, Cambridge, England

Elisabeth Rosser Consultant Clinical Geneticist, Great Ormond Street Hospital, London, England

David Rubinsztein Wellcome Senior Clinical Fellow, Cambridge Institute for Medical Research, Cambridge, England

Judy Rubinsztein Clinical Lecturer in Old Age Psychiatry, University of Cambridge, Cambridge, England

Richard Sandford Wellcome Trust Senior Fellow in Clinical Research and Honorary Consultant in Medical Genetics, University of Cambridge, Cambridge, England

David Savage Wellcome Trust Training Fellow, Department of Clinical Biochemistry, University of Cambridge, Cambridge, England

Ravi Savirirayan Professor, Murdoch Children's Research Institute and Department of Paediatrics, University of Melbourne, Parkville, Victoria, Australia

A. Schinzel Professor, Institute of Medical Genetics, University of Zurich, Schwerzenbach, Switzerland

Robert Semple Wellcome Clinical Research Training Fellow, Department of Clinical Biochemistry, University of Cambridge, Cambridge, England

S.M. Sisodiya Department of Clinical and Experimental Epilepsy, University College London Institute of Neurology, London, England

Roger Smith Honorary Metabolic Bone Physician, Nuffield Orthopaedic Centre, Oxford, England

Martin Snead Consultant Ophthalmologist, Addenbrooke's Hospital, Cambridge, England

Miranda P. Splitt Consultant in Clinical Genetics, Northern Genetics Service, Newcastle upon tyne, England

Robert Surtees Professor of Paediatric Neurology, Institute of Child Health, London, England

Malcolm Taylor Professor of Cancer Genetics, University of Birmingham, Birmingham, England

Karen Temple Consultant Clinical Geneticist, Wessex Regional Genetics Service, Southampton, England

Rajesh Thakker May Professor of Medicine, University of Oxford, Oxford, England

Susan Thomas Information Team, Breast Test Wales, Cardiff, Wales

Hugh Watkins Professor of Cardiovascular Medicine, University of Oxford, John Radcliffe Hospital, Oxford, England

A.O.M. Wilkie Nuffield Professor of Pathology and Honorary Consultant in Clinical Genetics, University of Oxford, England

David I. Wilson Professor of Medical Genetics, University of Southampton, Southampton, England

Louise Wilson Consultant Clinical Geneticist, Great Ormond Street Hospital, London, England

the late Robin Winter Former Professor of Clinical Genetics and Dysmorphology, Institute of Child Health, London, England

C. Geoff Woods Lecturer in Medical Genetics, University of Cambridge, Cambridge, England

Paul Wordsworth Professor of Rheumatology, University of Oxford, Oxford, England

Tim Wreghitt Consultant Virologist, Addenbrooke's Hospital, Cambridge, England

John R.W. Yates Professor of Clinical Genetics, University of Cambridge, Cambridge, England

Ian D. Young Consultant Clinical Geneticist, Leicester, England

Chapter 1

Introduction

Chapter contents

Adoption 2
Approach to the consultation with a child with dysmorphism, congenital malformation, or developmental delay 4
Autosomal dominant (AD) inheritance 6
Autosomal recessive (AR) inheritance 8
Communication skills 10
Confidentiality 12
Confirmation of diagnosis 14
Consent for genetic testing 16
The genetic code and mutations 18
Genomic imprinting 20
Mitochondrial inheritance 22
Multifactorial inheritance 24
Reproductive options 26
Testing for genetic status 28
Useful resources 30
X-linked dominant (XLD) inheritance 32
X-linked recessive (XLR) inheritance 34

Adoption

Adoption is the legal transfer of parental responsibility from the birth family to a new adoptive family. In the UK the Adoption Act 1976 states that to be eligible for adoption the child must be under the age of 18 years and there must be no possibility of continuing in the care of his/her birth parents. Should the child be married or have been married he cannot be adopted. In the UK, an Adoption Order severs all legal ties with the birth family and confers parental rights and responsibilities on the new adoptive family. The birth parents no longer have any legal rights over the child and they are not entitled to claim him/her back. The child becomes a full member of the adoptive family; he/she takes the surname and assumes the same rights and privileges as if he/she had been born to her adoptive parents, including the right of inheritance.

Adoption continues to provide an important service for children, offering a positive and beneficial outcome. Research shows that, generally, adopted children make very good progress through their childhood and into adulthood and do considerably better than children who have remained in the care system throughout most of their childhood (Department of Health, UK).

Fostering is an agreement to offer a temporary home to children whose parents are unable to care for them. It is usually organized by social workers working for local authorities. The authority pays for the children's accommodation and food.

Adoption agency. This is the organization that has arranged the adoption and has had contact with the birth and adoptive parents. The agency may be a state-run organization, a charity, or a profit-making company. The agencies have a statutory obligation to keep records of the adoption process.

Confidentiality. In the UK when an adopted individual reaches the age of 18 he/she can request the original birth certificate that will contain the mother's name and address at the time of the birth. A birth parent is not able to obtain details of the child's new family and name, though some contact between the birth and adoptive parents is more common now.

Genetic issues relating to adoption

(1) Genetic information given to adoptive parents

Family history

The birth parents are asked to give information about medical problems in the family. Often there is no contact with the father and this limits the information that can be given.

In the USA, the American Society of Human Genetics (1991) endorsed a statement concerning the importance of including a genetic history as part of the adoption process. Their recommendations are as follows and were written to encourage state and private agencies to collect helpful genetic histories.

- Every person should have the right to gain access to his or her medical record, including genetic data that may reside therein.
- A child entering foster care or the adoption process is at risk of losing access to relevant genetic facts about himself or herself.
- The compilation of an appropriate genetic history and the inclusion of genetic data in the adoptee's medical files should be a routine part of the adoption process.
- Genetic information should be obtained, organized, and stored in a manner that permits review, including periodic updating, by appropriate individuals.
- When medically appropriate, genetic data may be shared among the adoptive parents, biological parents, and adoptees. This should be done with the utmost respect for the right to privacy of the parties. The sharing of information should be bidirectional between the adoptive and biological parents until the child reaches an appropriate age to receive such information himself or herself.
- The right to privacy includes the right of any party to refuse to enter into or cease to participate in the process of gathering genetic information.

Known genetic disease prior to adoption

When there is a known genetic condition in the family (e.g. single gene or chromosomal disorder) the question of whether to test a healthy child for the condition may arise prior to adoption. 'It should not be assumed that genetic (predictive or carrier) testing will be required before a suitable placement can be achieved. In each case, we would advise discussion between the medical adviser to the adoption agency and a clinical geneticist. The important factors other than the possible laboratory test results need to be identified for future attention in advance of any test being performed' (Clinical Genetics Society 1994). See below (4) for a further discussion of issues relating to genetic testing and adoption.

(2) Genetic disorder diagnosed in child after adoption

The geneticist may be involved in the diagnosis of a genetic condition in an adopted individual that may be of importance to his/her birth family.

Some adopted adults are in contact with their birth families but in most the route to passing on this information is through the adoption agency. The geneticist may write a brief letter stating the name of the condition that has been diagnosed in the adopted child and that this is a condition that could have genetic implications for the biological family and recommending referral to their local genetic service. The medical advisor to the agency can assess the information and it may be feasible for them then to contact the birth family. Records made many years ago are less complete and for individuals >18 years these may not be adequate to enable contact to be made with the birth family.

(3) Genetic disorder diagnosed in birth family after a child has been adopted out

The geneticist may be involved in the diagnosis of a genetic condition or carrier status in the biological parent of a child who has been adopted out of the family. In most situations the route to passing on this information is through the adoption agency. The geneticist may write a brief letter stating the name of the condition that has been diagnosed in the biological family and that it could have genetic implications for the adopted child and recommending referral to their local genetic service. The medical adviser to the agency can assess the information and, for those who are still <18 years of age, should have the information to contact the parents of the adopted child. Records made many years ago are less complete and it may be more difficult to trace an individual, adopted as a child, who is now an adult.

(4) Genetic testing

When a child is being considered for adoption the guidelines for genetic testing should be followed as for other children. The American Society of Human Genetics (ASHG) and the American College of Medical Genetics (ACMG) recommend the following.

- All genetic testing of newborns and children in the adoption process should be consistent with the tests performed on all children of a similar age for the purposes of diagnosis or of identifying appropriate prevention strategies.
- Because the primary justification for genetic testing of any child is a timely medical benefit to the child, genetic testing of newborns and children in the adoption process should be limited to testing for conditions that manifest themselves during childhood or for which preventive measures or therapies may be undertaken during childhood.
- In the adoption process, it is not appropriate to test newborns and children for the purpose of detecting genetic variations of or predispositions to physical, mental, or behavioural traits within the normal range.

(Some dissent from this consensus view and argue that special ethical considerations arise in the pre-adoption context (Jansen and Ross 2001).)

Support group: Adoption UK <www.adoption. org.uk>.

Expert adviser: Angus Clarke, Professor in Clinical Genetics, University of Wales College of Medicine, Cardiff, Wales.

References

American Society of Human Genetics. American Society of Human Genetics Social Issues Committee report on genetics and adoption: points to consider. *Am J Hum Genet* 1991; **48**: 1009–10.

American Society of Human Genetics/American College of Medical Geneticists. Points to consider; ethical, legal, and psychological implications of genetic testing in children and adolescents. *Am J Hum Genet* 1995; **57**: 1233–41.

Clinical Genetics Society. The genetic testing of children. Report of a Working Party of the Clinical Genetics Society, Birmingham, England, March 1994. *J Med Genet* 1994; **31**: 785–97.

Department of Health (UK). <www.doh.gov.uk/adoption>.

Jansen LA, Ross LF. The ethics of preadoption genetic testing. *Am J Med Genet* 2001; **104**: 214–20.

Plumridge D, Burns J, et al. Heredity and adoption: a survey of state adoption agencies. *Am J Hum Genet* 1990; **46**: 208–14.

Turnpenny P (ed.). *Secrets in the genes. Adoption, inheritance and genetic disease*. British Agencies for Adoption and Fostering, 1995.

Approach to the consultation with a child with dysmorphism, congenital malformation, or developmental delay

Terminology

Dysmorphology is the recognition and study of birth defects and syndromes. The term was first used by David Smith from the USA in the 1960s to describe the study of human congenital malformations and patterns of birth defects.

Malformation is a morphological abnormality that arises because of an abnormal developmental process (a primary error in morphogenesis, e.g. cleft lip).

Syndrome is a particular set of developmental anomalies occurring together in a recognizable and consistent pattern (from the Greek 'running together') and known or assumed to be the result of a single aetiology.

Sequence is a pattern of developmental anomalies consequent upon a primary defect, often with heterogeneous aetiology, e.g. the oligohydramnios sequence in which renal aplasia leads to lack of fetal urine production leading to deformation (micrognathia and talipes) and pulmonary hypoplasia. Robin sequence describes the combination of micrognathia, a wide U-shaped cleft palate and upper airway obstruction, with the cleft palate and airway compromise consequent upon failure of normal mandibular growth in the 8th–11th weeks of embryonic development.

Association is a non-random collection of developmental anomalies not known to represent a sequence or syndrome that are seen together more frequently than would be expected by chance e.g. VACTERL (vertebral defects–anal atresia–cardiac anomalies–tracheo-oesophageal fistula–(o)esophageal atresia–renal anomalies–limb defects) associations.

Dysplasia is abnormal cellular organization within a tissue resulting in structural changes, e.g. within cartilage and bone in skeletal dysplasias.

Congenital anomalies

Approximately 2–3% of singleton neonates have an obvious major congenital anomaly. However, with follow-up this rate doubles. Results of several studies suggest that there is a 2–3-fold increase of congenital anomalies in monozygotic (MZ) twins, i.e. ~10% of MZ twins are born with a congenital anomaly. Congenital anomalies (birth defects) may arise due to a number of mechanisms:

1 **localized errors** in morphogenesis, e.g. cleft lip/palate;
2 **deformation**, i.e. distortion by physical force of normally programmed structures, e.g. oligohydramnios sequence;
3 **disruption**, i.e. destruction of normally programmed structures, e.g. limb defects caused by amniotic bands;
4 **teratogenic exposure** disturbing normally programmed morphogenesis, e.g. fetal alcohol syndrome, fetal anticonvulsant syndrome, diabetic embryopathy;
5 **germline genetic alterations affecting morphogenesis.** i.e. abnormal programming of development (Donnai and Read 2003). This may result in:
   - failure of structural integrity—qualitative or quantitative defects of structural molecules, e.g. mutations in *COL2A1* in Stickler syndrome;
   - failure to regulate cell numbers appropriately—e.g. mutations in *MCPH5* (*ASPM*) causing primary autosomal recessive (AR) microcephaly;
   - failure of cell migration such that cells do not reach their correct location, e.g. mutations in *MID1* in Opitz syndrome;
   - failure of a developmental switch—many developmental defects result from deficiencies in transcription factors or cell–cell signalling systems.

Very many genes may be involved, e.g. chromosomal aneuploidy, or a number of genes, e.g. chromosomal microdeletion disorders such as Williams syndrome, or a single gene. Some single gene mutations have devastating consequences for development, e.g. Lys650Glu mutations in *FGFR3* cause the perinatal lethal condition thanatophoric dysplasia type 2.

The term 'dysmorphic' is used to describe children whose physical features are not usually found in a child of the same age or ethnic background. Some features are abnormal in all circumstances, e.g. premature fusion of the cranial sutures, whereas other features may be a non-significant familial trait, e.g. 2/3 toe syndactyly. The recognition of which features are good diagnostic aids comes with experience, but most trainees will be able to come to a differential diagnosis, if not the exact diagnosis, by pursuing a plan such as we outline here.

Although 'dysmorphic' is generally used to refer to visible malformations or distinctive features, the term more correctly means the presence of an abnormality of structure. Internal organs may therefore be affected by the same mechanism as the visible malformations. Knowledge of normal fetal development is necessary to an understanding of dysmorphology.

Background

The clinical geneticist is asked to see children for the following reasons:

1 to give a diagnostic opinion;
2 to help understand the aetiology;
3 to discuss the genetic aspects of the condition;
4 to advise if there are other investigations pertinent to the diagnosis;
5 to advise about the prognosis and suggest various therapeutic options;
6 to discuss the risk of recurrence in another pregnancy;
7 to discuss if prenatal testing is available.

This chapter will deal primarily with the diagnostic aspects of the consultation and the gathering of clinical information necessary to answer the other questions.

The consultation

A consultation starts with a *referral* or a request for a *ward visit*. Use the information you have been given. Determine what questions are being asked by the referee. Ask for the hospital notes and X-rays. A call to the paediatrician, or indeed the family, may help your pre-clinic work-up.

A child will usually attend with his parents, but ask, not assume this, during introductions to save embarrassment later. Parents can give you the child's history and family history and also you are able to observe, and later ask, if they have features in common with their child. Family photographs may be helpful.

Structure of the consultation

This is dependent on the circumstances, place, and age of the child. Even if you recognize the diagnosis at first sight, hold back. Build up a rapport with the family and check that the history and examination support your diagnosis. Below is a suggested approach.

1 **Introductions.** Explain why you have been asked to see the child. Ask the parents about their main concerns and what they would like you to help with.

2 **Observation.** Watch the child during the consultation. Try to involve him/her in the history and take note of spontaneous language and interaction between the child and adults, as well as looking at the face.

3 **History**
- **Family history.** Draw the family tree, usually extending over three generations, but extend further if there are known affected individuals in one branch of the family. Photographs of family members may be helpful.
- **Pregnancy history.** Bleeding, fever, medication, investigations, alcohol/non-prescription drugs (ask with tact), fetal movements, liquor volume, gestation, mode of delivery.
- **Neonatal history.** Birthweight, length, head circumference. Resuscitation, feeding difficulties, ventilation, malformations, surgery, seizures, other medical problems?
- **Developmental milestones and current schooling provision** (e.g. mainstream school with 1:1 learning support assistant (LSA), special needs nursery). If developmentally delayed ask about agencies involved, e.g. physical therapist.
- **Photographs** of the child at various ages may be helpful, especially if assessing an older child/adult.
- **Behavioural phenotype.**
- **Vision, hearing, seizures.**
- **Other questions.** Any other questions that may be of relevance.

4 **Physical examination** including clinical photographs (face, profile of face, hands, and any unusual features. A photograph of the child with his/her parents is helpful in assessing any familial contribution to facial dysmorphology). See 'Dysmorphology examination checklist' in the Appendix, page 670.

5 **Further investigations.**

6 **Conclusions.** Assessment of genetic risk and counselling.

7 **Correspondence.**

8 **Follow-up.**

Normal variation

Without a thorough knowledge of normal pregnancy, delivery, developmental milestones, and usual infant/child behaviour you may miss many important diagnostic clues in the history. It is of equal importance to the physical examination in establishing the diagnosis.

Examination

In the examination, the key to good practice is meticulous and accurate observation, measurement, and documentation of your findings (*photography* is extremely helpful in providing an accurate record of unusual features). Syndrome features alter with age and the geneticist tries to overcome this problem by noting serial measurements, e.g. of head circumference, and by asking the parents to bring photographs of the child at different ages. A natural history of the condition can then be seen. Trainees may find it helpful to use an examination checklist, such as the one on page 670. The descriptive terms used may seem like a completely new language. The Glossary on page xvii describes these, but if in doubt use everyday words or draw a simple sketch in the notes.

Diagnostic 'handles'

Some features are more likely to be of diagnostic help. These are sometimes called good 'handles' and these are not found as normal or familial traits or variations but are only present in a small number of conditions. A poor handle may occur as a normal variant or be found in a large number of syndromes. Diagnostic databases assist you most when a child has one or more of these distinctive features.

Making a diagnosis

It takes several years to develop the confidence to come to a diagnosis and several more to know when you won't! Many senior colleagues talk about 'gestalt' diagnoses. Such a diagnosis is made on the basis of recognition of previously having seen the condition. Many syndromes have characteristic facial movements, e.g. Down syndrome. The trainee should be assisted by a senior colleague for the diagnostic conclusions and counselling, having first presented the history and demonstrated the physical signs. Further investigations are often necessary to establish a diagnosis. You will find these listed in the chapters of the book that refer to specific features, e.g. 'Short limbs' in Chapter 6, 'Pregnancy and fertility'.

Making an accurate diagnosis is central to the practice of clinical genetics. With a diagnosis, the genetic advice is usually accurate, the prognosis and natural history can be discussed, surveillance can be targeted appropriately, prenatal diagnosis may be possible, and the family can be given details of support groups and are empowered to access further information. Although it is satisfying to make a diagnosis, time spent ensuring that the diagnosis is correct and establishing a rapport with the parents and making an assessment of their state of readiness to receive a diagnosis will be valuable when you come to give this news to the family.

Expert adviser: Judith G. Hall, Professor of Pediatrics and Medical Genetics, University of British Columbia, Vancouver, British Columbia, Canada.

References

Aase JM. *Diagnostic dysmorphology*. Plenum, New York, 1990.

Donnai D, Read AP. How clinicians add to knowledge of development. *Lancet* 2003; **362**: 477–84.

Jones KL (ed.). *Smith's recognisable patterns of human malformation*, 5th edn. W.B. Saunders, Philadelphia, 1997.

Merks JHM, van Karnembeek CDM, *et al.* Phenotypic abnormalities: terminology and classification. *Am J Med Genet* 2003; **123A**: 211–30.

Shalev SA, Hall JG. Behavioural pattern profile: a tool for the description of behaviour to be used in the genetics clinic. *Am J Med Genet* 2004; **128A** (4): 389–95.

Winter RM, Baraitser M. *London Dysmorphology Database*. London Medical Databases, 2003.

Autosomal dominant (AD) inheritance

AD disorders are encoded on the autosomes and the disorder manifests in heterozygotes, i.e. when a single copy of the mutant allele is present. AD disorders are characterized by inter- and intrafamilial variability. Factors influencing this variability may include modifier genes, environmental exposure, and stochastic effects.

Some AD disorders such as retinoblastoma and von Hippel–Lindau (VHL) disease are recessive at the cellular level. The mutation confers increased susceptibility to tumours because of a heritable germline mutation in one allele, but cell behaviour appears normal in the heterozygous state. Tumorigenesis requires inactivation of the second allele ('second-hit').

Aspects of AD inheritance

Penetrance is the percentage of individuals expressing the disorder to any degree, from the most trivial to the most severe. Many dominant disorders show *age-dependent penetrance*, e.g. hereditary motor and sensory neuropathies (HMSN), hereditary spastic paresis (HSP), Huntington disease (HD). Features of the condition are not present at birth, but become evident over time. Some conditions show *incomplete penetrance*, i.e. not all mutation carriers will manifest the disorder during a natural lifespan, e.g. hereditary nonpolyposis colorectal cancer (HNPCC).

Expressivity is the variation in the severity of a disorder in individuals who have inherited the same disease alleles. Many AD conditions show quite striking variation in severity between families (interfamilial variation) and also within families carrying the same mutation (intrafamilial variation). A mildly affected parent can have a severely affected child and vice versa. For example, in tuberous sclerosis a parent with minimal cutaneous signs may have a child who develops infantile spasms and severe developmental delay.

Somatic mosaicism. A new mutation arising at an early stage in embryogenesis can give rise to a partial phenotype, often present in a dermatomal distribution, e.g. segmental neurofibromatosis type 1 (NF1). If the mutation is also present in the germline (*germline mosaicism*) it can be transmitted to future generations.

Germline mosaicism (gonadal mosaicism). A new mutation arising during oogenesis or spermatogenesis may cause no phenotype in the parent unless the somatic cells are involved as well (gonosomal mosaicism), but can be transmitted to the offspring. If a population of germ cells harbours the mutation there may be a significant recurrence risk, e.g. osteogenesis imperfecta types IIA and IIB.

Reproductive fitness. Some AD disorders, e.g. lissencephaly due to a *LIS1* mutation, have a reproductive fitness of zero, i.e. mutation carriers do not reproduce. Such a condition is maintained in the population entirely by new mutation. Many other AD disorders have only modest effects on reproductive fitness.

New mutation rate. The *de novo* mutation rate varies considerably between different AD conditions. It is high in NF1 with as many as 50% of cases representing new mutations; for other conditions, e.g. HD, new mutation is unusual.

Paternal age effect. For some AD disorders the chance of a new mutation increases with advancing paternal age. In Apert syndrome this observation is explained by germ cell selection for the pathogenic *FGFR2* mutation (Goriely *et al.* 2003).

Anticipation is worsening of disease severity in successive generations. This is a feature of a few AD conditions and characteristically occurs in triplet repeat disorders where there is expansion of the triplet repeat in the maternal or paternal germline, e.g. myotonic dystrophy (maternal), HD (paternal). In addition to variable expressivity the mutation itself is unstably transmitted and varies in size between different generations (dynamic mutation).

Typical family tree

Autosomal dominant inheritance

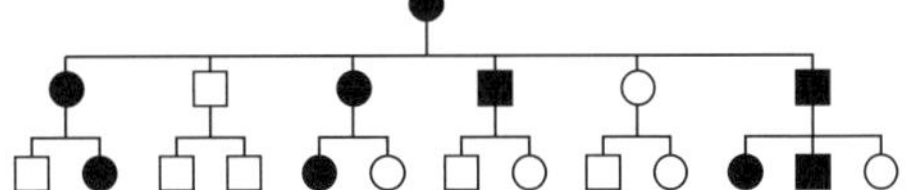

A typical family tree showing autosomal dominant inheritance. An affected parent has a 50% risk of transmitting the condition to each child whether they are male or female.

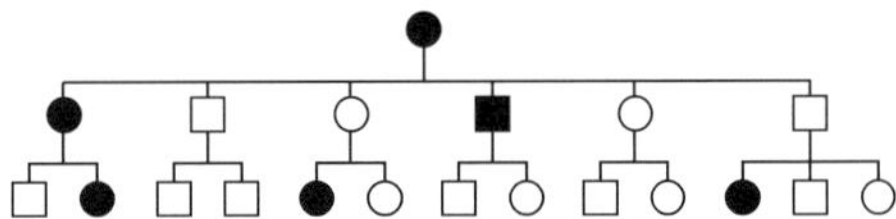

The same family tree showing AD inheritance with incomplete penetrance. In this example the penetrance is reduced from 100% to 67%.

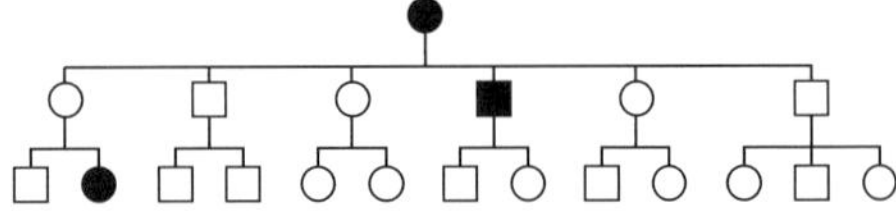

In this example the family tree still shows AD inheritance, but with the penetrance reduced to 33%. The family tree then begins to look suggestive of a disorder following multifactorial inheritance (see 'Multifactorial inheritance', this chapter for further discussion).

Some conditions show incomplete and age-dependent penetrance and these factors can make it difficult to give accurate genetic advice where the familial mutation is unknown.

Genetic advice

- Males and females are affected equally.
- Males and females can both transmit the disorder.
- There is a 50% risk to offspring in any pregnancy that they will inherit the mutation. (NB. Depending on penetrance and expressivity the risk of becoming symptomatic may be less than this.)
- The severity of the disorder in the offspring may vary, being similar, more severe, or less severe than in the parent.
- Examine parents very carefully before concluding that they are unaffected. For disorders with incomplete penetrance, apparently unaffected individuals will still be at some risk of transmitting the disorder (see above).

Autosomal dominant inheritance

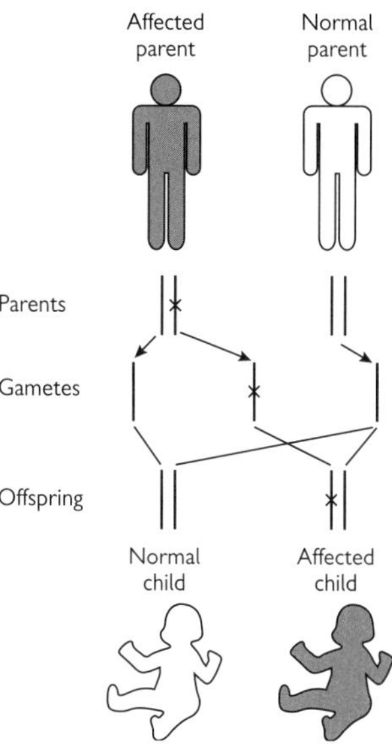

Expert adviser: Ian D. Young, Consultant Clinical Geneticist, Leicester, England.

References

Goriely A, McVean GA, *et al.* Evidence for selective advantage of pathogenic *FGFR2* mutations in the male germ line. *Science* 2003; **301**: 643–6.

Strachan T, Read AP. *Human molecular genetics*, 3rd edn. Garland Science, Philadelphia, 2003.

Young ID. *Introduction to risk calculation in genetic counselling*, 2nd edn. Oxford University Press, Oxford, 1999.

Autosomal recessive (AR) inheritance

See 'Carrier frequency and carrier testing for autosomal recessive disorders' in the Appendix, page 650.

AR disorders are encoded on the autosomes and the disorder manifests in homozygotes and compound heterozygotes, i.e. when both alleles at a given locus are mutated. Heterozygotes do not manifest a phenotype (e.g. cystic fibrosis (CF)), or if they do this is very mild in comparison with the disease state (e.g. sickle cell trait versus sickle cell disease). Affected siblings often follow a broadly similar clinical course which is more similar than for many autosomal dominant (AD) disorders.

Aspects of AR inheritance

Consanguinity. AR disorders are far more common in the offspring of consanguineous partnerships. See 'Consanguinity', page 284.

Heterozygote advantage. For common recessive conditions, heterozygote advantage is usually much more important than recurrent mutation for maintaining the disease gene at high frequency, e.g. sickle cell disease where heterozygotes are less susceptible than normal individuals to malaria.

Founder effect is a high prevalence of a genetic disorder in an isolated or inbred population due to the fact that many members of the population are derived from a common ancestor who harboured a disease-causing mutation. The affected individuals in a given population are all homozygous for the same mutation (founder mutation). Examples include the recessive disorders Meckel syndrome, hydrolethalus syndrome, Cohen syndrome, and congenital Finnish nephropathy, which all occur with disproportionately high incidence in Finland compared with other European populations.

Carrier determination for a relative of the proband is reasonably straightforward if the mutations in the proband are defined. Determining whether an unrelated partner is a carrier is usually more problematic. Unless the partner has a family history of the disorder, he/she will be at population risk for carrier status. If the disorder is rare, the risk of affected offspring will be low and equivalent to half the carrier risk in the general population. Carrier testing for those at population risk is possible for a few diseases, e.g. CF, spinal muscular atrophy (SMA), sickle cell disease, thalassaemia, but not for many others. Whereas inborn errors of metabolism often show a marked distinction in enzyme activity (or other biochemical markers) between normal and affected, there is often considerable overlap in levels between heterozygotes and normals making assignment of carrier status problematic. Tay–Sachs disease is a notable exception.

Deriving population risk for carrier status from disease frequency. See 'Carrier frequency and carrier testing for autosomal recessive disorders', page 650.

Family trees

Autosomal recessive inheritance

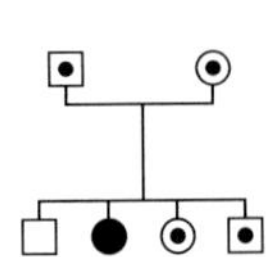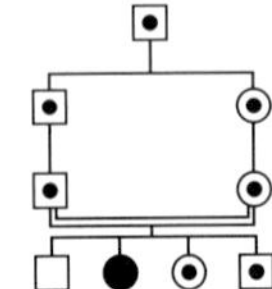

Family trees showing AR inheritance. If both parents are carriers, there is a 25% risk of an affected child in any pregnancy, independent of gender. The diagram on the right illustrates a consanguineous relationship between first cousins. A common ancestor is a carrier for a recessive mutation that may occur in homozygous form in a descendent as a consequence of consanguinity.

Genetic advice

- Disease expressed only in homozygotes and compound heterozygotes.
- Parents are obligate carriers (SMA is an exception to this rule as there is a significant new mutation rate of 1.7%).
- Risk to carrier parents for an affected child is 25% (1 in 4).
- Healthy siblings of affected individuals have a two-thirds risk of carrier status.
- Risk of carrier status diminishes by one-half with every degree of relationship distanced from parents of affected individual, e.g. second-degree relatives (grandparents and aunts/uncles) and third-degree relatives (first cousins, great-grandparents, great-aunts, and great-uncles).
- All offspring of an affected individual whose partner is a non-carrier are obligate carriers.

Autosomal recessive inheritance

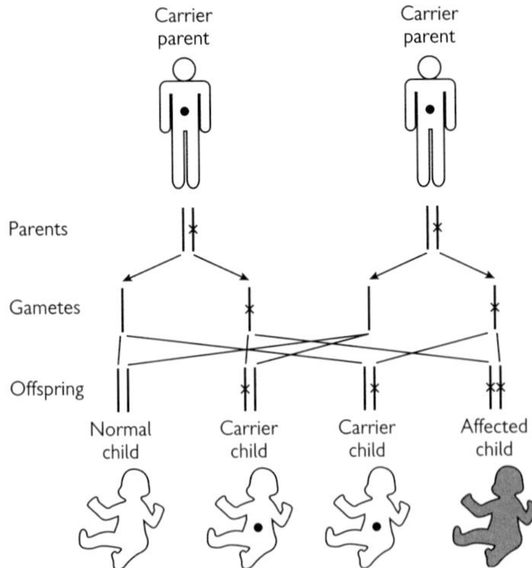

Expert adviser: Ian D. Young, Consultant Clinical Geneticist, Leicester, England.

References

Strachan T, Read AP. *Human molecular genetics*, 3rd edn. Garland Science, Philadelphia, 2003.

Young ID. *Introduction to risk calculation in genetic counselling*, 2nd edn. Oxford University Press, Oxford, 1999.

Communication skills

The genetics consultation

The success of any consultation depends on how well the patient and doctor communicate with each other. Time is limited so it is important to ensure that it is used as effectively as possible. It may be helpful to think of the consultation as divided into three separate phases:

1 establishing rapport and trust—building a relationship;
2 collecting data;
3 agreeing a plan of action (management plan).

Key skills

1 **Setting an agenda for the consultation.** Elicit the main issues at the outset of the consultation. Is the main issue finding a diagnosis, or determining whether an individual with a family history is themselves at risk of developing the condition, or reviewing the natural history if that is known? If the condition may have implications for future children, offer to discuss this. What do the family want to know?

2 **Determine the patients' perception.** What is their interpretation of the child's problems, or family history?

3 **Explain the genetic basis of the condition** if known or, if unknown, state whether you think it is likely to have a genetic basis or not. Check the family's understanding of the information you are giving as you go along. It is easier to change tack and alter the pitch of an explanation as you are going along.

4 **Assess the genetic risk to other family members.** Discuss whether or not there is a significant risk to other family members not present at the consultation and, if an appreciable risk exists, agree a strategy for offering genetic advice and investigation.

Breaking bad news

Geneticists are frequently called upon to give bad news to patients, whether it is a chorionic villus sampling (CVS) result indicating an affected fetus or an adverse result in a Huntington or *BRCA* predictive test, that the disorder just diagnosed has a progressive downhill course, or to tell parents that the disorder that has afflicted one of their children has a substantial recurrence risk.

When arranging prenatal or predictive tests careful plans should be laid for the giving of results. Care should be taken to ensure the following.

- The individual is aware of the possibility of an adverse result and has thought through how they might handle this information and is prepared for this eventuality.
- The result is given by a member of staff well known to the individual, usually the person who has undertaken the pre-test counselling.
- The individual has a choice in how they receive the result and know when to expect the result, e.g. by telephone, in a clinic visit, or by letter.
- Ongoing support is offered following receipt of the test result.

Studies show that patients take in and retain very little of the information that is given after receiving a bad-news result. Aim to keep discussion simple and focused on the patient's needs.

Communicating a diagnosis (after Unique–rare chromosome disorder support group)

Diagnosis and genetic counselling should be given:

- in private, in person, and with both partners present, or with a supporter;
- with sensitivity, respect, compassion, understanding, and honesty;
- without being rushed and without jargon, using positive, sensitive language;
- with the contact details of relevant support groups;
- with the offer of a follow-up appointment to answer new questions and discuss new issues;
- with the offer of ongoing support to help the family cope and adjust.

Sometimes, it can be helpful to remind the family that, although knowledge of the diagnosis is new, the genetic condition has in fact been present since conception and has always been a part of their child's life.

Expert adviser: Tony Hope, Professor, Director of Ethox, Institute of Health Sciences, University of Oxford, Oxford, England.

References

Gask L, Usherwood T. ABC of psychological medicine: the consultation. *Br Med J* 2002; **324**: 1567–9.

Maguire P, Pitceathly C. Key communication skills and how to acquire them. *Br Med J* 2002; **325**: 697–700.

Unique–rare chromosome disorder support group <www.rarechromo.org>. *Survey of 585 UK families.* Unique, 2003.

Confidentiality

Confidentiality is a major issue for all doctors. Medical geneticists must particularly be on their guard against the potential for breaching confidentiality when their advice is sought by different members of the same family.

The general duty to maintain the confidential nature of personal genetic information is, however, not an absolute one. The Human Genetics Commission note circumstances where it may be appropriate to disclose personal information. Wherever possible, this will be with the consent of the patient, and will be in the interest of the patient, of relatives, or of the wider public.

Disclosure

The Human Genetics Commission recognizes that, exceptionally, 'disclosure of sensitive personal genetic information without consent may be justified in rare cases where a patient refuses to consent to such disclosure but the benefit to other family members or the wider public substantially outweighs the need to respect confidentiality.'

If you decide to disclose confidential information you must be prepared to explain and justify your decision. In practice such cases are usually discussed within a professional forum such as a departmental meeting or with a group of consultant colleagues so that the subjective decision about the balance of interests is shared and agreed.

Children

In 1985, Gillick challenged the right of a doctor to prescribe contraception to a girl under the age of 16 years without obtaining the consent of the girl's parents. This became an important case in English law and Lord Scarman gave the following ruling in the House of Lords, 'As a matter of law the parental right to determine whether or not their minor child below the age of 16 will have medical treatment terminates if and when the child achieves sufficient understanding and intelligence to enable him to understand fully what is proposed.' It is a matter for a doctor to judge whether a child aged under 16 years is 'Gillick competent', i.e. is competent to make judgements about their own medical care. Furthermore, if a child is deemed 'Gillick competent' a doctor can only disclose information to the parent with the child's consent, regardless of parental responsibility.

In the non-Gillick competent child, authority must be given by whoever has parental responsibility under the provisions of the *Children's Act 1989*. In deciding whether to disclose information, the practitioner's overriding consideration must always be what is in the *best interests of the child*.

A child's biological parents both have parental responsibility if they were married at the time of the child's birth. In such circumstances a practitioner will normally disclose all information concerning a young child to either parent without the other's consent. When such parents are separated or divorced, information may still be disclosed to either parent irrespective of who has custody, unless a court has removed parental responsibility from one or other parent.

With parents who were unmarried at the time of the child's birth, only the mother automatically has legal parental responsibility. Her consent is therefore required before information may be disclosed to the father, unless he has been given parental responsibility either by agreement with the mother or by a court order.

Deceased patients

Seek consent from the next of kin. The Human Genetics Commission recognizes that 'There may be some clinical situations where genetic information about the dead is needed *in order to assess the risk to a living relative*. This information may be obtained by testing samples removed from an individual during life. The approach we favour is that a presumption should be made that the dead person would have consented in his or her lifetime to such testing and that this justifies post-mortem testing.'

Refusal of consent

Whilst privacy and the right to refuse consent is an important proposition it is not an absolute principle and it can be overridden if the harm to others outweighs the importance to the individual concerned, e.g. if the refusal of consent is capricious or vindictive.

Useful websites: General Medical Council (GMC) <www.gmc-uk.org/standards/consent.htm>; Joint Committee on Consent and Confidentiality in Medical Genetics <www.bshg.org.uk/JCMG/jcmg.htm>.

Expert adviser: Martin Bobrow, Professor of Medical Genetics, University of Cambridge, Cambridge, England.

References

General Medical Council (GMC). *Confidentiality: protecting and providing information*. GMC, London, April, 2004.

Gillick v. West Norfolk and Wisbech Area Health Authority [1985] 3 All ER 402 (HL).

Human Genetics Commission. *Inside information—balancing interests in the use of personal genetic data*. Human Genetics Commission, London, May 2002.

Lucassen AM, Parker M *et al*. Role of next of kin in accessing health records. *Br Med J* 2004, **328**: 952–3.

Confirmation of diagnosis

See also 'Confirmation of diagnosis of cancer', page 440.

In order to provide precise genetic advice it is *essential* to have an accurate diagnosis. If the diagnosis in your patient has been made by others, and the patient and his/her family are referred to you for genetic advice, you will need to seek confirmation of the diagnosis. If you are asked to give advice to a relative, without the opportunity to see and assess the proband, you will need to confirm the diagnosis in the proband before giving definitive genetic advice. The diagnosis is of such fundamental importance that there may be medico-legal implications if it turns out that the given diagnosis was wrong and appropriate steps were not taken to substantiate it. Some diagnoses such as 'cystic fibrosis' tend to be fairly reliable, whereas others such as 'achondroplasia' are notoriously unreliable. Depending on the circumstances, various options are available.

- **Clinical assessment.** Some genetic disorders have specific clinical features that enable a rapid confirmation of diagnosis. Take a history of the main features/symptoms and briefly examine the patient to confirm that you agree with the clinical diagnosis, e.g. neurofibromatosis type 1 (NF1), tuberous sclerosis (TS), etc., before giving genetic advice. Where possible follow this up by seeking results of various key investigations that were instrumental in making the diagnosis, e.g. cranial magnetic resonance imaging (MRI) result, mutation result.
- **Laboratory findings.** Many genetic diagnoses depend on specific laboratory results. These may be the results of molecular genetic testing, e.g. Huntington disease (HD), fragile X (FRAXA) syndrome, myotonic dystrophy, or the results of biochemical investigations, e.g. Zellweger syndrome, phenylketonuria (PKU), etc., or histological assessment. Ensure that you have sight of the critical result(s) (or a copy of the result(s)) and that these are from a reliable source (e.g. an accredited laboratory) before giving definitive advice.
- **Radiological investigations.** Some genetic disorders, e.g. skeletal dysplasias, depend on radiological studies for diagnosis. Ensure that you see either the images or the radiologist's report confirming the radiological findings before giving definitive genetic advice.
- **Death certificate.** For deceased relatives, the death certificate may lend some support to diagnosis. This is generally less reliable than laboratory results, but is helpful if, for example, hospital notes have been destroyed and it is otherwise difficult to obtain any confirmation of diagnosis.
- **Family photographs.** These are often helpful when determining familial involvement with a syndrome that has dysmorphic features, and when other avenues fail.

Seeking confirmation of diagnosis in relatives

When advice is sought about a family history (and the proband is not seen in clinic) it is usual practice to obtain consent from the proband (their parents/guardians) to approach their doctor/genetics department for confirmation of the diagnosis. Many departments have a standard form for obtaining consent from relatives in these circumstances. Taking the family history and talking about affected family members may be a sensitive area—ensure that there is adequate time for this as it is often crucial to the provision of accurate genetic advice. Sometimes the genetic disorder is not openly discussed in the family, and not all families are on good speaking terms, so it often takes a lot of sensitivity to get accurate information and even so it can be difficult on occasion to establish the diagnosis truly accurately. Under such circumstances you need to explain to the family the limits of the information that you have and document in the medical notes that you have done the best job possible under the circumstances. See also 'Confidentiality', page 12.

Expert adviser: Judith G. Hall, Professor of Pediatrics and Medical Genetics, University of British Columbia, Vancouver, British Columbia, Canada.

References
Douglas FS, O'Dair LC, *et al*. The accuracy of diagnoses as reported in families with cancer: a retrospective study. *J Med Genet* 1999; **36**: 309–12.

Consent for genetic testing

Consent is the agreement to an action based on knowledge of what the action involves and its likely consequences.

Private genetic information about a person (e.g. whether they are affected with a genetic disorder) should generally not be obtained, held, or communicated without that person's free and informed consent (Human Genetics Commission 2002).

The nature and extent of information that is required in seeking consent for a genetic test depend on whether the test in question is likely to reveal sensitive genetic information—information that has special significance for the patient or for the patient's relatives (Human Genetics Commission 2002).

Genetic testing may reveal unexpected information, e.g. about misattributed parentage. The wider implications of testing should therefore be considered and discussed before a genetic test is done.

Points to consider when obtaining consent for genetic testing (Human Genetics Commission 2002)

See also 'Testing for genetic status', this chapter.

- What is the purpose of the test?
- Is there a clear explanation of the nature and treatment of the condition and the way in which it is inherited (if appropriate)?
- Is there a clear explanation of the test, or tests, to be carried out?
- What potential benefits might there be from having the test?
- What might be the potential disadvantages?
- Are there any alternatives to having the test that would achieve the same benefits? Does the test have to be done now or can it be delayed?
- Could the test have implications for the person's:
  - future health;
  - reproductive choices;
  - relatives;
  - family relationships (e.g. information about parentage);
  - present or future employment;
  - insurance prospects?
- What is the method of communication of the result to the patient and how long will it take from sampling to result?
- What are the arrangements for ensuring the confidentiality of the test result, e.g. arrangements for storing of test result in patient's individual medical record? Is any accompanying written information, particularly where this substitutes for face to face consultation, written in clear, simple, understandable language, objective and without bias?
- Is there an awareness of the patient's level of understanding/cultural beliefs/language?
- Would the person like further information or access to other sources of advice (e.g. the opportunity to talk to an independent counsellor or other persons who have faced the same choice)?
- What provision is there for post-test support?

Competence

Competence to make decisions depends on three broad capacities:

- the capacity for understanding and communication;
- the capacity for reasoning and deliberation;
- the capacity to develop and sustain a set of moral values.

Competent adult

A competent adult is a person who has reached 18 years of age and has the capacity to make medical decisions on his/her own behalf. To demonstrate that capacity an individual must be able to (British Medical Association and Law Society 1995):

1 understand in simple language what genetic testing is, its purpose, and why it is being proposed;
2 understand its principal benefits, risks, and alternatives;
3 understand in broad terms what the consequences would be of not undergoing genetic testing;
4 retain the information long enough to make an effective decision; and
5 make a free choice (i.e. free from pressure).

Incompetent adults

Adults with dementia or severe learning disability are often not competent to give consent to genetic testing (see criteria above). The Law Commission's (1995) recommendations include a proposal to consider the following:

(1) The ascertainable past and present wishes and feelings of the person concerned and the factors which he or she would consider if able to do so;
(2) The need to permit and encourage the person concerned to participate, or to improve his or her ability to participate, in anything done for and any decision affecting him or her;
(3) If it is practicable and appropriate to consult them, the views as to that person's wishes and feelings and as to what would be in the best interests of that person of:
    (i) Any person named by him or her as someone to be consulted;
    (ii) Any person (such as a spouse, relative or friend or other person) engaged in caring for or interested in the person's welfare;
    (iii) The donee of a continuing power of attorney granted by him or her;
    (iv) Any manager appointed by the court; and
(4) Whether the purpose for which any action or decision is required can be as effectively achieved in a manner less restrictive of the person's freedom of action.

The Law Commission (1995) recommends that 'it should be lawful to do anything for the personal welfare or health care of a person who is, or is reasonably believed to be, without capacity in relation to the matter in question if it is in all the circumstances reasonable for it to be done by the person who does it and it is in the best interests for that person'.

Young people

The *Family Law Reform Act 1969* enables children of 16 and over to consent to medical treatment and, by inference, genetic testing undertaken in a medical context. In such circumstances there is no legal requirement to obtain consent from the parent or guardian.

Children

For young children and babies, the parents (or those with parental responsibility) give or withhold consent on behalf of the child. Children under 16 years can truly consent to treatment only if they understand its nature, purpose, and risks (see 'Confidentiality', page 12 for further discussion).

In practice, as children grow older and if they express an interest, competence, and desire to be involved in decision-making, they should participate in such decisions. The parent and child may choose to both sign the consent form indicating their joint involvement in the decision-making process. Usually genetic tests that will have no impact on health care before adult life are deferred until the individual reaches an age when he/she is legally competent to make his/her own decisions regarding health care.

Children in care

When a child is the subject of a care order, the local authority acquires 'parental responsibility' under the *Children Act 1989*. The order does not, however, deprive parents of their parental responsibility and they are not deprived of their ability to authorize or refuse treatment.

Useful websites: General Medical Council (GMC) <www.gmc-uk.org/standards/consent.htm>; Joint Committee on Consent and Confidentiality in Medical Genetics <www.bshg.org.uk/JCMG/jcmg.htm>.

Expert adviser: Martin Bobrow, Professor of Medical Genetics, University of Cambridge, Cambridge, England.

References

British Medical Association (BMA) and the Law Society (1995). *Assessment of mental capacity—guidance for doctors and lawyers.* BMA, London, 1995.

Department of Health. *Reference guide to consent for examination or treatment.* Department of Health, London, 2001. Available on <www.doh.gov.uk/consent>.

General Medical Council (GMC). *Seeking patients' consent; the ethical considerations.* GMC, London, 1998.

Human Genetics Commission. *Inside information—balancing interests in the use of personal genetic data.* Human Genetics Commission, London, May 2002. Law Commission. *Mental incapacity,* Law Commission report 231. HMSO, London, 1995.

The genetic code and mutations

DNA (deoxyribonucleic acid) contains four types of bases—two purines, adenine (A) and guanine (G), and two pyrimidines, cytosine (C) and thymine (T). RNA (ribonucleic acid) contains uracil (U) in place of thymine. The DNA double helix (Watson and Crick 1953) maintains a constant width and is faithfully replicated, because purines always face pyrimidines in the complementary A–T, and G–C base pairs. Thus it can: (1) serve as a template for replication that re-establishes the double helix and (2) open to be 'read' and 'copied' in the process of transcription for producing proteins.

Because there are more codons (61 plus 3 STOP codons) than there are amino acids (20), almost all amino acids are represented by more than one codon, i.e. the code is degenerate, particularly at the third base.

Triplet codons and their corresponding amino acids and STOP sequences

	T	C	A	G
T	TTT = Phe	TCT = Ser	TAT = Tyr	TGT = Cys
	TTC = Phe	TCC = Ser	TAC = Tyr	TGC = Cys
	TTA = Leu	TCA = Ser	TAA = STOP	TGA = STOP
	TTG = Leu	TCG = Ser	TAG = STOP	TGG = Trp
C	CTT = Leu	CCT = Pro	CAT = His	CGT = Arg
	CTC = Leu	CCC = Pro	CAC = His	CGC = Arg
	CTA = Leu	CCA = Pro	CAA = Gln	CGA = Arg
	CTG = Leu	CCG = Pro	CAG = Gln	CGG = Arg
A	ATT = Ile	ACT = Thr	AAT = Asn	AGT = Ser
	ATC = Ile	ACC = Thr	AAC = Asn	AGC = Ser
	ATA = Ile	ACA = Thr	AAA = Lys	AGA = Arg
	ATG = Met	ACG = Thr	AAG = Lys	AGG = Arg
G	GTT = Val	GCT = Ala	GAT = Asp	GGT = Gly
	GTC = Val	GCC = Ala	GAC = Asp	GGC = Gly
	GTA = Val	GCA = Ala	GAA = Glu	GGA = Gly
	GTG = Val	GCG = Ala	GAG = Glu	GGG = Gly

Amino acid	Characteristic
Alanine (A)	Neutral
Arginine (R)	Basic
Asparagine (N)	Polar
Aspartic acid (D)	Acidic
Cysteine (C)	Polar, forms disulphide cross-links
Glutamine (Q)	Polar
Glutamic acid (E)	Acidic
Glycine (G)	Small, neutral
Histidine (H)	Basic (weak)
Isoleucine (I)	Hydrophobic
Leucine (L)	Hydrophobic
Lysine (K)	Basic
Methionine (M)	Hydrophobic
Phenylalanine (F)	Hydrophobic, bulky
Proline (P)	Hydrophobic, helix-breaker
Serine (S)	Polar
Threonine (T)	Polar
Tryptophan (W)	Hydrophobic, bulky
Tyrosine (Y)	Polar, bulky
Valine (V)	Hydrophobic
Nonsense (X)	(Stop)

Physical basis of some mutations

Nucleotide substitutions

These are described by a number representing the nucleotide in the coding DNA sequence (cDNA), followed by a letter representing the original nucleotide (A, C, G, T) followed by > and the mutated nucleotide, e.g. in the β-globin gene (*HBB*) 17A>T means that adenine at nucleotide 17 is changed to thymine, while in the haemochromatosis gene (*HFE*) 845G>A means that guanine at nucleotide 845 is changed to adenine.

If this results in an amino acid substitution the mutation is termed a *missense mutation*. In protein annotation this is written with a number representing the amino acid in the translated protein product, the first letter preceding the number being the wild-type amino acid, and the letter after being the altered amino acid, e.g. in sickle cell disease E6V (glutamic acid at amino acid 6 is changed to valine); in *HFE*, C282Y (cysteine at amino acid 282 is changed to tyrosine) and H63D (histidine at amino acid 63 is changed to aspartic acid). If the nucleotide substitution does not alter the genetic code it is termed a *silent* or *synonymous substitution*, but note this could still cause problems by affecting splicing, etc.

Most *splice site mutations* occur in introns. Mutations in introns are referred to by the nearest nucleotide in an exon, e.g. in *CFTR* 621+1G>T, the first nucleotide (G) in the intron 3′ to nucleotide 621 in the cDNA is replaced by T and, in 1717–1G>A, the last nucleotide (G) in the intron 5′ to nucleotide 1717 in the cDNA is replaced by A.

Nucleotide deletions and insertions

The nucleotide number is followed by del/ins and the letter for the relevant nucleotide, e.g. 394delT means the nucleotide T at position 394 in the cDNA is deleted. 3905–3906insT means a T is inserted after nucleotide 3905 in the cDNA. Insertions/deletions involving single nucleotides or pairs of nucleotides cause a shift in the reading frame (*frameshift mutation*) and usually result in protein truncation.

In protein annotation, the term delta or a small triangle is used to denote a deletion, e.g. in *CFTR*, the ΔF508 mutation means a deletion of phenylalanine at amino acid 508 resulting from a three-nucleotide deletion. Although this particular terminology is not current, it is still in widespread use.

Types of mutation and assessment of their significance

Some mutations, e.g. ΔF508, are well known and clearly pathogenic and their interpretation is straightforward. On the other hand, interpreting the clinical significance of a newly identified 'private mutation' can be very difficult and, unless it is a truncating mutation, you are strongly advised to discuss the situation with a clinical molecular geneticist before using the result in clinical practice, e.g. in predictive or prenatal testing.

Missense mutations

A mutation that results in an altered amino acid sequence in the encoded protein is termed a missense mutation. Not all missense mutations are pathogenic as the nature of the amino acid change and its precise location in the three-dimensional protein structure will determine whether there is any effect on protein function. The following factors increase the likelihood that a missense mutation is pathogenic.

- It is a *de novo* change in the gene of interest (i.e. not present in either parent), or it segregates with the disease in the family.
- It causes a significant alteration in the predicted protein conformation, e.g. a hydrophobic amino acid is substituted for a polar one, or it occurs at a key site in the protein (e.g. a binding site).
- It has been reported previously on several occasions in a database of mutations for the gene in question.
- It is not present at significant levels in the general population. Some 'missense mutations' are in reality polymorphisms. It is necessary to look at control data in the unaffected population to evaluate significance.

Truncating mutations

Mutations that result in protein truncation are nearly always pathogenic. They include single nucleotide substitutions that encode STOP codons (*nonsense mutations*), frameshift mutations in which the reading frame is lost, and also large deletions/insertions.

Splice-site mutations

Splicing is the process by which the introns are removed from the primary transcript, and the exons are joined together. A splice acceptor site is the junction between the dinucleotide AG at the end of an intron and the start of the next exon. A splice donor site is the junction between the end of an exon and the dinucleotide GT at the start of the next intron.

Some genes have alternative splice variants, where a single gene gives rise to more than one mRNA sequence that may have different tissue distributions. Mutations may abolish a splice acceptor or donor site or impair the efficiency of splicing resulting in abnormal ratios of splice variants.

Triplet repeat mutations

A mutation caused by an increase above threshold in the number of copies of a tandemly repeated trinucleotide, e.g. $(CTG)_n$ in myotonic dystrophy, $(CAG)_n$ in *SCA2*.

Mechanisms by which mutations exert their effect on phenotype

Loss-of-function mutation ('inactivating' mutation). This term includes nucleotide substitutions that introduce a stop codon, out-of-frame deletions resulting in a truncated protein, or specific mutations that cause loss of function of the protein by disturbing the conformation or charge of a site critical in the interaction of the protein with other molecules. Most mutations in recessively inherited disease are loss-of-function.

Gain-of-function mutation ('activating' mutation). These mutations are site-specific and usually result in constitutive activation of a specific protein function. In achondroplasia, where *FGFR3* is a bone growth-suppressing gene, two common mutations, 1138G > A and 1138G > C, both encoding G380R account for 98% of mutations in affected individuals. When *FGFR3* is mutated at this site its normal signalling function is partially constitutively activated (i.e. activated even in the absence of bound fibroblast growth factor (FGF)) resulting in increased inhibition of growth of cartilage cells.

Dominant-negative mutation. This is a mutation in one copy of a gene resulting in a mutant protein that has not only lost its own function, but also prevents the heterozygously produced wild-type protein of the same gene from functioning normally. It commonly acts by producing an altered polypeptide (subunit) that prevents or impairs the assembly of a multimeric protein, e.g. assembly of collagen triple helices in osteogenesis imperfecta (OI).

Haploinsufficiency arises when the normal phenotype requires the protein product of two alleles, and reduction of 50% of gene product as a result of loss-of-function mutations results in an abnormal phenotype.

Expert adviser: A.O.M. Wilkie, Nuffield Professor of Pathology and Honorary Consultant in Clinical Genetics, Oxford University, Oxford, England.

References

den Dunnen JT, Antonarakis SE. Nomenclature for the description of human sequence variations. *Hum Genet* 2001; **109**: 121–4.

Lewin B. *Genes VII*. Oxford University Press, Oxford, 2000.

Strachan T, Read AP. *Human molecular genetics*, 3rd edn. Garland Science, Philadelphia, 2003.

Sudbery P. *Human molecular genetics*. Longman, Essex, 1998.

Wain HM, Bruford EA, *et al.* for the Human Gene Nomenclature Committee. Guidelines for human gene nomenclature. *Genomics* 2002; **79**: 464–70; available at <www.gene.ucl.ac.uk/cgi-bin/nomenclature/searchgenes.pl>.

Watson JD, Crick FHC. Molecular structure of nucleic acids: a structure for deoxyribose nucleic acid. *Nature* 1953; **171**: 737–8. <www.genomic.unimelb.edu.au/mdi/muthomen>.

Genomic imprinting

Genomic imprinting is a genetic mechanism by which genes are *selectively expressed* from the *maternal or paternal homologue* of a chromosome. Imprinting invokes a variety of mechanisms that distinguish the maternal and paternal homologue and affect the chromatin structures that determine transcriptionally silent and active states. The inactive allele is epigenetically marked by histone modification, cytosine methylation, or both. The imprint is maintained throughout the life of the organism. Imprints once established are erased during the early development of the male and female germ cells and then reset prior to germ cell maturation.

Map of known human genomic imprinting sites

Chromosome location		Gene	Maternally/paternally expressed gene	Disease association
1	1p31.2	ARH1/NOEY2	Paternally expressed	
	1p36.32	p73	Maternally expressed	
6	6q24.2	HYMA1	Paternally expressed	
	6q24.2	ZAC/PLAGL1	Paternally expressed	Transient neonatal diabetes
	6q25.3	M6P/IGFR2	Biallelic expression with maternally methylated IC	
7	7q21.3	PEG10	Paternally expressed	
	7q32.2	COPG2	Maternally expressed	
	7q32.2	PEG1/MEST	Paternally expressed	Russell-Silver syndrome
	7q32.2	PEG1/AS	Paternally expressed	
11	11p15.5	H19	Maternally expressed Paternally methylated IC	
	11p15.5	IGF2	Paternally expressed	Beckwith-Wiedemann syndrome
	11p15.5	IGF2-AS	Paternally expressed	
	11p15.5	INS	Paternally expressed	
	11p15.5	ASCL2	Maternally expressed	
	11p15.5	TRPM5	Paternally expressed	
	11p15.5	KCNQ1	Maternally expressed Maternally methylated IC	
	11p15.5	KCNQ1 QT1	Paternally expressed	
	11p15.5	p57kip2/CDkN1C	Maternally expressed	
	11p15.5	SCL22A1L/ITM	Maternally expressed	
	11p15.5	ZNF215	Maternally expressed	
14	14q32	DLK1	Paternally expressed Paternally methylated IC	
		MEG3	Maternally expressed	
15	15q11-q13	MKRN3	Paternally expressed	
	15q11-q13	MAGEL2	Paternally expressed	
	15q11-q13	NDN	Paternally expressed	
	15q11-q13		Maternally methylated IC	
	15q11-q13	SNRPN	Paternally expressed	Prader-Willi syndrome
	15q11-q13	UBE3A	Maternally expressed	Angelman syndrome
	15q11-q13	ATP10C	Maternally expressed	
	15q11-q13	GABRB3	Paternally expressed	
18	18q21.1	ELONGIN A3	Maternally expressed	
19	19q13.43	PEG3/ZIM2	Paternally expressed	
20	20q13.32	GNAS1-AS	Maternally expressed	
	20q13.32	GNAS	Maternal and paternal transcripts distinctly expressed depending on promoter usage or alternate splicing	Albright hereditary osteodystrophy
X	Xq13.2	XIST		

In humans about 50 genes are known to be imprinted, i.e. differentially expressed according to their origin in either the oocytes or spermatozoa. These imprinted genes have roles in growth and development as well as in tumour suppression.

Imprinted genes cause disease when the maternal/paternal gene that is usually expressed is mutated, silenced, or deleted such that there is no functional copy (since the other homologue is transcriptionally silent) or when, in the case of a paternally expressed gene, the organism has two maternal homologues as a consequence of uniparental disomy or vice versa.

Imprinting centre (IC). One mechanism involves an IC that seems to control the resetting of a cluster of closely linked imprinted genes during transmission through the opposite sex. Imprinting centres are differentially (paternally or maternally) methylated. Deletion of an imprinting centre, can cause disordered imprinting of several genes in a chromosomal domain, e.g. in Prader–Willi or Angelman syndrome.

Uniparental disomy (UPD) describes the karyotype of a euploid cell or organism in which one of the chromosome pairs has been inherited exclusively from one parent. If two identical homologues are inherited this is called *isodisomy*; if non-identical homologues are inherited the term *heterodisomy* is used. This occurs when non-disjunction during meiosis in one parent leads to formation of a disomic gamete. A trisomic zygote is formed and trisomic rescue with loss of the chromosome from the other parent occurs. If UPD occurs in an imprinted region this may cause disease.

Expert adviser: Eamonn Maher, Professor of Medical Genetics, University of Birmingham, Birmingham, England.

Reference

<www.geneimprint.com>.

Mitochondrial inheritance

Mitochondrial DNA (mtDNA) has unique genetic features that distinguish it from nuclear DNA, which follows a Mendelian pattern of inheritance. The mtDNA genome of humans is a double-stranded circular DNA, 16.6 kb in length and encoding 13 proteins (all subunits of respiratory chain complexes), two ribosomal RNAs, and 22 transfer RNAs. There are no introns and, except for the D loop region that is involved in the initiation of DNA replication and transcription, most of the mitochondrial genome is coding sequence. Mitochondria typically contain several copies of mtDNA and a typical human somatic cell can contain up to 1000 mitochondria (i.e. 5000–10 000 copies of mtDNA) representing >1% of the cell's total DNA. Mature oocytes contain a staggering ~100 000 copies of mtDNA, whereas sperm contain ~100.

The organs most often affected in mitochondrial disorders are highly energy-demanding tissues, such as the central nervous system (CNS), skeletal and cardiac muscle, pancreatic islets, liver, and kidney.

Aspects of mitochondrial inheritance

Maternal inheritance. Mitochondrial DNA (mtDNA) is exclusively maternally inherited with very rare exceptions (Schwartz and Vissing 2002). Paternal mitochondria enter the egg on fertilization where they constitute a miniscule fraction (0.1%) of the total mitochondria. The paternal mitochondria and their mtDNA are rapidly eliminated early in embryogenesis. For the purposes of genetic counselling the risk of paternal inheritance is essentially zero.

Homoplasmy is the existence of only one mtDNA type in the same cell, tissue, or individual, e.g. mitochondria containing only mtDNA carrying the A1555G sequence sensorineural deafness sequence.

Heteroplasmy is the existence of more than one mtDNA type in the same cell, tissue, or individual, e.g. mitochondria containing a mixture of mtDNA carrying the MELAS 3243 point mutation and mtDNA with the wild-type sequence. In mitochondrial disorders, because of the thousands of mitochondria in each cell, there are often variable percentages of mutant and wild-type mtDNAs between different cells and especially between different tissues. The different mtDNAs can vary between 0 and 100%.

Threshold effect. For some mtDNA mutations there is a relatively narrow threshold below which mitochondrial function is normal, but above which mitochondrial function is greatly impaired. For some mtDNA mutations, e.g. the 8993 mutation seen in neuropathy/ataxia/retinitis pigmentosa (NARP) syndrome and some patients with Leigh syndrome, the severity of clinical symptoms increases sharply above a threshold mutant load.

Mitochondrial bottleneck. A high variation in mutant load is sometimes seen in the offspring of heteroplasmic women. This is at variance with expectation based on random distribution of mutant and wild-type mtDNA in the cell. The bottleneck hypothesis states that the number of mtDNAs during oogenesis is either relatively small or that only a few mtDNAs are used as templates for amplification. Brown *et al.* (2001) measured the mutant mtDNA load in 82 oocytes from a woman harbouring the MELAS (mitochondrial myopathy–encephalopathy–lactic acidosis–stroke-like episodes) A3242G mutation who had an 18% mutant load in her skeletal muscle. The mutant load in oocytes ranged from 0 to 45% and the mean within individual oocytes was similar to that in the mother.

Tissue variation. In heteroplasmic disorders, the distribution of mutant load in tissues is often not uniform. In some tissues the level of mutant mtDNA changes successively with time, for instance falling in blood and accumulating in non-dividing cells such as muscle.

Selection. Preferential accumulation of mutant mtDNA in affected tissues appears to explain their progressive nature (Poulton *et al.* 2003). However, in some cell lines, e.g. blood, cells with high mutant loads appear to be selected against and the mutant load may fall over time.

Mutation rate. Human mtDNA has a mutation rate 10–20 times that of nuclear DNA, probably due to replication repair systems that are less stringent than those in the nucleus. This has been exploited in a study of the migration of human populations (Sykes 2001).

Typical family tree

Mitochondrial inheritance

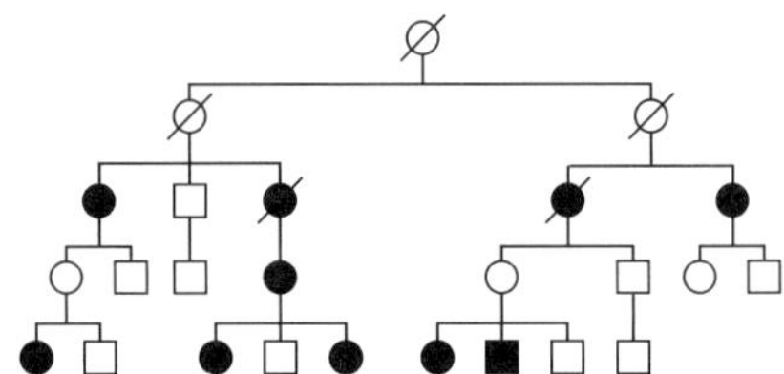

A typical family tree showing mitochondrial inheritance. Offspring of females in the maternal line are at risk; males do not transmit the condition.

Genetic advice

- Inheritance is matrilineal, i.e. the condition can only be transmitted by females in the maternal line.
- Males do not transmit mitochondrially inherited disorders with extremely rare exceptions (Schwartz and Vissing 2002).
- Typically a mitochondrially inherited condition can affect both sexes.
- Point mutations are commonly maternally inherited, whilst deletions and duplications are most often sporadic but see advice for specific mitochondrial disorders page 384.
- If the mother is heteroplasmic for a mutation, the proportion of mutant mtDNA in her offspring can vary considerably.

Mitochondrial inheritance

Homoplasmy

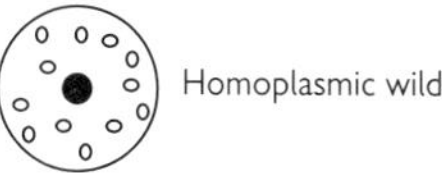

Homoplasmic wild-type mtDNA

Homoplasmic mutant mtDNA

Heteroplasmy

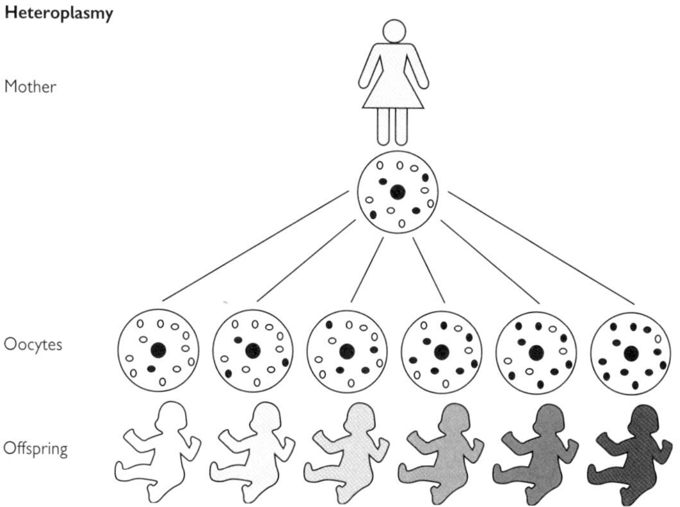

NB. Correlation between phenotypic severity and level of mutant mtDNA is poor in many mitochondrial diseases.

Expert adviser: Joanna Poulton, Professor of Mitochondrial Genetics, University of Oxford, Oxford, England.

References

Brown DT, Samuels DC, *et al.* Random genetic drift determines the level of mutant mtDNA in human primary oocytes. *Am J Hum Genet* 2001; **68**: 533–6.

Poulton J, Turnbull DM. 74th ENMC international workshop: mitochondrial diseases 19–20 November 1999, Naarden, the Netherlands. *Neuromuscul Disord* 2000; **10** (6): 460–2.

Poulton J, O'Rahilly S, *et al.* Mitochondrial DNA, diabetes and pancreatic pathology in Kearns–Sayre syndrome. *Diabetologia* 1995; **38**: 868–71.

Poulton J, Macaulay V, Marchington DR. Mitochondrial genetics '98: is the bottleneck cracked? *Am J Hum Genet* 1998; **62**: 752–7.

Poulton J, Macaulay V, Marchington DR. Transmission, genetic counselling and prenatal diagnosis of mitochondrial DNA disease. In *Genetics of mitochondrial disease* (ed. I. Holt), Oxford Monographs in Medical Genetics no. 47, pp. 309–26. Oxford University Press, Oxford, 2003.

Schwartz M, Vissing J. Paternal inheritance of mitochondrial DNA. *N Engl J Med* 2002; **347**: 576–80.

Sykes B. *The seven daughters of Eve.* Corgi Books, London, 2001.

Thorburn DR, Dahl HH. Mitochondrial disorders: genetics, counselling, prenatal diagnosis and reproductive options. *Am J Med Genet* 2001; **106**: 102–14.

Multifactorial inheritance

From a clinical perspective there is a continuous spectrum of disease from, at the one end, disorders that are strictly genetic and caused by fully penetrant mutations with minimal contribution from the environment to, at the other extreme, those caused predominantly by environmental factors (e.g. teratogens) with minimal contribution from genetic factors. Between these two extremes lie the incompletely penetrant, and the polygenic disorders, creating a smooth transition from strictly genetic to multifactorial illneses (Bomprezzi *et al.* 2003).

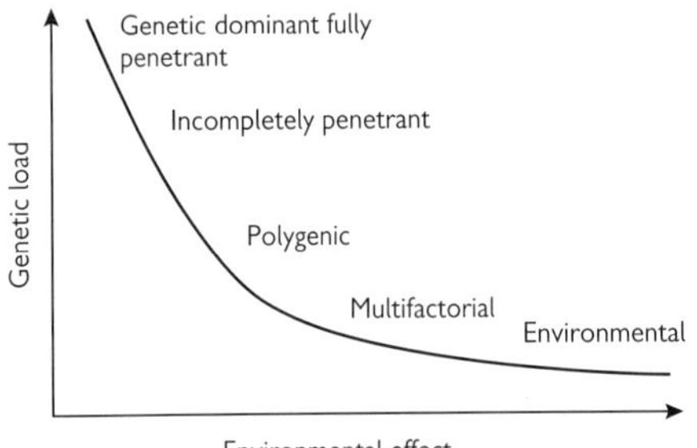

The progression from strictly genetic to strictly environmental causation in the aetiology of disease.

Genes and environment in the aetiology of disease (Bomprezzi *et al.* 2003)

Common birth defects such as cleft lip/palate, congenital dislocation of the hip, congenital heart disease, and neural tube defect do not generally follow a Mendelian pattern of inheritance. Nevertheless, a tendency for these conditions to cluster in families, more than would be expected by chance, is observed. The same is true for schizophrenia, ischaemic heart disease, and type 1 diabetes. Many of these conditions probably depend on a mixture of major and minor genetic determinants, together with environmental factors. This is termed multifactorial inheritance. Diseases inherited in this manner are termed complex diseases. Multifactorial inheritance may involve a small number of loci (oligogenic), many loci (polygenic), or a single major locus with a polygenic background.

In multifactorial inheritance, disease occurrence is attributable to the interaction of the environment with alleles at many loci interspersed throughout the genome. The mapping and identification of these genes is difficult because the disease-associated alleles occur almost as commonly in patients as in healthy individuals; even the highest-risk genotypes confer only modest risk of disease (Todd 1999).

Terminology

Polygenic traits are governed by the simultaneous action of many (>3) gene loci.

Oligogenic traits are governed by the simultaneous action of a few (e.g. 3) gene loci.

Digenic traits are governed by the simultaneous action of two gene loci.

Monogenic traits are governed by the individual action of a single gene (as in classical Mendelian disorders).

Modifier gene is a gene whose expression can influence a phenotype resulting from mutation at another locus.

Linkage is a physical relationship between a locus/loci and a trait/disease that lie on the same chromosome at a genetic distance of <50 centimorgans (cM).

Association is a statistical relationship between an allele(s) and a trait/disease.

Lambda (λ) is the ratio of the frequency of a multifactorial disease in the relative of an affected person compared with its rate in the general population, e.g. in sib pair studies λ_s is the ratio of the frequency of the disease in siblings compared with that in the general population. λ_s is a measure of relative risk and hence of disease heritability.

Aspects of multifactorial inheritance

Complex traits. Traits such as intelligence, behavioural traits, height, and weight approximate to a normal distribution in the general population. A large number of genes are involved in determining these characteristics together with environmental factors. For example, factors influencing height include parental height, nutrition, and chronic illness.

Falconer's polygenic threshold model. This is based on the assumption that liability to a condition is multifactorial and follows a normal distribution in the population and that the disease occurs when a particular threshold value is exceeded. The normal distribution for liability is shifted in close relatives of an affected individual; hence a greater proportion of them will exceed the critical threshold value and be affected (see figure at the end of this article). For first-degree relatives the expected incidence approximates to the square-root of the population incidence.

For a condition affecting 1/1000 individuals (0.1%), the risk to sibs, parents, and children is ~1/30 (3%), falling to 1/100 (1%) for second-degree relatives, and close to population risk for third-degree relatives. This is fairly close to the figures observed for neural tube defects and cleft palate.

Gender predisposition. For most multifactorial disorders males or females have a greater frequency. If the disorder does occur in the less likely gender then there is a greater recurrence risk implying more genes and/or environmental factors are present in that family.

Typical family tree

Multifactorial inheritance

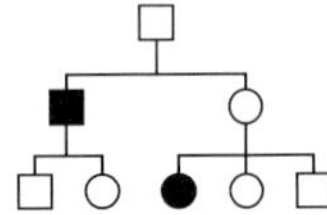

Genetic advice

This is based on *empiric data*. Refer to the individual tables of data for specific conditions.

Several general principles affect the risk.

- **Relationship to the affected individual.** The risk is greatest amongst close relatives and decreases rapidly with increasing distance of relationship (see above).
- **Severity of the disorder in the proband.** The risks to relatives are greater if the proband is severely affected, than if the proband is only mildly affected. The average liability in the siblings of affected individuals will be greater (further right-shifted) in such families (see figure at the end of this article).

- **The number of affected individuals in the family.** If there are two or more close relatives affected, then risks for other relatives are increased. If there are several affected close relatives, the possibility of an autosomal dominant (AD) disorder with incomplete penetrance should be carefully considered.

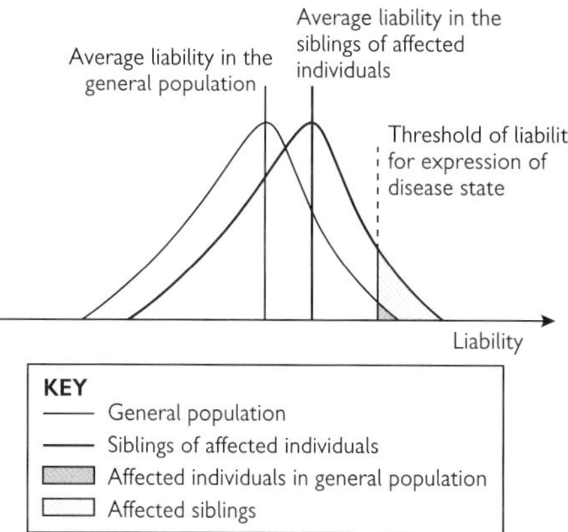

Figure showing the distribution of liability to a multifactorial trait/disease.

Expert adviser: Ian D. Young, Consultant Clinical Geneticist, Leicester, England.

References

Bomprezzi R, Kovanen PE, Martin R. New approaches to investigating heterogeneity in complex traits. *J Med Genet* 2003; **40**: 553–9.

Schliekelman P, Slatkin M. Multiplex relative risk and estimation of the number of loci underlying an inherited disease. *Am J Hum Genet* 2002; **71**: 1369–85.

Strachan T, Read AP. *Human molecular genetics*, 3rd edn. Garland Science, Philadelphia, 2003.

Todd JA. From genome to aetiology in a multifactorial disease, type 1 diabetes. *Bioessays* 1999; **21**: 164–74.

Young ID. *Introduction to risk calculation in genetic counselling*, 2nd edn. Oxford University Press, Oxford, 1999.

Reproductive options

After a genetic disorder that has a significant sibling or off-spring recurrence risk is diagnosed, many families are faced with a difficult choice about future pregnancies. It may be helpful for them to be introduced to the range of repro-ductive options available to them for future pregnancies. This is not always easy as such decisions are very personal. It may help to introduce the topic by explaining that some of the choices available may include options that they would not consider choosing.

Accepting the risk of another affected child. For some families this will be their option of choice; for others an option they cannot bear to contemplate.

Electing against further pregnancies. The burden of caring for a child with a severe genetic disorder may be such that the family feel that they do not wish to extend their family because all of their energy is channelled into caring for their existing child(ren).

Adoption. Although this process can be frustrating and lengthy, some couples are successful in locating a baby or child to join their family. (Some couples may choose to adopt another affected child as in achondroplasia and Down syndrome.)

Donor gamete. AID (artificial insemination by donor) is an option that can be used to minimize the risk of recurrence of an autosomal recessive (AR) disorder for which both parents are carriers, or to evade the risk of a dominant disorder present in the father, or the risk of unbalanced products of a balanced translocation present in the father. A donor ovum can also be used to minimize the risk of recurrence of an AR disorder and has the advantage that both parents play a biological role in bringing the baby into the world—technically this is much more demanding and the shortage of donor ova means that, in practice, AID is usually the more pragmatic option. A donor ovum is also an option to avoid the risk of a dominant disorder present in the mother, or a mitochondrial encoded disorder carried by the mother, or the risk of unbalanced products of a balanced translocation present in the mother.

Prenatal diagnosis. For many couples facing a high risk of recurrence for a serious disorder this is the option of choice, but for others (particularly those with religious or moral objections to termination of pregnancy) it is ethically unacceptable. Prenatal diagnosis by chorionic vil-lus sampling (CVS) or amniocentesis is possible for cytoge-netic disorders, monogenic disorders in which the pathogenic mutation is known, and the great majority of biochemical disorders. Prenatal diagnosis by ultrasound can be used in many conditions causing major structural malformations.

Pre-implantation genetic diagnosis (PGD). At first sight this seems the most attractive option to many couples. In reality, PGD is only available in a very few specialist centres and for a few severe genetic diseases (predominantly those in which single-cell diagnosis is technically feasible, e.g. fluorescent *in situ* hybridization (FISH)-diagnosable conditions such as chromosome translocations or trisomies, or where there is a commonly occurring mutation such as the exon 7, 8 deletion in spinal muscular atrophy (SMA)). PGD entails ovarian hyperstimulation (and its attendant risks), egg retrieval, *in vitro* fertilization, embryo biopsy, and implantation of screened embryos. For single gene disorders, a pregnancy rate of 21% per egg retrieval and 25% per embryo transfer procedure has been reported. The costs are often prohibitive (e.g. in the UK approximate current costs are £3500 for a first cycle plus the cost of the drugs (£800–£1200)). There are only limited data on safety and there may be unforeseen risks. See 'Assisted reproductive technology: *in vitro* fertilization (IVF), intra-cytoplasmic sperm injection (ICSI), and pre-implantation genetic diagnosis (PGD)' page 568.

Adopt-out or foster-out an affected child. If the family does not feel they can care for another affected child, but also have religious or other objections to contraception and prenatal diagnosis, this option may need to be considered.

Useful websites: British Association for Adoption and Fostering <www.baaf.org.uk>.

Testing for genetic status

The great expansion in the number of disease genes that are cloned and for which mutation analysis is available has led to a growth in the demand for genetic testing.

Genetic testing has some distinct differences from routine clinical investigation.

- The results are permanent for the individual concerned.
- The results may have important implications for other family members, usually offspring, but sometimes siblings or parents.
- Occasionally, some forms of genetic testing, e.g. linkage or testing of parents to confirm carrier status for an autosomal recessive (AR) condition present in the child, may reveal unwanted information about paternity.

These issues need to be carefully thought through before embarking on genetic testing. Particular issues arise with regard to genetic testing of children and monozygotic (MZ) twins and these are discussed further below.

Genetic testing for diagnostic indications

In this situation genetic testing is used as a diagnostic tool, e.g. in a preterm neonate with meconium ileus in whom sweat testing is not feasible molecular genetic testing for cystic fibrosis (CF) may enable a specific diagnosis of CF to be made and appropriate management to be instigated. Similarly, in a young boy presenting with delayed walking and a high creatine kinase (CK) level, genetic testing for Duchenne muscular dystrophy (DMD) may enable a specific diagnosis to be reached without the need to resort to an invasive test (muscle biopsy).

There are very few situations in which this is inappropriate in adults or in children, but those involved in the decision-making should be mindful that it does have genetic as well as therapeutic implications.

Genetic testing to confirm or refine an existing clinical diagnosis

In this situation there is a pre-existing clinical diagnosis and genetic testing serves to confirm and refine the diagnosis (but rarely to alter it). For example, an individual with tall stature, pectus carinatum, dilated aortic root, and dislocated lenses has a clinical diagnosis of Marfan syndrome (MFS). If a fibrillin mutation (*FBN1*) is identified on genetic testing this confirms the clinical diagnosis. For a child with sensorineural deafness diagnosed by audiometry the finding of homozygosity for the del 35G mutation in connexin 26 serves to further refine the clinical diagnosis. In hereditary motor and sensory neuropathies (HMSN) the finding of a duplication of *PMP22* serves to refine the diagnosis from HMSN type 1 to HMSN type 1A. There are very few situations in which this is inappropriate in adults or in children.

Predictive testing for disorders in which clinical management is affected by the test results

Examples of such disorders are familial adenomatous polyposis (FAP) and von Hippel–Lindau syndrome (VHL).

These are disorders where effective screening and/or treatments are available and yet where the burden of screening is sufficiently high that 'at risk' individuals may prefer to determine their risk in order to avoid unnecessary screening.

Testing should be offered in the context of a clinic consultation at which the following are discussed:

1 the natural history of the condition;
2 the implications of a 'high risk' result;
3 the screening programme/treatment available to individuals with a 'high risk' result (usually also available to 'at risk' individuals who elect not to discover their genetic status);
4 the possible implications of the test result for other family members;
5 the possibility that genetic testing may have implications for financial arrangements (e.g. mortgages, pensions, and insurance)—the patient may wish to take further advice from an independent financial adviser.

If the individual wishes to proceed with genetic testing *written consent* for predictive testing should usually be obtained, the expected time-scale for results should be discussed, and arrangements made for the giving of the results (e.g. letter, phone call, clinic appointment).

Predictive testing for disorders in which clinical management is not affected by the test result

Examples are Huntington disease (HD) and spinocerebellar ataxia (SCA).

Predictive testing for HD is usually only offered as part of a structured programme. There are usually a series of three or more meetings between the individual at risk and a geneticist/genetic counsellor to explore the reasons why they wish to have the test and to discuss possible outcomes and future management. Most programmes follow similar guidelines.

- The predictive programme extends over a period of months and includes a discussion of all points 1–5 raised above. Individuals are free to withdraw at any time.
- A 'supporter' (often a partner or friend) is nominated by the patient who attends all of the clinic visits and makes an ongoing commitment to support the individual undergoing testing.
- If the individual wishes to proceed with genetic testing, *written consent* for predictive testing should be obtained and the expected time-scale for results should be discussed. A clinic visit for the result is usually arranged so that this can be given in person by a member of the team known to the patient. (Alternative arrangements for giving the result may be considered in some circumstances, e.g. letter, phone call.)
- Testing for dominant disorders in individuals at 25% risk (in which the result may reveal the status of an individual in a previous generation) is only undertaken in exceptional cases in which every effort has been made to provide genetic counselling to the individual at 50% risk.
- Testing is not generally undertaken within 6 months of the individual first becoming aware of the diagnosis in the family

Formal programmes are less common for other dominantly inherited disorders for which there is no very effective treatment but, in general, a broadly similar approach is adopted in which individuals are discouraged from making a rushed decision about testing and encouraged to reflect on both the advantages and disadvantages and optimum timing of testing for them as individuals. Generally, this type of testing is not available to children/minors.

Testing for carrier status

Examples are in cases involving cystic fibrosis (CF) or chromosome translocations.

In general, testing for carrier status has potential implications for reproduction but not for the health of the individual being tested. Having explained the reproductive consequences if the individual is found to be a carrier it is reasonable to arrange testing for adults or younger adults who are able to give consent for themselves (Gillick competent) if this is requested.

Genetic testing of children

The best interests of the child need to direct genetic testing. In general, predictive genetic testing of children is only undertaken when the potential benefit of testing can reasonably be viewed as outweighing the disadvantages of testing (particularly removing the child's autonomy, when more mature, to be involved in decisions affecting his/her own future and the risk of stigmatization). It is usually undertaken when the child is at significant risk for a genetic disorder for which screening is burdensome and effective treatment is possible, e.g. retinoblastoma, FAP, and VHL. Please refer to the websites listed at the end of this section for a thorough discussion of the ethical, legal, and psychological issues.

The principal conclusions from the American Medical Association (1996) policy document are these.

1 When a child is at risk for a genetic condition for which preventative or other therapeutic measures are available, genetic testing should be offered or, in some cases, required.

2 When a child is at risk for a genetic condition with paediatric onset for which preventive therapeutic measures are not available, parents generally should have discretion to decide whether the child should undergo genetic testing.

3 When a child is at risk for a genetic condition with adult onset for which preventive or effective therapeutic measures are not available, genetic testing of children generally should not be performed. Families should still be informed of the existence of tests and given the opportunity to discuss the reasons why the tests are generally not offered for children.

4 Genetic testing for carrier status should be deferred until the child either reaches maturity or needs to make reproductive decisions or, in the case of children too immature to make the reproductive decisions, reproductive decisions need to be made for the child.

5 Genetic testing of children for the benefit of a family member should not be performed unless testing is necessary to prevent substantial harm to the family member.

Adoption

When a child is being considered for adoption the same guidelines for genetic testing should be followed as for other children.

The American Society of Human Genetics and the American College of Medical Genetics (1995) recommend the following .

1 All genetic testing of newborns and children in the adoption process should be consistent with the tests performed on all children of a similar age for the purposes of diagnosis or of identifying appropriate prevention strategies.

2 Because the primary justification for genetic testing of any child is a timely medical benefit to the child, genetic testing of newborns and children in the adoption process should be limited to testing for conditions that manifest themselves during childhood or for which preventive measures or therapies may be undertaken during childhood.

3 In the adoption process, it is not appropriate to test newborns and children for the purpose of detecting genetic variations of or predispositions to physical, mental, or behavioural traits within the normal range.

Testing for genetic status in MZ twins

Genetic testing of MZ twins raises special ethical issues, particularly with respect to predictive testing. Where possible, try to ascertain that both twins wish to proceed with predictive testing and arrange for them to proceed through the predictive testing process simultaneously (perhaps with parallel consultations). When a diagnostic test is contemplated in one twin, this may potentially be a predictive test for the other twin and that factor needs careful consideration and forethought. Usually, in the rare situation where one twin wishes to proceed with genetic testing and the other does not, the rights of the twin to seek a genetic test for him or herself as an individual will prevail (provided the test in question is part of routinely available health care to which other individuals would normally be entitled).

Paternity

Some genetic tests have the potential to reveal non-paternity. Unless this potential is recognized and discussed in advance of testing, a test result revealing non-paternity raises serious ethical dilemmas. (See Lucassen and Parker (2001) for a thorough discussion of this issue.)

In practice the geneticist should try to foresee situations where tests could potentially disclose non-paternity and include discussion of this topic in the pre-test counselling. Occasionally, unusual genetic mechanisms suggest non-paternity, e.g. *de novo* deletion of the SMN gene in spinal muscular atrophy (SMA), but more thorough analysis reveals parentage to be true.

Examples of genetic tests that may inadvertently reveal misattributed parentage include:

- analysis of triplet repeat size (alleles are often highly polymorphic), e.g. tests for myotonic dystrophy, HD, etc.;
- carrier testing where both mutations have been defined in the affected child;
- linkage-based tests where haplotypes are determined for different family members—when these results are collated discrepancies may be seen.

NB. In all these cases, it is imperative to consider that genetic mutation can also lead to discrepant findings in families.

Useful websites: British Society for Human Genetics 'Testing children' <www.bshg.org>; Canadian Paediatric Society 'Guidelines for genetic testing of healthy children' <www.cps.ca>; American Medical Association 'Testing children for genetic status' <www.ama-assn.org>; The American Society of Human Genetics (ASHG) and the American College of Medical Genetics (ACMG) 'Genetic testing in adoption' <www.faseb.org/genetics/acmg/pol-36.htm>.

Expert adviser: Martin Bobrow, Professor of Medical Genetics, University of Cambridge, Cambridge, England.

References

American Medical Association. *Genetic testing of children*, Policy document E-2.138, June 1996.

American Society of Human Genetics/American College of Medical Geneticists. Points to consider; ethical, legal, and psychological implications of genetic testing in children and adolescents. *Am J Hum Genet* 1995; **57**: 1233–41.

Clarke A (ed.). *The genetic testing of children*. BIOS Scientific Publishers Ltd, Oxford, 1998.

Codori AM, Zawacki KL, *et al.* Genetic testing for hereditary colorectal cancer in children: long-term psychological effects. *Am J Med Genet* 2003; **116A**: 117–28.

Lucassen A, Parker M. Revealing false paternity: some ethical considerations. *Lancet* 2001; **357**: 1033–5.

Useful resources

One of the frustrations in writing this handbook has been the brevity with which each topic can be discussed. Whilst this has been necessary in order to try to include the myriad of conditions that may be encountered in a general genetics clinic, we hope that we have included sufficient detail to enable the reader to make progress towards a diagnosis. Once a precise diagnosis is achieved, there is a wealth of sources from which further information can be obtained. Listed below is a selection of sources that we find particularly useful.

General

Books

Cassidy SB, Allanson JE (eds.). *Management of genetic syndromes*, 2nd edn, Wiley, New York, 2004.

Harper PS. *Practical genetic counselling*, 6th edn, revised reprint. Arnold, London, 2004.

Rimoin DL, Connor JM, Pyeritz RE, Korf BR. *Emery and Rimoin's principles and practice of medical genetics*, 4th edn. Churchill Livingstone, Edinburgh, 2002.

Strachan M, Read AP. *Human molecular genetics*, 3rd edn. Garland Science, Philadelphia, 2003.

Young ID. *Introduction to risk calculation in genetic counselling*, 2nd edn. Oxford University Press, Oxford, 1999.

Databases/websites

Pubmed <www.ncbi.nlm.nih.gov/PubMed>.

Support groups

Contact a Family (UK) <www.cafamily.org.uk>.

National Organization for Rare Disorders (US) <www.raredisease.org>.

Monogenic disorders

Databases/websites

Ensemble genome browser <www.ensembl.org>.

Geneclinics <www.geneclinics.org>.

Genew: Human Gene Nomenclature Database <www.gene.ucl.ac.uk>.

Online Mendelian Inheritance in Man (OMIM) <www.ncbi.nlm.nih.gov>.

The Frequency of Inherited Disorders Database (FIDD) http://archive.uwcm.ac.uk/uwcm/mg/fidd

Dysmorphology

Books

Aase JM. *Diagnostic dysmorphology*. Plenum Medical, New York, 1990.

Epstein CJ, Erickson RP, Wynshaw-Boris A (eds.). *Inborn errors of development—the molecular basis of clinical disorders of morphogenesis*. Oxford University Press, Oxford, 2004.

Gorlin RJ, Cohen MM, Hennekam RCM (eds.). *Syndromes of the head and neck*, 4th edn. Oxford University Press, Oxford, 1990.

Hall JG, Froster-Iskenius I, Allanson J. *Handbook of physical measurement*. Oxford University Press, Oxford, 1989.

Jones KL (ed.). *Smith's recognizable patterns of human malformations*, 5th edn. W.B. Saunders, Philadelphia, 1997.

Sadler TW. *Langman's medical embryology*, 8th edn. Lippincott Williams & Wilkins, Philadelphia, 2000.

Stevenson RE, Hall JG, Goodman RM (eds.). *Human malformations and related anomalies*. Oxford University Press, Oxford, 2003.

Databases/websites

POSSUM (Pictures of Standard Syndromes and Undiagnosed Malformations) version 5.5 Melbourne: The Murdoch Research Institute, 2001 <www.possum.net.au>.

Winter RM, Baraitser M (eds.) London Dysmorphology Database 2003 <www.lmdatabses.com>.

Chromosomes

Book

Gardner RJM, Sutherland GR. *Chromosome abnormalities and genetic counselling*, Oxford Monographs on Medical Genetics no. 31, 3rd edn. Oxford University Press, New York, 2004.

Databases/websites

Schinzel A. *Human cytogenetic database and catalogue of chromosome aberrations in man*, 2nd edn. Oxford University Press, Oxford, 2004.

Cancer

Book

Hodgson SV, Maher ER. *A practical guide to human cancer genetics*, 2nd edn. Cambridge University Press, Cambridge, 1999.

Neurogenetics

Books

Baraitser M. *The genetics of neurological disorders*, 3rd edn, Oxford Monographs on Medical Genetics no. 34. Oxford University Press, Oxford, 1997.

Dubovitz V. *Muscle disorders in childhood*, 2nd edn. W.B. Saunders, Philadelphia, 2000.

Databases/websites

Baraitser M, Winter R. London Neurogenetics Database (CD).

European Neuro Muscular Centre <www.enmc.org>.

Skin

Book

Sybert V. *Genetic skin disorders*, Oxford Monographs on Medical Genetics no. 33. Oxford University Press, Oxford, 1997.

Ear

Book

Toriello HV, Reardon W, Gorlin RJ. *Hereditary hearing loss and its syndromes*, 2nd edn, Oxford Monographs on Medical Genetics. Oxford University Press, New York, 2004.

Eye

Books

Moore, A (ed.). *Paediatric ophthalmology*, Fundamentals of Clinical Ophthalmology Series. BMJ Books, London, 2000.

Traboulsi EI (ed.). *Genetic diseases of the eye*, Oxford Monographs on Medical Genetics. Oxford University Press, New York, 1999.

Metabolic

Books

Clarke JTR. *A clinical guide to inherited metabolic diseases*, 2nd edn. Cambridge University Press, Cambridge, 2002.

Scriver CR, Beaudet AL, Sly WS, Valle D (eds.). *The metabolic and molecular bases of inherited disease*, 8th edn. McGraw-Hill, New York, 2001.

X-linked dominant (XLD) inheritance

XLD disorders are encoded on the X chromosome. An XLD disorder manifests very severely in males, often leading to spontaneous loss or neonatal death of affected male pregnancies. Typical examples include incontinentia pigmenti (IP) due to mutations in *NEMO*, Rett syndrome due to mutations in *MECP2*, oral–facial–digital syndrome type 1 (OFD-1) due to mutations in *CXORF5*, and otopalatodigital syndrome types 1 and 2 (OPD-1 and OPD-2) due to mutations in *FMNA* (filamin A).

An **X-linked semi-dominant disorder** manifests severely in males who are hemizygotes, and mildly or subclinically in females who have two X chromosomes (one normal and one mutated copy). Examples include Coffin–Lowry syndrome and X-linked hereditary motor and sensory neuropathy (X-HMSN) where a proportion of heterozygotes manifests features of the disorder. Where the disorder manifests only infrequently or not at all in heterozygotes it is said to follow X-linked recessive (XLR) inheritance (see the eponymous section, page 34).

Recombination between the X and Y chromosomes is limited to the **pseudoautosomal region** (PAR) and is necessary for proper segregation of the sex chromosomes during spermatogenesis. Cross-over between the sex chromosomes during male meiosis is restricted to the terminal pseudoautosomal pairing regions PAR1, a 2.6 Mb region on Xp/Yp, and PAR2, a 320 kb region on Xq/Yq. Genes in the PARs escape X-inactivation and exhibit pseudoautosomal inheritance. Genes encoded in PAR1 include *SHOX* which has an important role in growth. Under normal circumstances, the *SHOX* genes on both Xpters of a female are active, as are the *SHOX* genes on Xpter and Ypter in a male and hence the severity of the phenotype is not sex-dependent. Mutations in *SHOX* therefore show **pseudo-autosomal inheritance** rather than X-linked semi-dominant inheritance. Deletions or mutations causing haploinsufficiency of *SHOX* are a common cause of idiopathic short stature (4/56 cases ie ~7% in Morizio's series) and also cause Leri–Weill syndrome. Individuals homozygous for the deletion or homozygous or compound heterozygotes for inactivating mutations have the more severe Langer mesomelic dysplasia.

Aspects of X-linked dominant inheritance

Skewed X-inactivation. If there is complete skewing, the ratio is 100:0; often an intermediate value is found. Values <80:20 fall within values expected from normal variation in X-inactivation patterns in the general population; values >80:20 are suggestive of X-inactivation due to a selection bias due to a deleterious X-linked recessive (XLR) mutation, but are seen in ~9% of normal females (see 'X-linked recessive inheritance', page 34). This selection bias may not operate equally in all tissues and so variable degrees of skewing may be observed in different tissues.

Degree of manifestation in heterozygotes. Unfavourable skewing of X-inactivation in key tissues may be a major factor in determining the expression of an XLD disorder in heterozygotes. Skewing towards the X without the mutation may result in minimal features and it may not be clinically recognized that the individual is a heterozygote (and recurrence may be attributed erroneously to germline mosaicism).

Distribution of features in heterozygotes. The distribution of features in a female is a reflection of the X-inactivation pattern in specific tissues. Asymmetry is an important feature and this is well illustrated in X-linked chondrodysplasia punctata (XLCDP) where the limbs are shortened but not symmetrically. The skin lesions of IP are streaky and may follow the lines of Blashko.

Germline mosaicism. As with XLR disorders, the risk of germline mosaicism needs to be considered. For example, in Rett syndrome it is recommended that mothers and sisters of affected girls are tested for an *MECP2* mutation identified in the proband.

Typical family trees

X-linked dominant inheritance

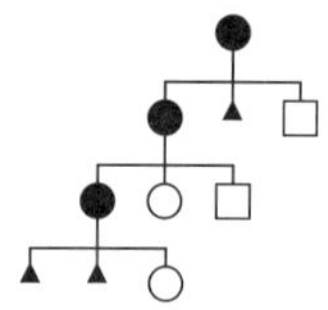

A typical family tree showing X-linked dominant inheritance. The condition is manifest in female heterozygotes and male hemizygotes. Many of these conditions cause spontaneous loss of affected male pregnancies.

X-linked semi-dominant inheritance

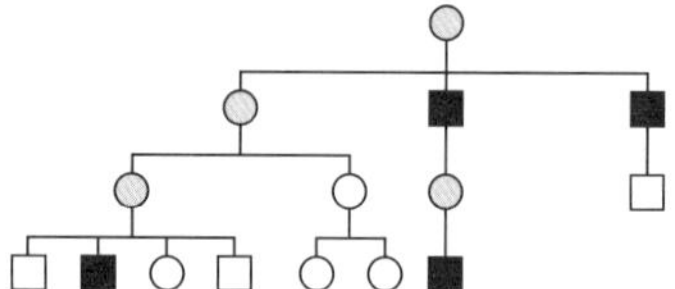

A typical family tree showing X-linked semi-dominant inheritance. The condition is expressed severely in males and mildly in females. For a mildly affected female, on average, 50% of her sons will be severely affected and 50% of her daughters will be mildly affected. Daughters of an affected male are mildly affected and none of his sons inherit the condition.

X-linked dominant inheritance

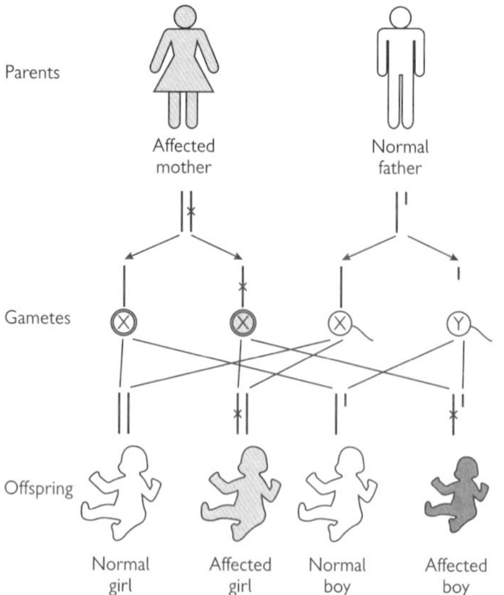

X-linked semi-dominant inheritance

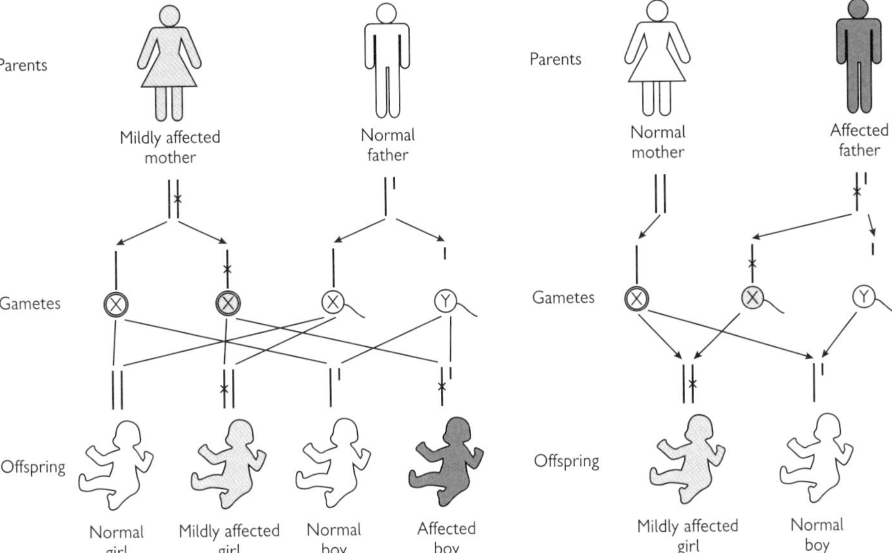

Genetic advice

- Males carrying the mutation are severely affected, often leading to spontaneous loss or neonatal death of affected male pregnancies in XLD conditions.
- Female heterozygotes are affected but have less severe features than males.
- The degree to which females express the disorder is largely governed by X-inactivation patterns.
- When a heterozygous affected female has a pregnancy there are four genetic possibilities at conception, each equally likely. These are: a normal daughter; an affected daughter; a normal son; and a severely affected son, e.g. X-linked hypophosphatasia (vitamin-D resistant rickets) where affected males are viable. For many XLD disorders, e.g. IP, affected males are typically lost in early pregnancy so at birth there are three possibilities: a normal daughter; an affected daughter; a normal son.
- When an affected male has a child, all of his daughters will inherit the mutation and none of his sons will be affected.
- The family tree shows no male-to-male transmission.
- If the mother of an affected female with a presumed *de novo* mutation does not herself carry the mutation in her blood, female siblings of the proband should still be offered carrier testing by mutation detection because of the small possibility of germline mosaicism in the parent.

- Males who are born with features of a severe and normally lethal XLD condition should have a karyotype to exclude Klinefelter syndrome.
- Females with unusually severe features of an XLD or an X-linked semi-dominant disorder may have this as a consequence of:
  - highly unfavourably skewed X-inactivation;
  - Turner syndrome, where the girl is a hemizygote;
  - X-autosome translocation.
  Hence a karyotype is indicated in these circumstances.

Expert adviser: Ian D. Young, Consultant Clinical Geneticist, Leicester, England.

References

Morizio E, Stuppia L *et al.* Deletion of the SHOX gene in patients with short stature of unknown cause. *Am J Med Genet A* 2003; **119**: 293–96.

Shears DJ, Guillen-Navaro E, *et al.* Pseudodominant inheritance of Langer mesomelic dysplasia caused by a *SHOX* homeobox missense mutation. *Am J Med Genet* 2002; **110**: 153–7.

Shi Q, Spriggs E, *et al.* Recombination between the X and Y chromosomes is limited to the pseudoautosomal region and is necessary for proper segregation of the sex chromosomes during spermatogenesis. *Am J Hum Genet* 2002; **71**: 254–61.

Strachan T, Read AP. *Human molecular genetics*, 3rd edn. Garland Science, Philadelphia, 2003.

Young ID. *Introduction to risk calculation in genetic counselling*, 2nd edn. Oxford University Press, 1999.

X-linked recessive (XLR) inheritance

XLR disorders are encoded on the X chromosome. An XLR disorder manifests in males who are hemizygotes, but generally not in carrier females who have two X chromosomes (one normal and one mutated copy). Some X-linked disorders are almost never expressed in females, e.g. alpha-thalassaemia/mental retardation syndrome (ATRX). In some disorders females have symptoms infrequently, e.g Duchenne muscular dystrophy (DMD)/Becker muscular dystrophy (BMD), whereas for others, e.g. X-linked hereditary motor and sensory neuropathy (X-HMSN) and fragile X syndrome (FRAXA), manifestation in female carriers is fairly common but is usually less severe than in affected males. Disorders in which heterozygotes commonly manifest, e.g. X-HMSN and Coffin–Lowry syndrome, may be said to follow **X-linked semi-dominant inheritance** (see 'X-linked dominant (XLD) inheritance', page 32).

X-inactivation is the process by which dosage compensation of X-linked genes in females is achieved by the transcriptional silencing of one of the two X chromosomes during early development (from day 9 post-fertilization when the inner cell mass of the blastocyst contains 64 cells). As a result of X-inactivation heterozygous females are mosaic for X-linked gene expression, with one population of cells expressing genes from the maternal X chromosome and the other population expressing genes from the paternal X chromosome (Nance 1964). The early events in X-inactivation are under the control of the X-chromosome inactivation centre (Xic). The *XIST* gene in the Xic at Xq13.2 is the only gene transcribed exclusively from the inactive X-chromosome and is known to play an essential role in the initiation of X-inactivation. Initiation of X-inactivation involves a counting step in which the number of X chromosomes in the cell is counted relative to cell ploidy so that only *a single X chromosome is functional per diploid adult cell.*

X-inactivation pattern	Frequency (%) of skewed X-inactivation in normal female controls (Plenge et al. 1999)
≥90:10	3
≥80:20	9
≥70:30	30

X inactivation in the embryo is a random process, with ~50% of cells containing the maternal X inactive and ~50% of cells containing the paternal X inactive. Significant deviation from a 50:50 inactivation pattern is occasionally observed among normal females in the population, a phenomenon referred to as **skewed X-inactivation** (see table). Skewing of X-inactivation is a feature of some X-linked disorders. In extra-embryonic tissues, e.g. placenta, there is imprinted inactivation of the paternal X-chromosome.

X-inactivation patterns may be assessed by comparing the ratio of the two alleles at a highly polymorphic site, e.g. the CA repeat in the androgen receptor gene, in a non-methylation-sensitive assay with the ratio of the same alleles in a methylation-sensitive assay. Usually the ratio approximates to 50%.

Aspects of XLR inheritance
Skewed X-inactivation. If there is complete skewing, the ratio is 100:0; often an intermediate value is found.

Values <80:20 fall within values expected from normal variation in X-inactivation patterns in the general population; values >80:20 are suggestive of X-inactivation due to a selection bias due to a deleterious XLR mutation, but are seen in ~9% of normal females (see above). This selection bias may not operate equally in all tissues and so variable degrees of skewing may be observed in different tissues. Maternal X-inactivation skewing may be used to suggest that a sporadic affected male has an X-linked disorder.

Manifesting carriers. Unfavourable skewing of X-inactivation in key tissues may be a major factor in determining whether or not an XLR disorder is expressed in heterozygotes. As noted above, the penetrance in heterozygotes shows wide variation between different XLR disorders.

Germline mosaicism. A number of XLR disorders have substantial germline mosaicism risks—most notably DMD/BMD. For the mother of an affected boy with a known mutation that is not present in the mother's genomic DNA, there is a suggested 1 in 5 (20%) risk to a future son who inherits the same X chromosome as his affected brother (i.e. there is an overall 5% risk to future pregnancies). For androgen insensitivity syndrome (AIS) this risk is much smaller, but nevertheless germline mosaicism has been observed.

Typical family tree
X-linked recessive inheritance

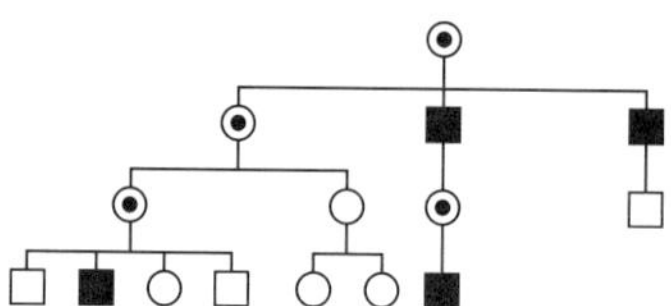

A typical family tree showing X-linked recessive inheritance. The condition is expressed in males, but not in females. For a carrier female, on average, 50% of her sons will be affected and 50% of her daughters will be carriers. All daughters of an affected male are obligate carriers and none of his sons inherit the condition.

Genetic advice
- Males carrying the mutation are severely affected; females carrying the mutation are generally either unaffected or more mildly affected than males.
- The degree to which females express the disorder is largely governed by X-inactivation patterns.
- When a carrier female has a pregnancy there are four possible outcomes, each equally likely. These are: a normal daughter; a carrier daughter; a normal son; an affected son. Another way of expressing this is that in a female pregnancy there is a 50% chance of a carrier daughter; in a male pregnancy there is a 50% chance of an affected son.
- When an affected male fathers a pregnancy, all of his daughters will be carriers and none of his sons will be affected.
- The family tree shows no male-to-male transmission.
- Even if the proband is the only affected member, it is generally more likely that the mother is a carrier than that the proband has the condition as the result of a *de novo* mutation. For XLR conditions where reproductive fitness is zero, there is a two-thirds chance that the mother is a mutation carrier and a one-third chance that the mutation is *de novo* for an apparently sporadic case.

X-linked recessive inheritance

- If the mother of a sporadic case with a presumed *de novo* mutation does not herself carry the mutation in her blood, female siblings of the proband should still be offered carrier testing by mutation detection because of the small possibility of germline mosaicism in the mother.
- Females with unusually severe features of an XLR disorder may have this as a consequence of:
  - highly unfavourably skewed X-inactivation;
  - Turner syndrome, where the girl is a hemizygote;
  - X-autosome translocation.
  Hence a karyotype is indicated in these circumstances.

Expert adviser: Ian D. Young, Consultant Clinical Geneticist, Leicester, England.

References

Nance WE. Genetic tests with a sex-linked marker: glucose-6-phosphate dehydrogenase. *Cold Spring Harbor Symp Quant Biol* 1964; **29**: 415–52.

Plenge RM, Tranebjaerg L, *et al.* Evidence that mutations in the X-linked DDP gene cause incompletely penetrant and variable skewed X inactivation. *Am J Hum Genet* 1999; **64**: 759–67.

Strachan T, Read AP. *Human molecular genetics*, 3rd edn. Garland Science, Philadelphia, 2003.

Young ID. *Introduction to risk calculation in genetic counselling*, 2nd edn. Oxford University Press, Oxford, 1999.

Chapter 2

Clinical approach

Chapter contents

Ambiguous genitalia (including sex reversal) 38
Anal anomalies (atresia, stenosis) 42
Anterior segment eye malformations 46
Arthrogryposis (arthrogryposis multiplex congenita) 48
Ataxic adult 50
Ataxic child 52
Brachydactyly 56
Broad thumbs 58
Cardiomyopathy in children under 10 years 60
Cataract 64
Cerebellar anomalies 66
Cerebral palsy 70
Chondrodysplasia punctata 72
Cleft lip and palate 74
Coarse facial features 78
Coloboma 82
Congenital heart disease 84
Corneal clouding 88
Severe deafness in early childhood 90
Developmental delay in the child with consanguineous parents 94
Developmental regression 96
Duane retraction syndrome 100
Dysmorphic child 102
Dystonia 106
Ear anomalies 108
Facial asymmetry 112
Failure to thrive (prenatal and postnatal growth failure) 116
Floppy infant 118
Fractures 122
Generalized disorders of skin pigmentation (including albinism) 126
Hemihypertrophy and limb asymmetry 128
Holoprosencephaly (HPE) 130
Hydrocephalus 134
Hypermobile joints 138
Hypoglycaemia in the neonate and infant 140
Hypospadias 142
Increased bone density 144
Large fontanelle 146
Laterality disorders including heterotaxy and isomerism 148
Leukodystrophy/leukoencephalopathy 150
Limb reduction defects 152
Lissencephaly and neuronal migration disorders 156
Lumps and bumps 160
Macrocephaly 162
Mental retardation with apparent X-linked inheritance 164
Mental retardation 168
Microcephaly 172
Micrognathia and Robin sequence 174
Microphthalmia and anophthalmia 176
Minor congenital anomalies 180
Nasal anomalies 182
Neonatal encephalopathy and intractable seizures in the neonate 186
Nystagmus 190
Obesity with and without developmental delay 192
Ocular hypertelorism 196
Oedema—generalized or puffy extremities 198
Oesophageal and intestinal atresia (including tracheo-oesophageal fistula) 200
Optic nerve hypoplasia 204
Overgrowth 206
Patchy hypomelanotic skin lesions 208
Patchy pigmented skin lesions (including café-au-lait spots) 210
Plagiocephaly and abnormalities of skull shape 212
Postaxial polydactyly 214
Preaxial polydactyly 218
Prolonged neonatal jaundice and jaundice in infants below 6 months 220
Ptosis, blepharophimosis, and other eyelid anomalies 224
Radial ray defects and thumb hypoplasia 228
Retinal dysplasia 230
Retinal receptor dystrophies 232
Scalp defects 236
Seizures with developmental delay/mental retardation 238
Short stature 242
Skeletal dysplasia 246
Structural intracranial anomalies (agenesis of the corpus callosum, septo-optic dysplasia, and arachnoid cysts) 248
Suspected non-accidental injury 252
Syndactyly (other than 2, 3 toe syndactyly) 254
Unusual hair, teeth, nails, and skin 256

Ambiguous genitalia (including sex reversal)

Genetic sex is determined at fertilization. In sex chromosome aneuploidy, presence of a Y chromosome promotes normal male sexual differentiation (e.g. 47,XXY and 47,XYY). Only a single X chromosome is required for female development as in 45,X (although complete ovarian development requires XX). Up to 12 weeks gestation the external genitalia appear the same in both sexes; even up to 20 weeks gestation it can occasionally be difficult to reliably determine the fetal sex from the appearances of the external genitalia.

Under normal circumstances genetic sex determines gonadal sex, which determines phenotypic sex. Before 7 weeks gestation the gonadal precursor tissues are histologically identical. Both sexes possess paired Wolffian (precursors of vas deferens and epididymis and seminal vesicles) and Müllerian ducts (precursors of Fallopian tubes and uterus). External genitalia are female in appearance. Towards the end of the first trimester the indifferent gonad in males is stimulated to differentiate into a testis by the product of the *SRY* gene. If the *SRY* gene is absent (as in normal females), deleted, or mutated the indifferent gonad fails to develop into a testis. The testis produces Müllerian inhibitory factor, which leads to Müllerian tract regression in males. The stabilization of Wolffian duct derivatives requires testosterone. Testosterone is important for the development of the internal genitalia and dihydrotestosterone (DHT) has a key role in the development of the external genitalia. In the absence of testosterone (as in normal females) the Wolffian ducts regress.

Clinical approach

Assessment and investigation of neonates with ambiguous genitalia is best done in close liaison with a paediatric endocrinologist.

History: key points

- Three-generation family tree (including consanguinity).
- Detailed enquiry about maternal health and drug exposure during pregnancy.
- Detailed documentation of pregnancy history.

Examination: key points

Document the findings carefully; clinical photographs may be helpful.

- The phallus—micropenis or clitoris; measure length of phallus.
- The labioscrotal folds—bifid scrotum or labial fusion.
- The gonads—palpable or impalpable (examine the labioscrotal folds and groins; if palpable they are likely to be testes, or possibly ovotestes). Measure length.
- The urethra—position, chordee (tethering of penis).
- Other anomalies.
- Birthweight—strong association between low birthweight and hypospadias.

Special investigations

The *initial screen* should include:

- karyotype to determine genetic sex (initial karyotype by interphase fluorescent *in situ* hybridization (FISH) if available);

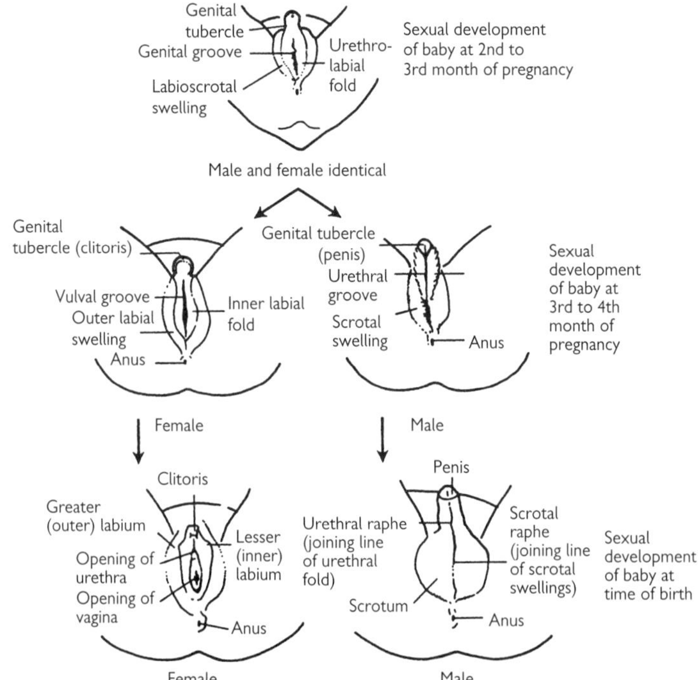

Differentiation of external genitalia in the human fetus. (Taken with permission from Hall *et al.* (1989), p. 315.)

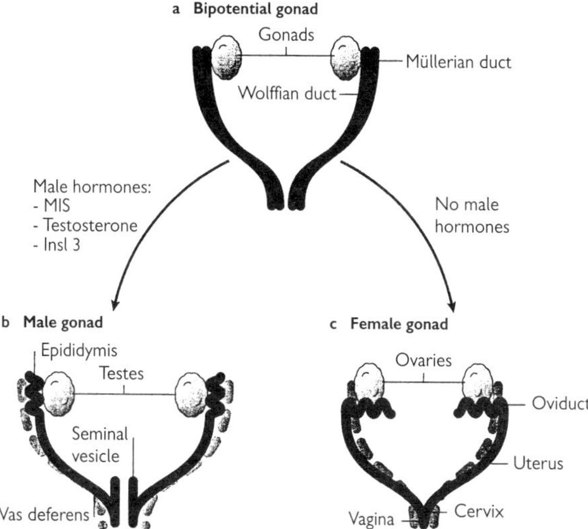

Sexual differentiation of the reproductive system. MIS, Müllerian inhibiting substance (also known as anti-Müllerian hormone (AMH); Insl3; insulin-like growth factor 3. (Taken with permission from Kobayashi and Behringer (2003), p. 972.)

- pelvic ultrasound scan (USS) to determine whether a uterus is present and whether the gonads can be visualized;
- electrolytes Na/K and blood glucose;
- plasma 17OH-progesterone (*urgent* analysis);
- testosterone.

If 46,XX: the most likely diagnosis is congenital adrenal hyperplasia (CAH). There is an urgent need to determine if this is a salt-losing variety and further investigations should include:
- 11-deoxycortisol;
- androstenedione;
- testosterone;
- renin;
- aldosterone;
- 24 hour urine collection for urine steroid profile by specific chromatography in a specialist lab;
- blood for DNA studies.

If 45X/46XY: 95% of those diagnosed prenatally are phenotypically normal males, but potential exists for gonadal dysgenesis if both cell lines are present in the gonad. Testosterone level in the normal range within the first 8 weeks of life (when the neonatal gonads are very active) would be indicative of normal male gonadal development and be reassuring. If not detected antenatally and expecially when ambiguous genitalia are present, the prognosis for normal masculinization is more guarded. Tests should include:
- testosterone level;
- consider follicle-stimulating hormone (FSH)/luteinizing hormone (LH) to see if gonad functional to suppress pituitary.

If 46,XY: specific diagnosis may be possible in only 25%. Testosterone implies the presence of testes. Measurement of testosterone, androstenedione, and DHT enables identification of the most common androgen biosynthetic defects, i.e. 17β-hydroxysteroid dehydrogenase and

5α-reductase. Proceed to a human chorionic gonadotropin (hCG) stimulation test and measure:
- plasma 17OH-progesterone;
- testosterone;
- androstenedione;
- DHT;
- dehydroepiandosterone (DHA);
- 24 hour urine for urine steroid profile;
- blood for DNA studies.

In some laboratories it may be possible to request anti-Müllerian hormone (AMH) and inhibin B.

Some diagnoses to consider

Congenital adrenal hyperplasia (CAH). The most common cause of ambiguous genitalia in infants with a 46,XX karyotype. See 'Congenital adrenal hyperplasia (CAH)', page 282.

Smith–Lemli–Opitz (SLO) disorder. An autosomal recessive (AR) disorder caused by deficiency of 7-dehydrocholesterol reductase. Males may have hypospadias, micropenis, and undescended testes, also Y-shaped 2,3 syndactyly, microcephaly, cleft palate, congenital heart disease, developmental delay, etc. See 'Hypospadias', page 142.

Camptomelic dysplasia (*SOX9*—an *SRY*-related gene on 17q23-ter). Often *de novo* autosomal dominant (AD) mutations. Bowing of femur and tibia, narrow chest, short first metacarpals, and sex reversal in the majority of 46,XY infants. Cleft palate is common and one-third have congenital heart disease.

WAGR (Wilms tumour–aniridia–genitourinary anomalies–(mental) retardation). A contiguous gene syndrome due to microscopic or submicroscopic interstitial deletion of 11p13. Specific FISH probes available. See 'Wilms tumour', page 486.

Drash syndrome or Wilms tumour and pseudohermaphroditism is caused by mutations in the Wilms tumour receptor gene *WT1* that abolish DNA-binding capacity.

Features are ambiguous genitalia, early onset hypertension, and proteinuria with nephritic syndrome and mesangial sclerosis leading to progressive renal failure. See 'Wilms tumour', page 486.

Frasier syndrome. Ambiguous genitalia and nephropathy as for Drash syndrome, with low risk of Wilms tumour, but risk of gonadoblastoma. Due to dominant mutations causing defective alternative splicing of *WTI* (Klamt *et al.* 1998). See 'Wilms tumour', page 486.

5α-reductase deficiency. AR defect in testosterone biosynthetic pathway that converts testosterone to the more potent androgen DHT. Mutations in this gene can cause perineoscrotal hypospadias. In some instances the genitalia may appear female with diagnosis made at puberty after presentation with primary amenorrhoea, lack of breast development, and deepening voice.

17β-hydroxysteroid dehydrogenase (17β-HSD) deficiency. An AR biosynthetic defect that impairs conversion of androstenedione to testosterone in the fetal testis. Defects in this conversion lead to a male form of pseudohermaphroditism with gynaecomastia. The *HSD 17β3* gene maps to 9q22, and ambiguous genitalia are seen in 9q22 deletions.

Partial androgen insensitivity syndrome (PAIS) caused by mutations in the androgen receptor gene which impair androgen binding and signalling see Androgen insensitivity syndrome, page 270.

Deletion of 9p24.3 or 10q26

Deletion of distal 9p has been reported in a number of cases to be associated with gonadal dysgenesis and XY sex reversal. This region contains the testic determining genes *DMR1* and *DMR2* (Raymond). Terminal 10q deletions appear to be associated with abnormal male genital development (Wilkie)

Genetic advice

Recurrence risk
Counsel for specific diagnosis.

Carrier detection
Counsel for specific diagnosis.

Prenatal diagnosis
Counsel for specific diagnosis.

Natural history and further management (preventative measures)
If the genitalia are truly ambiguous, the issue of gender assignment needs to be discussed with an expert team. Minto *et al.* (2003) have questioned whether surgical intervention in infancy is the best management, or whether a more conservative approach should be followed initially, deferring surgery to allow the individual themselves to be actively involved in decisions that have such a profound effect on their own future (see also Reiner and Gearhart 2004). It is crucial to work with a specialist team at a tertiary referral centre.

Dysgenetic gonads should be removed because of the risk of gonadoblastoma.

Sex reversal

Complete discordance between the phenotypic and karyotypic sex. Usually comes to light when there is a discrepancy between the karyotypic sex reported from chorionic villus sampling (CVS)/amniocentesis and the sex subsequently identified by prenatal USS or assessment of the newborn. Possibilities include:

- maternal contamination of CVS/amniocentesis (the most likely cause);
- sample mix-up;
- true discordance between phenotypic and genetic sex as in XX males and XY females (rare);
- chimerism from twin or lost twin (rare).

Previous bone marrow transplantation from a donor of the opposite sex may also give discrepant results between the phenotypic sex and the karyotypic sex as determined by a blood sample (lymphocytes) and may sometimes come to light during the investigation of infertility.

XX males

Prevalence is 1/20 000. This is usually due to:

- cryptic translocations involving SRY-bearing Y material and the X chromsomes (FISH for *SRY*);
- mosaicism for XX and cell lines involving Y chromosome material;
- true XX hermaphroditism where both testicular and ovarian tissues persist (findings are variable but may have ovary on one side and testis on the other) may be due to mosaicism or chimerism or to mutations in genes in the pathway downstream of SRY.

XY females

- *SRY* mutations or deletions of SRY (explains only 15–20% of XY females).
- Complete androgen insensitivity syndrome (AIS)—see eponymous section, page 270.
- Camptomelic dysplasia (see above).
- 9p24 monosomy can cause abnormalities of testicular development.
- dup Xp21.2-p22.2 can cause female differentiation—dosage-sensitive sex reversal.
- Approximately 80% of XY females with gonadal dysgenesis are of unknown aetiology. Often have uterus and streak gonads.

Support group contact: Androgen Insensitivity Syndrome Support Group <www.medhelp.org/www/ais>; Adrenal Hyperplasia Network <www.ahn.org.uk>.

Expert adviser: Ieuan Hughes, Professor of Paediatrics, University of Cambridge, Cambridge, England.

References

Hall JG, Froster-Iskenius UG, Allanson JE. *Handbook of normal physical measurements*. Oxford University Press, Oxford, 1989.

Klamt B, Koziell A, *et al*. Frasier syndrome is caused by defective alternative splicing of *WT1* leading to an altered ratio of WT1 ± KJS splice isoforms. *Hum Mol Genet* 1998; **7**: 709–14.

Kobayashi A, Behringer RR. Developmental genetics of the female reproductive tract in mammals. *Nature Rev Genet* 2003; **4**: 969–80.

MacLaughlin DT, Donahoe PK. Mechanisms of disease: sex determination and differentiation. *New Engl J Med* 2004; **350**: 367–78.

Minto CL, Liao L-M, *et al*. The effect of clitoral surgery on sexual outcome in individuals who have intersex conditions with ambiguous genitalia: a cross-sectional study. *Lancet* 2003; **361**: 1252–7.

Reiner WG, Gearhart JP. Discordant sexual identity in some genetic males with cloacal exstrophy assigned to female sex at birth. *New Engl J Med* 2004; **350**: 333–41.

Seminars in Medical Genetics. Sex determination and sex differentiation in humans. *Am J Med Genet* 1999; **89C** (4).

Hughes IA. Female development — all by default? (Perspective). *NEJM* 2004; **351**: 748–50.

Raymond CS, Parker ED, *et al*. A region of human chromosome 9p required for testis development contains two genes related to known sexual regulators. *Hum Mol Gen* 1999; **8**: 989–96.

Wilkie AO, Campbell FM, *et al*. Complete and partial XY sex reversal associated with terminal deletion of 10q: report of 2 cases and literature review. *Am J Med Genet* 1993; **46**: 567–600.

Anal anomalies (atresia, stenosis)

Anal anomalies affect 4/10 000 births. Only one-third are isolated anomalies; two-thirds occur with other anomalies. Most anorectal anomalies result from abnormal development of the urorectal septum, resulting in incomplete separation of the cloaca into urogenital and anorectal portions. In the London Dysmorphology Database (LDDB; Winter and Baraitser 2003), anal atresia/stenosis is a feature of 135 syndromes. Anal atresia also occurs in some chromosomal disorders (including trisomies). Of isolated anal anomalies, 75% are atresias, of which 10% are above and 90% below the level of the levator ani muscle ('high' and 'low' atresias). There is a predominance of males. The M:F ratio for high lesions is 6.7, and for low lesions it is 2.3. Findings on examination are absence of the anus or abnormal placement of the anus. Other anal anomalies include congenital anal fistula (15%), ectopic anus (3%), and persistent cloaca (1%). Heij et al. (1996) undertook routine lumbosacral magnetic resonance imaging (MRI) in patients presenting with anorectal malformations and identified anomalies in 30% of those with low anorectal malformations

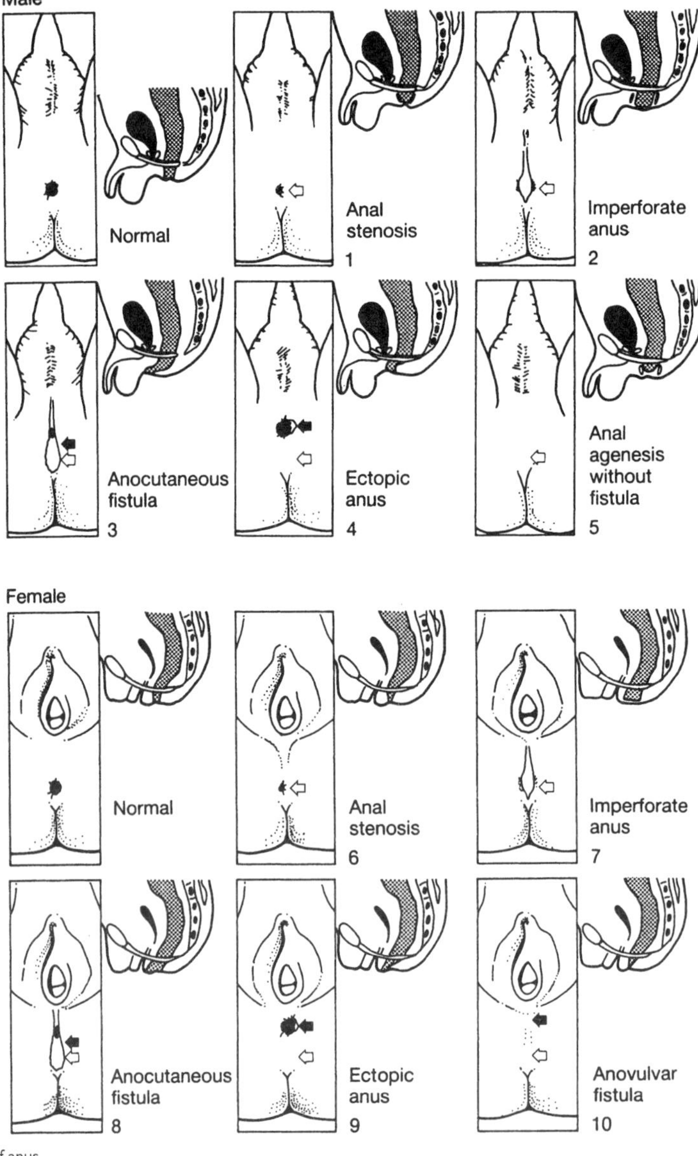

Anal anomalies. (From Santulli et al. (1970).).

and in 50% of those with high malformations. These included caudal regression syndrome, tethered cord, and other spinal anomalies.

Abnormalities of the external genitalia are often found in association with anal anomalies. In Heij *et al.*'s study urogenital anomalies were found in 49% of patients presenting with anorectal malformation.

Clinical approach

History: key points

- Three-generation family tree including specific enquiry regarding surgery in the neonatal period and history of colostomy.
- History of maternal diabetes, early bleeding.
- Feeding difficulties; any evidence of tracheo-oesphageal fistula or laryngeal cleft.
- Floppy baby, delayed motor milestones, or developmental delay (syndromes and chromosomal abnormalities).
- Visual or hearing problems (cat-eye syndrome, Townes–Brock syndrome (TBS)).

Examination: key points

- Carefully describe the anus and external genitalia and photograph prior to surgery.
- Bladder exstrophy (OEIS (omphalocele–exstrophy of the cloaca–imperforate anus–spinal defects); see below).
- Look carefully for other dysmorphic features but some, such as the anterior cowlicks of FG syndrome, are age-dependent.
- Carefully assess the external ear (TBS).
- Hypertelorism (Opitz G). Examine the heart (VACTERL (vertebral defects–anal atresia–cardiac anomalies–tracheo-oesophageal fistula–(o)esophageal atresia–renal anomalies–limb defects); see below).
- Examine the limbs: thumb deficiency, occasionally duplication, and radial ray anomalies (VACTERL), triphalangeal or hypoplastic thumbs (TBS), polydactyly (Pallister–Hall syndrome).

Special investigations

- Karyotype if associated anomalies.
- X-rays of spine, pelvis, and chest (VACTERL).
- Consider lumbosacral MRI.
- Renal ultrasound scan (USS; genitourinary anomalies constitute 49% of associated anomalies).
- Additional radiology if a fistula is suspected.
- Echocardiogram (cardiovascular anomalies constitute 27% of associated anomalies).
- Endocrine referral (Pallister–Hall syndrome).
- DNA analysis/storage.

Some diagnoses to consider

VATER/VACTERL association. Incidence 1.6/10 000. Most children usually have 3–4 features present. Hall *et al.* (1989) suggest at least one anomaly from limb, thorax, and pelvis/lower abdomen for a secure diagnosis and at least two anomalies in each of two of those regions for a probable diagnosis. Normal cognitive development expected. Usually sporadic with low recurrence risk. VATER/VACTERL denotes combinations of the following anomalies.

- V, Vertebral defects—usually upper to mid thoracic and lumbar regions. Usually hemivertebrae, but dyssegmented and fused vertebrae may occur—may be accompanying rib anomalies.
- A, Anal atresia—may be associated genital defects (hypospadias, bifid scrotum) or fistulae.
- C, Cardiac anomalies—present in ~80%; any type, any severity.
- T, Tracheo-oesophageal fistula.
- E, (O)esophageal atresia—80% have an associated tracheo-oesophageal fistula.
- R, Renal anomalies—present in 80%, e.g. renal agenesis/dysplasia.
- L, Limb (radial defects)—preaxial with underdevelopment or agenesis of thumbs and radial bones; usually bilateral defects, but asymmetric. Reduced thenar muscle mass is mildest end of spectrum. The lower limbs are not affected.

OEIS (omphalocele–exstrophy of the cloaca–imperforate anus–spinal defects) (Keppler-Noreuil 2001). Mostly sporadic.

Caudal regression. Most cases of caudal regression are sporadic or associated with maternal diabetes. The condition is thought to be part of a spectrum including imperforate anus, sacral agenesis, and sirenomelia.

Currarino syndrome. Autosomal dominant (AD) sacral agenesis is characterized by a partial agenesis of the sacrum typically involving sacral vertebrae S2–S5 only. Associated features include anorectal malformation, a presacral mass, and urogenital malformation. See 'Congenital cystic lung lesions, Currarino syndrome, and sacrococcygeal teratoma', page 576.

Townes-Brock syndrome (TBS) is an AD condition with imperforate anus, hand anomalies (triphalangeal thumb, hypoplastic thumb), and ear malformations (dysplastic ears and ear tags) with sensorineural hearing loss. Within and between families, the phenotype displays striking variability. *SALL1*, a zinc finger transcription factor, is the disease-causing gene. There is a high incidence of new mutations. Cardiac anomalies have been reported.

Cat-eye syndrome (CES). Anal anomalies (imperforate anus, anal atresia, or anteriorly placed anus), pre-auricular pits/tags, congenital heart defects, iris colobomata, renal anomalies, and variable learning disability. Results from a small marker chromosome containing a duplication of 22q11 resulting in tetrasomy 22q11. Can be an unbalanced product of the relatively common 11q23;22q11 reciprocal translocation. CES can occur in mosaic form and can also be inherited.

Pallister–Hall syndrome (anocerebrodigital syndrome) is characterized by imperforate anus, mesoaxial (or postaxial) polydactyly, hypopituitarism, and hypothalamic hamartoblastoma. Some have a cleft larynx or bifid epiglottis. An AD condition with very variable expression and caused by mutations in *GLI3* on 7p13 (allelic to Greig).

FG syndrome is difficult to diagnose without a strong family history. Hypotonia and constipation are common in infants. There may be a history of rectal biopsy to exclude short-segment Hirschsprung's disease. The anal defects reported are imperforate, stenotic, and anteriorly placed anus; also perianal skin tags. Agenesis of the corpus callosum may be present. There is macrocephaly with a frontal upsweep of the hair (cowlick). Some families are linked to Xq12–q21.3 but there is at least one other locus on the X. It is only possible to offer carrier testing or prenatal testing in families large enough to confirm linkage.

Opitz syndrome (also known as Opitz G or G/BBB). Hypospadias is the major anomaly of urorectal development, but imperforate and ectopic anus are reported. There is striking hypertelorism and swallowing problems due to laryngeal clefts. There is an X-linked and an autosomal (22q) locus. The X-linked gene is *MID1* at Xp22.

Genetic advice

Recurrence risk

After carefully excluding syndromic and chromosomal causes and those with a family history, isolated recto-anal malformations are rarely genetic. Both affected sibs and offspring have been reported but overall the recurrence risk is about 1%.

Carrier detection

In syndromic cases, clinical examination combined with mutation analysis, if available.

Prenatal diagnosis

Prenatal diagnosis is possible for some of these conditions on the basis of:

- USS for structural abnormalities;
- chromosomal or mutation analysis if an abnormality has been identified in the proband.

Natural history and further management (preventative measures)

Surgical management. A colostomy is usually performed in the neonatal period with anastamosis at a later stage, depending on the anatomy and prognosis for continence.

Support group contact: Many of the individual syndromes have their own support groups. See Contact a Family (UK) <www.cafamily.org.uk> and National Organization for Rare Disorders (US) <www.rarediseases.org>.

Expert adviser: Dian Donnai, Professor of Medical Genetics, University of Manchester, Manchester, England.

References

Cho S, Moore SP, Fangman T. One hundred three consecutive patients with anorectal malformations and their associated anomalies. *Arch Pediatr Adolesc Med* 2001; **155**: 587–91.

Cuschieri A, EUROCAT Working Group. Descriptive epidemiology of isolated anal anomalies: a survey of 4.6 million births in Europe. *Am J Med Genet* 2001; **103**: 207–15.

Hall JG, Froster-Iskenius UG, Allanson JE. *Handbook of normal physical measurements*. Oxford University Press, Oxford, 1989.

Heij HA, Nievelstein RA, *et al.* Abnormal anatomy of the lumbosacral region imaged by magnetic resonance in children with anorectal malformations. *Arch Dis Child* 1996; **74**: 441–4.

Keppler-Noreuil KM. OEIS complex (omphalocele–exstrophy–imperforate anus–spinal defects): a review of 14 cases. *Am J Med Genet* 2001; **99**: 271–9.

Santulli TV, Kiesewetter WB, Bill AH Jr. Anorectal anomalies: a suggested international classification. *J Pediatr Surg* 1970; **5** (3): 281–7.

Winter RM, Baraitser M. *London Dysmorphology Database*. London Medical Databases, London, 2003.

Anterior segment eye malformations

The cornea, iris, and the trabecular meshwork together are known as the anterior segment of the eye. Although genes predominantly control the development of one of these components, malformation of one structure can cause problems in the other components of the anterior segment. Additionally, different mutations of the same gene may lead to a different clinical phenotype. For example, truncating mutations in *PAX6* have been found in aniridia, whereas missense mutation in the paired box domain are found in some cases of Peter anomaly. Bilateral involvement may only be detected after careful examination of the apparently normal eye by an ophthalmologist.

A child may be referred to the geneticist for counselling after the identification of an anterior segment anomaly. The aim is to determine whether this is a purely ocular condition or if there are non-ocular features that suggest a syndrome diagnosis.

Clinical approach

History: key points

- Family history. At least three generations. Enquire about consanguinity. Ask about all visual difficulties. Affected individuals may be minimally affected.
- Exposure to teratogens, and infections during pregnancy.
- Growth (most chromosomal conditions show poor growth; Rieger syndrome is associated with pituitary abnormalities).
- Developmental progress (allowing for visual difficulties).
- Wilms tumour (WAGR: Wilms tumour–aniridia–genitourinary anomalies (hypospadias and cryptorchidism)–mental retardation).

Examination: key points

- **Eye.** Examination and photography of eye and surrounding structures (usually performed by the ophthalmologist). Anomalies detected may include: aniridia, sclerocornea, megalocornea, microphthalmia, and/or lens abnormality.
- **Growth parameters** (height, weight, and occipital-frontal circumference (OFC)):
  - short stature in Peter plus syndrome, SHORT syndrome, and Rieger syndrome.
- **Face and mouth:**
  - orofacial clefts (Peter plus syndrome, Kivlin syndrome);
  - abnormal dentition (Rieger syndrome).
- **Skin:**
  - lipoatrophy (SHORT syndrome);
  - patchy skin lesions with sclerocornea (Goltz syndrome, del Xp22);
  - redundant skin in umbilicus (Rieger syndrome).
- **Genitalia:**
  - hypospadias and cryptorchidism in WAGR; hypospadias in Rieger syndrome;
- **Neurological:**
  - cerebellar ataxia (Gillespie syndrome);
  - olfaction abnormalities may be found with *PAX6* mutations.

Special investigations

- Chromosome analysis and consider more detailed analysis if features are suggestive of a submicroscopic deletion, e.g. fluorescent *in situ* hybridization (FISH) for 11p13, Xp22.

- Store DNA for possible genetic testing.
- Renal ultrasound scan (USS) in children with aniridia who have 11p– syndrome of loss of *WT1* suppressor gene on FISH, or mutations in *WT1*.
- Consider brain imaging (*PAX 6* and Rieger syndrome).

Some diagnoses to consider

Peter anomaly

Absence of the central corneal endothelium and Descemet's membrane leads to congenital central corneal opacities. 80% are bilateral, but may be very asymmetrical. Lens abnormalities and microphthalmia are common. If short stature and clefts, consider **Peter plus** and **Kivlin syndrome** (autosomal recessive (AR)).

- Ensure a karyotype is performed if there are other congenital anomalies or developmental delay.
- Mutations of *PAX6* (aniridia gene) and *PITX2* (Axenfeld-Reiger syndromes) have been identified in some individuals.
- Recessive and dominant inheritance are both reported in isolated Peter anomaly.

Axenfeld–Rieger syndromes

A number of previously distinct eye phenotypes have now been grouped together under the heading of Axenfeld–Rieger malformation syndromes to eliminate arbitrary and confusing subclassification. They are associated with dominant mutation in the transcription factor genes *FOXC1* and *PITX2*. There are also loci on 13q14 and 16q24. Most Axenfeld–Rieger syndromes have autosomal dominant (AD) inheritance. There is a ~50% risk of developing glaucoma.

Although now grouped together the following may help in interpreting the literature:

- Axenfeld anomaly: defects limited to the peripheral anterior segment.
- Rieger anomaly: defects of the peripheral anterior segment and changes in the iris.
- Rieger syndrome: eye abnormalities and non-ocular defects (dental anomalies, midface hypoplasia, redundant periumbilical skin, hypospadias, and pituitary abnormalities):
  - type 1 Rieger syndrome: *RIEG1* mutations have been found in both *FOXC1* and *PITX2*;
  - type 2 Rieger syndrome: *RIEG2* is linked to 13q14.
- Posterior embryotoxon and Axenfeld anomaly can be found in apparently normal mutation carriers of Peter anomaly, and Alagille syndrome.

SHORT syndrome is the association of Rieger anomaly with short stature, deep-set eyes, and lipoatrophy. Previously thought to be AR, recent reports suggest AD inheritance is more likely.

Aniridia

Iris hypoplasia. 1 in 60–100 000 population frequency. Associated eye anomalies may include: corneal and lens opacities, cataract, foveal hypoplasia (100%), optic nerve hypoplasia, and glaucoma. 65% are familial (AD); extremely variable both within and between families.

- Arrange for examination of parents of sporadic cases.
- Karyotype with screen for 11p13 deletions (WAGR locus) in *all* sporadic and familial cases. Use a panel of

cosmids, encompassing the aniridia-associated *PAX6* gene, the Wilms tumor predisposition gene *WT1*, and flanking markers, in distal chromosome 11p13 to exclude a submicroscopic deletion (Crolla and van Heyningen 2002). These authors found a high frequency (~40%) of chromosomal rearrangements in a cohort of 77 patients with sporadic and familial aniridia. Ensure follow-up and screening for Wilms tumour risk if a deletion present.

- *PAX6* gene mutations at 11p13 causes aniridia. Arrange mutation analysis if FISH studies are negative. Prenatal diagnosis may be possible if the mutation is identified but counsel that this would not give guidance as to the clinical manifestations.

Gillespie syndrome. Aniridia plus cerebellar ataxia and mental retardation. Inheritance uncertain.

Corneal malformations

Megalocornea is defined as a cornea of greater than or equal to 13 mm at birth, but which is still clear with normal other parameters. Exclude buphthalmos (congenital glaucoma) where the corner is hazy. Developmental delay, cerebellar abnormalities, and short stature with megalocornea is sometimes known as **Neuhauser syndrome** and inherited as AR. Megalocornea can follow an X-linked or occasionally dominant, pattern of inheritance.

Sclerocornea is congenital nonprogressive corneal opacification with vascularization and can be associated with glaucoma. It is commonly found in conjunction with other abnormalities of the anterior segment such as Peter anomaly microphthalmia, coloboma and cataract formation and also in hypomelanosis of Ito and incontinentia pigmenti. It is a feature of del Xp22 in females who also have linear skin pigmentation on the face and neck. Sclerocornea in its mildst form is just peripheral corneal opacification, but if more extensive is sometimes referred to as microcornea (see below).

Microcornea. The cornea is less than 9–10 mm diameter at birth. It may be associated with a normal-sized globe on ultrasound or microphthalmia. It may follow AD/AR inheritance. Microcornea may be a feature of Nance-Horan syndrome (XLR), see Clinical approach to 'Cataracts', page 64.

Corneal clouding

The cornea is opacified. It is important to exclude glaucoma (and rubella embryopathy in centres where this is common). Many of the causes are progressive metabolic conditions rather than malformations. See 'Corneal clouding', page 88.

Genetic advice

Recurrence risk

- Arrange parental ophthalmological assessment of the anterior segment. Variability is well described for most of the anterior segment disorders and parents may have subtle features that are only detectable on careful assessment by a specialist.
- Check literature for recent gene localizations. At present, known genes include *PAX6*, *PITX2*, *PITX3*, *FOXC1*, and *CHX10*. Most are transcription factor genes with AD inheritance. *CYPIB1* has been found to be a cause of AR glaucoma.

Carrier detection

- By ophthalmological examination.
- Is possible in families where a causative mutation has been identified.

Prenatal diagnosis

- By genetic testing where there is molecular or chromosomal confirmation of diagnosis.
- USS in mid-trimester can visualize the eye and lens but is unlikely to be sensitive enough to detect recurrence.

Natural history and further management (preventative measures)

Long-term ophthalmological follow-up is indicated, particularly to screen for glaucoma.

Support group contact: Many of the individual syndromes have their own support groups. See Contact a Family (UK) <www.cafamily.org.uk> and National Organization for Rare Disorders (US) <www.rarediseases.org>.

Expert adviser: Nicola Ragge, Consultant Paediatric Ophthalmologist, Moorfields Eye Hospital, London, UK.

References

Alward WL. Axenfeld–Rieger syndrome in the age of molecular genetics. *Am J Ophthalmol* 2000; **130**: 107–15.

Crolla JA, van Heyningen V. Frequent chromosome aberrations revealed by molecular cytogenetic studies in patients with aniridia. *Am J Hum Genet* 2002; **71** (5): 1138–49.

Genetic diseases of the eye. Ed Elias Traboulsi. Chapter 5 Malformations of the anterior segment of the Eye, pp81-98. OUP 1998

Gregory-Evans K. Developmental disorders of the eye. In *Paediatric ophthalmology*, Fundamentals of Clinical Ophthalmology series (ed. A. Moore), pp. 53–61. BMJ Books, London, 2000.

Lines MA, Kozlowski K, Walter MA. Molecular genetics of Axenfeld–Rieger malformations. *Hum Mol Genet* 2002; **11**: 1177–84.

Schimmenti LA, de la Cruz, *et al.* Novel mutations in sonic hedgehog in non-syndromic colobomatous micropthalmia. *Am J Med Genet* 2003; **116A**: 215–21.

Van Heyningen V, Williamson KA. PAX6 in sensory development. *Hum Mol Genet* 2002; **11**: 1161–7.

Arthrogryposis (arthrogryposis multiplex congenita)

Arthrogryposis is a term used to describe non-progressive multiple congenital joint contractures that generally result from lack of fetal movement in utero. Its incidence is 1/3000 livebirths. In general, more than one type of joint is involved—bilateral talipes in the absence of other joint involvement does not constitute arthrogryposis. Any condition that causes decreased fetal movement may lead to congenital contractures. Over the past year an exciting start has been made in elucidating the genetic basis of some of the dominant arthrogryposis syndromes. It seems likely that specific types of arthrogryposis result from unique spatiotemporal patterns of expression of sarcomeric proteins in embryonic and fetal life. Mutations in contractile proteins have been found to underlie some distal arthrogryposis syndromes eg. troponins I and T in type 2B, β-tropomyosin in type 1 (Sung), myosin IIa in inclusion-body myopathy which is sometimes associated with joint contractures and perinatal myosin heavy chain *(MYH8)* in trismus-pseudocamptodactyly syndrome (Veugelers). Arthrogryposis is immensely heterogeneous, and achieving a specific diagnosis is often difficult (possible in 50% after careful assessment). During clinical assessment try to classify your patient into one or more of the following aetiological groups:

- muscle (5–10%), e.g. congenital myopathy, congenital myasthaenia
- neurological (90%), e.g. central nervous system (CNS) anomaly;
- abnormal connective tissue, e.g. diastrophic dysplasia;
- uterine constraint, e.g. bicornuate uterus;
- maternal illness, e.g. myasthaenia, myotonic dystrophy, fever >39 °C;
- environmental, e.g. early amniocentesis (<14 gestational weeks); drugs, e.g. misoprostol.

Clinical approach

History: key points

- Three-generation family tree. Enquire specifically for club-feet, joint dislocation, congenital hip dislocation, contractures, hyperextensibility.
- Enquire about maternal illness (myotonic dystrophy, myasthaenia gravis, diabetes mellitus, etc.) and uterine anomaly.
- Detailed pregnancy history. Enquire about infection, and fever (>39°C), fetal movement, polyhydramnios (may be secondary to poor fetal swallowing), oligohydramnios, or amniotic fluid leak.
- Detailed history of the delivery, e.g. abnormal presentation or difficulty in delivery due to fixed joints; fracture may occur (5–10%).
- Detailed history of the position of the baby after delivery (obtain photos if available).

Examination: key points

- Photographs are extremely helpful in documenting the position of contractures.
- Examine the rest position and the range of passive and active movement in each joint—take great care to avoid causing a fracture!

- Document carefully which joints are involved (this may be helpful in achieving a specific diagnosis).
- Look for skin dimples overlying contractures and document flexion creases.
- Look for skin webs across joints with joint limitation.
- Examine for limitation of jaw opening (trismus). NB. intubation.
- Detailed neurological assessment—level of alertness, tone, reflexes.
- Feel muscle texture (fibrous band, firm, soft).
- Examine carefully for other anomalies, e.g. cleft palate or jaundice (ARC syndrome).
- Examine both parents carefully for joint contractures and lack of flexion creases.
- Examine mother for features of myotonic dystrophy or myasthenia.

Special investigations

- Karyotype—unless older child with normal intelligence and no dysmorphic features (if child has developmental delay and deep furrows on palms/soles consider skin biopsy for trisomy 8).
- Store DNA (the list of arthrogryposis syndromes for which the causative gene has been defined is growing rapidly)
- Consider hip ultrasound scan (USS) in neonate if clinical suspicion of hip involvement.
- Consider TORCH (toxoplasmosis, other (including syphilis, varicella zoster, parvovirus), rubella, cytomegalovirus, and herpes simplex virus) screen if neonate or <6 months old; include viral studies for enterovirus and Cocksackie.
- Consider creatine kinase (CK) if clinical assessment compatible with primary muscle aetiology.
- Consider electromyography (EMG) and nerve conduction velocity (NCV) tests to clarify whether lower motor neuron involvement or primary muscle pathology are likely.
- Consider muscle biopsy if primary muscle pathology seems likely (biopsy both involved and apparently uninvolved muscle and do electron microscopy (EM) and multiple stains).
- Consider radiographs if suspicion of chondrodysplasia or other skeletal dysplasia.
- Consider muscle magnetic resonance imaging (MRI) of affected limb if considering diagnosis of amyoplasia (muscle is replaced by fat/fibrous tissue).
- Consider cranial MRI scan if CNS involvement with normal chromosomes.
- Consider testing mother for myotonic dystrophy (DNA for triplet repeat expansion).
- Consider testing mother for myasthaenia (anti-cholinesterase receptor antibodies). Rarely, the mother generates antibodies against fetal receptor which affect fetus in absence of maternal disease). Inexpensive test, positive in 1–2% of mothers ascertained through a single affected infant (Polizzi).

For lethal forms of arthrogryposis an autopsy with detailed neuropathology and muscle biopsy and storage of DNA will offer the best chance of making a specific diagnosis.

Some diagnoses to consider

Fetal akinesia sequence. Multiple joint contractures, pulmonary hypoplasia, micrognathia, intrauterine growth retardation (IUGR), short umbilical cord, and polyhydramnios. A consequence (deformation) of severely reduced fetal movement.

Amyoplasia. 'Classical arthrogryposis'. The most common condition with severe multiple congenital contractures (one-third of all cases). Characterized by very specific positioning with symmetrical limb involvement. Muscle tissue is replaced by fibrous bands/fatty tissue; firmly fixed joints with fusiform shape to the limbs in the neonate. Flexion creases shallow/absent. Feet in equinovarus, wrists, flexed, shoulders internally rotated, elbows in fixed extension at birth, but may later develop some flexion with growth. Hips may be flexed or extended and are often dislocated. Knees fixed in extension/flexion. No sensory loss. Deep dimples often present over joints. Vascular birthmarks over midface are common. Mild syndactyly is often found. Normal intelligence quotient (IQ). Sporadic (possibly due to vascular disruption). Increased occurrence in one of monozygotic (MZ) twins. Recurrence risk <1%.

Distal arthrogryposis type 1. Autosomal dominant (AD) with marked variability. Characteristic positioning of hands (+18 like with clenched fist and overlapping fingers) in newborn period with primarily distal contractures of the limbs. Responds well to physiotherapy, and generally improves with time. Feet may be in equinovarus or calcaneovalgus. Both the hand and foot anomalies appear to be due to misplaced tendons.

Congenital contractural arachnodactyly (CCA, Beal's syndrome). AD disorder characterized by congenital contractures, long thin extremities, crumpled ear helix, and kyphoscoliosis. May have cardiac involvement, e.g. mitral valve prolapse (MVP), but generally less severe than in Marfan. Due to mutations in fibrillin 2 (*FBN2*) on 5q.

Multiple pterygium syndromes. Specific diagnosis should be possible—see Hall (2001).

COFS (cerebro-oculo-facial-skeletal syndrome). Lethal condition with contractures, structural brain anomalies, microphthalmia/cataracts. Some are due to mutations in DNA-repair genes, as in Cockayne. See 'DNA repair defects', page 304.

Arthrogryposis multiplex congenita–spinal muscular atrophy association. Approximately 50% are homozygous for *SMN* deletions. Most *SMN* abnormalities are hypotonic at birth. Larger deletions of 5q are associated with contractures. See 'Spinal muscular atrophy (SMA)', page 412.

ARC syndrome (Arthrogryposis multiplex congenita, Renal dysfunction and neonatal Cholestasis) AR condition characterised by arthrogryposis and cholestasis with bile duct hypoplasia (see Clinical approach to 'Prolonged neonatal jaundice and jaundice in infants below 6 months, page 220).

Genetic advice

Recurrence risk

As for specific diagnosis. If specific diagnosis is not possible consider the following.

- Distal forms of arthrogryposis are often AD.
- In arthrogryposis with CNS involvement many cases are autosomal recessive (AR), so recurrence risk for subsequent pregnancies after one affected child is 10–15%.
- If no specific diagnosis, empiric recurrence risk for unaffected parents of an affected child is 3–5%.
- If no specific diagnosis, empiric risk to the child of an affected individual is 3–5% (but beware AD forms).
- Amyoplasia is sporadic with no appreciable recurrence risk; however, care should be used when making this diagnosis and this recurrence risk is given only if there are classical features.

Prenatal diagnosis

Prenatal diagnosis is possible in many types of arthrogryposis by real-time USS to assess fetal movement. Studies at 16, 20, 24, and 32 weeks are recommended. Care must be taken to look at each major joint for range of movement. Need to discuss limitations of USS and small possibility of failure to detect significant joint contracture.

Natural history and further management (preventative measures)

This varies depending on specific diagnosis. Physiotherapy with passive stretching is often useful (but avoid in diastrophic dysplasia). Surgery may be required as an adjunct to physiotherapy in most children with amyoplasia.

If there is primary muscle pathology, you need to be cautious about anaesthesia. NB. Multiple pterygium with malignant hyperthermia (scoliosis, torticollis, myopathic facies, cleft palate).

Support group: The Arthrogryposis Group <www.tagonline.org.uk>.

Expert adviser: Judith G. Hall, Emeritus Professor of Paediatrics and Medical Genetics, University of British Columbia, Vancouver, British Columbia, Canada.

References

Hall JG. Arthrogryposes (multiple congenital contractures). In *Emery and Rimoin's principles and practice of medical genetics*, 3rd edn (ed. D.L. Rimoin), pp. 4182–225. Churchill Livingstone, Edinburgh, 2001.

Sung SS, Brassington AM, *et al*. Mutations in genes encoding fast-twitch contractile proteins cause distal arthrogryposis syndromes. *Am J Hum Genet* 2003; **72** :681–90.

Sung SS, Brassington AM, *et al*. Mutations in TNNT3 cause multiple congenital contractures: a second locus for distal arthrogryposis type 2B. *Am J Hum Genet* 2003; **73**: 212–14.

Veugelers M, Bressan M, *et al*. Mutation of perinatal myosin heavy chain associated with a carney complex variant. *NEJM* 2004; **351**: 460–69.

Polizzi A, Huson SM, Vincent A. Teratogen update: maternal myasthenia gravis as a cause of congenital arthrogryposis (Review). Teratology, 2000; **62**: 332–41.

Ataxic adult

An individual with ataxia has poor coordination of his/her movements. This affects walking. The gait is wide-based and unsteady. Speech and movement of the eyes may also be affected.

Ataxia may be caused by abnormalities that affect the function of the cerebellum, spinal cord, and the peripheral sensory system.

The neurologist will investigate to determine the likely aetiology and particularly to differentiate acquired from genetic causes of ataxia. The geneticist may be involved in the diagnostic process when there is no definitive diagnosis or otherwise at a later stage to counsel an individual and the family.

Clinical approach

The approach here is primarily to distinguish between the hereditary ataxias.

History: key points

- Three-generation pedigree. Ask about signs of a similar problem in parents and sibs. Note if they have been investigated and if there is consent to ask for results.
- Consanguinity in parents may indicate an autosomal recessive (AR) ataxia.
- Ethnic origin. Some ataxias are found in specific geographical areas.
- Onset and description of symptoms; document disability stage.
- Visual loss.
- Cognitive disturbance (dementia).

Examination: key points

- There is an overlap in the clinical features of spinocerebellar ataxia (SCA) genes SCA 1–25.
- Gait ataxia. Observe the patient walking. Ataxic patients typically have a wide-based gait.
- Tremor/parkinsonian features (SCA3). Titubation.
- Eye movement disorder. Slow saccadic eye movement (SCA2). Oculomotor apraxia.
- Examine with finger–nose test, heel–shin test, and test ability to perform rapid alternating movements.
- Reflexes. Increased in SCA1 and 3. Decreased in SCA2.
- Sensory signs. Sensory axonal neuropathy may occur in some dominant families.
- Eyes and fundus. Retinopathy in SCA7. Cataract in Marinesco–Sjögren syndrome.
- Cardiac. Cardiomyopathy in Friedreich's ataxia (FRDA).

Special investigations

Prioritizing investigations depends on the family history and clinical features. In individuals with a family history proceed to genetic testing.

- Magnetic resonance imaging (MRI) brain scan. eg. for Cerebellar atrophy (SCA), other structural abnormalities, tumours (bilateral acoustic neuromas indicate a diagnosis of neurofibromatosis type 2 (NF2)), white matter abnormalities (found in metabolic disorders as well as acquired conditions such as multiple sclerosis).
- Peripheral nerve conduction studies.
- Ophthalmic assessment, including electroretinography (ERG).

- Electrocardiogram (ECG)/cardiac echo (cardiomyopathy in FRDA).
- Consider further biochemical screening, such as alpha-fetoprotein (AFP), vitamin E, cholesterol, and albumin, and additional tests for metabolic disorders such as white-cell enzymes (late-onset GM2 gangliosidosis).
- Antigliadin antibodies. A positive antibody test is found in 10–15% of patients with ataxia but it is uncertain whether this is a consequence rather than a cause of cerebellar degeneration.
- DNA analysis: *SCA 1, 2, 3, 6, 7* frataxin *(FRDA)*, DRPLA, mitochondrial DNA analysis. Consider Huntington disease (HD) and Gerstmann–Straussler Disease (GSD); if proband is male and >50 years old, consider fragile X tremor/ataxia syndrome (FXTAS) syndrome (test for *FRAXA* premutation).
- Consider DNA storage for future testing.
- Consider cytogenetic analysis for breakage disorders. These more typically have a childhood presentation.

Some diagnoses to consider

In individuals in whom acquired, non-genetic conditions have been excluded as far as possible, a genetic aetiology needs to be considered even in the absence of a family history. Moseley *et al.* (1998) report a 2–5% probability that an individual with a sporadically occurring ataxia has SCA1, SCA2, SCA3, SCA6, SCA7, or FRDA. For young adults see also 'Ataxic child', page 52.

Autosomal dominant (AD) disorders

Spinocerebellar ataxia (SCA). The most likely diagnostic group for adult cerebellar ataxias. It is extremely genetically heterogeneous. All have gait ataxia and are slowly progressive. There is overlap in the clinical features but some of the useful differentiating features are listed in the key points. <www.geneclinics.org> has useful reviews of many of the individual SCA types.

- Because of the clinical overlap, laboratories usually perform testing for several SCA genes, unless the familial type is known. Molecular testing is available for SCA 1, 2, 3, 6, 7. In the absence of a known type, testing is done in a step-wise fashion excluding the most common first.
- They are $(CAG)_n$ trinucleotide expansion disorders.
- Intermediate alleles may cause problems in genetic counselling and predictive testing of relatives.
- Anticipation. SCA7 has a particularly unstable $(CAG)_n$ repeat and children may have early-onset disease that presents prior to any signs in the parent. Except for SCA 8, expansion of the $(CAG)_n$ is more likely with paternal transmission.

Episodic ataxia. This is caused by mutations in ion channel genes. *EA2* is allelic to *SCA6* and to familial hemiplegic migraine.

Huntington disease (HD). AD neurodegenerative disorder characterized by a progressive involuntary movement disorder, psychiatric disturbance, and dementia. See 'Huntington disease (HD)', page 354.

Dentatorubro-pallidoluysian atrophy (DRPLA). An AD neurodegenerative disorder that causes symptoms and signs very like those of HD.

Gerstmann–Straussler disease (GSD). A rare AD familial prion disorder characterized by cerebellar ataxia, progressive dementia, and absent reflexes in the legs and, pathologically, by amyloid plaques throughout the central nervous system (CNS). Onset is usually in the fifth decade and in the early phase ataxia is predominant. Dementia develops later. The course ranges from 2 to 10 years. The disorder is caused by mutations in the prion protein gene (*PRNP*) on 20pter–p12.

Autosomal recessive (AR) disorders
Particularly important is a history of parental consanguinity and/or affected sibs.

Friedreich's ataxia (FRDA). FRDA is caused by a GAA repeat in the *FRDA* gene coding for frataxin protein. The usual presentation is in childhood but the disease may be mild with later presentation. Some patients present in adulthood. Prior to molecular genetic testing there were strict diagnostic criteria for FRDA that included onset prior to age 20 years. Since genetic testing became possible many patients have been diagnosed with FRDA where onset has occurred at ages >20 years. There is no evidence for anticipation.

Typical clinical features are absent or reduced reflexes with up-going plantars, loss of vibration sense and proprioception, and cardiomyopathy. Adult-onset patients may have retained reflexes and a much milder clinical course. See section on 'Ataxic child' in this chapter, page 52.

Ataxia with vitamin E deficiency. It is important to recognize this as the disorder can be treated with vitamin E supplements. It has clinical features similar to those of FRDA.

AR cerebellar ataxia. This is found in specific populations; enquire about ethnic origin.

Metabolic disorders
- Refsum disease.
- Tay–Sachs (GM2 gangliosidosis).

Ataxia telangiectasia (AT). AR condition usually presenting in childhood. See 'DNA repair defects', page 304.

Ataxia with oculomotor apraxia (AOA). Ataxia, and oculomotor apraxia, may have mild choreoathetosis or dystonia. See section on the 'Ataxic child', page 52.

X-linked (XL) disorders

Fragile X pre-mutation tremor/ataxia syndrome (FXTAS). A recently defined syndrome in which a small percentage of male carriers of a *FRAXA* permutation are affected by a multisystem progressive neurological disorder characterized by cerebellar ataxia and/or intention tremor, with a variety of other neurological features, e.g. cognitive decline, parkinsonism, etc. Symmetrical regions of increased T2 signal intensity in the middle cerebellar peduncles and adjacent cerebellar white matter on cranial MRI are thought to be highly sensitive for this neurological condition. Van Esch found ~3% of male patients >50 yrs presenting with ataxia had FXTAS.

Mitochondrial disorders
Ataxia is found in association with other organ involvement. Note if deafness or diabetes mellitus are present.
- MERRF (myoclonic epilepsy with ragged red fibres).
- NARP (neuropathy, ataxia, and retinitis pigmentosa).
See 'Mitochondrial DNA diseases', page 384.

Genetic advice
Recurrence risk

Offspring and sibling risk, sporadic progressive cerebellar ataxia. If testing to exclude syndromic and acquired causes is negative:
- The inheritance pattern may be found from close questioning of the family history, for example, if there is parental consanguinity, then an AR aetiology is possible.
- Consider if non-paternity is a possibility.

Offspring risks in sporadic adult-onset ataxia are unknown, but it is likely that some are due to unknown genetic mutations. Abele *et al.* (2002) conclude from their study that this does not account for many patients. A 5% offspring risk is usually given but there is no firm data to support this.

Pre-symptomatic, predictive testing in AD ataxia families (mainly SCA)
Confirm the mutation in an affected family member before arranging predictive testing. It is not of use in predicting the age of onset or the severity and progression of the disease. Follow the guidelines for predictive testing of asymptomatic at-risk individuals. See 'Testing for genetic status', page 28.

Carrier detection in AR/XL ataxia
- By molecular testing in families in which a causative mutation has been identified.
- Analysis of the family history in XL ataxia.

Prenatal diagnosis
By molecular analysis of a chorionic villus sampling (CVS) or amniocytes in families with a known mutation.

Natural history and further management (preventative measures)
Management is essentially supportive; affected individuals should be under the care of a neurological team with expertise in disability.

Support group: National Ataxia Foundation, 2600 Fernbrook Lane, Suite 119, Minneapolis, MN 55447, USA <www.ataxia.org>; Ataxia UK <www.ataxia.uk.org>.

Expert adviser: Andrea Németh, Consultant and Lecturer in Clincal Genetics, University of Oxford, Oxford, England.

References
Abele M, Bürk K, *et al.* The aetiology of sporadic adult-onset ataxia. *Brain* 2002; **125**: 961–8.

Bird TD. Hereditary ataxia overview. *GeneReviews* <www.geneclinics.org>.

Jacquemont S, Hagerman RJ. Fragile X premutation tremor/ataxia syndrome: molecular, clinical, and neuroimaging correlates. *Am J Hum Genet* 2003; **72** (4): 869–78.

Moseley ML, *et al.* Incidence of dominant spinocerebellar and Friedreich triplet repeats among 361 ataxia families. *Neurology* 1998; **51**: 1661–71.

Nagafuchi S, Yanagisawa H, *et al.* Dentatorubral and pallidoluysian atrophy expansion of an unstable CAG trinucleotide on chromosome 12p. *Nature Genet* 1994; **6**: 14–18.

Van Esch H, Dom R, *et al.* Screening for FMR-1 premutations in 122 older Flemish males presenting with ataxia. *Eur J Hum Geneti* 2005; **13**: 121–23.

Ataxic child

Individuals with ataxia have poor coordination of their movements. This affects walking and the gait is wide-based and unsteady. In children it is important to distinguish ataxia from an unsteady gait due to immaturity or muscle weakness. Speech and movement of the eyes may also be affected. Ataxia may be caused by abnormalities that affect the function of the cerebellum, spinal cord, and the peripheral sensory system, such as structural lesions, metabolic disturbance, and inherited genetic disorders.

In congenital ataxia, clinical features of ataxia do not become apparent until between 1 and 2 years of age. Infants are hypotonic with poor sucking and delayed motor milestones; ataxia becomes apparent once the child is walking. To test for ataxia in an older child, assess heel–toe walking (gait ataxia), finger–nose and heel–shin test (dysmetria), rapid alternating movements (dysdiadochokinesis), and observe for a wide-based gait and unsteady walking (e.g. chair walking or walking with support). A significant proportion of children with congenital ataxia have a degree of learning disability.

The child requires assessment by a paediatric neurologist who will investigate to determine the likely aetiology. The geneticist may be involved in the diagnostic process when there is no definitive diagnosis or otherwise at a later stage to counsel the family. The approach here is to consider the differential diagnosis of the genetic causes of ataxia based on the age of presentation.

Clinical approach

History: key points

- Three-generation pedigree. Ask about signs of a similar problem in parents and sibs. Some of the autosomal dominant (AD) ataxias caused by spinocerebellar ataxia (SCA) can present in childhood, particularly SCA7. For more detail on the adult ataxias see 'Ataxic adult', page 50.
- Consanguinity in parents may indicate an autosomal recessive (AR) ataxia or metabolic condition.
- Ethnic origin. Some ataxias are found in specific geographical areas.
- Pregnancy history with detailed account of delivery and perinatal period.
- Developmental milestones, in particular early motor milestones and the age at which the child walked, in order to try to distinguish between congenital and later onset ataxias.
- Speech and swallowing difficulties. Dysarthria. Language is very delayed in Angelman syndrome (AS) and affected children usually have fewer than six words.
- Visual loss.
- Intermittent ataxia is suggestive of metabolic decompensation, particularly:
  - urea cycle defects (dietary protein intolerance is a feature of the manifesting female carriers of the X-linked urea cycle defect ornithine transcarbamylase (OTC) deficiency);
  - organic acidaemia;
  - maple syrup urine disease;
  - pyruvate dehydrogenase (PDH) deficiency.

Examination: key points

- Head circumference, note any change in the rate of growth.
- Gait ataxia.

- Hand flapping, jerky limb movement, laughter (AS).
- Reflexes. Classically absent in Friedreich's ataxia (FRDA) and Vitamin E deficiency with extensor plantars.
- Sensory signs. Vibration sense and joint position sense usually impaired in FRDA.
- Eyes and fundus. Conjunctival telangiectasia in ataxia telangiectasia (AT). Retinopathy in SCA7, abetalipoproteinaemia, and the mitochondrial disorder NARP (neuropathy–ataxia– retinitis pigmentosa). Cataract in Marinesco–Sjögren syndrome. Optic atrophy in FRDA.
- Eye movement disorder in AT and Gaucher disease. Oculomotor apraxia ('head thrusts') in ataxia with oculomotor apraxia (AOA).
- Cardiac. Cardiomyopathy in FRDA.
- Muscle weakness in NARP.
- Extrapyramidal signs (seen in AOA).

Special investigations

Investigate in conjunction with a paediatric neurologist, who will have investigated the child for acquired as well as genetic causes for the ataxia (unless there is a strong family history of an inherited form of ataxia presenting at a similar age).

- Biochemical screening. Basic biochemical screening has usually already been performed but should include plasma electrolytes, liver function tests, acid/base status, fasting glucose, pyruvate and lactate, ammonium, amino acids, and a urine screen for amino and organic acids.
- Further biochemical testing to consider: white cell enzymes (metachromatic leukodystrophy, Krabbes, gangliosidoses, galactosialodosis); very long chain fatty acids and phytanic acid (Refsum disease); alpha-fetoprotein (AFP; elevated in ataxia telangiectasia (AT)); vitamin E; cholesterol and albumin; abetalipoprotein B (abetalipoproteinaemia), transferrin isoelectrophoresis (congenital disorders of glycosylation).
- Lysosomal inclusions if there is a suspected metabolic aetiology, e.g. infantile neuronal ceroid lipofuscinosis (NCL).
- Magnetic resonance imaging (MRI) brain scan. Cerebellar hypoplasia suggests a congenital cause. White matter abnormalities are found in metabolic disorders (see 'Developmental regression', page 96).
- Peripheral nerve conduction studies (FRDA, Charlevois–Saguenay syndrome, Roussy–Levy syndrome).
- Ophthalmic assessment, including electroretinography (ERG).
- Electrocardiogram (ECG) and cardiac echo (cardiomyopathy in FRDA).
- Electroencephalography (EEG) in children with suspected AS.
- Endocrinology; exclude hypogonadotrophic hypogonadism.
- DNA analysis: frataxin (FRDA), mitochondrial DNA analysis (NARP). Storage for future testing. In the older child consider SCA and dentatorubro-pallidoluysian atrophy (DRPLA; see 'Ataxic adult', page 50).
- Cytogenetic analysis:
  - for breakage disorders if there are signs of AT or xeroderma pigmentosum (XP).
  - SNRP methylation studies for AS if there is severe developmental delay.

Some diagnoses to consider
Presumed congenital ataxia

Structural abnormalities of the cerebellum. See 'Cerebellar anomalies', page 66.

Ataxic cerebral palsy. A descriptive term for a heterogeneous group of disorders where the child presents with ataxia but degrees of global developmental delay and hypotonia are often present. It is a diagnosis of exclusion of other causes of a congenital ataxia. Take a careful birth history to assess if there is a history of hypoxia or injury to account for the problems. A high-resolution brain MRI scan is mandatory prior to definitive counselling. Congenital structural lesions of the cerebellum, such as hypoplasia or a Dandy–Walker cyst, may be found and aid estimation of recurrence risks. See 'Cerebral palsy', page 70.

Angelman syndrome (AS). See 'Angelman syndrome', page 272.

Inborn errors of metabolism. 'Small molecule disorders' such as urea cycle disorders, maple syrup urine disease, and PDH deficiency have ataxia along with other manifestations of metabolic decompensation such as altered consciousness/encephalopathy.

Childhood onset disorders
Friedreich's ataxia (FRDA). This is the most common inherited ataxia. The mean age at onset is 15.5 years ± 8 years with range 2–51 years. It is autosomal recessive (AR) and caused by mutations in frataxin (*FRDA*) on 9q. Frataxin is a nuclear-encoded mitochondrial protein. It is characterized by a dying back from the periphery of the longest and largest myelinated fibres (e.g. large fibres arising in dorsal root ganglia). The carrier frequency in the Caucasian population is ~1:85 with a disease prevalence of 1/29 000; FRDA is rare in Africans and Asians. 98% of mutations are triplet repeat expansions of $(GAA)_n$ in intron 1 and 2% are point mutations or deletions. Normal triplet repeat allele size is 6–34; mutations have 67–1700 repeats. Repeat size is unstable with a tendency to decrease in size when paternally transmitted and increase or decrease when maternally transmitted. The disease is slowly but relentlessly progressive with loss of walking ~15 years after onset and the mean age of death is ~37.5 years (usual cause is cardiomyopathy). Late-onset FRDA (onset >25 years) has been recognized since the onset of molecular testing.

The clinical features of FRDA are:
- progressive gait and limb ataxia;
- dysarthria;
- absent lower limb reflexes;
- extensor plantar responses;
- reduced vibration sense and proprioception (posterior columns);
- cardiomyopathy (hypertrophic cardiomyopathy (HCM) usually), diabetes, scoliosis, pes cavus, and optic atrophy are common features;
- nerve conduction velocity (NCV) studies show absent sensory nerve action potentials. Motor conduction velocities are reduced but > 40m/s.

Carrier testing is possible for relatives and their partners. If the partner of a carrier does not have a $(GAA)_n$ expansion, then, since only 2% of mutations are point mutations, carrier risk falls to ~1/5000. Prenatal diagnosis is possible by chorionic villus sampling (CVS) if mutations in parents are both defined.

Ataxia with vitamin E deficiency. Clinical picture very similar to that for FRDA. It is AR resulting from mutations in alpha-tocopherol transfer protein gene on chromosome 8. It is *treatable*, and it is therefore important to exclude this diagnosis by measurement of vitamin E levels if molecular testing for FRDA is negative.

Charlevoix–Saguenay syndrome (SACS). This is AR with hypermyelinated retinal nerve fibres and mixed peripheral neuropathy. It presents with ataxia, dysarthria, and nystagmus with spasticity in lower limbs. Consider in differential diagnosis of FRDA if genetic tests for FRDA are negative. SACS is common in north-eastern Quebec, where the carrier frequency reaches 1/22 in one region. SACS is caused by mutations in a gene encoding the protein sacsin on 13q11 (Engert *et al.* 2000).

Ataxia with oculomotor apraxia (AOA). AOA type 1 is the most frequent cause of AR ataxia in Japan and is second only to Friedreich ataxia in Portugal. It shares several neurological features with AT, including early-onset ataxia, oculomotor apraxia, and cerebellar atrophy, but does not share its extraneurological features (immune deficiency, chromosomal instability, and hypersensitivity to X-rays). AOA1 is also characterized by axonal motor neuropathy and decrease of serum albumin levels and elevation of total cholesterol. Caused by mutations in *AOA1* on 9p encoding aprataxin. The gene has a DNA single-strand break repair domain. A second gene, senataxin on 9q causes AOA2 characterised by onset between 11–22 years (Moreira).

Inborn errors of metabolism. Progressive ataxia is one of the features of a number of inborn errors. Consider hypobetalipoproteinaemia and abetalipoproteinaemia, Refsum disease, L-2 hydroxyglutaric aciduria, NCL, GM2 (Tay–Sachs), and investigate further if necessary.

Mitochondrial disorders. See 'Mitochondrial DNA diseases' in Chapter 3, 'Common consultations', page 384.

Ataxia is found in association with other organ involvement. Note if deafness or diabetes mellitus are features in the family history.
- MERFF (myoclonic epilepsy with ragged red fibres).
- NARP.
- Kearns–Sayre syndrome.

DNA repair disorders. See 'DNA repair defects', page 304.
- AT (ataxia usually evident from 1 year of age; telangiectasia from 4–8 years).
- XP.

Hereditary spastic paraplegia (HSP). See 'Hereditary spastic paraplegia (HSP)' page 348.

Roussy–Levy syndrome. AD form of hereditary motor and sensory neuropathy type 1 (HMSN1) with ataxia and tremor. See 'Hereditary motor and sensory neuropathy (HMSN)' page 344.

Spinocerebellar ataxia (SCA). The triplet repeat in SCA7 is particularly unstable and large expansions in the triplet repeat can occur. SCA7 can present in childhood before signs appear in the parent. See 'Ataxic adult', page 50.

Genetic advice
Recurrence risk
If after investigation there is no known aetiology, the precise genetic risks are unknown.

- Assume AR inheritance is likely if there is an affected sib or parental consanguinity.
- Progressive ataxia suggests a metabolic or genetic aetiology with a high recurrence risk.
- Ataxic cerebral palsy. There is a genetic subgroup within this disorder and the recurrence risk may be as high as 25%. An estimate of 10–15% may be used if there is no family history or parental consanguinity. See 'Cerebral palsy', page 70.

Carrier detection

This is possible where there is a known mutation with the usual restrictions on the genetic testing of children. See 'Testing for genetic status', page 28.

Prenatal diagnosis

Prenatal diagnosis by CVS can be offered to families at risk for some of the syndromic causes of ataxia if the causative familial mutations are known. Prenatal testing for mitochondrial disorders is rarely straightforward—see 'Mitochondrial DNA diseases', page 384'. Ultrasound scan (USS) or fetal MRI may be of some value if there are structural abnormalities of the cerebellum. (See 'Cerebellar anomalies', page 66.

Natural history and further management (preventative measures)

These are dependent on the diagnosis. Most are progressive conditions so follow-up by a paediatric neurologist and childhood disability team is appropriate.

Support groups: National Ataxia Foundation, 2600 Fernbrook Lane, Suite 119, Minneapolis, MN 55447, USA <www.ataxia.org>; Ataxia UK <www.ataxia.uk.org>.

Expert adviser: Andrea Németh, Consultant and Lecturer in Clincal Genetics, University of Oxford, Oxford, England.

References

Bird TD. Hereditary ataxia overview. *GeneReviews* <www.geneclinics.org>.

Delataycki MB, Williamson R, *et al.* Friedreich's ataxia: an overview. *J Med Genet* 2000; **37**: 1–8.

Engert JC, Berube P, *et al.* ARSACS, a spastic ataxia common in northeastern Quebec, is caused by mutations in a new gene encoding an 11.5-kb ORF. *Nat Genet* 2000; **24**: 120–5.

Moreira MC, Barbot C, *et al.* The gene mutated in ataxia–ocular apraxia 1 encodes the new HIT/Zn-finger protein aprataxin. *Nat Genet* 2001; **29**: 189–93.

Moreira MC, Klur S, *et al.* Senataxin, the ortholog of a yeast RNA helicase, is mutant in ataxia-ocular apraxia 2. *Nat Genet* 2004; **36**: 225–7.

Brachydactyly

Brachydactyly is shortening of the digits due to anomalous development of the phalanges or metacarpals.

Brachydactyly can be divided into the following categories:

- predominantly isolated brachydactyly;
- brachydactyly as part of a skeletal dysplasia;
- brachydactyly as part of a syndrome. In particular we will discuss those syndromes where brachydactyly is a distinctive diagnostic feature, e.g. Albright, de Lange, Robinow.

Brachydactyly should be distinguished from small but structurally normal hands and feet (as seen in Prader–Willi syndrome, Smith–Magenis syndrome, and uniparental disomy 14 (UPD14)).

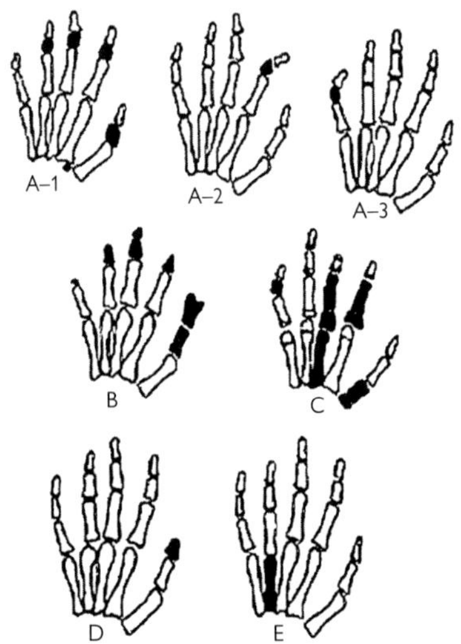

Bell's classification of brachydactyly (see accompanying table). The black bones are those affected. (Reprinted from Poznanski ©1984 with permission from Elsevier.)

Brachydactyly was the first human trait to be interpreted as a Mendelian dominant by Farabee in 1903. The most commonly used classification is the clinical descriptive system devised by Julia Bell (1951). She classified the published pedigrees into seven groups on the basis of the anatomy (see table and figure). Molecular analysis has shown that many are genetically heterogeneous. It has also been found that one gene produces several different phenotypes depending on the action of the mutation, e.g. the *ROR2* gene, where heterozygous truncating mutations thought to produce a specific gain-of-function cause autosomal dominant (AD) brachydactyly B (which predominantly affects the distal phalanges and nails) and homozygous loss-of-function mutations lead to autosomal recessive (AR) Robinow syndrome.

Clinical approach

History: key points

- At least three-generation family tree. The phenotype may vary in severity (variable expressivity) and gene-carriers may be non-penetrant.
- Parental stature.
- Developmental delay.
- Other medical problems.

Examination: key points

- Measure height, arm span, and upper and lower body length. Assess for short stature and disproportion. If limbs are short is the shortening rhizomelic or mesomelic?
- Make measurements of hands: total length (tip of middle finger to the distal wrist crease), middle finger length (tip of middle finger to proximal crease at the base of the finger), and palm length (proximal crease at the base of the middle finger to the distal wrist crease).
- Observe and document palmar creases, finger contractures (camptodactyly), nail morphology/absence, and syndactyly (bony and skin).
- Carefully examine both feet.
- Dysmorphic features (syndromal causes of brachdactyly).
- Measure blood pressure (brachydactyly/hypertension).

Classification of isolated brachydactylies (all autosomal dominant)*

Type A Shortening confined mainly to middle phalanges
- **A1** (MIM 112500 & 607004) Short/absent middle phalanges in all digits. May be short proximal phalanges in thumbs and halluces, plus short stature. Genetically heterogeneous. Can be caused by heterozygous missense mutations in the *IHH* gene. (Homozygous *IHH* mutations cause acrocapitofemoral dysplasia.)
- **A2** (MIM 112600) Short middle phalanges in the 2nd fingers and toes only. Caused by heterozygous mutations in the *BMPR1B* gene
- **A3** (MIM 112700) Short middle phalanges in 5th fingers only

Type B (MIM 113000) Hypoplastic/absent nails, short/absent distal phalanges and short middle phalanges in 2nd–5th digits. May be broad/bifid thumbs and halluces, central syndactyly, and characteristic face. Genetically heterogeneous. Can be caused by heterozygous truncating mutations in the *ROR2* gene

Type C (MIM 113100) Short middle phalanges in 2nd, 3rd, & 5th fingers; hyperphalangism (extra phalanges) in 2nd and 3rd fingers; relative sparing of 4th fingers; short 1st metacarpals. May be short stature. Genetically homogeneous. Caused by heterozygous mutations in the *GDF5* gene—probably loss-of-function mutations. (Homozygous *GDF5* mutations cause two very similar recessive chondrodysplasias—Grebe type and Hunter–Thompson type.)

Type D (MIM 113200) Short broad distal phalanges in thumbs and halluces

Type E (MIM 113300) Shortening of one or more metacarpals/metatarsals. May be short stature. Genetically heterogeneous. Specific heterozygous missense mutations in the *HOXD13* gene can cause phenotypes overlapping with brachydactylies types D and E

* MIM numbers are taken from the Mendelian Inheritance in Man database.

Special investigations
- Photography.
- X-rays of hands and feet are required to investigate the structure of the bones. This is important in classification as there are recognizable patterns of malformation.
- Skeletal survey, if indicated from clinical assessment.
- DNA investigations may be possible to confirm the diagnosis.
- Cytogenetic investigations (e.g. del2q37) if there is developmental delay or additional malformations.

Some diagnoses to consider

Predominantly isolated brachydactyly
See below for genetic advice.

Brachydactyly, hypertension. This AD condition characterized by brachydactyly, severe essential hypertension, and mild short stature has been mapped to 12p (Gong *et al.* 2003).

Skeletal dysplasias
Here are some that should be considered.

Achondroplasia. A 'starfish' or 'trident' configuration to hands is found as the metacarpals are of an even size. See 'Achondroplasia', page 260.

Acrodysostosis. Short snub nose. Not thought to be allelic to Albright as no GNAS1 mutations have been identified in acrodysostosis.

Acromesomelic dysplasia (AMD). Broad hands with short stubby fingers. AMD Maroteaux type (AMDM) is AR; some but not all families are linked to chromosome 9. AMD Grebe type (AMDG) and AMD Hunter–Thompson type (AMDH) are similar very rare AR conditions both caused by *GDF5* mutations.

Geleophysic dysplasia. Heart valve thickening, tip-toe gait, developmental delay.

Hypochondroplasia. Clinical features resemble those of achondroplasia, but are milder with less involvement of the face, skull, and spine. See 'Achondroplasia', page 260.

Pseudoachondroplasia. Early arthritic problems with joint pain. AD and caused by mutations in the *COMP* gene.

Syndromic diagnoses
Aarskog syndrome. Short stature (rhizomelic), ptosis in some, hypermetropia, shawl scrotum, brachydactyly with hyperextendable proximal interphalangeal (PIP) joints. Facial features tend to normalize with age. X-linked inheritance, caused by mutations in the *FGD1* gene.

Albright hereditary osteodystrophy (AHO). This term describes a phenotype characterized by short adult stature with generalized obesity and relative microcephaly, brachydactyly particularly involving the distal phalanges (especially of the thumbs) and metacarpals/metatarsals, mild to moderate learning disability, and cutaneous ossifications (subcutaneous or intradermal lumps or flakes) in around 60%. The facial features are subtle, but usually these patients have a round face with a short neck, short nose, and mild midface hypoplasia. The obesity is not usually associated with hyperphagia. The brachydactyly is associated with cone-epiphyses and disharmonic bone age. Stature may be normal or above average in childhood but there is reduced longitudinal growth and early epiphyseal closure. The condition tends to be overdiagnosed largely because, with the exception of the cutaneous ossifications, the physical findings are non-specific. See 'Obesity with and without developmental delay', page 192.

NB. Some patients with an AHO-like phenotype, including brachydactyly type E and developmental delay, have a 2q37 deletion.

Hand–foot–genital syndrome is an AD condition caused by mutations in *HOXA13* on 7p15. Hands are small with hypoplastic proximally placed thumbs, and feet are small with short halluces. Males have hypospadias and females have duplication of the uterus and sometimes of the cervix and may have a septate vagina. Urinary tract malformations are common in both sexes.

Smith–Magenis syndrome (SMS). Some patients are short and obese with small hands and feet, as well as square, rather heavy facies. They may have a history of hypotonia in infancy, developmental delay, behaviour disturbance (especially sleep), and sometimes food-searching behaviour. Some individuals with SMS have mutations in *RAI1* a gene encompassed by the common 17p11.2 microdeletion.

Robinow syndrome. Mesomelia (short limbs), characteristic facies (fetal face), vertebral abnormalities, small penis. The AR form is due to homozygous loss-of-function mutations in the *ROR2* gene.

Small hands and feet are found in Prader-Willi syndrome and maternal UPD14.

Genetic advice

Recurrence risk
- **Isolated brachydactyly** is inherited as an AD trait and in the majority of affected individuals there is a family history. Mild short stature is frequently part of the phenotype. After classifying the form of brachydactyly counsel appropriately.
- **Syndromic brachydactyly.** Counsel as appropriate for the specific syndrome diagnosed.

Carrier detection
Note that in dominant kindreds there is often marked variability in expression and sometimes incomplete penetrance.

Prenatal diagnosis
This is technically feasible if the familial mutation is known, but not usually requested or appropriate for isolated forms of brachydactyly.

Support group: Many of the syndromes have their own support groups. See <www.cafamily.org.uk>.

Expert adviser: Frances R. Goodman, previously Honorary Clinical Lecturer, Molecular Medicine Unit, Institute of Child Health, London, England.

References
Bell J. On brachydactyly and symphalangism. In *The treasury of human inheritance* (ed. L.S. Penrose), Vol. 5, part 1, pp. 1–31. Cambridge University Press, Cambridge, 1951.

Everman DB, *et al.* The mutational spectrum of brachydactyly type C. *Am J Med Genet* 2002; **112**: 291–6.

Fitch N. Classification and identification of inherited brachydactylies. *J Med Genet* 1979; **16**: 36–44.

Gong M, Zhang H, *et al.* Genome-wide linkage reveals a locus for human essential (primary) hypertension on chromosome 12p. *Hum Mol Genet* 2003; **12** (11): 1273–7.

Patton M, *et al.* Robinow syndrome. *Am J Med Genet* 2002; **39**: 305–10.

Poznanski AK. *The hand in radiologic diagnosis with gamuts and pattern profiles.* Saunders, Philadelphia, 1984.

Temtamy S, McKusick VA. The genetics of hand malformation. *Birth Defects Orig Art Series* 1978; **14** (3): 187–225.

Broad thumbs

There are some distinctive syndromes with broad thumbs as a key diagnostic feature. If there is difficulty in deciding whether the thumb is significantly broad, then it is unlikely to be a good diagnostic 'handle'. The degree of thumb involvement may be variable, especially in the autosomal dominant (AD) syndromes.

A bifid thumb may be described as broad, and X-ray examination is necessary in most affected individuals unless they clearly have a syndromic cause such as Rubinstein–Taybi syndrome (RTS). There is considerable overlap between some of these syndromes and those described in 'Preaxial polydactyly', page 218.

Clinical approach

History: key points

- At least three-generation pedigree; explain to parents about the minimal signs that could indicate a gene carrier.
- Consanguinity.
- Neurological/developmental problems (RTS).

Examination: key points

- Thumb. Document structure and function:
  - number of phalanges (three phalanges known as 'triphalangeal');
  - if duplicated;
  - if broad;
  - opposition.
- Hallux (great or big toe). Document structure as above.
- Hands and feet. Examine for anomalies affecting the other digits such as syndactyly, brachydactyly, or pre/postaxial polydactyly (refer to these sections, pages 254, 56, 218 and 214 respectively).
- Head and skull shape: macrocephaly and broad/high forehead (Greig syndrome); craniosynostosis (Pfeiffer syndrome).
- Features suggestive of any other skeletal abnormalities, talipes, or limb shortening (diastrophic dysplasia).
- Prominent nose (RTS).
- Cysts within the ear pinnae (diastrophic dysplasia).
- Atresia of the lacrimal puntae causing overflow tears (lacrimo-auriculo-dental-digital (LADD) syndrome).
- Cardiac murmurs (RTS and Townes–Brock syndrome (TBS)).
- Genital and renal anomalies (TBS).
- *Remember to examine the parents!*

Special investigations

- X-rays of the hands and feet are essential to assess the skeletal elements and to detect minor features not seen on clinical examination. The X-ray will assist in the process of definition.
- Skull X-rays and further skeletal films, if indicated from clinical assessment.
- Renal scan or cardiac echo, if indicated.
- Blood for DNA storage or genetic analysis if available.

Some diagnoses to consider

Brachydactyly type B

The thumbs and halluces may be broad or bifid. There is central syndactyly and a characteristic face. Hypoplastic/absent nails, short/absent distal phalanges, and short middle phalanges in 2nd–5th digits are other digital anomalies. AD but genetically heterogeneous. Can be caused by heterozygous truncating mutations in the *ROR2* gene.

Brachydactyly types D and E

Type D (MIM 113200). Short broad distal phalanges in thumbs and halluces.

Type E (MIM 113300). Shortening of one or more metacarpals/metatarsals. May be short stature. Genetically heterogeneous. Specific heterozygous missense mutations in the *HOXD13* gene can cause phenotypes overlapping with brachydactylies types D and E.

Greig cephalopolysyndactyly

AD condition characterized by a high forehead with frontal bossing, macrocephaly, hypertelorism, and a broad base to the nose. In the hands, both postaxial polydactyly (type B) and, less commonly, preaxial polydactyly (broad thumbs with bifid nails and distal phalanges) can occur; also often central syndactyly. In the feet, usually preaxial polydactyly (duplicated hallux) with syndactyly in toes 1–3. Caused by mutations in *GLI3* on 7p13. The facial features of Greig can be subtle, especially in infancy. It is generally considered that *type IV preaxial polydactyly* is part of the spectrum of Greig syndrome and caused by mutations in *GLI 3*. Mutation analysis will help to determine if the cause is a new mutation in situations where there is clinical doubt.

Lacrimo-auriculo-dental-digital (LADD) syndrome

AD condition characterized by absence or atresia of the lacrimal puntae causing overflow of tears (epiphora) and recurrent eye infection, simple, cup-shaped ears with sensorineural or conductive deafness, and hypoplastic teeth. The thumbs are usually bifid or triphalangeal with clinodactyly.

Otopalatodigital syndrome type 1 (Taybi syndrome)

Otopalatodigital syndrome type 1 (OPD-1) is a rare X-linked disease with diagnostic skeletal features, conductive deafness, cleft palate, and mild mental retardation. Affected individuals have a 'pugilistic facies'. The thumbs are broad. The feet have a particularly characteristic appearance with a large sandal gap, a short hallux, and lateral curvature of the toes. Caused by mutation in the *FLNA* gene on Xq 28 (Robertson).

Pfeiffer syndrome

AD condition with coronal craniosynostosis, broad thumbs and halluces, and soft-tissue syndactyly. The halluces are usually in the varus position, and a variety of anomalies are found including broad halluces, bifid halluces, and preaxial polydactyly. The face is similar to that in Crouzon syndrome but clover leaf skull is a more frequent complication. Sometimes the thumbs and halluces are broad and there may be a degree of skin syndactyly. Mutations are found in either *FGFR1* or *FGFR2*. *FGFR2* mutations may lead to a more severe craniofacial phenotype.

Robinow syndrome

Both AD and autosomal recessive (AR) types. Skeletal survey to assess mesomelia, costovertebral abnormalities, and distinctive phalangeal changes. There is brachydactyly with abnormal orientation of the thumbs and occasional bifid thumbs. Large mouth and tongue, gingival hypertrophy, micropenis, and congenital heart defects. The AR type is due to homozygous abnormality in the *ROR2* gene. Different heterozygous mutations in *ROR2* cause brachydactyly type B.

Rubinstein–Taybi syndrome (RTS)

Children with RTS usually have a normal birthweight, but subsequent growth is poor, with most children being of short stature with microcephaly. Mental retardation is usually moderate to severe, but some have mild learning difficulties. The most striking physical feature is broad, sometimes angulated thumbs and first toes. The facial features vary with age and include a prominent beaked nose with the columella below the alae nasae and downslanting eyes. Cryptorchidism occurs in males. Other variable features include congenital heart disease (~30%) and kidney abnormalities, eye and hearing problems, feeding difficulties in infancy, and constipation. Seizures may occur. Most people with RTS are very sociable, even over-friendly, and enjoy adult attention. See Wiley et al. (2003) for medical guidelines for individuals with RTS.

The gene for RTS is at 16p13.3. Petrij et al. (2000) concluded that microdeletions and truncating mutations in CBP account for approximately 20% of mutations in individuals with the RTS phenotype.

Teunissen–Cremers (congenital ankylosis of the stapes with broad thumbs)

AD condition with conductive deafness due to ankylosis of the auditory ossicles together with mild skeletal anomalies, e.g. broad thumbs and halluces, short distal phalanges, fused cervical vertebrae, and syndactyly. Hypermetropia is a common feature.

Genetic advice

Recurrence risk

Counsel as appropriate for the underlying syndrome.

Prenatal diagnosis

- Genetic testing for some of these syndromes may be available.
- Ultrasound scans. Ultrasound markers additional to the broad thumbs should be used to confirm a diagnosis.

Support group contact: Many of the syndromes have their own support groups. See <www.cafamily.org.uk>.

Expert adviser: late Robin Winter, previously Professor of Clinical Genetics and Dysmorphology, Institute of Child Health, London, England.

References

Petrij F, Dauwerse HG, Blough RI, et al. Diagnostic analysis of the Rubinstein–Taybi syndrome: five cosmids should be used for microdeletion detection and low number of protein truncating mutations. J Med Genet 2000; **37**: 168–76.

Robertson SP, Twigg SR, et al. Localised mutations in the gene encoding the cytoskeletal protein filamin A cause diverse malformations in humans. Nat Genet 2004; **33**: 487–91.

Temtamy SA, McKusick VA. The genetics of hand malformations. Alan R. Liss, New York, 1978.

Wiley S, Swayne S, et al. Rubinstein–Taybi syndrome medical guidelines. Am J Med Genet 2003; **119A** (2): 101–10.

Cardiomyopathy in children under 10 years

Cardiomyopathies are defined as diseases of the myocardium associated with cardiac dysfunction. Severe peripartum asphyxia can cause an ischaemic cardiomyopathy, 'transient myocardial ischaemia of the newborn'. These neonates usually do not have ischaemic encephalopathy or serious renal problems—the dilated heart with impaired function is the major manifestation. Usually these infants have some degree of intrauterine growth retardation (IUGR) and are small-for-dates, and usually there has been a hypoglycaemic episode as well as asphyxial stress.

Infants of diabetic mothers may have asymmetric septal hypertrophy (ASH) or left ventricular hypertrophy in the neonatal period. ASH is present in 38.8% of large for gestational age (LGA) infants of diabetic mothers compared with 7.1% of LGA infants of non-diabetics. Hypertrophic cardiomyopathy in infants of diabetic mothers is generally transient and benign.

In utero ritodrine exposure may cause neonatal ventricular hypertrophy.

The annual incidence of cardiomyopathy in Australian children is 1.2 per 100 000 and it is over 10 times higher in children aged <1 year compared to 1–18 years (0.7 per 100 000 versus 8.3 per 100 000; Nugent *et al.* 2003). Arola *et al.* (1997) estimated an incidence of 0.65/100 000 in the 0–20 year old population in Finland. Dilated cardiomyopathy is the most frequently found type and hypertrophic cardiomyopathy the second most common. The differential diagnosis in infants is different from that in adults, mainly due to the contribution of metabolic disease and dysmorphic syndromes.

The geneticist is asked to see children in whom there is no evidence of an infective, or other environmental cause, and to discuss recurrence risks with parents after a genetic aetiology has been identified.

Clinical approach

Carefully review the child's notes and the results of cardiac investigations, e.g. echocardiogram and electrocardiogram (ECG). Attempt to classify the cardiomyopathy into:

1 dilated cardiomyopathy (DCM);
2 hypertrophic cardiomyopathy (HCM) with normal to increased systolic function;
3 HCM with decreased function (the latter patients are much more likely to have a metabolic disorder or a storage disorder).

History: key points

- Three-generation family tree with special note of congenital heart disease and neonatal or infant deaths. Any evidence for X-linkage or mitochondrial inheritance?
- Consanguinity (metabolic conditions, autosomal recessive (AR) conditions).
- Pregnancy, diabetes, medication, infections, polyhydramnios.
- Birth asphyxia.
- Valvular heart defect (pulmonary stenosis in Noonan and LEOPARD (lentigines–ECG abnormalities–ocular hypertelorism–pulmonary stenosis–abnormal genitalia–retardation of growth–deafness) syndromes).
- Muscle weakness (skeletal muscle involvement, e.g. muscular dystrophies and mitochondrial myopathy).

- Developmental delay—differentiate between motor delay (muscular weakness) and global developmental delay.
- Fluctuation in level of consciousness especially with intercurrent infections.
- Regression (multiple acyl-CoA dehydrogenation deficiency (MADD), mitochondrial disorders).
- Deafness (LEOPARD, Alstrom syndrome).
- Visual problems (mitochondrial disorders, though unlikely in infants).

Examination: key points

- Look carefully for facial features of Noonan, cardio-facio-cutaneous, Costello, and LEOPARD syndromes.
- Hypotonia or weakness (skeletal muscle involvement).
- Skin, acanthosis nigricans (Alstrom syndrome), lentigines (LEOPARD syndrome).

Special investigations

- 24-hour tape to investigate heart rhythm disturbances.
- Creatine kinase (CK; skeletal muscle involvement, e.g. muscular dystrophies).
- Plasma carnitine.
- Dried blood spot on Guthrie card for acyl carnitine profile (fatty acid oxidation defects).
- Glucose (to exclude hypoglycaemia). Controlled and monitored fasting studies may be required.
- Blood lactate.
- Ammonia (raised in carnitine deficiency and disorders of fatty acid oxidation).
- Enzyme analysis (α-glucosidase deficiency, type II glycogen storage disease).
- Full blood count (FBC) and differential count: neutropenia (Barth syndrome).
- Lactate dehydrogenase (LDH) is often markedly raised in fatty acid oxidation defects and low cholesterol with high uric acid is typical for Barth syndrome (see below).
- Urine organic acids (methylmalonic aciduria, malonyl-CoA decarboxylase, 3-methylglutaconic aciduria)—preferably early morning urine before any diuretic dose.
- Urine dicarboxylic acids.
- Magnetic resonance imaging (MRI) brain scan if there are central nervous system (CNS) features or regression (mitochondrial disorders, MADD).
- DNA for analysis or storage. Consider medium-chain acyl-CoA dehydrogenase (MCAD) deficiency.
- Consider skeletal muscle biopsy—may be informative in the absence of clinical skeletal muscle weakness. Do histochemistry and histology and assay mitochondrial enzyme function.

Some diagnoses to consider

Dysmorphic syndromes

Noonan syndrome. HCM, pulmonary valve stenosis, and secundum atrial septal defect (ASD) are the most frequently found cardiac anomalies. Short stature and a characteristic facies with hypertelorism, coarse features, and short webbed neck are characteristic. 50% have mutations in *PTPN11*, but there is locus heterogeneity and other genes are not yet defined. In Nugent *et al.*'s (2003) study, 30% of children diagnosed with HCM at <10 years had Noonan syndrome. See 'Noonan syndrome (NS)', page 402.

LEOPARD (lentigines–ECG abnormalities–ocular hypertelorism–pulmonary stenosis–abnormal genitalia–retardation of growth–deafness) syndrome is caused by mutations in the *PTPN11* gene, which also causes Noonan syndrome.

Cardiofaciocutaneous syndrome. The hair is sparse, there is relative macrocephaly, and there can be cardiac defects, most commonly pulmonary stenosis and HCM. The skin is rough, dry, and hyperkeratotic. Polyhydramnios in pregnancy is common, perhaps a prenatal presentation of the severe feeding problems and failure to thrive that are common in the first year of life. Development is usually delayed.

Costello syndrome is characterized by prenatally increased growth, postnatal growth retardation, coarse face, loose skin resembling cutis laxa, non-progressive cardiomyopathy (sometimes with arrhythmia), developmental delay, and an outgoing, friendly behaviour. There are very characteristic wrinkled palms and ulnar deviation of the hands. Patients can develop papillomas, especially around the mouth, and have a predisposition for malignancies (mainly abdominal and pelvic rhabdomyosarcoma in childhood). Consider ultrasound scan (USS) surveillance. Costello syndrome is likely to be an autosomal dominant (AD) disorder. The pathogenesis is unclear, but there are many clues implicating disturbed elastogenesis (Hennekam 2003).

Beckwith–Wiedemann syndrome (BWS). HCM is a rare component of BWS. In Nugent *et al.*'s (2003) study it accounted for only ~1% of HCM presenting before the age of 10 years. See 'Beckwith–Wiedemann syndrome (BWS)' in Chapter 3, 'Common consultations', page 278.

Metabolic disorders
Carnitine deficiency. Systemic carnitine deficiency is autosomal recessive (AR) and due to mutation in *SLC22A5*. The cardiac features are cardiomyopathy, often with striking T-wave abnormalities on ECG, and endocardial fibroelastosis. Hypoglycaemia may be found and it is a cause of sudden infant death. It is important to recognize as therapeutic treatment with L-carnitine is life-saving. Many other conditions have moderately low carnitine and may benefit from carnitine even though they do not have *SLC22A5* mutations.

Fatty acid oxidation abnormalities.
• **HADHB** (hydroxyacyl-CoA dehydrogenase/3-ketoacyl-coa thiolase/enoyl-CoA hydratase, β-subunit). Also known as LCHAD (long-chain hydroxy acyl-CoA dehydrogenase) deficiency.
• **Mutiple acyl-coA dehydrogenase deficiency (MADD).** Cardiomyopathy and leukodystrophy.
• **MCAD.** Sudden death due to hypoglycaemia rather than cardiomyopathy is the typical serious complication.

Glycogen storage disease. Hepatomegaly is an important feature. Typically the ECG shows large voltages and prolonged activation time.
• Type II, alpha glucosidase deficiency, was previously known as acid maltase deficiency (Pompe disease). Infants are breathless and floppy due to skeletal muscle

involvement and cardiac failure. AR due to mutations in the gene *GAA* on 17q23.
• Type IIb. X-linked *LAMP2* gene at Xq24.

Methylmalonic aciduria. AR methmethylmalonic aciduria (cobalamin deficiency). Type A is caused by mutations in *MMAA* on 4q31.1 and type B is caused by mutations in *MMAB* on 12q24. Toxic metabolites accumulating in methylmalonic acidurias can inhibit adenosine triphosphate (ATP)-synthase, which is normally actively regulated in cardiac muscle in response to cellular energy demand (Das 2003).

Malonyl-CoA decarboxylase deficiency. This AR disorder may present with sudden cardiac failure or death in the first year. Dietary manipulation is unlikely to prevent the development of cardiomyopathy. Mutation in *MLYCD*.

Barth syndrome. Cardioskeletal myopathy with neutropenia occurring in males. An X-linked cause of a dilated cardiomyopathy due to mutation in 'taffazin' the *TAZ* gene at Xq28. Affected boys have hypocholesterolaemia, hyperuricaemia, and methylglutaconic aciduria. (NB. Carnitine supplementation can cause rapid deterioration in cardiac function, but pantothenic acid supplementation may substantially improve cardiac function in some cases (Ostman-Smith).)

Alstrom syndrome. Rare AR syndrome caused by mutations in *ALMS1* on 2p13. Alstrom syndrome is characterized by childhood obesity with type 2 diabetes mellitus (hyperinsulinism and chronic hyperglycaemia) and neurosensory deficits, e.g. cone–rod retinal dystrophy. A subset of individuals have dilated cardiomyopathy, hepatic dysfunction, hypothyroidism, male hypogonadism, short stature, and mild/moderate developmental delay.

Mitochondrial disorders (usually HCM)
A number of mitochondrial disorders such as complex 1 (mitochondrial respiratory chain) deficiency (DCM), Kearns–Sayre syndrome (KSS), cytochrome C deficiency, and Leigh's disease may have cardiac involvement. The mitochondrial mutation may be difficult to confirm and in some instances may only be detected in the myocardium. There is overlap between these conditions and the disorders of fatty acid oxidation. See 'Mitochondrial DNA diseases', page 384.

Friedreich's ataxia (FRDA). Sometimes the characteristically hypertrophic cardiomyopathy is fortuitously diagnosed before the neurological symptoms present. See 'Ataxic child', page 52.

Muscular dystrophies (usually DCM)
Duchenne and Becker muscular dystrophy, Emery–Dreifuss muscular dystrophy, and limb-girdle muscular dystrophy all have an associated cardiomyopathy. Typically, the cardiomyopathy becomes apparent in adolescence or later. See 'Duchenne and Becker muscular dystrophy (DMD and BMD)' and 'Limb girdle muscular dystrophies', page 308 and page 374.

Genetic advice
Recurrence risk
There will be a genetic aetiology in some children who have an isolated cardiomyopathy in whom there is no clear aetiology. The presentation, family history, and the cardiac features may give guidance as to the likelihood of a genetic condition. Mitochondrial conditions may have matrilineal inheritance, AR inheritance, or may be sporadic.

Overall, approximately one-third of HCM cases detected in childhood have familial AD HCM with mutations in the usual sarcomere protein gene.

Carrier detection

Both parents of a child with cardiomyopathy should have an ECG and an echocardiogram. (There is a considerable risk of HCM, and even DCM, being familial with AD inheritance.)

Carrier detection is possible in families where a causative mutation has been defined and may be possible for some biochemical abnormalities.

Prenatal diagnosis

This is available to those families where there is molecular or biochemical confirmation of the diagnosis.

Natural history and further management (preventative measures)

Prevent hypoglycaemia in children with carnitine deficiency or MCAD with dietary advice and a management plan for adequate carbohydrate intake during intercurrent illnesses.

Lay group contact: Cardiomyopathy Association <www.cardiomyopathy.org>.

Expert adviser: Ingegerd Östman-Smith, Professor of Paediatric Cardiology, Gothenburg University, Gothenburg, Sweden.

References

Arola A, Jokinen E, et al. Epidemiology of idiopathic cardiomyopathies in children and adolescents. A nationwide study in Finland. Am J Epidemiol 1997; **146**: 385–93.

Das AM. Regulation of the mitochondrial ATP-synthase in health and disease. Mol Genet Metab 2003; **79**: 71–82.

Hennekam RC. Costello syndrome: an overview. Am J Med Genet 2003; **117C** (1): 42–8.

Lipshultz SE, et al. The incidence of pediatric cardiomyopathy in two regions of the United States. New Engl J Med 2003; **348**: 1647–55.

Nugent AW, et al. The National Australian Childhood Cardiomyopathy Study. The epidemiology of childhood cardiomyopathy in Australia. New Engl J Med 2003; **348**: 1639–46.

Ostman-Smith I, Brown G, et al. Dilated cardiomyopathy due to type II X-linked 3-methylglutaconic aciduria: successful treatment with pantothenic acid. Br Heart J 1994; **72**: 349–53.

Vela-Huerta MM, Vargas-Origel A, et al. Assymmetrical septal hypertrophy in newborn infants of diabetic mothers. Am J Perinatol 2000; **17**: 89–94.

Cataract

A cataract is an opacity of the lens of the eye. The birth incidence is 6 per 10 000 births and about 50% of congenital cataracts are genetic. Cataracts may be isolated or associated with other anterior segment malformations, e.g. aniridia or congenital glaucoma, or be associated with syndromes. Lens opacities develop as part of the natural ageing process and cataracts are common in the elderly and conditions with premature ageing or DNA repair defects.

Ophthalmologists describe the type of cataract by its morphology and position in the lens and this will help with the differential diagnosis and classification. A totally opaque lens is the end point of all the pathological types and classification is not then possible. Screening for cataracts is part of the routine neonatal examination. Even after early detection about 20% of infants with bilateral cataracts will be registered blind.

The geneticist is asked to see infants with cataract to assess if it is part of a metabolic or genetic condition. In adults the indication is usually to estimate offspring risks.

Clinical approach

History: key points

- Three-generation family tree with specific enquiry about cataract, visual impairment, and consanguinity.
- At what age were the cataracts first detected?
- Are there other eye anomalies?
- Are there other congenital anomalies or a known chromosomal condition?
- Non-genetic factors: congenital and acquired infections, drugs, radiation, diabetes mellitus.
- Sun sensitivity (DNA repair defects, e.g. Cockayne syndrome).
- Deafness (Cockayne syndrome, type 2 neurofibromatosis (NF2)).
- Developmental milestones. Is there any evidence of developmental delay?

Examination: key points

- **Eyes.** Detailed assessment for additional ophthalmological features or malformations including photographs.
- **Growth parameters** including head occipital-frontal circumference (OFC). Investigate:
  - any evidence of deceleration (metabolic disease);
  - failure to thrive (metabolic disease, cerebro-oculo-facial-skeletal (COFS) syndrome, Cockayne syndrome);
  - short stature (skeletal conditions, e.g. Stickler syndrome, Kniest syndrome, chondrodysplasia punctata (CDP)).
- **Head and face:**
  - large fontanelle (Wiedemann–Rautenstrauch syndrome (WRS));
  - hair (hypotrichosis in Hallermann–Streiff syndrome);
  - deep-set eyes (Cockayne syndrome);
  - 'beaked nose' (Hallermann–Streiff syndrome, WRS).
- **Mouth:**
  - cleft palate (Stickler and Kniest syndromes);
  - teeth ('screwdriver' incisors in Nance–Horan syndrome).
- **Skin:**
  - blisters (incontinentia pigmenti (IP));
  - sun sensitivity (Cockayne);
  - poikiloderma (Rothmund Thomson);

- ichthyosis (CDP);
- premature ageing (progeria).
- lipoatrophy (WRS).
- **Limbs:**
  - asymmetry of limb lengths in a female (Conradi–Humerman–Happle type of CDP);
  - talipes, myotonia (myotonic dystophy).

Special investigations

In an *otherwise normal child*, the basic screen is:

- TORCH (toxoplasmosis, other (including syphilis, varicella zoster, parvovirus), rubella, cytomegalovirus, and herpes simplex virus) screen;
- urinary reducing substances (e.g. galactosaemia);
- urinary amino and organic acids;
- *examine parents and siblings*. Many gene carriers are asymptomatic because of variable expression and mild involvement. Female carriers for Lowe syndrome have characteristic punctate lens opacities; carriers for Nance–Horan syndrome have posterior sutural lens opacities.

Other investigations as dictated by systemic findings include the following.

- **Metabolic:**
  - urine reducing substances. If reducing substances are found proceed to enzyme analysis (galactosaemia);
  - urine protein. Proteinuria may indicate renal Fanconi syndrome which is found in Lowe syndrome. If present investigate further with urine osmololality, phosphate, and urine and plasma amino acids;
  - urinary amino acids. May need repeating as sometimes in Lowe syndrome very early screen is negative;
  - serum calcium and phosphate;
  - peroxisomal analysis (plasma very-long-chain fatty acids (VLCFAs)) if features suggest rhizomelic CDP or Zellweger syndrome;
  - sterol analysis (Connradi–Humermann–Happle or X-linked dominant (XLD) CDP due to emopamil binding protein (EBP) mutation).
- **Radiological investigations.** Consider a skeletal survey to exclude:
  - rickets (Lowe syndrome);
  - epiphyseal stippling (CDP);
  - skeletal dysplasia (Kniest and Stickler syndromes).
- **Chromosome analysis.** 60% of children with trisomy 21 develop cataracts.
- **DNA analysis:**
  - myotonic dystrophy;
  - known familial genetic cataract;
  - consider blood sample to store DNA for future genetic analysis.
- **TORCH** screen in congenital or early infancy cataracts.
- **Audiology** (Cockayne syndrome, NF2).
- **Skin biopsy.** Consider a skin biopsy to detect DNA repair defects if the clinical picture is suggestive.

Some diagnoses to consider

Congenital or early infancy cataracts

Galactosaemia. Classic galactosaemia is an autosomal recessive (AR) condition caused by a deficiency of galactose-1-phosphate uridyl-transferase (*GALT*). The infants are unwell and fail to thrive. See 'Prolonged neonatal jaundice and jaundice in infants below 6 months', page 220.

Galactokinase deficiency. AR condition caused by mutations in *GALK1* on 17q24. They may develop cataracts (as in galactosaemia due to accumulation of galactitol in the lenses, which may resolve with dietary management).

Lowe oculo-cerebro-renal syndrome. There is renal dysfunction and a generalized aminoaciduria. Failure to thrive, developmental delay, and rickets are features. Affected males have dense cataracts present from birth. Glaucoma may be a later feature that follows cataract surgery. Inheritance is X-linked recessive (XLR). Mutation testing of *OCRL* on Xq25–26.1 is available. Carrier females typically have characteristic punctate lens opacities. If the familial mutation is known, mutation analysis enables definitive assignment of carrier status.

Peroxisomal disorders. Rhizomelic CDP and Zellweger syndrome are both AR disorders that present in infancy with a poor prognosis. See 'Floppy infant', page 118.

Cerebro-oculo-facio-skeletal syndrome (COFS). An AR rapidly progressive neurological disorder leading to brain atrophy with calcifications, cataracts, microcornea, optic atrophy, progressive joint contractures, and growth failure. See 'DNA repair defects', page 304.

Hallermann–Streiff syndrome. Microcornea is present. The nose is thin, the mandible small, and there is hypotrichosis.

Wiedemann–Rautenstrauch syndrome (WRS). This condition is also known as neonatal progeria. The facial features can be confused with those of Hallermann–Streiff syndrome but WRS is a progressive condition leading to early death. Lipoatrophy, prominent veins, and wide fontanelles are features. The inheritance is AR.

Nance–Horan syndrome. Nance–Horan is a very rare XLsemi-dominant syndromic cause of cataract due to mutations in the *NHS* gene on Xp22.13 (Burdon 2003) Males have severe cataracts from birth; other features include screwdriver incisors and dental anomalies of shape and number, long face with prominent chin. Variable mental retardation is seen in ~30% of males. ~5% of carrier females have no ocular signs.

Infancy or childhood onset cataract

In a fit child with normal development and stature the likelihood of finding a syndromic cause is much less than in a neonate. Screening of children with syndromes known to have a cataract as a component will lead to detection in this age group.

Stickler syndrome. Short stature, joint pain (especially the hip), deafness (sensorineural and conductive), and myopia are features (see 'Stickler syndrome', page 414).

Chondrodysplasia punctata (CDP). Milder types of CDP (autosomal dominant (AD), XLD, and XLR) See 'Chondrodysplasia punctata', page 72.

Premature ageing and/or DNA repair defects. Examples are progeria and Cockayne syndrome. A skin biopsy will be required to confirm DNA repair defects by ultraviolet (UV) irradiation of cultured fibroblasts. DNA mutation analysis may also be available. See 'DNA repair defects', page 304.

Juvenile onset cataract

Neurofibromatosis type 2 (NF2). Individuals with NF2 have posterior subcapsular lenticular opacities but this is rarely the mode of presentation.

Adult onset cataract

Age-related cataract is a common finding in elderly. In cross-sectional studies the prevalence of cataracts is 50% in people aged 65–74 years increasing to 70% in the over 75s.

Myotonic dystrophy. Cataracts are found in otherwise asymptomatic individuals with myotonic dystrophy, so test for this condition if any clinical suspicion or positive family history.

Genetic advice

Recurrence risk

If, after careful exclusion of syndromic and environmental causes of cataract, the cataracts appear to be isolated, consider the following.

- Ophthalmological examination of first-degree relatives may detect cataracts and determine the mode of inheritance.
- There are many different forms of inherited cataract and the morphology is not always the same within a family.
- The most common mode of inheritance of familial cataract is AD and these are generally caused by mutations in the structural proteins such as crystallins. Mutations in the γ-crystallin encoding genes are the most frequent cause of isolated congenital cataract; mutations in the β-crystallin gene cluster on 22q11.2 also cause familial cataract. Abnormalities in the gap junction connexin genes 50 and 46 have also been shown to lead to familial cataract.
- Consanguinity suggests AR and metabolic abnormalities.
- X-linked inheritance has been reported.

If the cataracts are a component of a syndrome or chromosomal anomaly, counsel as appropriate for the specific diagnosis.

Carrier detection

- Identification of early cataracts by slit lamp examination.
- Possible by DNA analysis in families where a causative mutation has been identified.
- May be possible for some biochemical abnormalities.

Prenatal diagnosis

This is technically feasible in those families where there is molecular or biochemical confirmation of diagnosis.

Natural history and further management (preventative measures)

Long-term ophthalmological follow-up and surgery where appropriate. Patients with isolated inherited congenital cataract have a better visual and surgical outcome than those with coexisting ocular and systemic abnormalities (Francis *et al.* 2001).

Support group contact: CLIMB (Children Living With Inherited Metabolic Diseases) <www.climb.org.uk.>; Lowe (oculo-cerebro-renal) syndrome <www.lowesyndrome.org>.

Expert adviser: Nicola Ragge, Consultant Paediatric Ophthalmologist, Moorfields Eye Hospital, London, UK.

References

Bermejo E, Martinez-Frias ML. Congenital eye malformations: clinical–epidemiological analysis of 1,124,654 conseutive births in Spain. *Am J Med Genet* 1998; **75**: 497–504.

Burdon KP, McKay JD, *et al.* Mutations in a novel gene, NHS, cause the pleiotropic effects of Nance-Horan syndrome, including severe congenital cataract, dental anomalies, and mental retardation. *Am J Hum Genet* 2003; **73**: 1120–30.

Francis PJ, Ionides A, *et al.* Visual outcome in patients with isolated autosomal dominant congenital cataract. *Ophthalmology* 2001; **108**: 1104–8.

Francis PJ, Berry V, Bhattacharya SS, Moore AT. The genetics of childhood cataract. *J Med Genet* 2002; **37**: 481–8.

He W, Li S. Congenital cataracts: gene mapping. *Hum Genet* 2000; **106**: 1–13.

Cerebellar anomalies

This section addresses the diagnostic approach to structural abnormality of the cerebellum. As in practice it is difficult to differentiate between primary non-development and an atrophic process, conditions that have magnetic resonance imaging (MRI) evidence of a small or structurally abnormal cerebellum in infancy are included. The terminology of other posterior fossa abnormalities is listed in the table. For more details on Dandy–Walker malformation see 'Dandy–Walker malformation', page 582 and for Chiari malformation see the table.

Always try to get hold of both the MRI (or computerized tomography (CT)) report and the images, and make an effort to understand the terminology used in the report so you have a clear anatomical picture of the abnormality. Determine whether the structural abnormality of the brain is restricted to the cerebellum, or also involves the cerebral cortex or other neural tissues. Similarly, within the cerebellum, is the hypoplasia restricted to the vermis, or are the cerebellar hemispheres also involved?

The role of the geneticist is to try to establish a specific diagnosis and to offer genetic advice.

Clinical approach

History: key points

- Detailed three-generation family tree with specific enquiry about consanguinity.
- Pregnancy: exposure to retinoic acid, cytomegalovirus (CMV), excess alcohol.
- History of episodic ventilation (hyperventilation alternating with hypoventilation).
- Developmental milestones, any loss of skills, hypotonia.
- Visual problems (chorioretinitis, retinal dystrophy, retinitis pigmentosa).
- Recurrent infections (Hoyerall–Hreidarsson syndrome (HHS)).

Examination: key points

- Occipital-frontal circumference (OFC). Macrocephaly and microcephaly may be found, but each has different syndromic associations.
- Neurological examination: tone; posture; ataxia.
- Muscle weakness (muscular dystrophy in muscle–eye–brain (MEB) disease).
- Nystagmus.
- Tongue cysts and excessive oral frenulae (oral–facial–digital (OFD) syndromes, Joubert syndrome).

- Aniridia (Gillespie syndrome).
- Polydactyly (OFD, Joubert syndrome).

Special investigations

- Blood count (aplastic anaemia in HHS; also consider immunological investigations).
- Liver function tests (hepatic fibrosis in COACH (cerebellar vermian hypoplasia–oligophrenia–ataxia–coloboma–hepatic fibrosis) syndrome).
- Creatine kinase (CK; muscular dystrophy and myopathy).
- Renal function and ultrasound scan (Joubert syndrome).
- Ophthalmology referral (retinal dystrophy or dysplasia in Joubert syndrome, retinal dysplasia in MEB, aniridia in Gillespie syndrome).
- Karyotype if there are dysmorphic features.
- 7-dehydrocholesterol (Smith–Lemli–Opitz (SLO) syndrome).
- Isoelectric focusing of transferrins (carbohydrate-deficient glycoprotein syndrome).
- Metabolic testing (lactate, pyruvate, etc.) if a respiratory chain disorder is suspected.
- DNA for storage or analysis.

Some diagnoses to consider

Joubert syndrome

Autosomal recessive (AR) disorder with diagnosis based on:
- hypotonia: present in all patients, moderately severe in infancy with frog-leg posture and lack of spontaneous movement;
- ataxia: 75% learn to sit (average 19 months) and 50% to walk (average 4 years). Gait is unstable and tandem walking is poor;
- developmental delay: often severe, but very variable;
- neuroradiology shows cerebellar vermis hypoplasia and molar tooth sign.

Associated anomalies include: episodic hyperpnoea and/or apnoea in 50–75% especially in infancy; distinctive facial features (high rounded eyebrows, broad nasal bridge and mild epicanthus, anteverted nostrils, triangular shaped open mouth with irregular tongue protrusion, low-set and coarse ears); eye anomalies (retinal dysplasia, colobomas, nytagmus, strabismus, and ptosis); oculomotor apraxia; microcystic renal disease; occasionally polydactyly; and a variety of other features. Joubert syndrome is genetically heterogeneous. Mutations have been identified in *AHI1*, encoding

Glossary of terms

Dandy–Walker malformation (DWM) describes a triad of findings including cystic dilatation of the fourth ventricle, complete or partial agenesis of the cerebellar vermis, and an enlarged posterior fossa with displacement of the tentorium

Cerebellar vermis aplasia. Neuroradiology demonstrates a midline defect between the cerebellar hemispheres but the posterior fossa is not enlarged

Molar-tooth sign is seen on axial neuroimaging (MR or CT) in Joubert syndrome, but is not specific for this condition as it is also seen in the cerebello-oculo-renal syndromes. It is characterized by a deep posterior interpeduncular fossa (best seen on transverse section), thick and elongated superior cerebellar peduncles (best seen on parasaggital section), and hypoplastic or aplastic superior cerebellar vermis

Chiari malformations

- **Chiari I.** Downward displacement of the lower cerebellum, including the tonsils; rarely causes symptoms in childhood, but may be associated with hydrocephalus and syringomyelia
- **Chiari II.** Usually associated with myelomeningocele (see 'Neural tube defects', page 392)
- **Chiari III.** Downward displacement of the cerebellum into a posterior encephalocele
- **Chiari IV.** A form of cerebellar hypoplasia

jouberin, on 6q23 in some families (Ferland) and in Joubert syndrome with cortical polymicrogyria (Dixon–Salazar).

Syndromes with overlapping features to Joubert
Cerebello-oculo-renal syndromes (Arima, Senior–Loken, and COACH). These forms of Joubert syndrome includes retinal dysplasia and cystic dysplastic kidneys. Some patients with Senior–Loken have mutations in *NPHP5* on 3q.

Leber congenital amaurosis (LCA). LCA presents with nystagmus and variable neurological involvement, the patient may have seizures. Fundus is normal in infancy but the electroretinograph (ERG) is very subnormal or, more usually, non-recordable. Later there are signs of retinal degeneration. Genetic heterogeneity with 8 genes identified to date. Mostly AR. See 'Nystagmus', page 190.

Oral-facial-digital (OFD) syndromes type Mohr (II) and Varadi (VI). OFD type II and VI are AR malformation syndromes. The features in the hands are syndactyly (usually skin syndactyly affecting variable digits), brachydactyly, and postaxial polydactyly. Craniofacial anomalies are midline cleft lip, tongue cysts, and excess oral frenulae; the nasal tip may be bifid in type II. A central Y-shaped metacarpal is typically found in type VI.

Isolated cerebellar vermis aplasia
This may be found in children with a presentation of ataxic cerebral palsy. Carefully exclude AR syndromes with vermian aplasia. Sibling recurrence and autosomal dominant (AD) inheritance have been reported.

Other neuroradiological features and neuronal migration defects
Lissencephaly with cerebellar hypoplasia (LCH) is genetically heterogeneous. *DCX-* and *LIS1*-related lissencephaly can be associated with cerebellar hypoplasia (usually mild).

Microlissencephaly with severe cerebellar abnormality and hippocampal involvement suggests an AR condition with mutation in *RELN* in some affected infants.

Walker–Warburg syndrome (WWS) and **muscle-eye– brain disease** (MEB) are AR disorders that share the combination of cerebral neuronal migration defects (cobblestone lissencephaly) and cerebellar abnormalities, ocular abnormalities, and a congenital muscular dystrophy. Mutations in *POMT1* (WWS) and *POMGnT1* (MEB) have been identified. See 'Floppy infant', page 118.

Respiratory chain disorders
These are conditions that reduce the amount of energy available to the developing brain and this may lead to structural defects of the brain. Examples include complex 1 deficiency, pyruvate dehydrogenase (PDH) deficiency, and MELAS (mitochondrial myopathy–encephalopathy–lactic acidosis–stroke-like episodes).

Smith–Lemli–Opitz (SLO) syndrome
Cerebellar hypoplasia may be a feature of SLO, which is an AR syndrome characterized by microcephaly, prenatal onset growth deficiency, cleft palate, thickened alveolar ridges, 2, 3 syndactyly of toes, small proximally placed thumbs, and sometimes postaxial polydactyly. Males have ambiguous genitalia or hypospadias with hypoplastic scrotum. See 'Hypospadias', page 142.

PEHO (progressive encephalopathy–(o)edema–hypsarrhythmia–optic atrophy) syndrome
AR disorder originally described in Finland, but there are reports from other parts of Europe. Progressive cerebellar atrophy is a key MRI feature.

3C (craniocerebellocardiac) syndrome
Also called Ritscher–Schinzel syndrome, this is an AR condition characterized by abnormalities of the cranium (large head with prominent forehead), cerebellum (Dandy–Walker malformation (DWM) with vermis hypoplasia), heart (primarily septal defects), and also short stature.

Diagnostic criteria for chromosomally normal sporadic case (Leonardi *et al.* 2001):
- cardiac malformation other than isolated patent ductus arteriosus (PDA);
- cerebellar malformation;
- cleft palate *or* ocular coloboma *or* four of the following seven findings: prominent forehead; prominent occiput; hypertelorism; down-slanting palpebral fissures; low-set ears; depressed nasal bridge; and micrognathia.

Carbohydrate-deficient glycoprotein syndrome
Congenital disorders of glycosylation (CDG) are a group of AR metabolic disorders that are characterized biochemically by defective glycosylation of proteins (abnormal transferrin isoelectrophoresis). The most common type is CDG-Ia, which is a multisytem disorder affecting the nervous system (cerebellar atrophy and encephalopathy), liver, kidney, heart, adipose tissue (lipodystrophy and abnormal fat pads), bone, and genitalia. It is caused by phosphomannomutase (PMM) deficiency, and mutations have been identified in the gene *PMM2*.

Hoyerall–Hreidarsson syndrome (HHS)
X-linked recessive (XLR) and due to mutation in *DKC1* (the same gene as dyskeratosis congenita). Features include microcephaly, growth retardation, aplastic anaemia, and immunodeficiency. Death can occur in early childhood.

Gillespie syndrome
An AR syndrome with aniridia, cerebellar ataxia, and mental retardation.

Genetic advice

Recurrence risk
After careful evaluation and exclusion of syndromic conditions consider the following.
- Many of the syndromic causes of cerebellar structural abnormalities have AR inheritance. For apparently isolated cerebellar hypoplasia or vermian agenesis the recurrence risk may be as high as 25%. Empiric risk data is not available.
- Autosomal dominant (AD) inheritance of vermis aplasia is also reported; scan any parent with ataxia, nystagmus, or other neurological abnormalities.
- DWM. When the evidence suggests that DWM has not occurred as part of a Mendelian or chromosomal disorder then the recurrence risk is relatively low at 1–5% (Murray *et al.* 1985).

Carrier detection
This is possible in families with a known mutation.

Prenatal diagnosis
- This is possible by chorionic villus sampling (CVS) in families with a known mutation.
- Prenatal diagnosis of cerebellar hypoplasia based on early ultrasound scan (USS) is not reliable. Detailed USS is often offered in a subsequent pregnancy, but these limitations must be carefully discussed with the parents.
- DWM. Refer to 'Dandy–Walker malformation', page 582.

Support group contact: Many of the syndromes have their own support groups. See <www.cafamily.org.uk>.

Expert adviser: Daniela Pilz, Consultant Clinical Geneticist, Institute of Medical Genetics, University Hospital of Wales, Cardiff, Wales.

References

Dixon–Salazar T, Silhavy JL, *et al*. Mutations in the AHI1 gene, encoding jouberin, cause Joubert syndrome with cortical poly-microgyria. *Am J Hum Genet* 2004; **75**: 979–87.

Drouin-Garraud V, Belgrand M, *et al*. Neurological presentation of a congenital disorder of glycosylation CDG-Ia: implications for diagnosis and genetic counseling. *Am J Med Genet* 2001; **101**: 46–9.

Ferland RJ, Eyaid W, *et al*. Abnormal cerebellar development and axonal decussation due to mutations in AHI1 in Joubert syndrome. *Nat Genet* 2004; **36**: 1008–13.

Keeler LC, Marsh SE, *et al*. Linkage analysis in families with Joubert syndrome plus oculo-renal involvement identifies the CORS2 locus on chromosome 11p12–q13.3. *Am J Hum Genet* 2003; **73**: 656–62.

Leonardi ML, Pai GS, Wilkes B, Lebel RR. Ritscher–Schinzel cranio-cerebello-cardiac (3C) syndrome: report of four new cases and review. *Am J Med Genet* 2001; **102** (3): 237–42.

Maria BL, Boltshauser E, Plamer SC, Tran TX. Clinical features and revised diagnostic criteria in Joubert syndrome. *J Child Neurol* 1999; **14**: 583–90.

Murray JC, Johnson JA, Bird TD. Dandy–Walker malformation: etiologic heterogeneity and empiric recurrence risks. *Clin Genet* 1985; **28**: 272–83.

Parisi MA, Dobyns WB. Human malformations of the midbrain and hindbrain: review and proposed classification scheme. *Mol Genet Metab* 2003; **80**: 36–53.

Ross ME, Swanson K, Dobyns WB. Lissencephaly with cerebellar hypoplasia (LCH): a heterogeneous group of cortical malforma-tions. *Neuropediatrics* 2001; **32**: 256–63.

Satran D, Pierpont ME, Dobyns WB. Cerebello-oculo-renal syn-dromes including Arima, Senior–Loken and COACH syndromes: more than just variants of Joubert syndrome. *Am J Med Genet* 1999; **86**: 459–69.

Cerebral palsy

Cerebral palsy (CP) is a term used to describe a non-progressive physical disorder that affects movement. CP is not a progressive disorder because there is no on-going pathological process. The features do alter with the age of the child and brain maturity, e.g.children who later develop spasticity may be very floppy as neonates.

- **Spastic CP.** The muscle tone is increased and the reflexes are brisk. Muscle strength is reduced.
  - Hemiplegic CP: non-symmetrical. The contralateral limbs are affected.
  - Diplegic CP: symmetrical. The legs are affected more than the arms.
  - Quadriplegic CP: all four limbs are affected.
- **Athetoid (extrapyramidal, dystonic, choreoathetoid, dyskinetic) CP.** Involuntary movements and loss of control of posture.
- **Ataxic CP.** There is poor coordination of movements with balance difficulties. These patients have a wide-based gait and a tremor may be observed.

CP affects about 1 in 400 births. This figure is not reducing with better obstetric care because more premature infants are surviving. Prematurity, low birthweight, abnormal birth history, infections (pre- and postnatal), and vascular events are considered as aetiological factors when paediatricians assess children with CP. Birth trauma is not a frequent cause; perinatal asphyxia is a major factor in <5%. CP is more common in the first child and then from the fifth or subsequent child and in twins. The aetiology is unknown for most children with CP. There may be predisposing genetic factors, e.g. thrombophilia.

The challenge for the geneticist is to ensure that genetic conditions are detected, whilst recognizing that in the majority of children with CP there is a non-genetic aetiology. Some clinical features are more closely associated with a genetic aetiology and it is important to recognize these.

Clinical approach

History: key points

- Family history. Enquire about consanguinity, previously affected sibs. Birth order.
- Paternal age. A raised paternal age has been associated with athetoid CP in one study.
- Pregnancy: bleeding in the first trimester (vascular event, loss of twin), invasive testing, infections, drug exposure, twinning, fetal movements.
- Birth history risk factors:
  - prematurity—the lower the gestational age, the greater the risk of CP;
  - birthweight <1500 g;
  - twins;
  - birth history suggestive of anoxia, e.g. low Apgar scores, resuscitation and admission to a neonatal intensive care unit (NICU), seizures, irritability, and poor feeding in the neonatal period (see 'Neonatal encephalopathy and intractable seizures in the neonate', page 186).
- Occipital-frontal circumference (OFC) measurement at birth and subsequent records.
- Seizures. Found in 25–30% of children and 10% of adults. Could indicate an underlying structural brain malformation with genetic implications.

- Developmental milestones. Global delay or, particularly, motor problems.
- Evidence of regression. CP by definition is a non-progressive disorder.

Examination: key points

- Head circumference. Plot and compare with previous readings.
- Neurological signs:
  - muscle power and tone;
  - reflexes are brisk in association with spasticity;
  - are the signs symmetrical?
  - movement disorder—athetosis, dystonia;
  - ataxia: assess for both fine and gross motor ataxia.
- Dysmorphic features, other congenital anomalies, skin pigmentary disturbances (investigate for genetic and chromosomal conditions), icthyosis (Sjögren–Larsen syndrome).

Investigation

- Brain imaging, preferably magnetic resonance imaging (MRI) scan, to:
  - **(1)** confirm that any lesions are compatible with asphyxia, prematurity, etc.;
  - **(2)** exclude possibly genetically determined structural brain malformations such as migrational abnormalities;
  - **(3)** assess for features of metabolic or mitochondrial disease (e.g. basal ganglia lesions, agenesis of the corpus callosum);
  - **(4)** may be helpful in establishing the timing of the insult.
- Basic screen of biochemistry to include creatine phosphokinase (CPK; muscle–eye–brain (MEB) disease).
- Urine for amino and organic acids. Organic acidaemias can present with a spastic diplegia.
- Karyotype on all children with any features in addition to uncomplicated CP with no intellectual impairment.
- DNA. Conditions with specific diagnostic tests have been confused with CP even though the features of these conditions are not classical for CP. These include Angelman syndrome, Rett syndrome, Batten disease, lissencephalies, and X-linked mental retardation conditions, e.g. ARX mutations.
- Thrombophilia screen and factor V Leiden in children with a perinatal stroke as the cause of the CP.
- Consider investigating mother for lupus.

Some diagnoses to consider

Maternal factors. Mothers with medical problems are at higher risk in each pregnancy. Make sure that maternal phenylketonuria (PKU) is not a possibility. Teratogens, placental dysfunction, and autoimmune factors may need to be considered, particularly systemic lupus erythematosus (SLE).

Genetic advice

For all types of CP, the following features have been described in familial cases:

- microcephaly;
- significant and symmetrical spasticity;

- progression of symptoms;
- seizures;
- mental retardation;
- other congenital anomalies;
- a positive family history;
- a *lack* of significant perinatal asphyxia and other known environmental risk factors.

Recurrence risk

If there is consanguinity, a sibling recurrence risk of 25% may be advised. Where there are two affected children, a 25% recurrence risk to further siblings may be appropriate.

Spastic CP

Bundey and Griffiths (1977) confirmed earlier studies that established that the major determinants of genetic risk were symmetry of the spasticity and microcephaly. The 1977 study gave a recurrence risk of 9% to siblings of a child with symmetrical CP and a normal birth history. Some of these children may have had recognized genetically determined conditions if MRI scans had been available to screen for structural brain malformations and signs suggestive of metabolic disorders. This risk figure may overestimate the risk but it does highlight the children with a potential (autosomal recessive (AR) or X-linked (XL)) genetic risk.

Children without an abnormal pregnancy, birth, or perinatal history should be investigated thoroughly to exclude genetic conditions. If there is significant microcephaly, see 'Microcephaly', page 172.

Athetoid CP

Within the CP syndromes, athetosis is most commonly causally associated with serious perinatal complications. It can follow hypoxic ischaemic encephalopathy and, in these children, the brain MRI shows characteristic features with atrophy in the caudate and putamen. Genetic disorders to consider are:

- mitochondrial disorders;
- organic acidaemias;
- dopa-responsive dystonia (DRD; Segawa syndrome). The phenotype in childhood may resemble athetoid CP and all children with this condition should have a trial of L-dopa. See 'Dystonia', page 106;
- *MECP2* mutations, Rett syndrome;
- X-linked *ARX* mutations.

Genetic factors are thought to play a lesser role, although the risk of recurrence in siblings has been suggested to be as high as 10%. However, Amor *et al.* (2001) state that the genetic contribution to athetoid CP is small with an overall recurrence risk of 1%; many geneticists consider this risk is too low to use for counselling purposes. The actual risk figure given in any individual case will depend on how compelling the evidence is for serious perinatal

complications, and how thoroughly genetic factors have been considered and excluded.

Ataxic CP

If there is no evidence of birth asphyxia, this is a diagnosis made after exclusion of other causes of a congenital ataxia, (please refer to 'Ataxic child', page 52). A high-resolution brain MRI scan is mandatory prior to definitive counselling as congenital structural lesions of the cerebellum, such as hypoplasia or a Dandy–Walker cyst, may be found and aid estimation of recurrence risks.

Conflicting recurrence risk figures are found in the literature. There are undoubtedly a number of AR conditions with congenital ataxia and these require careful consideration. Most authors and geneticists advise an up to 10% recurrence risk but Miller (1988) states that the genetic risks are low.

CP with dysmorphic features and no diagnosis

Accurate empiric figures are not available for this heterogeneous group. Unless there are factors suggesting a high recurrence risk (e.g. consanguinity), the risk is probably small (Baraitser, personal communication 2003).

Carrier detection

Not possible unless a specific biochemical or genetic cause has been identified.

Prenatal diagnosis

Not possible unless a specific biochemical or genetic cause has been identified

Natural history and further management (preventative measures)

Children should be under the care of a neurodevelopmental multidisciplinary team.

Lay support: Scope, PO Box 833, Milton Keynes, MK12 5NY, UK <www.scope.org.uk>; Cerebral Palsy Research Foundation, USA.

Expert adviser: Michael Baraitser, Emeritus Consultant Clinical Geneticist, Great Ormond Street Hospital, London, England.

References

Amor DJ, Craig JE, Delatycki MB, Reddihough D. Genetic factors in athetoid cerebral palsy. *J Child Neurol* 2001; **16**: 793–7.

Bundey S, Griffiths MI. Recurrence risks in families of children with symmetrical spasticity. *Dev Med Child Neurol* 1977; **19**: 179–91.

Hoon AH Jr, *et al.* Brain imaging in suspected extrapyramidal cerebral palsy: observations in distinguishing genetic–metabolic from acquired causes. *J Pediatr* 1997; **131**: 240–5.

Lynch JK, Nelson KB, Curry CJ, Grether JK. Cerebrovascular accidents in children with factor V Leiden mutation. *J Child Neurol* 2001; **16**: 735–44.

Miller G. Ataxic cerebral palsy and genetic predisposition. *Arch Dis Child* 1988; **63**: 1260–1.

Chondrodysplasia punctata

In chondrodysplasia punctata (CDP) there is punctiform calcification (stippling) of bones, especially the epiphyses of the long tubular bones, patellae, and carpal and tarsal bones. Sites to look at specifically on a radiograph are the spine, knee joint, and shoulder. The larynx and tracheal rings may be affected. There may be paravertebral stippling. Stippling represents aberrant calcification of cartilage in the bones. Stippling is seen in fetuses, babies, and infants but in older children, >2 years, it is no longer present. It seems to be incorporated into the growing bone, but may lead to disharmonic growth as in Conradi–Hünermann syndrome. It is important to request the early films when children and adults are referred for counselling.

CDP is a heterogeneous condition involving:

- genetic defects in:
    - (1) peroxisomal metabolism;
    - (2) cholesterol metabolism; or
    - (3) vitamin K metabolism;
- acquired embryopathies caused by:
    - (1) maternal malabsorption of vitamin K;
    - (2) maternal use of warfarin;
    - (3) maternal use of phenytoin; or
    - (4) maternal systemic lupus erythematosus (SLE).

The table gives a classification of the various CDPs.

Clinical approach

History: key points

- Three-generation family tree with specific enquiry for consanguinity (autosomal recessive (AR) types of CDP).
- Pregnancy loss of males in second trimester (X-linked dominant (XLD) CDP).
- Male proband; consider X-linked recessive (XLR) CDP.
- Detailed enquiry about maternal health, e.g. malabsorption, maternal SLE.
- Detailed enquiry re pregnancy history, e.g. fetal exposure to warfarin or phenytoin.
- Bleeding in the neonatal period (vitamin K deficiency).
- Growth delay (associated with failure to thrive in rhizomelic CDP (RCDP)).
- Developmental progress. Seizures?

Examination: key points

- Height or length, arm span, upper and lower body lengths.
- Limb shortening. Is it predominantly proximal (rhizomelic)?
- Asymmetry of limb shortening (XL CDP).
- Scoliosis.
- Congenital contractures.
- Flat nasal bridge/nasal hypoplasia (more severe in XLR CDP and acquired embryopathies).
- Cataracts.
- Hyperkeratosis and ichthyosis. Patchy or generalized?
- Alopecia (patchy in XLD CDP).
- Hands (hypoplasia of the distal phalanges in XLR CDP and warfarin embryopathy).
- Neurological signs of spinal stenosis.

Special investigations

- Full radiological survey including lateral of foot. Look for other characteristic features, e.g. vertebral coronal clefts in RCDP, hypoplasia of distal phalanges in XLR CDP, and warfarin embryopathy. These additional diagnostic features are important in children of age 3 years and over when the stippling may no longer be seen. Patterns of stippling are characteristic for different disorders.
- Abnormalities of plasmalogen biosynthesis such as elevated phytanic acid.
- Very-long-chain fatty acids (VLCFAs; Zellweger syndrome).
- Sterol analysis: elevation of 8-dehydrocholesterol and 8(9)-cholestenol in XLD CDP. Elevated 7-dehydrocholesterol in Smith–Lemli–Opitz (SLO) syndrome.
- Arylsulphatase E analysis.
- DNA for diagnostic testing or storage.
- Cytogenetic. Particularly to exclude deletions of Xp. Consider fluorescent *in situ* hybridization (FISH) for steroid sulphatase or *SHOX* as these are located close to *ARSE* and may be involved in a contiguous gene sequence.
- Investigation of mother for SLE (antinuclear factor (ANF) and antibodies to double-stranded DNA).

Classification of the various types of CDP. (Modified from International Working Group on Constitutional Diseases of Bone (1998).)

Diagnosis*	Inheritance	MIM no.†	Chromosome	Gene
Rhizomelic CDP				
Type 1	AR	215100	6q22–q24	PEX7
Type 2	AR	222765	1q42	DHPAT
Type 3	AR	600121	2q31	AGPS
CDP				
Conradi–Hünermann type	XLD	302960	Xp11.23–11.22	EBP
XLR type (brachytelephalangic)	XLR	302940 302950	Xp22.3	ARSE
Tibia–metacarpal type	AD	118651		
CHILD (limb-reduction–icthyosis)	XLD	308050	Xq28	NSDHL
HEM (Greenberg dysplasia)	AR	215140	1q42	LBR
Dappled diaphyseal dysplasia	AR			

* CHILD, Congenital hemidysplasia–ichythiosiform erythroderma–limb defects; HEM, hydrops–ectopic calcification–moth-eaten appearance.
† MIM, Mendelian Inheritance in Man (database).

Some diagnoses to consider

Rhizomelic chondrodysplasia punctata (RCDP). This is divided into three types. Classical RCDP is associated with mutation in *PEX7* that encodes peroxin 7. There is a correlation between low gene activity and a more severe clinical phenotype. Congenital contractures, typical facial features, symmetrical, predominantly proximal limb shortening, and cataracts. Failure to thrive, developmental delay, and seizures become apparent in the first year.

X-linked chondrodysplasia punctata.

- **XLR** (ARSE deficiency, brachytelephalangic). Males are affected. The nose is very flat and there is hypoplasia of the distal phalanges. The condition is caused by mutations in *ARSE* leading to arylsulphatase E deficiency. In children with additional features, consider a contiguous gene deletion syndrome of Xp22.
- **XLD** (Conradi–Hunnerman or Conradi–Hunnerman–Happle syndrome). Asymmetry of limb involvement is a useful diagnostic feature. Scoliosis can be a serious problem. Most affected females have hair and skin signs, which are patchy in keeping with X-inactivation. The condition can be confirmed by sterol analysis: there is elevation of 8 dehydrocholesterol and 8(9)-cholestenol. The gene, *EPB*, is at Xp11.

Autosomal dominant (AD) CDP (tibia–metacarpal type). In adults the radiological features show improvement compared to early films. Surveillance required for spinal stenosis.

Binder syndrome. The main feature is a hypoplastic nose with flattening of the tip and alae nasi and relative prognathism. There is debate as to whether this is a distinct entity, or if it represents the adult phenotype of milder forms of CDP.

CHILD syndrome (congenital hemidysplasia–ichthiosiform erythroderma–limb defects). An XLD disorder with clinical similarities to XLD CDP; indeed some patients originally thought to have CHILD had mutation in *EPB*. CHILD syndrome has been found to be due to mutation in NSDHL, another gene involved in cholesterol biosynthesis.

Zellweger syndrome. AR persoxisomal disorder often presenting in the neonatal period with central hypotonia ± seizures. The fontanelle is large and the forehead high. Punctate calcification is typically seen in the patellae. The stippled epiphyses are most commonly seen at the knees. See 'Floppy infant', page 118.

Smith–Lemli–Opitz (SLO) syndrome. Failure to thrive, microcephaly, hypospadias in males, and 2/3 toe syndactyly are important features. Stippled epiphyses are not a constant feature. See 'Hypospadias', page 142.

Stickler syndrome. There is no stippling in Stickler syndrome, but there may be some diagnostic difficulties as the facies of Stickler is similar to that of CDP. See 'Stickler syndrome', page 414.

Acquired embryopathies

Warfarin embryopathy. Warfarin and other coumarin derivatives are vitamin K antagonists that cross the placenta and, after exposure at 6–12/40 weeks gestation, can cause an embryopathy (CDP with nasal hypoplasia and/or stippled epiphyses). The nasal hypoplasia may be severe.

Maternal malabsorption leading to vitamin K deficiency. This can cause an embryopathy clinically indistinguishable from warfarin embryopathy.

Pseudo-warfarin embryopathy. This is due to an inborn deficiency of vitamin K epoxide reductase. Phenotype includes hypoplasia of the distal phalanges, which is a characteristic feature of XLR CDP due to arylsulphatase E deficiency, and helped establish that there is a common metabolic aetiology for XLR CDP, pseudo-warfarin embryopathy, and the acquired embryopathies.

Maternal SLE. This has been associated with a similar phenotype to that of warfarin embryopathy.

Genetic advice

Recurrence and offspring risk

If the cause of the stippling is unknown after careful investigation and expert analysis of the radiological features, consider:

- the possibility of mildly affected parents. X-rays of adults will not show stippling, but may show irregular bone growth;
- the need to investigate the mother for evidence of malabsorption or SLE;
- the adult asking for offspring risks may be unaware of his/her own mother's pregnancy history.

Carrier detection

Possible where there is a causative mutation, biochemical test, or radiological features.

Prenatal diagnosis

The two main techniques are ultrasound scan (USS) and chorionic villus sampling (CVS)/amniocentesis.

- Early prenatal testing may be possible using molecular or biochemical analysis.
- USS examination of the epiphyses combined with limb measurements may be used in pregnancies at risk due to maternal medication or SLE.

Natural history and further management (preventative measures)

- Arrange for on-going medical supervision with particular attention to the spine (scoliosis and spinal stenosis).
- **Rhizomelic CDP.** In the study of White *et al.* (2003), 90% survived to 1.5–2 years and 50% to 6–6.5 years. They discuss surveillance based on the medical complications of the children studied.

Support group: Many of the syndromes have their own support groups. See <www.cafamily.org.uk.>

Expert advisers: Ravi Savarirayan, Professor, Murdoch Children's Research Institute and Department of Paediatrics, University of Melbourne, Parkville, Victoria, Australia and Dian Donnai, Professor of Medical Genetics, University of Manchester, Manchester, England.

References

Hall JG, Pauli RM, Wilson KM. Maternal and fetal sequelae of anticoagulation therapy during pregnancy. *Am J Med* 1980; **68**: 122–40.

International Working Group on Constitutional Diseases of Bone. International nomenclature and classification of the osteochondrodysplasias. *Am J Med Genet* 1998; **79**: 376–82.

Savarirayan R, Boyle RJ, et al. Longterm follow up in chondrodysplasia punctata, tibia–metacarpal type, demonstrating natural history. Am J Med Genet 2004; **124A** (2): 148–57.

White AL, Modaff P, Holland-Morris F, Pauli RM. Natural history of rhizomelic chondrodysplasia punctata. *Am J Med Genet* 2003; **118A**: 332–42.

Cleft lip and palate

The development of the facial structures requires migration of cells and then fusion of adjacent areas. Clefts of the lip and palate occur at the place where this fusion naturally occurs. At ~7 weeks gestation the maxillary prominences on each sides of the face move into close proximity with the fused medial nasal prominences forming the labial grooves. Normally this groove is infilled by mesenchyme. When this process is impaired the labial groove persists and over time the thin residual tissue in the floor of the groove breaks down forming a complete unilateral cleft. Cleft palate occurs when there is failure of the mesenchymal masses in the lateral palatine processes to meet and fuse with each other, with the nasal septum, and/or with the posterior margin of the median palatine process. In the female, palatal processes fuse approximately 1 week later than in the male. Formation of the upper lip and palate is complete by 12 weeks gestation.

Cleft lip, with or without cleft palate is found in 1/700–1/1000 births. It is unilateral in 80%, with the left side more commonly affected, and bilateral in 20%. Males are more likely to have severe disease with alveolar (gum) and palatal involvement. There is a spectrum of abnormality ranging from a small notch in the upper lip lateral to the midline to a bilateral cleft extending up to the nostrils and into the gums and palate. Midline cleft lip is rare and may be a feature of oral-facial-digital (OFD) syndrome and Ellis van Creveld syndrome and holoprosencephaly.

Cleft palate occurs in 4 per 10 000 births. The spectrum goes from a bifid uvula, to submucous cleft palate (palatal mucosa intact but underlying muscle deficiency) with velopharyngeal insufficiency (regurgitation of milk through nose in babies and nasal speech in older children), to cleft soft palate, narrow V-shaped cleft, and, finally, wide U-shaped central cleft involving the hard palate.

Isolated midline cleft palate appears to represent a different malformation process to that of cleft lip and palate with different syndrome associations. We have attempted to show this by using the abbreviation CL/P for cleft lip and palate and CP for cleft palate.

In the majority of children the cleft is an isolated malformation. In the newborn surveys of Stoll, 37% of children born with clefts had an associated malformation (47% CP; 37% CL/P; 13% CL) and Milerad's figures were 22% with CP, 28% CL/P, and 8% in association with CL.

There are many syndromes that may have a cleft as a feature, and the aim of the clinic visit is to exclude these as far as possible prior to genetic counselling.

Pierre–Robin or Robin sequence: The Robin sequence is defined as a U-shaped palatal cleft in association with micrognathia and glossoptosis (retrodisplacement of the tongue in the pharynx) causing upper airway obstruction. It occurs with a frequency of 1/8500 births. In Robin sequence, micrognathia is present at the time that palate fusion is programmed to begin. Because of the mandibular anomaly, the tongue is not free to descend from between the vertical palatal shelves and prevents them from orientating horizontally and fusing in the midline. See 'Micrognathia and Robin sequence', page 174.

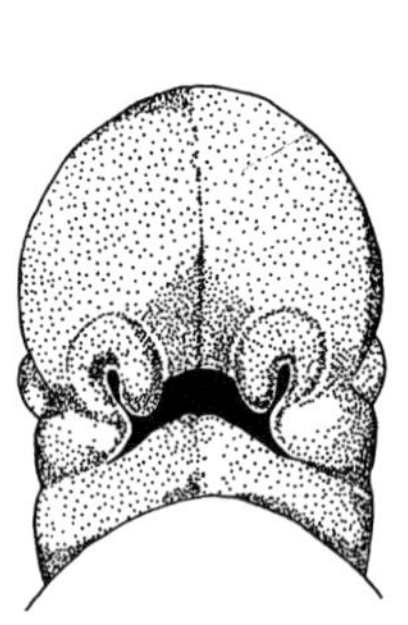
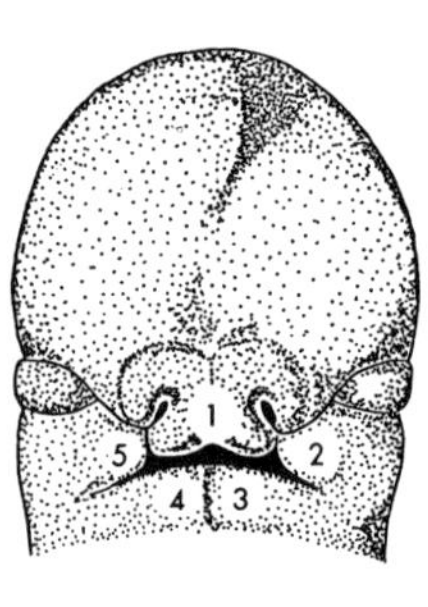
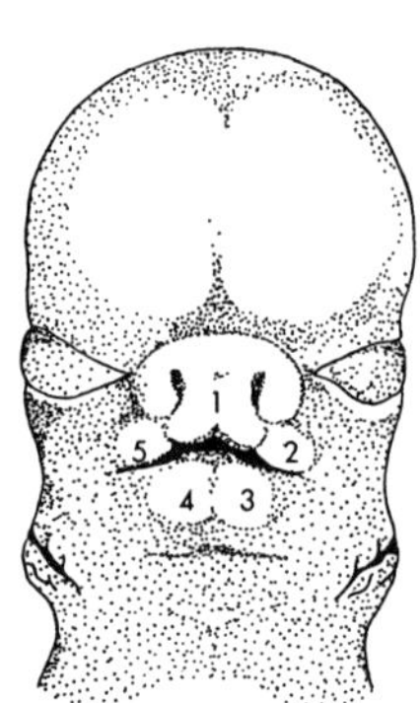
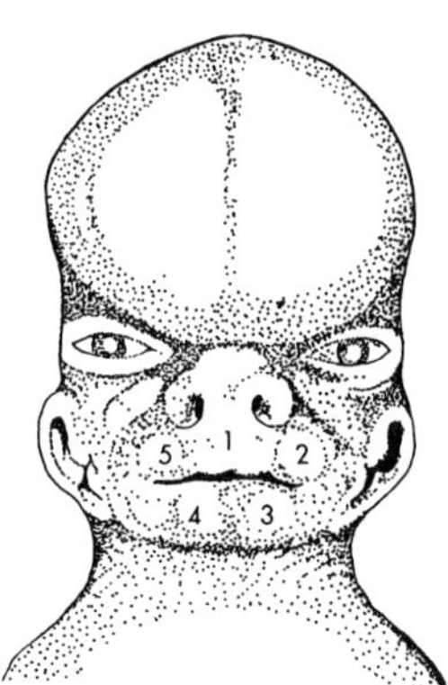

Schematic of facial features of embryos at stages 15 (33 days), 18 (45 days), 21 (52 days), and 23+ (60 days). The lip is a mosaic structure composed of the frontonasal (1), left maxillary (2), left mandibular (3), right mandibular (4), and right maxillary (5) processes. (Adapted from Tuchmann-Duplessis H, Haegel P: *Illustrated Human Embryology*, Vol 2. Springer-Verlag, New York, 1972, and from Patten BM: *Human Embryology*, ed 3. McGraw-Hill, New York, 1968.)

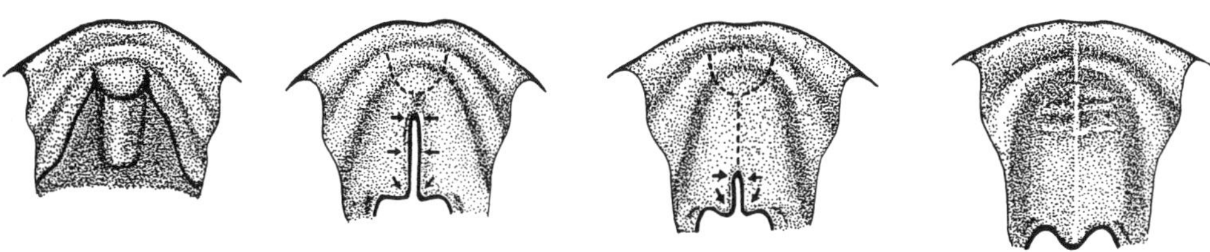

Schematic of closure of secondary palate. (Reprinted with permission from Moore KL: *The Developing Human*, ed 4. CV Mosby Co, St. Louis, 1988.)

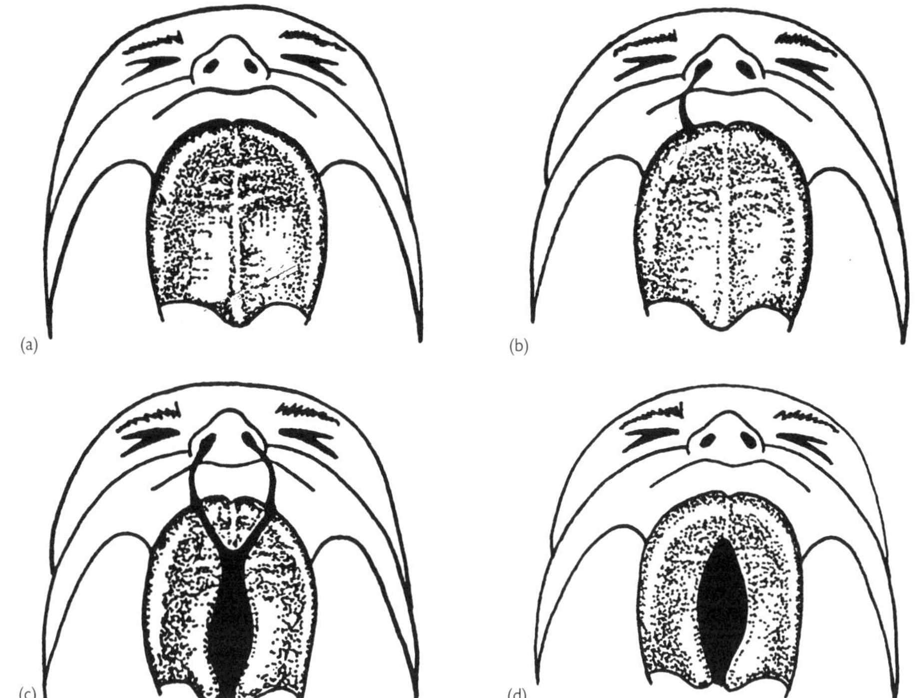

Schematics of various types cleft lip with and without cleft palate. Orientation is from the tongue looking upward.
(a) Normal (b) Unilateral cleft lip (c) Bilateral cleft lip and palate (d) Cleft palate.

Clinical approach

History: key points

- Three-generation family tree with specific enquiry about clefts and missing teeth.
- Pregnancy. Anticonvulsant medication, steroid treatment.
- Oligohydramnios (CP in Pierre–Robin or with micrognathia).
- Maternal diabetes.
- Vision (CP and myopia in Stickler syndrome).
- Delayed speech development and schooling difficulties (CP del 22q11).
- Hypocalcaemia, immune deficiency, cardiac abnomality (CP del 22q11).

Examination: key points

- **Stature** (short stature in 22q11, Stickler syndrome, bone dysplasia, e.g. Kniest)
- **Skeletal abnormalities** (skeletal dysplasias, otopalatodigital (OPD) syndrome).
- **Mouth:**
  - lip pits (CL/P and CP/van der Woude (VWS) syndrome, popliteal pterygium syndrome);
  - oral frenulae (OFD).
  - Ankyloglossia (X-linked cleft palate and ankyloglossia)
- **Face:**
  - 'pugilistic' facies (OPD);

- absent lacrimal punctae (ectrodactyly–ectodermal dysplasia–clefting (EEC) syndrome);
- flat midface (Stickler syndrome).
- **Chin.** Robin sequence (CP, Stickler syndrome, del(22q); spondyloepiphyseal dysplasia congenital type (SEDC); abnormal fetal position pushing the tongue up on to the developing palate).
- **Hands/feet:**
  - polydactyly (OFD syndromes, Smith–Lemli–Opitz (SLO) syndrome);
  - 'tree-frog' abnormality of the feet (OPD syndrome);
  - ectrodactyly (CL/P–ectrodactyly—EEC syndrome).
- **Limbs.** Contractures and webbing of knees, elbows (popliteal pterygium syndrome).
- **Heart.** Cardiac murmur/defects (22q11, other chromosomal conditions, SLO).
- **Genital anomalies** (SLO, popliteal pterygium syndrome).
- **Examine parents** for submucous cleft, bifid uvula, and lip pits.

Special investigations

- Routine chromosomes if CL/P or CP plus another abnormality.
- Fluorescent *in situ* hybridization (FISH) for del 22q11 for CP plus another abnormality or speech delay.
- Consider FISH for del 4p or 1q terminal deletions if cardiac defects are present.
- Skull and/or skeletal survey if indicated from examination or pedigree.
- 7 Dehydrocholesterol if any other features of SLO (e.g. growth deficiency, 2,3 syndactyly, cardiac defects, polydactyly, hypospadias).
- Cardiac echo if murmur present.
- Renal ultrasound scan (USS) in OFD syndrome.
- Ophthalmology assessment in children with possible Stickler syndrome.
- DNA for *IRF6* analysis in VWS, *p63* in EEC, MSX1 mutation analysis if autosomal dominant (AD) family history or family history of tooth agenesis and CL ± CP or for *TBX22* mutation analysis if X-linked (XL) CP with ankyloglossia.

Some diagnoses to consider

CL/P and CP are features of a large number of syndromes. Those listed below are selected because they are comparatively common and the presenting feature may be a cleft. In some individuals the other features may be quite subtle.

Van der Woude syndrome (VWS—CL/P and CP).

This is the most common syndromic form of CL/P and a condition where CL/P and CP can occur. It is a dominantly inherited condition caused in some families by mutations in the interferon regulatory factor 6 gene (*IRF6*). Mutation detection rate in IRF6 is ~50%. Between 30% and 50% represent new mutations. It is characterized by bilateral indentations on the lower lips known as lip pits. Some gene carriers have missing teeth. Penetrance ranges between 89% and 99%, but expression can be *very* variable within a family and gene carriers may have lip pits as the only manifestation of the condition. Risks for clefts are less than the genetic risks and this is an example of a condition where prenatal genetic testing would not accurately predict phenotype. Popliteal pterygium syndrome is allelic.

Stickler syndrome (CP). AD condition characterized by congenital and non-progressive myopia with abnormality of the vitreous gel, flat midface and depressed nasal bridge, midline clefting ranging from a cleft of the soft palate to Pierre–Robin sequence, deafness, and hypermobility in youth with early degenerative arthritis in older individuals. See 'Stickler syndrome', page 414.

22q del (CP). Conotruncal heart defects, cleft palate, or palatal insufficiency with nasal speech, speech delay, mild learning disability, immunodeficiency (usually mild), and hypocalcaemia in some. See '22q11 deletion syndrome', page 490.

Treacher–Collins syndrome (CP). AD due to mutations in *TCOF1 on* 5q31. Severe micrognathia, ear anomalies including microtia, conductive deafness, malar hypoplasia, inferior lid colobomata. See 'Micrognathia and Robin sequence', page 174.

Opitz syndrome (CL/P). X-linked recessive (XLR) due to mutations in *MID1*. Associated features include hypertelorism, hypospadias. See 'Ocular hypertelorism', page 196.

Kabuki syndrome is characterized by facial dysmorphism with long palpebral fissures and eversion of the lateral one-third of the lower lid, postnatal growth retardation. skeletal anomalies, mental retardation, and persistent fetal finger pads. Joint laxity, highly arched palate or cleft palate, dental anomalies, and recurrent otitis media are very common. Breast development in female infants is common. Congenital heart defects are seen in ~42% (Matsumoto).

Smith–Lemli–Opitz (SLO) syndrome (CP). The alveolar ridges are thickened. Prenatal onset growth deficiency, failure to thrive, microcephaly, postaxial polydactyly, small proximally placed thumbs, and Y-shaped 2,3 toe syndactyly. See 'Hypospadias', page 142.

X-linked cleft palate and ankyloglossia. X-linked semi-dominant disorder caused by mutations in the T-box transcription factor gene *TBX22* on Xq21 (Braybrook).

Ectrodactyly, ectodermal dysplasia, and clefting syndrome (EEC; CL/P). Due to mutations in *p63*. See 'Unusual hair, teeth, nails, and skin', page 256.

Non-syndromic CL/P due to MSX1. *MSX1* mutations are found in 2% of cases of non-syndromic CL/P (Jezewski *et al.* 2003) and should be considered in those families in which AD inheritance patterns or dental anomalies appear to be co-segregating with the clefting phenotype.

Genetic advice

Recurrence risk

Isolated cleft lip and palate. The aetiology of isolated clefts, when syndromes and dominant families have been excluded, is a combination of genetic and environmental factors. A number of candidate genes have been identified, some of which appear to play a major role in cleft development. Schliekelman estimates that 3–6 major genetic loci may contribute to clefting. *IRF6* plays a substantial role with an attributable risk of 12% (Zucchero). See the table for the recurrence risks.

Isolated cleft palate. Infants with CP are more likely to have associated malformations and syndromes than those with CL/P. Examine and investigate carefully to exclude these prior to counselling. See the table for the recurrence risk.

Recurrence risks for isolated **CL** and isolated **CL/P**

Relationship to index case	Recurrence risk (%)
Sibling unilateral CL	2–3
Sibling unilateral CL/P	4
Sibling bilateral CL/P	5–6
Two affected siblings	10
Affected sibling and parent	10*
Affected parent	4

* Consider dominant risks with reduced penetrance.

Recurrence risk for isolated **CP**

Relationship to index case	Recurrence risk (%)
Sibling	2–3
Affected parent	4

Older studies gave a 5–15% risk for offspring of an affected parent. This may not truly represent isolated cleft palate as some affected individuals may have a dominant condition or del(22q11) that would now be detected, and a lower risk is likely.

Cleft palate is difficult to detect on ultrasound scan (USS) in pregnancy. The small jaw of Pierre–Robin sequence can be visualized on specialist scanning.

Identified syndromal cause. Counsel as indicated

Carrier detection
Examine parents carefully for lip pits and a bifid uvula. If there is nasal speech, carefully examine for a submucous cleft palate and ensure that del(22q11) has been excluded.

Prenatal diagnosis
Prenatal detection of cleft lip is possible on USS at 20 weeks gestation. It may not be detected on routine obstetric scans and a small cleft may be missed even with expert scanning. Cleft palate is difficult to detect on USS in pregnancy. The small jaw of Pierre–Robin sequence may be visualized with specialist scanning.

Pre-conceptual folic acid
A recent case-control study has shown that periconceptual folate supplementation gave a 47% risk reduction in CL/P in the offspring when compared with no maternal folate supplementation (van Rooij). Currently there is conflicting evidence as to whether or not high-dose pre-conceptual folic acid (5 mg/day rather than the conventional 400 micrograms per day) further reduces the risk of clefting.

Natural history and further management

- **Feeding** is a priority in the neonatal period. Involvement of a specialist cleft team should ensure that appropriate support and advice is available with provision of specially adapted nipple shields and teats as required. Babies with Robin syndrome and significant upper airway obstruction may require nasogastric feeding initially. The nasogastric tube may be sufficient to stent the tongue forward and the airway open, allowing the baby to breathe and gain weight by nasogastric feeding for several days/weeks.
- **Surgery** is usually undertaken at 3 months of age for a primary repair of cleft lip, alveolus, and anterior palate and at 6–8 months of age for a primary repair of the posterior palate. Further palate surgery may be required later to optimize speech production.
- **Hearing.** Children with cleft palate have a high incidence of 'glue ear'.
- **Orthodontics.** Children with a cleft lip involving the alveolus often have missing teeth. Orthodontic treatment is not typically initiated until the early mixed dentition stage at 7–8 years of age.

Support group: Cleft Lip and Palate Association (CLAPA), <www.clapa.com>; American Cleft Palate–Craniofacial Association (ACPA), <www.cleftpalate-craniofacial.org>.

Expert adviser: late Robin Winter, previously Professor of Clinical Genetics and Dysmorphology, Institute of Child Health, London, England and David FitzPatrick, Consultant Clinical Geneticist, Western General Hospital, Edinburgh, UK.

References

Braybrook C, Dondney K *et al*. The T-box transcription factor gene TBX22 is mutated in X-linked cleft palate and ankyloglossia. *Nat Genet* 2001; **29**: 179–83.

Jezewski PA, Vieira AR, *et al*. Complete sequencing shows a role for MSX1 in non-syndromic cleft lip and palate. *J Med Genet* 2003; **40** (6): 399–407.

Matsumoto N, Niikawa N. Kabuki make-up syndrome: a review, *Am J Med Genet C* 2003; **117**: 57–65.

Schutte BC, Murray JC. The many faces and factors of orofacial clefts. *Hum Mol Genet* 1999; **8**: 1853–9.

Schliekelman P, Slatkin M. Multiplex relative risk and estimation of the number of loci underlying an inherited disease. Am J Hum Genet 2002; **71**: 1369-85

Shprintzen RJ. Robin sequence. In *Management of genetic syndromes* (ed. S.B. Cassidy and J.E. Allanson), Chapter 19. Wiley-Liss, New York, 2001.

Tolarova MM, Cervenka J. Classification and birth prevalence of orofacial clefts. *Am J Med Genet* 1998; **75**: 126–37.

van Rooij IA, Ocke MC, *et al*. Periconceptual folate intake by supplement and food intake reduces the risk of non-syndromic left lip with or without cleft palate. Prev Med 2004; **39**: 689–94.

Zucchero TM, Cooper ME, *et al*. Interferon regulatory factor 6 (*IRF6*) gene variants and the risk of isolated cleft lip and palate. *NEJM* 2004; **351**: 769–80.

Coarse facial features

The facial features appear thickened and heavy. The fleshy parts of the nose, the mouth, lips, and gums are enlarged There may be periorbital oedema. In disorders such as the mucopolysaccharidoses, the progressive coarsening is due to deposition of material in the tissues, but there are syndromal causes for which, at present, there is no metabolic explanation.

The history and photographic evidence are particularly important when dealing with a progressive condition, and to establish when the signs were first apparent.

One approach to this difficult diagnostic problem is to consider the following.

1 Have the investigations for known metabolic disorders been performed?

2 Do the features fit with any of the known presumed metabolic conditions that do not have a confirmatory test? Would additional investigations such as skeletal survey, histochemistry of skin biopsy be helpful?

3 Does the child have one of the syndromal causes of a coarse face such as Noonan syndrome?

Clinical approach

History: key points

- Three-generation family tree with specific enquiry for consanguinity (many of the conditions have recessive inheritance) and for ethnic background (many of the conditions are more common in certain areas, e.g. Salla disease in Finland).
- When were the facial features first considered coarse? Explain the term to the parents. Establish who first noticed the feature and if there has been progression.
- Development. Any slow down in progress or loss of skills?
- Visual difficulties.
- Hearing loss.
- Seizures. Are they becoming more difficult to control?
- Upper respiratory and respiratory infections (enlargement of tonsils and adenoids, tracheal involvement).
- Medication. Anti-epileptic medication can change the facial features and lead to gum hypertrophy.

Examination: key points

- **Growth parameters.** Height, weight, and occipital-frontal circumference (OFC). Children with storage disorders may develop macrocephaly.
- **Hair.** Coarse? Thick or sparse? Hypertrichosis and hirsuitism?
- **Face:**
  - describe the facial features carefully;
  - Are there horizontal creases of the ear lobules (Beckwith-Wiedemann syndrome (BWS))?
- **Mouth.** Is there gum hypertrophy?
- **Skin.** Does it feel as though there is deposition of an abnormal metabolite in the subcutaneous layers? Is it stiff or ichthyotic? Are there any papillomas (Costello syndrome)? Is there acanthosis nigricans (Donohue syndrome)? Is there pigment in Blashko's lines (Pallister-Killian)?
- **Hands:**
  - contractures (storage disorders);
  - nail hypoplasia (Coffin–Siris syndrome).

- **Heart.** Is there a cardiac murmur?
- **Abdomen:**
  - enlargement of liver and spleen;
  - umbilical hernia (storage diseases and Beckwith syndrome).
- **Neurological examination.**
- **Eyes.** Fundi, for lesions such as cherry red spots, corneal clouding.

Special investigations

If the diagnosis seems likely on the basis of your examination, e.g. Hurler syndrome, then proceed directly to the confirmatory enzymatic and molecular analysis. If the diagnosis is uncertain start with baseline tests and then more targeted testing can follow on when these results are through. These children should be under the care of a paediatrician with an interest in metabolic conditions and investigations should be done under his or her guidance. The investigations here have a bias towards rarer conditions, of unknown aetiology, and syndromal causes, which are the usual reasons for the involvement of a geneticist in the diagnostic process.

- **Baseline:**
  - thyroid function;
  - urine metabolic screen (mucopolysaccharides, oligosaccharides, amino and organic acids);
  - plasma amino acids; basic biochemistry including creatine kinase (CK) and glucose;
  - vacuolated lymphocytes.
- **Photography** to document features over time—this can be valuable in determining whether there is progression.
- **Ophthalmology assessment.** Consider conjunctival biopsy for storage deposits.
- **Cranial magnetic resonance imaging (MRI) scan.** In practice, brain imaging is performed on most children to clarify diagnosis and prognosis.
- **White cell enzymes.** These need to arrive in the laboratory within a few hours. Please discuss your differential diagnosis with the lab so that the correct analyses are performed. Relatively large volumes are required.
- **Skeletal survey.** This is a useful investigation to assess if there are features of a storage disease such as abnormal bone modelling. A feature such as rib thickening may suggest a rare syndrome such as Cantu syndrome. (see 'Skeletal dysplasia', page 246, for list of films to arrange).
- **Skin biopsy.** To assess if there is deposition of an abnormal compound. Storage of tissue for possible future analysis. Also to investigate for Pallister–Killian syndrome (mosaic 12p tetrasomy).
- **Echocardiogram** to asses for cardiomyopathies and valvular abnormalities.
- **Abdominal ultrasound scan** (USS; organomegaly, renal enlargement, or structural abnormality).
- **Chromosome analysis.** Include specific fluorescent *in situ* hybridization (FISH) testing, e.g. for Williams syndrome 7q11.23 and Smith–Magenis syndrome (17p11.2). Also consider FISH for 1p36 cryptic deletions (facial features become coarser with age).
- **DNA** testing/storage.

- **Endocrine studies.** Insulin level if Donahue syndrome suspected.
- **Very long chain fatty acids (VLCFAs).**

Some diagnoses to consider
Confirmed metabolic conditions
- Mucopolysaccharide (MPS) disorders (typically present with glue ear, coarse facial features and finger contractures)
- Gangliosidoses
- Sialic acid storage diseases

With short stature
Noonan syndrome. Typically, pulmonary valve stenosis, peripheral pulmonary artery stenosis, or hypertrophic cardiomyopathy with short stature and characteristic facies (*PTPN11* mutations are found in ~40%). A stenotic and often dysplastic pulmonary valve is found in 20–50% of affected individuals. See page 402.

Williams syndrome. Microdeletion on 7q11.23, which encompasses the elastin gene (*ELN*). Congenital heart disease occurs in 80%. Infants and young children have peri-orbital fullness, bulbous nasal tip, long philtrum, wide mouth, full lips, full cheeks, and small widely spaced teeth. Older children and adults have a more gaunt appearance with coarser facial features. Very variable mental retardation, overfriendly personality, short attention span, and anxiety. See 'Congenital heart disease', page 84.

Smith–Magenis syndrome (SMS). Some patients have square, rather heavy facies and are short and obese with small hands and feet. They may have a history of hypotonia in infancy, developmental delay, behaviour disturbance (especially sleep), and sometimes food-searching behaviour. Some individuals with SMS have mutations in *RAI1*, a gene encompassed by the common 17p11.2 microdeletion.

Nicolaides–Baraitser syndrome. Seizures, sparse hair. X-ray and clinical abnormalities of the phalanges with brachydactyly and swelling of the interphalangeal (IP) joints.

Pallister–Killian syndrome (tetrasomy 12p). Individuals with Pallister–Killian syndrome are mosaic for an isochromosome of 12p that is present in skin fibroblasts but not in blood lymphocytes; hence skin biopsy is necessary to make the diagnosis. They tend to have coarse features, with a broad forehead, normal OFC, apparent hypertelorism, sagging cheeks, and a prominent full philtrum. There may be additional folds of skin around the neck. Hair seems sparse especially over the temporal areas. Birthweight is often normal or above average. Mental retardation is usually severe.

With failure to thrive
See 'Failure to thrive', page 116.

Donohue syndrome (leprechaunism). Autosomal recessive (AR) disorder due to mutations in the insulin receptor gene. Pre- and postnatal failure to thrive, hirsutism, aged face with thick lips and prominent ears, enlargement of breast and genitalia; acanthosis nigricans may be present. The serum insulin level is grossly elevated.

Costello syndrome. Macrosomia, coarse facial features, and cardiac defects usually presenting in the neonatal period or early infancy. With time, failure to thrive may supervene and papillomas develop around the nose and periorally. There are very characteristic wrinkled palms and ulnar deviation of the hands. See 'Failure to thrive', page 116.

With overgrowth
Beckwith–Wiedemann syndrome (BWS). Macrosomia, anterior abdominal wall defects, macroglossia, anterior ear lobe creases, and posterior helical pits. Complex genetics—see 'Beckwith–Wiedemann syndrome (BWS)', page 278.

Simpson–Golabi–Behmel (SGB) syndrome. X-linked recessive (XLR) disorder due to mutations in *glypican 3* (Xq26). Overgrowth is of prenatal onset and continues postnatally. Birthweight and birth OFC of affected males are usually both >97th centile. Other findings include hypertelorism, macroglossia, central groove of lower lip, supernumerary nipples, advanced bone age, vertebral segmentation defects, coarse facies in adults; most have normal IQ. May have cardiac/gastrointestinal malformations; refer for echo/electrocardiogram (ECG). Diagnostic overlap with BWS, but combination of minor facial anomalies, skeletal/hand anomalies, and supernumerary nipples only occurs in SGB. Small risk of Wilms tumour—consider periodic renal USS as for BWS, i.e. USS of kidneys, liver, and adrenals at 4-monthly intervals (triannually) until 8 years of age.

With severe developmental delay (without regression)
Coffin–Lowry syndrome. Mutation in the *Rsk-2* gene. The facial features become more pronounced with time and can also be recognized in some female carriers. Examine the hands as these are large and 'soft' with tapering of the distal phalanges. Scoliosis and kyphosis develop. X-rays of the hands, chest, and spine may help confirm the diagnosis.

Nicolaides–Baraitser syndrome. Seizures, sparse hair. X-ray and clinical abnormalities of the phalanges with brachydactyly and swelling of the IP joints.

With hypertrichosis
Coffin–Siris syndrome. A possibly AR malformation syndrome with sparse hair, coarse facial features, and nail hypoplasia, especially of the fifth finger. Carefully exclude chromosomal abnormalities.

Cantu syndrome. AR condition with slightly coarse facial features. Facial hair is abundant and there is generalized hypertrichosis. Growth and development are normal. Dilated cardiomyopathy may be a feature.

Genetic advice
Recurrence risk
When a diagnosis remains unknown, counselling is difficult. If there is clear progression of the signs and symptoms, an AR risk should be considered. When the condition is non-progressive and there are other malformations, the cause may be a syndrome with a lower risk of recurrence.

Carrier detection
This can be performed for some of the metabolic conditions by DNA and enzymatic methods. General population testing, i.e. for the partners of siblings of the parents, may not be possible.

Prenatal diagnosis
This can be offered to those parents in whom a diagnosis has been confirmed. Consult closely with the laboratory to ascertain the type of sample (direct or cultured chorionic villus sampling (CVS), amniocytes, etc.) that is required.

Natural history and further management (preventative measures)

Therapy such as enzymatic replacement therapy (ERT) and bone marrow transplant may be possible and these children should be under the care of a paediatrician to ensure up to date advice. ERT is currently under trial for mucopolysaccharide (MPS) I (Hurler), MPS II (Hunter), MPS VI, and infantile Pompe disease.

Support group contact: CLIMB (Children Living with Inherited Metabolic Diseases) <www.climb.org.uk>, 0870 770 0326; and <www.cafamily.org.uk.> The Society for Mucopolysaccharide Diseases Tel: 01494 434156 www.mpssociety.co.uk

Expert advisers: Robert Surtees, Professor of Paediatric Neurology, Institute of Child Health, London and Dian Donnai, Professor of Medical Genetics, University of Manchester, Manchester, England.

References

Gorlin R, *et al. Syndromes of the head and neck*, 4th edn. Oxford University Press, Oxford, 2001.

Clarke JTR. *A clinical guide to inherited metabolic diseases*, 2nd edn. Cambridge University Press, Cambridge, 2002.

Coloboma

A coloboma is a segmental ocular defect, most commonly a 'keyhole' deficiency in the iris. A typical coloboma arises from defective closure of the optic fissure during the sixth week post-conception. The line of closure of the primitive fissure is along the inferior and medial side of the optic cup; iris colobomata are usually seen in the inferior 6 o'clock position of the iris giving the pupil a 'keyhole' appearance. True colobomata only occur in this position. The gap or notch may be limited to the iris or may extend deeper and involve the ciliary body and retina. If the coloboma affects the retina, this may give rise to a visual field defect. Optic nerve involvement is associated with visual impairment.

Ocular (uveoretinal) colobomata occur in ~1/10 000 individuals. Ocular colobomata may be unilateral or bilateral and are most commonly seen in otherwise normal children. A family history is uncommon. Colobomata are a common finding in some chromosomal disorders and a number of dysmorphic syndromes.

Coloboma of the eyelid. Defects in the eyelid are seen in Treacher–Collins syndrome, Nager syndrome, and oculo-auriculovertebral (OAV) syndrome (Goldenhar)—see 'Ear anomalies', page 108. They also occur in some rare facial clefting syndromes and occasionally in amnion disruption sequence.

Clinical approach

History: key points

- Three-generation family tree with specific enquiry regarding coloboma and visual difficulties and renal failure.
- Developmental milestones.

Examination: key points

- Growth parameters including occipital-frontal circumference (OFC).
- Careful assessment for dysmorphic features.
- Look carefully for subtle microphthalmia.
- Detailed examination of both eyes by an ophthalmologist.
- Examine the ears carefully for pits/tags/abnormal morphology (CHARGE (coloboma–heart defects–atresia choanae–retardation of growth and/or development–genital defect–ear anomalies and/or deafness) association, cat-eye syndrome (CES), branchio-oculo-facial (BOF) syndrome).
- Examine for anal anomalies (CHARGE, CES).

Special investigations

- Arrange ophthalmological examination for parents (even in apparently sporadic cases). Subtle retinal colobomata may be easily missed by a non-specialist.
- Chromosome analysis—babies and young children or if there is associated developmental delay or other congenital anomalies. Consider 4p. Fluorescent *in situ* hybridization (FISH) if Wolf–Hirschorn syndrome is a possibility.
- DNA for mutation analysis or storage
- Consider renal function tests, e.g. plasma creatinine if optic nerve coloboma (renal-coloboma syndrome).

Some diagnoses to consider

CHARGE (coloboma – heart defects – atresia choanae – retardation of growth and/or development – genital defect – ear anomalies and/or deafness) syndrome. CHARGE has a prevalence of ~1/12,000. It is caused by mutation in the gene *CHD7* on 8q12 which acts in early embryonic development by affecting chromatin structure and gene expression (Vissers). Some children have a whole gene deletion (detection may require FISH or dosage sensitive analysis). Empiric data suggests that most are sporadic with a low recurrence risk (2–3%), but if a mutation is identified this risk can be clarified. Note that chromosomal imbalance can mimic CHARGE syndome—ensure high quality chromosome analysis including telomere screen/array-CGH in mutation negative individuals.

Cat-eye syndrome (CES). Anal anomalies (imperforate anus, anal atresia, or anteriorly placed anus), pre-auricular pits/tags, congenital heart defects, iris colobomata, renal anomalies, and variable learning disability. Only 41% of CES patients have the combination of iris coloboma, anal anomalies, and pre-auricular anomalies (Berends *et al.* 2001). The remainder of CES patients are hard to recognize by their phenotype alone. Mild to moderate mental retardation is found in 32%; mental retardation occurs more frequently in male CES patients. There is no apparent phenotypic difference between mentally retarded and mentally normal CES patients. CES results from a small marker chromosome containing a duplication of 22q11 resulting in tetrasomy 22q11. It can be an unbalanced product of the relatively common 11q23;22q11 reciprocal translocation.

Kabuki syndrome. Kabuki (Niikawa–Kuroki) syndrome is associated with growth retardation, developmental delay, congenital heart disease, cleft palate, and characteristic facial features. The incidence of coloboma is greatly increased in Kabuki syndrome. Phenotypic overlap, including congenital heart, ear, and renal defects, can lead to the misdiagnosis of CHARGE association, especially since the typical facial features of Kabuki syndrome may not be apparent in early infancy (Ming *et al.* 2003). See 'Ptosis, blepharophimosis, and other eyelid anomalies', page 224.

4p–(Wolf–Hirschorn syndrome) is characterized by low birthweight and postnatal failure to thrive, microcephaly, developmental delay, and hypotonia. There is a characteristic facial appearance with sagging everted lower eyelids, a 'Greek-helmet' profile, a short nose, and very short philtrum. Patients may have iris colobomata. Seizures are common. Some have a visible deletion with varying breakpoints on 4p; others have a cryptic deletion requiring FISH to make the diagnosis.

Colobomatous microphthalmia. Mild degrees of microphthalmia are difficult to detect. This has been reported in families so consider the possibility of autosomal dominant (AD) inheritance with variable penetrance. A novel mutation in the sonic hedgehog gene (*SHH*) has recently been reported in one family with non-syndromic colobomatous microphthalmia (Schimmenti *et al.* 2003).

Focal dermal hypoplasia (Goltz syndrome). X-linked dominant (due to mutations in, or deletions encompassing, the *PORCN* gene at Xp11.23). Areas of focal dermal hypoplasia may be found on the trunk and limbs, where there may be fat herniation through the skin deficiency. The eyes are frequently affected, mostly asymmetrically, with chorioretinal or iris colobomata, but unilateral anophthalmos has been reported.

Branchio-oculo-facial syndrome (BOF; haemangiomatous branchial clefts). An AD condition with distinctive areas of thin, erythematous wrinkled skin in the neck or infra/supraauricular regions in addition to craniofacial, auricular, ophthalmologic (coloboma of the iris and/or retina), and oral anomalies. Some phenotypic overlap with branchio-oto-renal (BOR) syndrome since both can have nasolacrimal duct stenosis, deafness, prehelical pits, malformed pinna, and renal anomalies, but the two conditions are not allelic.

Renal coloboma syndrome (papillorenal syndrome). An AD condition caused by mutations in *PAX2* characterized by colobomata of the optic nerve (and occasionally retina) together with renal anomalies (vesicoureteral reflux (VUR) and renal hypoplasia with loss of corticomedullary differentiation). Ophthalmic and renal characteristics of the renal coloboma syndrome are highly variable. The need for dialysis or renal transplantation can occur early in life or several years later. A wide range of ocular abnormalities located in the posterior segment can be observed. Mild optic disc dysplasia or pit have no functional consequence and can be underdiagnosed. More severe colobomata or related abnormalities, such as morning glory anomaly, often lead to poor visual acuity.

Aicardi syndrome. Optic nerve colobomata, retinal lacunae, central nervous system (CNS) abnormalities, and seizures. X-linked dominant.

Genetic advice

Recurrence risk

Isolated bilateral colobomata of the iris may follow an AD pattern of inheritance. The empiric recurrence risk is ~10% (~5% if the parents have a normal ocular examination) (Morrison).

Carrier detection

Careful ophthalmological examination of parents is essential.

Prenatal diagnosis

If the proband has a chromosomal disorder or a single gene mutation, prenatal diagnosis by chorionic villus sampling (CVS) or amniocentesis is possible.

Natural history and further management (preventative measures)

Chorioretinal colobomata are associated with a significant risk of rhegmatogenous retinal detachment. Retinal tears can occur in the thinned retina overlying the colobomatous defect. Lens colobomata may also be associated with giant retinal tears. Children with large defects should be under the care of a paediatric ophthalmologist.

Support group contact: MACS (Micro and Anophthalmic Children's Society) <www.macs.org.uk>, tel: 0870 600 6227.

Expert adviser: David FitzPatrick, Consultant Clinical Geneticist, Western General Hospital, Edinburgh, Scotland.

References

Berends MJ, Tan-Sindhunata G, *et al.* Phenotypic variability of cat-eye syndrome. *Genet Couns* 2001; **12** (1): 23–34.

Dureau P, Attie-Bitach T, *et al.* Renal coloboma syndrome. *Ophthalmology* 2001; **108** (10): 1912–16.

Ford B, Rupps R, *et al.* Renal-coloboma syndrome: prenatal detection and clinical spectrum in a large family. *Am J Med Genet* 2001; **99**: 137–41.

Lin AE, Semina EV, *et al.* Exclusion of the branchio-oto-renal syndrome locus (EYA1) from patients with branchio-oculo-facial syndrome. *Am J Med Genet* 2000; **91** (5): 387–90.

Ming JE, Russell KL, *et al.* Coloboma and other ophthalmologic anomalies in Kabuki syndrome: distinction from charge association. *Am J Med Genet* 2003; **123A** (3): 249–52.

Morrison, *et al.* A national study of microphthalmia, coloboma and anophthalmia in Scotland. *J Med Genet* 2002; **39**: 16–22.

Schimmenti LA, de la Cruz J, *et al.* Novel mutation in sonic hedgehog in non-syndromic colobomatous microphthalmia. *Am J Med Genet* 2003; **116A** (3): 215–21.

Stoll C, Viville B, *et al.* A family with dominant oculoauriculovertebral spectrum. *Am J Med Genet* 1998; **78** (4): 345–9.

Vissers LE, van Ravenswaajj CM, *et al.* Mutations in a new member of the chromodomain gene family cause CHARGE syndrome. *Nat Genet* 2004; **36**: 955–57.

Congenital heart disease

Structural heart malformations (see table for nomenclature) occur in 7/1000 livebirths (0.7%). An echocardiogram is the single most useful investigation to define the cardiac anatomy.Most commonly, congenital heart disease (CHD) occurs as an isolated finding in an otherwise normal individual. However, CHD can occur as part of an enormous number of chromosomal disorders or specific syndromes, or as a consequence of teratogenic exposure. Where a second anomaly is identified, this should increase the chance of making a specific diagnosis.

The task of the geneticist is to determine whether the CHD is:

1 isolated;

2 isolated, but with a significant family history (other close relatives with similar CHD);

3 syndromic;

4 chromosomal;

5 the result of a teratogenic exposure or maternal illness (see tables).

Clinical approach

History: key points

- Three-generation family tree with special note of CHD and neonatal or infant deaths.

- History of twinning (monozygotic (MZ) twins have a ~threefold excess risk for CHD compared with singletons; dizygotic (DZ) twins have a slight excess risk, ~1.3-fold).
- History of alcohol or drug exposure in pregnancy (e.g. anticonvulsants or lithium).
- History of chronic maternal illness (e.g. maternal diabetes, maternal phenylketonuria (PKU); maternal systemic lupus erythematosus (SLE) may cause congenital heart block).
- History of maternal infection (e.g. rubella).
- History of prematurity (patent ductus arteriosus (PDA)), birth, and subsequent development.

Examination: key points

- Growth parameters. Height, weight, and occipital-frontal circumference (OFC). Abnormal growth parameters raise concerns that the cardiac defect is not isolated, provided the infant/child is not in heart failure or cyanosed which may both cause failure to thrive.
- Assess index case carefully for any dysmorphic features, or facies suggestive of Noonan, Williams, Turner, 22q, trisomies, etc.

Nomenclature

ASD	Atrial septal defect
AVSD	Atrioventricular septal defect (AV canal defect)—an endocardial cushion defect. 76% are syndromic (e.g. Down syndrome). A 'complete AVSD' involves underdevelopment of the lower part of the atrial septum and the upper part of the ventricular septum with a single common AV valve resulting in unrestricted communication between the atria and ventricles. A 'partial AVSD' or 'ostium primum ASD' has a deficiency of the atrial septum. Defects of the inlet muscular ventricular septum and isolated cleft mitral valve are also part of the clinical spectrum
Coarct	Coarctation of the aorta
DORV	Double-outlet right ventricle (aorta lies predominantly over the right ventricle)
Fallot's tetralogy	Aorta overriding a VSD with RVOT (e.g. pulmonary stenosis) and RV hypertrophy
HLH	Hypoplastic left heart
MVP	Mitral valve prolapse
PDA	Patent ductus arteriosus (common in preterm infants)
PFO	Persistent foramen ovale
RVOT	Right ventricular outflow tract obstruction
SVAS	Supravalvular aortic stenosis
TAPVD	Total anomalous pulmonary venous drainage
TGA	Transposition of the great arteries
VSD	Ventricular septal defect

Teratogens and the risk of congenital heart disease

Alcohol (fetal alcohol syndrome)	Up to 25–30%	Mainly VSD and/or ASD; also Fallot's tetralogy
Anticonvulsants	1.8%	3-fold increased risk over baseline
Lithium	Small	Ebstein anomaly, tricuspid atresia, ASD
Retinoic acid	10–20%	Conotruncal heart defects
Rubella	35%	PDA, peripheral pulmonary artery stenosis, septal defects

Maternal illness and the risk of congenital heart disease*

Maternal diabetes	3–5%	VSD, coarct, TGA, truncus arteriosus, tricuspid atresia, and a variety of other defects including L isomerism sequence
Maternal phenylketonuria (PKU)	~15%	Fallot's tetralogy, coarctation of aorta
Maternal systemic lupus erythematosus (SLE)	20–40%	Complete heart block

* See 'Maternal diabetes mellitus and diabetic embryopathy' and 'Maternal phenylketonuria (PKU)', pages 612 and 614.

- Assess index case for nasal speech, submucous palate (22q deletion).
- Examine index case for limb anomalies, e.g. hypoplastic thumb and thenar eminence (Holt-Oram), radial ray defects (VACTERL and Fanconi), or polydactyly (Ellis–van Creveld).
- Examine both parents. Detailed clinical examination of the cardiovascular systems of both parents

Special investigations
- Karyotype for all complex defects, or if any accompanying learning disability or congenital anomaly. (Consider telomere screen (and microarray/comparative genomic hybridization (CGH)) if there is developmental delay and dysmorphism.)
- 22q11 fluorescent *in situ* hybridization (FISH) for all outflow tract anomalies, e.g. Fallot's, truncus arteriosus, interrupted aortic arch, also pulmonary atresia/stenosis, tricuspid atresia, transposition of the great arteries (TGA), vascular rings, aberrant major vessels, e.g. right-sided aorta. Ventricular septal defect (VSD) is common in 22q11 deletion but, since VSD is such a common anomaly, pick-up rate would be tiny in apparently normal children with isolated VSD. Atrial septal defect (ASD) and PDA also occur in 22q but, as above, a 22q screen is not usually indicated in otherwise normal children.
- Echocardiogram and electrocardiogram (ECG) for parent if any abnormality noted on cardiovascular history or examination; cardiological referral if abnormality detected.

Some diagnoses to consider (see table)

Trisomies. 40–50% of individuals with Down syndrome have a CHD, with perimembranous VSD the most common defect, followed by PDA and ASD. At least 90% of individuals with trisomy 18 have CHD, usually VSD with/without valve dysplasia. 80% of individuals with trisomy 13 have a cardiac malformation, e.g. ASD or VSD. See 'Down syndrome (trisomy 21)', 'Edwards syndrome (trisomy 18)' and 'Patau syndrome (trisomy 13)', pages 524, 526 and 534.

22q11 deletion. CHD with short stature, cleft palate, or velopharyngeal insufficiency (nasal speech) and speech delay may have low calcium, mild learning disability, and immunodeficiency (typically reduced T-cell subsets). The single most common cardiac anomaly amongst children with 22q is VSD. Aortic arch anomalies such as interrupted aortic arch or truncus arteriosus are characteristic. A significant proportion of children with Fallot's tetralogy have 22q11 deletions. See '22q11 deletion syndrome', page 490.

Chromosomal deletions/microdeletion with recognizable phenotypes. Examples are 4p– (Wolf–Hirschorn syndrome), 5p– (cri-du-chat), and del(1p36). See 'Deletions and duplications' and 'Submicroscopic chromosomal rearrangements and the chromosomal phenotype', pages 520 and 546.

Noonan syndrome. Typically, pulmonary valve stenosis, peripheral pulmonary artery stenosis, or hypertrophic cardiomyopathy with short stature and characteristic facies. (*PTPN11* mutations are found in ~40%.) A stenotic and often dysplastic pulmonary valve is found in 20–50% of affected individuals. 7% of children with pulmonary stenosis have Noonan syndrome. See page 402.

Smith–Lemli–Opitz (SLO). Cardiac defects are present in just <40%, especially atrioventricular septal defect (AVSD) and total anomalous pulmonary venous drainage (TAPVD). Prenatal and postnatal growth deficiency, developmental delay (almost all), cleft palate (37–52%), hypospadias and/or cryptorchidism (90–100%) in affected males, Y-shaped 2,3 toe syndactyly (>95%), and postaxial polydactyly (~50%). Facial features include: narrow bifrontal diameter, ptosis (50%), down-slanting palpebral fissures, and a short nose with depressed nasal bridge and anteverted nares. See 'Hypospadias', page 142.

Turner syndrome (45, X). CHD occurs in 17–45%. Coarctation of the aorta and bicuspid aortic valve or other aortic valve anomaly, e.g. stenosis. See 'Turner syndrome, 45, X and variants', page 558.

Williams syndrome. Microdeletion on 7q11.23 which encompasses the elastin gene (*ELN*). CHD occurs in 80%: 75% have supravalvular aortic stenosis (SVAS) and ~25% have a discrete supravalvular pulmonary stenosis. Peripheral pulmonic stenosis is found in 50–75% of infants, but improves with time. The elastin anomaly is generalized and almost any artery can be narrowed, e.g. renal artery stenosis (40%). Aortic insufficiency (20%) and mitral valve prolapse (MVP; 15%) may occur in some adults. As to characteristic facial features, infants and young children

Congenital heart disease with dysmorphic features, developmental delay, or other congenital anomalies—syndromic diagnoses to consider

VSD	Perimembranous VSD is the most common cardiac defect seen in Down; VSD is also common in trisomy 18 and trisomy 13. Also seen in del 22q11, fetal alcohol syndrome (FAS), maternal diabetes
ASD	Down, trisomy 13, FAS
AVSD	60% have Down syndrome; next most common is isomerism sequence; also Smith–Lemli–Opitz, Smith–Magenis, Ellis–van Creveld, CHARGE syndrome, hydrolethalus, Kaufman–McKusick, Holt–Oram, 3C syndrome (craniocerebellocardiac syndrome), oral–facial–digital (OFD) II (Mohr syndrome), and 3p– syndrome
Aortic stenosis	Williams syndrome (supravalvular aortic stenosis), Turner syndrome
Coarctation of aorta	Turner syndrome, Kabuki syndrome
Ebstein/tricuspid valve	del 1p36
Fallot's tetralogy	del 22q11, Alagille syndrome
Interrupted aortic arch	del 22q11
Pulmonary stenosis	Noonan syndrome, Nf-Noonan syndrome, Williams (supravalvular PS), del 22q11
Peripheral pulmonary artery stenosis	Williams, Alagille
Truncus arteriosus	del 22q11

have periorbital fullness, bulbous nasal tip, long philtrum, wide mouth, full lips, full cheeks, and small widely spaced teeth; older children and adults have a more gaunt appearance with coarser facial features. Developmental delay with very variable mental retardation from severe to low-average with most having mild mental retardation, strengths in language but poor visuospatial skills, over-friendly personality, short attention span, and anxiety. Approximately 15% of infants have hypercalcaemia.

Alagille syndrome. Caused by haploinsufficiency of *JAGGED1* on 20p11.2–20p12. Characterized by hypoplasia of the intrahepatic bile ducts (often presenting with prolonged neonatal jaundice). Approximately 90% have single or multiple areas of peripheral pulmonary artery stenosis, and ~ one-third have other cardiac malformations, especially Fallot's tetralogy. Other features include butterfly vertebrae and posterior embryotoxon (slit-lamp examination). Facial features are subtle with a prominent forehead, deep-set eyes, and long nose; adults have a prominent chin. See 'Prolonged neonatal jaundice and jaundice in infants below 6 months', page 220.

Holt–Oram syndrome. AD heart–hand syndrome caused by mutations in TBX5. Penetrance is 100%. *Cardiac defects* include ASD (34%), VSD (25%), MVP (7%), with ECG changes only in 39% (long PR interval, bradycardia, and left or right axis deviation being the most frequent). Pectus deformity occurs in 40%. Cardiac defects (including minimal ECG changes) occur in 95%. *Skeletal defects* affect the upper limbs exclusively and are invariably bilateral and usually asymmetrical. They range from clinodactyly, limited supination, and narrow, sloping shoulders to absent, hypoplastic, or triphalangeal thumb and severe reduction deformities of the upper arm (4.5%). See 'Radial ray defects and thumb hypoplasia', page 228.

Kabuki syndrome. Characterized by facial dysmorphism with long palpebral fissures and eversion of the lateral one-third of the lower lid, postnatal growth retardation, skeletal anomalies, mental retardation, and persistent fetal finger pads. Joint laxity, highly arched palate or cleft palate, dental anomalies, and recurrent otitis media are very common. Breast development in female infants is common.

CHD are seen in ~42% (Matsumoto *et al.* 2003). Aortic coarctation, ASD, and VSD are the most common defects (Digilio *et al.* 2001).

VACTERL (vertebral defects–anal atresia–cardiac anomalies–tracheo-oesophageal fistula–(o)esophageal atresia– renal anomalies–limb defects) association. Secure diagnosis requires at least one anomaly in each of the three anatomical domains (limb, thorax, and pelvis/lower abdomen), and at least two anomalies in each of two domains for a probable diagnosis. Sporadic with a low recurrence risk (2–3%).

CHARGE (coloboma – heart defects – atresia choanae – retardation of growth and/or development – genital defect – ear anomalies and/or deafness). CHARGE syndrome (coloboma–heart defects etc...) is caused by heterozygous mutations of the *CHD7* gene on 8q12.N. 50% of affected individuals have congenitial heart disease eg. ASD, AVSD. See 'Colomboma', page 82.

Isomerism sequence. See 'Laterality disorders including heterotaxy and isomerism', page 148.

Genetic advice

Isolated heart malformations are usually sporadic, but occasionally particular defects can be shown to be inherited as a simple Mendelian trait. The risks quoted in the table are not appropriate in the latter case, when advice should be given according to the apparent inheritance in the family, with reference to Online Mendelian Inheritance in Man (OMIM).

Prenatal diagnosis

Fetal echocardiography can be used for antenatal diagnosis of most complex CHD (not TGA) with scans at 14, 19, and 22 weeks gestation.

Pre-conceptual folic acid

Currently there is conflicting evidence as to whether or not high-dose pre-conceptual folic acid (5 mg/day rather than the conventional 400 micrograms per day) reduces the risk of CHD. The higher dose is of unproven benefit.

Recurrence risk for isolated non-syndromic defects (after Burn and Goodship 2001)
In general the risks are greater in the offspring of affected mothers (overall risk 6.5%) than in the offspring of affected fathers (overall risk 2.2%).

Cardiac malformation	Risk in siblings (%)	Risk in offspring (%)*
Situs inversus (check for Kartagener)	3	
Isomerism sequence—non-syndromic	5–10	
Tricuspid atresia	1	
Mitral atresia	2	
Transposition of great arteries	2	
Truncus arteriosus	1	
Pulmonary atresia	1	
Secundum ASD	3	
AVSD	2	7.7 (m); 7.9 (f)
Ebstein anomaly (check for fetal exposure to lithium)	1	
VSD	3	
Pulmonary stenosis	2	
Tetralogy of Fallot	2	1.6 (m); 4.7 (f)
Aortic stenosis	3	
Coarctation of aorta	2	
Patent ductus arteriosus (PDA)	2.5	
Hypoplastic left heart	Low (1/77 in Birmingham study)	

* (m), Risk to offspring of affected father; (f), risk to offspring of an affected mother.

Natural history and further management (preventative measures)

If an affected individual is contemplating pregnancy it may be appropriate to refer her to a GUCH (grown-up congenital heart disease) clinic or a cardiologist for assessment prior to pregnancy. Also offer prenatal diagnosis by fetal echocardiography. Note increased miscarriage in mothers with CHD (20% with maternal proband, compared with 10% with paternal proband).

Lay group contact: Children's Heart Federation <www.childrens-heart-fed.org.uk>; Grown up Congenital Heart Patients' Association <www.guch.demon.co.uk>.

Expert adviser: Judith Goodship, Professor of Medical Genetics, University of Newcastle, Newcastle-upon-Tyne, England.

References

Burn J, Goodship J. Congenital heart disease. In *Emery and Rimoin's principles and practice of medical genetics*, 4th edn (ed. D. Rimoin), pp. 1239–326. Churchill Livingstone, Edinburgh, 2001.

Burn J, *et al.* Recurrence risks in offspring of adults with major heart defects. *Lancet* 1998; **351**: 311–15.

Digilio MC, Marino B, *et al.* Congenital heart defects in Kabuki syndrome. *Am J Med Genet* 2001; **100** (4): 269–74.

Eldadal ZA, Hamosh A, *et al.* Familial tetralogy of Fallot caused by mutation in the jagged 1 gene. *Hum Mol Genet* 2001; **10**: 163–9.

Goldmuntz E, Bamford R, *et al.* CFC1 mutations in patients with transposition of the great arteries and double-outlet right ventricle. *Am J Hum Genet* 2002; **70**: 776–80.

Matsumoto N, Niikawa N. Kabuki make-up syndrome: a review. *Am J Med Genet* 2003; **117C** (1): 57–65.

Robinson SW, Morris CD, *et al.* Missense mutations in *CRELD1* are associated with cardiac atrioventricular septal defects. *Am J Hum Genet* 2003; **72**: 1047–52.

Sanlaville D, Romana SP, *et al.* A CGH study of 27 patients with CHARGE association. *Clin Genet* 2002; **61** (2): 135–8.

Seminars in Medical Genetics. Heart Development and the genetic aspects of cardiovascular malformations. *Am J Med Genet* 2000; **97C** (4).

Wren C, Birrell G, *et al.* Cardiovascular malformations in infants of diabetic mothers. *Heart* 2003; **89**: 1217–20.

Corneal clouding

Corneal clouding is opacification of the cornea. It is a sign of several different systemic disorders, many of which are inherited metabolic conditions. Corneal clarity is maintained by the endothelium, which functions abnormally in the endothelial dystrophies leading to corneal opacification. The corneal dystrophies are classified according to the corneal layer which is predominantly affected. The cornea has 5 layers: epithelium (outermost), Bowman's membrane, stroma, Descemet's membrane and endothelium (innermost). The geneticist may be asked for advice during the diagnostic process, in particular to consider rare conditions of unknown aetiology and syndromic causes of corneal clouding.

Clinical approach

History: key points

- Family history. At least three generations, consider all forms of autosomal inheritance and with specific enquiry for consanguinity.
- Exposure to teratogens, and infections during pregnancy.
- Growth (syndromic conditions).
- Developmental progress. Evidence of loss of skill/ regression (metabolic disorders)?
- Polyuria, polydipsia, renal disease (cystinosis).

Examination: key points

- Eyes. Ophthalmological confirmation and examination with fundoscopy for lesions such as cherry red spots (mucolipidoses). It is essential to exclude glaucoma.
- Head circumference. Macrocephaly in storage disorders.
- Height. Assess for disproportion.
- Hands. Contractures (storage disorders, Winchester syndrome).
- Hair. Coarse? Thick or sparse? Hypertrichosis and hirsuitism?
- Skin. Does it feel as though there is deposition of an abnormal metabolite in the subcutaneous layers? Is it stiff or ichthyotic?
- Cardiac murmur.
- Enlargement of liver and spleen, umbilical hernia (storage diseases).
- Nail hypoplasia (Fryn syndrome).
- Neurological examination.

Special investigations

If a diagnosis seems likely on the basis of your examination, e.g. Hurler syndrome, then proceed directly to the confirmatory enzymatic and molecular analysis. If the diagnosis is uncertain start with baseline tests and then more targeted testing can follow on when these results are through.

- Baseline: thyroid function; urine metabolic screen (mucopolysaccharides, oligosaccharides, amino and organic acids); plasma amino acids; basic biochemistry; vacuolated lymphocytes.
- Congenital infection screen.
- White cell enzymes. These need to arrive in the laboratory within a few hours. Please discuss your differential diagnosis with the laboratory so that the correct analyses are performed.
- Skeletal survey. This is a useful investigation to assess if there are features of a storage disease such as abnormal

bone modelling or if there are features of a skeletal dysplasia.
- Very long chain fatty acids (VLCFAs).
- Abdominal ultrasound scan (USS; organomegaly, renal enlargement, or structural abnormality).
- Chromosome analysis in infants and children with malformations or mental retardation.
- DNA testing/storage.
- Skin or muscle biopsy to assess if there is deposition of an abnormal compound. Storage of tissue for possible future analysis.

Some diagnoses to consider
Congenital

- Structural malformation of the eye (see particularly 'Microphthalmia and anophthalmia' and 'Anterior segment eye malformations', pages 176 and 46).
- Fryn syndrome. A rare lethal autosomal recessive (AR) condition with nail/digital hypoplasia and diaphragmatic hernia.
- Zellweger syndrome. An AR disorder of peroxisome metabolism.
- Rare congenital corneal dystrophies. eg. congenital endothelial dystrophies (CHED) and congenital stromal dystrophy. CHED has AD and AR forms, CHED1 and CHED2 respectively. CHED2 is also called Maumenee corneal dystrophy. In view of the degree of corneal clouding in CHED, vision is often surprisingly good. CHED1 and CHED2 map to distinct loci on chromosome 20. Congenital stromal dystrophy can be caused by mutations in the decorin gene on 12q22 (Bedrup).
- Congenital infection and trauma.

Childhood

Arrange for thorough metabolic investigations.
- Mucopolysaccharidoses (MPS):
  - type I. Hurler, Hurler/Scheie and Scheie syndromes;
  - type II. Hunter syndrome;
  - type IV. Morquoi syndrome;
  - type VI. Maroteax–Lamy;
  - type VII. Sly;
  - but *not* type III. Sanfilippo.
- Mucoliposes (other eye findings include cherry-red spot).
- Cystinosis. AR. Check for renal and thyroid involvement
- Fabry disease, X-linked semi-dominant with manifestation in females. Mutation in the alpha-galactosidase A gene. In addition to a corneal dystrophy ('cornea verticillata') there are tortuous retinal vessels. The cutaneous signs are angiokeratoderma (vascular skin lesions) in a truncal distribution. Neuropathic pain with acroparaesthesia and abdominal pain, fatigue, autonomic dysfunction, and renal failure are additional features. Treatment with enzyme replacement therapy currently under clinical trial. See 'Hypertrophic cardiomyopathy (HCM)', page 360.
- Skeletal dysplasia.
- Winchester syndrome.

Adult-corneal dystrophy

The corneal dystrophies are bilateral, genetic, and usually slowly progressive conditions. Many manifest in adulthood.

They rarely present to the geneticist, but families may be seen in genetic eye clinics. Most are dominantly inherited and have a family history.
- Several clinical subtypes are caused by mutations in the *BIGH3* gene at 5q31. Fuchs endothelial dystrophy of the cornea (FCED) and posterior polymorphous dystrophy (PPCD) are AD disorders. Missense mutations in *COL8A2* (which may be 'de novo') are found in some individuals (Biswas).
- Check the precise type of dystrophy and inheritance prior to counselling.
- The disease may recur after corneal grafting.
- Most are limited to the cornea.
- Exclude Fabry disease and adult cystinosis.

Genetic advice

Recurrence risk
Dependent on the aetiology. For adult corneal dystrophy see above.

Carrier detection
- By ophthalmological examination (corneal dystrophy, Fabry disease).
- Is possible in families where a causative mutation has been identified also within families with enzyme deficiencies.

Prenatal diagnosis
- By chorionic villus sampling (CVS) or amniocentesis where there is molecular or biochemical confirmation of diagnosis.
- USS in mid-trimester for syndromes with structural abnormalities, e.g. Fryn syndrome.

Natural history and further management (preventative measures)
- Long-term ophthalmological and/or medical follow-up.
- Corneal grafting may be possible.

Lay group contact: CLIMB (Children Living With Inherited Metabolic Diseases) <www.climb.org.uk>.

Expert adviser: Nicola Ragge, Consultant Paediatric Ophthalmologist, Moorfields Eye Hospital, London, UK.

References

Bedrup C, Knappskog PM, *et al.* Congenital stromal dystrophy of the cornea caused by a mutation in the decorin gene. *Invet Ophthalmol Vis Sci* 2005; **46**: 420–26.

Biswas S, Munier FL, *et al.* Missense mutations in COL8A2, the gene encoding the alpha2 chain of type VIII collagen, cause two forms of corneal endothelial dystrophy. *Hum Mol Genet* 2001; **10**: 2415–23.

Bron AJ. Genetics of the corneal dystrophies: What we have learned in the past 25 years. *Cornea* 2000; **19**: 699–711.

Severe deafness in early childhood

Severe or profound deafness affects approximately 1/1000 infants at birth or during early childhood (pre-lingual period). Acquisition of speech is a major difficulty for these children, and some may be considered for cochlear implantation. A further 2–3/1000 children have moderate/progressive deafness requiring aiding. In developed countries, deafness has an important genetic origin and at least 60% of cases are inherited. The pattern of inheritance can be autosomal dominant (AD), autosomal recessive (AR), X-linked recessive (XLR), or mitochondrial.

- In **sensorineural deafness** (neural or nerve deafness, perceptive deafness) the abnormality lies between the hair-cells of the cochlea and the auditory regions of the brain. . Most sensorineural hearing loss is due to dysfunction of the hair cells themselves but rarely may be caused by pathology of the auditory nerve itself (auditory neuropathy). This is diagnosed by the presence of otoacoustic emissions (intact outer hair cells) in the presence of deafness ie. Absent auditory brainstem responses. Auditory neuropathy may be syndromic (often as part of a generalised neuropathic process) or non-syndromic and is rare.
- In **conductive deafness** the abnormality lies in the external or middle ear.

Causes of severe deafness are the following.
- Environmental (35%):
  - congenital infection (rubella, cytomegalovirus (CMV));
  - perinatal asphyxia;
  - hyperbilirubinaemia (serum bilirubin (SB) >250 micromole per litre for prolonged period);
  - infection, e.g. meningitis;
  - drugs, e.g. aminoglycosides.
- Genetic—syndromic (35%).
- Genetic—non-syndromic (30%). There is huge genetic heterogeneity with >50 AD loci and >30 AR. The majority (~80–85%) follow AR inheritance.

Aim to identify syndromic causes of deafness in order to enable assessment for associated problems (e.g. visual impairment) and to permit accurate genetic counselling.

Methods of assessing deafness include the following.
- **Pure tone audiogram.** Comprehensive test of the auditory pathway from tympanic membrane to auditory cortex.
- **Otoacoustic emissions (newborn hearing test).** Outer hair cell function (possible for this to be normal neonatally and yet the baby is unable to hear due to a problem with the VIIIth nerve). Mutations in *otoferlin* can give an auditory neuropathy.
- **BAER (brainstem auditory evoked response).** Testing nerve and brainstem pathways.
- **MRI or CT scan.** Some genetic conditions may give rise to characteristic malformations of the inner ear which may aid diagnosis (in Pendred syndrome there are often dilated vestibular aqueducts and enlarged endolymphatic sacs and in BOR syndrome there may be a Mondini cochlea dysplasia with or without dilated vestibular aqueducts).

Connexin 26 and connexin 30 (*DFNB1* locus). Connexins are transmembrane proteins that form channels allowing rapid transport of ions or small molecules between cells. There are two types, named GJA or GJB followed by a number. Mutations in the gap-junction protein connexin 26 *Cx26* (*GJB2*) on 13q12 may account for up to 50% of all cases of prelingual AR non-syndromic hearing loss and 10–40% of sporadic cases. GJB2 which encodes *Cx26* has a single coding exon. The carrier frequency in European, North American, and Mediterranean populations is approx 1/50. A hotspot at 35delG accounts for 70% of *Cx 26* mutations in these populations; 167delT accounts for 3–4% in Ashkenazi Jews. Cx26 deafness is less common in Asian populations, but 235delC is the most common mutation among Japanese and W77X, Q124X are the most common in the Asian subcontinent.

There is no structural abnormality of the inner ear in *Cx26* deafness and no vestibular pathology. It usually causes severe to profound prelingual sensorineural deafness, but there is considerable variation particularly with missense and non-truncating mutations. 20% of sib pairs may show significant variation in the degree of hearing loss, differing by two or more classes of severity (mild/moderate/severe/profound).

Connexin 30 *Cx30* (*GJB6*) is a gene lying adjacent to *GJB2* at the DFNB1 locus on 13q12. *Cx30* encodes a protein that is co-expressed with connexin 26 in the inner ear. A 342-kb deletion in *Cx30* is the second most common mutation causing prelingual deafness among Mediterranean populations. The deletion extends distally to *GJB2* the coding region of which remains intact. Mutations in the complex locus containing the genes for *Cx26* and *Cx30* can result in deafness which may be due to a digenic effect or secondary to deletion of a distant regulatory element for GJB2 lying with GJB6. Sensorineural deafness is found in individuals who are homozygotes or compound heterozygotes for mutations in *GJB2*, homozygotes for the deletion in *GJB6*, and heterozygotes for both *GJB2* and *GJB6*. See <www.crg.es/deafness> for more information.

Deafness due to mutations in mitochondrial DNA (mtDNA). A1555G is the most common mutation but usually only causes hearing impairment in early life if there has been exposure to aminoglycosides (e.g. gentamicin), A74445G is the second most common mitochondrial mutation (sometimes associated with palmoplantar keratoderma). 7472insC can cause isolated progressive deafness or deafness with ataxia/dysarthria/myoclonus. Overall, mitochondrial mutations are found in up to 30% of families with affected members in two or more generations related through the maternal line, but only 1% of sporadic early-onset non-syndromic deafness. The age of onset of deafness can be very variable (Estivill *et al.* 1998). A1555G is homoplasmic in nearly all pedigrees.

Clinical approach

Prior to the consultation try to obtain the child's audiograms to determine whether the deafness is sensorineural or conductive, and the severity, i.e. mild (20–40 dB), moderate (40–60 dB), severe (60–80 dB), or profound >80 dB and which frequencies are affected. Occasionally an audiometric pattern may be the key diagnostic clue (low frequency hearing loss is unusual and may be caused by mutations in *WFS1* or *HDIA1*; 'U' shaped or 'cookie-bite' hearing losses are usually dominant and may be caused by mutations in *COL11A2* or mutations in *TECTA*). If not available, you may need to repeat the audiogram; it is difficult to provide accurate advice without this information. The level of conversational speech is 45–60 dB.

If either parent is deaf you may need to arrange for a communicator skilled in sign language to facilitate the consultation.

History: key points

- Family history. Three-generation (or more) family tree with specific enquiry about:
  - hearing loss—age of onset, unilateral/bilateral, progressive/not;
  - sudden death or fainting (Jervell–Nielson), goitre (Pendred), renal disease (Alport, branchio-oto-renal (BOR)), poor vision (Usher, peroxisomal, mitochondrial), pigmentary anomalies (Waardenburg, piebaldism);
  - consanguinity (if present, counsel as for AR inheritance if rest of assessment is negative).
- Pre- and peri- and postnatal history:
  - Viral infections (CMV, rubella)—enquire about rash, arthralgia;
  - Severe jaundice, meningitis, aminoglycosides. Aminoglycosides tend to cause a steep high frequency hearing loss; hearing loss secondary to jaundice and perinatal factors would be expected to cause neurological problems and learning difficulties in addition to deafness ie. the brain is more sensitive to hypoxia and jaundice than the inner ear).
- Developmental delay (mild delay in motor milestones is common in deaf children who are otherwise neurologically normal probably due to involvement of the vestibular system). The vestibular system is frequently involved in Usher type 1, Jervell and Lange–Nielsen syndrome, Pendred syndrome, and sometimes BOR. Thus a history of profound congenital hearing loss in association with vestibular problems/delayed motor milestones, should prompt the specific investigations to exclude these syndromes (ECG, ERG, MRI/CT etc).
- Vestibular symptoms (Meniere-like symptoms are seen in families with COCH mutations; clues to this are the autosomal dominant family history of hearing loss, which is mainly high frequency, in contrast to the hearing loss in 'sporadic Meniere's which is predominantly low frequency, and the association with Meniere-like symptoms). *MYO7A* mutations have also been reported in families with dominant deafness and mild vestibular symptoms.

Examination: key points

- **Ear.** Look for external ear malformations, e.g. tags, pits, atretic ear canal (BOR, Treacher–Collins).
- **Eyes.** Look for dystopia canthorum and heterochromia or hypoplastic irides (Waardenberg), coloboma in lower eye lid (Treacher–Collins), retinal pigmentation (Usher and peroxisomal disorders). Retinal pigmentation in Usher syndrome is unlikely to be visible before puberty.
- **Neck.** Look for branchial cysts (BOR); check for goitre (Pendred).
- **Hair.** Look for pigmentary disturbance (white forelock).
- **Skin.** Piebaldism and subtle pigmentary disturbances seen in Waardenburg.
- Abnormal neurological signs.

Special investigations

- **Parental audiograms** in all and sibling audiograms if any clinical suspicion of hearing loss.
- **Mutation analysis in connexin 26 and connexin 30.**

- **Consider mitochondrial mutation analysis** if progressive sensorineural deafness in families consistent with maternal inheritance, i.e. without male–male transmission. Also if there has been a sudden deterioration or diagnosis of deafness following aminoglycoside exposure.
- **Ophthalmology referral** for refractive errors and fundoscopy in all cases (fundal assessment for retinitis pigmentosa, optic atrophy). Electroretinography (ERG) if delayed motor milestones have raised suspicion of Usher type I. Individuals with severe hearing impairment will rely heavily on visual function so comprehensive ophthalmology assessment is important in all. If normal, suggest annual optician review with return to ophthalmologist if any abnormality is detected.
- **TORCH** (toxoplasmosis–other (including syphilis, varicella zoster virus, parvovirus)–rubella–cytomegalovirus screen for congenital infections. CMV can be cultured from urine in first few weeks of life; rubella serology may be useful in children <6 months old.
- **Computerized tomography (CT)/magnetic resonance imaging (MRI) scan of temporal bone** in children (80% of those with Pendred have structural cochlear malformations, e.g. enlarged vestibular aqueducts and some, especially in childhood do not have goitre and therefore appear non-syndromal.
- **Renal ultrasound scan** (USS) if abnormalities of pinna, ear pits or tags, or branchial sinus (BOR), or multiple congenital anomalies, or low serum calcium (hypoparathyroidism–sensorineural deafness–renal dysplasia (HDR) syndrome).
- **Urine dipstick** for glucose (DIDMOAD (diabetes mellitus–optic atrophy–deafness) and MELAS (mitochondrial myopathy–encephalopathy–lactic acidosis–stroke-like episodes) 3243) and blood (Alport); send to lab if positive for confirmation.
- **Electrocardiogram (ECG)** for QT interval if severe/profound deafness (Jervell and Lange–Nielson long QT syndromes). Only in children with severe/profound deafness. If there is a suggestion of QT prolongation, assessment by a cardiologist is indicated. (See 'Long QT and Brugada syndromes' in Chapter 3, 'Common consultations'.)
- Thyroid function (thyroxine (T4)/thyroid-stimulating hormone (TSH)), if goitre present (Pendred syndrome—but diagnosis not excluded by normal results). Goitre is rare in children before puberty.

Some diagnoses to consider

Waardenburg syndrome. Waardenburg syndrome (WS) accounts for >2% of childhood deafness and typically follows AD inheritance (see below for exceptions). Auditory–pigmentary syndromes are caused by physical absence of melanocytes from the skin, hair, eyes, and the stria vascularis of the cochlea. All forms of Waardenburg show marked variability from minor pigmentary changes to profound deafness even within families, and at present it is not possible to predict the severity, even when a mutation is detected.

- **WS1.** In type 1 there is dystopia canthorum and 25% of patients have deafness. Type 1 patients tend to have the distinctive facial features of a high nasal bridge, synophrys, and hypoplasia of the alae nasi. Type 1 is caused by loss-of-function mutations in *PAX3* on 2q35.
- **WS2.** In type 2 there is no dystopia canthorum and over 50% of patients have deafness (Liu *et al.* 1995). It is a

heterogeneous group, 20% are caused by mutations in the micropthalmia associated transcription factor gene (*MITF*) (type 2A) and others by genes including homozygous mutations in *SNAI2*. Risk for clinically important deafness in *MITF* mutation carriers is around 1/3. The remainder have minor pigmentary anomalies, and some have mild hearing impairment which is not clinically significant. Deafness is thought to be non-progressive. There is little or no risk of Hirschsprung's in *MITF* mutation carriers.

- **WS3 (Klein–Waardenburg (rare))** with upper limb anomalies including flexion contractures of the fingers is an extreme presentation of type 1; caused by mutations in PAX3. Some but not all patients are homozygotes; at least two parent–child transmissions are reported in the literature.
- **WS4 (Shah–Waardenburg syndrome with Hirschsprung disease)** is genetically heterogeneous and can be caused by homozygous endothelin pathway mutations (genes for endothelin-3 or one of its receptors, *EDNRB*) and heterozygous *SOX10* mutations. In the latter case, various neurological symptoms with demyelinization might occur (Inoue). Some of these *SOX10* patients have been reported to have dysplastic semicircular canals).

Pendred syndrome. Pendrin (*SLC26A4*). AR congenital severe/profound deafness particularly affecting high frequencies with step-wise progressive fluctuating hearing loss. Speech/language is usually well developed for the degree of deafness identified on the audiogram. CT/MRI may show dilated vestibular aqueducts in ~80%. Goitre develops from puberty, so imaging is important in making the diagnosis in childhood. Approximately 5% of all severe/profound deafness in childhood.

Branchio-oto-renal syndrome (BOR). AD disorder with variable expressivity but high penetrance caused by mutations in *EYA1* and also rarely, *SIX1*. Branchial, otic, and renal anomalies. Ear pits are a common feature. Hearing loss can be mixed or sensorineural and those with hearing impairment may have characterisitic changes on their cochlear CT (Mondini dysplasia (fewer turns—normal is 21/2)). BOR affects an estimated 2% of profoundly deaf children. Point mutations in *EYA1* are present in ~50%. Complex rearrangements such as inversions or large deletions appear to be common and evade detection by direct sequencing methods (Vervoort *et al.* 2002). Renal anomalies vary from normal to mild dysplasia to agenesis. Branchial clefts or sinuses are less common than the otic or renal features.

Hypoparathyroidism, sensorineural deafness, renal dysplasia syndrome (HDR). AD disorder caused by mutations in a transcription factor *GATA3* on 10p. Renal spectrum varies from normal through mild dysplasia to aplasia. HDR syndrome is primarily caused by *GATA3* haploinsufficiency and is associated with a wide phenotypic spectrum (Muroya *et al.* 2001).

Treacher–Collins syndrome is caused by mutations in *TCOF1*. Deafness is mixed or sensorineural. Abnormal external ear, malar hypoplasia, inferior lid colobomata and down-slanting palpebral fissures, cleft palate, Pierre–Robin sequence. AD; very variable expressivity but fairly high penetrance. See 'Ear anomalies', page 108.

Usher syndrome is characterized by sensorineural hearing loss and progressive retinitis pigmentosa (RP). There are three clinical types (all AR) each with underlying molecular heterogeneity.

- Type 1. Congenital severe/profound deafness with absent vestibular function. Delayed motor milestones, poor head control, late sitting, rarely walk before 18 months of age.
  - Type 1B is the most common type and is caused by mutation in *myosin 7A*.
  - There are patients described with type 1D who have normal motor milestones.
- Type 2. Also congenital moderate/severe with sloping audiogram. Patients wear aids and develop speech.
- Type 3. Common in Finland, usually postlingual and progressive. Vestibular function may be normal or absent. Also common among Ashkenazi Jews (specific mutations).

RP is usually not visible until the teenage years by which time symptoms will be present (night-blindness and loss of peripheral vision). The ERG is abnormal years before. In type 1 the ERG is likely to be abnormal within the first few years of life. For types 2 and 3 there is little data on when ERGs become abnormal.

KID syndrome (Keratosis-Icthyosis-Deafness) syndrome Dominant mutations in the *Cx26* gene *GJB2* have been shown to cause keratitis-ichthyosis-deafness (KID) syndrome (skin thickening & fissuring with multiple hyperkeratotic plaques), palmoplantar keratoderma associated with hearing loss, and Vohwinkel syndrome. Missense mutations in the closely related *Cx30* gene *GJB6* underlie Clouston syndrome (autosomal dominant hidrotic ectodermal dysplasia).

Genetic advice

Many genes are involved in the different types of deafness (syndromic and non-syndromic). Non-syndromic hereditary deafness in early childhood is mainly (80%) due to recessive genes.

Recurrence risk

- If sporadic case and all the above are normal, i.e. no environmental or syndromic diagnosis can be made, recurrence risk for future pregnancies is 10% (empiric figure; in reality some families will have 25% recurrence risk, and others much lower risks, but it is not possible to discriminate).
- If two affected sibs or consanguinity, assume AR—25% risk in future pregnancies.
- If affected parent and child, assume AD—50% risk in future pregnancies.
- If parent has severe congenital hearing loss and environmental and syndromic forms have been excluded as far as possible, empiric risk to offspring is 5%.
- If both parents have severe congenital hearing loss (neither with environmental or syndromic form) and there is no consanguinity or likelihood of consanguinity, empiric risk to offspring is 10%. NB. If first child is deaf consider the possibility that both parents have allellic AR deafness (risk to offspring 100%), as well as the possibility of one or other or both parents having AD deafness.

Carrier detection

- Parental audiograms in all and sibling audiograms if any clinical suspicion of hearing loss.
- For connexin 26 deafness and other types where the mutations are defined it is possible to offer accurate carrier detection to family members.

Prenatal diagnosis

Prenatal diagnosis for hearing loss is highly contentious but is technically feasible by chorionic villus sampling (CVS) if the causative mutations are known.

Natural history and further management (preventative measures)

- **Hearing aids.** Skilled assessment by an audiologist is required to ensure good results. In young children the ear moulds need to be changed periodically as the ear canal grows.
- **Cochlear implants.** These represent an exciting advance in the management of very young children with profound hearing loss. They are best suited to children in the pre-school years who with optimal hearing aid correction still have a loss >65 dB.
- **Education.** Provision needs to be carefully matched to the child's level of hearing loss.

Support group: <www.ndcs.org.uk>; <www.rnid.org.uk>; <www.deafplus.org>.

Expert adviser: Maria Bitner-Glindzicz, Senior Lecturer and Honorary Consultant Geneticist, Institute of Child Health, London, England.

References

Bitner-Glindzicz M. Hereditary deafness and phenotyping in humans. *Br Med Bull.* 2002; **63**: 73–94.

Connexin-deafness homepage <www.crg.es/deafness> (a resource for clinicians incorporating mutation databases for the various connexin genes involved in deafness).

Del Castillo I, Villamar M, *et al*. A deletion involving the connexion 30 gene in nonsyndromic hearing impairment. *New Engl J Med* 2002; **346**: 243–9.

Estivill X, Govea N, *et al*. Familial progressive sensorineural deafness is mainly due to the mtDNA A1555G mutation and is enhanced by treatment of amnioglycosides. *Am J Hum Genet* 1998; **62**: 27–35.

Fraser GR. *The causes of profound deafness in children*. John Hopkins University Press, Baltimore, 1976.

Hereditary hearing loss homepage <www.uia.ac.be/dnalab/hhh> (a resource for clinicians).

Hutchin TP, Thompson KR, *et al*. Prevalence of mitochondrial DNA mutations in childhood/congenital onset non-syndromal sensorineural hearing impairment. *J Med Genet* 2001; **38**: 229–31.

Inoue K, Khajavi M, *et al*. Molecular mechanism for distinct neurological phenotypes conveyed by allelic truncating mutations. *Nat Genet*. 2004; **36**: 361–9.

Kalatzis V, Petit C. The fundamental and medical impacts of recent progress in research on hereditary hearing loss. *Hum Mol Genet* 1998; **7**: 1589–97.

Liu XZ, Newton VE, Read AP. Waardenburg syndrome type II: phenotypic findings and diagnostic criteria. *Am J Med Genet* 1995; **55** (1): 95–100.

Muroya K, Hasegawa T, *et al*. GATA3 abnormalities and the phenotypic spectrum of HDR syndrome. *J Med Genet* 2001; **38** (6): 374–80.

Parker MJ, Fortnum H, Young ID, Davis AC. Variations in genetic assessment and recurrence risks quoted for childhood deafness: a survey of clinical geneticists. *J Med Genet* 1999; **36**: 125–30.

Read AP, Newton VE. Waardenburg syndrome. *J Med Genet* 1997; **34**: 656–65.

Sanchez-Martin M, Rodriguez-Garcia A, *et al*. SLUG (SNAI2) deletions in patients with Waardenburg disease. *Hum Mol Genet* 2002; **11**: 3231–6.

Seminars in Medical Genetics. Hereditary deafness. *Am J Med Genet* 1999; **89C** (3).

Smith RJH, Bale JF Jr, White KR. Sensorineural hearing loss in children (Seminar). *Lancet* 2005; **365**: 879–90.

Steel K. Science, medicine, and the future: new interventions in hearing impairment. *Br Med J* 2000; **320**: 622–5.

Tekin M, Arnos K, Pandya A. Advances in hereditary deafness. *Lancet* 2001; **358**: 1082–90.

Vervoort VS, Smith RJ, *et al*. Genomic rearrangements of EYA1 account for a large fraction of families with BOR syndrome. *Eur J Hum Genet* 2002; **10** (11): 757–66.

Willems PJ. Genetic causes of hearing loss (review). *NEJM* 2000; **342**: 1101–9

Developmental delay in the child with consanguineous parents

See also 'Consanguinity' and 'Incest', pages 284 and 370. The presence of consanguinity increases the probability of an autosomal recessive (AR) condition. Whilst it is important not to forget that non-genetic, chromosomal, autosomal dominant (AD), and X-linked conditions also occur in consanguineous populations, there is strong evidence for an increased risk for developmental delay, chronic disease, and neonatal death in the children of related parents. This risk increases when there are multiple consanguineous marriages within the same kindred. The genetic conditions are well described in the work of Mc Kusick and colleagues (Khoury *et al.* 1987) in the American Amish community and Bundey and Aslam (1993) within the British Pakistani community (see 'Consanguinity', page 284.)

Clinical approach

History: key points

- It may be necessary to arrange for an interpreter to help obtain a full history.
- Three-generation family tree. Ask specifically about consanguinity and define the relationships. Ask specifically if any child has/had schooling difficulties and about pregnancy, deaths in childhood, and early adult life as proxy markers for malformations and neurological disability.
- Developmental history. Remember especially to ask about any loss of skills.
- Seizures?
- Occipital-frontal circumference (OFC) from birth to the present time
- Visual or hearing problems.
- Additional medical problems.

Examination: key points

A complete physical and neurological examination is required.

- **Growth parameters.** Height, span, weight, and OFC; plot centile. Note any disproportion.
- **Neurological exam.** Spasticity, hypotonia, ataxia, reflexes.
- **Face.** Coarse features (storage disorders).
- **Abdomen.** Organomegaly (storage disorders).
- **Eyes.** Fundal examination particularly for pigmentary retinopathy.
- **Skin.** Pigmentation abnormalities, sun sensitivity, premature ageing (DNA repair defects).
- **Skeletal** and limbs (skeletal dysplasia, radial defects).
- Other features and malformations.

Special investigations

In this group of patients, with a higher prior risk of metabolic disease, more extensive metabolic screening is indicated. If the karyotype is normal there is a better chance of diagnostic yield in this group of patients from investigating to exclude metabolic/AR single gene conditions than proceeding straight to specialized chromosome analysis, e.g. telomere/microarray studies.

- Chromosomes. Consider if there are any signs of AR conditions that can be confirmed by cytogenetic testing, e.g. Fanconi anaemia, ataxia telangiectasia, Bloom syndrome, Roberts syndrome.
- Consider AR conditions with a high carrier frequency within the population and exclude, e.g. Tay–Sachs disease.

- DNA for *FRAXA* and storage.
- Baseline biochemistry plus fasting lactate and pyruvate.
- Urine for amino and organic acids. Plasma amino acids. Some children will have been born in area of no neonatal screening for phenylketonuria (PKU).
- Urine mucopolysaccharide (MPS) screen; when there are coarse features add oligosaccharides.
- Vacuolated lymphocytes.
- White cell enzymes, DNA testing for neuronal ceroid lipofuscinosis (NCL; Battens): often not done as a first-line investigation unless evidence for regression or other neurological features. Discuss with paediatric neurologists if in doubt.
- Consider very long chain fatty acids (VLCFAs) to exclude a peroxisomal disorder.
- Consider 7-dehydrocholesterol (Smith–Lemli–Opitz (SLO) syndrome).
- If there are significant dysmorphic features look in the appropriate section of this chapter.
- Magnetic resonance imaging (MRI) brain imaging to look for structural genetic brain abnormality, e.g. neuronal migration abnormalities.
- Additional radiological investigations if clinically indicated (cardiac, renal, skeletal).
- Ophthalmological referral for detailed assessment including fundoscopy in children with regression, syndromes with eye involvement, and in the presence of visual difficulties and squint.
- Children with undiagnosed neurological disorder: refer to a paediatric neurologist.

Some diagnoses to consider

Known AR conditions

- Metabolic disorders: Late onset milder phenotypes more difficult. Carefully review all metabolic investigations in children with any evidence of regression, deteriorating behaviour, or an increased frequency of seizures.
- Recognizable syndromes with known AR inheritance. Each ethnic group will have particular syndromes and conditions that are more common.

Probable AR conditions

- The same phenotype in two affected sibs of different sexes or two female sibs.
- Developmental regression (See page 96).

Possible AR

- Similar features to those of a known recessive condition.
- Severe mental retardation with no environmental risk factors.

Genetic advice

Recurrence risk

When a diagnosis remains unknown counselling is difficult. Consider if the diagnosis falls into the probable or possible AR group and advise accordingly.

When the condition is non-progressive and there are other malformations, remember that chromosome anomalies and dysmorphic syndromes which do not follow AR inheritance can also occur in consanguineous families.

Carrier detection
- This can be performed for some of the metabolic conditions by DNA and enzymatic methods. General population testing, i.e. for the partners of the parents' sibs, may not be possible.
- Mutational or linkage analysis may be possible.
- Pedigree analysis

Prenatal diagnosis
- Biochemical or molecular testing by chorionic villus sampling (CVS) or amniocentesis can be offered to those parents in whom a diagnosis has been confirmed. Consult closely with the laboratory to ascertain the type of sample (direct or cultured CVS, amniocytes, etc. that is required).
- Ultrasound for structural anomalies.

Natural history and further management (preventative measures)
Information, education, and the offer of genetic advice to members of the extended family. Dual language information.

Support group contact: CLIMB (Children Living With Inherited Metabolic Diseases) <www.climb.org.uk>. National Organisation for Rare Disorders (US) <www.raredisease.org>

Expert adviser: Dian Donnai, Professor of Medical Genetics, University of Manchester, Manchester, England.

References
Bundey S, Aslam H. A five-year prospective study of the health of children in different ethnic groups, with particular reference to the effect of inbreeding. *Eur J Hum Genet* 1993; **1**: 206–19.
Khoury MJ, Cohen BH, Diamond EL, Chase GA, McKusick VA. Inbreeding and prereproductive mortality in the Old Order Amish. III. Direct and indirect effects of imbreeding. *Am J Epidemiol* 1987; **125**: 473–83.

Developmental regression

This typically presents with a loss of previously learned skills. Other signs such as behavioural changes or the onset of seizures usually accompany it. In older children the presentation may be schooling difficulties with emotional lability and immaturity.

These children should primarily be under the care of a paediatric neurologist, who will work closely with a child development team for the assessment of developmental skills. It may take some months of observation to determine the pattern of developmental loss and to diagnose conditions such as autism. Geneticists become involved:

- as many of the neurodegenerative conditions have a genetic aetiology;
- during the period of investigation to help establish the diagnosis;
- with ethical discussions such as whether to offer pre-symptomatic testing to siblings and how much intensive support to give to the child;
- to give genetic advice after the diagnosis has been made.

Clinical approach

History: key points

- Three-generation family tree with specific enquiry about consanguinity and other similarly affected relatives.
- Family history of neurological disease. Consider that conditions usually found in adults such as Huntington disease (HD) can present in childhood due to anticipation.
- Full developmental history. Obtain copies of assessments.
- Age of onset and mode of presentation.
- Sex of child. Females: consider Rett syndrome; males: consider X-linked conditions such as adrenoleukodystrophy (X-ALD), Pelizaeus–Merzbacher disease.
- Ethnic group, e.g. Tay–Sachs in Ashkenazi Jewish population, Salla disease and PEHO (progressive encephalopathy–(o)edema–hypsarrhythmia–optic atrophy) syndrome in Finns, megalencephalic leukoencephalopathy with subcortical cysts (MLC) in Turks.
- Fluctuation with intercurrent illnesses may indicate an underlying metabolic disturbance.
- Seizures. Poorly controlled seizures can lead to apparent regression that is reversed on good control. This is a difficult assessment area because the development of seizures may be part of the progressive nature of a neurodegenerative process.
- Loss of vision and hearing and timing of this in relation to the course of regression.

Examination: key points

- Head circumference and note any change in the rate of growth.
- Deceleration of head growth (Rett, Cockayne syndromes).
- Macrocephaly (Canavan, Alexander disease, other storage diseases, MLC).
- Hypotonia or spasticity.
- Ataxia, a useful diagnostic feature.
- Coarsening of facial features (see 'Coarse facial features', page 78).
- Deep set eyes (Cockayne syndrome).
- Optic fundi: optic atrophy, cherry red spots, pigmentary changes (Refsum disease, GM2-gangliosidosis, mitochondrial disorders).
- Stereotypical hand movements such as wringing (Rett syndrome).
- Skin: increased pigment (Addison disease in adrenoleukodystrophy), chilblain lesions (Aicardi–Goutieres syndrome).
- Hepatosplenomegaly (storage disorders).
- Scoliosis (Rett syndrome).

Special investigations

The list of investigations will differ depending on the differential diagnosis. This list is a guide but is not comprehensive.

- Baseline biochemistry: glucose, lactate, pyruvate, creatine kinase (CK), and urine metabolic screen for mucopolysaccharide (MPS) disorders and urinary oligosaccharides. Also amino and organic acid screens.
- Vacuolated lymphocytes.
- Immunoglobulins (ataxia telangiectasia).
- Adrenal function.
- Very long chain fatty acids (VLCFAs; peroxisomal disorders).
- White cell enzymes (lysosomal enzyme and storage diseases, infantile and late-infantile NCL).
- Electron microscope (EM) studies of tissue (storage disorders; particularly used in the investigation of the NCLs).
- Magnetic resonance imaging (MRI) brain scan. An expert paediatric neuroradiologist will be able to interpret, for example, the pattern of white matter disease, to establish a small list of differential diagnoses. Conditions like MLC have a characteristic appearance.
- Electroencephalography (EEG). Specific patterns may be associated with certain conditions.
- Ophthalmological assessment including visual evoked responses.
- Brainstem evoked potentials and other electrophysiological studies.
- DNA analysis and storage. Consider any specific tests such as *MeCP2* for Rett syndrome, *CLNC3* in Battens disease, mitochondrial DNA analysis. Also, in children with a proven enzyme defect, enquire if mutation analysis would make prenatal testing easier and offer the potential of carrier detection.
- Chromosome analysis: consider need for special techniques such as irradiation for DNA repair defects (Cockayne syndrome).
- Electrocardiogram (ECG) and cardiac echo: mitochondrial diseases.
- Lumbar puncture (lactate level as a marker for disorders of respiratory chain, Aicardi–Goutieres syndrome has a cerebrospinal fluid (CSF) lymphocytosis).
- Skeletal survey for signs of dysostosis multiplex.

Some diagnoses to consider

Non-genetic conditions

Non-genetic conditions where *the diagnosis should not be made by a geneticist* include environmental factors such as severe emotional deprivation, psychiatric conditions such as disintegrative psychosis, vascular disorders, tumours, and infections.

Autism
Another condition where the diagnosis is not within the expertise of a geneticist is autism. Disintegrative psychosis can be difficult to differentiate from developmental regression and some baseline investigations, e.g. MRI, will probably be needed. There are genetic issues in this condition and these are discussed in 'Autism and autistic spectrum disorders', page 274.

Metabolic and storage disorders
The group of conditions that are known as the neuronal ceroid lipofuscinoses have particular diagnostic difficulties and are discussed in more detail.

Neuronal ceroid lipofuscinoses (NCL). These are lysosomal storage disorders characterized by mental and motor deterioration, seizures, and visual loss. The juvenile form is *Battens disease.* Until recently confirmation of these diagnoses depended on EM detection of specific lysosomal storage material in tissue, a rectal or skin biopsy, or conjunctival tissue. It is now possible for most neurologists and geneticists to have access to molecular testing for the genes *CLCN 1, 2,* and *3* and enzyme analysis of palmitoyl-protein thioesterase (PPT)-1 and tripeptidyl-peptidase (TPP)-1.

- Infantile NCL (INCL). Gene *CLCN1.* Movement disorder, dementia, and retinal blindness by 2 years. The enzyme PPT-1 is encoded by *CLCN1.*
- Late infantile NCL (LINCL). Gene *CLCN1* (8%) and *CLCN2* (80%). TPP-1 is encoded by *CLCN2.* Presents at age 2–4 years with epilepsy and regression.
- Juvenile NCL (JNCL). Battens disease. Gene *CLCN1* (21%), *CLCN2* (7%), *CLCN3* (72%). Presents with visual loss between the ages of 4 and 10 years. Myoclonic seizures and regression. Vacuolated lymphocytes are seen. Common 1 kb deletion in *CLCN3* removes exon 7 and 8, which is offered as a diagnostic service to most clinicians.
- Adult NCL (ANCL). Onset around 30 years.
- Northern epilepsy (NE). Onset 5–10 years.

Sanfilippo syndrome (mucopolysaccharidoses (MPS) III). Sanfilippo A and B syndromes are lysosomal storage disorders caused by the deficiency of heparin sulphaminidase and alpha-*N*-acetylglucosaminidase, respectively, which are enzymes involved in the degradation of heparan sulphate. Accumulation of the substrate in lysosomes leads to degeneration of the central nervous system (CNS) with progressive dementia often combined with hyperactivity and aggressive behaviour. Age of onset and rate of progression vary considerably, whilst diagnosis is often delayed due to the absence of the pronounced skeletal changes observed in other MPSs (Weber *et al.* 1999).

Progressive myoclonic epilepsy (PME)
PME is the triad of: stimulus sensitive myoclonus; grand mal and absence epilepsy; and progressive neurological deterioration/regression.

Most causes of PME are rare AR conditions; exclude NCLs (e.g. Battens), Unverricht–Lunborg disease (cystatin B), Lafora disease (laforin gene), sialodosis. Other genetic conditions to consider are mitochondrial encephalopathy with ragged red fibres (MERFF) and dentatorubro-pallidoluysian atrophy (DRPLA).

Rett syndrome
The clinical criteria for classic Rett syndrome are:
- normal development to 6 months;
- regression 6 months–2 years;
- deceleration of head growth;

- stereotypical hand movements develop;
- acquisition of severe developmental delay;
- gait ataxia and apraxia.

MECP2 mutations are detected in ~80% of girls with classical Rett syndrome. See 'Rett syndrome', page 408.

Macrocephaly
Alexander disease. The most notable features of the infantile form of Alexander disease, which begins during the first 2 years of life, are macrocephaly and sometimes hydrocephaly (either of which may develop later in the course of the disease), psychomotor regression, seizures, and spasticity. See 'Macrocephaly', page 162.

Canavan disease. Clinical features of the disease are macrocephaly, head lag, progressive severe mental retardation, and hypotonia in early life, which later changes to spasticity. See 'Macrocephaly', page 162.

Rare AR disorders
PEHO (progressive encephalopathy–(o)edema–hypsarrhythmia–optic atrophy) syndrome. AR. Originally described in Finland, there are reports from other parts of Europe. Progressive cerebellar atrophy is a key MRI feature.

Cockayne syndrome. An AR condition with progressive microcephaly, deep set eyes, retinal pigmentary abnormalities and cataract, sun sensitivity, and deafness. Confirmed by abnormal DNA repair to ultraviolet (UV) irradiation of fibroblasts. See 'DNA repair defects', page 304.

Mitochondrial disorders
These may follow a mitochondrial, sporadic, or AR pattern of inheritance. See 'Mitochondrial DNA diseases' page 384.

X-linked disorders
Adrenoleukodystrophy. X-linked recessive (XLR) inheritance. Known to show variability within families of the age of onset ranging from childhood to adult males. Although the diagnosis can be made on the basis of biochemical testing, this is not reliable for carrier testing. See 'Adrenoleukodystrophy, X-linked (X-ALD)', page 264.

Genetic advice
Recurrence risk
- For those families in whom a definitive diagnosis has not been made after thorough investigation, there is a high recurrence risk and AR inheritance is the most likely mode of inheritance.
- X-linked conditions should be considered if there have been two or more affected boys and/or there is a family history compatible with X-linkage.
- Mitochondrial conditions pose difficult counselling problems; see 'Mitochondrial DNA diseases', page 384.
- Store DNA and/or fibroblast cell line for future diagnostic use.

Carrier detection
This is possible in those families in whom a causative mutation has been identified. It may be possible for some biochemical abnormalities.

Prenatal diagnosis
This is available to those families in whom there is molecular or biochemical confirmation of diagnosis.

Pre-symptomatic testing of other siblings

Parents may wish to have apparently unaffected siblings tested for the condition that has been diagnosed in the child. Expert psychological help is needed to explain the pros and cons of such testing and the issue of consent. Please refer to the guidelines on the genetic testing of children. If there is a therapeutic intervention then the issues are somewhat clearer.

Natural history and further management (preventative measures)

Unfortunately, there is usually progression of these conditions with early death. Symptomatic treatment of epilepsy and maintenance of adequate nutrition help. Hospice care and family support are very important.

Support group contact: CLIMB (Children Living with Inherited Metabolic Diseases) <www.climb.org.uk>, tel. 0870 770 0326. NORD (National Organisation for Rare Disorders <www.rarediseases.org>

Expert adviser: Robert Surtees, Professor of Paediatric Neurology, Institute of Child Health, London, England.

References

Aicardi J. Paediatric Neurology

Clarke JTR. *A clinical guide to inherited metabolic diseases*, 2nd edn. Cambridge University Press, Cambridge 2002.

Neuronal ceroid lipofuscinoses: <www.gene clinics.org>.

Surtees R. Understanding neurodegenerative disorders. *Curr Paediatr* 2002; 12: 191–98.

Weber B, Guo XH, Kleijer WJ, *et al.* Sanfilippo type B syndrome (mucopolysaccharidosis III B): allelic heterogeneity corresponds to the wide spectrum of clinical phenotypes. *Eur J Hum Genet* 1999; **7** (1): 34–44.

Winter R, Baraitser M. *Dysmorphology Photo Library 2.2 and London Neurogenetics Database 2.2 and London Dysmorphology Database 2.2.* Oxford University Press, Oxford, 2000.

Duane retraction syndrome

This is also known as the Duane anomaly.

Strabismus is a misalignment of the visual axes. It is found in 4–5% of children and a much higher frequency is seen in children with neurodevelopmental delay. Duane anomaly accounts for 1% of strabismus. There is aberrant innervation of the horizontal external ocular muscles.

- **Duane 1.** Marked or complete limitation of abduction with minimal or no limitation of adduction.
- **Duane 2.** Marked or complete limitation of adduction with minimal or no limitation of abduction.
- **Duane 3.** Marked or complete limitation of adduction *and* abduction.

In addition there is retraction of the globe and narrowing of the palpebral fissure on adduction on the affected side(s). The condition is bilateral in 20%.

Clinical approach

History: key points

- Family history, particularly for evidence of autosomal dominant (AD) inheritance.
- Developmental delay (chromosome abnormalities).
- Other central nervous system (CNS) features, e.g. seizures.
- Hearing loss (Wilderwank syndrome, Okihiro syndrome).
- May be associated with other miswiring symptoms, e.g. crocodile tears.

Examination: key points

- Exclude congenital cranial nerve palsies (Moebius syndrome).
- Ear tags and malformation of the external ear.
- Short neck (Klippel–Feil anomaly, Wilderwank syndrome).
- Thumb: structural abnormalities and hypoplasia; radial ray deficiencies (Okihiro syndrome).

Special investigations

- X-ray of cervical spine for fusion abnormalities in children with a short neck (Klippel–Feil anomaly).
- Abdominal ultrasound scan (USS; renal abnormalities in del (8)(q13), inv dup(22)(q11), Wilderwank syndrome, and Klippel–Feil anomaly).
- Hearing test.
- Consider imaging of the inner ear in the presence of a hearing loss.
- Chromosome analysis if there are additional features and/or mental retardation (see below) with telomere screen or microarray/comparative genomic hybridization (CGH) if multiple anomalies suggestive of a 'chromosomal phenotype'.

Some diagnoses to consider

Klippel–Feil anomaly. Klippel–Feil anomaly of the cervical spine (fusion of one or more cervical vertebrae).

Wildervank syndrome. Wildervank syndrome is the triad of Duane retraction syndrome, Klippel–Feil anomaly, and sensorineural deafness. More females are affected than males. The inheritance pattern is unclear. Most cases are sporadic, but there are reports of other affected family members having one or more component of the condition.

Okihiro syndrome (Duane radial ray syndrome). This is an AD condition with degrees of radial ray hypoplasia and Duane anomaly. It results from mutation in the *SALL4* gene.

Chromosomal anomalies. Duane has been associated with a number of cytogenetic anomalies. In particular consider cat-eye syndrome due to an inv dup (22)(q11) and a contiguous gene deletion syndrome at 8q13 that results in type 1 Duane anomaly and branchio-oto-renal (BOR) syndrome.

Moebius syndrome. The congenital cranial nerve palsies of Moebius syndrome may be confused with Duane retraction syndrome.

Other.

- Absence of external ocular muscles may occur in craniosynostosis syndromes.
- The squint caused by thalidomide embryopathy is similar to Duane anomaly.

Genetic advice

Recurrence risk

Most cases are sporadic. Approximately 10% of isolated Duane anomaly is familial with AD inheritance. Type 1 is linked to 8q13 and type 2 to 2q31.

Carrier detection

This may be available when Duane anomaly is part of a syndrome with a known mutation or cytogenetic abnormality.

Prenatal diagnosis

This may be available when Duane anomaly is part of a syndrome with a known mutation or cytogenetic abnormality.

Natural history and further management (preventative measures)

Amblyopia is a common complication.

Lay group contact: Many of the individual syndromes have their own support groups. See <www.cafamily.org.uk>.

Expert adviser: Anonymous.

References

Al Baradie R, *et al.* Duane radial ray syndrome (Okihiro syndrome) maps to 20q13 and results from mutation in SALL4 a new member of the SAL family. *Am J Hum Genet* 2002; **71**: 1195–9.

Chung M, *et al.* Clinical diversity of hereditary Duane's retraction syndrome. *Ophthalmology* 2000; **107**: 500–3.

Dysmorphic child

This section describes the clinical approach to the infant/child/adult with dysmorphic features of unknown cause so that the useful and significant diagnostic signs can be documented. Other sections in this chapter and diagnostic databases will be of help when the dysmorphic features have been carefully assessed.

The term 'dysmorphic' is used to describe children whose physical features, particularly facial, are not usually found in a child of the same age or ethnic background. Some features are abnormal in all circumstances, e.g. premature fusion of the cranial sutures. These are called good diagnostic 'handles' as they are not found as normal or familial traits or variations, and are only present in a small number of conditions. In contrast, a feature such as 2,3 toe syndactyly may be a useful diagnostic tool, or be a non-significant familial trait. The recognition of which features are good diagnostic aids comes with experience.

Clinical approach

The key points of the history are of equal importance to the physical examination in establishing the diagnosis.

History: key points

- **Three-generation family tree.** Enquire specifically for consanguinity and other members of the family with similar problems.
- **Pregnancy history.** Bleeding, fever, medication, investigations, alcohol/non-prescription drugs (ask with tact), fetal movements, liquor volume, gestation, mode of delivery.
- **Neonatal history.** Birthweight, length, head circumference. Resuscitation, feeding difficulties, ventilation, malformations, surgery, seizures, other medical problems.
- **Developmental milestones and current schooling provision** (e.g. mainstream school with 1:1 learning support assistant (LSA), special needs nursery). If developmentally delayed, ask about agencies involved, e.g. physical therapist.
- Any specific difficulties with **vision** or **hearing**.
- **Past medical and surgical history** (previous hospital admissions) and current medication.
- **Behavioural phenotype.** Ask about unusual patterns of behaviour.

Examination: key points

- **Observation.** Look carefully at the child. Some conditions are immediately recognizable, e.g. Down syndrome. Watch the child during the consultation. Try to involve him/her in the history and take note of spontaneous language and interaction between the child and adults, as well as looking at the face.
- **Growth parameters.** Height, weight, and occipital-frontal circumference (OFC). In general, the further measurements deviate from the normal centile ranges the greater the chance of making a genetic diagnosis. Plot measurements on a centile chart. For measurements outside the normal ranges, estimate by how many standard deviations. The statement 'the OFC is <0.4th centile at −5.5 SD' conveys far more information than simply noting that 'the OFC is <0.4th centile'.
- Use an **examination checklist** to ensure that all the systems have been adequately examined and the findings

documented. See 'Dysmorphology examination checklist', page 670.
- Enquire specifically about 'birthmarks' and examine for skin pigmentary abnormalities (chromosomal mosaicism).
- Assess the need for more extensive investigation of systems, e.g. of the skeletal system in an individual with short or tall stature.
- Review any photographs of the child that are in the notes, or supplied by the family.

Special investigations

- **Chromosome analysis.** Standard Giemsa-banded karyotype of good quality. Consider a repeat analysis if the report is ≥5 years old. Additional cytogenetic testing is indicated in the following circumstances.
  1. In the presence of features suggestive of a known microdeletion syndrome, e.g. Williams syndrome, arrange specific fluorescent *in situ* hybridization (FISH) test.
  2. When the features are suggestive of a chromosomal anomaly, but the routine karyotype is normal, arrange telomere screen or microarray/ comparative genomic hybridization (CGH). See 'Submicroscopic chromosomal rearrangements and the chromosomal phenotype', page 546. The prevalence of subtelomeric abnormalities in idiopathic mental retardation is 5.1%, but the figure is higher (6.8%) in individuals with moderate to severe mental retardation (Flint and Knight 2003).
- **Molecular genetic analysis.** Fragile X (FRAXA) in children with developmental delay. Other specific testing, as indicated.
- **Clinical photography.** Document any significant features and use the photos to observe the evolution of the features with age (natural history). Photographs of the child with both parents can be useful in determining which of the distinctive features are potentially significant and which may just be family characteristics. Consider making a video record of movement. Many syndromes, particularly microdeletion disorders, have unusual expression of facial movement (trisomy 18 and trisomy 21 have been shown to have abnormal facial muscle attachments).
- **Metabolic testing.** Curry *et al.* (1997) found an extremely low pick-up of abnormalities when metabolic screening was performed without specific signs of a metabolic disorder. However, many children with a dysmorphic appearance and developmental delay are offered testing for thyroid function and urine amino and organic acid abnormalities. If a child is microcephalic with no normal sibs, test the mother for phenylketonuria (PKU) and organic acid abnormalities.
- **Brain imaging.** This is not routinely performed in children with a normal head circumference and no abnormal neurological signs, but the number having such scans is increasing since magnetic resonance imaging (MRI) is better than computerized tomography (CT) in detecting more subtle features that can be of diagnostic significance. Neuroimaging should be considered in patients without a known diagnosis especially in the presence of neurological symptoms, cranial contour abnormalities, microcephaly, or macrocephaly (Curry *et al.* 1997). In most situations MRI is the testing modality of choice.

- Further investigations to help establish a diagnosis and to evaluate the significance of a physical feature, e.g. echocardiogram if a heart murmur is noted.
- **Skin biopsy.** Consider a skin biopsy for karyotype if the following features are present:
  - streaky skin pigmentation, especially if following lines of Blashko (hypomelanosis of Ito);
  - asymmetry;
  - 3,4 finger syndactyly with 2,3 finger syndactyly and bulbous finger tips (diploid/triploid mosaicism).

Making a diagnosis

It is useful in these situations to have a diagnostic framework.

1 Ask some basic questions.
  - Are you dealing with a single malformation or multiple malformations?
  - Is the child likely to have a multiple anomaly syndrome?
  - Are there deformations that might tie in with the pregnancy history?
  - Does the family history help?

2 Think about the various mechanisms by which birth defects come about.
  - Chromosomal anomalies.
  - Single gene defects (consider different types of genes, e.g. those encoding structural proteins, transcription factors, etc.). Also consider disturbances in gene expression, e.g. imprinted genes.
  - Effects of multiple gene mutations/polymorphisms, e.g. Hirschsprung disease.
  - Multifactorial disorder (a combination of genetic predisposition and environmental factors, e.g. neural tube defects (NTD)).
  - Mainly environmental, e.g. mechanical compression and teratogens (although in the latter genetic predisposition may play a part, e.g. in drug metabolism).
  - Mosaicism: chromosomal, single gene mutation, or in gene expression.

3 Think whether you have seen this before.
  - Personal experience is helpful and people get better and more experienced at dysmorphology over time. You may be able to recognize a 'gestalt' that is familiar to you from a previous consultation or from the literature.

4 Seek help from the literature.
  - See 'Useful resources', page 30.

5 Search the London Dysmorphology Database and OMIM (Online Mendelian Inheritance in Man) database.
  - Databases are most useful if you search on distinctive features ('hard' diagnostic handles), e.g. midline cleft lip, rather than common or subjective features such as 'low-set ears'. With experience it becomes easier to 'sift out' syndromes that are least likely matches with your patient.

6 Seek help from colleagues.
  - Share information and photographs/images with other colleagues in your department and with specialists in the field.

Genetic advice for a known diagnosis

If you are able to make a specific diagnosis, take steps to confirm it where possible by suitable laboratory tests. Genetic advice about recurrence risk or offspring risk is usually relatively straightforward in this situation.

Genetic advice for an unknown diagnosis

The clinical geneticist may need to give advice in the absence of a specific diagnosis. Studies have shown that follow-up of children may lead to a diagnosis as genetic and biochemical testing improves and syndrome delineation is clearer. The practice of sharing knowledge within a genetics department by the use of clinical photography sessions ensures that expertise and experience of rare syndromes are shared for the benefit of the patients and the training of junior staff.

When a diagnosis remains unknown, it is important to spend time in the counselling session explaining the reasons for this and the fact that genetic advice is derived from the probability that the child's problems have a genetic cause.

Recurrence risk

Certain features, or patterns of features, suggest a high recurrence risk of up to 25%. These include (but this is *not* a complete list):

- previous affected child;
- previous stillbirth/late miscarriages due to fetal abnormalities;
- family history of a similarly affected individual (X-linked, chromosomal, variable dominant condition);
- consanguinity;
- neurodevelopmental regression;
- coarsening of facial features;
- symmetrical structural defects previously noted in autosomal recessive (AR) conditions;
- maternal influences such as immunological conditions like myasthenia where the antibodies cross the placenta have a very high risk in a subsequent pregnancies.

In the absence of features suggesting a high risk (see above), an *empiric risk* of ~5% may be advised. Explain that this is a composite risk—for the majority of families the risks are very low, but for some they will be high (25%). Also emphasize that this risk figure could change substantially if a specific diagnosis is subsequently made.

Carrier detection

Individuals at high risk may be determined from the pedigree, e.g. where there is evidence of X-linked inheritance.

Prenatal diagnosis

In the absence of a specific diagnosis it is not usually possible to offer prenatal diagnosis unless there are congenital malformations, e.g. congenital heart disease, polydactyly. If malformations are present (and these are thought to be part of the child's condition, rather than coincidental) it may be possible to look for structural abnormalities in the fetus by USS in the second trimester. Consult a fetal medicine specialist if there is any doubt over the timing of scanning, or the ease with which the specific structural anomalies in question can be visualized. Explain the limitations of this approach.

Natural history and further management

Observation of the natural history is an extremely important part of the management of the child with an undiagnosed dysmorphic syndrome. Follow-up the first consultation with another to establish that the investigations are complete and that all of this information has been exchanged.

Subsequent follow-up at 1 year is suggested and thereafter by discussion with the family depending on such issues as their plans to have more children.

Surveillance and follow-up

Review appointments can help in the following ways:

- to offer newly available diagnostic tests;
- to establish that there are no additional medical problems and that there is forward developmental progress;
- to increase the chance of syndrome recognition. Some dysmorphic syndromes are not easy to diagnose until a few years of age;
- to discuss recurrence risks.

Support group: Contact a family, `<www.cafamily.org.uk>`. Puts families in touch with others with similar features.

Expert advisers: Karen Temple, Consultant Clinical Geneticist, Wessex Regional Genetics Service, Southampton, Dian Donnai, Professor of Medical Genetics, University of Manchester, Manchester, and Jill Clayton-Smith, Consultant Clinical Geneticist, St Mary's Hospital, Manchester, England.

References

Aase JM. *Diagnostic dysmorphology*. Plenum, New York, 1990.

Biesecker LG. The end of the beginning of chromosome ends. *Am J Med Genet* 2002; **107**: 263–6.

Bundey S, Carter C. Recurrence risks in severe undiagnosed mental deficiency. *J Ment Defic Res* 1974; **18**: 115–34.

Curry CJ, Stevenson RE, *et al.* Evaluation of mental retardation: recommendations of a Consensus Conference: American College of Medical Genetics. *Am J Med Genet* 1997; **72**: 468–77.

Flint J, Knight S. The use of telomere probes to investigate submicroscopic rearrangements associated with mental retardation. *Curr Opin Genet Dev* 2003; **13**: 310–16.

Jones KL (ed.). *Smith's recognizable patterns of human malformation*, 5th edn. W.B. Saunders, Philadelphia, 1997.

Knight SJ, Flint J. Screening chromosome ends for learning disability. *Br Med J* 2000; **321**: 1240.

Knight SJ, Regan R, *et al.* Subtle chromosomal rearrangments in children with unexplained mental retardation. *Lancet* 1999; **354**: 1666–81.

Kotzot D. Review and meta-analysis of systematic searches for uniparental disomy (UPD). *Am J Med Genet* 2002; **111**: 366–75.

Ness GO, Lybaek H, Houge G. Usefulness of high-resolution comparative genomic hybridization (CGH) for detecting and characterizing constitutional chromosome abnormalities. *Am J Med Genet* 2002; **113** (2): 125–36.

Rosenthal ET, Biesecker LG, Biesecker BB. Parental attitudes toward a diagnosis in children with unidentified multiple congenital anomaly syndromes. *Am J Med Genet* 2001; **103**: 106–14.

Turner G, Partington M. Recurrence risks in undiagnosed mental retardation. *J Med Genet* 2000; **37**: E45.

Winter RM, Baraitser M. London Dysmorphology Database 2003. `<www.lmdatabses.com>`.

Dystonia

Dystonia is defined as a disorder of movement caused by involuntary sustained muscle contractions affecting one or more sites of the body, frequently causing twisting and repetitive movements or abnormal postures.

Prevalence figures have varied between 127 and 329 per million, but it is probably more common than this. Focal dystonia, which affects a single body part, is the most common type.

The method of classification of dystonia (see table) by aetiology is useful when considering the differential diagnosis.

Clinical approach

The investigation of the child/adult with dystonia is primarily by a neurologist and the clinical approach of this section is primarily to detect genetic forms of dystonia.

History: key points

- Three-generation family tree. consider autosomal dominant (AD), autosomal recessive (AR), X-linked (XL), and mitochondrial forms of inheritance.
- Ethnic origin. AD early-onset torsion dystonia is 5 to 10 times more common in Ashkenazi Jews. XL dystonia–parkinsonism is found mainly in Filipinos.
- Age of onset.
- Site of onset and progression, both in severity and to other parts of the body. Presentation with dystonia involving the legs is more likely to progress.
- Reaction to alcohol. (Alcohol can improve the symptoms and signs in myoclonic dystonia.)
- Constant or paroxysmal?
- Other neurological features (epilepsy, mental retardation, regression, or loss of acquired skills).
- Exposure to neuroleptic medication.

Examination: key points

- Abnormal posturing. Distribution of dystonia—is it predominantly focal or generalized?
- Myoclonus.
- Parkinsonism (tremor, rigidity).
- Choreoathetosis (some heredodegenerative dystonias).
- Brisk or reduced reflexes, extensor plantars?
- Eyes. Eye movement disorder and nystagmus. Kaiser–Fleischer rings (Wilson disease).
- Fundal examination. Pigmentary retinopathy (Hallervorden–Spatz syndrome (HSS), mitochondrial disorders), optic atrophy (HSS, XL deafness–dystonia–optic atrophy syndrome, mitochondrial disorders).
- Muscle or cardiac involvement?
- Dementia.

- Hearing.
- Ataxia (patients with Friedreich's ataxia (FRDA) may have dystonia).

Special investigations

- Brain imaging, preferably magnetic resonance imaging (MRI) scan. Basal ganglia calcification (Fahr disease, Aicardi–Goutieres disease, mitochondrial disorders), 'eye of the tiger' sign in HSS.
- Electrophysiology (myoclonus).
- Molecular DNA analysis: In patients with an age of onset <26 years with any site of involvement, test for the *DYT1* mutation. Store with consent for future testing when there is no genetic testing available.
- Response to L-dopa—if positive consider specialist neurometabolic tests.

For **heredodegenerative dystonia** consider the following.

- Metabolic investigations amino acids in plasma and urine, urine organic acids (L-2 hydroxyglutaric aciduria, glutaric aciduria), white cell enzymes (GM2, Niemann–Pick type C, Krabbe disease), lipoproteins (hypobetalipoproteinaemia and abetalipoproteinaemia), neuronal ceroid lipofuscinosis, cerebrospinal fluid (CSF) pyruvate/lactate, and investigate further if necessary. See 'Developmental regression', page 96, on the investigation of metabolic disorders.
- Acanthocytes (neuroacanthocytosis).
- Copper studies to exclude Wilson disease.
- Consider ataxia telangiectasia (AT). See 'DNA repair defects', page 304.
- Consider Huntington disease (HD), spinocerebellar ataxias (SCAs), dentatorubro-pallidoluysian atrophy (DRPLA), Gerstmann–Straussler disease (GSD), especially if there is a dominant family history or if other neurological features develop.

Some diagnoses to consider

The primary dystonias

AD early-onset torsion dystonia (idiopathic torsion dystonia, dystonia 1). A predominantly generalized dystonia, it typically presents in children and young adults. The arms or legs are often the primary focus of dystonia and it then spreads to affect other areas. It is an extremely variable condition and some obligate carriers have minimal symptoms. The gene locus is DYT1. The GAG deletion mutation, which leads to a loss of glutamic acid, accounts for all known mutations and is usually referred to as the '*DYT1* mutation'. Penetrance is 30–40%.

Classification of dystonia

Primary torsion dystonia	Dystonia is the only symptom
'Dystonia-plus'	Dystonia is one of only two neurological conditions present; the other is usually myoclonus or parkinsonism
Heredodegenerative dystonia	Dystonia is part of a more widespread neurodegenerative syndrome, often of genetic aetiology
Secondary ('symptomatic') dystonia	Caused by environmental insults such as drugs (especially neuroleptics), infections, strokes, and tumours

Empirical recurrence risks were calculated prior to the availability of *DYT1* testing. The sib recurrence risk given in familial cases was 21% and for an isolated case 14%. Observed risks are slightly lower. There is no figure for the risk of a severely affected child.

Adult-onset idiopathic torsion dystonia. A predominantly focal or segmental dystonia. The main differentiating features from the early-onset idiopathic torsion dystonia are:

- later presentation, typically mid adult life;
- the symptoms do not usually spread to become generalized.

The genetic contribution to this condition is uncertain but there has been an estimate that 25% of affected individuals have a significant family history.

Genetic testing is not possible unless there is a family history of early-onset in which cases arrange *DYT1* analysis.

'Dystonia-plus'

Dopa-responsive dystonia (DRD; Segawa syndrome). This is a rare condition (prevalence 0.5–1.0 per million) but important to recognize as it is treatable. Onset is usually in childhood/adolescence and dystonia is the presenting feature. Parkinsonism may also occur. Reflexes may become brisk with extensor plantars.

The phenotype in childhood may resemble athetoid cerebral palsy and all children with this condition should have a trial of L-dopa.

Inheritance is usually AD with reduced penetrance. The gene *GCH1* codes for an enzyme in the tetrahydrobiopterin pathway. An AR type is due to mutation in the tyrosine hydroxylase gene.

Myoclonic dystonia. This group includes patients with variable degrees of dystonia and myoclonus. An important feature in the history is that there may be a dramatic improvement in symptoms with alcohol.

Inheritance is AD with reduced penetrance. There is more than one locus and one gene have been characterized (E. sarcoglycan).

Heredodegenerative dystonia

Investigate for metabolic and mitochondrial disorders. In addition the following have recognizable phenotypes and should be considered:

- **Krabbe disease.** Krabbe disease or globoid cell leukodystrophy is an AR disorder involving the white matter of the peripheral and central nervous systems. Mutations in the gene for the lysosomal enzyme galactocerebrosidase (*GALC*) result in low enzymatic activity and decreased ability to degrade galactolipids found almost exclusively in myelin. While most patients present with symptoms within the first 6 months of life, others present later in life including adulthood. Infantile Krabbe disease can present with dystonia (lead-pipe rigidity of the limbs and abnormal posturing) together with irritability, poor feeding, motor regression, and seizures. The MRI may show white matter changes and calcification particularly affecting the basal ganglia.
- **Fahr disease.** Basal ganglia calcification. Adult-onset, AD.
- **Aicardi–Goutieres syndrome.** Rapidly fatal encephalopathy of infancy with intracerebral calcification and white matter disease.

- **Pantothenate kinase-associated neurodegeneration syndrome (Hallervorden–Spatz syndrome (HSS)).** AR. Characteristic MRI features.
- **X-linked dystonia parkinsonism**. Mainly found in the Philippines.
- **X-linked deafness–dystonia–optic atrophy syndrome** (Mohr–Tranebjaerg syndrome). *DDP* gene.
- **Neuroacanthocytosis.** Distinguish between McLeod syndrome (X-linked recessive (XLR)) and choreoacanthocytosis (AR).

Paroxysmal dystonia/dyskinesia

Intermittent episodes of dystonia or dyskinesia, usually with no neurological features in between attacks. As for episodic ataxia and some forms of epilepsy, mutations in ion channel genes may be the underlying cause.

Genetic advice

If the exact diagnosis is unknown, aim to place into one of the above groups.

- Most of the primary dystonias and 'dystonia-plus' syndromes show AD inheritance, often with reduced penetrance and clinical variability.
- Heredodegenerative conditions may have AD, AR, XL, or mitochondrial inheritance.

Recurrence risk

As for the underlying diagnosis.

Carrier detection

Pedigee analysis or using a specific biochemical or genetic test.

Prenatal diagnosis

Not possible unless a specific biochemical or genetic cause has been identified.

Natural history and further management (preventative measures)

- Specific treatment for DRD and Wilson disease.
- Medication may help the symptoms.
- Injection of the affected muscles with botulinum toxin.
- Peripheral or central stereotatic surgery.

Lay group contact: The Dystonia Society <www.dystonia.org.uk>.

Expert adviser: Andrea Németh, Consultant and Lecturer in Clinical Genetics, University of Oxford, Oxford, England.

References

Bressman SB, *et al*. The DYT1 phenotype and guidelines for diagnostic testing. *Neurology* 2000; **54**: 1746–52.

Fahn S, Marsden CD, Calne DB. Classification and investigation of dystonia. In *Movement disorders*, Vol. 2 (ed. C.D. Marsden and S. Fahn), pp. 332–58. Butterworths, London, 1987.

Fletcher NA. The genetics of idiopathic torsion dystonia [review]. *J Med Genet* 1990; **27**: 409–12.

Németh AH. The genetics of primary dystonia and related disorders. *Brain* 2002; **125**: 695–721.

Wenger DA, Rafi MA, *et al*. Krabbe disease: genetic aspects and progress toward therapy. *Mol Genet Metab* 2000; **70**: 1–9.

Ear anomalies

The external auricle (pinna) develops from the six auricular hillocks that arise as mesenchymal derivatives of the first and second branchial arches. The external ears begin to develop around the first branchial groove and ascend up to the level of the eyes during embryonic and early fetal life.

Accurate description of ear anomalies (see table for terminology used) is not always straightforward—photography provides the best documentation. The ear of newborns, especially in premature babies, is sometimes rather 'crumpled' and the helix may appear deficient. If there is a major anomaly this is usually obvious, but otherwise it may be best to review when the infant is a few weeks older.

This section describes the approach to the diagnosis in children where the ear anomalies are a major diagnostic feature. There are many syndromes where the abnormality of the ear is a component of the condition, e.g. low-set and posteriorly rotated ears in Noonan syndrome and ear creases in Beckwith syndrome, but is not the presenting or main diagnostic feature, nor always present.

Clinical approach
History: key points
- Three-generation family tree including specific enquiry regarding ear anomalies, deafness, renal problems, unusual facial appearance.
- History of maternal diabetes, early bleeding, teratogenic agents, e.g. retinoic acid, alcohol.
- Delayed motor milestones or developmental delay.
- Visual or hearing problems.

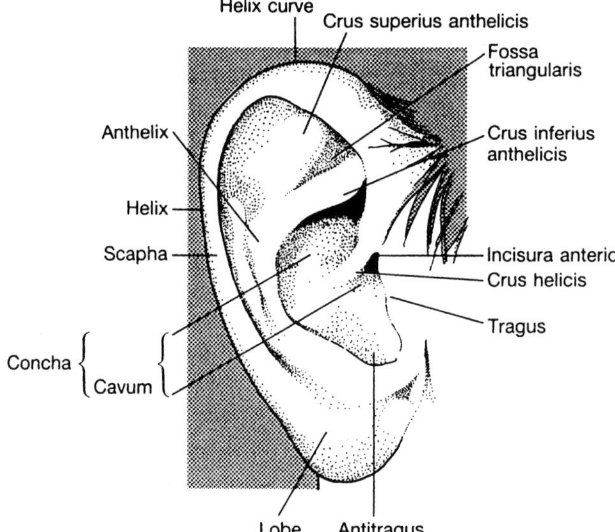

Landmarks of the external ear. (Reproduced from Hall *et al.* (1989) by permission of Oxford University Press.)

Terminology

Anomaly	Description
Simple ear	Lack of interior detail such as anthelix and crus inferius anthelicus rather than showing the sculpting and moulding usually seen. The pinna is largely flat and the helix may be partly deficient
Dysplastic ear	Loosely used to describe any form of ear malformation
Microtia	Vestiges of the external ear are present, but it is very small. Complete absence of the external ear (anotia) is very rare
Ear tags	These result from the development of accessory auricular hillocks. Usually fleshy, but may contain cartilage, may be sessile or pedunculated. In OAV they occur in the line between the tragus and angle of the mouth (line of junction of the mandibular and maxillary processes)
'Cupped ear'	Caused by deficiency of the posterior auricular muscle
'Lop ear'	Caused by deficiency of the superior auricular muscle
'Ear pits'	Blind-ending pits typically found in the pre-auricular region
'Ear creases'	Usually found on the ear lobe and on the back of the ear, particularly along the rim
'Low-set ear'	The upper attachment of the ear is below a line connecting the outer canthus of the eye and the occiput
'Posteriorly rotated ear'	The longitudinal axis of the ear is rotated towards the occiput

Examination: key points
- Carefully describe the ear morphology and photograph if appropriate.
- Look carefully for ear pits.
- Carefully assess the external auditory meatus. Is it normal in diameter or atretic?
- Examine the eyes for lower lid colobomata (Treacher Collins syndrome (TCS)) or epibulbar dermoid (oculo-auriculo-vertebral (OAV) syndrome), upper lid colobomata (OAV), iris and retinal colobomata (CHARGE (coloboma–heart defects–atresia choanae– retardation of growth and/or development–genital defect–ear anomalies and/or deafness) association).
- Assess the face for malar hypoplasia (TCS, Nager, and Miller syndromes).
- Examine the neck for branchial sinuses/cysts (branchio-oto-renal (BOR) syndrome)
- Examine the heart (CHARGE).
- Examine the limbs: thumb duplications and deficiency (OAV syndrome), triphalangeal or hypoplastic thumbs (Townes–Brock syndrome (TBS)), radial ray anomalies (Nager syndrome), ulnar ray anomalies (Miller syndrome).

Special investigations
- Karyotype eg. abnormalities of 22, del 4p, del 5p (include telomeres/comparative genomic hybridization (CGH) for apparent CHARGE association).
- Store blood for DNA if diagnosis of TCS, TBS, or BOR is possible.
- Audiogram.
- Ophthalmology opinion, epibulbar dermoid (OAV syndrome), coloboma of choroids and/or retina (CHARGE).
- Renal ultrasound scan (USS) unless clear diagnosis of TCS in which renal anomalies are not found; renal anomalies are rare in OAV.
- Chest X-ray, electrocardiogram (ECG), cardiac echo in suspected CHARGE or if signs of a cardiac abnormality.
- Consider cervical spine films if diagnosis of OAV is possible (cervical vertebral fusion in 20–35%).

Some diagnoses to consider

Treacher Collins syndrome (TCS; mandibulofacial dysostosis). An autosomal dominant (AD) disorder with extremely variable expressivity caused by mutations in the *TCOF1* gene at 5q32–33.1. The ear anomalies are bilateral. They are malformed and displaced towards the angle of the mandible. One-third have atresia of the external auditory meatus and abnormality of the ossicles. The facial features tend to be symmetrical. Conductive hearing loss is common but also screen for sensorineural deafness. Malar hypoplasia, coloboma (V-shaped notch) of inferior eyelid at junction of medial two-thirds and lateral one-third. Choanal atresia may be a feature of severe TCS. Intelligence is normal. Consider mutation analysis of *TCS1*. Approximately 17% have a 5 nucleotide deletion towards the 3' end of the gene. 60–70% are the result of *de novo* mutations.

Oculo-auriculo-vertebral spectrum (OAV). Also known as Goldenhar syndrome, hemifacial microsomia, first and second arch syndrome, and craniofacial microsomia.

In the majority of children the disorder is unilateral. When bilateral, there is a difference in severity between the right and left sides. The right is more often involved than the left. OAV syndrome is extremely variable ranging from isolated, unilateral ear anomalies as the mildest form to an expanded form with malformations in the central nervous system (CNS), vertebrae, heart, and kidneys. Ear abnormalities are present in 65%. Microtia with preauricular skin tags and additional skin tags in the line between the tragus and the angle of the mouth. The ear abnormalities may be bilateral but are asymmetric. See 'Facial asymmetry', page 112.

CHARGE (coloboma – heart defects – atresia choanae – retardation of growth and/or development – genital defect – ear anomalies and/or deafness) syndrome. Distinctive ear anomalies and/or deafness occur in 85–100%. Usually bilateral but asymmetrical, with low-set, prominent, posteriorly rotated ears with deficient cartilage and hypoplastic lobes. The ears may be 'cup-shaped' or lop, but the variation in morphology is very wide and often quite marked between the two ears of an individual patient. Deafness is variable, most usually a moderate to severe progressive mixed loss, with defects of the ossicles and 'glue-ear' causing the conductive component. Absent or hypoplastic semicircular canals appear to be a common and important feature.

CHARGE has a prevalence of ~1/12,000. It is caused by mutation in the gene *CHD7* which acts in early embryonic development by affecting chromatin structure and gene expression (Vissers). See 'Coloboma', page 82 for further details.

Branchio-oto-renal (BOR) syndrome. An AD disorder caused by mutations in *EYA1* on 8q13. Ear anomalies include ear pits, dysplastic pinnae, and conductive, sensorineural, or mixed hearing loss. Branchial fistulae or cysts (60%) usually found on the medial border of the sternomastoid muscle. Renal anomalies include duplex collecting system, hydronephrosis, cystic kidneys, and unilateral or bilateral renal agenesis. The nasolacrimal duct may be blocked.

Townes–Brock syndrome (TBS). An AD disorder caused by mutations in the *SALL1* transcription factor gene, which is expressed in the developing ear, limb buds, and excretory organs. Phenotypic expression is extremely variable but includes two or more of: bilateral ear malformation, e.g. dysplastic ears; ear tags; sensorineural hearing loss (71%); hand malformations, e.g. triphalangeal or hypoplastic thumbs (56%); and imperforate anus or recto-vaginal/rectourethral fistula (47%); and renal anomalies. High incidence of new mutations. Cardiac anomalies have been reported.

Nager acrofacial dysostosis. TCS-like facial features with marked micrognathia. Radial ray anomalies (hypoplastic or absent thumbs and radii) are the main distinguishing features. 95% have hearing impairment.

Miller syndrome. An autosomal recessive (AR) condition with TCS-like facial features with lower lid colobomata, malar hypoplasia, micrognathia. Ulnar ray hypoplasia (ulnar hypoplasia or fifth finger hypoplasia/aplasia) is the key distinguishing feature. 20% have hearing impairment.

Cat-eye syndrome (CES). Variable pattern of multiple anomalies including iris colobomata, anal atresia, and pre-auricular anomalies (triad only present in 40%). Mild to moderate mental retardation in 32%. Bisatellite marker chromosome derived from inverted dicentric duplication of 22q. Occasionally inherited. See 'Supernumerary marker chromosomes (SMCs)—postnatal' and 'Supernumerary marker chromosomes (SMCs)—prenatal', pages 552 and 554.

18q–. Patients with subtelomeric deletions of 18q typically have narrow slit-like ear canals together with mental retardation, midface hypoplasia, and a carp-shaped mouth.

Genetic advice

Recurrence risk
As for specific condition.

Carrier detection
Clinical examination combined with mutation analysis, if available.

Prenatal diagnosis
Is possible for some of these conditions, e.g.
- ultrasound scans for structural abnormalities;
- chromosomal or mutation analysis if an abnormality has been identified in the proband.

Lay group contact: Many of the conditions have their own support group. See <www.cafamily.org.uk>.

Expert adviser: Maria Bitner-Glindzicz, Senior Lecturer and Honorary Consultant Geneticist, Institute of Child Health, London, England.

References

Gorlin RJ. Oculo-auriculo-vertebral spectrum. In *Management of genetic syndromes* (ed. S.B. Cassidy and J.E. Allanson), Chapter 16. Wiley-Liss, New York, 2001.

Hall, JG, *et al. Handbook of normal physical measurements.* Oxford University Press, Oxford, 1989.

Ogilvy-Stuart AL, Parsons AC. Miller syndrome (postaxial acrofacial dysostosis): further evidence for autosomal recessive inheritance and expansion of the phenotype. *J Med Genet* 1992; **28**: 695–700.

Oley CA. CHARGE association. In *Management of genetic syndromes* (ed. S.B. Cassidy and J.E. Allanson), Chapter 5. Wiley-Liss, New York, 2001.

Powell CM, Michaelis RC. Townes–Brock syndrome. *J Med Genet* 1999; **36**: 89–93.

Sanlaville D, Romana SP, *et al.* A CGH study pf 27 patients with CHARGE association. *Clin Genet* 2002; **61**: 135–8.

Vissers L, Ravenswaaij C, *et al.* Mutations in a new member of the chromodomain gene family cause CHARGE syndrome. *Nat Gen* 2004; **36**: 955–57.

Wang RY, Earl DL, *et al.* Syndromic ear anomalies and renal ultrasounds. *Pediatrics* 2001; **108**: E32.

Facial asymmetry

Although all faces show some asymmetry, significant facial asymmetry is a well-recognized feature of a number of distinctive conditions including the oculo-auriculo-vertebral spectrum (OAVS), which is one of the most common malformations seen in babies.

If there is a size difference without malformation, a common difficulty is distinguishing which side is 'normal'.

Please also refer to 'Ear anomalies' and 'Plagiocephaly and abnormalities of skull shape', pages 108 and 212.

Clinical approach

History: key points

- Family history, particularly to exclude autosomal dominant (AD) conditions with variable expression.
- Pregnancy. Diabetes, early bleeding, teratogenic agents e.g. retinoic acid, alcohol (OAVS), bleeding, placental abnormality (disruption), decreased liquor, abnormal fetal presentation, persistent discomfort and sensation of 'head being stuck', twin pregnancy (deformation).
- Uterine abnormalities such as bicornuate uterus, precipitate delivery, sleeping position (deformation).
- Obstructed labour (pre-existing craniosynostosis, syndromes with macrocephaly).
- Was asymmetry noted at birth? If not at what age?
- Progression of deformity.
- Delayed motor milestones or developmental delay.
- Visual or hearing problems.
- Seizures (structural brain malformations, hemimegalencephaly, raised intracranial pressure from craniosynostosis).

Examination: key points

Careful measurements and clinical photography should be used to document the visual impression.

- Overall shape of the face and supraorbital area. Is any abnormality unilateral or is it bilateral with asymmetry?
- Is it possible to differentiate the normal from the affected side of the face?
- Are all the structures normally formed or are malformations present?
- Ears. Shape, size, symmetry.
- Ear malformations: accessory auricles, skin tags between the tragus and the angle of the mouth (OAVS), preauricular ear pits (branchio-oto-renal (BOR) syndrome).
- Midfacial (malar) flattening?
- Mandibular asymmetry.
- Eye spacing (measure) and/or exorbitism.
- Eye malformations: epibulbar dermoid (OAVS), microphthalmia (OAVS), coloboma or notch in the outer third of the lower eyelid (Treacher–Collins syndrome (TCS)).
- Mouth. Macrostomia in OAVS, facial clefting.
- Facial weakness/palsy gives an asymmetric appearance (CHARGE syndrome).
- Fontanelle. Position, size, and tension.
- Palpable sutures, compensatory bulging/bossing (craniosynostosis).
- Describe skull shape. Examine the head from both sides, above and from the front (differentiating postural plagiocephaly and craniosynostosis). Ear position, used in conjunction with the skull shape to assess if deformation is likely.

- Facial clefts (developmental disruptions, malformation syndromes) and cleft palate (deformations, OAVS).
- Neck: torticollis, branchial cyst (BOR).
- Skin pigmentary abnormalities and haemangiomas.
- Cardiac murmur.
- Hands and feet:
  - Thumb duplications and deficiency (OAVS), triphalangeal or hypoplastic thumbs (Townes–Brocks syndrome (TBS)).
  - Minor degrees of syndactyly in Saethre–Chotzen syndrome.
- Movement asymmetric?

Special investigations

- Clinical photographs are valuable, especially for documenting changes over time.
- Audiology in children with ear anomalies.
- Ophthalmology review: delineate structural lesions, epibulbar dermoid (OAVS), coloboma of choroid and/or retina (CHARGE).
- Cervical X-rays in children with OAVS (cervical vertebral fusion in 20–35%).
- Skull X-ray. Posteroanterior (PA); lateral if there is cranial asymmetry:
  - orbital asymmetry (OAVS);
  - sphenoid wing dysplasia (neurofibromatosis type 1 (NF1));
  - the signs of synostosis are partial or total absence of the suture, indistinct zones along the suture, and perisutural sclerosis. Assess for evidence of a harlequin sign (elevation of the lesser wing of sphenoid) in coronal synostosis. Interpretation is difficult in infants and requires good quality films and expert reporting.
- Consider cranial ultrasound scan (USS) in infants.
- Chest X-ray, electrocardiogram (ECG), cardiac echo in syndromes with a high incidence of cardiac abnormality.
- Consider the need for a renal USS.
- Referral to specialist surgical centre if appropriate for detailed assessment and further imaging.
- Assessment of parents.
- Chromosomal analysis. Routine cytogenetic analysis in the normally developing infant with no features other than facial asymmetry is not indicated. The presence of developmental delay would be sufficient to warrant investigation. Consider fluorescent *in situ* hybridization (FISH) tests for *TWIST* (Saethre–Chotzen syndrome).
- Molecular analysis in infants with TBS, BOR, and Saethre–Chotzen syndrome and *FGFR3* for Muenke syndrome.
- Consider video to demonstrate asymmetric facial movement.

Some diagnoses to consider

With features that usually lead to presentation at birth or during infancy

Oculo-auriculo-vertebral spectrum (OAVS). Also known as Goldenhar syndrome, hemifacial microsomia, first and second arch syndrome, and craniofacial microsomia. Gorlin (2001) recommends the use of the term oculo-auricular-vertebral spectrum for this heterogeneous condition that affects primarily the development of the ear, oral structures, and mandible. In the majority of children the disorder is unilateral. When bilateral, there is a difference in severity between the right and left sides. The right is more often involved than the left. OAVS is extremely variable ranging from isolated, unilateral ear anomalies as the mildest form to an expanded form with malformations in the central nervous system (CNS), vertebrae, heart, and kidneys.

Facial asymmetry is severe in 20%, but evident to some extent in 65%. This is due to a combination of hypoplasia of the bony structures of the face and abnormality of the ear. The ear abnormalities are more fully described in 'Ear anomalies', page 108.

Gorlin (2001) estimates the frequency to be about 1 in 5600 births. OAVS is usually a sporadic disorder, and a vascular event in early pregnancy is a possible mechanism. There are some dominant families, so it is important to examine parents.

Syndromes with overlapping features of OAVS. Asymmetry may be present but the bilateral features help differentiate these from OAVS.

- **Treacher Collins syndrome (TCS).** An AD condition characterised by a distinctive facial appearance with ear anomalies, malar hypoplasia and micrognathia and caused by mutations in the TCS1 gene on 5q32-33.1. The symmetry of TCS is not found in OAVS (for more detail, see 'Ear anomalies', page 108.)
- **Townes–Brocks syndrome (TBS).** Caused by mutation in the SALL1 transcription factor gene, which is expressed in the developing ear, limb buds, and excretory organs. Phenotypic expression is extremely variable but includes two or more of: bilateral ear malformation, eg. dysplastic ears; ear tags; sensorineural hearing loss (71%); hand malformations, e.g.triphalangeal or hypoplastic thumbs (56%); and imperforate anus or rectovaginal/rectourethral fistula (47%); and renal anomalies. High incidence of new mutations. Cardiac anomalies have been reported. Consider screening patients with overlapping features of OAVS for mutations in SALL1.
- **Branchio-oto-renal syndrome (BOR).** AD disorder caused by mutations in *EYA1* on 8q13. Pre-auricular pits and branchial fistulae are useful diagnostic craniofacial features. (See 'Ear anomalies', page 108.)
- **CHARGE syndrome** (coloboma – heart defects – atresia choanae – retardation of growth and/or development – genital defect – ear anomalies and/or deafness). Asymmetry of the ears is commonly seen in CHARGE syndrome. Facial asymmetry and unilateral facial palsy are also common in this condition which is caused by mutations in the gene *CHD7*. See Clinical approach to Coloboma for further details.
- **Oculocerebrocutaneous (Delleman) syndrome.** A rare syndrome with orbital cysts, focal dermal malformations, periorbital skin tags, and agenesis of the corpus callosum.

Moebius syndrome. The face is asymmetric if there is unilateral weakness of the VIIth (facial) nerve. Moebius sequence/syndrome is a rare disorder characterized by congenital palsy of the VIth and VIIth cranial nerves. Other cranial nerves may be affected, together with skeletal and orofacial anomalies. In Stromland *et al.*'s (2002) survey of 25 patients with Moebius syndrome, associated anomalies included: limb malformations (10); Poland anomaly (2); hypodontia (7); microglossia (6); cleft palate (4); hearing impairment (5); and external ear malformation (1). Pronounced functional abnormalities were observed involving facial expression (16); speech (13); eating and swallowing (12); and difficulty in sucking in infancy (11). Six patients had an autistic syndrome, one an autistic-like condition, and mental retardation was found in all these patients. Bouwes-Bavinck *et al.* (1986) propose that Moebius syndrome results from vascular disruption of the primitive trigeminal arteries before the establishment of sufficient blood supply for the brainstem by the vertebral arteries. Moebius is usually sporadic (especially when there are accompanying limb defects), but there are some reports of dominant transmission in the literature.

Deformation. See 'Plagiocephaly and abnormalities of skull shape', this chapter.

Disruptions. Unusual facial clefts, possibly associated with amniotic bands.

Craniosynostosis. See 'Craniosynostosis' in Chapter 3, page 288.

- Unilateral coronal craniosynostosis.
- Saethre–Chotzen syndrome (SCS): facial asymmetry is a major feature of SCS, unlike the other syndromal craniosynostosis syndromes.
- *FGFR3*-associated coronal synostosis (Muenke syndrome). The mutation Pro250Arg in *FGFR3* causes AD inheritance of unilateral or bilateral craniosynostosis (Reardon *et al.* 1997).

Chromosomal abnormalities.

- Abnormalities of chromosome 22, including trisomy 22, del 22q, ring and duplication (cat eye syndrome) are particularly associated with ear tags and facial asymmetry.
- Mosaic chromosome abnormalities.

Vascular anomalies. Arteriovenous malformations and haemangiomas.

With features that usually lead to presentation in childhood

Hemihyperplasia or overgrowth (and tumours).

- Encephalocraniocutaneous lipomatosis and Proteus syndrome. There is disagreement as whether to classify these as separate disorders. Features are multiple lipomas of the head and neck, hyperostosis of the skull, macrocephaly, and streaks of yellow-brown pigmentation.
- NF1 sphenoid wing dysplasia, plexiform neurofibromata.
- Isolated hemihypertrophy. Examine for features of Beckwith–Wiedemann and Silver–Russell syndromes.

Hemiatrophy is less common than hyperplasia.

- Consider mosaicism for single gene and chromosomal disorders.
- Progressive hemiatrophy/Parry–Romberg syndrome in older children.
- Post-radiation damage.

Genetic advice

Recurrence risk
As for specific condition.

Carrier detection
Clinical examination combined with mutation analysis, if available.

Prenatal diagnosis
This is possible for conditions for some of these conditions
- USS for structural abnormalities.
- Chromosomal or mutation analysis.

Natural history and further management (preventative measures)

- Deformational disorders improve with time once the deformational force has been lost.
- Specialist surgical assessment by a craniofacial centre.

Support group: Many of the syndromes have their own support groups. See <www.cafamily.org.uk>.

Expert adviser: Robert J. Gorlin, Department of Oral Pathology and Genetics, University of Minnesota, Minneapolis, Minnesota, USA.

References

Bouwes-Bavinck J, Weaver D. Subclavian artery disruption sequence—hypothesis of vascular aetiology for Poland, Klippel–Feil and Moebius anomalies. *Am J Med Genet* 1986; **23**: 903–18.

Gorlin RJ. Oculo-auriculo-vertebral spectrum. In *Management of genetic syndromes* (ed. S.B. Cassidy and J.E. Allanson), Chapter 16. Wiley-Liss, New York, 2001.

Keegan CE, Mulliken JB, *et al.* Townes–Brocks syndrome versus expanded spectrum hemifacial microsomia: review of eight patients and further evidence of a 'hot spot' for mutation in the *SALL1* gene. *Genet Med* 2001; **3**: 310–13.

Kelberman D, *et al.* Hemifacial microsomia: progress in understanding the genetic basis of a complex malformation syndrome. *Hum Genet* 2001; **109**: 638–45.

Reardon W, *et al.* Craniosynostosis associated with *FGFR3* Pro250Arg mutation results in a range of clinical presentations including unilateral sporadic craniosynostosis. *J Med Genet* 1997; **34**: 632–6.

Sanlaville D, Romana SP, *et al.* A CGH study of 27 patients with CHARGE association. *Clin Genet* 2002; **61**: 135–8.

Stromland K, Sjogreen L, *et al.* Mobius sequence—a Swedish multidiscipline study. *Eur J Paediatr Neurol* 2002; **6** (1): 35–45.

Failure to thrive (prenatal and postnatal growth failure)

The section describes the genetic investigation of babies who are small at birth and infants who fail to gain weight normally and are relatively proportionate, but small and thin with a weight below the 0.4th centile. They are usually short, though their height/length centile may be slightly better than the weight centile. Their head size may be normal for age, or in proportion to their body size. If the child's weight is on a similar or higher centile to the height/length centile, use 'Short stature', page 242.

One of the most useful features is the differentiation between pre- and postnatal onset of growth retardation. Early embryonic growth is largely driven by insulin-like growth factors 1 & 2 (1GF-1 and 1GF-2) fetal and early neonatal growth by IGF-1, and growth in later childhood by growth hormone (GH) and IGF-1.

It is assumed that a paediatrician has excluded the most common medical causes of failure to thrive (coeliac disease, cows-milk protein intolerance, etc.). Often the referral letter will query whether the child has Silver–Russell (Russell–Silver) syndrome (SRS).

Clinical approach

History: key points

- Three-generation family tree with specific enquiry for consanguinity, parental heights, and birthweights and current size (in relation to their peers) of other children in the family.
- Pregnancy.
  - Did ultrasound scans (USS) indicate growth problems and at what gestation was it noted?
  - Liquor volume. Oligohydramnios (placental insufficiency), polyhydramnios (cardiofaciocutaneous (CFC) syndrome, Costello and Bartter syndromes).
- Birthweight, length, and head circumference. Copy the growth record chart into the genetic files.
- Feeding history.
- Developmental milestones. Children with SRS may have some delay in motor milestones because of the relatively large head size compared to body size and strength. Also allow for prematurity.
- Medical history. Recurrent infections?

Examination: key points

- Accurate measurement of weight, length, and head circumference. Note any disproportion.
- Limb or body asymmetry (SRS). Compare the length and circumference of the limbs (align thumbs and feet for comparison).
- Skin pigmentation abnormalities. Café-au-lait patches (SRS), telangiectasias (Bloom), acanthosis nigricans (lipoatrophic conditions and Donohue syndrome).
- Dry or lax skin (CFC syndrome and Costello syndrome).
- Polyps and papillomas around mucous membranes (Costello syndrome).
- Coarse facial features (Costello, CFC syndrome, Donohue syndrome, and other metabolic disorders).
- Blue sclerae (SRS).
- Sparse, curly hair (CFC syndrome).
- Fifth finger clinodactyly (SRS).
- Cardiac murmurs (pulmonary stenosis is the most common lesion in CFC and Costello syndromes).

Special investigations

- Basic investigations (usually performed by paediatrician): serum urea and electrolytes, thyroid function, antigliadin antibodies, full blood count, and erythrocyte sedimentation rate (ESR).
- Bone age (wrist X-ray) and other skeletal films if a skeletal dysplasia is a possibility.
- Cytogenetic. Consider additional testing for DNA repair defects and chromosome breakage if clinically indicated and fluorescent *in situ* hybridization (FISH) for Williams del 7q11.23 if clinically indicated.
- DNA for uniparental disomy 7 (UPD-7; see below). Consider Prader–Willi syndrome (PWS) methylation assay if hypotonic. Consider cystic fibrosis (CF) screen.
- Cardiac echo for valvular and heart muscle abnormalities.
- Metabolic investigations. Ensure a basic screen has been performed. Further specific testing, e.g. insulin levels (Donohue syndrome), if clinically indicated.
- Consider tests of exocrine pancreatic function, e.g. faecal elastase 1 (FE1; Shwachman–Diamond and Johanssen–Blizzard syndromes). FE1 is a simple, non-invasive, highly specific, and sensitive test for determining pancreatic function. FE1 levels in meconium are low, and reach normal levels by day 3 in term newborns and by 2 weeks in infants born before 28 weeks gestation (Kori *et al.* 2003).
- Consider plasma aldosterone level if history of polyhydramnios (Bartter syndrome).
- Consider lymphocyte subsets and immunoglobulins to exclude a primary immunodeficiency.

Some syndromes/conditions to consider

With prenatal onset of growth retardation

Non-syndromic, or idiopathic intrauterine growth retardation (IUGR). These children may remain below the 2nd or 0.4th centile throughout childhood, though some catch-up is usual after birth. This group includes infants whose mothers had significant medical problems, as well as babies who are undernourished for a variety of non-genetic causes such as deprivation and drug and/or alcohol abuse.

Silver–Russell syndrome (SRS). The head is proportionately large, but usually between the 3rd and 25th centiles. The face is triangular and the mouth downturned. Asymmetry is a key diagnostic feature. The children are notoriously fussy eaters. Parents may comment on excessive sweating. There have been some dominant families described with a milder phenotype but the condition is generally sporadic. Discordant identical twins have been described. The development is usually within normal limits, but about one-third have late cognitive impairment. Approximately 10% of children have maternal UPD 7.

Uniparental disomy. This phenomenon may account for up to 5% of apparently idiopathic IUGR. Maternal UPD 7 is a recognized phenotype, which is similar to SRS. Maternal UPD studies were performed on 205 children with pre- and postnatal growth failure by Hannula *et al.* (2002), and only those with an SRS phenotype had positive results. DNA samples from parents and child are required.

Fetal alcohol syndrome (FAS). Growth retardation is a cardinal feature of FAS. Affected children have a low birthweight for gestational age (less than 2.5 centile), with decelerating weight over time not due to nutrition and disproportionately low weight to height. See 'Fetal alcohol syndrome (FAS)', page 588.

Dubowitz syndrome is an autosomal recessive (AR) condition characterized by pre- and postnatal growth retardation, eczema, telecanthus, epicanthal folds, blepharophimosis, ptosis, and broadening of the bridge and tip of the nose.

Bartter syndrome. AR condition characterized by hypokalaemic alkalosis with hypercalciuria. Genetically heterogeneous with mutations in *SLC12A1, KCNJ1*, and *SLC12A3*. History of polyhydramnios and often of preterm delivery with low birthweight and severe failure to thrive. Large head with prominent forehead, triangular face, large pinnae, and large eyes. Plasma K may be normal.

Donohue syndrome (leprechaunism). AR disorder due to mutations in the insulin receptor gene. Pre- and postnatal failure to thrive, hirsutism, aged face with thick lips and prominent ears, enlargement of breast and genitalia; acanthosis nigricans may be present. The serum insulin is grossly elevated. The prognosis is poor.

DNA repair defects. Rare syndromes with chromosome breaks, etc., e.g. Bloom syndrome and Cockayne syndrome. Patients have short stature and microcephaly and developmental delay. See 'DNA repair defects', page 304.

With predominantly postnatal failure to thrive and developmental delay/learning disability

Williams syndrome. These children may have terrible feeding difficulties and it is worth considering the diagnosis. See 'Congenital heart disease', page 84.

Prader–Willi syndrome (PWS). Central hypotonia and feeding difficulties with failure to thrive in infancy. See 'Obesity with and without developmental delay', page 192.

Metabolic and mitochondrial disorders. Assess for other features of these conditions and investigate accordingly in close collaboration with paediatric colleagues.

Cardiofaciocutaneous (CFC) syndrome. The hair is sparse, there is relative macrocephaly, and there can be cardiac defects, most commonly pulmonary stenosis and cardiomyopathy. The skin is rough, dry, and hyperkeratotic. Noonan-like facies. Polyhydramnios in pregnancy is common, perhaps a prenatal presentation of the severe feeding problems and failure to thrive that are common in the first year of life. Development is delayed. *PTPN11* mutations are not found.

Costello syndrome. Costello syndrome is characterized by prenatally increased growth, postnatal growth retardation, coarse face, loose skin resembling cutis laxa, nonprogressive cardiomyopathy (sometimes with arrhythmia), developmental delay, and an outgoing, friendly behaviour. There are very characteristic wrinkled palms and ulnar deviation of the hands.Patients can develop papillomata, especially around the mouth, and have a predisposition for malignancies (mainly abdominal and pelvic rhabdomyosarcoma in childhood). Consider USS surveillance. Costello syndrome is likely to be an autosomal dominant (AD) disorder. The pathogenesis is unclear, but there are many clues for implicating disturbed elastogenesis (Hennekam 2003).

Johanson–Blizzard syndrome. An AR condition with IUGR, scalp defects, and exocrine pancreatic insufficiency (FE1 is a useful screen) combined with dysmorphic features, notably a 'pinched' nose and notching of the alae nasi. Congenital heart disease and deafness may occur. The hair is often spiky. Usually associated with some learning disability, but not in all cases.

DNA repair defects. See above.

With predominantly postnatal failure to thrive and normal cognitive development

Metabolic and mitochondrial disorders. Assess for other features of these conditions and investigate accordingly in close collaboration with paediatric colleagues.

Lipodystrophies. There is loss of subcutaneous fat. Insulin resistance is common. Syndromic diagnoses include Beradinelli and SHORT syndromes. See 'Diabetes mellitus', page 298.

Schwachman–Diamond syndrome. AR condition characterized by pancreatic exocrine insufficiency, haematological dysfunction, and skeletal anomalies (metaphyseal dysplasia). Caused by mutations in *SBDS* on 7q11 (Boocock *et al.* 2003).

Genetic advice
Recurrence risk

When the diagnosis is unknown consult carefully with the paediatricians to establish the likelihood of non-genetic factors. If there has been severe IUGR this may recur in the absence of a known cause. The presence of significant developmental delay and other dysmorphic features would suggest a syndromal cause. Beware that some of the conditions listed above have recessive inheritance and try to exclude these.

Prenatal diagnosis

Ultrasound growth scans, but growth retardation is rarely detectable before ~28 weeks gestation.

Natural history and further management (preventative measures)

Children should remain under the care of a paediatrician or paediatric endocrinologist to ensure optimal nutrition and growth.

Lay group contact: Child Growth Foundation, Tel. 020 8994 7625, <costellokids.org.uk>.

Expert advisers: Sue Price, Consultant Geneticist, Oxford Regional Genetics Service, Oxford and David Dunger, Professor of Paediatrics, University of Cambridge, Cambridge, England.

References

Boocock GR, Morrison JA, *et al.* Mutations in SBDS are associated with Schwachman–Diamond syndrome. *Nat Genet* 2003; **33**: 97–101.

Eggermann T, Klaus Z, *et al.* Uniparental disomy; clinical indications for testing in growth retardation. *Eur J Paediatr* 2002; **161**: 305–12.

Hannula K, Lipsanen-Nyman M, Kristo P, Katila I, Simola KO, Lenko HL, Tapinainen P, Holmberg C, Kere J. Genetic screening for maternal uniparental disomy of chromosome 7 in prenatal and postnatal growth retardation of unknown cause. *Pediatrics* 2002; **109** (3): 441–8.

Hennekam RC. Costello syndrome: an overview. *Am J Med Genet* 2003; **117C** (1): 42–8.

Kofoed EM, Hwa V, *et al.* Growth hormone insensitivity associated with a *STAT5b* mutation. *New Engl J Med* 2003; **349**: 1139–47.

Kori M, Maayan-Metzger A, *et al.* Faecal elastase 1 levels in premature and full term infants. *Arch Dis Child Fetal Neonatal Ed* 2003; **88**: F106–8.

Price SM, Stanhope R, *et al.* The spectrum of Silver–Russell syndrome: a clinical and molecular genetic study. *J Med Genet* 1999; **36**: 837–42.

Floppy infant

You may be asked to see a baby on a neonatal intensive care unit (NICU) or on the postnatal wards who appears floppy. The paediatricians will usually have already excluded sepsis and hypoglycaemia as possible causes and are asking your opinion because they are considering a metabolic or neuromuscular cause. Central hypotonia is much more common than peripheral neuromuscular disease as a cause for presentation as a floppy infant. The most common neuromuscular cause of floppiness in the neonatal period is congenital myotonic dystrophy. Other causes include neonatal myasthenia, congenital muscular dystrophy, and congenital myopathies (nemaline or myotubular). Rarely severe cases of type 1 spinal muscular atrophy (SMA) may present neonatally. Other types of SMA may also present in the neonatal period.

General points

- **Distribution of weakness.** In truncal hypotonia of central origin there is relative sparing of the face and limbs. Although the baby may appear very floppy when picked up, with exaggerated head lag, when laid supine it will be able to kick quite powerfully.
- **Facial muscle involvement.** This is common in some of the congenital myopathies and congenital myotonic dystrophy, but not SMA.
- **Sucking and swallowing difficulty.** This presents with poor feeding. If swallowing is impaired there is a risk of aspiration. Sucking and swallowing difficulty are common features of severe SMA (with bulbar involvement), congenital myotonic dystrophy, myotubular myopathy, nemaline myopathy, and neonatal myasthenia as well as Prader–Willi syndrome (PWS) and hypoxic ischaemic encephalopathy (HIE).
- **Respiratory difficulty.** Respiratory problems soon after birth are rare in type 1 SMA, but common in congenital myotonic dystrophy, severe nemaline myopathy, and myotubular myopathy. Diaphragmatic weakness may be an early feature of SMA with respiratory distress (SMARD).

Clinical approach

History: key points

- Three-generation family history with specific enquiry for consanguinity and for any neuromuscular problems, e.g. muscle weakness, and for features suggestive of myotonic dystrophy, e.g. cataracts, diabetes, sudden cardiac death, unexplained infant deaths in offspring of other relatives (autosomal dominant (AD) pattern for myotonic dystrophy, X-linked for myotubular myopathy).
- Normal fetal movements in pregnancy?
- Was there polyhydramnios (poor fetal swallowing)?
- Normal labour and delivery or is there evidence of asphyxia and poor Apgars?
- Term or preterm delivery?
- When was the baby first noted to be floppy; did the baby handle normally immediately after delivery? Did it cry and kick?
- Is the floppiness getting worse or remaining static?
- Is the baby able to feed?

Examination: key points

If the labour was prolonged and/or the delivery traumatic and if there is an impression that the situation is improving, it may be appropriate to observe closely before launching into extensive investigations. If there is any hint that the situation is deteriorating it is important to initiate investigations and to work in conjunction with your paediatric colleagues who will need to decide if the baby needs transfer to the NICU.

- Peripheral neuromuscular cause more likely if the baby is alert and responsive and the floppiness appears static over a period of hours/days. In SMA type 1 there is preservation of facial movement compared to limb movement. The presence of reflexes does not exclude SMA.
- A strikingly myopathic face is characteristic of myotonic dystrophy or myotubular myopathy. The face is generally less myopathic in babies with congenital muscular dystrophy.
- Central or metabolic cause more likely if the baby is not alert, but lethargic and sleepy. Progression of floppiness over a period of hours/days is suggestive of a metabolic cause.
- Describe the posture of the baby. Is it frog-legged?
- Look carefully for fasciculation: tongue and limbs (SMA type I can present in the neonatal period, but more usually evolves over a period of weeks).
- Examine for contractures and talipes, suggestive of reduced fetal movement *in utero*.
- Observe spontaneous movements. Does the baby make any; does the baby grimace or cry?
- Check for head lag, usually present in the newborn, but can be very marked truncal hypotonia in some conditions of central origin.
- Check deep tendon reflexes (DTRs). Are they present? If absent suggests peripheral neuromuscular cause (but may be reduced in PWS and can be present in SMA).
- Occipital-frontal circumference (OFC), cry, drooling, swallowing, facial and eye movement, level of alertness.
- Document muscle strength and changes over time.
- *Examine the mother* for features of myotonic dystrophy or myasthaenia gravis.

Special investigations

The paediatric team will probably have completed glucose, ammonia, blood gas (to check for metabolic or respiratory acidosis) before you are asked to assess the baby. A paediatric neurologist should also be involved in the diagnosis and ongoing care of the infant.

1 **Clinical picture suggestive of central cause for hypotonia.**
   - Karyotype.
   - Urine for amino and organic acids.
   - Consider lactate.
   - Very long chain fatty acids (VLCFAs).
   - DNA for SNRP (small nuclear ribonuclear protein) methylation status (Prader–Willi syndrome) if central hypotonia, poor suck, and no other cause likely. Typical facies include delicate features, thin upper lip.
   - DNA for myotonic dystrophy expansion (usually >1000 (CTG) repeats) especially if face is myopathic and examination of the mother is suggestive. Rarely a baby can have congenital myotonic dystrophy when examination of the mother is apparently normal.

- Creatine kinase (CK). Should be normal in all central causes of hypotonia. Re-evaluate if raised and consider congenital muscular dystrophies, e.g. Walker–Warburg syndrome (WWS) and muscle–eye–brain (MEB) syndrome, where the hypotonia is of mixed origin.

2 **Clinical picture suggestive of peripheral cause for hypotonia.**

- CK (will be elevated in most forms of congenital muscular dystrophy, but normal or only slightly elevated in SMA or congenital myopathies).
- Electromyography (EMG) and nerve conduction velocities (NCVs). Fibrillation in SMA; if myopathic proceed to muscle biopsy.
- DNA for *SMN1* exons 7 and 8 deletion for type I SMA if peripheral cause evident.

When most of these results are available you should be in a position to decide whether this is likely to be a peripheral neuromuscular, central, or metabolic problem and proceed with further investigations accordingly.

For a central cause for hypotonia consider:

- magnetic resonance imaging (MRI) brain scan.
- DNA storage.

For a peripheral cause for hypotonia consider:

- muscle biopsy with histology and immunohistochemistry.
- echocardiogram to exclude cardiomyopathy if suggestive of primary muscle disorder.
- DNA storage.

Some diagnoses to consider

Prader–Willi syndrome (PWS)

The neonatal period is dominated by hypotonia, lethargy, and weak suck leading to feeding difficulties. The central hypotonia may manifest as reduced fetal movement, abnormal fetal position, e.g. breech, and difficulty at the time of delivery, often necessitating delivery by lower segment Caesarean section (LSCS). Reflexes may be reduced. The baby has to be awakened for feeds, sucks poorly, and frequently nasogastric feeeding or other special feeding techniques may be needed in the early weeks of life. Breastfeeding is rarely possible. The facial features are delicate with a thin upper lip. The baby is quiet and sleeps for long periods and has a weak cry. Birthweight and length are usually within normal limits. See 'Obesity with and without developmental delay', page 192 for further details.

Congenital myotonic dystrophy

Pregnancy often complicated by polyhydramnios. At delivery severely affected infants are floppy and often have respiratory problems with diaphragmatic hypoplasia and may require ventilatory support. There is a confusing combination of central and peripheral hypotonia. The diagnosis is usually apparent following a careful history and examination of the mother for signs of myotonic dystrophy (typical facies, weak sternomastoids, grip myotonia, etc.). See 'Myotonic dystrophy (DM)', page 388, for further details.

Spinal muscular atrophy (SMA)

See 'Spinal muscular atrophy (SMA)', page 412.

Zellweger syndrome

Autosomal recessive (AR) persoxisomal disorder often presenting in the neonatal period with central hypotonia ± seizures. The fontanelle is large and the forehead high. There may be stippled epiphyses (especially knees). VLCFAs are elevated. Prognosis is poor and most die in the first year of life. Zellweger syndrome is genetically heterogeneous and is caused by mutations in any of several genes involved in peroxisome biogenesis, e.g. peroxin-1, 2, 3, 5, 6, and 12 (*PEX1, 2, 3, 5, 6,* and 12). Prenatal diagnosis is possible by analysis of VLCFAs in tissue from chorionic villus sampling (CVS).

Pompe disease

AR acid maltase deficiency—cardiomyopathy. See page 61.

Congenital myopathy

Types of congenital myopathy typically presenting at birth include severe nemaline myopathy and myotubular myopathy (which may clinically resemble congenital myotonic dystrophy). CK levels are normal or marginally raised. Diagnosis requires muscle biopsy, which shows no necrosis or degenerative changes, but may have characteristic structural features. Specialized examination of the muscle biopsy is indicated if a congenital myopathy is suspected.

Congenital muscular dystrophy (CMD)

These are a heterogeneous group of severely disabling AR disorders that affect skeletal muscle and have an overall frequency of ~1/10 000 livebirths. Affected children present with muscle weakness and hypotonia at birth, or within the first 6 months of life, and progressive joint contractures. Motor development is delayed. The progression of the disease is variable and dependent on the disease subtype, and some children never achieve the ability to walk without support and remain wheelchair-dependent for life. Brain involvement in the form of mental retardation and abnormal formation of different parts of the brain is a feature of several forms of CMD. The prognosis varies and some die early of respiratory failure. CK is variable in these disorders and diagnosis requires muscle biopsy, and often also cranial MRI.

CMD without brain involvement. Of cases without intellectual impairment or major structural brain abnormalities, half of the cases show deficiency of laminin alpha-2 (merosin) due to mutations of the laminin alpha-2 chain gene. These children typically have a very high CK and white matter changes visible on brain MRI from the age of six months. Mutations in the fukutin-related protein (FKRP) gene can cause a secondary deficiency of laminin alpha-2 and a severe form of congenital muscular dystrophy 1C (MDC1C), also associated with a very high CK. Other causes of secondary laminin alpha-2 deficiency are yet to be elucidated. Of the types of CMD with normal laminin alpha-2, the best defined is **Ullrich congenital muscular dystrophy**, due to AR mutations in the collagen 6A genes. These children typically have distal joint laxity and proximal contractures. Most have absence of collagen VI in their muscle biopsies.

With brain involvement—lissencephaly. Fukuyama CMD, MEB, and WWS are associated with eye abnormalities and neuronal migration defects, and result from mutations in fukutin, POMGnT1, and POMT1, respectively. (See 'Lissencephaly and neuronal migration disorders', page 156.) Abnormalities of α-dystroglycan are a common feature, reflecting the role of these proteins in glycosylation.

- **White matter changes**. Another glycosyltransferase, encoded by the gene *LARGE*, causes CMD and profound mental retardation, with white matter changes and subtle structural abnormalities on brain MRI (MDC1D). In several cases, the gene localization remains unknown.

Genetic advice

Recurrence risk

This is dependent on the diagnosis—see appropriate section.

Carrier detection

This may be possible if the causative mutation is defined in the proband.

Prenatal diagnosis

This may be possible if the causative mutation is defined in the proband.

Natural history and further management (preventative measures)

Babies should be under the care of a paediatric neurologist for ongoing care.

Lay group contact: Many of the individual conditions have their own support groups. See <www.cafamily.org.uk>.

Expert advisor: Kate Bushby, Professor of Neuromuscular Genetics, University of Newcastle, Newcastle-upon-Tyne, England.

References

Dubowitz V. The floppy infant syndrome. In *Muscle disorders in childhood*, 2nd edn, Chapter 12, pp. 457–72. W.B. Saunders, Philadelphia, 1995.

Gunay-Aygun M, Schwartz S, *et al.* The changing purpose of Prader–Willi syndrome clinical diagnostic criteria and proposed revised criteria. *Pediatrics* 2001; **108**: E92.

Longman C, Brockington M, *et al.* Mutations in the human LARGE gene cause MDC1D, a novel form of congenital muscular dystrophy with severe mental retardation and abnormal glycosylation of alpha-dystroglycan. *Hum Mol Genet* 2003; **12**: 2853–61.

Miller SP, Riley P, *et al.* The neonatal presentation of Prader–Willi syndrome revisited. *Pediatrics* 1999; **134**: 226–8.

Tubridy N, Fontaine B, Eymard B. Congenital myopathies and congenital muscular dystrophies. *Curr Opin Neurol* 2001; **14**: 575–82.

Fractures

Many children have one fracture during childhood, but a few have more and a geneticist may be asked to see the child, usually to determine if the cause is osteogenesis imperfecta (OI; brittle bone disease). The severe forms of OI have marked clinical and radiological changes that present either prenatally on ultrasound scan (USS) or in the neonatal period. Most patients harbour heterozygote germline mutations in the *COL1A1* or *COL1A2* genes that encode the chains of type I procollagen, the major protein in bone.

The clinical approach described here is to assist in the diagnosis of milder forms of OI. Sometimes the possibility of non-accidental injury has been raised, so sensitive questioning is appropriate.

History: key points

- Three-generation family tree with specific enquiry about fractures, blue sclerae, dental problems, hearing loss, short stature, and osteoporosis; age at walking.
- Child's age at each fracture. Were fractures present at birth? (Babies with arthrogryposis often sustain fractures during delivery.)
- Number of fractures and which bones were fractured.
- The cause of the fracture. Was the injury appropriate for the degree of trauma?
- Did anyone observe the events; is the story consistent? (Non-accidental injury has to be considered.)
- Did the fracture heal normally? (Occasionally children with OI have a large mass of callus at the site of a healing fracture that is mistaken for a malignant lesion; this is now recognized as a specific form of OI, type V.)
- Is there any limb deformity?
- Joint dislocations (ligamentous laxity is a feature of OI) or joint contractures.
- Hearing loss (stapedial fixation occurs in OI, as does sensorineural deafness).

Examination: key points, mainly for features of OI

- Height (reduced in OI).
- Limb deformity (often none with mild OI).
- Blue sclerae (often said to be more striking when the fractures occur; note young infants often have blue sclerae).
- Scoliosis (due to lax ligaments and osteoporosis in older children and adults).
- Ligamentous laxity; estimate 'Beighton score'. See Clinical approach to 'Hypermobile joints', page 138.
- Skin. Is it smooth, soft, easily bruised; does it show poor wound healing or scarring?
- Teeth for dentinogenesis imperfecta (discoloration, poor growth, defective enamel).
- Heart (mitral valve prolapse more common).
- Neurological if spinal abnormality or basilar impression.

Special investigations

Osteogenesis imperfecta (OI). The presence of Wormian bones is the main diagnostic feature in type 1 OI, as the rest of the skeletal survey may be normal. Bone density may be reduced but is often normal. In type III there are progressive bony deformities and in type IV there may be occipital overhang and platybasia. There is considerable debate whether clinical differentiation between types I and IV is possible.

- Radiology:
  - a full radiological survey is used to document old fractures and is important in distinguishing between genetic conditions and child abuse;
  - Skull X-ray (SXR) is useful to look for Wormian bones if mild OI is suspected in a child with a known family history (teeth with poor roots may also be visible on the SXR);
  - lateral spine X-ray has a role in the assessment of a baby <12 months old with OI: looking for biconcavity of vertebral bodies, and wedge fractures, prior to consideration of biphosphonate therapy.
- Hearing test.
- Bone biochemistry including alkaline phosphatase (reduced/absent in hypophosphatasia, normal or increased in OI).
- Urine, for amino acids (homocystinuria) and/or markers of collagen breakdown (*N*-telopeptide of type 1 collagen (NTx) is the most useful).
- Blood for DNA storage. Molecular confirmation especially useful in prenatal situations rather than in an older child. Testing for collagen mutations on genomic DNA is now available.
- Skin biopsy for collagen studies may be useful to confirm a suspected diagnosis or to help with prenatal diagnosis, but there is limited availability of collagen protein analysis.
- Bone density scans may help to determine if osteoporotic complications are likely. This should be done in conjunction with a physician with a special interest in bone metabolic disorders.

Some diagnoses to consider

Osteogenesis imperfecta (OI). See below for more details.

Non-accidental injury. See 'Suspected non-accidental injury', page 252.

Juvenile osteoporosis. Reduced bone density; can resolve spontaneously and may rarely be familial.

Premature osteoporosis. Search for endocrine causes. The increased use of bone density scanning in young women has resulted in the identification of some individuals who have such reduced density that they may have a mild form of OI.

Hypophosphatasia. Hypophosphatasia is an inherited disorder characterized by defective bone mineralization and a deficiency of tissue-non-specific alkaline phosphatase (*TNSALP*) activity. The disease is highly variable in its clinical expression, depending on the specific mutation in *TNSALP*. Levels of alkaline phophatase in blood are very low. The disease usually follows autosomal recessive (AR) inheritance, but Lia-Baldini *et al.* (2002) provide evidence that some mutations may have a dominant negative effect, and so be transmitted in an autosomal dominant (AD) rather than an AR pattern. Expression of the disease may be highly variable, with parents of even severely affected children showing no or extremely mild symptoms of the disease. Parental molecular genetic analysis and parental alkaline phosphatase levels may be helpful.

Skeletal dysplasias with Wormian bones. Distinguished on the basis of their other features.

Osteoporosis–pseudoglioma syndrome. Rare AR disorder characterized by severe juvenile-onset osteoporosis and congenital or early-onset blindness. Other manifestations include muscular hypotonia, ligamentous laxity, mild mental retardation, and seizures. The gene responsible is *LRP5* on chromosome 11q11–12.

Bruck syndrome (BS). An AR syndrome presenting with OI (blue sclerae and Wormian bones are found) and congenital contractures of the large joints often with bilateral talipes equinovarus. Webbing (pterygia) is seen at the elbow and knee. Bank *et al.* (1999) reported that the molecular defect underlying Bruck syndrome is a deficiency of bone-specific telopeptide lysyl hydroxylase that results in aberrant crosslinking of bone collagen. BS is caused by mutations at a locus on 17p12 (BS1) or by mutations in the *PLOD2* gene on 3q23-q24 (BS2).

Arthrogryposis. Multiple congenital contractures, often with gracile long bones that are poorly ossified and so frequently fracture during delivery (8–10%) or iatrogenically when trying to move limbs with contractures. See 'Arthrogryposis (arthrogryposis multiplex congenita)', page 48.

Genetic advice: osteogenesis imperfecta (OI)

In types I–IV OI, excessive bone fragility is caused by mutations in the α1 and α2 chains of type 1 collagen (Ward *et al.* 2001). Type I OI is the most common and has a frequency of 2–5 per 100 000. In *type I* there may be mutations that cause non-functional alleles (null alleles) giving a 50% reduction in collagen (reduced amount of normal collagen), whereas in *type II and other severe forms* there are often glycine substitutions that disturb the helical structure and stability of collagen (dominant–negative) and thus lead to a more severe phenotype.

The clinical classification of Sillence is used to describe Types I–IV OI, and more recently Rauch and Glorieux (2004) have described three new types (V–VII) that are not associated with mutations in type I collagen genes (see table).

Recurrence risks
- Type I and IV: AD inheritance.
- Most type II is caused by *de novo* dominant mutations and recurrences are due to germline mosaicism. Recurrence risk is given as 7% (Cole) suggesting a high rate of mosaicism. There are reports of possible AR inheritance in 'milder' forms of type II and AR inheritance due to homozygosity for *COL1A1α1* mutation has been described (Bonadio *et al.* 1990), so consult the literature prior to counselling.
- Type III: mostly AD except for southern African where there is an AR form that is also reported in an Irish kindred and in several other consanguineous families. Germline mosaicism risk is likely to be similar to that of type II.
- Types V–VII are not caused by mutations in collagen 1. Type V follows AD inheritance, type VI has unknown inheritance, and type VII is AR.

Prenatal diagnosis
This is mostly requested by couples who have a child with type II or type III OI.
- USS will detect recurrence of type II and most of type III in the second trimester. Safe, effective, but relatively late diagnosis.
- Chorionic villus sampling (CVS) is possible when the diagnosis has been confirmed by molecular methods or collagen studies.
- Amniocentesis is not suitable for collagen studies.

Expanded Sillence classification of osteogenesis imperfecta* (after Rauch and Glorieux 2004)

Type	Severity	Clinical description	Genetic basis
I	Mild non-deforming	Normal height, or mild short stature; blue sclera; no dentinogenesis imperfecta	AD; premature stop codon in *COL1A1*
II	Perinatal lethal	Multiple rib and long-bone fractures are present at birth. Deformities. Dark sclera. Radiographs show low density of skull bones and broad long bones. Lethal in perinatal period usually due to respiratory failure from multiple rib fractures	Glycine substitutions in *COL1A1* or *COL1A2*
IIA	Lethal	Broad crumpled long bones, broad ribs with continuous beading	
IIB	Lethal	Broad, crumpled long bones but ribs have discontinuous or no beading	
IIC	Lethal	Thin fractured long bones and thin beaded ribs	
III	Severely deforming	Very short stature; limb and spine deformity due to multiple fractures. Severe scoliosis can lead to respiratory difficulty which is a leading cause of death in type III OI; greyish sclera; dentinogenesis imperfecta; triangular facies	Mostly *de novo* AD due to glycine substitutions in *COL1A1* or *COL1A2*
IV	Moderately deforming	Moderate short stature; mild/moderate scoliosis; greyish/white sclera; dentinogenesis imperfecta	AD, glycine substitutions in *COL1A1* or *COL1A2*
V	Moderately deforming	Mild/moderate short stature; interosseous membrane of forearm calcifies early in life limiting hand movement and sometimes causing dislocation of the radial head; hyperplastic callus; white sclera; no dentinogenesis imperfecta	AD, gene unknown
VI	Moderately/severely deforming	Moderately short; scoliosis; accumulation of osteoid in bone tissue, 'fish-scale' pattern of bone lamellation; white sclera; no dentinogenesis imperfecta	Inheritance unknown; gene unknown
VII	Moderately deforming	Mild short stature; proximal shortening of limbs; coxa vara; white sclera. No dentinogenesis imperfecta. Rare.	AR, gene at 3p22–24.1

* The range of clinical severity in OI is a continuum; however, categorization of patients is helpful in determining prognosis and assessing treatment.

Management of delivery

Cubert *et al.* (2001) reviewed the records of 167 babies affected by OI. There was an unusually high incidence of breech presentation at term (37%). In infants with non-lethal forms of OI, 40% delivered by lower segment Caesarean section (LSCS) and 32% delivered vaginally had new fractures. LSCS did not decrease fracture rate at birth in infants with non-lethal OI nor did it prolong survival for those with lethal forms. If a baby is diagnosed to have OI antenatally it may be best to avoid an instrumental delivery and proceed with LSCS (unless progress through the second stage is normal, but delivery needs to be expedited because of fetal distress when a lift-out delivery may be feasible).

Natural history and further management

Children should be under the care of a specialist in bone disorders. Physiotherapy, rehabilitation, and orthopaedic surgery are the mainstay of treatment for patients with OI (Glorieux 2000). Biphosphonates, e.g. pamidronate, are a relatively new therapeutic option in OI and these drugs are currently undergoing clinical trial in those with moderate/severe forms of OI. They are used to reduce osteoclast-mediated bone resorption and trials are showing an increase in bone density and a reduced fracture rate in treated children.

Lay group: Brittle Bone Society of the UK, <www.brittlebone.org>; Osteogenesis Imperfecta Foundation (US), <www.oif.org>.

Expert advisers: Roger Smith, Honorary Metabolic Bone Physician, Nuffield Orthopaedic Centre, Oxford and Nick Bishop, Professor of Paediatric Bone Disease, University of Sheffield, Sheffield, England.

References

Bank RA, Robins SP, Wijmenga C, Breslau-Siderius LJ, Bardoel AFJ, Van der Sluijs HA, Pruijs HEH, TeKoppele JM. Defective collagen crosslinking in bone, but not in ligament or cartilage, in Bruck syndrome: indications for a bone-specific telopeptide lysyl hydroxylase on chromosome 17. *Proc Natl Acad Sci, USA* 1999; **96**: 1054–8.

Bonadio J, Ramirez F, Barr M. An intron mutation in the human alpha 1(I) collagen gene alters the efficiency of pre-mRNA splicing and is associated with osteogenesis imperfecta type II. *J Biol Chem* 1990; **265** (4): 2262–8.

Byers PH, Cole WG. Osteogenesis imperfecta. In *Connective tissue and its heritable disorders*, 2nd edn (ed. P.M. Royce and B. Steinmann), pp. 385–430. Wiley-Liss, New York, 2002.

Cole WG, Dalgleish R. Perinatal lethal osteogenesis imperfecta. *J Med Genet* 1995; **32**: 284–89.

Cubert R, Cheng EY, et al. Osteogenesis imperfecta: mode of delivery and neonatal outcome. *Obstet Gynecol* 2001; **97**: 66–9.

Glorieux FH. Bisphosphonate therapy in severe osteogenesis imperfecta. *J Pediatr Endocrinol Metab* 2000; **Suppl. 2**: 989–92.

Ha-Vinh R, Alanay Y, et al. phenotypic and molecular characterisation of Bruck syndrome (osteogenesis imperfecta with contractures of the large joints) caused by a recessive mutation in *PLOD2. Am J Med genet* 2004; **131A**: 115–20.

Lia-Baldini AS, Muller F, et al. A molecular approach to dominance in hypophosphatasia. *Hum Genet* 2001; **109** (1): 99–108.

Plotkin H, Rauch F, Bishop NJ, et al. Pamidronate treatment of severe osteogenesis imperfecta in children under 3 years of age. *J Clin Endocrinol Metab* 2000; **85**: 1846–50.

Rauch F, Glorieux FH. Osteogenesis imperfecta [seminar]. *Lancet* 2004; **363**: 1377–85.

Rauch F, Plotkin H, Zeitlin L, Glorieux F. Bone mass, size, and density in children and adolescents with osteogenesis imperfecta: effect of intravenous pamidronate therapy. *Bone Miner Res* 2003; **18**: 610–14.

Roughley PJ, Rauch F, Glorieux FH. Osteogenesis imperfecta—clinical and molecular diversity. *Eur Cell Mater* 2003; **5**: 41–7; discussion, 47.

Sillence DO, Senn A, Danks DM. Genetic heterogeneity in osteogenesis imperfecta. *J Med Genet* 1979; **16**: 101–16.

Tsipouras P. Osteogenesis imperfecta. In *McKusick's heritable disorders of collagen*, 5th edn (ed. P. Beighton), pp. 281–314. Mosby, St Louis, 1993.

Ward LM, Lalic L, et al. Thirty-three novel COL1A1 and COL1A2 mutations in patients with osteogenesis imperfecta types I–IV. *Hum Mutat* 2001; **17**: 434.

Zeitlin L, Fassier F, Glorieux FH. Modern approach to children with osteogenesis imperfecta. *J Pediatr Orthop B* 2003; **12**: 77–87.

Ha-Vinh R, Alamay Y et al. phenotypeic and Molecules characterisation of bruck syndrome (Osteogenesis imperfection with contractures of the large joints) caused by a necesive mutation in PLoo2. *Am J Med genet* 2004; **131A**: 115–20.

Generalized disorders of skin pigmentation (including albinism)

The skin pigments (eumelanin and phaeomelanin) are produced in melanosomes by melanocytes, which are large cells found among the basal cells of the epidermis. The melanosomes are then transferred to keratinocytes. Melanocytes are of neural crest origin.

The first part of an assessment of skin pigmentation is to classify it as *generalized* or *only affecting a portion of the body* and then to decide whether the abnormality is of *hypo-* or *hyperpigmentation*. The non-generalized disorders are discussed elsewhere in this chapter in 'Patchy pigmented skin lesions (including café-au-lait spots)', page 210 and 'Patchy hypomelanotic lesions', page 208. In many instances the differentiation between hypo- and hyperpigmentation is not easy, and it may not be possible to establish which is the 'normal' skin colour.

Generalized hyperpigmentation

This is defined as an increased degree of skin pigmentation affecting the whole body.

Clinical approach
History: key points
- Three-generation family tree. Enquire specifically for ethnicity and consanguinity.
- Always consider familial and racial background as well as sun exposure and normal variation in skin tones (e.g. Futcher's line).

Examination: key points
- Hair and eye colour.
- Skin on the palms and soles for pigmentation in the creases (endocrine abnormalities, e.g. Addison's).
- If appropriate, genital skin and areola of nipple.
- Assess if there are any non-cutaneous features.

Some diagnoses to consider
- **Endocrine causes** such as Addison's disease, adrenoleukodystrophy, congenital adrenal hyperplasia.
- **Metabolic disorders**, including Wilson's disease, alkaptonuria, haemachromatosis.
- **Syndromic conditions:** Fanconi syndrome, Patterson syndrome, neurofibromatosis type 1 (NF-1).

Generalized hypopigmentation

Decreased pigmentation of the whole body.
- **Albinism.** Skin, hair, and eye pigment is absent, or much reduced. The terms tyrosinase-positive (a milder phenotype) and tyrosinase-negative are older terms that have been replaced by OCA1A, OCA1B since the genetic causes of oculocutaneous albinism (OCA) have been established.
- **Albinoidism.** The eye problems are not present. There may be features of other syndromes (see below).
- **Generalized vitiligo.** Common generalized vitiligo is an acquired depigmenting disorder characterized by a chronic and progressive loss of melanocytes from the epidermis and follicular reservoir. It sometimes clusters in families together with autoimmune thyroid disease, pernicious anaemia, lupus, Addison's disease, and adult-onset autoimmune diabetes.

Clinical approach
History: key points
- Three-generation family tree with specific enquiry regarding consanguinity (OCA) and other affected family members.
- Visual problems.
- Easy bruising from toddlerhood (Hermansky–Pudlak syndrome (HPS)).
- Serious or recurrent infections (Chediak–Higashi syndrome (CHS)).
- Global developmental delay is not a feature of OCA.

Examination: key points
- Skin, hair, and eye colour.
- Iris transillumination.
- Nystagmus and other indicators of poor visual acuity.
- Features of syndromes associated with reduced pigmentation.

Special investigations
- Molecular testing for OCA syndromes is available but is rarely required for diagnostic reasons. It may have utility in carrier detection.
- Ophthalmology referral for visual assessment, looking for albinism of the retina, and follow-up.
- Platelet testing if there are features to suggest HPS.
- Vacuolations in white cells in CHS.
- Additional diagnostic tests in presence of albinoid features rather than OCA.

Some diagnoses to consider
Oculocutaneous albinism (OCA)
OCA affects about 1 in 20 000. All types have generalized hypopigmentation (affecting skin, hair, and eyes). There are abnormalities in the decussation of the optic nerves. The visual problems are reduced acuity, nystagmus, and alternating strabismus (squint). The skin is more at risk from damage due to exposure to ultraviolet (UV) light.

OCA1A and OCA1B. Autosomal recessive (AR) and caused by mutations in *TYR* gene encoding tyrosinase on 11q14–21. Mutation detection rate is ~70–80%. OCA1 is divided into two types: type 1A, characterized by complete lack of tyrosinase activity due to production of an inactive enzyme; and type 1B (OCA1B), characterized by reduced activity of tyrosinase. Temperature-sensitive albinism is a subtype of OCA1B. Compound heterozygosity is common. OCA1 is the most common type of OCA in Caucasians, but is uncommon in African-Americans and Africans. Together OCA1A and OCA1B account for 40% of OCA. Most babies with tyrosine-deficient OCA have completely white hair at birth, even though in type 1B a certain amount of pigment may develop later.

OCA2. This causes AR tyrosine-positive OCA and is caused by mutations in the *P* gene at 15q11–2. It accounts for about 50% of OCA worldwide. In OCA2 some pigment is present at birth and is lost later. Pigmented naevi may be another clue that the OCA is tyrosine-positive. OCA2 is common throughout subSaharan Africa where it is responsible for a high morbidity with skin cancer and visual impairment being important sequelae. OCA2 is uncommon in Caucasians. In blacks with this form of albinism, the hair is yellow and many pigmented spots develop in the skin. The occurrence of both brown oculocutaneous albinism (BOCA) and OCA2 within the same family suggested that these disorders are allelic. The 2.7-kb deletion on one allele in the *P* gene is the most frequent cause of OCA2 among southern African blacks.

OCA3. This is often called rufous or red albinism due to reddish hair and skin colour. Some retinal pigment may be present on fundoscopy and sun-sensitivity is less marked. In dark-skinned races the diagnosis may not be obvious and signs such as nystagmus and red-reflex on transillumination of the iris are important clues. AR and caused by mutations in *TYRP1* (tyrosinase-related protein 1) on 9p23.

OCA4 (rare). Mutations have been reported in *MATP* gene on 5p. AR
It is thought that other OCA loci may be identified.

Albinoid syndromes

Phenylketonuria (PKU). PKU is a treatable AR inborn error of metabolism resulting from a deficiency of phenylalanine hydroxylase and characterized by mental retardation. It is caused by mutations in the *PAH* gene on 12q24.1. In the UK neonates are screened for PKU using the Guthrie test ('heel-prick') on day 6 of life.

Homocystinuria is an AR metabolic disorder due to deficiency of cystathionine beta-synthase producing increased urinary homocystine and methionine. Major clinical manifestations involve the eyes (lens discolcation) and the central nervous (mental retardation in untreated individuals), skeletal (Marfanoid habitus with long limbs and pectus excavatum, osteoporosis), and vascular systems (thrombotic lesions of arteries and veins, premature strokes).

Prader–Willi syndrome (PWS) and Angelman syndrome (AS). Albinism occurs in association with PWS and AS where a del 15q11–12 has deleted one copy of the *P* gene and the child has an inherited *P* mutation on the other chromosome 15.

Menkes syndrome. X-linked recessive disorder of copper metabolism. Main features are sparse, steely hair (with pili torti on microscopy) and progressive neurological impairment often with seizures and spasticity.

Chediak-Higashi syndrome (CHS). Rare AR disorder characterized by OCA, bleeding tendency, recurrent bacterial infections, and various neurological symptoms. This is a life-limiting condition with children dying from infection or lymphoma, usually by 10 years. Intracellular vesicle formation is deficient, resulting in giant granules in many cells, e.g. giant melanosomes in the melanocytes. Diagnosis is by staining for giant lysosomal granules in the peripheral granulocytes, or by mutation analysis of the *LYST* gene.

Hermansky–Pudlack syndrome (HPS). Very rare AR disorder characterized by variable OCA, excessive bruising, nose bleeding and bleeding after dental extraction, progressive pulmonary fibrosis leading to death in the 4th or 5th decade, and granulomatous colitis. It is caused by mutations in *HPS* on 10q23. There is a founder effect in Puerto Ricans where the carrier rate is 1/18. Diagnosis is by electron microscopy of platelets which show absent platelet dense bodies.

Cross syndrome. Oculocerebral syndrome with hypopigmentation

Griscelli syndrome. Rare AR disorder caused by mutations in the gene *myosin-Va* on 15q21. The disorder is similar to CHS. Infants have silver-grey hair and generalized hypo- or hyperpigmentation of the skin, immunodeficiency with recurrent infections, and lymphadenopathy, neutropenia, and low immunoglobulins.

Cystinosis. Cystinosis presents in the first year of life with severe failure to thrive and photophobia with corneal crystals. There is renal tubular dysfunction with proteinuria, glycosuria, and a generalized aminoaciduria progressing to end-stage renal failure. Affected individuals have lighter skin and hair pigmentation than their unaffected siblings. Incidence 1/100 000–1/200 000 live births. AR condition caused by mutations in the cystinosin gene (*CTNS*) on 17p13. A 65-kb deletion is present in either the homozygous or the heterozygous state in 76% of cystinotic patients of European origin. Three types of cystinosis are recognized: (1) infantile nephropathic; (2) juvenile or adolescent nephropathic; and (3) adult non-nephropathic.

Genetic advice

Recurrence risk
All the above-mentioned forms of OCA plus CHS and HPS follow AR inheritance.

Carrier detection
Some carriers of OCA type 1 are fairer than the population norm. Strabismus may be more prevalent, but generally carriers do not have problems.

Prenatal diagnosis
Potentially possible by chorionic villus sampling (CVS) if familial mutations are known.

Natural history and further management (preventative measures)

- Use of sun block is critical for individuals with OCA—risk of cutaneous malignancy with UV exposure.
- Protect the skin from UV damage by using broad spectrum sunscreens with a sun protection factor of 45 or greater.
- Protect the eyes with sunglasses and hats with broad brims or peaks.

Support group contact: Albinism Fellowship <www.albinism.org.uk>.

Expert adviser: Anonymous.

Reference

Sybert VP. *Genetic skin disorders*, Oxford Monographs in Medical Genetics. Oxford University Press, New York, 1997.

Hemihypertrophy and limb asymmetry

Hemihyperplasia, hematrophy, hemihypoplasia.
This may affect the face, or a single limb, or half the body. If facial asymmetry is the only feature, refer to 'Facial asymmetry', page 112. Some degree of asymmetry is not unusual in the general population. A small percentage of normal children have a minor discrepancy of foot size when measured for shoes, but a difference sufficient to require differently sized shoes for each foot is unusual. Similarly leg-length discrepancy is a not an uncommon referral to a paediatric orthopaedic clinic. A discrepancy of >1 cm in limb length together with a measurable difference in limb circumference should be regarded as abnormal.

It is often not that easy to decide which side is normal and whether the fundamental abnormality is hyperplasia or hypoplasia. Hemihypertrophy is more common in a developmentally normal or large child; hemiatrophy is more likely in a child with a mosaic chromosome problem who may have developmental delay, growth retardation, and dysmorphic features.

Making limb measurements (see figure)
- **To measure total upper limb length.** With arms hanging loosely down, measure between the acromion (most prominent posterior lateral bony prominence of the shoulder joint) and the tip of the middle finger.
- **To measure total lower limb length.** If the child can stand, measure between the greater trochanter and the floor (with measure perpendicular to the floor); for a baby, measure between the greater trochanter and the lateral malleolus of the ankle.
- **To measure limb circumference.** Circumference measurements are taken at the widest diameter of the limb, or from a fixed bony point, e.g. 10 cm distal to lower edge of patella. In the upper arm, the widest point is at the middle of the biceps, just below the insertion of the deltoid. In the upper leg (thigh), the widest point is usually just below the gluteal crease. In the lower leg (calf), the widest point is in the mid-upper calf muscle.

Clinical approach
History: key points
- Three-generation family tree with specific enquiry about birthweights, height, and cancer.
- Pregnancy, neonatal, and developmental history.

Examination: key points
- Growth parameters. Height, weight, and occipital-frontal circumference (OFC).
- Observe upper limbs with both arms hanging loosely by the child's side and compare sides. Photograph and measure as above.
- Observe lower limbs with child sitting with legs outstretched on bed and compare sides. Photograph and measure as above.
- Look carefully for café-au-lait patches, abnormal skin pigmentation, vascular birthmarks, connective tissue, and epidermal naevi (Proteus syndrome), lymphatic malformations, lipomas.
- Assess tongue size and symmetry.
- Look for syndactyly, macrodactyly.

Special investigations
1 **Hemihypertrophy**.
- Chromosome analysis (looking especially for 11p15dup).
- DNA for uniparental disomy (UPD)11p15 analysis (anecdotal reports of patients with hemihypertrophy and no other features of Beckwith–Wiedemann syndrome (BWS) with UPD11p15).
- Renal ultrasound for Wilms tumour surveillance every 3–4 months until 7 years, only if abnormality of 11p15 identified.

2 **Hemiatrophy**.
- Chromosome analysis with mosaicism screen.
- Skin biopsy for chromosome analysis if developmental delay (especially with syndactyly or hypomelanosis of Ito) if blood karyotype is normal.

Some diagnoses to consider
Beckwith–Wiedemann syndrome (BWS). Macrosomia (prenatal and/or postnatal), hemihypertrophy, macroglossia, abdominal wall defect (omphalocele, umbilical hernia, diastasis recti), ear anomalies. See 'Beckwith–Wiedemann syndrome (BWS)' in Chapter 3, 'Common consultations'.

Neurofibromatosis type 1 (NF1). See 'Neurofibromatosis type 1 (NF1)', page 396.

McCune–Albright syndrome. A syndromic association between polyostotic fibrous dysplasia, cutaneous pigmentation (coast of Maine areas of café-au-lait coloured pigmentation), and precocious puberty (50% of affected girls and some affected boys). Caused by mosaicism for somatic activating mutation in the *GNAS* gene. Recurrence risks are very low.

Klippel–Trenaunay syndrome (KTS). Combined capillary, lymphatic, and venous malformation, varicosities, and limb enlargement. Lower limb involved in 95%; upper limb in 5%. 15% have combined upper and lower limb involvement. Trunk involvement is not common. Capillary malformations of the skin are purplish in colour. Lymphoedema is common. Lower limb enlargement is present in nearly all cases—the limb being thicker and longer. Macrodactyly may involve toes on the affected foot.

Proteus syndrome. A complex and variable disorder characterized by limb asymmetry, disproportionate overgrowth of hands and/or feet and especially digits, vascular and lymphatic malformations, and cranial hyperostosis (see table). Proteus is mostly sporadic and presumed due to somatic mosaicism. Most babies show comparatively little asymmetry at birth, although they may have vascular or lymphatic malformations. The condition is very progressive in early childhood, but tends to change little after adolescence. Intelligence quotient (IQ) is usually normal.

Isolated hemihypertrophy. Isolated finding in an otherwise normal individual who after careful assessment has none of the features of the above conditions. Cause unknown, but may represent mosaic overexpression of *IGF2* due to an imprinting defect. In Hoyme *et al.*'s (1998) multicentre study, tumours developed in 9/168 patients (5.9%). Tumours were of embryonal origin (similar to those noted for other overgrowth disorders including Wilms tumour, hepatoblastoma, adrenal cell carcinoma, and leiomyosarcoma of the small bowel (in one case)). Estimated prevalence 1/86 000.

Diagnostic criteria for Proteus syndrome (modified from Biesecker et al. 1999)

Proteus syndrome = Mosaic distribution of lesions + progressive course + sporadic + 1 from A, or 2 from B or 3 from C		
A		Connective tissue naevus (fibrous connective tissue with gyral pattern occurring most frequently on soles, but also found on palms and abdomen)
B	i	Epidermal naevus (linear, whorled, or verrucous and usually found on neck, trunk, or extremities). Appear like areas of leathery discoloured skin and are present from infancy
	ii	Disproportionate overgrowth of limbs (arms/legs/hands/feet/digits), skull, external auditory meatus, vertebrae, or viscera (spleen/thymus)
	iii	Specific tumours <20 years (bilateral ovarian cystadenomas, parotid monomorphic adenoma)
C	i	Dysregulated adipose tissue (lipomas, or regional absence of fat)
	ii	Vascular malformations (capillary malformation, venous malformation, lymphatic malformation)
	iii	Facial phenotype (dolicocephaly, long face, minor downslanting palpebral fissures and/or minor ptosis, wide or anteverted nares, open mouth appearance)

Silver-Russell syndrome (SRS) Failure to thrive, proportionately large head, but usually between 3rd and 25th centile, triangular face, and downturned mouth. Asymmetry is a key diagnostic feature. See 'Failure to thrive', page 116.

Genetic advice

Recurrence risk

As for underlying disgnosis. If isolated hemihypertrophy, recurrence risk is likely to be low.

Prenatal diagnosis

As for underlying diagnosis.

Natural history and further management (preventative measures)

- 3-4 monthly renal USS surveillance for Wilms tumor during first 7 years of life for BWS due to 11p15 uniparental disomy.
- Regular clinical surveillance and imaging if Proteus syndrome.
- Otherwise manage as for specific diagnosis.

Lay group contact: Many of the individual syndromes have their own support groups. See <www.cafamily.org.uk>.

Expert adviser: Eamonn Maher, Professor of Medical Genetics, University of Birmingham, Birmingham, England. Nazneen Rahman, Senior Lecturer and Honorary Consultant in Clinical Genetics, Institute of Cancer Research, Sutton, Surrey, England

References

Biesecker LG, Happle R, Mulliken JB. Proteus syndrome: diagnostic criteria, differential diagnosis, and patient evaluation. *Am J Med Genet* 1999; **84** (5): 389–95.

Cohen MM Jr, Neri G, Weksberg R. *Overgrowth syndromes*, Oxford Monographs on Medical Genetics no. 43. Oxford University Press, Oxford, 2002.

Hoyme HE, Seaver LH, Jones KL, et al. Isolated hemihyperplasia (hemihypertrophy): report of a prospective multicenter study of the incidence of neoplasia and review. *Am J Med Genet* 1998; **79**: 274–8.

Weksberg R, Shuman C. Beckwith–Wiedemann syndrome. In *Management of genetic syndromes* (ed. S.B. Cassidy and J.E. Allanson), Chapter 4. Wiley-Liss, New York, 2001.

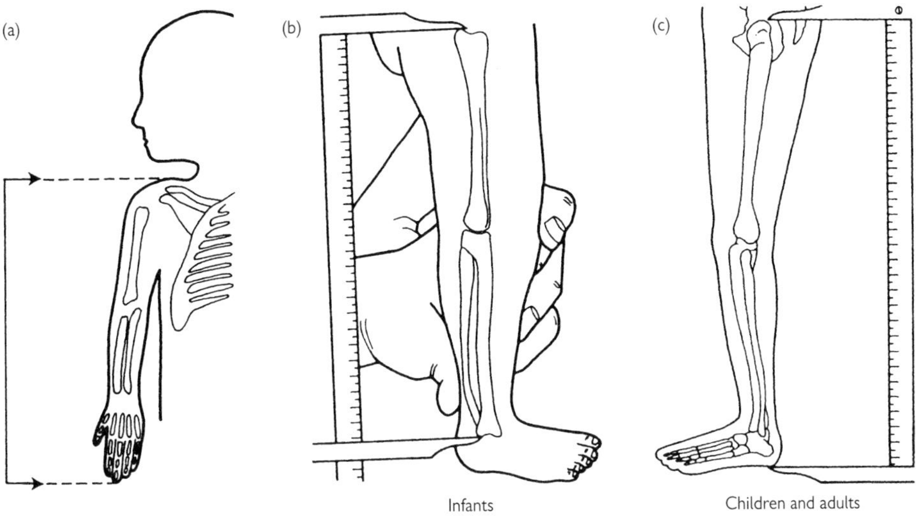

Measurement of limb length. (a) Total upper limb length. Measure between the acromim (the most prominent posterior lateral bony prominence of the shoulder joint) and the tip of the middle finger. (b) Total lower limb length. In infant measure between the greater trochanter of the femur to the lateral malleolus of the ankle. (c) In older children and adults measure from the greater trochanter to the plan of the sole of the foot (floor). Reprinted from Hall et al. *Handbook of Normal Physical Measurements*, with permission of Oxford University Press, 1989.

Holoprosencephaly (HPE)

During embryonic life the forebrain vesicle divides along the dorsal midline to form the cerebral hemispheres. Failure, or partial failure, of this cleavage result in, respectively, *alobar holoprosencephaly* where the two lateral ventricles are replaced by a single midline ventricle (which is often greatly enlarged) and part fusion of the frontal lobes (*lobar holoprosencephaly*). Other midline forebrain structures, including the olfactory bulbs and tracts, optic bulbs and tracts, corpus callosus, thalamus, hypothalamus, and pituitary, are frequently also affected.

The development of the midface is related to that of the forebrain and there is a range of anomalies, particularly affecting the midfacial structures (eyes, nose, midline cleft lip) associated with HPE. Cyclopia, where there is a single midline orbit with abnormal eye tissue, is the most severe malformation. The nose in cyclopic babies is usually represented by a proboscis that is sited above the orbit.

HPE occurs in approximately 1/10 000–15 000 livebirths, but in 1/250 during early embryogenesis, since most affected fetuses are miscarried. It is genetically heterogeneous—chromosomal in up to 50% (especially +13, and many other small deletions (including 7q36) and duplications), recognizable syndrome in 15%, familial autosomal dominant (AD) in some, *de novo* AD mutation in some of the remainder. Twelve loci contain genes implicated in pathogenesis of HPE, of which five are known (see table).

Some of the gene loci implicated in the pathogenesis of holoprosencephaly

HPE1	21q22.3	
HPE2	2p21	*SIX3*
HPE3	7q36	*SHH**
HPE4	18p11.3	*TG1F*
HPE5	13q32	*ZIC2*
HPE6	3p24-pter	
HPE7	9q22	*PTCH*

* Sonic hedgehog: heterozygous mutations reported in >30 unrelated patients and in one-third of familial cases.

Associated facial features. HPE may be identified on ultrasound scan (USS) in pregnancy, or a neonate is born with *hypotelorism* and *median* (*midline*) *cleft lip* in whom cranial USS or magnetic resonance imaging (MRI) reveals HPE. The most extreme form of craniofacial malformation is cyclopia (a single central eye) with a nose-like structure (proboscis) above it. More commonly there is severe hypotelorism, a flat nose with a single nostril and median clefting of the upper lip. Milder cases can have bilateral or unilateral cleft lip/palate, slight hypotelorism, and a single central upper incisor. Up to 20% of children with major brain malformations have only minor dysmorphic features.

Alobar holoprosencephaly. In alobar HPE, the cerebrum is a single U-shaped mass, without division into right and left hemispheres. Most affected children die before, during, or soon after birth. 50% of livebirths with alobar HPE will have died by 4 months of age, but survival for several years is possible (such children have profound learning disability, seizures, feeding difficulties often requiring gastrostomy). Pituitary and hypothalamic dysfunction is common.

Semilobar and lobar holoprosencephaly. In semilobar and lobar HPE there is more complete development of the right and left cerebral hemispheres (see figure). Many affected children live into adulthood, although early death is also common. Some degree of learning disability is usual. There is a spectrum of severity from children with severe semilobar HPE having problems similar to those seen in alobar HPE through to minimal disability and a normal lifespan in the mildest forms of lobar HPE.

Clinical approach

History: key points

- Three-generation family history.
- History of HPE, microcephaly, anosmia, or single central incisor tooth in other family members may indicate that this is a family with AD HPE.

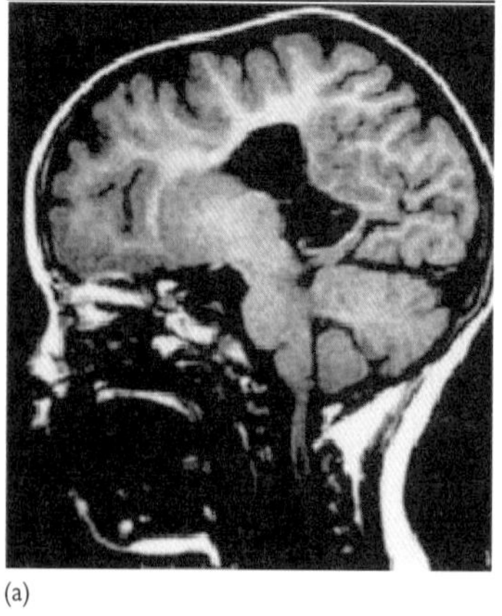

(a)

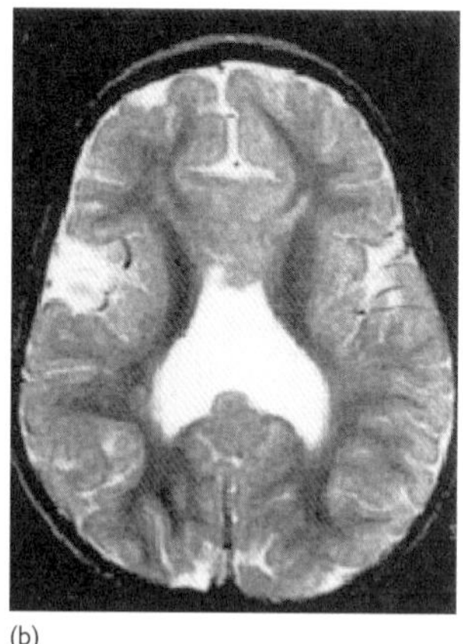

(b)

(a) Semilobar holoprosencephaly in a girl aged 2 years imaged with T_1-weighted sagittal MRI. This midline view shows absence of the corpus callosum and fusion of the frontal lobes. (b) Semilobar holoprosencephaly in the same patient using T_2-weighted axial MRI. There is fusion of the frontal lobes of both central hemispheres and a common central ventricle. (Taken from Warrell (2003), p. 1205, by permission of Oxford University Press.)

- Maternal diabetes mellitus (infants of diabetic mothers have an overall ~1% risk for holoprosencephaly—a 200-fold risk compared with the general population).
- Raised maternal age (increased risk for trisomy 13).

Examination: key points
- Birthweight (reduced in most chromosomal imbalance).
- Occipital-frontal circumference (OFC). Shape of cranium, microcephaly, trigonocephaly.
- Eyes. Spectrum from hypotelorism through to cyclopia.
- Nose. Spectrum from midline proboscis through absence of anterior nasal spine and nasal septum and single nostril.
- Mouth. Spectrum ranging from poorly defined cupid's bow and absent labial frenulum through to midline clefting of the upper lip with associated cleft palate (sometimes referred to as premaxillary agenesis).
- Agnathia (agnathia–HPE).
- Other midline anomalies, e.g. congenital heart disease, anal anomalies.
- Limbs. Polydactyly (Pallister–Hall syndrome, pseudotrisomy 13), 2,3 toe syndactyly (Smith–Lemli–Opitz (SLO) syndrome).
- Examine parents, including testing for anosmia.

Special investigations
- Chromosomes, looking for trisomy 13, del(18p), del(7q), and other known HPE loci.
- MRI scan for better delineation of cranial anatomy if diagnosis based on cranial USS.
- Store DNA, consider looking for mutations in SHH (sonic hedgehog gene at 7q36)—detectable in 37% of families with AD HPE.
- Sporadic cases; screening of genes not routinely offered.
- 7 dehydrocholesterol to exclude SLO syndrome.

Some diagnoses to consider

Chromosomal imbalance. up to 50% of HPE has a chromosomal aetiology. Trisomy 13 is the most common abnormality but many other anomalies have been described. Particularly exclude loci known to have been associated with HPE. Triploidy may be found in fetuses with HPE. Consider telomere analysis in babies with HPE and other malformations/low birthweight.

AD HPE. AD HPE is characterized by incomplete penetrance and extreme intrafamilial variability. The transmitting parent may have a single central incisor as their only manifestation, or even be clinically normal. When a mutation is identified in an affected child, it is not uncommon to find that it is inherited from an unaffected parent.

The most common single gene associated with HPE is sonic hedgehog, *SHH*.

Environmental causes. Maternal diabetes: 200-fold increased risk for HPE.

Pallister–Hall syndrome. AD with mutation in *GLI3* at 7p13 which is a major downstream effector of SHH signalling. Hypothalamic hamartoblastoma, postaxial polydactyly, imperforate anus, hypospadias. Highly variable. Examine parents for features.

Smith-Lemli-Opitz (SLO) syndrome. A rare, but testable, cause of HPE. The diagnostic test is measurement of 7-dehydrocholesterol in the blood. Postaxial polydactyly, cleft palate, hypospadias, and 2,3 syndactyly are features

that may suggest the diagnosis in a neonate. The frequency is approximately 1 in 20 000–30 000. HPE occurs in ~5% of patients with SLO. See 'Hypospadias', page 142.

Rubinstein–Taybi syndrome (RTS). Normal birthweight, postnatal short stature and microcephaly, moderate–severe learning difficulties in most, broad thumbs and halluces; ~25% have deletions of *CREBBP* on 16p13. See 'Broad thumbs', page 58.

Pseudotrisomy 13 or HPE polydactyly syndrome. Autosomal recessive (AR). Postaxial polydactyly and heart defects. Similarities to hydrolethalus syndrome.

Agnathia–HPE. Carefully exclude chromosomal imbalance. One report of possible dominant inheritance.

Fetal akinesia sequence. Features are microcephaly, poor fetal movement, and contractures. There are reports of families with X-linked inheritance.

Genetic advice

Recurrence risk

If after careful assessment the diagnosis is isolated HPE, consider if either parent could be minimally affected. Enquire about family history. Enquire about missing teeth or anosmia. Careful clinical examination of both parents looking for hypotelorism, poorly defined Cupid's bow, absent labial frenulum, and single central incisor. Arrange MRI scan of both parents for any evidence of a midline lesion.

- For sporadic case with no family history and normal parents, recurrence risk counselling is difficult if the underlying cause has not been identified. Recurrence risk can range from as low as 0% to as high as 50% (but see comment below regarding risk for severely affected child with AD inheritance).
- For AD families the risk of an obligate carrier having a severely affected child is 16–21%; the risk of milder effects is 13–14%. Males may be at greater risk than females for major malformations outside the central nervous system (CNS).
- For chromosomal and syndromic cases, counsel as for the specific diagnosis.

Prenatal diagnosis

If a specific chromosomal defect or gene mutation has been identified, prenatal diagnosis by chorionic villus sampling (CVS) or amniocentesis would be possible.

If not, prenatal diagnosis by detailed USS should enable detection of a severely affected fetus. Scanning could begin at 16 weeks when it should be possible to visualize the lateral ventricles, although repeat later scans will be required to exclude recurrence.

Prognosis

HPE is a serious developmental disorder but the prognosis depends on the severity of the abnormality and the presence of other malformations. See Barr and Cohen (1999).

Support group: Many of the individual syndromes have their own support groups. See <www.cafamily.org.uk>.

Expert adviser: Maximilian Muenke, Chief, Medical Genetics Branch, National Institutes of Health, Bethesda, Maryland, USA.

References

Barr M Jr, Cohen MM Jr. Holoprosencephaly survival and performance. *Am J Med Genet* 1999; **89**: 116–20.

Goodman FR. Congenital abnormalities of body patterning: embryology revisited. *Lancet* 2003; **362**: 651–62.

Moog U, De Die-Smulders CE, *et al.* Holoprosencephaly: the Maastricht experience. *Genet Counsel* 2001; **12**: 287–98.

Nanni L, Ming JE, *et al.* The mutational spectrum of the sonic hedgehog gene in holoprosencephaly: SHH mutations cause a significant proportion of autosomal dominant holoprosencephaly. *Hum Mol Genet* 1999; **8**: 2479–88.

Odent S, Le Marec B, Munnich A, Le Merrer M, Bonaiti-Pellie C. Segregation analysis in non syndromic holoprosencephaly. *Am J Med Genet* 1998; **77**: 139–43.

Roessler E, Muenke M. How a hedgehog might see HPE. *Hum Mol Genet* 2003; **12** (Suppl.): 1215–25.

Roessler E, Belloni E, *et al.* Mutations in the human sonic hedgehog gene cause holoprosencephaly. *Nat Genet* 1996; **14**: 357–60.

Suthers G, Smith S. Springbett S. Skewed sex ratios in familial holoprosencephaly and in people with isolated single maxillary central incisor. *J Med Genet* 1999; **36**: 924–6.

Walsh C. Genetic malformations of the human cerebral cortex. *Neuron* 1999; **23**: 19–29.

Warrell D. (ed.). *Oxford textbook of medicine*, 4th edn. Oxford University Press, Oxford, 2003.

Whiteford M, Tolmie JL. Holoprosencephaly in the West of Scotland 1975–1994. *J Med Genet* 1996; **33**: 578–84.

Hydrocephalus

Congenital hydrocephalus comprises a diverse group of conditions in which there are impaired circulation and absorption of cerebrospinal fluid (CSF). The incidence is 4–8/10 000 livebirths and stillbirths. Congenital malformations of the central nervous system (CNS), e.g spina bifida, infections, e.g. congenital infection or meningitis, and haemorrhage can all give rise to hydrocephalus.

The CSF flows from the lateral ventricles into the third ventricle through the foramina of Monro, and then into the fourth ventricle via the aqueduct of Sylvius. CSF leaves the ventricular system through the foramen of Magendie (into the cisterna magna) and the foramina of Luschka (into the pontine cistern). See figure.

Hydrocephalus usually refers to *obstructive* or *non-communicating* hydrocephalus, where all or part of the ventricular system is enlarged. In *aqueduct stenosis* the lateral and third ventricles are enlarged, but not the fourth ventricle (see figure on p135). Bleeding into the ventricles may block the foramina causing obstructive hydrocephalus, whereas bleeding into the subarachnoid space may impair resorption of CSF by the arachnoid villi causing *non-obstructive* or *communicating* hydrocephalus.

Hydrocephalus causing increased intracranial pressure and progressive hydrocephalus are treated by insertion of a ventriculo-peritoneal (VP) shunt.

Clinical approach

History: key points

- Detailed three-generation family tree. Extend further on maternal side if possible. Enquire specifically for other relatives with hydrocephalus, unexplained stillbirths, spasticity, mental handicap, or neural tube defects. (Neural tube defects and hydrocephalus can occur in the same family.)
- Enquire about infections in pregnancy.
- Was ventriculomegaly noted on antenatal scans? What was the occipital-frontal circumference (OFC) at birth?
- Detailed perinatal history enquiring for secondary causes of hydrocephalus. Was there intracranial haemorrhage,

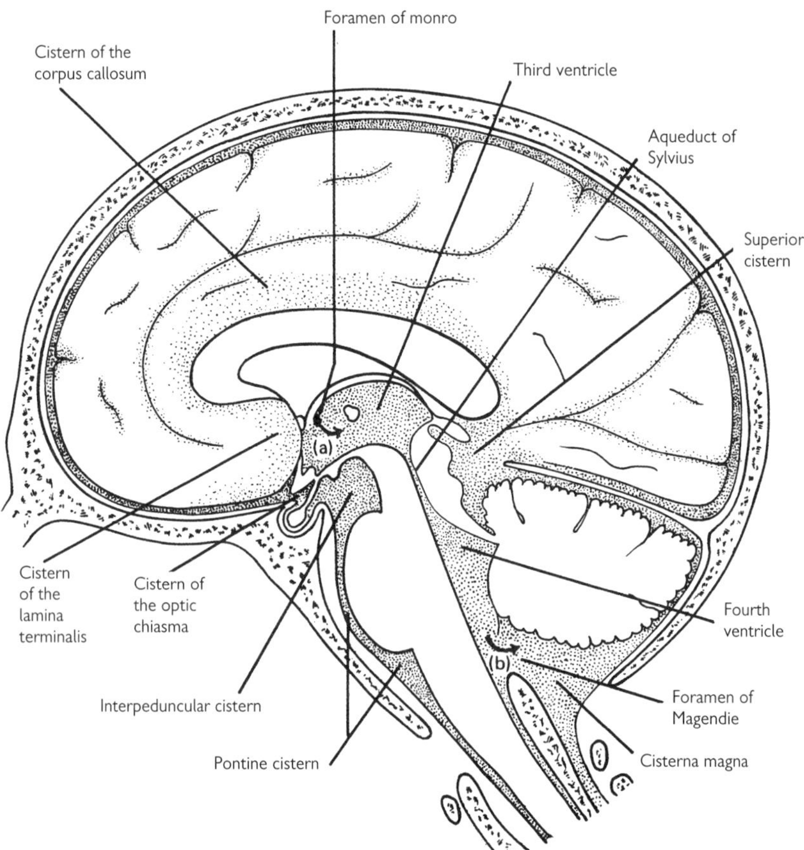

Subarachnoid cisterns. (a) Cerebrospinal fluid entering the third ventricle from the lateral ventricle through the foramen of Monro. (b) Cerebrospinal fluid entering the cisterna magna from the fourth ventricle through the foramen of Magendie. (Taken from Barr, p. 369, with the permission of Lippincott Williams and Wilkins.)

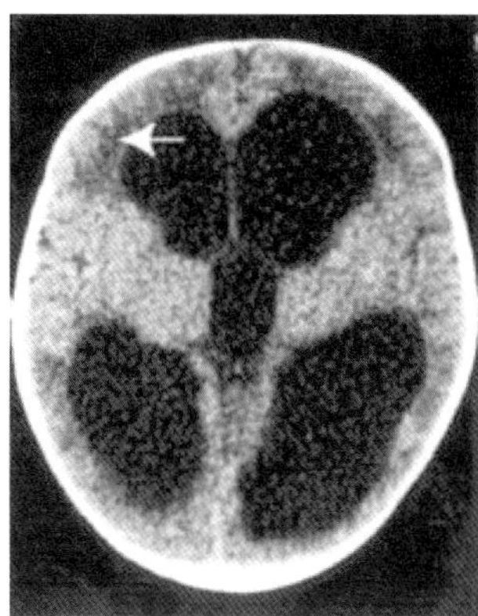

Aqueduct stenosis in a boy aged 1 month with a bulging anterior fontanelle and increasing head circumference. Axial CT shows a gross dilatation of the third and lateral ventricles (the fourth ventricle is not shown but was normal in size). Note the periventricular low density due to transependymal exudation of cerebrospinal fluid under pressure (arrow). (Taken from Warrell (2003), p. 1213, by permission of Oxford University Press.)

e.g. intraventricular haemorrhage (IVH), following premature delivery? Was there neonatal meningitis?
- Developmental milestones.
- Seizures.
- Exclude clinical features of raised intracranial pressure.

Examination: key points
- Height, OFC, and fontanelle size and tension. (Has the OFC crossed centiles?)
- Head shape.
- Palpate VP shunt if present.
- Eyes. 'Setting sun' sign.
- Spina bifida?
- Other congenital malformations and dysmorphic features (syndromic and chromosomal conditions).
- In a male infant look carefully for congenitally adducted thumbs.
- In a male infant detailed neurological exam looking for spasticity (increased tone, exaggerated deep tendon reflexes (DTRs), and extensor plantar response).
- Café-au-lait skin lesions (neurofibromatosis type 1 (NF1)).

Special investigations
- Review MRI scan for:
  - complications associated with prematurity, e.g. periventricular leucomalacia;
  - tumours and cysts;
  - structural malformations like aqueduct stenosis, Chiari malformation, Dandy–Walker malformation;
  - cortical abnormality such as cobblestone (type II) lissencephaly;
  - intracranial calcification (congenital infections and autosomal recessive (AR) 'pseudoTORCH');
  - differentiation from hydranencephaly;
  - to look for evidence of cerebral atrophy.
- Skull X-ray if there are features suggestive of premature cranial suture closure.

- Creatine kinase (CK; Walker–Warburg syndrome (WWS) and muscle–eye–brain (MEB) disease).
- Ophthalmology opinion (papilloedema, optic atrophy, oculomotor palsy).
- Chromosomes (unless development is entirely normal and there are no dysmorphic features).
- TORCH (toxoplasmosis–other (including syphilis, varicella zoster virus, parvovirus)–rubella virus–cytomegalovirus) screen for congenital infection in babies <6 months of age.
- Consider *L1CAM* mutation analysis if male infant with aqueduct stenosis and positive family history or suggestive clinical features (e.g. adducted thumbs, spasticity, agenesis or hypoplasia of corpus callosum). Mutation detection rate is 75% in families with three affected male members, and 15% with a negative family history.
- Review brain histology of any affected individuals.

Some diagnoses to consider
Arnold–Chiari malformation.
- **Type I.** Downward displacement of the lower cerebellum, including the tonsils; rarely causes symptoms in childhood but may be associated with hydrocephalus and syringomyelia.
- **Type II.** Downward displacement of the cerebellar vermis, tonsils, and medulla through the foramen magnum and associated with myelomeningocele (see 'Neural tube defects', page 392). Counsel as for neural tube defect.

Hydranencephaly. Scans show a small rim of cerebral cortex but the cerebellum and brainstem may be normal. Distruption to the carotid artery supply is one cause. Enquire about early pregnancy. May be confused with holoprosencephaly (HPE).

Arachnoid cyst is a cystic cavity within the arachnoid membrane. Hydrocephalus can occur by obstruction and reduced CSF resorption. The majority of arachnoid cysts are sporadic. See 'Structural intracranial anomalies (agenesis of the corpus callosum, septic-optic dysplasia, and arachnoid cysts)', page 248.

X-linked hydrocephalus. The neural cell adhesion molecule L1CAM plays a key role during neurodevelopment. The gene encoding *L1CAM* maps to Xq28, and males with mutation in this gene have a phenotype characterized by a combination of corpus callosum hypoplasia, mental retardation, adducted thumbs, spastic paraplegia, and hydrocephalus. There is a high degree of intra- and interfamilial variability.

Walker–Warburg syndrome (WWS) and muscle–eye–brain disease (MEB). These are AR disorders that share the combination of cerebral neuronal migration defects (cobblestone lissencephaly), ocular abnormalities, and a congenital muscular dystrophy. The features of WWS are hydrocephalus, agyria, retinal dystrophy, and sometimes an encephalocele—thus its alternate name of HARD ± E. Both are due to genes in the O-mannosylation pathway (*POMT1* gene in WWS and *POMGNT1* in MEB). See 'Lissencephaly and neuronal migration disorders', page 156.

PseudoTORCH. An AR condition with intracranial calcification therefore mimicking congenital infection.

Neurofibromatosis type 1 (NF1). Aqueduct stenosis is a rare but well recognized complication in infancy. See 'Neurofibromatosis type 1 (NF1)', page 396.

Achondroplasia. Most infants with achondroplasia are macrocephalic. OFC should be plotted on achondroplasia-specific charts and monitored serially (every 1–2 months) during the first years of life. Hydrocephalus is usually communicating but can also be due to cervicomedullary compression (small foramen magnum, displacement of the brainstem). See 'Achondroplasia', page 260.

Craniosynostosis syndromes. Affected infants may have raised intracranial pressure from the synostosis but ventricular dilatation is an additional reason. See 'Craniosynostosis', page 288.

Genetic advice

The extent to which some degree of neurological impairment or abnormal neurological signs are attributed to sequelae of sustained hydrocephalus *in utero* may determine how exhaustive a search is made for an underlying cause. Discussion with a paediatric neurologist may be very helpful in making this judgement.

Recurrence risk.
Review babies and young infants when older to exclude other signs of a genetic disorder, e.g. NF1.

After careful evaluation and exclusion of syndromic conditions:
- the empiric risk for sibs of an isolated case is up to 5%, all studies showing a higher risk for male sibs of an affected male;
- the risk for male sibs of an isolated male case with aqueduct stenosis is higher (5–10%) unless *L1CAM* has been excluded;
- children of consanguineous parents may have hydrocephalus as part of an AR condition.

Carrier detection
This is possible in families with a known mutation or by linked markers in X-linked families.

Prenatal diagnosis
Prenatal diagnosis based on early ultrasound scan (USS) is often not reliable as ventriculomegaly usually starts after 20 weeks of gestation, and may not appear until near term or after delivery. Serial USS is often offered in a subsequent pregnancy, but these limitations must be carefully discussed with the parents. See 'Ventriculomegaly', page 642.

Support group: Support and advice about hydrocephalus are available from Association for Spina Bifida and Hydrocephalus (ASBAH) <www.asbah.org>, Tel. 01733 555988.

Expert adviser: Daniela Pilz, Consultant Clinical Geneticist, Institute of Medical Genetics, University Hospital of Wales, Cardiff, Wales.

References

Barr ML. *The human nervous system: an anatomical viewpoint*, 2nd edn. Harper and Row, Hagerstown, Maryland.

Burton BK. Recurrence risks for congenital hydrocephalus. *Clin Genet* 1979; **16**: 47–53.

Fransen E, Van Camp G, D'Hooge R, *et al*. Genotype–phenotype correlation in L1 associated diseases. *J Med Genet* 1998; **35**: 399–404.

Howard FM, Till K, Carter CO. A family study of hydrocephalus. *J Med Genet* 1981; **18**: 252–5.

Kenwrick S, Jouet M, Donnai D. X-linked hydrocephalus and MASA syndrome. *J Med Genet* 1996; **33**: 59–65.

Schrander-Stumpel C, Fryns JP. Congenital hydrocephalus: nosology and guidelines for clinical approach and genetic counselling. *Eur J Pediatr* 1998; **157**: 355–62.

Varadi V, Toth A, Torok O. Heterogeneity and recurrence risk for congenital hydrocephalus (ventriculomegaly): a prospective study, *Am J Med Genet* 1988; **29**: 305–10.

Warrell D. (ed.). *Oxford textbook of medicine*, 4th edn. Oxford University Press, Oxford, 2003.

Hypermobile joints

Joint hypermobility, ligamentous laxity, joint laxity, loose jointed, double jointed.

Hypermobile joints have an excessive range of movement due to lack of support from the soft tissues that surround the joint. The ligaments consist principally of collagen but elastic tissue containing fibrillin and elastin is also important. Hypermobility is evaluated using a scoring system described below. Approximately 5–10% of school age children are hypermobile, but the percentage decreases with age. It is more common in females at all ages. There is considerable variation between different ethnic groups in the range of joint movement that is normal for a given population.

Hypermobility is a diagnostic feature of Ehlers–Danlos syndrome (EDS), but also occurs in about 25% of patients with Marfan syndrome. The benign joint hypermobility syndrome (EDS hypermobility type) is heterogeneous and generally differs from the other forms of EDS in that the skin involvement is less pronounced. Hypermobility needs to be differentiated from hypotonia of central or peripheral origin.

The 'Beighton scoring system (see table) assesses the degree to which specific joints can be hyperextended or hyperflexed. A point is given if an individual is able to perform the manoeuvre and the left and right are scored independently giving a maximum score of 9.

Clinical approach

History: key points

A child may be referred by a paediatrician or a bone and joint specialist who has noted the excessive hypermobility and asks if there are other conditions or associated features.

- Three-generation family tree. Ask about congenital hip dislocation, joint pain, and joint replacement surgery.
- Joint pain, dislocation, effusions.
- Abnormal skin scarring after trauma. Easy bruising.
- Fractures after minor trauma (osteogenesis imperfecta (OI)).
- Motor milestones are often delayed but global developmental delay indicates the possibility of a central neurological problem.

Examination: key points

- Assessment of joint mobility. Beighton score.
- Skin: excessive stretching and abnormal scars that are often described as like tissue paper; excessive bruising (EDS). Cutis laxa can sometimes be confused with EDS.
- Skeletal signs associated with joint hypermobility: flat feet (pes planus), knock knees (genu valgum), scoliosis.

- Heart murmurs. Floppy mitral valves are particularly common. Aortic root dilatation and rupture in Marfan syndrome and rupture of blood vessels and internal viscera in EDS vascular type.
- Hernias.
- Eyes. Retinal detachment (EDS), dislocated lenses (Marfan syndrome), myopia (Marfan and Stickler syndromes), blue sclerae (OI).
- Palate. High (Marfan), cleft (Stickler syndrome, Larsen syndrome).
- Many skeletal dysplasias are caused by collagen mutations and also have joint laxity. Milder dysplasias such as Stickler syndrome may be missed unless specifically considered.
- Muscle strength to exclude myopathies and other causes of peripheral hypotonia.

Special investigations

Individuals with benign hypermobility do not usually require special investigations.

- Molecular testing is available for some forms of EDS—see 'Ehlers–Danlos syndrome (EDS)', page 312.
- Radiology if congenital hip dislocation or other orthopaedic complications are present.
- Skeletal survey or limited skeletal survey for diagnostic reasons, e.g in the presence of features of Stickler syndrome or OI.
- Cardiac echo if there is a murmur or clinical suspicion of Marfan syndrome.

Some diagnoses to consider

The differential diagnosis will depend on the age of presentation and the presence of other features.

Ehlers Danlos syndrome (EDS)—hypermobility type (benign joint hypermobility syndrome). In this condition there is isolated joint hypermobility and the diagnosis is made after excluding other syndromic causes of hypermobility. The child may present with delayed motor milestones. Labels such as poor muscle tone may have used to describe the signs as the condition may be severe enough to cause floppiness in infancy. Fine, as well as gross, motor milestones may be delayed and the older child may be described as clumsy. There is no intellectual impairment. There is often a dominant family history. Early onset osteoarthritis in the major weight-bearing joints may be found in adults. Examine parents and assess their joint mobility. The condition is variable but girls are usually more affected than boys. Carefully exclude congenital dislocation of the hip (CDH) in subsequent children. Chronic

Beighton scoring system (Beighton)

Type of hypermobility	Score
Passive extension of the little finger metacarpophalangeal (MCP) joint to $\geq 90°$ (1 point for each hand)	2
Passive apposition of the thumb to the flexor aspect of the forearm (1 point for each hand)	2
Hyperextension of the elbow by $>10°$ (1 point for each elbow)	2
Hyperextension of the knee by $>10°$ (1 point for each knee)	2
Bend forward and flex the spine. Palms of the hands touch the floor with the knees extended	1
Total score	9

joint pain is a possible troublesome complication for some individuals in the absence of obvious structural joint damage.

Ehlers–Danlos syndrome (EDS) except EDS hypermobility type. There are several other types of Ehlers–Danlos syndrome: joint hypermobility, hyperextensible skin, and tissue fragility with abnormal scarring and easy bruising are the major features. See 'Ehlers–Danlos syndrome (EDS)', page 312.

Marfan syndrome (MFS). Autosomal dominant (AD) systemic disorder of connective tissue with a high degree of clinical variability. Cardinal manifestations involve the ocular (myopia, lens dislocation), skeletal (pectus excavatum, pectus carinatum, scoliosis, long limbs, arachnodactyly, high palate), and cardiovascular systems (aortic root dilatation and dissection, mitral and aortic regurgitation). Caused by mutations in FBN1, the gene encoding fibrillin, a component of the extracellular matrix. Use the Ghent criteria to establish the diagnosis. See 'Marfan syndrome', page 380.

Floppy infant. Floppiness in infancy can be caused by many disorders of the central nervous system (CNS) that are associated with hypotonia; also myopathies, dystrophies, and peripheral nerve problems such as spinal muscular atrophy. See 'Floppy infant', page 118.

Skeletal dysplasias.
- In **Larsen syndrome** there are multiple joint dislocations. There are both AD and autosomal recessive (AR) types. A skeletal survey is required to establish the diagnosis. One of the characteristic features is that the tarsal bones show a bifid calcaneus in childhood.
- In **Stickler syndrome**, cleft palate, myopia, retinal detachment, and epiphyseal dysplasia are 'harder' diagnostic handles than joint hypermobility. See 'Stickler syndrome', page 414.

- **Osteogenesis imperfecta.** The cardinal features are fractures and reduced bone density. See 'Fractures', page 122.

Genetic advice
Recurrence risk

Counsel for the specific condition diagnosed. Specific diagnosis is not always possible for some of the milder phenotypes. Many of the milder connective tissue disorders follow AD inheritance with a 50% risk to offspring, and typically show quite wide inter- and intrafamilial variation.

Prenatal diagnosis

Possible only if the pathogenic mutation has been defined in a given family.

Natural history and further management (preventative measures)

The condition can be aggravated by excessive weight-bearing, exercise, and obesity. A physiotherapist can advise about posture and the benefit of orthoses, such as insoles to support the arches of the feet, and suggest a beneficial exercise regime (swimming, cycling, walking).

High impact activities, e.g. trampolining, that place a severe stress on the joints are probably best avoided.

Support group: Hypermobility Syndrome Association <www.hypermobility.org>.

Expert adviser: Paul Wordsworth, Professor of Rheumatology, University of Oxford, Oxford, England.

References

Beighton P, McKusick VA. McKusick's heutable disorders of connective tissue 5th edn. St Louis Mosby 1993.

Grahame R. Joint hypermobility and genetic collagen disorders: are they related? *Arch Dis Child* **199**; 80: 188–91.

Raff ML, Byers PH. Joint hypermobility syndromes. *Curr Opin Rheumatol* 1996; **8**: 459–66.

Hypoglycaemia in the neonate and infant

After 72 hours in term babies and after the first week in pre-term babies, hypoglycaemia may be defined as a plasma or whole blood glucose of <2.6 mmol/l, although a stricter definition is used by some (<2.5 mmol/l; Saudubray *et al.* 2000) and definition is a contentious area (Cornblath *et al.* 2000). After feeding, the liver builds up stores of glycogen and triglyceride. During fasting, glucose and ketones are released to provide energy.

To maintain a normal blood glucose level there must be:

- intact hepatic glycogenolytic and gluconeogenic enzymes systems to produce glucose from stored glycogen (impaired in glycogen storage disorders);
- adequate supply of amino acids, glycerol, and lactate;
- adequate energy from beta-oxidation of fatty acids to produce glucose and ketones (impaired in fatty acid oxidation disorders);
- a normal endocrine system (impaired in hyperinsulinism, growth hormone deficiency, and Laron syndrome).

In normal neonates, hypoglycaemia immediately after birth is associated with developmental immaturity of hepatic gluconeogenesis and ketogenesis. In the majority of babies with hypoglycaemia there is a non-genetic aetiology (prematurity, low birthweight, sepsis, infant of diabetic mother, etc). This section is an approach to some of the genetic causes of hypoglycaemia.

Clinical approach

History: key points

- Three-generation family history with specific enquiry for consanguinity and unexplained infant/neonatal death or Reyes syndrome.
- Gestational diabetes.
- Birthweight (increased in persistent hyperinsulinaemic hypoglycaemia of infancy (PHHI) and Beckwith–Wiedemann syndrome (BWS)).
- Apgar scores at delivery and was resuscitation required?
- Was the baby handling normally and feeding well before the onset of symptoms? Babies who appear normal at birth and handle and feed well and subsequently deteriorate are more likely to have an inborn error of metabolism.
- How old was the infant when hypoglycaemia was noted? Was it after a period of fasting? Was there any additional metabolic stress?
- Seizures.

Examination: key points

- Weight, length, and occipito-frontal head circumference (OFC).
- Assess the posture and tone of the infant and note any abnormal movements.
- Dysmorphic features and macrosomia (BWS).
- Hepatomegaly (moderate in PHHI and fatty acid oxidation (FAO) disorders; severe in glycogen storage disease (GSD) I and III).
- Cardiomyopathy and arrhythmia: FAO defects (see also 'Cardiomyopathy in children under 10 years', page 60).
- Micropenis (pituitary dysfunction).

Special investigations

Ensure that non-genetic causes of hypoglycaemia are being concurrently investigated. Usually by the time the geneticist is called a basic screen for glucose, calcium, sodium, metabolic acidosis (pH, base excess, and HCO_3^-), liver function, ammonia, uric acid, blood count, and urine dipstick for pH, ketones, and reducing substances will have been completed.

NB. The list below covers many of the likely causes, but is not an exhaustive list of diagnostic investigations.

- Urine:
  - urine ketones. If there is significant ketonuria with no acidosis in a sick neonate, exclude maple syrup urine disease (MSUD). Ketosis is not an important fuel source in the normal neonate, due to liver immaturity. In the infant or older child, ketonuria is typically absent in hyperinsulinaemia and FAO disorders, moderate in association with fasting hypoglycaemia in GSD types I and III, and raised in idiopathic ketotic hypoglycaemia (but this does not present until 1–2 years). If ketonuria occurs in conjunction with metabolic acidosis, consider GSD type III;
  - urine organic acids and amino acids to pick up abnormal metabolites suggestive of an inborn error of metabolism.
- Blood:
  - DNA for storage and analysis. For further investigation of BWS, e.g uniparental disomy (UPD) 11p studies, parental samples will be required;
  - cytogenetic analysis on babies with dysmorphic features;
  - acyl carnitines (dried blood spot on Guthrie card), total and free carnitine (FAO and carnitine transporter defects);
  - insulin level (record blood glucose level at time sample is taken);
  - growth hormone;
  - lactate: lactic acidosis in GSD type III (and see below);
  - ammonia: raised ammonia and lactate in hyperinsulinism/hyperammonaemic syndrome, FAO, organic acidaemias, and mitochondrial cytopathies;
  - free fatty acids in the blood and ketone bodies (disorders of beta oxidation and hyperinsulinism);
  - neutropenia is a feature of GSD Ib.
- Imaging:
  - cardiac echo to exclude cardiomyopathy and electrocardiogram (ECG) for arrhythmia: FAO (see also 'Cardiomyopathy in children under 10 years', page 60);
  - imaging of liver and pancreas;
  - cranial ultrasound scan (USS)/magnetic resonance imaging (MRI) of the brain for panhypopituitarism, agenesis of the corpus callosum.

Under the supervision of a paediatrician with expertise in metabolic/endocrine disease:

- glucose requirements (high in PHHI; low in other causes);
- response to glucagons (dramatic in PHHI, absent in GSD, variable in FAO and endocrine disorders);

- response to diazoxide and hydrochlorothiazide (PHHI);
- consider liver biopsy for specific enzyme abnormality (may not be necessary to perform liver biopsy to confirm diagnosis).

Some diagnoses to consider

Neonate

Persistent hyperinsulinaemic hypoglycaemia of infancy (PHHI). This is the most common cause of recurrent hypoglycaemia in early infancy. This term is now preferred to nesidioblastosis. It is characterized by dysregulation of insulin secretion. It occurs in ~1/50 000 livebirths. Approximately 95% of cases are sporadic; some cases are autosomal recessive (AR) (Cohen 2003). Birthweights are >90th centile in at least 45%. Most present in the first 72 hours with hypoglycaemia. A small number present later and these have adenomas. In the neonate, the diagnosis is made on the high glucose requirement. Response to glucagon is dramatic. There may be focal or diffuse abnormalities of the β-cells of the pancreas.

There is molecular heterogeneity in the sporadic forms of PHHI; some patients with the focal type have somatic loss of maternal alleles at the imprinted domain on 11p15. AR PHHI can be caused by mutations in the high-affinity sulfonylurea receptor (*SUR1*) and by mutations in the K$^+$ channel *Kir6.2*, which both encode subunits of the K$_{ATP}$ channels of the pancreatic β-cells. This channel is involved in glucose-mediated insulin secretion, promoting insulin release when intracellular glucose levels are high and preventing it when intracellular insulin levels fall. When this channel is faulty, insulin release is unregulated leading to profound hypoglycaemia.

Early recognition of hypoglycaemia, correct differentiation between histological types (focal or diffuse), and maintenance of adequate glucose levels are of critical importance for the outcome of these patients. If medical therapy is not effective, surgical removal of the pancreas (either partial or complete) is performed. Discuss management with a centre with expertise in PHHI.

Beckwith–Wiedemann syndrome (BWS). BWS is a somatic overgrowth and cancer-predisposition syndrome estimated to affect ~1/13 700 individuals. 85% of cases are sporadic and 15% are the result of vertical transmission. The genetic basis of BWS is complex but involves genes at 11p15. (See 'Beckwith–Wiedemann syndrome (BWS)', page 278.)

Fatty acid oxidation (FAO) and ketogenesis disorders. Hypoketotic hypoglycaemia and cardiac abnormalities. In infants the presentation may resemble Reyes syndrome. It is important to recognize primary carnitine deficiencies, as therapeutic treatment with L-carnitine is life-saving. (Secondary causes of carnitine deficiency include malnutrition and renal failure.)

Endocrine abnormalities. Exclude growth hormone deficiency in neonates, panhypopituitarism, disorders of cortisol metabolism, etc.

Infant and older child

Autosomal dominant (AD) hyperinsulinism. Median age of onset is 1 year. Normal birthweight. May present with a seizure, or seizure-like disorder. Caused by mutation in the glucokinase gene (*GCK*) or mutations in the glutamate dehydrogenase gene (*GDH*). Hyperammonaemia is also found in the latter. In some families the molecular cause is unknown.

Endocrine abnormalities. Laron syndrome (mutation in growth hormone-releasing hormone receptor) can present with hypoglycaemia in infants. Short stature, micropenis, and obesity are additional features.

Abnormalities of glycogen synthesis and degradation. Glycogen synthase deficiency and GSD IV prevent synthesis of glycogen but these do not present in neonates. GSD IV typically causes hypogylcaemia and hyperketonuria in the mornings after night feeds are discontinued. Deficiencies of the enzymes involved in the degradation of glycogen cause hypoglycaemia 2–3 hours after a meal and present in infancy rather than in neonates.

Genetic advice

Recurrence risk

As for given diagnosis. Thorough testing usually gives a clue to the aetiological group even if a precise diagnosis is not possible.

For infants with sudden death in whom hypoglycaemia was suspected, the possibility of a genetic condition needs to be considered with a risk of up to 25% for recurrence.

Carrier detection

This is possible in families where a causative mutation has been identified. May be possible for some biochemical abnormalities.

Prenatal diagnosis

This is available to those families where there is molecular or biochemical confirmation of the diagnosis.

Natural history and further management (preventative measures)

Children with these problems require close medical and dietetic supervision to prevent death and neurological disability as a consequence of hypoglycaemia.

Lay group contact: CLIMB (Children Living with Inherited Metabolic Diseases) <www.climb.org.uk>.

Expert adviser: Uma Ramaswami, Consultant Paediatrician (Metabolic Disorders), Addenbrookes Hospital, Cambridge, England and Derek Applegarth, Emeritus Professor of Pediatrics University of British Columbia, Vancorner, British Columbia, Canada.

References

Cohen MM Jr. Persistent hyperinsulinemic hypoglycaemia of infancy. *Am J Med Genet* 2003; **122A**; 351–3.

Cornblath M, Hawdon JM, *et al.* Controversies regarding definition of neonatal hypoglycemia: suggested operational thresholds. *Pediatrics* 2000; **105** (5): 1141–5.

Meissner T, Mayatepek E. Clinical and genetic heterogeneity in congenital hyperinsulinism. *Eur J Pediatr* 2002; **161** (1): 6–20.

Saudubray JM, de Lonlay P, Touati G, Martin D, Nassogne MC, Castelnau P, Sevin C, Baussan C, Brivet M, Vassault A, Rabier D, Bonnefont JP, Kamoin P. Genetic hypoglcaemia in infancy and childhood: pathophysiology and diagnosis. *J Inherit Metab Dis* 2000; **23**: 197–214.

Saudubray JM, Nassogne MC, de Lonlay P, Touati G. Clinical approach to inherited metabolic disorders in neonates: an overview. *Semin Neonatol* 2002; **7**: 3–15.

Society for the Study of Inborn Errors of Metabolism <www.ssiem.org.uk>.

Hypospadias

In hypospadias, the urethral meatus is abnormally located and is displaced proximally on to the ventral surface of the penis—in mild cases on the glans itself and in more severe cases at some point along the ventral surface of the penile shaft. The foreskin is also almost always affected, being imperfectly formed beneath, and this deformity may be more obvious than the hypospadias itself. In a proportion of cases, there is also a downward bend on the shaft of the penis (chordee) which becomes exaggerated during penile erections and, as a general rule, the more severe the hypospadias the greater the chance of significant chordee. It is classified as shown in the table and figure.

Classification of hypospadias*

Severity	Position of urethral meatus
Mild	Glandular or coronal
Moderate	Penile (along the length of the shaft)
Severe	Perineal/scrotal

* NB. The presence of chordee (ventral curvature of the penis due to fibrous tethering) may make it difficult to estimate the severity and extent of the hypospadias until the chordee are released at the first repair.

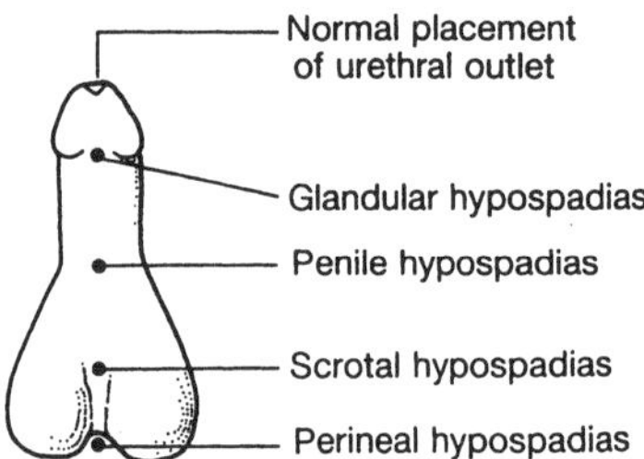

Types of hypospadias. (From Alken and Soekeland (1976), by permission.)

The male external genitalia develop from 8 weeks in the presence of dihydrotestosterone which is produced by the action of the enzyme 5α-reductase on testosterone. Hypospadias is found in 6.4/1000 live male births. Stoll *et al.* (1990) established that 80% are of the mild phenotype and over 90% of these do not have any other malformations. The incidence of associated malformations is higher in the severe group and studies have established the aetiology in about one-third of these. In severely affected infants the gender may be in doubt and careful counselling is required. A stepwise diagnostic approach is recommended to avoid unnecessary invasive and expensive testing.

Epispadias. This occurs in ~1/117 000 livebirths and is much more common in boys (5M:1F). The urethral meatus is abnormally located and is displaced on to the dorsal surface of the penis. The penis is short and broad.

Clinical approach

History: key points
- Three-generation family tree.
- Birthweight (hypospadias is more common in low-birthweight babies).
- Medication during pregnancy, e.g. anti-epilepsy drugs.
- Developmental delay (syndromes and chromosomal conditions).

Examination: key points
- Position of urethral meatus to classify severity.
- Presence of chordee, bifid scrotum, position of testes.
- Blood pressure and renal masses (Wilms tumour).
- Growth parameters and head circumference.
- Hypertelorism, swallowing and laryngeal problems (Opitz G/BBB syndrome).
- Cleft palate (Smith–Lemli–Opitz (SLO) syndrome and chromosomal anomalies).
- Postaxial poyldactyly and syndactyly between 2nd and 3rd toes (SLO).

Special investigations
Step-wise diagnostic studies usually coordinated by a paediatric endocrinologist working with a paediatric urologist.
- Ultrasound scans (USS) of renal and urogenital (UG) system in all affected boys.
- Karyotype (additional X chromosomes, XX males, triploidy, trisomy 13 and 18, many other visible cytogenetic abnormalities). This is an essential investigation in infants with additional malformations and ambiguous genitalia but not routine for the boy with isolated mild hypospadias. Fluorescent *in situ* hybridization (FISH) investigation for del 11p in presence of aniridia or Wilms tumour.
- Human chorionic gonadotrophin (hCG) stimulation to measure testosterone and dihydrotestosterone (5α-reductase deficiency) in boys with moderate or severe hypospadias.
- Genital skin sample for androgen-binding studies at time of surgical repair.
- Consider molecular genetic analysis of the androgen receptor gene or 5α-reductase gene if endocrine studies indicate an abnormality.
- 7-dehydrocholesterol if there are other features of SLO syndrome.

Some diagnoses to consider

In the Albers *et al.*'s (1990) study, 33 patients with severe hypospadias were investigated and in 12 the cause was found. The diagnoses were Drash syndrome (3 patients), androgen receptor mutations leading to partial androgen insensitivity (2), true hermaphrodite (2), chromosome abnormality (1), deficiency of anti-Müllerian hormone (AMH; 1), gonadal dysgenesis (1), partial 5 alpha-reductase deficiency (1), XX male (1). Boehmer *et al.* (2001) investigated 63 children with severe hypospadias and were able to find the underlying aetiology in about one-third. Of these, 17% had a complex genetic syndrome and 10% chromosomal anomalies.

Smith–Lemli–Opitz syndrome (SLO). Hypospadias and/or cryptorchidism are found in 90–100% of males with SLO. The genitalia may be ambiguous with a hypoplastic scrotum. Other features are prenatal and postnatal growth deficiency (almost all), microcephaly, cleft palate (37–52%), thickened alveolar ridges, cardiac defects (36–38%; especially atrioventricular septal defect (AVSD) and total anomalous pulmonary venous drainage (TAPVD)), Y-shaped 2,3 toe syndactyly (>95%), and postaxial polydactyly (~50%). Facial features include narrow bifrontal diameter, ptosis (50%), down-slanting palpebral fissures, and a short nose with depressed nasal bridge and anteverted nares. It is an autosomal recessive (AR) condition. Plasma 7-dehydrocholesterol levels are elevated because mutations in the *DHCR7* gene on 11q13 lead to deficient activity of 7-dehydrocholesterol reductase (*DHCR7*); the final enzyme of the cholesterol biosynthetic pathway (Jira *et al.* 2003). The frequency is ~1 in 20 000–30 000.

WAGR (Wilms tumour–aniridia–genitourinary anomalies–mental retardation). A contiguous gene syndrome due to microscopic or submicroscopic deletion of 11p13. Specific FISH probes available. See 'Wilms tumour', page 486.

Drash syndrome or Wilms tumour and pseudohermaphrodism and Frasier syndrome. Usually have ambiguous genitalia. Caused by mutations in *WT1*. See 'Ambiguous genitalia (including sex reversal)', page 38.

Opitz syndrome. The key features of hypertelorism, hypospadias, swallowing difficulties, and developmental delay are found in both the autosomal dominant (AD) and X-linked (XL) conditions. Anteverted nares and laryngeal clefts appear to be features found in the XL type. The AD locus is on 22q11.2 and the XL locus is on Xp22.3 (*MID1* gene).

Mowat–Wilson syndrome. Characteristic facial appearance (hypertelorism, pointed chin, prominent columella, open-mouthed expression, broad, medial flared eyebrows and uplifted earlobes) together with severe mental retardation. Microcephaly, seizures, congenital heart defects, aplasia/hypoplasia of corpus callosum and urogenital anomalies (especially hypospadias in boys) are frequent findings. Caused by 'de novo' truncating mutations in *ZFHX1B* on 2q22.

Hand–foot–genital syndrome. AD condition caused by mutations in *HOXA13* on 7p15. Males have hypospadias and females have duplication of the uterus and sometimes of the cervix and may have a septate vagina. Hands are small with hypoplastic proximally placed thumbs, and feet are small with short halluces. Urinary tract malformations are common in both sexes.

Genetic advice

Recurrence risk

- **Syndromic hypospadias.** Counsel as appropriate for specific diagnosis.

- **Isolated hypospadias.** Stoll *et al.*'s (1990) study of births in northeastern France found a 17%, or 1 in 6 recurrence risk for brothers. There have been reports of dominant transmission and a couple of reports of recessive inheritance in consanguineous kindreds. Androgen receptor gene mutations are a rare cause of isolated hypospadias.

Prenatal diagnosis

A severe hypospadias may be detected if there is severe chordee or ambiguous genitalia by combining USS information with cytogenetic analysis showing a male karyotype.

Natural history and further management

Surgical treatment for the hypospadias as necessary. Moderate or severe hypospadias is usually repaired as a staged procedure. As a rule, the repair is undertaken some time between 12 months and 2 years of age or after toilet-training, between 3 and 4 years of age. Although repair is usually successful, there is an appreciable (15–30%) rate of complications requiring further surgery. Because the foreskin may be needed for the repair, the child should not be circumcized. In severe cases gender assignment is a difficult problem. Patients at risk of malignancy or hormonal imbalance require long-term surveillance.

Support group: Hypospadias Support Group <www.hypospadias.co.uk>, Tel. 01925 496510.

Expert adviser: Ieuan Hughes, Professor of Paediatrics, University of Cambridge, Cambridge, England.

References

Albers N, Ulrichs C, Gluer S, Hiort O, Sinnecker GH, Mildenberger H, Broedehl J. Etiological classification of severe hypospadias: implications for prognosis and management. *J Pediatr* 1997; **131**: 386–92.

Boehmer AL, *et al.* Etiological studies of severe or familial hypospadias. *J Urol* 2001; **165**: 1246–54.

Jira PE, Waterham HR, *et al.* Smith–Lemli–Opitz syndrome and the *DHCR7* gene. *Am J Hum Genet* 2003; **67**: 269–80.

Klamt B, Koziell A, *et al.* Frasier syndrome is caused by defective alternative splicing of *WT1* leading to an altered ratio of WT1 ± KJS splice isoforms. *Hum Mol Genet* 1998; **7**: 709–14.

Stoll C, Alembik Y, Roth MP, Dott B. Genetic and environmental factors in hypospadias. *J Med Genet* 1990; **27**: 559–63.

Increased bone density

Skeletal X-rays may reveal increased bone density and generalized skeletal changes consistent with a skeletal dysplasia. These disorders are known as sclerosing skeletal dysplasias. The International Nomenclature of Constitutional Disorders of Bone divides these conditions into four groups:

1 increased bone density without modification of bone shape;

2 increased bone density with diaphyseal involvement;

3 increased bone density with metaphyseal involvement;

4 neonatal severe osteosclerotic disorders.

There is an underlying disturbance of bone metabolism and many of these conditions have a progressive natural history. They are rare, and expert radiological advice is extremely important. As this is such a diverse group of conditions, the radiological findings need to be interpreted along with the clinical and biochemical data.

Sclerosis refers to a generalized disturbance with increased bone density. Hyperostosis refers to an overgrowth process localized to a part of the bone. In osteopetrosis, the bone cortex and the cancellous bone cannot be differentiated radiologically.

Clinical approach

History: key points

- Three-generation family history with enquiry about consanguinity and affected relatives.
- Age of onset of symptoms and signs.
- Progression of symptoms and signs.
- Ethnic group (van Buchem disease in Holland, sclerosteosis in Afrikaaners).
- Muscle weakness (Cammurati–Engelmann syndrome)
- Visual and hearing problems, headaches (cranial nerve compression).
- Osteomyelitis of the mandible (osteopetrosis).
- Developmental delay.

Examination: key points

- Height (reduced in pyknodysostosis, increased in sclerosteosis).
- Head circumference (increased in many of these conditions).
- Bony overgrowth of the nasal bridge, forehead, and upper face (craniometaphyseal dysplasia, craniodiaphyseal dysplasia, and frontometaphyseal dysplasia).
- Overgrowth of the mandible (infantile cortical hyperostosis; in adults van Buchem disease, sclerosteosis, and Worth type dominant endosteal hyperostosis).
- Prominent eyes and large fontanelle (Melnick–Needles syndrome and pyknodysostosis).
- Teeth. Eruption or retention of primary dentition.
- Choanal stenosis.
- Cranial nerves for evidence of compression.
- Fundal examination for papilloedema.
- Digits for contractures and expansion.
- Limb and joint abnormalities due to bone expansion and modelling anomalies.
- Secondary sexual development (pituitary compression).
- Hepatosplenomegaly (autosomal recessive (AR) osteopetrosis due to extramedullary haematopoiesis).

- Non-skeletal anomalies in rare syndromes, e.g. Raine, Schinzel–Giedion, Lenz–Makewski, oculodentodigital syndrome.
- Torus palatinus. High bone mass phenotype families with activating mutations of *LRP5*.

Special investigations

- Bone biochemistry will often be normal but the following may help with classification:
  - alkaline phosphatase, increased in Van Buchem disease but not in Worth endosteal hyperostosis;
  - acid phosphatase increased in autosomal dominant (AD) osteopetrosis.
- Blood count (anaemia and bone marrow failure due to loss of bone marrow).
- Urinalysis, renal function (AR type of osteopetrosis due to carbonic anhydrase deficiency).
- Visual assessment (optic atrophy, papilloedema, squints).
- Hearing tests.
- Consider endocrine investigations.
- Exclude raised intracranial pressure due to medullary compression.
- Genetic analysis (see below).

Some diagnoses to consider

The age of onset, severity of the condition, and the presence of non-skeletal features should all be considered.

From the neonatal period–2 years

Severe precocious AR osteopetrosis is rapidly progressive with bone marrow failure with distinctive clinical and skeletal features. Infants may present with macrocephaly, hepatosplenomegaly, and visual inattention. It is a heterogeneous disorder and homozygous/compound heterozygous mutations have been described in the chloride channel gene *CLCN7* and also the gene *TCIRG1*. An intermediate type osteopetrosis has been described with a mutation in *CLCN7*.

Carbonic anhydrase type. AR, gene *CA2*.

Pycnodysostosis. AR, gene *CTSK*, cathepsin K. Large fontanelles, facial dysmorphic features, and short limbs.

Severe craniometaphyseal dysplasia. AR. There is progressive bony overgrowth of the nasal bridge and forehead.

Craniodiaphyseal dysplasia. Inheritance uncertain, probably AR. Non-skeletal features include raised intracranial pressure and developmental delay.

Rare osteosclerotic conditions. Conditions in which the other non-skeletal features will aid the diagnosis.

- **Blomstrand dysplasia.** AR. Advanced skeletal maturation. Inactivating mutations in *PTHR1* gene.
- **Raine syndrome.** AR intracranial calcification. Choanal stenosis, cleft palate, usually lethal.
- **Schinzel–Giedion syndrome.** AR. Wide open fontanelle, midface hypoplasia, choanal stenosis, hydronephrosis, genital anomalies. May be a milder form of Raine syndrome.
- **Lenz–Majewski syndrome.** Wide cranial sutures, loose skin, choanal stenosis, developmental delay.
- **Severe Melnick–Needles syndrome.** Skull base sclerosis; features overlap with oto-palato-digital (OPD)

syndrome. Caused by gain-of-function mutations in the gene encoding filamin A (*FLNA*) on Xq28 (Robertson). X-linked dominant (XLD). Most cases occur in females; usually lethal in males.

- **Otopalatodigital (OPD) syndrome.** XL. Skull base sclerosis is seen. Allelic conditions due to gain-of-function mutation in *FLNA* on Xq28.

2–12 years

Craniometaphyseal dysplasia. AR and AD forms. Cranial nerve compression occurs as the child grows older with optic atrophy and facial nerve palsy. The AD form is caused by mutations in the *ANKH* gene.

Frontometaphyseal dysplasia. XL. Enlarged foramen magnum and cervical vertebral abnormalities. Features overlap with type 1 OPD and it has also been shown to be due to *FLNA* mutation.

Engelmann or Camurati–Engelmann syndrome. AD, *TGFB1* gene. Diaphyseal dysplasia, muscular weakness, anaemia.

Pyle dysplasia. AR. Metaphyseal dysplasia distinguished from craniometaphyseal dysplasia by mild involvement of the skull.

Sclerosteosis. AR, *SOST* gene. Endosteal hyperostosis, Afrikaaner population.

Juvenile Paget Disease and Idiopathic Hyperphosphatasia. The condition is characterised by rapidly remodelling woven bone, osteopenia, fractures, progressive long bone deformities, vertebral collapse, skull enlargement and deafness. It follows AR inheritance and is caused by variable expression of mutations in the *TNFRSF11B* gene encoding osteoprotogerin. AR. Bowing, hyperostosis but osteoporosis.

Osteopathia striata. AD. Cranial stenosis; usually female.

Dysosteosclerosis. AR, XL. Short stature; may fracture.

Osteopetrosis. Mild AD type; see below for details.

Kenny–Caffey syndrome. Probably most are AD, also AR; hypocalcaemia and hypophosphataemia.

Melnick–Needles syndrome. Skull base sclerosis; features overlap with those of OPD. Caused by gain-of-function mutations in the gene encoding filamin A (*FLNA*; Robertson *et al.* 2003). XLD. Most cases occur in females; usually lethal in males.

12 years–adult

Camurati–Engelmann syndrome. See above.

Pyle dysplasia. See above.

Van Buchem disease. AR. Elevated alkaline phosphatase; slowly progressive enlargement of the mandible and other cranial bones.

Endosteal hyperostosis, Worth type. AD. Usually no cranial nerve compression.

Osteopetrosis. Mild AD type. There is elevation of serum acid phosphatase. In type 1 mutations have been found in *LRP5* and in type II they have been found in *CLCN7*.

Otopalatodigital syndrome (OPD). XL. Skull base sclerosis is seen. Allelic conditions due to gain-of-function mutations in *FLNA* on Xq28. OPD is allelic in frontometaphyseal dysplasia and Melnick Needles Syndrome.

Genetic advice

These conditions are rare and genetic mutation analysis may only be available on a research basis.

A number of different conditions and phenotypes with increased bone density have been associated with mutation in the low-density lipoprotein (LDL) receptor protein 5 (*LRP5*). Please see Van Westenbeeck *et al.* (2003) for additional information.

Recurrence or offspring risk

As appropriate for each diagnosis.

Carrier detection

- Possible in families in whom causative mutations have been identified in the proband.
- Clinical and radiological examination may be informative in the XL and AD conditions.

Prenatal diagnosis

- By mutation analysis if a causative mutation has been identified in the proband.
- Ultrasound may detect increased bone density and other skeletal features, but usually not until the second or third trimester. Please check the literature carefully relating to the specific condition prior to counselling.

Support group: Many of the syndromes have their own support groups. See <www.cafamily.org.uk>.

Expert advisers: Roger Smith, Honorary Metabolic Bone Physician, Nuffield Orthopaedic Centre, Oxford and Nick Bishop, Professor of Paediatric Bone Disease, University of Sheffield, Sheffield, England.

References

International Skeletal Dysplasia Registry. Nomenclature and genetic information. <www.csmc.edu/genetics/skeldys>.

Janssens K, Van Hul W. Molecular medicine of too much bone. *Hum Mol Genet* 2002; **11**: 2385–93.

Nurnberg P, Thiele H, *et al.* Heterozygous mutations in ANKH, the human ortholog of the mouse progressive ankylosis gene, result in craniometaphyseal dysplasia. *Nat Genet* 2001; **28** (1): 37–41.

Robertson SA, *et al.* Localised mutations in the gene encoding cytoskeletal protein filamin A can cause diverse malformations in humans. *Nat Genet* 2003; **33**: 487–91.

Teitelbaum SL, Ross FP. Genetic regulation of osteoclast development and function (Review). *Nat Rev Genet.* 2003; **4**: 638–49.

Van Westenbeeck L, *et al.* Six novel missense mutations in the LDL receptor related protein 5 (LRP5) gene in different conditions with increased bone density. *Am J Med Genet* 2003; **72**: 763–71.

Whyte P. Osteopetrosis. In *Connective tissue and its heritable disorders*, 2nd edn (ed. P.M. Royce and B. Steinmann), pp. 789–807. Wiley-Liss, New York, 2002.

Large fontanelle

The fontanelles are the spaces in the immature and incompletely ossified skulls of babies and infants that permit brain growth. They lie in the sutures between the bones of the skull. The bones of the skull base and vault are known as the neurocranium. There are intricate processes that control the pre- and postnatal growth of the neurocranium and coordinate it to brain growth.

At birth the anterior fontanelle should always be patent and is known as a constant fontanelle. Those not always present are known as accessory fontanelles. Charts are available showing age-related sizes for the anterior and posterior fontanelles (see figure; Hall *et al.* 1989). The anterior fontanelle normally closes at 12 ± 4 months. The posterior fontanelle normally closes at birth ±2 months.

Very delayed and/or deficient ossification of the skull leads to cranium bifidum and parietal foramina. Parietal foramina have also been called Caitlin marks after the name of an affected family. They are defects in the parietal bone found on each side of the sagittal suture.

The first diagnostic step is to exclude raised intracranial pressure and hydrocephalus. Paediatric conditions to exclude are hypothyroidism and congenital infections. The geneticist is usually called once structural brain lesions have been excluded and this chapter concentrates on:

- syndromic causes of fontanelle enlargement due to abnormalities of the neurocranium;
- genetic and chromosomal disorders that characteristically have enlarged fontanelles.

A mildly enlarged fontanelle with no other craniofacial features is not a good diagnostic handle, but the cause of gross enlargement is usually found.

Clinical approach

History: key points

- Three-generation family tree with specific enquiry about consanguinity (pyknodysostosis, autosomal recessive (AR) Robinow) and other affected family members (cleidocranial dysplasia, parietal foramina).
- Pregnancy. Congenital infection, aminopterin or angiotensin-converting enzyme (ACE) inhibitor exposure.
- Occipital-frontal circumference (OFC) at birth (hydrocephalus).
- Neonatal screening, to exclude hypothyroidism.
- Developmental delay (chromosomal abnormalities, hypothyroidism, congenital infections).

Examination: key points

- Measurement of the OFC and fontanelles.
- Palpation of the cranial sutures; assess if open or closed. Remember to feel over the metopic region and on either side of the midline back to the occiput for parietal foramina.
- Scalp defects.
- Asymmetry of the cranium and face.
- Orofacial clefts can delay midline suture closure.
- Spina bifida (hydrocephalus).
- In floppy neonates look for dysmorphic features of Down and Zellweger syndromes and monosomy 1p36.
- Height, span, and limbs (skeletal dysplasias).
- Clavicles (cleidocranial dysplasia).
- Hands and feet (in Apert and Pfeiffer syndromes the metopic and sagittal sutures remain patent to allow the brain to grow).

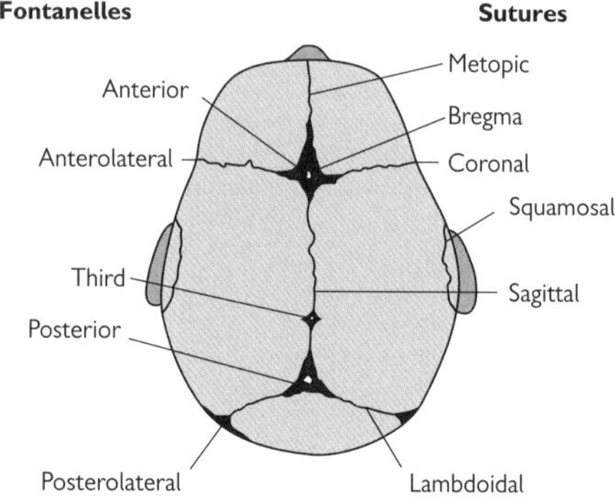

- Bony exostoses (proximal 11p deletion syndrome).
- Features of a chronic medical or metabolic condition (organomegaly, failure to thrive, developmental delay).

Special investigations
- Radiology:
  - skull X-rays;
  - consider full skeletal survey;
  - a delayed bone age may be an indicator of a generalized condition delaying skull maturation.
- In conjunction with a craniofacial team the following are often performed:
  - brain imaging;
  - computerized tomographic (CT) reconstruction of the skull bones;
  - exclusion of raised intracranial pressure.
- Cytogenetics:
  - routine analysis;
  - fluorescent *in situ* hybridization (FISH) 11p11.2 and 7p21 (*TWIST* duplication) and a careful check of 5q34–35 (contains gene *MSX2* but no visible cytogenetic deletions of this area have been found).
- Molecular genetics. Specific genetic testing or DNA storage for future analysis.
- Very long chain fatty acids (VLCFAs; Zellweger syndrome).

Check that medical conditions such as hypothyroidism and congenital infections have been excluded.

Some diagnoses to consider

Craniosynostosis, epecially Saethre–Chotzen syndrome, may be associated with parietal foramina. Do not confuse with multiple craniolacunae related to dysplastic skull vault.

Cleidocranial dysostosis. Autosomal dominant (AD) caused by mutations in *CBFA1*. In some families there is severely delayed skull ossification with a cranium bifidum. Careful examination of relatives is required. In addition to the widely patent anterior fontanelle, the clavicles are either absent or severely hypoplastic and there is delayed eruption of the dentition with dental enamel abnormalities. Skull X-ray may show wormian bones, and chest X-ray displays the hypoplastic or absent clavicles.

Pycnodysostosis. Autosomal recessive (AR) condition caused by mutations in the gene cathepsin K (*CTSK*). Large fontanelles, increased bone density, facial dysmorphic features, and short limbs.

AR Robinow syndrome. Caused by mutations in *ROR2* and characterized by a prominent forehead, large fontanelle, hypertelorism, a wide mouth, and a small nose with anteverted nostrils. There may be a cleft lip/palate and significant gum hypertrophy. Some affected individuals have congenital heart disease. There is mesomelic shortening of the limbs.

Hypophosphatasia. There are two forms, one presenting *in utero* or in infancy that is usually lethal, and the other presenting in childhood or adulthood. Both have reduced chondro-osseous mineralization with undermineralization of the skull and low levels of alkaline phosphatase in blood.

Mutations in *TNSALP* on 1p36.1 are found in both severe and mild cases. The severe form is AR.

Zellweger syndrome. An AR peroxisomal disorder often presenting in the neonatal period with central hypotonia ± seizures. The fontanelle is large and the forehead high. There may be stippled epiphyses (especially knees). VLCFAs are elevated. See 'Floppy infant', page 118.

Parietal foramina syndrome. AD with variable penetrance due to haploinsufficiency of *MSX2*. Parental skull X-rays are helpful in evaluating possible mutation carriers.

Proximal 11p deletion syndrome. Parietal foramina associated with exostoses, developmental delay, and mildly dysmorphic facial features may occur as part of a microdeletion syndrome at 11p11.2 that incorporates haploinsufficiency of *ALX4*. Parental karyotypes necessary.

Vascular malformations. Vascular malformations of the brain have been associated with scalp defects and parietal foramina as well as brain malformation.

Other rare syndromes. Skull ossification defects are a good handle for some rare syndromes including Schinzel phocomelia, ASSA (aminopterin syndrome sine amniopterin) or 'pseudoaminopterin' syndrome, and renal tubular dysgenesis.

Genetic advice

This is dependent on the diagnosis, but the following points may be useful for counselling.

Recurrence risk and carrier detection

It is important to consider the possibility that other family members may be affected in all the AD conditions described above. Examine parents and siblings and ask whether they were known to have any soft areas in the skull as a child. Radiology may help to detect parietal foramina or other skeletal features.

Prenatal diagnosis

May be requested by families at risk of the conditions with mental retardation where molecular, cytogenetic, or molecular genetic testing is available.

Natural history and further management (preventative measures)

The fontanelles usually close during childhood. Parents are concerned about the risk of trauma and advice from a craniofacial surgeon is reassuring. Surgical intervention is usually contraindicated.

Support group contact: Headlines Craniofacial support <info@headlines.org.uk>.

Expert adviser: A.O.M. Wilkie, Nuffield Professor of Pathology and Honorary Consultant in Clinical Genetics, Churchill Hospital, Oxford, England.

References

Hall JG, Froster-Iskenius I, Allanson J. *Handbook of normal physical measurements*. Oxford University Press, Oxford, 1989.

Mavrogiannis LA, *et al*. Haploinsufficiency of the human homeobox gene *ALX4* causes skull ossification defects. *Nat Genet* 2001; **27**: 17–18.

Wilkie AOM, *et al*. Functional haploinsufficiency of the human homeobox gene MSX2 causes defects in skull ossification. *Nat Genet* 2000; **24**: 387–90.

Laterality disorders including heterotaxy and isomerism

The left–right (L–R) axis of the embryo is defined as soon as the rostrocaudal and dorsoventral axes are established. Curvature of the heart loop to the right is the first morphological sign of asymmetry in embryogenesis.

- **Terminology:**
  - **situs solitus.** The usual L–R body plan with the heart, spleen, and stomach on the left and the liver and gall bladder on the right;
  - **situs inversus.** Approximately 1/10 000 individuals have a mirror image arrangement of the L–R body plan, with the heart, spleen, and stomach on the right and the liver and gall-bladder on the left. There is an increased incidence of congenital heart disease (3–9%) compared with 0.6% in situs solitus;
  - **situs ambiguus/visceral heterotaxy.** Discordance between situs of asymmetric organs often accompanied by complex cardiovascular malformation;
  - **R isomerism sequence. Asplenia syndrome, Ivemark syndrome, right atrial isomerism.** Right isomerism sequence is the consequence of bilateral right sided signalling pathways in early development which invariably leads to complex congenital heart disease. There are two morphogically right atria, often with a single ventricle, atrioventricular septal defect (AVSD), and transposition of the great arteries (TGA) and anomalous pulmonary venous drainage. The spleen is absent and there may be abnormal folding of the intestines that may present as intestinal obstruction.
  - **L isomerism sequence. (Polysplenia syndrome)** Left isomerism sequence is the consequence of bilateral left sided signalling pathways in early development. Absence of the sinoatrial (SA) node may cause complete heart block. There are two morphologically left atria. There may be an atrial septal defect (ASD) or AVSD, but usually the heart defects are not as severe as in R isomerism sequence. Multiple small spleens may be found and there may be abnormal folding of the intestines, which may present as intestinal obstruction.

Isomerism sequence (see table) accounts for ~1% of congenital heart disease and occurs with an incidence of ~1/24 000. In humans relatively few genes have been associated with a small percentage of human situs defects. These include: *ZIC3, LEFTB, ACVR2B* (activin binding receptor2), and *CFC1* encoding the cryptic protein.

Twins. There are several reports of R isomerism in the right twin of conjoined twin pairs. There is evidence for a left lead in determination of the L–R gradient. In conjoined twin pairs, separation of the right side of the early embryo from the left results in the left half producing an embryo with normal situs, while the right half, having lost its point of reference, is at risk of a major disturbance of laterality, with R isomerism sequence as its most extreme manifestation (Burn 1991).

Clinical approach

History: key points

- Detailed three-generation family tree with specific enquiry for consanguinity and congenital heart disease.
- Enquire for maternal diabetes. (In Splitt *et al.*'s (1999) study, 50% of cases of L isomerism occurred in infants of diabetic mothers).

Examination: key points

Careful cardiovascular assessment.

Special investigations

- Echocardiogram to define cardiac anatomy.
- Ultrasound (USS) scan to define position of liver and presence/absence of spleen.
- DNA to store or, if the family tree is suggestive of X-linked inheritance, for ZIC3 mutation analysis.

Some diagnoses to consider

Kartagener's syndrome. Primary ciliary dyskinesia with situs inversus, nasal polyps, and bronchiectasis. A genetically heterogeneous autosomal recessive (AR) disorder. All affected individuals have ciliary dyskinesia and half of affected individuals have situs inversus.

X-linked laterality sequence. A rare X-linked condition in which laterality disturbance may be combined with sacral agenesis or neural tube defects caused by mutations in *ZIC3* on Xq28.

Genetic advice

Recurrence risk

Overall, an empiric 5–10% sibling recurrence risk is given where no specific diagnosis is possible (if there is no family history and no consanguinity). If there is consanguinity, a sibling recurrence risk of 25% may be appropriate.

Prenatal diagnosis

Fetal echocardiography can be used for antenatal diagnosis of most laterality disorders with scans at 14, 19, and 22 weeks gestation.

Natural history and further management (preventative measures)

If the spleen is absent, prophylactic penicillin should be prescribed.

Support group: Children's Heart Federation <www.childrens-heart-fed.org.uk.>.

Heart defects in patients with isomerism sequence (after Burn and Goodship 2001)

Principal heart defect* (%)	Left isomerism (%)	Right isomerism (%)
Interruption of IVC with azygos continuation	75	7
TAPVD	0	35
Common atrium	47	67
Single ventricle	30	70
AVSD	68	93
DORV	7	47
Pulmonary stenosis/atresia	48	78

* IVC, Inferior vena cava; TAPVD, total anomalous pulmonary venous drainage; AVSD, atrioventricular septal defect; DORV, double-outlet right ventricle.

Expert advisers: Judith Goodship, Professor of Medical Genetics, University of Newcastle, Newcastle-upon-Tyne and Miranda P. Splitt, Consultant in Clinical Genetics, Northern genetics service, Newcastle-upon-Type, England.

References

Bamford RN, Roessler E, *et al.* Loss-of-function mutations in the EGF-CFC gene CFC1 are associated with human left–right laterality defects. *Nat Genet* 2000; **26**: 501.

Burn J. Disturbance of morphological laterality in humans. In *Biological asymmetry and handedness* (ed. G.R. Bock and J. Marsh), pp. 282–99. Wiley, Chichester, 1991.

Burn J, Goodship J. Congenital heart disease. In *Emery and Rimoin's principles and practice of medical genetics*, 4th edn (ed. D. Rimoin), pp. 1239–326. Churchill Livingstone, Edinburgh, 2001.

Gebbia M, Ferrara GB, *et al.* X-linked situs abnormalities result from mutations in *ZIC3*. *Nat Genet* 1997; **17**: 305–9.

Splitt M, Wright C, *et al.* Left-isomerism sequence and maternal type-1 diabetes. *Lancet* 1999; **354**: 305–6.

Leukodystrophy/leukoencephalopathy

A leukodystrophy is a genetic condition affecting mainly the white matter of the brain. The term leukoencephalopathy is used to reflect the broader number of diseases that may cause either primary or secondary changes in myelin development. All leukodystrophies (by definition) have an underlying genetic or metabolic basis and a thorough metabolic work-up is mandatory. Other causes of white matter disease have an environmental basis such as asphyxia and congenital infection (particularly cytomegalovirus (CMV)). Magnetic resonance imaging (MRI) brain scanning is an essential part of the diagnostic process and the pattern of white matter abnormality seen on MRI can be used to target further testing.

The clinical geneticist may be asked to see an affected child after the diagnosis has been established to offer counseling, prenatal diagnosis, and carrier detection.

In about 50% of children with white matter disease, a precise aetiology is not found. Many of these children are seen by a geneticist for a diagnostic opinion and to determine genetic risks.

Clinical approach

History: key points

- Family history of a previous affected child.
- Parental consanguinity.
- Ethnicity, e.g. Canavan disease in Ashkenazi Jews.
- Pregnancy and labour (congenital infections, perinatal or prenatal birth asphyxia).
- Birthweight and occipital-frontal circumference (OFC).
- Early developmental milestones. How long did the period of normal development last? This can help with the differential diagnosis.
- Regression/loss of skills/dementia, e.g. deteriorating school performance.
- Seizures.
- Psychiatric disturbance.
- Vision and hearing loss.
- Motor abnormalities: weakness, incoordination.

Examination: key points

- Macrocephaly (Canavan disease, Alexander disease).
- Peripheral nerve involvement (metachromatic leukodystrophy, infantile Krabbe disease).
- Eyes (rotatory eye movements in Pelizaeus–Merzbacher disease (PMD), macular cherry red spots, visual loss).
- Gait abnormalities.
- Dysarthria, dystonia, ataxia.
- Hypotonia early in disease can progress to spasticity later.
- Increased skin pigmentation due to adrenal insufficiency in X-linked adrenoleukodystrophy (X-ALD).
- Cognitive/developmental assessment.

Special investigations

Initial investigations.

- Brain imaging, preferably MRI. Pattern of white matter disturbance gives diagnostic information.
- Urine mucopolysaccharide and oligosaccharide screen, amino and organic acids.
- Plasma lactate, ammonium, amino acids, vacuolated lymphocytes.

- Electrophysiology. Visual evoked potentials (VEPs), auditory evoked potentials, nerve conduction test, electromyography (EMG).
- Consider skeletal X-rays to look for evidence of dysostosis caused by abnormal metabolites.
- Store DNA.

Secondary investigations (depending on above results and clinical presentation).

- White cell enyme assay.
- Peroxisomal analysis, very long chain fatty acids (VLCFAs; X-ALD).
- Adrenal hormone analysis if X-ALD suspected.
- Mitochondrial disorders (more grey than white matter involvement, multiorgan involvement).
- Cerebrospinal (CSF) protein raised in metachromatic leukodystrophy (MLD); interferon alpha raised in Aicardi–Goutieres disease.
- DNA for specific genetic testing.

Some diagnoses to consider

With macrocephaly

Canavan disease. Canavan disease is a rare autosomal recessive (AR) condition that presents in the first year of life with hypotonia, which changes to spasticity, macrocephaly, head lag, and progressive severe mental retardation. There is an excess of N-acetylaspartate in CSF, blood, and urine, and it is caused by mutations in the aspartoacetylase gene (*ASPA*). Canavan disease occurs worldwide, but is most prevalent in the Ashkenazi Jewish population, where the E285A mutation accounts for 80–85% of mutant alleles.

Alexander disease. In infants and young children, it causes developmental delay, psychomotor retardation, paraparesis, feeding problems, usually megalencephaly, often seizures, and sometimes hydrocephalus. The diagnosis was previously made at post mortem by the identification of Rosenthal fibres in the brain. It has now been shown to be due to *de novo* heterozygous mutations in the *GFAP* gene (glial fibrillary acidic protein). Recurrence has been reported in sibs, which may be due to germline mosaicism; therefore prenatal diagnosis has been recommended even when the child has a *de novo* mutation.

AR lysosomal disorders

Metachromatic leukodystrophy. Arylsulphatase A deficiency with accumulation of the myelin lipid called sulfatide in the brain and peripheral nerves. Juvenile and adult onset forms.

Late onset types of GM1 gangliosidosis (β-galactosidase-1 deficiency). The typical presentation of GM1 is soon after birth with coarse facial features, feeding difficulties, failure to thrive. Dysostosis is striking. Later-onset GM1 may present as an ataxia with leukodystrophy.

GM2 gangliosidoses. Tay–Sachs disease, Sandhoff disease, and variants are AR disorders caused by mutations in the genes encoding the α-subunit of the lysosomal enzymes hexosaminidase A (*HEXA*) and the β-subunit (*HEXB*), respectively. These lead to the accumulation of GM2 ganglioside in neurons. In both disorders, a virtually identical course of neurodegeneration begins in infancy and leads to demise generally by 4–6 years of age. Typically, infants show developmental regression, increased startle to sound, and a cherry-red spot is visible in the macula. The carrier frequency in Ashkenazim is 1/30.

In males

X-linked adrenoleukodystrophy (X-ALD). Due to mutations in the *ALDP* gene. Late-onset disease is called adrenomyeloneuropathy (AMN) and carrier females may also develop AMN in middle-age. Even within the same family there may be extreme variation in the clinical presentation though biochemical testing will detect those at risk. See 'X-linked adrenoleukodystrophy (X-ALD)', page 264.

Pelizaeus–Merzbacher disease (PMD). An X-linked recessive condition due to duplication or mutation in the *PLP1* gene that codes for proteolipid protein. Fluorescent *in situ* hybridization (FISH)-based test for the duplication available. The MRI scan shows very delayed, or even absent, myelination.

With basal ganglia calcification

Krabbe disease. Krabbe disease or globoid cell leukodystrophy is an AR disorder involving the white matter of the peripheral and central nervous systems. Mutations in the gene for the lysosomal enzyme galactocerebrosidase (*GALC*) result in low enzymatic activity and decreased ability to degrade galactolipids found almost exclusively in myelin. While most patients present with symptoms within the first 6 months of life, others present later in life including adulthood. Infantile Krabbe disease can present with dystonia (lead-pipe rigidity of the limbs and abnormal posturing) together with irritability, poor feeding, motor regression, and seizures. The MRI may show white matter changes and calcification particularly affecting the basal ganglia.

Aicardi–Goutieres syndrome. AR disorder with onset in the first 4 months of life. The main clinical symptoms are pyramidal and extrapyramidal symptoms, psychomotor delay, microcephaly, and neuroradiological features (basal ganglia calcification, atrophy, white matter alterations). There is a CSF lymphocytosis and a raised CSF level of interferon alpha. The clinical picture may mimic a congenital infection. Chilblain-like lesions are a feature.

With ataxia

Childhood ataxia with central hypomyelination (CACH) / Vanishing white matter disease (VWM). Recently described leukoencephalopathy with vanishing white matter. It is caused by recessive mutations in genes encoding the 5 eucaryotic initiation factor 2B subunits ($\alpha,\beta,\gamma,\delta,\epsilon$). A wide clinical spectrum is observed from rapidly fatal infantile to asymptomatic adult forms (Fogli). Disease severity is correlated strongly with age of onset. eIF2B is involved in the regulation of protein synthesis during cellular stress.

Genetic advice, known diagnosis

Recurrence risk
Counsel as appropriate.

Carrier detection
Within a family, carrier testing by genetic testing is possible when there is a known mutation. Screening of the partners of known carriers may present problems except in populations where there are common mutations.

Enzyme testing within families can often detect carriers but is rarely discriminatory enough to use for partners of carriers.

Prenatal diagnosis
Chorionic villus sampling (CVS) and amniocentesis measuring enzyme levels or mutation analysis. Please check with your laboratory to ensure that the correct samples are taken.

Genetic advice, undiagnosed leukodystrophy
The recognition of characteristic MRI abnormalities has led to an increasing number of newly recognized conditions, such as megalencephalic leukoencephalopathy with subcortical cysts and 'vanishing white matter' disease. Therefore, a recent and expert opinion on the MRI is important. If, despite this, there is no known cause, counselling is given on the basis of the probability that the condition is genetic.

Recurrence risk
1 If there is parental consanguinity, an AR aetiology is probable and recurrence risks are likely to be 25%.
2 If there is a history of a previous affected sibling then recurrence risks are likely to be 25%. AR inheritance is more likely than X-linked or germline mosaicism.
3 If neither of the above apply, then consider the possibility of environmental factors, or non-recurring genetic conditions such as *de novo* mutations, but counsel that the risk may be as high as 25%.

Carrier detection
Not available, other than a pedigree-based risk.

Prenatal diagnosis
Not possible.

Natural history and further management (preventative measures)
These conditions are progressive and in the undiagnosed group the progression over a period of review may give guidance. Review may bring about a diagnosis based on the features or after repeat testing, e.g MRI, or by recent delineation of a phenotype.

Support group: CLIMB (Children Living with Inherited Metabolic Diseases) <www.climb.org.uk>, Tel. 0870 770 0326; and <www.cafamily.org.uk>.

Expert adviser: Robert Surtees, Professor of Paediatric Neurology, Institute of Child Health, London, England.

References

Fogli A, Schiffmann R, *et al.* The effect of genotype on the natural history of eIF2B-related leukodystrophy. *Neurology* 2004; **62**: 1509–17.

Johnson AB, Brenner M. Alexander's disease: clinical, pathologic, and genetic features. *J Child Neurol* 2003; **18**: 625–32.

Kaye EM. Update on genetic disorders affecting white matter. *Pediatr Neurol* 2001; **24**: 11–24.

Leegwater PA, Pronk JC, van der Knaap MS. Leukoencephalopathy with vanishing white matter: from magnetic resonance imaging pattern to five genes. *J Child Neurol* 2003; **18**: 639–45.

Myerowitz R, Lawson D, *et al.* Molecular pathophysiology in Tay–Sachs and Sandhoff diseases as revealed by gene expression profiling. *Hum Mol Genet* 2002; **11**: 1343–50.

Schiffmann R, Boespflug-Tanguy O. An update on the leukodsytrophies. *Curr Opin Neurol* 2001; **14**: 789–94.

Surendran S, Matalon KM, *et al.* Molecular basis of Canavan's disease: from human to mouse. *J Child Neurol* 2003; **18**: 604–10.

Schiffmann R, van der Knaap MS. The latest on leukodystrophies. *Curr Opinion Neurol* 2004; **17**: 187–92.

Limb reduction defects

See also 'Radial ray and thumb hypoplasia', page 228. Congenital limb reduction defects are more common at the extremes of maternal age, but the age association is not a strong one. Matsunaga and Shiota (1979) found that the prevalence of limb reduction defects was 15 times greater where there was a history of first trimester bleeding. Most major malformations are more common in multiple births than singletons. One small study reported a prevalence of limb anomalies as 1/252 twins (40/10 000) and 2/287 triplets (60/10 000). Possible mechanisms include amniotic bands, inequalities of blood supply in monozygotic (MZ) twins, vascular disruption from a deceased co-twin. Malformations such as sirenomelia (fusion of the lower extremities) are increased in MZ twins (risk 100–150 times greater than for singletons). The table outlines the stages in human limb development.

The fact that different aetiologies can cause a similar result makes the analysis of limb defects particularly challenging, e.g. *TBX5* mutations in Holt–Oram syndrome and thalidomide exposure can cause limb and cardiac defects that are clinically indistinguishable.

Overall, the minimum prevalence of limb reduction defects is ~5.6/10 000 livebirths (higher rates in miscarriages, intrauterine deaths (IUDs), and stillbirths (SBs)). About half of the defects are transverse. There are many ways of classifying limb defects (see table).

Teratogens. Limb abnormalities are one of the most common and visible phenotypic effects of several human teratogens. The specific effects are different for most teratogens and include effects on limb morphogenesis (thalidomide, warfarin, phenytoin, valproic acid) and the effect of vascular disruption on a limb that had formed normally (misoprostol, chorionic villus sampling (CVS), and phenytoin). Procedures during pregnancy, including CVS and dilatation and curettage (D & C), produce defects of vascular disruption (Holmes 2003).

Clinical approach

History: key points

- Three-generation family tree with detailed enquiry regarding limb defects, congenital heart disease, deafness, or eye problems, e.g. squint/Duane (Okihiro), thalassaemia.
- Is there a history of maternal diabetes?
- Detailed history of pregnancy from 5–11 weeks gestation:
  - vaginal bleeding;
  - drug exposure, e.g. misoprostol, vitamin A or other retinoids, cocaine;
  - twinning;
  - trauma, e.g. road traffic accident (RTA);
  - invasive procedures, e.g. CVS, D & C.
- Were fibrous bands attached to the affected limb(s) noted at delivery; did the placenta and membranes show amniotic bands?

Examination: key points

- Examine all four limbs. If the defect appears to be limited to a single limb, make certain that the other three limbs are truly normal (is there nail hypoplasia?). Defects are best documented with photos, supplemented with a sketch and written description.
- Examine the limbs for constriction bands.
- Examine the scalp for scalp defects (Adams–Oliver syndrome).
- Examine the tongue and mandible (oromandibular–limb–hypogenesis (OMLH) syndrome).

Outline of stages in human limb development (after Brown et al. 1996)

Days from fertilisation	Gestation	Upper limb	Lower limb
27 days	5 weeks, 6days	Arm buds begin to appear	
28–30 days	6 weeks–6 weeks, 2days	Well-developed arm bud	Lower limb bud appears
34–36 days	6 weeks, 6 days–7 weeks, 1 day	Elongated arm bud	
34–38 days	6 weeks, 6 days–7 weeks 3 days	Hand paddle formed	
38–40 days	7 weeks, 3days–7 weeks, 5 days	Fingers begin to separate	
41–43 days	7 weeks, 6 days–8 weeks, 1 day	Fingers distinct	
44–46 days	8 weeks, 2 days–8 weeks, 4 days	Fingers separated	Toes distinguishable
52–53 days	9 weeks, 3 days–9 weeks, 4 days	Fingers fully separated	
54–55 days	9 weeks, 5 days–9 weeks, 6 days		Toes fully separated

Eurocat classification of congenital limb defects (after Stoll et al. 1988)

Terminal transverse defects* Absence of distal structures of the limb with proximal structures more or less normal, e.g. absent hand. May vary from absence of a nail or distal phalange or finger through to absence of a whole limb

Proximal intercalary defect Absence or severe hypoplasia of proximal intercalary parts of the limb when the distal structures (i.e. the digits), whether normal or malformed, are present, e.g. radial aplasia with intact thumb, femoral hypoplasia

Longitudinal absence or severe hypoplasia of lateral part of the limb e.g. Radial aplasia with absent thumb, or ulnar aplasia with absent 5th finger

Split hand/foot Absence of central digits with or without absence of central metacarpal/metatarsal bones usually associated with syndactyly of other digits (e.g. ectrodactyly–ectodermal dysplasia–clefting (EEC) syndrome)

Multiple types of reduction defect Infants with more than one type of reduction according to the classification given above

* Not infrequently some soft tissue nubbins (rudimentary digits) are seen at the end of a proximal transverse limb defect. Only if there are significant skeletal elements present should this lead to classification as an intercalary defect.

- Examine the eyes and face for VIth or VII cranial nerve palsy (very easily missed in a young baby).
- If there is an upper limb defect, examine the pectoral muscle and chest (Poland anomaly).
- Examine the heart.
- If there is a major limb reduction defect affecting the lower limb(s), examine the anus (anorectal malformation) and male genitalia (e.g. splenogonadal fusion-limb defect).
- Examine the hands and feet of the parents. If there is any suspicion of Holt–Oram syndrome (HOS), examine the parents' hearts as well.

Special investigations
- Radiograph of both upper or both lower limbs including the affected limb (also any other limbs where there is clinical suspicion of abnormality).
- Echocardiogram and ECG. Always indicated in babies and young children. Also indicated in adults if you suspect HOS or another hand–heart syndrome. Note that 15% of children with limb reduction defects have congenital heart disease.
- Karyotype if there are other associated malformations or developmental delay and for chromosome 'puffing' if features of Roberts syndrome.
- DNA if a syndromic diagnosis with a known gene seems likely (e.g. HOS).

Some diagnoses to consider

NB. For many of these syndromes, the limb defect may fit into one of several types.

Terminal transverse defects

Amniotic bands. Early rupture of the amnion may lead to the production of fibrous mesodermal cords that constrict or cleave parts of the fetus, causing disruption of otherwise normal development. Another possible causal mechanism is the modification of fetal blood flow—the bands being a secondary phenomenon. Sometimes amniotic bands can be visualized by ultrasound scan (USS). There may be a clear history that at delivery fibrous cords were wrapped tightly round the affected digit(s). Recurrence risk is very small (<2%).

Adams–Oliver syndrome. Autosomal dominant (AD) characterized by terminal transverse limb defects and scalp defects (cutis aplasa). Small defects underlying the scalp defect are sometimes seen. Most affected individuals have relatively minor limb defects (usually affecting fingers and toes), but considerable variability is seen and occasionally severe limb defects can be present. Serious bleeding from the scalp defects can occur in neonates. Cardiac malformations also form part of the syndrome.

Moebius syndrome. Congenital cranial nerve palsies affecting VI (abduction of the eye) and VII (facial movement) in conjunction with terminal transverse defects and/or Poland anomaly. See 'Facial asymmetry', page 112.

Poland anomaly. There is congenital absence of the sternal head of pectoralis major, often in association with hypoplasia of the breast on the ipsilateral side and sometimes with shortening of phalanges and other elements of the digits in association with cutaneous syndactyly. Poland anomaly is usually sporadic and is thought to have a multifactorial basis involving vascular disruption in early development. Occasional parent–child occurrences are reported (Shalev and Hall 2003).

Oromandibular-limb-hypogenesis (OMLH) syndrome. This group of disorders includes hypoglossia–hypodactyly, splenogonadal fusion–limb defects, and Hanhart syndrome. The clinical expression is variable and the limb abnormalities can vary from absence of digits to absence of the distal part of a whole limb. The jaw is small (micrognathia) and the tongue may also be small. Those who survive usually have normal intelligence. There is a definite association with the Moebius syndrome, in which there are bilateral facial and abducens nerve palsies. Most cases are sporadic and attributed to vascular disruption. OMLH has been reported after exposure to misoprostol in the first trimester of pregnancy and after very early CVS (prior to the tenth week).

Proximal intercalary defect

Thrombocytopenia–absent radius (TAR). TAR syndrome is characterized by bilateral absence of the radii and a thrombocytopenia; the thumbs are present. The lower limbs, gastrointestinal, cardiovascular, and other systems may also be involved. In a survey of 34 cases, Greenhalgh *et al.* (2002) found that all cases had a documented thrombocytopenia and bilateral radial aplasia, 47% had lower limb anomalies, 47% cow's milk intolerance, 23% renal anomalies, and 15% cardiac anomalies. The inheritance is unclear. Autosomal recessive (AR) inheritance is possible but there have been fewer affected siblings than expected and a rarity of consanguinity.

Longitudinal absence or severe hypoplasia of lateral part of the limb

See 'Radial ray defects and thumb hypoplasia', page 228.

Holt–Oram syndrome (HOS). AD heart–hand syndrome caused by mutations in *TBX5*. Penetrance is 100%. *Skeletal defects* affect the upper limbs exclusively and are invariably bilateral and usually asymmetrical. They range from clinodactyly, limited supination, and narrow, sloping shoulders to absent, hypoplastic, or triphalangeal thumb and severe reduction deformities of the upper arm (4.5%). Hypoplasia of the thenar eminence accompanies thumb hypoplasia. The radial ray is predominantly affected and the left side is usually more severely affected than the right. *Cardiac defects* (including minimal ECG changes) occur in 95%. See 'Radial ray defects and thumb hypoplasia', page 228.

VACTERL (vertebral defects – anal atresia – cardiac anomalies – tracheo-oesophageal fistula – (o)esophageal atresia – renal anomalies – limb defects) association. Preaxial limb defects with underdevelopment or agenesis of thumbs and radial bones; usually bilateral defects, but may be asymmetric. Reduced thenar muscle mass is mildest end of spectrum. The lower limbs are not affected. Sporadic with low recurrence risk (2–3%). See 'Anal anomalies (atresia, stenosis)', page 42, for further details.

Okihiro syndrome (Duane radial ray syndrome). This is an AD condition with degrees of radial ray hypoplasia and Duane anomaly. It results from mutation in the *SALL4* gene.

Acrofacial dysostosis with limb defects (Miller syndrome, postaxial acrofacial dysostosis syndrome (POADS)). AR condition characterized by hypoplasia of the 5th ray of all limbs together with malar hypoplasia and micrognathia ± cleft palate.

Ulnar–mammary syndrome. AD with variable penetrance. Ulnar ray defects varying from hypoplasia of the 5th digit to absence of the ulna and ulnar ray (occasionally may have postaxial polydactyly). In addition, females have small/absent breast with hypoplastic nipples and males have small penises and delayed puberty and reduced fertility. Due to mutations in *TBX3* on 12q23.

Split hand/foot

AD ectrodactyly. AD with high penetrance but variable expressivity. Locus on 7q.

Ectrodactyly–ectodermal dysplasia–clefting (EEC) syndrome. AD condition caused by mutations in *p63* on 7q21–22. Cleft lip and/or palate is common. Dry skin with variable hypohidrosis. Sparse fair dry hair often with absent eyebrows and eyelashes. Tear duct anomalies are common. Often have hypodontia. Nails are thin, brittle, and ridged. Mental development is usually normal. The middle rays of the limbs are affected to a variable degree ranging from no obvious defect to absence of the middle three rays.

Multiple types of reduction defect

Cornelia de Lange syndrome. Birth incidence ~1/50 000. The syndrome is characterized by mental retardation, short stature (often with intrauterine growth retardation (IUGR)), limb anomalies, and distinctive craniofacial features (microbrachycephaly with a low anterior and posterior hairline, neat arched eyebrows often with synophyrys, depressed nasal bridge with anteverted nares, long smooth philtrum and thin lips often with downturned corners to the mouth, micrognathia). Cardiac septal defects, hirsutism and feeding problems are common. The limb anomalies range from short forearms with small hands and tapering fingers to severe limb reduction defects with missing fingers, hands, and forearms. More minor hand anomalies include proximally placed thumbs, single palmar creases, and clinodactyly of the 5th finger. Occasionally fusion of two fingers or polydactyly may be seen. Upper limb defects are very much more common than lower limb defects. Most cases are sporadic and a recurrence risk of 1% is usually given. (NB. A milder form of the condition is recognized, which may follow a dominant pattern of inheritance.) A gene for de Lange syndrome was recently identified as *NIPBL* on 5p13.1 (Krantz) and mutations are reported in 47% of affected individuals (Gillis) suggesting possible genetic heterogeneity.

Femur–fibula–ulna complex. A poorly defined condition with a spectrum of abnormalities affecting the ulnar ray, the femur, and the fibular ray. Upper limb anomalies are more common than lower limb anomalies. Overall, sibling recurrence risks seem to be low, but beware of the limitation of diagnostic uncertainty.

Roberts syndrome. AR disorder characterised by craniofacial anomalies, limb reduction defects and loss of cohesion at heterochromatic regions of centromeres (chromosome 'puffing'). Limb defects vary from tetraphocomelia to radial ray defects. Caused by mutations in ESCO2 (Vega). See 'Radial ray defects' page 228.

Genetic advice

Work systematically to try to establish an accurate diagnosis. Ask yourself the following questions.

- How many limbs are affected?
- What is the pattern of the limb defect (according to Stoll *et al.*'s (1988) classification)?
- Are there any other malformations or associated developmental delay?

You should then be in a position to reach a diagnosis and assess the recurrence risk.

Recurrence risk

Isolated transverse defects affecting only one limb are most likely to be sporadic with a low recurrence risk for both siblings and offspring. *Think very carefully about a genetic aetiology for defects affecting more than one limb, especially if they are symmetrical.* (Defects affecting the middle ray of more than one limb are highly likely to be genetic.)

Carrier detection

Examine the hands and feet of the parents for subtle anomalies. Consider the possibility of incomplete penetrance and variable expressivity for an AD condition.

Prenatal diagnosis

Detailed fetal anomaly USS is the mainstay of prenatal diagnosis. The limbs can be visualized on scan by 13–14 weeks gestation. It is usually not possible to visualize the digits clearly before ~20 weeks gestation.

Support group contact: REACH (for upper limb defects) <www.reach.org.uk>, Tel. 08451 306225; STEPS (for lower limb defects) <www.steps-charity.org.uk>, Tel. 0871 717 0045.

Expert adviser: Ruth Newbury-Ecob, Consultant in Clinical Genetics, St Michael's Hospital, Bristol, England.

References

Brown N, Lumley J, *et al. Congenital limb reduction defects—clues from developmental biology, teratology and epidemiology.* The Stationery Office, London, 1996.

Duijf PH, Van Bokhoven H, Brunner HG. Pathogenesis of split-hand/split-foot malformation. *Hum Mol Genet* 2003; **12** (Suppl. 1): R51–60.

Gillis LA, McCallum J, *et al. NIPBL* mutational analysis in 120 individuals with Cornelia deLange syndrome and evaluation of genotype–phenotype correlations. *Am J Hum Genet* 2004; **75**: 610–23.

Gonzalez C, Vargas F, *et al.* Limb deficiency with or without Moebius sequence in seven Brazilian children associated with misoprostol use in the first trimester of pregnancy. *Am J Med Genet* 1993; **47**: 59–64.

Greenhalgh KL, Howell RT, *et al.* Thrombocytopenia–absent radius syndrome: a clinical genetic study. *J Med Genet* 2002; **39** (12): 876–81.

Holmes LB. Teratogen-induced limb defects. *Am J Med Genet* 2003; **112**: 297–303.

Ireland M. Cornelia de Lange syndrome. In *Management of genetic syndromes* (ed. S.B. Cassidy and J.E. Allanson), Chapter 6. Wiley-Liss, New York, 2001.

Krantz ID, McCallum J, *et al.* Cornelia de Lange syndrome is caused by mutations in *NIPBL*, the human homolog of Drosophila melanogaster Nipped-B. *Nat Genet* 2004; **36**: 631–35.

Matsunaga E, Shiota K. Threatened abortion, hormone therapy and malformed embryos. *Teratology* 1979; **20**: 469–80.

Newbury-Ecob RA, Leanage R, Raeburn JA, Young ID. Holt–Oram syndrome: a clinical genetic study. *J Med Genet* 1996; **33**: 300–7.

Shalev SA, Hall JG. Poland anomaly—report of an unusual family. *Am J Med Genet* 2003; **118A**; 180–3.

Stoll C, Mastroiacovo P, *et al. Eurocat guide 3: for the description and classification of congenital limb defects.* Department of Epidemiology University of Louvain, Brussels, 1988.

Vega H, Waisfisz Q *et al.* Roberts syndrome is caused by mutations in ESCO2, a human homolog of yeast ECO1 that is essential for the establishment of sister chromatid cohesion. *Nat Genet.* 2005; **37**: 468–70.

Lissencephaly and neuronal migration disorders

Lissencephaly may be identified on a cranial ultrasound scan (USS) of a neonate with poor feeding and hypotonia or seizures. A magnetic resonance imaging (MRI) scan is the investigation of choice to confirm the diagnosis. Most children with lissencephaly have severe developmental delay and epilepsy. They often present with infantile spasms early in life.

Lissencephaly (Greek for 'smooth brain') is a genetically heterogeneous group of disorders characterized by lack of normal gyri and sulci of the cerebral cortex (see figure). The abnormalities of gyration are a consequence of abnormal neuronal migration. In a normally developing brain, cells in the developing cortex migrate from the inner ventricular zone to the outer cortical plate. The contour of the normal fetal brain as seen on USS appears smooth until about 24 weeks of gestation; thereafter the first sulcal and gyral folds become visible and increase in number throughout the remainder of pregnancy. Various descriptive terms are used to describe the macroscopic appearance of the cortex. **Agyria** is an absence of gyral folds. **Pachygria** describes a reduced number of very thick gyral folds. The disturbance

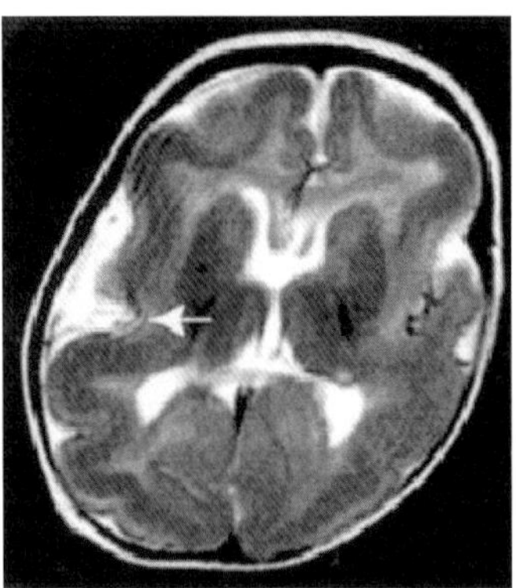

Lissencephaly type I in a girl aged 5 months who is visually and socially unresponsive, displays poor feeding, and increased tone. The T_2-weighted axial MRI shows a smooth cerebral cortex with absence of normal gyri and sulci. A vertically orientated shallow Sylvian fissure is seen (arrow). (Taken from Warrell (2003), fig. 3a, p. 1206 by permission of Oxford University Press.)

Types of lissencephaly

MRI appearances	Gene(s) to consider
Classical lissencephaly with posteriorly more severe gyral abnormality	LIS1
Classical lissencephaly with anterior predominant gyral abnromality in males	DCX
Subcortical band heterotopia (SBH) in females	DCX
Subcortical band heterotopia (SBH) in males (likely somatic mosaicism)	DCX/LIS1
Lissencephaly with cerebellar hypoplasia	RELN/DCX (very few cases)
Bilateral periventricular nodular heterotopia in females	FLNA
Lissencephaly with agenesis of corpus callosum and abnormal genitalia (XLAG)	ARX

of neuronal migration can create partially overlapping phenotypes ranging from pachygyria to agyria. If the abnormal neuronal migration only affects a subset of neurons this may be evident as subcortical band heterotopia (SBH).

The types of lissencephaly can be summarized as follows (see table).

- **'Classical' lissencephaly** (type I lissencephaly) is characterized by agyria and pachygyria and a thickened cortex. Subcortical band heterotopia is seen at the milder end of the spectrum. The genes involved are *LIS1* (17p13.3) and *DCX* (Xq22.3). The proteins are associated with the cytoskeleton; however their exact mechanism in neuronal migration remains to be defined.

- **'Cobblestone' lissencephaly** (type II lissencephaly) is characterized by a disorganized cortex, with migration of cortical cells through defects in the pia. Deficiency of α-dystroglycan, which functions as a link between the cytoskeleton and the extracellular matrix, has been identified with genes mutated in conditions associated with this type of lissencephaly (*POMT1, POMGnT1, Fukutin*).

- **Lissencephaly variants.** Lissencephaly with cerebellar hypoplasia (LCH) is genetically heterogeneous, but may be caused by mutations in 'reelin' (*RELN*), which encodes an extracellular protein that regulates neuronal migration. X-linked lissencephaly with abnormal genitalia (XLAG) is associated with absence of the corpus callosum, ambiguous genitalia, and neonatal seizures. Mutations in the *ARX* gene have been identified.

Clinical approach

History: key points

- Three-generation family tree with specific enquiry regarding consanguinity, seizures, and developmental delay.
- History of pregnancy and delivery and neonatal period (feeding difficulties, level of alertness).
- Developmental milestones.
- Seizure activity: onset and type of seizures.

Examination: key points

- Measure occipital-frontal circumference (OFC; microcephaly is common), length, and weight.
- Examine for dysmorphic facial features (Miller–Dieker syndrome (MDS)) and other associated anomalies
- Examine for ocular abnormalities (Walker–Warburg syndrome (WWS)).
- Assess for hypotonia or hypertonia.
- Examine genitalia of males (XLAG).

Special investigations

- MRI scan if assessment based on cranial USS or CT scan
- Ophthalmic examination for retinal dysplasia, cataracts, myopia (WWS, muscle–eye–brain (MEB) disease, Fukayama congenital muscular dystrophy (FCMD)).
- Plasma creatine kinase (CK; WWS, MEB, FCMD).
- Chromosomes. (Consider fluorescent *in situ* hybridization (FISH) 22q11 in polymicrogyria and FISH 17p13.3 in classical lissencephaly).
- In classical lissencephaly FISH with a *LIS1* specific probe—if normal, consider *DCX* mutation analysis in males, particularly if gyral abnormality is more severe-anteriorly; consider *LIS1* mutation analysis if former investigations normal.

	Media Type	Title / Author	Seller List Price	Order Date
76523826-66	SONG0192628968B083659892	BOOK	Oxford Desk Reference Clinical Genetics Firth, Helen V (Editor), and Hurst, Jane A, and Ha	$54.96	Jul, 6 2026

Good. Trade paperback Trade paperback (US). Glued binding. 752 p. Contains: Illustrations. Oxford Desk Reference.

76523826-66

alibris

ERGODEBOOKS
14932 KUYKENDAHL ROAD
HOUSTON, TX 77090
UNITED STATES

To: **ALIBRIS APEX DC 76523826-66**
APEX
800 AVONDALE AVE.
GRANDVIEW HEIGHTS, OH 43212-3473

Shipping Instructions for AVIBOOKS

Print this Packing Slip and enclose inside the front cover of the book.

Please ship this item no later than Thu Jul 16, 2026.

Ship to:

ALIBRIS APEX DC 76523826-66
APEX
800 AVONDALE AVE.
GRANDVIEW HEIGHTS, OH 43212-3473
UNITED STATES

- If isolated affected male with apparent isolated lissencephaly sequence (ILS) and normal *DCX* mutation analysis, consider MRI scan in mother to look for subcortical band heterotopia (SBH). Band heterotopia in female gene-carriers usually cause seizures and learning difficulties, but may be clinically unapparent. Note, however, that female *DCX* mutation carriers can have normal MRI scans; therefore always consider *DCX* analysis first.
- Consider *ARX* mutation analysis in males with lissencephaly and abnormal genitalia.

Some diagnoses to consider

Lissencephalies

Isolated lissencephaly sequence (ILS). If lissencephaly is the only abnormality after careful clinical assessment and the MRI is typical of classical (type 1) lissencephaly, a diagnosis of ILS is made. About 64% of patients with ILS have a deletion or mutation of *LIS1*, and 12% (males) of *DCX*.

Miller–Dieker syndrome (MDS). Lissencephaly with dysmorphic features (see list below) due to a deletion at 17p13.3 that includes the *LIS1* gene. In about 12% the deletion is due to a familial chromosome rearrangement.
- Tall prominent forehead with vertical furrowing, bitemporal narrowing.
- Hypertelorism; upslanting palpebral fissures.
- Short nose with anteverted nares.
- Inverted vermilion border of upper lip with long, broad, and thick upper lip.
- Associated anomalies such as congenital heart disease, omphalocele, joint contractures.

Doublecortin (DCX/XLIS). X-linked semi-dominant. X-linked isolated lissencephaly sequence (XLIS) and subcortical band heterotopia (SBH) are allelic disorders caused by mutations in the doublecortin (*DCX*) gene. Most patients with SBH or XLIS are sporadic, representing *de novo* doublecortin mutations. Females are functionally mosaic for the DCX mutation due to X inactivation. A proportion of cortical neurons arrest early in migration forming a subcortical band, whereas the remainder migrate normally to the cortical surface (hence 'double cortex').

Males with sporadic SBH may be somatic mosaics for DCX. There is a high rate of somatic mosaicism in male and female patients with variable penetrance of bilateral SBH. Incomplete penetrance (normal MRI scan) has been reported in a woman with a germline mutation in DCX who had three affected sons (Demelas *et al.* 2001).

X-linked lissencephaly with abnormal genitalia (XLAG). Caused by loss of function mutations in the homeobox gene *ARX*. All affected individuals are genotypic males, with severe congenital or postnatal microcephaly, lissencephaly, agenesis of the corpus callosum, neonatal-onset intractable epilepsy, poor temperature regulation, chronic diarrhoea, and ambiguous or underdeveloped genitalia (Kitamura *et al.* 2002). In XLAG the cortical thickness is only 6–7 mm, rather than the 15–20 mm cortical thickness seen in classical lissencephaly associated with mutations in *LIS1* or *DCX*. (In addition, mutations in *ARX* are associated with a wide range of phenotypes including X-linked infantile spasms (polyA tract expansions), X-linked myoclonic epilepsy with spasticity and intellectual disability, and mild/moderate mental retardation with or without dystonia, ataxia, or autism.)

Lissencephaly with cerebellar hypoplasia (LCH). Features include small head circumference (OFC) and cortical malformation ranging from agyria to simplification of the gyral pattern and from near normal cortical thickness to marked thickening of the cortical grey matter. Cerebellar manifestations range from midline hypoplasia to diffuse volume reduction and disturbed foliation. LCH is within the spectrum of malformations caused by mutations in *DCX*. LCH caused by mutations in 'reelin' (*RLN*) is distinguished by the severity of cerebellar and hippocampal involvement. When due to mutations in *RELN*, inheritance is autosomal recessive (AR).

Walker–Warburg syndrome (WWS), muscle–eye–brain disease (MEB), and Fukayama congental muscular dystrophy (FCMD). WWS, MEB, and FCMD are all associated with cobblestone lissencephaly and mental retardation. They are all AR. Interference in O-mannosyl glycosylation appears to be the common pathological mechanism underlying both the muscular dystrophy and the neuronal migration disorder.
- **WWS** is the most severe form of these conditions, and is associated with ocular anomalies like retinal dysplasia, and a markedly elevated CK. The prognosis is usually poor. Mutations in the POMT1 gene account for 20% of patients.
- **MEB** is comparatively common in Finland and is characterized by ocular anomalies and muscular dystrophy with an elevated CK. The gene is a glycosyl transferase *POMGnT1*.
- **FCMD** is characterized by congenital muscular dystrophy and myopia. It is comparatively common in Japan and is due to mutations in the Fukutin gene at 9q31–33. There is a founder effect with a common 3 kb insertion.

Microlissencephaly. Microlissencephaly encompasses a wide range of cerebrocortical malformations, including simplified gyration, lissencephaly, and polymicrogyria. It is associated with severe congenital microcephaly (−3 SD and more below the mean). AR inheritance has been commonly reported.

Other cortical dysplasias

Polymicrogyria is characterized by the formation of multiple small gyri. The exact pathogenesis is yet unknown. A cleft from the cortex to the ventricle is known as **schizencephaly** (see below). The cleft is usually lined with polymicrogyria.

Polymicrogyria (PMG). This is aetiologically heterogeneous. PMG has been associated with intrauterine infection especially cytomegalovirus (CMV), intrauterine hypoperfusion, and other teratogenic exposures in pregnancy (e.g. alcohol). A substantial proportion is genetic with genetic heterogeneity including AR, X-linked, and autosomal dominant (AD) PMG. PMG has been reported in several children with 22q11 deletions and a number of other chromosomal anomalies such as 1p36 deletions. A karyotype and 22q11 deletions analysis should be considered when assessing individuals with PMG.

Schizencephaly. Schizencephaly has a wide anatomoclinical spectrum, including focal epilepsy in most patients. Association with an intrauterine CMV infection has been reported. Heterozygous mutations in *EMX2* have been seen in a very small subset of patients.

Periventricular nodular heterotopia

In periventricular nodular heterotopia, a subset of neurons destined for the cerebral cortex fail to migrate due to loss of function mutations in the gene FLNA on Xq28. Severe mutations in males lead to fetal death and usually cause epilepsy in females (sometimes with learning disability) (X-linked dominant inheritance). ~10% of males with periventricular heterotopia also have mutations in FLNA, but these are mild mutations causing only partial loss of function (Sheen).

Genetic advice

Recurrence risk

ILS. In the absence of a *LIS1* or *DCX* mutation the recurrence risk is ~5% (note possibility of AR inheritance if severe microcephaly).

- All intragenic mutations reported to date were *de novo*. If an *LIS1* mutation is identified in the affected child, there is very little risk of recurrence in a future pregnancy. (The only documented recurrences have been in the setting of a balanced translocation involving chromosome 17.)
- If the ILS is caused by a *DCX* mutation (XLIS) the mother may be a carrier, in which case 50% of daughters will have SBH and 50% of sons will have XLIS. However in an apparent *de novo* case, maternal germline mosaicism needs to be taken into account, with a possible recurrence risk of 10%, and prenatal diagnosis should be offered (see below).

MDS. If parental chromosomes are normal, recurrence risk is very low, <1%.

SBH. If an affected female carries a *DCX* mutation, 50% of daughters will have SBH and 50% of sons will have XLIS. Somatic and gonadal mosaicism is not uncommon. For a woman whose child has an apparently *de novo* DCX mutation there is a significant (up to 10%) risk of recurrence on the basis of gonadal mosaicism and prenatal diagnosis should be offered.

WWS, MEB, and FCMD. All follow AR inheritance with 25% sibling recurrence risk.

LCH. When caused by mutations in *DCX*, counsel as above; when caused by mutations in *RELN*, inheritance is AR with a 25% sibling recurrence risk.

PMG. Familial recurrence has been reported with PMG on a number of occasions. An intrauterine infection, abnormal karyotype, e.g. del 22q11, should be excluded. In the absence of a family history the recurrence risk is uncertain. There appears to be a higher risk with perisylvian PMG, particularly in males, which has been quoted as up to 30%. However, there is so far very little published data, and many cases appear to be sporadic.

Schizencephaly. Familial occurrence is rare; heterozygous *EMX2* mutations have been reported in some patients.

Periventricular nodular heterotopia

X-linked inheritance – women with a FLNA mutation will transmit the mutation to 50% of their daughters. At conception, 50% of male pregnancies will carry the FLNA mutation, but these will usually be lost prenatally or early in the postnatal period.

Carrier detection

DCX mutation analysis in mothers of patients (XLIS, SBH) with DCX mutations. In the absence of a mutation, MRI scanning should be considered in mothers who have children with these conditions.

Prenatal diagnosis

If a specific diagnosis has been possible, and the familial mutation(s) is known, prenatal diagnosis by CVS at 11 weeks gestation may be possible.

Prenatal diagnosis of lissencephaly by USS is *not reliable* and does not become possible before about 28 weeks gestation; fetal MRI scanning in these cases is more accurate. However, there may be associated features, such as congenital microcephaly, hydrocephalus, or cerebellar hypoplasia, that may be a useful guide earlier in pregnancy.

Natural history and further management (preventative measures)

The child should be under the care of a paediatric neurologist.

Support group contact: Lissencephaly Contact Group <www.lissencephaly.org.uk>.

Expert adviser: Daniela Pilz, Consultant Clinical Geneticist, Institute of Medical Genetics, University Hospital of Wales, Cardiff, Wales.

References

Aigner L, Uyanik G, *et al.* Somatic mosaicism and variable penetrance in doublecortin-associated migration disorders. *Neurology* 2003; **60**: 329–32.

Allanson JE, Ledbetter DH, Dobyns WB. Classical lissencephaly syndromes: does the face reflect the brain? *J Med Genet* 1998; **35**: 920–3.

Allen KM, Walsh CA. Genes that regulate neuronal migration in the cerebral cortex. *Epilepsy Res* 1999; **36**: 143–54.

Barkovich AJ. Neuroimaging manifestations and classification of congenital muscular dystrophies. *Am J Neuroradiol* 1998; **19**: 1386–96.

Cardoso C, Leventre RJ, *et al.* Clinical and molecular basis of classical lissencephaly: mutations in the LIS1 gene (*PAFAH1B1*). *Hum Mutat* 2002; **19**: 4–15.

Demelas L, Serra G, *et al.* Incomplete penetrance with normal MRI in a woman with germline mutation of the DCX gene. *Neurology* 2001; **57**: 327–30

Ehara H, Maegaki Y, *et al.* Pachygyria and polymicrogyria in 22q11 deletion syndrome. *Am J Med Genet* 2003; **117A**: 80–2.

Gleeson JG, Minnerath S, *et al.* Somatic and germline mosaic mutations in the doublecortin gene are associated with variable phenotypes. *Am J Hum Genet* 2000; **67**: 574–81.

Guerrini R, Carrozzo R. Epileptogenic brain malformations: clinical presentation, malformative patterns and indications for genetic testing. *Seizure* 2002; **11** (Suppl. A): 532–43.

Kato M, Dobyns WB. Lissencephaly and the molecular basis of neuronal migration. *Hum Mol Gen* 2003; **12** (Suppl.): R89–96.

Kitamura K, Yanazawa M, *et al.* Mutation of ARX causes abnormal development of forebrain and testes in mice and X-linked lissencephaly with abnormal genitalia in humans. *Nat Genet* 2002; **32**: 359–69.

Olson EC, Walsh CA. Smooth, rough and upside-down neocortical development. *Curr Opin Genet Dev* 2002; **12**: 320–7.

Parrini E, Mei D, *et al.* Neurrogenetics 2004; **5**: 191–96

Ross ME, Swanson K, *et al.* Lissencephaly with cerebellar hypoplasia (LCH): a heterogeneous group of cortical malformations. *Neuropaediatrics* 2001; **32**: 256–63.

Sheen VL, Dixon PH, *et al.* Mutations in the X-linked filamin 1 gene cause periventricular nodular heterotopia in males as well as in females. Hum Mol Genet. 2001; **10**: 1775-83.

Walsh CA. Genetic malformations of the human cerebral cortex. *Neuron* 1999; **23**: 19–29.

Warrell D. (ed.). *Oxford textbook of medicine*, 4th edn. Oxford University Press, Oxford, 2003.

Lumps and bumps

Children and adults may be referred to geneticist to determine if a 'lump or bump' is a marker for an inherited condition. There is often a dominant family history of similar lesions.

The history may be the first clue as to the underlying diagnosis, but the new mutation rate is significant and there is variability and incomplete penetrance for many of the dominantly inherited conditions.

Clinical approach

History: key points

- Three-generation family tree. Enquire whether any other family members have similar lesions.
- Family history of malignancy.
- At what age did the lesions first appear?
- Take a full medical history to identify any other problems.

Examination: key points

- Document the approximate number and location of the lesions (photographs if possible).
- Examine a typical lesion carefully and describe in detail.
- Is the lump in the soft tissues or is it hard and bony?
- If there is more than one type of lesion, record the various types.
- Examine carefully for other clues, e.g. café au lait (CAL) spots.

Special investigations

If the diagnosis is not evident consider referring to a dermatologist or surgeon for consideration of biopsy of one of the lesions to obtain a histological diagnosis.

Some diagnoses to consider

Predominantly cutaneous syndromes

Autosomal dominant (AD) lipomas. These usually appear in adults predominantly in a central distribution. They rarely affect the face. Usually the lipomas are benign, though progression to mixoid liposarcoma may rarely occur. Advise patients to report enlarging lesions.

Neurofibromatosis type 1 (NF1). Dermal neurofibromas are a characteristic feature of NF1 and occur in the majority of NF1 patients from early adolescence. They increase in number with time especially during puberty and during pregnancy. See 'Neurofibromatosis type 1 (NF1)', page 396.

Multiple cutaneous and uterine leiomyomatosis (MCUL). AD condition that causes multiple small skin lumps (cutaneous leiomyomata), associated with uterine fibroids. Heterozygous mutations of the fumarate hydratase (*FH*) gene can readily be found in about 75% of MCUL cases (Alam *et al.* 2003). Renal cancer (with papillary or collecting duct morphology) is sometimes part of the MCUL spectrum. Homozygosity or compound heterozygosity for mutations of the fumarate hydratase (*FH*) gene cause fumarase deficiency, a rare autosomal recessive (AR) disorder of the citric acid cycle causing severe neurological impairment.

Steatocystoma multiplex. AD condition characterized by multiple sebaceous cysts. Due to mutations in keratin 17.

Autosomal dominant glomus tumours. These present as small soft blue swellings particularly on the limbs. They can be tender and ache and may increase in size. Mutations may be detected in glomulin on 1p21-22. (They should not be confused with paraganglionomas, which are sometimes called 'glomus tumours'.)

Familial angiolipomatosis. Familial angiolipomatosis is a rare syndrome that may be confused clinically with NF1. Usually AD, but AR inheritance has been described. It is characterised by subcutaneous tumours at wrists, knees and ankles. There may be bone deformity near affected joints. Onset is usually in early adult life.

Proteus syndrome. Can be confused with NF1. Lipomas, pigmentary skin changes. Localized overgrowth of limbs and digits. Deep creases on the soles of the feet. See 'Overgrowth', page 207.

Juvenile hyaline fibromatosis (JHF) and infantile systemic hyalinosis (ISH) are AR conditions characterized by multiple subcutaneous skin nodules, gingival hypertrophy, joint contractures, and hyaline deposition. Allelic conditions caused by mutations in capillary morphogenesis protein 2 (*CMG2*) on 4q21.

Cancer syndromes

Neurofibromatosis type 2 (NF2). Cutaneous neurofibromas are found in nearly 30% of NF2 patients. See 'Neurofibromatosis type 2 (NF2)', page 470.

Familial adenomatous polyposis (FAP). Multiple sebaceous cysts, especially over the scalp and occurring in young individuals, may be a feature of FAP. It is caused by mutations in the *APC* gene. Mutations 3′ of codon 1400 are especially associated with desmoid tumours. See 'Familial adenomatous polyposis (FAP)' page 444.

Muir–Torre syndrome (MTS) is the co-occurrence of skin sebaceous tumours, adenomas, epitheliomas, or carcinomas with internal malignancy. A subset (probably most) of MTS is due to hereditary nonpolyposis colorectal cancer (HNPCC), but the literature abounds with an association with breast cancer, so HNPCC may not be the sole cause of MTS. Other skin tumours, such as keratoacanthomas, are associated with MTS, but there can often be a fine histological distinction between keratoacanthomas and squamous carcinomas, which may account for the latter also being associated with MTS.

Bannayan–Riley–Ruvalcaba/Cowden syndrome. An AD disorder consisting of macrocephaly, vascular malformations, lipomas, and pigmented macules on the shaft of the penis associated with malignancies (breast, thyroid, endometrial, and gut hamartomas). Birthweight usually >4000 g, occipito-frontal circumference (OFC) often >4.5 SD. Hypotonia, gross motor delay (60% have a mild proximal myopathy), learning disability, and speech delay occur in 70%. 25% have seizures. They may have mild hypertelorism. 60% have mutations in *PTEN*. See 'Cowden syndrome (CS)' page 442.

Carney complex. An AD condition characterised by skin pigmentary anomalies, cardiac and cutaneous myxomas, endocrine tumours and schwannomas. Cutaneous myxomas are pale, smooth papules or subcutaneous nodules that appear between birth and middle age on any part of the body eg. eyelid, except the hands and feet. See 'Multiple endocrine neoplasia' page 446.

Bony lumps
Hereditary multiple exostoses (HME). HME is an AD disorder characterized by multiple exostoses most commonly arising from the juxtaepiphyseal region of the long bones. These start as cartilaginous lesions and then ossify. Other bones that can be involved include the pectoral and pelvic girdles and ribs. The skull is not usually involved. Abnormal bone modelling, particularly of the long bones, causes bowing, shortness, cortical irregularities, and metaphyseal widening of the involved bones, leading to the deformities of the forearms and disproportionate short stature in severe cases. Malignant transformation to sarcoma is uncommon (0.5–2% of cases) and usually occurs between the ages of 10 and 50 years (Hennekam 1991); families should be told to report any enlarging or painful lesions. HME is genetically heterogeneous; most families have mutations in *EXT1* (8q24) or *EXT2* (11p12–p11). Hall *et al.* (2002) found evidence of loss of heterozygosity (LOH) in exostoses providing limited support for Knudson's two-hit hypothesis involving the *EXT1* and *EXT2* genes for the development of an exostosis. Penetrance is 100%. Males have more severe and frequent complications.

NB. **Langer–Giedion syndrome** is due to a microdeletion at 8q24 involving the genes for multiple exostoses 1 and trichorhinophalangeal syndrome.

Enchondromatosis (multiple enchondromatosis, Ollier disease, Maffucci syndrome). Enchondromas are common benign cartilage tumours of bone. They can occur as solitary lesions or as multiple lesions in enchondromatosis (Ollier and Maffucci diseases). Clinical problems caused by enchondromas include skeletal deformity and the potential for malignant change to chondrosarcoma. The extent of skeletal involvement is variable in enchondromatosis and may include dysplasia that is not directly attributable to enchondromas. When haemangiomata are associated, the condition is known as Maffucci syndrome. Neither condition seems to be genetically determined in a simple Mendelian manner. There are a few instances of familial occurrence of Ollier disease, however. Enchondromatosis can be caused by a mutation in the PTH/PTHRP type I receptor (*PTHR1*; Hopyan *et al.* 2002).

Albright hereditary osteodystrophy (pseudohypoparathyroidism, pseudopseudohypoparathyroidism). Subcutaneous gritty deposits of calcification, predominantly affecting the scalp, hands, and feet. Shortness of the 4th and 5th metacarpals, short distal phalanges of the thumb, cone-shaped epiphyses. AD but with imprinting effect. Gs alpha (*GNAS*) gene. See 'Obesity with and without developmental delay', page 192.

Fibrodysplasia ossificans progressiva (FOP). FOP is an extremely rare and disabling genetic disorder characterized by ectopic ossification of the soft tissues. The hallux is short. Avoid surgery and dental work as these lead to significant acceleration of the ossification. Most arise as new dominant mutations in the Noggin gene (*NOG*) whose product is a powerful antagonist of bone morphogenetic protein 4 (BMP4).

Other syndromes
Myotonic dystrophy. Rarely patients with myotonic dystrophy may develop pilomatrixomas, benign tumours of the hair matrix. (See 'Myotonic dystrophy (DM)' page 388.)

Genetic advice
Recurrence risk
As for specific disorder.

Carrier detection
Clinical examination combined with mutation analysis, if available.

Prenatal diagnosis
This is possible for some of these conditions.

Natural history and further management (preventative measures)
Many of the conditions require long-term medical surveillance.

Support group contact: Many of the individual syndromes have their own support groups. See <www.cafamily.org.uk>.

Expert adviser: Amanda Collins, Consultant Clinical Geneticist, Wessex Regional Genetics Service, Southampton, England.

References
Alam NA, Rowan AJ, *et al.* Genetic and functional analyses of FH mutations in multiple cutaneous and uterine leiomyomatosis, hereditary leiomyomatosis and renal cancer, and fumarate hydratase deficiency. *Hum Mol Genet* 2003; **12**: 1241–52.

Hall CR, Cole WG, *et al.* Reevaluation of a genetic model for the development of exostosis in hereditary multiple exostosis. *Am J Med Genet* 2002; **112** (1): 1–5.

Hanks S, Adams S, *et al.* Mutations in the gene encoding capillary morphogenesis protein 2 cause juvenile hyaline fibromatosis and infantile systemic hyalinosis. *Am J Hum Genet* 2003; **73**: 791–800.

Hennekam RC. Hereditary multiple exostoses. *J Med Genet* 1991; **28** (4): 262–6.

Hopyan S, Gokgoz N, *et al.* A mutant PTH/PTHrP type I receptor in enchondromatosis. *Nat Genet* 2002; **30** (3): 306–10.

Sybert VP. *Genetic skin disorders*, Oxford Monographs in Medical Genetics. Oxford University Press, New York, 1997.

Macrocephaly

Megalencephaly, megacephaly.
Macrocephaly is the term used to describe a head circumference more than 3 standard deviations (SD) above the mean for chronological age. It is compared with the length/height to determine if it is proportionate. Macrocephaly associated with large stature is found in the overgrowth syndromes (see 'Overgrowth', page 206). Here we address the problem of a head circumference disproportionately large in relation to stature. Neuroimaging has an especially important role in patients with developmental delay and macrocephaly. Large ventricles are frequently reported in children with macrocephaly; the ventricular volume needs to be assessed in relation to the degree of megalencephaly. If the predominant abnomality is hydrocephalus, please refer to 'Hydrocephalus', page 134.

Bolton *et al.* (2001) found that idiopathic infantile macrocephaly was associated with an increased risk of developing autism spectrum disorders (odds ratio 5.44). In Nevo *et al.*'s (2002) community-based study of >4000 children with neurodevelopmental disability in Israel, 1.4% of children had macrocephaly (occipito-frontal circumference (OFC) >98th centile). Children with developmental disability and macrocephaly had an increased risk of seizures (odds ratio (OR), 7.7).

Clinical approach

History: key points

- Three-generation family history with specific enquiry about family history of large head circumference and family history of malignancy (especially breast and thyroid disorders in Bannayan–Riley–Ruvalcaba/Cowden syndrome (BRR-CS)) and skin disorders in Gorlin syndrome). Enquire specifically about consanguinity.
- Head circumference at birth.
- Developmental milestones.
- Regression.
- Seizures.

Examination: key points

- Measurement of head circumference, height/length, and weight. Exclude causes of a spuriously large head size such as hair arrangements, craniosynostosis, or other abnormalities of head shape.
- Coarse facial features (storage disorders).
- Large jaw (Sotos syndrome).
- Neurocutaneous lesions: café au lait spots (CALs), capillary haemangiomata, depigmented lesions.
- Other skin lesions: lipomata (Bannayan–Riley–Ruvalcaba (BRR) syndrome), cutis marmorata (macrocephaly–cutis marmorata–telangiectatica congenita (M-CMTC)), basal cell carcinoma (Gorlin syndrome), papillomata around nose and mouth and behind ears (Cowden syndrome).
- Limb asymmetry and syndactyly, philtral haemangioma (M-CMTC).
- Organomegaly.
- Penile or vulval freckling (BRR syndrome).
- Parental head circumferences (page 660).

Special investigations

- Brain imaging. Magnetic resonance imaging (MRI) preferable to identify white matter changes.
- Neurodevelopmental assessment.
- Metabolic screen. Urine organic acids and mucopolysaccharide screen.
- Chromosomes. Some duplications are associated with macrocephaly.
- Fragile X.
- Consider *PTEN* mutation analysis if consistent with BRR-CS.

Some diagnoses to consider

Structurally normal brain

Large ventricles are frequently reported in children with macrocephaly. **Virchow–Robin spaces** are perivascular extensions of the subarachnoid space. They are found normally and frequently seen on modern MRI scans. There are some individuals, especially those with macrocephaly, in whom these spaces are prominent and widespread.

Familial macrocephaly. Diagnosis based on parental OFC and absence of any associated features or developmental delay; may follow autosomal dominant (AD) inheritance.

Neurofibromatosis type 1 (NF1). AD condition characterized by CALs, axillary freckling, dermal neurofibroma, short stature. See 'Neurofibromatosis type 1 (NF1)' page 396.

Fragile X syndrome. X-linked recessive (XLR) condition characterized by developmental delay. The head circumference, though relatively large, is usually nearer to 75th centile size. See 'Fragile X syndrome' page 324.

Sotos syndrome. Overgrowth from the prenatal stage through childhood, with advanced bone age, an unusual face with large skull and pointed chin, occasional seizures, and mild learning problems. Mutations in *NSD1*. See 'Overgrowth', page 206.

Simpson-Golabi-Behmel syndrome. XLR disorder with high birthweight, heavy facies, supernumerary nipples, bilateral UDT, mild/moderate learning disability. Mutations in glypican3. See 'Overgrowth', page 206.

Storage disorders. In association with developmental delay and regression. Mucopolysaccharidosis type III (Sanfilippo). Dysmorphic features may be less pronounced than in other mucopolysaccharidoses. See 'Developmental regression', page 96.

Glutaric aciduria type 1. Detectable on urine organic acid screen.

Bannayan–Riley–Ruvalcaba/Cowden syndrome (BRR-CS). AD disorder consisting of macrocephaly, vascular malformations, lipomas, pigmented macules on the shaft of the penis. It is associated with malignancies (breast, thyroid, endometrial, and gut hamartomas). Birthweight usually >4000 g; OFC often >4.5 SD. Hypotonia, gross motor delay (60% have a mild proximal myopathy), learning disability, and speech delay occur in 70%. 25% have seizures. May have mild hypertelorism. 60% have mutations in *PTEN*. See 'Cowden syndrome (CS)', page 442.

Gorlin syndrome (basal cell naevus syndrome). AD condition characterized in older individuals by basal cell carcinomas and jaw cysts, mutations in *PATCH* (see 'Gorlin syndrome', page 452.)

Cardiofaciocutaneous (CFC) and Costello syndromes. Feeding difficulties in infancy and Noonan-like features. See 'Noonan syndrome' page 402.

Macrocephaly–cutis maramorata–telangiectatica congenita (M-CMTC). Macrocephaly (often with hydrocephalus that may require shunting), macrosomia, philtral haemangioma, cutis marmorata (vascular mottling of skin), syndactyly toes 2,3 and/or fingers 3,4; may have postaxial polydactyly and asymmetry. Variable developmental delay. The expressivity of the syndrome is variable. All cases reported to date are sporadic. The genetic basis of the syndrome is not yet defined and is likely to be heterogeneous.

Diagnostic criteria for M-CMTC (Franceschini *et al.* 2000):

- Macrocephaly *and*
- Two features out of:
  - overgrowth;
  - cutis marmorata;
  - angiomata;
  - polydactyly/syndactyly;
  - asymmetry.

Macrocephaly–autism syndrome. Stevenson *et al.* (1997) found macrocephaly in 24% of 100 patients with autism. A family history of macrocephaly occurred in 62% of macrocephaly–autism cases. Poorly defined syndrome entity. Genetic basis not determined.

Structurally abnormal brain

The structural abnormality may guide further investigation, eg. lissencephaly, pachygyria, or other migration anomaly.

If a diagnosis is suggested on the basis of brain imaging, ensure that any other investigations that may support the diagnosis are performed. Genetic counselling is as appropriate for the diagnosis.

Neurofibromatosis type 1 (NF1). UBOs (unidentified bright objects) may be seen on a T_2-weighted MRI scan in children with NF-1 as may optic tract gliomas (seen in up to 15%, but only symptomatic in ~1.5%). See 'Neurofibromatosis type 1 (NF1)' page 396.

Canavan disease. Canavan disease (CD) is an inherited autosomal recessive (AR) leukodystrophy with an increased prevalence in Ashkenazim (carrier frequency ~1/40). The clinical features of the disease are macrocephaly, head lag, progressive severe mental retardation, and hypotonia in early life, which later changes to spasticity. It is caused by aspartoacylase (ASPA) deficiency and accumulation of *N*-acetylaspartic acid (NAA) in the brain that result in disruption of myelin and spongiform degeneration of the white matter of the brain. The gene for ASPA has been cloned and there are two founder mutations in the Ashkenazi Jewish population.

Alexander disease. Regression and megalencephaly with leukodystrophy. The most notable features of the infantile form of Alexander disease, which begins during the first 2 years of life, are macrocephaly (and sometimes hydrocephaly), psychomotor regression, seizures, and spasticity. MRI shows signal changes in white matter with frontal predominance. The patient dies within the first decade. Caused by heterozygous *de novo* mutations in the glial fibrillary acidic protein gene (*GFAP*).

Genetic advice

Recurrence risk

As appropriate for each identified condition.

For an isolated female with learning difficulties in whom all the above investigations do not reveal a diagnosis, a recurrence risk for sibs of approx 3–5% may be appropriate. For an isolated male a recurrence risk of 5–10% may be used to cover the possibility of an X-linked condition.

Carrier detection

Not possible unless familial mutation is identified.

Prenatal diagnosis

Not possible unless familial mutation is identified.

Natural history and further management (preventative measures)

If there are seizures or abnormal features on MRI the child should be assessed by a paediatric neurologist. If there are associated developmental problems the child should be under the care of a child development team.

Support group: M-CMTC Network `<www.Macrocephaly-cmtc.com>`, Tel. 0808 808 3555. Many of the individual syndromes have their own support groups. See `<www.cafamily.org.uk>`.

Expert advisers: Trevor Cole, Consultant Clinical Geneticist, Birmingham and Nazneen Rahman, Senior Lecturer and Honorary Consultant in Clinical Genetics, Institute of Cancer Research, Sutton, Surrey, England.

References

Bolton PF, Roobol M, *et al.* Association between idiopathic infantile macrocephaly and autism spectrum disorders. *Lancet* 2001; **358**: 726–7.

Brenner M, Lampel K, *et al.* Mutations in GFAP, encoding glial fibrillary acidic protein, are associated with Alexander disease. *Nat Genet* 2001; **27**: 117–20.

Franceschini P, Licata D, *et al.* Macrocephaly–cutis marmorata telangiectatica congenital without cutis maramorata? *Am J Med Genet* 2000; **90**: 265–9.

Nevo Y, Kramer U, *et al.* Macrocephaly in children with developmental disabilities. *Pediatr Neurol* 2002; **27**: 363–8.

Stevenson RE, Schroer RJ, Skinner C, Fender D, Simensen RJ. Autism and macrocephaly. *Lancet* 1997; **349**: 1744–5.

Mental retardation with apparent X-linked inheritance

Mental retardation (MR) and learning difficulties are more prevalent in males. Studies show a 20–40% excess of males with MR. Assuming this excess was caused by genes on the X chromosomes, X-linked MR (XLMR) would account for about 14% of MR. This has not been proven in clinical surveys of individuals with MR, which may be due to the paucity of distinctive features in many of the conditions, the lack of confirmatory tests, and the presence of new mutations.

Fragile X syndrome (*FRAXA*) is the most common form of XLMR, accounting for 30–40%.

This section addresses the approach to the investigation of the family where only males are affected by MR (or males are much more severely affected than females) and there is no evidence of male-to-male transmission, i.e. a family history consistent with an X-linked (XL) mode of inheritance.

The number of genes that have been identified as causing XLMR syndromes is rapidly growing. Most of the genetic defects that underlie syndromic XLMR (which is associated with additional phenotypes) are either known or have been mapped to small regions of the X chromosome. In 2005, <50% of the genes underlying non-syndromic XLMR (mental retardation is the only phenotype) have been mapped (Ropers). Additionally, it is becoming apparent that different mutations in one gene may give a spectrum of phenotypes; thus some XLMR syndromes that were considered to be distinct are now known to be allelic. The distinction between syndromic XLMR and non-syndromic XLMR is becoming increasingly blurred.

This is a very fast moving field. The review by Ropers & Hamel (2005) provides an excellent overview. Readers may need to supplement this by reference to the current literature and the XLMR update **www.ggc.org/xlmr.htm**

The approach is to:

- assess the affected individuals in the family;
- confirm that the inheritance is compatible with X-linkage;
- divide into syndromic or non-syndromic XLMR;
- in syndromic XLMR, compare the features with known XLMR syndromes;
- not to forget that other mechanisms of inheritance, such as the segregation of an unbalanced chromosome rearrangement, could mimic apparent XL inheritance in small families.

Clinical approach

History: key points

- Family history. Look carefully at the family tree for evidence of XL inheritance. Aim to expand further than a three-generation pedigree, especially concentrating on the maternal line and the children of maternal aunts and the maternal grandmother.
- Establish if either parent had special educational needs. Is there evidence of girls with milder degrees of learning difficulties than boys? Ask about the developmental and educational progress of siblings, uncles, and aunts.
- Pregnancy, labour, delivery. Note if there have been any previous pregnancy losses that might indicate a subtle chromosomal re-arrangement rather than an XL genetic aetiology for the problems.

- Developmental progress. Education/schooling.
- Assess if there is loss of skills (regression).
- Seizure disorder in males and females (*ARX* mutations, bilateral periventricular nodular heterotopia (BPNH) in carrier females of filamin A gene, subcortical band heterotopia (SBH) in carrier females with *XLIS/DCX*).
- Is there a recognizable behavioural phenotype (*FRAXA*, autism)?
- Severe constipation (Opitz FG syndrome).
- Other medical and neurological problems including enquiry about vision and hearing.

Examination: key points

- Head:
  - macrocephaly/relatively large occipital-frontal circumference (OFC; FRAXA, Opitz FG, SGB, mucopolysaccharidosis (MPS) IIA, Aitkin–Flaitz syndrome);
  - hydrocephalus (XL hydrocephalus);
  - microcephaly (Börjeson–Forssman–Lehmann syndrome, Renpenning syndrome, XL alpha-thalassaemia-mental retardation syndrome (ATR-X));
  - hair: cowlicks (Opitz FG syndrome);
- Eyes:
  - hypertelorism (Coffin–Lowry syndrome ATRX, Opitz G);
  - structural abnormalities in Lenz microphthalmia, Norrie disease.
- Face:
  - coarse facial features with full/thick lips (CLS, Aitkin–Flaitz syndrome, SGB);
  - flat nasal bridge with small triangular nose (ATRX);
  - mouth: tented/arched upper lip (ATRX, Chudley–Lowry syndrome). Wide mouth with midline groove of the lower lip and tongue (SGB).
  - Long narrow face with prognathism (Renpenning)
- Hands:
  - tapering fingers (CLS);
  - fetal finger tip pads (Opitz FG syndrome);
  - adducted thumbs (mental retardation–aphasia–shuffling gait–adducted thumbs (MASA) and XL hydrocephalus due to *L1CAM* mutations);
  - postaxial polydactyly (SGB).
- Chest:
  - accessory nipples (SGB).
- Abnormalities of the male genitalia:
  - macroorchidism (FRAXA, XL psychosis–pyramidal signs–macroorchidism (PPM-X) syndrome);
  - spectrum from undescended testes to apparently female external genitalia in males in ATRX and XLAG;
  - hypospadias (Opitz G);
  - small genitalia with hypogonadism (Börjeson–Forssman–Lehmann syndrome).
- Neurological signs (*L1CAM* mutations, Pelizaeus–Merzbacher disease and X-linked spastic paraplegia 2):
  - hypotonia (FG);
  - dystonia (*ARX* gene abnormalities).
- If there are minor dysmorphic features, are these familial?

Special investigations

- **Baseline general investigations** including electrolytes, uric acid, liver function tests, full blood count (FBC) with indices and blood film, creatinine phosphokinase (CPK), and urine metabolic screen (reducing substances, amino and organic acids, and mucopolysaccharides). Consider measurement of free T_3 (elevated free T_3 levels are found in XLMR due to mutations in *SLC16A2*) and urinary creatine (increased urinary creatine to creatinine ratio is found in XLMR due to mutations in *SLC6A8*).
- Further **biochemical screening** is necessary if there is neurodevelopmental regression. (See 'Developmental regression', page 96):
  - very long chain fatty acid (VLCFA) abnormalities in adrenoleukodystrophy;
  - exclude MPS IIA.
- **Cytogenetic analysis:**
  - routine cytogenetic analysis to the 500 band level. Consider a repeat analysis if not done in the past 5 years. Routine testing is indicated even in non-dysmorphic boys;
  - fragile sites. If molecular analysis for FMR2 (FRAXE) is not easily available, the cytogenetic laboratory may look for fragile sites;
  - consider high resolution cytogenetic analysis eg. X-tiling array (Veltman) if there are unusual features which do not fit with a known XLMR syndrome .
- **Molecular genetic analysis:**
  - FRAXA. *FMR1* molecular testing in all individuals;
  - *FMR2* analysis to exclude FRAXE;
  - specific mutation testing may be available for other conditions, e.g *Rsk-2* in CLS, ATRX;
  - store DNA for future analysis (obtain consent).
- **Brain imaging.** (preferably MRI) Should be performed on individuals with:
  - microcephaly or macrocephaly, except those with an established diagnosis such as FRAXA;
  - neurological signs;
  - seizures.
- **Electroencephalogram (EEG).** If any suspicion of seizures.
- Haemoglobin H (HbH) inclusions in erythrocytes (males with abnormal genitalia to exclude ATRX).
- Consider X-inactivation studies in female carriers from large kindreds but note that, unless there is consistent almost complete skewing in all obligate carriers in a large kindred, then using this information for carrier testing is risky. See 'X-linked recessive (XLR) inheritance', page 34.

Diagnoses to consider

Syndromic XLMR

Coffin–Lowry syndrome (CLS). Males with CLS show mental retardation (usually severe) with characteristic dysmorphism, most notably affecting the face and hands. The typical facial features consist of a prominent forehead, hypertelorism, a flat nasal bridge, downward sloping palpebral fissures, and a wide mouth with full lips. Mild progression in facial coarsening occurs during childhood and adult life. The hands are broad with soft, stubby, tapering fingers. Other clinical findings include short stature (95%), a pectus deformity (80%), a kyphosis and/or scoliosis (80%), mitral valve dysfunction, and sensorineural hearing loss. The facial

features become more pronounced with time and can also be recognized in some female carriers. X-rays of the hands, chest, and spine may help confirm the diagnosis. CLS is caused by mutations in the *Rsk-2* gene. See Hunter (2002) for information on long-term outcome in CLS.

Simpson–Golabi–Behmel (SGB) syndrome. There is prenatal and postnatal overgrowth. The facial features appear coarse with wide thick lips. Macrocephaly is present. The development can vary from normal to mildly delayed. Other physical features are described above. Surveillance for malignancy (Wilms tumour, neuroblastoma, and others have been described) should be considered. Mutations in glypican 3 (*GPC3*). See page 206.

X-linked alpha-thalassaemia mental retardation (ATRX). Mutations in the *ATRX* gene. The key facial features are the characteristic tenting of the upper lip associated with a small triangular-shaped nose and a flat nasal bridge. Abnormalities of the genitalia in males ranging from hypoplasia of the external genitalia to ambiguous genitalia are found (these are not seen in CLS). Search carefully for HbH inclusions in erythrocytes stained with brilliant cresyl blue. The facial features have been confused with those of CLS, but in ATRX carrier females do *not* have physical or intellectual manifestations of the condition. Carrier women may have some HbH inclusions, but it is not a reliable method of carrier detection (Gibbons and Higgs 2000).

Opitz FG syndrome. This syndrome is difficult to diagnose without a strong family history. Hypotonia and constipation are common in infants. Agenesis of the corpus callosum may be present. There is macrocephaly with a frontal upsweep of the hair (cowlick). Some families are linked to Xq12–q21.3 but there is at least one other locus on the X. It is only possible to offer carrier testing or prenatal testing in families large enough to confirm linkage.

Opitz syndrome (also known as Opitz G or G/BBB). These families are usually referred for a dysmorphology opinion rather than because of a family history of MR. There is striking hypertelorism, swallowing problems due to laryngeal clefts, and hypospadias. There is an an XL and an autosomal (22q) locus. The XL gene is *MID1* at Xp22.

Börjeson–Forssman–Lehmann syndrome. Mutations in the *PHF6* gene. Affected males are short with microcephaly, deep-set eyes, obesity, and hypogonadism. Carrier females have milder physical features with some impairment of cognitive function.

Renpenning syndrome. This term was previously used to describe all types of *XLMR*. Stevenson *et al.* (2000) consider that Renpenning syndrome should be reserved for the condition caused by mutations in *PQBP1* on Xp11.2-11.4 (Lenski). Renpenning syndrome is characterized by severe mental impairment, microcephaly, and a tendency to short stature and small testes. Patients have a striking facial appearance with a long narrow face, malar hypoplasia, prognathism and nasal speech.

ARX (Aristaless related homeobox) gene abnormalities. A spectrum of clinical phenotypes have been described with mutation in *ARX*.

- X-linked lissencephaly with abnormal genitalia in males (XLAG) and agenesis of the corpus callosum in females.
- X-linked infantile spasms (West syndrome).
- X-linked mental retardation.
- Partington syndrome (XLMR with dystonia).

Pelizaeus–Merzbacher disease (PMD) and X-linked spastic paraplegia 2. These two conditions are caused by mutations in the proteolipid protein gene, *PLD*. There is striking hypomyelination in PMD. A duplication within the gene can be detected with a specific fluorescent *in situ* hybridization (FISH) probe.

X-linked isolated lissencephaly XLIS (or DCX). Mutations leading to SBH in heterozygous females and predominantly anterior lissencephaly in hemizygous males.

Bilateral periventricular nodular heterotopia (BPNH). Lethal in the perinatal period in males; focal epilepsy in carrier females who have BPNH on magnetic resonance imaging (MRI) scan. Filamin A (*FLNA*) gene at Xq28.

MECP2. A number of phenotypes have now been associated with *MECP2* mutations.

- Rett syndrome. See 'Rett syndrome', page 408.
- Neonatal encephalopathy in males. See 'Neonatal encephalopathy and intractable seizures in the neonate', page 186.
- XL Psychosis–pyramidal signs–macroorchidism syndrome (PPM-X). Parkinsonian features are also found. An A140V mutation in *MECP2* has been identified.

Additional clinical features found in syndromic XLMR (adapted from Raymond 2006)

Absent speech	*ATRX, SLC16A2, SLC6A8*
Abnormal genitalia	*ATRX*
Autistic behaviour	*NLGN3, NLGN4, AGTR2, SLC6A8*
Cerebellar hypoplasia	*OPHN1*
Cleft lip and palate	*PQBP1, PHF8*
Congenital heart disease	*PQBP1*
Dystonia	*ARX*
Free T3 elevated	*SLC16A2*
Hypertelorism	*RSK2*
Infantile spasms	*ARX*
Microcephaly	*ATRX, MECP2, PQBP1, SMCX*
Scoliosis	*RSK2, ATRX*
Seizures	*AGTR2, SYN1, ATRX, SLC6A8, ARX, PQBP1, KIAA1202*
Short stature	*PQBP1, SMCX*
Spastic paraplegia	*SLC16A2, ATRX, SMCX, MECP2*
Tapering fingers	*RSK2*

Non-syndromic XLMR

Fragile X syndrome (FRAXA). See 'Fragile X syndrome', page 324.

FRAXE. Caused by an unstable CGC repeat in the *FMR2* gene. Affected boys are not dysmorphic and the degree of MR is variable but speech and behavioural problems are usually present.

X-linked autism. Mutations have been found in neuroligins 3 and 4 (*NLGN3* and *NLGN4*) in some families with both autism and Asperger syndrome affecting males and where the family tree is consistent with X-linked recessive (XLR) inheritance (Jamain *et al.* 2003).

Oligophrenin-1. Moderate/severe MR with neonatal hypotonia and variable cerebellar hypoplasia. Cranial MRI shows some degree of vermic hypoplasia and cystic dilatation of the cisterna magna (Philip).

Genetic advice

Recurrence risk

- Carefully exclude other causes for the apparent XLMR.
- For families with established XL inheritance (affected males in more than one generation linked through the maternal line) but no diagnosis, calculate the carrier risk and counsel as appropriate. Assess the likelihood of females manifesting signs and symptoms, particularly the MR, by careful family history questioning (but note the vagaries of X-inactivation and the wide variation seen, for example, in women with FRAXA who carry a full mutation). Consider if the family is large enough for linkage analysis. Discuss the fact that prenatal sexing will not differentiate between an affected and unaffected male. Ensure that DNA is stored from affected members of the family.
- The offspring risk to sisters of two affected boys, but no other affected male relatives, is ~10% (see 'Mental retardation', page 168). (This family structure is consistent with both XLR and autosomal recessive (AR) inheritance.)

Carrier detection

- Possible where the causative mutation has been established.
- The carrier risk may be calculated from the pedigree.
- Carriers may be detectable on the basis of similarities in phenotype to the affected males.

Prenatal diagnosis

- If the causative mutation in the family has been defined, prenatal diagnosis by chorionic villus sampling (CVS) is possible.
- Where there is no defined mutation, sex determination by CVS or amniocentesis can be offered. This approach necessitates stringent evidence that the disorder is X-linked, e.g. affected males in more than one generation linked through the maternal line, and cannot distinguish between affected and unaffected male pregnancies.
- If there is a definite diagnosis of an XLMR syndrome and the familial mutation is unknown, prenatal diagnosis by linkage may be an option.
- Ultrasound scan (USS) for associated anomalies and biochemical markers may give additional information.

Lay group contact: Mencap (England and Wales) <www.mencap.org.uk>, Tel. 020 7454 0454; Enable (Scotland) <www.enable.org.uk>, Tel. 0141 226 4541.

Expert adviser: Richard Gibbons, Lecturer in Clinical Biochemistry and Honorary Consultant in Clinical Genetics, Oxford, England.

References

Frints SGM, Froyen G, Marynen P, Fryns J-P. X-linked mental retardation: vanishing boundaries between non-specific (MRX) and syndromic (MRXS) forms. *Clin Genet* 2002; **62**: 423–32.

Gibbons RJ, Higgs DR. Molecular-clinical spectrum of the ATR-X syndrome. *Am J Med Genet* 2000; **97**: 204–12.

Greenwood Genetic Center XLMR Update http://www.ggc.org/xlmr.htm

Hanauer A, Young ID. Coffin–Lowry syndrome: clinical and molecular features. *J Med Genet* 2002; **39**: 705–13.

Hunter AGW. Coffin–Lowry syndrome: a 20-year follow-up of long-term outcomes. *Am J Med Genet* 2002; **111**: 345–55.

Jamain S, Quach H, *et al.* Mutations of the X-linked genes encoding neuroligins NLGN3 and NLGN4 are associated with autism. *Nat Genet* 2003; **34**: 27–8.

Klank SM, Lindsay S, *et al.* A mutation hot spot for non-specific X-linked mental retardation in the MECP2 gene causes PPM-X syndrome. *Am J Hum Genet* 2002; **70**: 1034–7.

Lenski C, Abidid F, *et al.* Novel truncating mutations in the polyglutamine tract binding protein 1 gene (PQBP1) cause Renpenning syndrome and X-linked mental retardation in another family with microcephaly. *Am J Hum Genet.* 2004; **74**: 777–80.

Lowe KM, *et al.* Mutations in *PHF6* are associated with Börjeson–Forssman–Lehmann syndrome. *Nat Genet* 2002; **32**: 661–5.

Philip N, Chabrol B, *et al.* Mutations, in the oligophrenin-1 gene (OPHNI) cause X-linked congenitial cerebellar hypoplasia. *J Med Genet* 2003; **40**: 441–46.

Raymond FL. X-linked Mental Retardation: a clinical guide. *J Med Genet* 2005; Aug23 Epub ahead of print due March 2006.

Ropers HH, Hamel BC. X-linked mental retardation. *Nat Rev Genet* 2005; **6**: 46–57.

Seminars in Medical Genetics. X-linked mental retardation. *Am J Med Genet* 2000; **97C** (Issue 3).

Stevenson RE, Schwartz CE, Schroer RJ. *X-linked mental retardation*, Oxford Monographs on Medical Genetics, no. 39. Oxford University Press, Oxford, 2000.

Turner G. Intelligence and the X chromosome [essay]. *Lancet* 1996; **347**: 1814–15.

Veltman JA, Yntema HG, *et al.* High resolution profiling of X chromosomal aberrations by array comparative genomic hybridisation. *J Med Genet* 2004; **41**: 425–32.

Mental retardation

Mental handicap, intellectual disability, intellectual handicap, learning difficulty, learning disability, developmental delay. Mental retardation (MR) is the preferred term in the USA but the Department of Health in the UK uses 'learning disability' and the Department of Education term is 'learning difficulties'.

The reported frequency of learning disability varies substantially across studies. Most studies report overall rates of 1–2.5% for intelligence quotient (IQ) <70, and 0.3–0.5% for IQ <50. Population studies show a preponderance of males (M:F, 1.3:1), mainly attributable to X-linked MR (XLMR).

Definitions

There are two categories of definition: one is IQ-based where MR is divided into groups based on IQ; the other is based on definition of functional deficits (see table). The older literature describes four degrees of retardation, whereas more recently this has been simplified into 'mild', IQ range 50–70, and 'severe', IQ less than 50.

Definition and coding of learning disability according to the *Diagnostic and statistical manual for mental disorders*, 4th edn (DSM-IV) of the American Psychiatric Association (1994)

Definition of learning disability

IQ <70 on the basis of an individually administered IQ test

Dysfunction or impairment in >2 areas of: communication, self-care, home living, social/interpersonal skills, use of community resources, self direction, functional academic skills, work, leisure, health, and safety

Onset during childhood

Coding of learning disability (using IQ) IQ

Mild	50–55 to ~70
Moderate	35–40 to 50–55
Severe	20–25 to 35–40
Profound	<20 or 25

The definition of mental retardation given by the American Association on Mental Retardation (1992) is 'Mental retardation refers to substantial limitations in present functioning. It is characterized by significantly subaverage intellectual functioning, existing concurrently with related limitations in two or more of the applicable adaptive skill areas: communication, self-care, home living, social skills, community use, self-direction, health and safety, functional academics, leisure and work.'

The *ICD-10 classification of mental and behavioural disorders* defines it as follows 'Mental retardation is a condition of arrested or incomplete development of the mind, which is especially characterised by impairment of skills manifested during the developmental period, contributing to the overall level of intelligence—i.e. cognitive, language, motor and social abilities' (World Health Organisation 1992).

Idiopathic MR is MR of no known cause. Within this group is the subgroup of non-specific MR that refers to the normally grown, non-dysmorphic child with no problems other than MR. In this subgroup there is an excess of males.

Mental retardation usually presents with delay in the developmental milestones but those with complex medical problems will present accordingly.

Mild mental retardation. The prevalence figures for mild mental retardation do vary from study to study with an average of about 3% of the population. There is a higher rate in socially disadvantaged groups. Those with an IQ in the top of the range for this group live a relatively independent life. Some of this group represent individuals at the lower end of the normal distribution for IQ. The aetiology is unknown in about 70–80% (see table).

Causes of mild mental retardation (from Bundey et al. 1989)*

Cause	Number (%)
Down syndrome	25 (5.7)
Fragile X	20 (4.6)
Other chromosome abnormalities	2 (0.6)
Cerebral palsy, neonatal illness, intrauterine infection	12 (2.7)
Postnatal trauma and illness	14 (3.2)
Malformation or genetic syndrome	15 (3.4)
Unknown	88 (80)

* N = 439. In 88 (20%) a cause for the MR was identified.

Severe mental retardation. In the moderate, severe, and profound groups there is a more equal social class distribution. This group has special educational needs and will require long-term care as adults. Many have serious long-term health problems. The life expectancy is reduced by a combination of these health problems and the delay in getting appropriate and prompt treatment of acute problems due to communication difficulties. The cause of the mental retardation can be established in about 50%, with Down syndrome as the most common condition (see table). It is hoped that new technologies such as fluorescence *in situ* hybridization (FISH)-based cytogenetic assays will increase the diagnostic rate. The improving resolution of brain imaging, especially magnetic resonance imaging (MRI), will reveal structural brain abnormalities in more children, especially those with neurological signs and epilepsy.

Causes of severe mental retardation (adapted from Curry et al. 1997)

Cause	Percentage of cases
Chromosomal, including Down syndrome	4–28
Fragile X	2–6
Central nervous system anomalies	7–17
Environmental causes, prematurity	5–13
Malformation or genetic syndrome	10–20
Unknown	30–50

Clinical approach

The aim is to try and establish the aetiology so that precise rather than empiric recurrence risks can be discussed as well as giving information about the natural history. Spend time making certain that the child is continuing to make forward progress and find out if there are areas of development where the child has particular difficulties. When dysmorphic features accompany MR, these should be used to help establish the diagnosis. Recognition of a specific syndrome may prevent further extensive and invasive testing. This section is primarily addressing the counselling problem of the child with no, or minor, dysmorphic features.

History: key points
- Three-generation family tree with enquiry about consanguinity. Try to establish if either parent had special educational needs. In other words, is the child's educational attainment similar to, or very different from, that of the rest of the family? Ask about the developmental and educational progress of siblings, uncles, and aunts. Look carefully at the family tree for evidence of X-linked inheritance.
- Pregnancy, labour, delivery. Note any adverse events. Ask about alcohol, prescription medications, and recreational drugs. Note if there have been any previous pregnancy losses that might indicate a subtle chromosomal re-arrangement.
- Developmental progress. Education/schooling. Exclude loss of skills (regression), autism, seizure disorder.
- Does he/she have a recognizable behavioural phenotype?
- Other medical and neurological problems.

Examination: key points
- Measure occipital-frontal circumference (OFC) to establish if microcephalic or macrocephalic. Refer also to 'Macrocephaly' and 'Microcephaly', pages 162 and 172.
- Focal neurological signs such as hemiplegia.
- Neurocutaneous signs, particularly pigmentary changes (to exclude tuberous sclerosis and type 1 neurofibromatosis (NF1) and chromosomal/genetic mosaicism).
- Presence of dysmorphic features. When there are minor dysmorphic features, are these familial?

Investigation
- Debate continues as to the usefulness of baseline general investigations including electrolytes, uric acid, liver function tests, full blood count with indices and blood film, creatinine phosphokinase (CPK), and urine metabolic screen (reducing substances, amino and organic acids, and mucopolysaccharides). Curry *et al.* (1997) recommend targeted rather than routine metabolic screening.
- Routine cytogenetic analysis to the 500 band level. Consider a repeat analysis if not done in the past 5 years. Routine testing is indicated even in non-dysmorphic children.
- Fragile X (FRAXA). FMR1 molecular testing is considered in all individuals. In children over 6 and adults a clinical checklist for the signs of FRAXA can reduce the number of tests.
- FRAXE in the presence of an X-linked mode of inheritance.
- Molecular cytogenetic techniques:
  - microdeletion screen. Consider if the child has features of a syndrome that can be confirmed by specific FISH studies such as Williams syndrome or del 22q11;
  - telomere analysis and other new techniques, e.g. microarray-based comparative genomic hybridization (array-CGH) to search for submicroscopic chromosomal abnormalities. Knight and Flint (2000) reported a 7.4% frequency of subtelomeric abnormality in children with severe mental retardation. Most of the children with subtelomeric rearrangements have severe MR and dysmorphic features and 50% had a family history, but there are

some exceptions. A history of recurrent miscarriage may also be relevant (Joyce *et al.* 2002). de Vries *et al.* (2003) in a recent literature review report a detection rate of 4.8% in individuals with idiopathic mental retardation. Preliminary data from Ness *et al.* (2002) using high resolution CGH and Vissers *et al.* (2003) using array-CGH suggest that the yield from CGH in children with mental retardation with/without dysmorphic features may be higher (~10%);
  - uniparental disomy (UPD) screening. There are a few recognizable phenotypes associated with UPD.
- Brain imaging. Indicated in individuals with micro- or macrocephaly and/or neurological signs. There is currently no consensus on whether to arrange imaging in patients without neurological signs. MRI is preferred except in cases of suspected craniosynostosis or congenital infection when computerized tomography (CT) is preferable.
- Electroencephalography (EEG):
  - if any suspicion of seizures.
  - if neurodevelopmental regression. Rett analysis in females with regression and also consider in X-linked pedigrees. (See 'Developmental regression', page 96)
- Consider creatine kinase (CK) in young males with developmental delay. Approximately one-third of boys with Duchenne muscular dystrophy (DMD) will present with developmental delay in the first instance.
- Haemoglobin H (HbH) inclusions in males with abnormal genitalia (X-linked alpha-thalassaemia/mental retardation (ATR-X) syndrome).

Some diagnoses to consider
- **Chromosomal abnormalities.** See 'Submicroscopic chromosomal rearrangements and the chromosomal phenotype', page 546.
- **X-linked mental retardation syndromes,** including Fragile X. See 'Mental retardation with apparent X-linked inheritance', page 164.
- **Structural brain lesion.**
- **Environmental factors,** e.g. fetal alcohol syndrome (FAS). (See 'Fetal alcohol syndrome (FAS)', page 588)

Genetic advice: non-specific mental retardation
Inheritance and recurrence risk
All studies have shown a risk of recurrence but with widely different rates. Older studies did not include routine cytogenetic analysis or molecular testing for fragileX. When the condition has recurred, all modes of Mendelian inheritance have been documented but special mention needs to be made of the possibility of an X-linked condition. There is an excess of males with MR but conflicting data about the contribution of XLMR conditions. Turner and Partington (2000) have reviewed the data from a cohort of 429 subjects with MR. In about two-thirds the IQ was <50, 8% had no IQ assessment, and in the remainder the IQ was >50. 28% were undiagnosed and recurrence risks in these families were ascertained (see table). The male to female ratio was 1.76.

Turner and Partington's (2000) figures support the hypothesis that genes on the X chromosome contribute to MR. They also state that submicroscopic chromosomal rearrangements can be found in non-dysmorphic children.

Observed recurrence risks for mental retardation in the sibs of index cases (Turner and Partington 2000)

Index case				
Gender	Number	Affected brothers	Affected sisters	All affected sibs
Male	69	11/83 (1 in 7.5) (13%)	3/60 (1 in 20) (5%)	14/43 (1 in 10) (10%)
Female	32	3/36 (1 in 12) (8%)	2/30 (1 in 15) (6.5%)	5/66 (1 in 13) (7.5%)

Estimated risks for severe MR to the offspring of sibs of index cases (assuming normal intelligence and no learning difficulties in the consultand or the consultand's mother). Table derived from data given in Turner and Partington 2000 to incorporate estimated risks after negative telomere screening.

NB. Use this table with caution, it is based on extrapolations from data from a small sample (101 families) and is not suitable for use in consanguineous families.

Index	Offspring risk (%)			
	Brother (cryptic translocation risk)	Brother (telomere screen negative)*	Sister (XLMR and cryptic translocation risk)	Sister (telomere screen negative)*
1 affected male sib	1–2	~1	2–5	1.5–3
1 affected female sib				
mild MR	~1[†]	~1	1.5–3[†]	1.5–3
severe MR	1–2	~1	1–2	~1
2 affected male sibs	1–2	~1	11–12[‡]	10
2 affected female sibs	Not known	Not known[§]	Not known	Not known[§]

* Telomere screen must be done in proband, unless using a FISH-based assay. (Dosage-based techniques eg MLPA or away-CGH will give normal results in carriers of a balanced crypictranslocation.)

[†] Assuming that telomeric deletions are only very rarely a cause of mild MR.

[‡] Sister has 40% risk of carrier status for XLMR (since her mother has an 80% risk of being a carrier with 2 affected sons).

[§] Likely to be low if no consanguinity, once translocation risk excluded.

Variability and penetrance

There may be variability in the severity of problems, especially in the context of X-linked inheritance. Turner and Partington (2000) believe that, if the mother or maternal aunt of an affected male has learning and educational difficulties, this is strongly suggestive of XLMR.

Offspring risk to the siblings of MR individuals

The data of Bundey et al. (1989) probably overestimated the proportion of MR caused by FRAXA. For various counselling situations and further explanation please refer to Turner and Partington (2000; see table). Their calculations estimate the likelihood of XLMR, as against other mechanisms of inheritance and then add the risk that the MR is caused by a familial occult chromosomal abnormality, using the data of Knight et al. (1999).

Prenatal diagnosis

Unless a specific laboratory-based diagnosis has been made in the proband, no specific diagnostic tests are available. Parents may ask about sex selection or termination of males. Inform them of the risks of an affected female child and that such testing cannot distinguish between normal and affected boys.

Surveillance and follow-up

Review appointments can help:

- to offer newly available diagnostic tests;
- to establish that there are no additional medical problems and that there is forward developmental progress;
- to increase the chance of syndrome recognition;
- to discuss recurrence risks.

There are no absolute guidelines for review but a reasonable approach would be a review 1 year after the initial completed consultation (which may involve more than one appointment) and another 2 years after this.

Genetic advice: mild mental retardation

The study of Bundey et al. (1989) investigated a group of 439 school children with mild MR. Although there were 274 boys and 165 girls in the group the recurrence risks were not higher for male sibs. There were considerable contributions from familial, environmental, and cultural factors that make individual risks vary. The overall recurrence risk was high at between 1 in 4 and 1 in 5 (i.e. 20–25%).

Support groups: Mencap <www.mencap.org.uk>, Tel. 0808 808 1111 (England and Wales); American Association on Mental Retardation (AAMR); The ARC—Association of Retarded Citizens of the US.

Expert advisers: John M Opitz, Professor of Human Genetics, Pediatrics, Obstetrics & Gynaecology and Pathology, University of Utah, Salt Lake City, Utah, USA and Samantha J.L. Knight, University Research Lecturer and Wellcome Trust Research Fellow, Wellcome Trust Centre for Human Genetics, Oxford, England.

References

American Association on Mental Retardation (AAMR). *Mental retardation: definition, classification and systems of support*, 9th edn. AAMR, Annapolis, Maryland, 1992.

American Psychiatric Association (APA). *Diagnostic and statistical manual of mental disorders*, 4th edn. APA, Washington DC, 1994.

Biesecker LG. The end of the beginning of chromosome ends. *Am J Med Genet* 2002; **107**: 263–6.

Bundey S, Thake A, Todd J. The recurrence risks for mild idiopathic mental retardation. *J Med Genet* 1989; **26**: 260–6.

Crow YJ, Tolmie JL. Recurrence risks in mental retardation. *J Med Genet* 1998; **35**: 177–82.

Curry CJ, et al. Evaluation of mental retardation: recommendations of a consensus conference. *Am J Med Genet* 1997; **72**: 468–72.

De Vries BBA, Winter R, et al. Telomere: a diagnosis at the end of the chromosomes. *J Med Genet* 2003; **40**: 385–98.

Gillberg C, Soderstrom H. Learning disability [seminar]. *Lancet* 2003; **362**: 811–21.

Joyce CA, Dennis NR, *et al.* An 11p;17p telomeric translocation in two families associated with recurrent miscarriages and Miller–Dieker syndrome. *Eur J Hum Genet* 2002; **10** (11): 707–14.

Knight SJL, Flint J. Screening chromosome ends for learning disability. *Br Med J* 2000; **321**: 1240.

Knight SJL, Regan R, *et al.* Subtle chromosomal rearrangements in children with unexplained mental retardation. *Lancet* 1999; **354**: 1666–81.

Ness GO, Lybaek H, Houge G. Usefulness of high-resolution comparative genomic hybridization (CGH) for detecting and characterizing constitutional chromosome abnormalities. *Am J Med Genet* 2002; **113** (2): 125–36.

Roelveld N, Zeilhuis GA, Gabreels F. The prevalence of mental retardation: a recent critical review of the literature. *Dev Med Child Neurol* 1997; **39**: 125–32.

Seminars in Medical Genetics. Genetics of mental retardation. *Am J Med Genet* 2003; **117C** (Issue1).

Turner G, Partington M. Recurrence risks in undiagnosed mental retardation. *J Med Genet* 2000; **37**: E45.

Vissers LE, De Vries BB, *et al.* Array-based comparative genomic hybridization for the genomewide detection of submicroscopic chromosomal abnormalities. *Am J Hum Genet* 2003; **73**: 1261–70.

Wilson HL, Wong AC, *et al.* Molecular characterisation of the 22q13 deletion syndrome supports the role of haploinsufficiency of *SHANK3/PROSAP2* in the major neurological symptoms. *J Med Genet* 2003; **40**: 575–84.

World Health Organisation (WHO). *The ICD-10 classification of mental and behavioural disorders. Clinical descriptions and diagnostic guidelines.* WHO, Geneva, 1992.

Xu J, Chen Z. Advances in molecular cytogenetics for the evaluation of mental retardation. *Am J Med Genet* 2003; **117C** (1): 15–24.

Microcephaly

The clinical finding of an abnormally small head that is disproportionately small in relation to the rest of the body. In practice the term is applied if the occipital-frontal circumference (OFC) is -3 standard deviations (SD) or <0.4th centile. Primary microcephaly occurs prior to 36 weeks gestation. When the birth OFC is within normal limits but falls away from the centiles subsequently, the term secondary microcephaly is used. Current work suggests that primary microcephaly is caused by a decrease in the number of neurones generated during neurogenesis, but that in secondary microcephaly it is the number of dendritic processes and synaptic connections that is reduced.

Microcephaly is caused by a very heterogeneous group of conditions. The role of the geneticist is to exclude chromosomal and environmental causes and to attempt to identify syndromic associations. Microcephaly is a feature in more than 450 syndromes listed in the London Dysmorphology Database so the number of possible diagnoses is frighteningly large; fortunately most will have other features that are obvious on careful clinical assessment.

Clinical approach

History: key points

- Three-generation family tree.
- History of infection, drug exposure, radiation, or excess alcohol during pregnancy.
- Enquire carefully for possible consanguinity.
- If antenatal ultrasound scanning (USS) was performed, was the estimated date of delivery (EDD) revised because the biparietal diameter (BPD) was smaller than expected?
- Birthweight (average birthweight in Seckel syndrome is 1500 g at birth).
- Ascertain OFC at birth or earliest record in infancy and plot longitudinally. Is the microcephaly static or progressive (primary or secondary)?
- Developmental progress.
- Does the child have seizures?

Examination: key points

- Plot the OFC, height (or length), and weight accurately, and estimate how small the head is e.g. -5 SD; exclude craniosynostosis. If the microcephaly is borderline (turricephaly or -2–3 SD), ensure that this is not a dominant family trait by measuring parental OFCs.
- Assess carefully for dysmorphic features. Assessment of the facies is particularly difficult as these are distorted by severe microcephaly.
- Examine carefully for other congenital anomalies, e.g. congenital heart disease.
- Detailed neurological exam? Spasticity?

Special investigations

- Detailed karyotype and telomere screen (especially 1p–, 4p–, 5p–, 8p subtelomeres). Consider microarray/comparative genomic hybridization (CGH) if available.
- Magnetic resonance imaging (MRI) scan (look carefully for migration abnormalities).
- Urine for organic and amino acids.
- Ophthalmology referral.
- TORCH (toxoplasmosis–other (including syphilis, varicella zoster, parvovirus)–rubella–cytomegalovirus–herpes simplex virus) screen. Consider congenital infection.
- Maternal urine biochemistry to exclude maternal phenylketonuria (PKU) if first child. Not necessary if the mother has an existing child with normal OFC.
- Consider testing for Angelman syndrome (may present with mild microcephaly in first year of life, before seizures or characteristic facies and movement become apparent).
- Consider lactate, very long chain fatty acids (VLCFAs) if hypotonic.
- Consider plasma 7-dehydrocholesterol to exclude Smith–Lemli–Opitz (SLO) syndrome if one additional suggestive feature, e.g. syndactyly, cleft palate.
- Consider parental chromosomes if telomere screen not available to exclude subtle rearrangement, especially if there is a history of previous miscarriages.
- DNA (EDTA (ethylenedinitrilotetraacetate) sample) for *MCPH1* and *MCPH5* mutation analysis in primary autosomal recessive (AR) microcephaly.

Some diagnoses to consider

AR conditions

Primary AR microcephaly. Characterized by relatively normal development in the first year of life, but later moderate mental retardation. Head size is usually <4 SD at birth and growth is along the same centile thereafter. Remainder of examination and investigations are normal. Neuroimaging shows a small but structurally normal cerebral cortex. Four genes, including *MCPH1* (microcephalin) and *MCPH5* (*ASPM*), have been recently cloned and three other loci identified. (Woods, 2005)

Seckel syndrome and the osteodysplastic dwarfisms. Seckel syndrome is characterized by severe intrauterine growth retardation (IUGR; average birthweight at term 1500 g), severe microcephaly (average OFC, -8.7 SD), short stature (average, -7 SD), delayed bone age, and moderate to severe learning difficulties with sociable personality, characteristic facies with sloping forehead, large-appearing eyes, and beaked nose. Genetically heterogeneous with some cases due to mutations in the gene encoding ataxia–telangiectasia and Rad3-related protein (*ATR*) at 3q11.1-q24 (O'Driscoll *et al.* 2003) and others mapped to another locus on chromosome 18. Majewski *et al.* (1982) have defined three types of osteodysplastic primordial dwarfism and distinguished these from Seckel syndrome, although they share severe microcephaly, pre- and postnatal dwarfism, and a beaked nose.

Smith–Lemli–Opitz (SLO) syndrome. Prenatal and postnatal growth deficiency, developmental delay (almost all), cleft palate (37–52%), cardiac defects (36–38%), especially atrioventricular septal defect (AVSD) and total anomalous pulmonary venous drainage (TAPVD), hypospadias and/or cryptorchidism (90–100%) in affected males, Y-shaped 2,3 toe syndactyly (>95%), and postaxial polydactyly (~50%). See 'Hypospadias', page 142.

pseudo-TORCH syndrome. AR condition characterized by congenital microcephaly, congenital cerebral calcification, spasticity, and seizures

DNA repair defects (Fanconi, Cockayne syndrome, Nijmegan breakage syndrome, etc.). Growth retardation is a feature of most of these conditions with proportionate microcephaly or minor microcephaly. Nijmegan breakage syndrome is an extremely rare AR condition, but affected children have moderate microcephaly with IUGR, short stature, prominent midface, growth retardation, mild learning difficulties, and susceptibility to infections with panhypogammaglobulinaemia, and susceptibility to lymphoma and other tumours. See 'DNA repair defects', page 304.

Chromosomal deletions/microdeletion with recognizable phenotypes

Examples are 5p– (Cri-du-chat) and del(1p36). See 'Deletions and duplications' and 'Submicroscopic chromosomal rearrangements and the chromosomal phenotype', page 546.

Wolf–Hirschhorn syndrome (4p–). Prevalence is 1/50 000. 58% are detectable with routine G-banded karyotype; the remainder require fluorescent *in situ* hybridization (FISH). Microcephaly, growth retardation, and mental retardation with dysmorphic features. Prominent nasal bridge with 'Greek-helmet' profile in children and adults. They may have iris colobomata. Seizures are common, as is congenital heart disease. Frequent infections are common in infancy.

Mowat–Wilson syndrome. Pre- or postnatal microcephaly with severe intellectual disability and seizures associated with hypospadias, Hirschsprung's (67%), congenital heart disease, genitourinary anomalies, agenesis of the corpus callosum (35%), and short stature (see Zweier *et al.* 2003). Affected individuals have a typical facies with upturned ear lobules. 82% have seizures. Results from large-scale deletions or truncating mutations in *ZFHX1B* (*SMAD1P1*) on 2q22.

Other syndromes

Angelman syndrome. Severe mental retardation with little expressive language, seizures, ataxia, and wide-based gait. Characteristic jerky movement disorder with hand-flapping and episodic laughter. Facial features include a wide mouth and prominent chin. Severe microcephaly is not a feature, but most have OFC <25th centile by 3 years of age. See 'Angelman syndrome', page 272.

Rubenstein–Taybi syndrome (RTS). Normal birthweight, postnatal short stature and microcephaly, moderate–severe learning difficulties in most, broad thumbs and halluces. Approximately 25% have deletions of *CREBBP* on 16p13. See 'Broad thumbs', page 58.

Metabolic conditions

The OFC may be normal at birth. Regression of skills may be a feature. See other sections of this chapter, especially 'Developmental regression', page 96.

Environmental aetiology

Infections, trauma, teratogens (both pre- and postnatal). See other sections of this chapter, especially 'Cerebral palsy', page 70.

Genetic advice

Recurrence risk

- After careful exclusion of syndromic and environmental causes, and if the MRI brain scan is normal, there is a high proportion of primary AR microcephaly amongst the remainder and so, for primary microcephaly, a recurrence risk of 15–20% is appropriate for future pregnancies.
- If there is consanguinity, assume AR inheritance and advise a recurrence risk of 25%.
- Beware of genetic conditions mimicking environmental ones, e.g. pseudo-TORCH.
- If structural brain abnormality seen on MRI, investigate and counsel appropriately.

Carrier detection

Possible in families in whom causative mutations have been identified in the proband (currently a tiny minority).

Prenatal diagnosis

With recurrence of primary microcephaly, head size often falls off only late in pregnancy, sometimes as late as 32–36 weeks gestation. Prenatal diagnosis by USS is therefore unreliable, although in practice most subsequent pregnancies are scanned. Only conditions causing severe primary microcephaly (<12 SD) are likely to be diagnosed prior to 20 weeks gestation.

Support group: Microcephaly Support Group <info@cafamily.org.uk>, Tel. 0808 808 3555.

Expert adviser: C. Geoff Woods, University Lecturer in Medical Genetics, University of Cambridge, Cambridge, England.

References

Bond J, Roberts E, *et al.* ASPM is a major determinant of cerebral cortical size. *Nat Genet* 2002; **32**: 316–20.

Jackson AP, Eastwood H, *et al.* Identification of microcephalin, a protein implicated in determining the size of the human brain. *Am J Hum Genet* 2002; **71**: 136–42.

Majewski F, *et al.* Studies of osetodysplastic primordial dwarfism I, II and III. *Am J Med Genet* 1982; **12**: 7–42.

Mowat DR, Wilson MJ, Goossens M. Mowat–Wilson syndrome. *J Med Genet* 2003; **40**: 305–10.

O'Driscoll M, Ruiz-Perez VL, *et al.* A splicing mutation affecting expression of ataxia–telangiectasia and Rad3-related protein (ATR) results in Seckel syndrome. *Nat Genet* 2003; **33**: 467–501.

Rouse B, Matalon R, *et al.* Maternal phenylketonuria syndrome: congenital heart defects, microcephaly, and developmental outcomes. *J Pediatr* 2000; **136**: 57–61.

Tolmie J. Prenatal diagnosis of microcephaly. *Prenat Diag* 1991; **11**: 347.

Vivarelli R, Grosso S, *et al.* Pseudo-TORCH syndrome or Baraitser–Reardon syndrome: diagnostic criteria. *Brain Dev* 2001; **23**: 18–23.

Woods CG. Human microcephaly. *Curr Opin Neurobiol* 2004; **14**: 112–17.

Woods CG, Bond J *et al.* Autosomal recessive primary microcephaly (MCPH): A review of clinical, molecular, and evolutionary findings. *Am J Hum Genet* 2005; **76**: 717–28.

Zweier C, Templet IK, *et al.* Characterisation of deletions of the *ZFHX1B* region and genotype–phenotype analysis in Mowat–Wilson syndrome. *J Med Genet* 2003; **40**: 601–5.

Micrognathia and Robin sequence

Micrognathia is the term used to describe a small mandible or small chin. Mild micrognathia is seen in a large number of conditions and is rarely useful as a diagnostic handle. In some conditions marked micrognathia is a major feature and can be a useful aid to diagnosis.

Micrognathia may occur as a deformation as in oligohydramnios (e.g. Potter sequence: renal agenesis, micrognathia, pulmonary hypoplasia, talipes, crumpled ears) or as part of a genetically determined restriction of mandibular growth as in Treacher–Collins syndrome (TCS), or 22q11 deletion, or certain skeletal dysplasias.

Robin sequence (also termed Pierre–Robin sequence, Robin anomaly) describes a triad of micrognathia, cleft palate, and upper airway obstruction. In practice many clinicians use the term when only two of these three features are present. In Robin sequence, micrognathia is present at the time that palate fusion is programmed to begin. Because of the mandibular anomaly, the tongue is not free to descend from between the vertical palatal shelves and prevents them from orientating horizontally and fusing in the midline.

Typically, the cleft in Robin sequence is U-shaped, but the term is still often used when a V-shaped cleft is present (see figure). Infants with Robin sequence may have airway and feeding problems in infancy and need specialist care as neonates. A deep pectus excavatum is commonly seen with each inspiration and may be accompanied by suprasternal and intercoastal retraction. Careful monitoring by pulse oximetry is important. Management should be in conjunction with a neonatologist and paediatric ear, nose, and throat (ENT) specialist.

In a retrospective survey of 74 patients with Robin sequence, van den Elzen *et al.* (2001) found that Robin sequence was the only anomaly in two-thirds, but was part of a more complex phenotype in the remaining one-third. Stickler syndrome and 22q11 deletions were the most common diagnoses in the complex group. However, in Shprintzen's (2001) large case series <20% were isolated. A 'diagnosis' of Robin sequence should therefore prompt a very careful search for an underlying aetiology.

- Stickler syndrome was the most common associated diagnosis (34%).
- Del(22q11) accounted for 11%.
- Deformation caused by restriction of fetal movement and growth due to oligohydramnios.
- Neurological problems such as central nervous system (CNS) malformations and hypotonia where poor fetal movement and fetal akinesia are features, e.g. myotonic dystrophy.

Normal mandibular growth is not typical for Robin sequence unless it is secondary to mechanical constraint (deformation sequence) in which case the mandible has usually achieved normal size by 2 years of age. In syndromes that have intrinsic mandibular anomalies, mandibular growth remains deficient. In some syndromes, such as Stickler where there is also maxillary hypoplasia, the mandible and maxilla may become proportionate with time.

Clinical approach

History: key points

- Three-generation family tree with specific enquiry about small chin, cleft palate, osteoarthritis.
- Pregnancy history. Was there normal liquor volume on ultrasound scan (USS) and at delivery?
- Neonatal history. Were there feeding problems?
- Developmental milestones.
- Specific enquiry regarding vision and hearing.

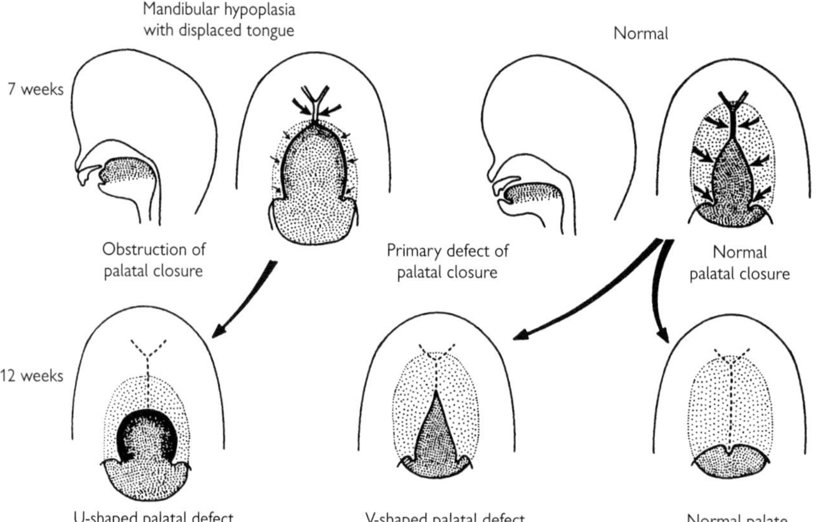

Robin sequence. At left, small mandible results in posteriorly placed tongue partially interposed between palatal shelves. This prevents closure and posterior growth of soft palate, producing U-shaped cleft palate. V-shaped defect at right is frequently seen in primary defects of palatal closure not secondary to mandibular involvement. (From Hanson and Smith (1975).)

Examination: key points

If the baby has respiratory compromise, be careful not to disturb the position of the head and neck during your examination.

- Growth parameters. Height, weight, and occipital-frontal circumference (OFC).
- Observe carefully for a cleft palate and consider the possibility of a submucous cleft.
- Heart. Listen for a murmur (22q).
- Limbs. Examine digits and nails carefully for transverse limb deficiency.
- Ophthalmological assessment for features of Stickler syndrome (vitreoretinal and high myopia).

Special investigations

- Karyotype with 22q11 fluorescent *in situ* hybridization (FISH).
- DNA if mutation analysis is possible for specific syndromes, e.g. TCS.
- Consider chest X-ray or skeletal suvey to look for rib gaps or signs of skeletal dysplasia.

Some diagnoses to consider

Stickler syndrome is a dominantly inherited disorder of collagen, resulting in a congenital vitreous gel anomaly, myopia, variable oro-facial features, deafness, and arthropathy. Stickler syndrome is caused by mutations in either *COL2A1* or *COL11A1*. See 'Stickler syndrome', page 414.

22q11 deletion. Congenital heart disease (CHD) with short stature, cleft palate or velopharyngeal insufficiency (nasal speech), and speech delay. Patients may have low calcium, mild learning disability, and immunodeficiency (typically reduced T-cell subsets). The single most common cardiac anomaly amongst children with 22q is ventricular septal defect (VSD). Aortic arch anomalies such as interrupted aortic arch or truncus arteriosus are characteristic. A significant proportion of children with Fallot's tetralogy have 22q11 deletions. See '22q11 deletion syndrome', page 490.

Treacher–Collins syndrome (TCS; mandibulofacial dysostosis). An autosomal dominant (AD) disorder with extremely variable expressivity caused by mutations in the *TCOF1* gene at 5q32–33.1. The ear anomalies are bilateral. They are malformed and displaced towards the angle of the mandible. One-third have atresia of the external auditory meatus and abnormality of the ossicles. Conductive hearing loss is common, but also screen for sensorineural deafness. Malar hypoplasia, coloboma (V-shaped notch) of inferior eyelid at junction of medial two-thirds and lateral one-third. Intelligence is normal. Consider mutation analysis of *TSC1*. Approximately 17% have a 5 nucleotide deletion towards the 3′ end of the gene. 60–70% are the result of *de novo* mutations.

Nager syndrome (acrofacial dysostosis). AD condition with TCS-like facies combined with radial ray limb defects, e.g. absent/hypoplastic thumbs and radial hypoplasia.

Potter sequence. Deformation sequence arising from severe oligo- or anhydramnios—typically resulting from bilateral renal agenesis. In addition to severe micrognathia

the baby has talipes and severe pulmonary hypoplasia usually resulting in neonatal death.

Oromandibular–limb–hypogenesis syndromes. Combination of micrognathia and/or hypoglossia (small tongue) with transverse limb reduction defects. Sometimes a U-shaped cleft palate is seen. Moebius syndrome (VI and VII nerve palsies) is sometimes associated. Most are sporadic and attributed to vascular disruption.

Oculo-auriculo-vertebral (OAV) spectrum. Also known as Goldenhar syndrome, hemifacial microsomia, first and second arch syndrome, and craniofacial microsomia. OAV spectrum is a heterogeneous condition that affects primarily the development of the ear, oral structures, and mandible. In the majority of children the disorder is unilateral. When bilateral, there is a difference in severity between the right and left sides. The chin is often small. See 'Facial asymmetry', page 112.

Cerebrocostomandibular syndrome (CCMS). CCMS, also known as 'rib-gap syndrome', is characterized by Robin sequence, multiple rib defects, and the occasional occurrence of intellectual impairment. Over 60 cases have been reported, nearly half of which are familial. Families suggestive of autosomal recessive (AR) and AD inheritance are both reported and are not distinguishable on the basis of clinical manifestations.

Genetic advice

Recurrence risk

Counsel as for specific syndrome. When Robin syndrome is truly an isolated defect, the recurrence risk is low.

Carrier detection

TCS is highly variable and on occasion virtually nonpenetrant. If a mutation is identified, mutation detection can be offered to the parents to help in determining the risk to future pregnancies

Prenatal diagnosis

Very severe micrognathia can be visualized on USS from ~12–14 weeks gestation.

Lay group contact: Cleft Lip and Palate Association (CLAPA)   <www.clapa.com>;   American   Cleft Palate–Craniofacial Association (ACPA) <www.cleftpalate-craniofacial.org>. Many of the individual syndromes   have   their   own   support   groups.   See <www.cafamily.org.uk>;   Pierre   Robin   Network <www.pierrerobin.org>.

Expert adviser: Dian Donnai, Professor of Medical Genetics, University of Manchester, Manchester, England.

References

Hanson JW, Smith DW. U-shaped palatal defect in the Robin anomalad: developmental and clinical relevance. *J Pediatr* 1975; **87** (1): 30–3.

James PA, Aftimos S. Familial cerebro-costo-mandibular syndrome: a case with unusual prenatal findings and review. *Clin Dysmorphol* 2003; **12** (1): 63–8.

Shprintzen RJ. Robin sequence. In *Management of genetic syndromes* (ed. S.B. Cassidy and J.E. Allanson), Chapter 19, pp. 323–36. Wiley-Liss, New York, 2001.

van den Elzen AP, Semmekrot BA, *et al.* Diagnosis and treatment of the Pierre Robin sequence: results of a retrospective clinical study and review of the literature. *Eur J Pediatr* 2001; **160**: 47–53.

Microphthalmia and anophthalmia

The embryological development of the eye is complex, controlled by many developmental genes and very sensitive to teratogens. The lens is derived from surface ectoderm, the retina from neural ectoderm, the extraocular muscles from the mesoderm, and the cornea, iris, and connective tissue of the extraocular muscles are neural crest derivatives. It is not surprising that eye anomalies are common and the eye is second only to the brain in its sensitivity to damage. The Scottish study of microphthalmia, anophthalmia, and coloboma over a 16-year period gave a minimum birth prevalence of 14/100 000 for microphthalmia and 3/100 000 for anophthalmia. (Morrison *et al.* 2002).

Microphthalmia is a small eye, and it is usually associated with other ocular malformation. Even when it is thought to be unilateral, there is often mild abnormality in the apparently normal eye. The eye volume is reduced.The normal mean axis length of an eye is 22.5 mm in a child of 2 years, and in microphthalmia this is usually less than 18.5 mm. There is a spectrum of abnormality from microphthalmos to complete absence of the globe (**anophthalmos**). The term 'clinical anophthalmos' is a useful term to mean the clinical absence of eyes (there may be rudimentary eye vestiges histopathologically).

A small eye with no structural abnormality is **nanophthalmos** or simple microphthalmia. The nanophthalmic eye has a proportionately thicker sclera. The lens is usually of normal size that leads to a narrow anterior chamber and glaucoma may develop.

Cryptophthalmos is the presence of microphthalmos with skin covering the globe; the lids are attached to the cornea.

You may be asked to see a baby of child with microphthalmos as part of a more generalized condition or may be asked to counsel recurrence or offspring risks for isolated microphthalmia. Obtain a detailed examination and report from an ophthalmologist prior to genetic counselling.

Clinical approach

History: key points

- Exposure to teratogens, alcohol, and infections during pregnancy.
- Family history. At least three generations. Ask about all visual difficulties. Affected individuals may be minimally affected.
- Consanguinity.
- Growth (most chromosomal conditions show poor growth, association with pituitary abnormalities).
- Abnormalities of renal structure and/or function (Fraser syndrome, *PAX2* mutations, del 14q22).
- Developmental progress (allowing for visual difficulties).

Examination: key points

- Growth parameters including occipital-frontal circumference (OFC).
- Eye:
  - measurement and photography of eye and surrounding structures and ultrasound scan (USS) of the eye to measure axial length and to exclude retinal detachment or retinal dysplasia (usually performed by the ophthalmologist);

- coloboma in addition to micro- or anophthalmia (colobomatous microphthalmia, CHARGE (coloboma–heart defects–atresia choanae–retardation of growth and/or development–genital defect–ear anomalies and/or deafness) association);
  - eye lid fusion (Fraser syndrome).
- Face:
  - facial asymmetry, skin tags, external ear anomalies (Goldenhar syndrome);
  - oro-facial clefts (trisomy 13, colobomatous microphthalmia, Fryns 'anophthalmia plus' syndrome);
  - nasal shape and sparse hair (Hallerman–Strieff syndrome);
  - abnormal dentition (Hallerman-Strieff syndrome, Lenz syndrome).
- Hands:
  - polydactyly (trisomy 13, Meckel syndrome);
  - nail hypoplasia (fetal alcohol syndrome (FAS)).
- Oesophageal atresia (AEG (anophthalmia–(o)esophageal atresia–genital anomalies) syndrome).
- Patchy skin lesions (Goltz syndrome, del Xp).
- Genital abnormalities (chromosomal abnormalities, Fraser syndrome, AEG syndrome, CHARGE association).

Special investigations

- Chromosome analysis and consider more detailed analysis (e.g. fluorescent *in situ* hybridization (FISH)) if features are suggestive of a microscopic deletion (16% of children with microphthalmia and anophthalmia have a chromosomal anomaly (EUROCAT Registry).
- Save DNA for possible genetic testing. In Fantes *et al.*'s (2003) study, *de novo* truncating mutations of *SOX2* were found in 4/35 (11%) individuals with anophthalmia, and up to 20% of patients with bilateral anophthalmia (Fitzpatrick, personal communication, 2004). Both eyes were affected in all cases with an identified mutation. Some children with truncating mutations in *SOX2* have associated learning difficulties.
- Renal USS in children with genital anomalies.
- Magnetic resonance imaging (MRI) scan of head and orbits is indicated for all children with clinical anophthalmos or severe microphthalmos.
- TORCH (toxoplasmosis–other (including syphilis, varicella zoster, parvovirus)–rubella–cytomegalovirus–herpes simplex virus) screen.
- Consider maternal phenylketonuria (PKU).
- *Examine parents and sibs for subtle colobomata.*

Some diagnoses to consider

Chromosomal syndromes

- **Trisomy 13** in the neonate. See 'Patau syndrome (trisomy 13)', page 534.
- Deletions involving **3q26.3.** The observation that deletions in this area cause microphthalmia/anophthalmia led to the identification of truncating heterozygous *SOX2* mutations in 4/35 (11%) of individuals with anophthalmia overall (Fantes *et al.* 2003).
- Deletions of **14q22** and *SIX6* hemizygosity. Panhypopituitarism and early-onset renal failure.
- Females with deletions of **Xp22** have microphthalmia and linear skin pigmentary abnormalities of the face.

- **Cat-eye syndrome (CES).** Anal anomalies (imperforate anus, anal atresia, or anteriorly placed anus), pre-auricular pits/tags, congenital heart defects, iris colobomata, renal anomalies, and variable learning disability. Microphthalmia is a less common feature (Schinzel *et al.* 1981). CES results from small marker chromosome containing a duplication of 22q11 resulting in tetrasomy 22q11. See 'Coloboma', page 82.

Neonatal lethal syndromes

- **Fraser syndrome.** Not all cases are lethal. Cryptophthalmos, syndactyly, renal and genital abnormalities, laryngeal stenosis. Autosomal recessive (AR). *FRAS 1* and *FRAS 2* genes (see 'Ptosis, blepharophimosis, and other eyelid anomalies', page 224).
- **Meckel syndrome.** Stillborn. Huge renal cystic enlargement, postaxial polydactyly, occipital encephalocele. AR with more than one locus. See 'Neural tube defects', page 392.
- **Cerebro-oculo-facio-skeletal (COFS) syndrome, Pena–Shokeir syndrome, and Walker–Warburg syndrome (WWS).** AR syndromes with major central nervous system (CNS) abnormalities. WWS cases usually show retinal dysplasia on USS. See 'DNA repair defects', page 304 for further information on COFS and 'Lissencephaly and neuronal migration disorders', page 156 for more information on WWS.

Other recognizable syndromes

- **Goldenhar syndrome.** Asymmetry of face and ear anomalies. See 'Facial asymmetry', page 112.
- **CHARGE (coloboma – heart defects – atresia choanae – retardation of growth and/or development – genital defect – ear anomalies and/or deafness) syndrome.** See 'Facial asymmetry', page 112.
- **Hallerman–Streiff syndrome.** Microcornea is present. The nose is thin, the mandible small, and there is hypotrichosis.
- **Colobomatous microphthalmia and clefting.** This has been reported in families so consider the possibility of variable autosomal dominant (AD) inheritance.
- **Non-syndromic colobomatous microphthalmia.** An intragenic deletion in the sonic hedgehog gene (*SHH*) has recently been reported in a three-generation family with iris and uveoretinal colobomata without optic nerve involvement (Schimmenti *et al.* 2003).
- **Goltz syndrome.** Focal dermal hypoplasia, limb deficiencies. X-linked dominant (XLD). See 'Coloboma' page 82.
- **Fryns 'anophthalmia plus' syndrome.** Facial cleft, nasal deformity, neural tube defect. Possibly AR as there was a recurrence in the original report, but a small chromosomal rearrangement would be an alterative mechanism.
- **Branchio-oculo-facial (BOF) syndrome (haemangiomatous branchial clefts).** An AD condition with distinctive areas of thin, erythematous wrinkled skin in the neck or infra/supraauricular regions in addition to craniofacial, auricular, ophthalmologic (coloboma of the iris and/or retina), and oral anomalies. See 'Coloboma', page 82.
- **AEG syndrome.** Anophthalmia with oesophageal atresia and genital abnormalities (cryptorchidism and hypospadias in males). Neuronal migation defects in the CNS are probably part of the syndrome. See page 201.
- **Lenz microphthalmia syndrome.** A very rare X-linked condition with mental retardation, highly arched or cleft palate and skeletal anomalies, genetically heterogeneous with one locus on Xp and another on Xq (Ng *et al.* 2002).

Environmental effects

- **Fetal alcohol syndrome (FAS).** Ask about alcohol intake. Low birthweight, developmental delay, microcephaly, cardiac abnormalities, digital hypoplasia, and craniofacial features.
- **Congenital infections.** Rubella and varicella.
- **Maternal PKU.** see 'Maternal phenylketonuria (PKU)', page 614.

Genetic counselling

Simple microphthalmia and colobomatous microphthalmia and anophthalmia

This diagnosis is made after excluding syndromal and chromosomal causes of microphthalmia.

Recurrence risk

- Bilateral involvement increases the probability of a genetic or chromosomal aetiology, but inherited microphthalmia may be unilateral as is very often the case.
- As parents have sometimes been shown to be affected after the birth of a second child, arrange parental ophthalmological assessment of eye size and structure. In particular, small retinal colobomata may be unrecognized without a specialist examination.
- The Scottish group (Morrison *et al.* 2002) proposed a robust classification of the eye phenotype based on the absence or presence of a defect in closure of the optic (choroidal) fissure. *All recurrences in first-degree relatives occurred in the optic fissure closure defect group.* The recurrence risk was between 8 and 13% depending on the statistical method used. Recurrences occurred with both unilateral and bilateral involvement.
- Sibling risks following the birth of a child with anophthalmia where both parents have normal eyes on detailed ophthalmological assessment may be of the order of 5%, but offspring risks for an affected individual may be considerably higher (a high proportion of SOX2 mutations are *de novo* nonsense mutations; D. Fitzpatrick, personal communication 2004).
- Spectrum of normal vision to complete blindness in a future affected child.
- All forms of Mendelian inheritance have been reported.
- Check literature for recent gene localizations. At present, known autosomal genes include *PAX2*, *SOX2*, and the sine oculis homeobox cluster at 14q22 (AD) and *CHX10* (AR locus at 14q32) and *SHH* when AD microphthalmia occurs in association with coloboma. AR mutations in the RAX homeobox gene have been reported in a patient with anophthalmia and sclerocornea (Voronina).

Carrier detection

- By ophthalmological examination.
- Is possible in families where a causative mutation has been identified.

Prenatal diagnosis

- By genetic testing where there is molecular or chromosomal confirmation of diagnosis.

- USS in mid-trimester can visualize the eye and lens but may not be sensitive enough to detect recurrence of microphthalmia although anophthalmia should be detectable with specialist scanning.

Natural history and further management (preventative measures)

Hornby *et al.* (2000) describe a classification system that helps predict the likely visual prognosis. Long-term ophthalmological follow-up is indicated for children with microphthalmos. Babies with anophthalmos require insertion of orbital expanders to encourage the eye socket to grow to enable prostheses to be fitted in childhood.

Support group contact: MACS (Micro and Anophthalmic Children's Society) <www.macs.org.uk>, tel. 0870 600 6227.

Expert adviser: David FitzPatrick, Consultant Clinical Geneticist, Western General Hospital, Edinburgh, Scotland.

References

Fantes J, Ragge NK, *et al.* Mutations in SOX2 cause anophthalmia. *Nat Genet* 2003; **33**: 461–3.

Gregory-Evans K. Developmental disorders of the globe. In *Pediatric ophthalmology* (ed. A. Moore), Chapter 5, pp. 53–61. BMJ Books, London, 2000.

Hornby SJ, *et al.* Visual acuity in children with coloboma: clinical features and a new phenotypic classification system. *Ophthalmology* 2000; **107**: 511–20.

Morrison D, Fitzpatrick D, *et al.* National study of microphthalmia, anophthalmia and coloboma (MAC) in Scotland: investigation of genetic aetiology. *J Med Genet* 2002; **39**: 16–22.

Ng D, Hadley DW, Tifft CJ, Biesecker LG. Genetic heterogeneity of syndromic X-linked recessive microphthalmia–anophthalmia: is Lenz microphthalmia a single disorder? *Am J Med Genet* 2002; **110**: 308–14.

Schimmenti LA, de la Cruz J, *et al.* Novel mutations in sonic hedgehog in non-syndromic colobomatous microphthalmia. *Am J Med Genet* 2003; **116A**: 215–21.

Schinzel A, Schmid W, *et al.* The 'cat eye syndrome': dicentric small marker chromosome probably derived from a no. 22 (tetrasomy 22pter to q11) associated with a characteristic phenotype. Report of 11 patients and delineation of the clinical picture. *Hum Genet* 1981; **57** (2): 148–58.

Voronina VA, Kozhemyakina EA, *et al.* Mutations in the human RAX homeobox gene in a patient with anophthalmia and sclerocornea. *Hum Mol Genet.* 2004;**13**: 315–22.

Minor congenital anomalies

Aase (1990) subdivides phenotypic anomalies into abnormalities and minor variants. Abnormalities are further subdivided into malformations, deformations, disruptions, and dysplasias (see 'Approach to consultatin with a child with dysmorphism, congenital malformation, or developmental delay', page 4). Minor variants can be subdivided into minor anomalies (prevalence ≤4%) and common variants (prevalence >4%) in the general population.

Ear tags and/or pits

Pre-auricular skin tags or pits are present in 0.5–1% of newborns. Of these, 20% have associated anomalies so a careful assessment of the external ear and a search for other dysmorphic features is warranted before the ear tag/pit is regarded as an isolated anomaly.

- Hearing assessment is indicated as 17% of infants with isolated tags/pits have conductive and/or sensorineural hearing impairment.
- Renal ultrasound scan (USS) should be performed in patients with bilateral pre-auricular pits/tags or isolated pre-auricular pits/tags accompanied by one or more of the following: other malformations or dysmorphic features; a family history of deafness; auricular and/or renal malformations; maternal diabetes. In the absence of these findings renal USS is not indicated.

Syndromic diagnoses to consider include oculo-auriculo-vertebral (OAV; Goldenhar) syndrome, Treacher–Collins syndrome (TCS), branchio-oto-renal (BOR) syndrome. See 'Ear anomalies', page 108.

Epicanthic folds

Epicanthic folds are seen in only ~3% of the Caucasian population in teenage and young adult life (12–25 years), but are very common in infancy (<6 months) when ~30% of Caucasian babies have epicanthic folds. Epicanthic folds are lateral extensions of the skin of the nasal bridge that extend down over the inner canthus of the eye, covering the medial angle of the orbital fissure. In young babies, the nasal root is low and hence epicanthic folds are common, but become less so with age as the root of the nose becomes less depressed and the nasal bridge becomes more prominent. Epicanthic folds are common in Down syndrome and other conditions where the nasal bridge remains hypoplastic.

Inverted nipples

Inverted nipples are seen in ~3% of the normal female population. If inverted nipples occur in a child with hypotonia and developmental problems, consider carbohydrate glycoprotein deficiency (transferrin isoelectric focusing) and propionic acidaemia (elevated glycine in blood and urine). Carbohydrate deficient glycoprotein disorders are autosomal recessive (AR) disorders of glycosylation characterized by a variable degree of mental retardation, liver dysfunction, and intestinal disorder. Propionic acidaemia is an AR organic acidaemia characterized by high NH_3, metabolic acidosis, and low platelets and white cell count.

Sacral pits and dimples

Small blind-ending sacral pits or dimples occur in 2% of neonates. In one study of 75 babies, each with a sacral dimple or pit, none had an abnormality on spinal USS suggesting that these skin lesions (if blind-ending and not accompanied by skin pigmentation or a hairy patch or subcutaneous lumbosacral mass) do not indicate a high risk for occult spinal dysraphism. In the absence of additional features, regard as a normal variant.

If other features are present, there may be a dorsal dermal sinus connecting the skin surface to the dura or to an intradural dermoid cyst. Arrange imaging and seek input from a paediatric neurologist or neurosurgeon.

Transverse palmar crease

A single palmar crease (simian crease) is present in 4% of the normal population—twice as common in males as females. 1% of the normal population have bilateral single palmar creases.

2,3 syndactyly of toes

When isolated, this is a common autosomal dominant (AD) condition with variable expressivity.

Y-shaped 2,3 syndactyly of the toes is found in ~95% of infants with Smith–Lemli–Opitz (SLO) syndrome, an AR syndrome with prenatal and postnatal growth deficiency, developmental delay (almost all), cleft palate (37–52%), cardiac defects (36–38%), hypospadias and/or cryptorchidism (90–100%) in affected males, and postaxial polydactyly (~50%). See 'Hypospadias', page 142.

Expert adviser: Judith G. Hall, Professor of Pediatrics and Medical Genetics, University of British Columbia, Vancouver, British Columbia, Canada.

References

Aase JM. *Diagnostic dysmorphology*. Plenum, New York, 1990.

Gibson PJ, Britton J, Hall DM, Hill CR. Lumbosacral skin markers and identification of occult spinal dysraphism in neonates. *Acta Paediatr* 1995; **84**: 208–9.

Kugelman A, Hadad B, *et al*. Preauricular tags and pits in the newborn: the role of hearing tests. *Acta Paediatr* 1997; **86**: 170–2.

Merks JHM, van Karnembeek CDM, *et al*. Phenotypic abnormalities: terminology and classification. *Am J Med Genet* 2003; **123A**: 211–30.

Park HS, Yoon CH, *et al*. The prevalence of congenital inverted nipple. *Aesthetic Plast Surg* 1999; **23**: 144–6.

Wang RY, Earl DL, *et al*. Syndromic ear anomalies and renal ultrasounds. *Pediatrics* 2001; **108** (2): E32.

Nasal anomalies

The nose is a variable structure but there are times when the shape of the nose may be the feature that is the key to syndrome recognition. This is most likely to be the case when the nasal structures (see figure) have an appearance that is not found within normal variation.

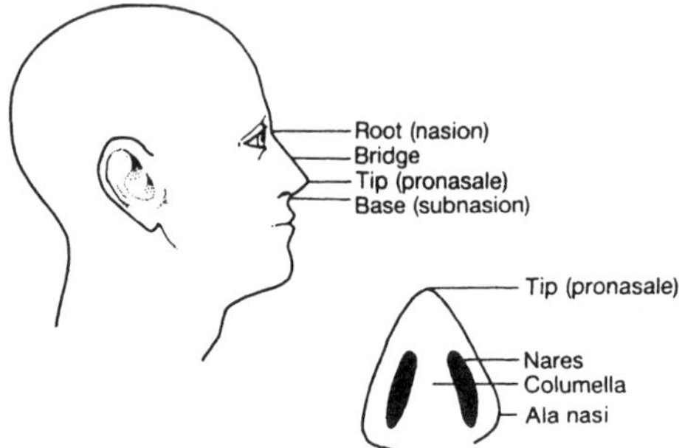

Landmarks of the nose. (Taken from Hall *et al.* (1989), fig. 7.63a, p. 176, by permission of Oxford University Press.)

- **Root of the nose** (nasion). The point where the nose meets the forehead.
- **Nasal bridge.** This forms the profile of the nose and is between the root and the tip. Flatter in infancy compared to its appearance in adults. In isolation it not a good discriminatory feature except for extreme cases.
- **Nasal tip.** The most anterior point of the nose.
- **Nares.** Nostrils.
- **Columella.** Fleshy inferior border of the nasal septum.
- **Ala nasi.** The lateral part of the nose forming the outer side of each nostril.
- **Nasal choanae.** The posterior nasal openings that are used for nasal breathing.

Clinical approach

History: key points

- Three-generation family tree with enquiry for similar features in relatives.
- Pregnancy history. Any drug exposure?
- Low birthweight, other congenital malformations (del 4p).
- Developmental milestones, schooling, and education.
- Expressive speech delay (Floating Harbor syndrome (FHS)).

Examination: key points

- Growth parameters. Short stature (FHS).
- Head:
  - scalp defects (Johanson–Blizzard syndrome (JBS));
  - skull shape asymmetry (craniosynostosis syndromes);
  - sparse hair (trichorhinophalangeal syndrome (TRPS)).
- Nose:
  - root of the nose (nasion). High with a 'Greek helmet' appearance in del 4p;
  - nasal bridge. Flat in many syndromes. Is it bulbous or beaked or wide and built-up?
  - nasal tip. Bifid, deficient (Majewski osteodysplastic primordial dwarfism II (MOPDII)), bulbous (TRPS)?
  - nares. Single opening (trisomy 13, holoprosencephaly);

- columella: Is it lower than the ala nasi (Rubinstein–Taybi syndrome (RTS))?
  - ala nasi. Hypoplastic (JBS).
- Mouth:
  - oral frenulae (oral-facial-digital type 1 (OFD1));
  - cleft palate (Stickler syndrome, OFD1, 22q11, Opitz syndrome).
- Hands:
  - syndactyly (oculodentodigital dysplasia, OFD1);
  - polydactyly (OFD1);
  - broad thumbs (RTS, Pfeiffer);
  - progressively bent fingers (TRPS).
- Genitalia:
  - hypospadias (Opitz syndrome);
  - genital hypoplasia (X-linked alpha-thalassaemia/mental retardation syndrome (ATR-X).

Special investigations

- Karyotype; consider 22q or 4p fluorescent *in situ* hybridization (FISH).
- Blood for DNA storage or genetic analysis if available.
- Skull X-rays and further skeletal films, if indicated from clinical assessment, e.g. left wrist for bone age (FHS).

Some diagnoses to consider

Flat nasal bridge

Binder syndrome (maxillonasal dysplasia). Binder syndrome or maxillonasal dysplasia is characterized by maxillary hypoplasia and a flat, vertical nose. The main feature is a hypoplastic nose with flattening of the tip and alae nasi, and absence of the nasal septum/spine. The maxillary hypoplasia creates the impression of relative prognathism. Inheritance is uncertain. There is debate as to whether Binder syndrome is a distinct entity, or if it represents the adult phenotype of milder forms of chondrodysplasia punctata (CDP). See 'Chondrodysplasia punctata', page 72.

Warfarin embryopathy. Warfarin and other coumarin derivatives are vitamin K antagonists that cross the placenta and, after exposure at 6–12 weeks gestation, can cause an embryopathy (CDP with nasal hypoplasia and/or stippled epiphyses). The nasal hypoplasia may be severe. See 'Chondrodysplasia punctata', page 72.

Stickler syndrome. Stickler syndrome is a dominantly inherited disorder of collagen. In infants the nose is hypoplastic with a flat nasal bridge. This grows out well during childhood. Ophthalmic complications include a congenital vitreous gel anomaly and myopia. There may be a cleft palate with micrognathia, deafness, and an arthropathy that is due to epiphyseal changes. See 'Stickler syndrome', page 414.

X-linked alpha-thalassaemia/mental retardation syndrome (ATR-X). The key facial features are the characteristic tenting of the upper lip associated with a small triangular-shaped nose and a flat nasal bridge. Abnormalities of the genitalia in males ranging from hypoplasia of the external genitalia to ambiguous genitalia are found. Caused by mutations in the *ATRX* gene. See 'Mental retardation with apparent X-linked inheritance', page 164.

High nasal root

Del 4p (Wolf–Hirschhorn syndrome). Characterized by low birthweight and postnatal failure to thrive, microcephaly, developmental delay, and hypotonia. There is a characteristic facial appearance with sagging everted lower eyelids, a 'Greek-helmet' profile, a short nose, and very short philtrum. Patients may have iris colobomata. Seizures are common. See 'Deletions and duplications', page 548.

Bulbous nose

Trichorhinophalangeal syndrome (TRPS). Autosomal dominant (AD) disorder characterized by fine, sparse growing scalp hair, dystrophic brittle nails, brachyphalangia with cone-shaped epiphyses on X-ray, and a pear-shaped bulbous nose. *TRPS1* is on 8q24. TRPS may be caused by intragenic mutations (TRPS1) or be part of a contiguous gene deletion syndrome that includes multiple exostosis (TRPS2). Specific FISH analysis is available for the microdeletion.

Floating Harbor syndrome (FHS). Predominantly postnatal short stature with growth −4 to −5 standard deviations (SD). The nose is broad, the mouth is large, and the ears are low-set and posteriorly rotated. The skull is long from front to back and affected children have mild developmental delay, especially of expressive language. The eyes are deep-set. Bone age is markedly delayed.

Velocardiofacial syndrome/del 22q11. Wide and prominent nasal bridge and root. Other dysmorphic features include: short palpebral fissures with telecanthus, wide and prominent nasal bridge and root, small mouth; ears are round in shape with deficient upper helices. See '22q11 deletion syndromes', page 490.

Beaked nose

Rubinstein–Taybi syndrome (RTS). The facial features vary with age and include a prominent beaked nose with the columella below the alae nasi and downslanting eyes The other striking physical feature is broad, sometimes angulated thumbs and first toes. The gene for RTS is at 16p13.3. Petrij *et al.* (2000) concluded that microdeletions and truncating mutations in *CREBBP* account for approximately 20% of mutations in individuals with the RTS phenotype. See 'Broad thumbs', page 58.

Crouzon syndrome. Shallow orbits leading to exorbitism and a hooked nose are characteristic features. Molecular testing can help to establish if there is a recurrence risk to parents as the clinical features in an affected parent can be mild. Caused by mutations in *FGFR2*.

Saethre–Chotzen syndrome (SCS). Asymmetric coronal suture involvement gives facial asymmetry. The nose is prominent and may continue in a straight profile from the sloping forehead. A low frontal hairline, ptosis, and small ears with a prominent crus are other helpful facial features. Examine for evidence of skin syndactyly and broad halluces. The majority of patients with SCS have mutations in the *TWIST* gene. See 'Craniosynostosis', page 288.

Majewski osteodysplastic primordial dwarfism II (MOPDII). Severe intrauterine growth restriction (IUGR) with proportionate head size that becomes more microcephalic with age. Beaked prominent nose, progressive hyperextensibility and bony dysplasia, high squeaky voice, prominent eyes, small teeth.

Hypoplastic alae nasi

Johanson–Blizzard syndrome (JBS). There is hypoplasia and notching of the alae nasi. An autosomal recessive (AR) condition with IUGR, scalp defects, and exocrine pancreatic insufficiency combined with dysmorphic features. Congenital heart disease and deafness may occur. Faecal elastase is a useful test of pancreatic exocrine function. Caused by mutations in *UBR1* on 15q (Zenker).

Oral-facial-digital type 1 (OFD1) is an X-linked dominant (XLD) malformation syndrome caused by mutation in *OFD1*. The features in the hands are syndactyly, usually skin syndactyly affecting variable digits, brachydactyly, and postaxial polydactyly. Other craniofacial anomalies are clefts, tongue cysts, and excess oral frenulae caused by mutations in the *CXORF5* gene on Xp22 (Ferrante).

Oculodentodigital dysplasia. An AD syndrome with a thin pinched nose with hypoplastic alae nasi, syndactyly of the 3rd, 4th, and 5th digits, dental anomalies, and neurodegeneration. Caused by mutations in connexin 43, *GJA1*, at 6q22–23. See clinical approach to 'Syndactyly', page 254.

Bifid nasal tip

Frontonasal dysplasia is a malformation. It is usually sporadic and more common in twins. Severely affected infants have a midline facial cleft with encephalocele; those mildly affected have hypertelorism and bifid nasal tip.

Craniofrontonasal dysplasia (CFNS). The presence of coronal synostosis and facial asymmetry helps distinguish this condition. Seen from above, the nasal tip is broad with a shallow groove. Ridged nails, syndactyly, sloping shoulders, and cleft lip are other features. X-linked but females are more severely affected caused by mutations in ephrin-B1 (*EFNB1*) on Xq13.1 (Twigg).

Opitz syndrome. Previously known as Opitz G/BBB and named after the initials of the original families. A gene *MID1* on the X chromosome at Xp22 does not account for all cases and there is a second locus on 22q with AD inheritance. Ocular hypertelorism is the most characteristic facial feature but the nasal tip may be bifid and, in addition, affected individuals may have hypospadias, cleft lip, and/or palate and some have a laryngeal cleft that may cause feeding/respiratory problems.

Oral-facial-digital syndrome type 2 (OFD2). AR malformation syndrome. Affected individuals may have a bifid nasal tip, together with syndactyly and polydactyly and midline cleft lip, oral frenulae, and tongue hamartoma.

Choanal atresia.

CHARGE syndrome C = coloboma, H = heart defects, A = atresia choanae, R = retardation of growth and/or development, G = genital defect, E = ear anomalies and/or deafness. It is caused my mutation in the gene *CHD7* which acts in early embryonic development by affecting chromatin structure and gene expression (Vissers). Some children have a whole gene deletion (detection may require FISH or dosage sensitive analysis). See also Coloboma section, page 82.

Carbimazole/methimazole embryopathy Choanal atresia, hypoplastic nipples, scalp defects and developmental delay have been reported in infants exposed to these drugs to treat maternal hyperthyroidism. For choanal atresia the critical period of exposure is days 35–38.

Genetic advice

Carefully examine parents.

Recurrence risk

Counsel for individual syndrome as appropriate.

Carrier detection

May be possible by molecular testing (see above) or by clinical examination.

Prenatal diagnosis

Although ultrasound scans (USS) can provide details of the phenotype from the second trimester onwards, only very significant nasal hypoplasia could be confidently predicted from prenatal scans.

Natural history and further management (preventative measures)

In some conditions, e.g. 22q11 deletion, a hypoplastic nasal bridge in infancy may grow into a high nasal bridge in older children and adults.

Lay group contact: Many of the individual syndromes have their own support groups. See <www.cafamily.org.uk>.

Expert adviser: A.O.M. Wilkie, Nuffield Professor of Pathology and Honorary Consultant in Clinical Genetics, University of Oxford, Oxford, England.

References

Ferrante ML, Giorgio G, *et al.* Identification of the gene for oral-facial-digital I syndrome. *Am J Hum Genet* 2001; **68**: 569–76.

Foulds N, Walpole I, *et al.* Carbimazole embryopathy: An emerging phenotype. *Am J Med Genet* 2005; **132A**: 130–35.

Gorlin RJ, Cohen MM, Hennekam RCM. (ed.). *Syndromes of the head and neck*, 4th edn. Oxford University Press, Oxford, 2001.

Hall JG, Froster-Iskenius UG, Allanson JE. *Handbook of normal physical measurements*. Oxford University Press, Oxford, 1989.

Petrij F, Dauwerse HG, Blough RI, *et al.* Diagnostic analysis of the Rubinstein–Taybi syndrome: five cosmids should be used for microdeletion detection and low number of protein truncating mutations. *J Med Genet* 2000; **37**: 168–76.

Roy-Doray B, Geraudel A, *et al.* Binder syndrome in a mother and her son. *Genet Couns* 1997; **8** (3): 227–33.

Twigg SRF, Kan R, *et al.* Mutations of ephrin-B1 (*EFNB1*), a marker of tissue boundary formation, cause craniofrontonasal syndrome. *PNAS* 2004; **101**: 8652–57.

Vissers L, Ravenswaaij C, *et al.* Mutations in a new members of the gene family cannot charge syndrome. *Not great* 2004: **36**: 955–57.

Zenker M, Mayerle J, *et al.* Deficiency of UBR1, a ubiquitin ligase of the N-end rule pathway, causes pancreatic dysfunction, malformations and mental retardation (Johanson-Blizzard syndrome). *Nat Genet.* 2005; **37**: 1345–50.

Neonatal encephalopathy and intractable seizures in the neonate

The main difficulty facing the neonatologist and geneticist in this situation is to differentiate metabolic or genetic causes of neonatal encephalopathy and seizures from those arising as part of hypoxic ischaemic encephalopathy (HIE). It is important to note that seizures may occur without features of an encephalopathy and that encephalopathy may be present but without seizures.

The features of neonatal encephalopathy

Neonatal encephalopathy in an infant of >36 weeks gestation may be defined as:

- Abnormal tone pattern
- Feeding difficulties
- Altered alertness (usually sleepiness, not waking for feeds, or excessive startle response)
- Three of the following features:
  (1) late decelerations on fetal monitoring or meconium staining
  (2) delayed onset of respiration
  (3) arterial cord blood pH <7.1
  (4) Apgar score <7 at 5 minutes
  (5) multiorgan failure

Usually, by the time the geneticist is called, a basic screen for glucose, calcium, sodium, metabolic acidosis (pH, base excess, and HCO_3^-), liver function, ammonia, uric acid, blood count, and urine dipstick for pH, ketones, and reducing substances will have been completed. Hypoglycaemia, metabolic acidosis, and high levels of ammonia are all features of metabolic conditions and require further investigation. In addition, investigations to exclude sepsis and other non-genetic causes will be in progress (see table).

Cowan et al. (2003) studied 261 infants of >36 weeks gestation with neonatal encephalopathy who were referred to a tertiary referral neonatal intensive care unit (NICU). The fact that the study was not population-based limits the epidemiological conclusions that can be reached, and the possibility of referral bias is another limitation. In Cowan et al.'s (2003) study, cranial magnetic resonance imaging (MRI) scan in 80% showed evidence of acutely evolving lesions that were compatible with a hypoxic ischaemic insult. These lesions were mostly bilateral abnormalities in basal ganglia, thalami, cortex, or white matter (see below). Of the remaining 20%, 16% had normal scans, and the remainder showed either additional findings or had other diagnoses as well as HIE (e.g. absent corpus callosum in non-ketotic hyperglycinaemia (NKH), basal ganglia cysts in a mitochondrial disorder, cerebellar hypoplasia in Walker–Warburg syndrome (WWS), and complex 1 deficiency of the mitochondrial respiratory chain).

Neonatal seizures may be a manifestation of neonatal encephalopathy when they occur in conjunction with abnormal tone, poor feeding, altered alertness, plus signs of fetal distress (see table). They may be difficult to recognize and may take a variey of forms such as episodes of bradycardia with desaturation, repetitive sucking movements of the lips, episodes of hiccoughing, subtle jerking, or twitching movements of the limbs. If there is frequent seizure activity, the baby may also have been treated with anticonvulsants (e.g. phenobarbitone) and possibly paralysed and ventilated making it difficult to complete a neurological assessment.

Cowan et al.'s (2003) study found a high rate of focal infarctions or haemorrhages in infants with seizures who did not meet other criteria for encephalopathy. She studied 90 infants of >36 weeks gestation who had seizures within 72 hours of birth, but not neonatal encephalopathy and who were referred to a tertiary referral NICU. Cranial MRI scan in most infants (69%) had evidence of an acutely developing region of focal infarction in an arterial territory or in a parasagittal distribution. A substantial proportion (31%) had an identifiable metabolic, neurocutaneous, vascular, or developmental disorder that was clearly of genetic or congenital origin, e.g. tuberous sclerosis (TS), incontinentia pigmenti (IP), Zellweger syndrome, neonatal adrenoleukodystrophy, non-ketotic hyperglycaemia, cortical dysplasia.

MRI scans in neonatal encephalopathy or seizures give results according to the timing of the scan.

- Scans within the first 24 hours of life may give a false-negative result.
- The most abnormal scan results, indicating very recent insult, arise in the first 1–5 days of life.
- Evidence of atrophy associated with perinatal insults does not appear within 2 weeks of birth (if present, it suggests an antenatal cause).

Clinical approach

History: key points

- Three-generation family history with specific enquiry for consanguinity and seizures or illness or infant/neonatal death.
- Were fetal movements normal or reduced? Were there periodic bursts of repetitive fetal activity or hiccoughs *in utero* suggestive of antenatal seizure activity?
- Is there a history of maternal drug ingestion making it possible that the infant is suffering from drug withdrawal, e.g. opiates, valproate?
- Detailed account of events in pregnancy. Were there any events in the third trimester that may have resulted in neurological damage (e.g. ante-partum haemorrhage, death of an identical co-twin)?
- Detailed account of the labour and delivery. Was there any suggestion of fetal distress?
- What were the Apgar scores at delivery and was resuscitation required?
- Was the baby handling normally and feeding well before the onset of symptoms (babies who appear normal at birth and handle and feed well and subsequently deteriorate are more likely to have a metabolic cause)? Organic acidaemias and urea cycle defects tend to present on days 2–3 (protein load from feeding).
- How old was the infant when the first abnormalities were noted?

Examination: key points

- Is the occipital-frontal circumference (OFC) within normal limits?
- Assess the posture and tone of the infant and note any abnormal movements such as tremor or myoclonic jerks.
- Is the anterior fontanelle large? (Consider Zellweger syndrome.)

- Are there dysmorphic features?
- Does the baby have an unusual odour (e.g. maple syrup urine disease (MSUD), isovaleric acidaemia)?
- Hepatomegaly or liver failure (see 'Prolonged neonatal jaundice and jaundice in infants below 6 months', page 220.
- Cardiomyopathy (see 'Cardiomyopathy in children under 10 years', page 60).

Special investigations
Check that non-genetic causes of encephalopathy are being concurrently investigated, e.g. infection, meningitis, infarction.
- Cranial ultrasound scan (USS) to identify structural brain anomalies.
- Computerized tomography (CT) and MRI scans will demonstrate cortical abnormalities better than USS. The hazards of transporting a ventilated neonate to the scanner need to be balanced against the need to make a diagnosis. This is an important investigation that should be considered if initial rapidly available blood tests are normal and there is still no diagnosis in the face of continuing seizures or encephalopathy. Non-contrast CT should be performed to detect haemorrhagic lesions in the encephalopathic term infant with a history of birth trauma, low haematocrit, or coagulopathy. If CT findings are inconclusive, MRI should be performed between days 2 and 8 to assess the location and extent of injury. The pattern of injury identified with conventional MRI may provide diagnostic and prognostic information for term infants with evidence of encephalopathy. In particular, basal ganglia and thalamic lesions detected by conventional MRI are associated with poor neurodevelopmental outcome (Ment *et al.* 2002).
- Electroencephalography (EEG).
- Cardiac echo and electrocardiography (ECG).
- Plasma amino acids and urine amino and organic acids.
- Two blood spot cards for tandem mass spectrometric analyses. (Diseases diagnosable by these techniques will probably vary between centres.)
- Urine dinitrophenylhydrazine (DPNH); test for the presence of alpha-keto acids (MSUD).
- Sulfitest (sulphite oxidase deficiency).
- Clotting studies (liver dysfunction).
- 3OH-butyrate and acetoacetate (plasma samples) done at the same time as the lactate and pyruvate (respiratory chain disorders).
- Acyl carnitine (can be measured on a dried blood spot, e.g. Guthrie card).
- Cerebrospinal fluid (CSF) glycine and lactate (NB. CSF lactate may be high after asphyxia and takes longer to fall than blood lactate; it is also affected by fitting).
- Ophthalmological opinion (looking for cataracts, optic atrophy).
- Karyotype; consider fluorescent *in situ* hybridization (FISH) for Miller–Dieker microdeletion 17p13.3.
- Consider coagulation studies, e.g. thrombophilia screen, if the MRI scan is suggestive of an arterial stroke.
- *If the neonate seems likely not to survive*, consider arranging for DNA to be saved (EDTA sample), 2 spots of blood on filter paper, plasma (heparinized sample) and urine to be frozen at −20°C, CSF (1 ml) frozen, a skin biopsy for fibroblast culture, a muscle and liver biopsy frozen at −70°C, clinical photographs, and a skeletal and chest X-ray.

In infants with dysmorphic features and/or seizures, consider the following additional investigations.
- Mg level.
- Biotinidase (plasma).
- Very long chain fatty acids (VLCFAs).
- Transferrin isoelectrophoresis (chronic granulomatous disease (CGD)).
- Cholesterol, 7-dehydrocholesterol (Smith–Lemli–Opitz (SLO) syndrome).
- Enzyme analysis for lysosomal disorders.
- Has the infant had a trial of pyridoxine under EEG monitoring?
- In males consider *MeCP2* and *ARX* analysis as both may present as severe neonatal encephalopathy.

Some diagnoses to consider
Note that pyridoxine-dependent seizures, folinic acid responsive seizures, biotin-responsive multicarboxylase deficiency, and congenital malabsorption of magnesium are *treatable* conditions.

Hypoxic ischaemic encephalopathy (HIE). The main issue is to determine whether the degree of asphyxia at delivery correlates with the subsequent clinical course. In HIE fits usually start after 6–12 hours.

Germinal matrix haemorrhage/intraventricular haemorrhage and cortical intraparenchymal haemorrhage are usually seen on neuroimaging of infants with HIE. MRI and CT are more sensitive for identifying intraparenchymal haemorrhage than USS. Consider getting an expert opinion as to whether the MRI/CT scan findings are supportive of a diagnosis of HIE (see table).

MRI scan abnormalities suggestive of an acute perinatal insult (after Cowan *et al.* 2003)

Brain swelling

Cortical highlighting

Focal or global loss of grey–white matter differentiation

Abnormal signal density in the basal ganglia and thalami—typically the posterior putamen and venterolateral nucleus of the thalamus (VLNT) but could include the caudate nucles and globus pallidus

Loss of normal signal intensity in the posterior limb of the internal capsule (PLIC) associated with the above cortical, white matter or basal ganglia and thalami abnormality

Acute and subacute parenchymal, intraventricular, or extracerebral haemorrhage

Acutely evolving focal infarction in an arterial territory or in a parasaggital or watershed distribution

The geneticist should be wary of this diagnosis if the above features are not present.

With neurological deterioration and seizures
Non-ketotic hyperglycinaemia (NKH). NKH is an autosomal recessive (AR) disorder due to abnormality of the glycine-cleavage enzyme. The incidence of NKH is 1/50 000–1/100 000, except in Finland where the incidence is higher. Characteristically fits begin in the first 24 hours of life and are accompanied by bursts of hiccoughing. The baby becomes profoundly floppy and compromised requiring ventilatory support. CSF glycine levels are typically increased out of proportion to the increases in plasma levels. In order to offer prenatal diagnosis in a subsequent pregnancy it is advisable to confirm the glycine cleavage enzyme activity in a liver biopsy. This can be taken immediately post-mortem and snap-frozen in a plain tube

without medium and placed in liquid nitrogen. Enzyme activity can be assayed in liver (100–300 mg tissue) and trophoblast, but is not present in fibroblasts. The glycine cleavage enzyme comprises four subunits, each encoded by a different gene. Mutation analysis is complicated by the fact that most mutations are likely to be rare or private except in Finnish patients where there is a founder effect. Unless the causative mutations are known, prenatal diagnosis depends upon assay of enzyme activity in uncultured chorionic villi.

With predominantly neurological deterioration

Maple syrup urine disease (MSUD), organic acidaemias, and urea cycle disorders. Babies with these conditions rarely have seizures in the absence of encephalopathy or hypoglycaemia. The EEG shows a periodic pattern with bursts of intense activity alternating with almost flat readings.

Multiple carboxylase deficiency (MCD). Holocarboxylase synthetase (HLCS) deficiency is a rare AR disorder of biotin metabolism. The diagnosis is made by analysis of urine organic acids. The *HLCS* gene encodes an enzyme that catalyses the biotinylation of the four human biotin-dependent carboxylases. The clinical findings, the age of onset, and response to biotin treatment are variable, but this is a treatable condition.

With predominantly intractable seizures

Non-genetic environmental and infective causes.

Pyridoxine-dependent seizures. Incidence is 1/150, 1 in 150,000. AR disorder. One-third had atypical presentations and one-third had features and/or initial diagnosis of birth asphyxia and HIE. A trial of pyridoxine is justified in all cases of early-onset intractable seizures, whatever the suspected cause, as pyridoxine-dependent seizures are treatable.

Biotinidase deficiency (late-onset MCD). Biotin is an essential water-soluble vitamin and is the coenzyme for four carboxylases necessary for normal metabolism in humans (see 'Multiple carboxylase deficiency (MCD)' above). Biotinidase (*BTD*) recycles biotin in the body by cleaving biocytin, a normal product of carboxylase degradation, resulting in regeneration of free biotin. The baby is born with presumably normal stores of free biotin but, once dependent on dietary biotin, becomes deficient with some delay in onset of symptoms (as compared to the neonatal onset in MCD). Age of onset usually 1 week–2 years. Seizures, either alone or with other neurological or cutaneous findings (skin rash and alopecia), are the most frequent initial symptom. Metabolic ketoacidosis and organic aciduria are also features. This condition is treatable.

Folinic acid-responsive seizures. Presents with seizures with onset within a few hours of birth to onset in the first week of life. May be responsive initially to phenobarbitone, but later breakthrough seizures occur. Seizures stop within 24 hours of starting folinic acid. Untreated intractable seizures develop. Torres *et al.* (1999) suggest that trial of folinic acid be considered in neonates with unexplained early-onset intractable seizures. Sibling recurrence has been reported (Torres *et al.* 1999).

Congenital magnesium malabsorption. Primary infantile hypomagnesaemia is an infrequent cause of neonatal hypocalcaemic seizures but one that responds well to magnesium supplementation.

Sulphite oxidase deficiency. Molybdenum cofactor deficiency and isolated sulphite oxidase deficiency are AR inborn errors of metabolism. The phenotype is severe, with progressive neurological damage leading in most cases to early childhood death, and results primarily from the deficiency of sulphite oxidase. The deficiencies can be diagnosed prenatally by monitoring sulphite oxidase activity in chorionic villus sampling (CVS) tissue. In those families in which the specific defects have been identified, diagnosis can be achieved by mutation analysis or linkage studies directed at affected genes. These include *MOCS1*, *MOCS2*, or *GEPH*, in cases of molybdenum cofactor deficiency, or *SUOX* in patients with isolated sulphite oxidase deficiency (Johnson 2003).

Cerebral malformations. Refer to Lissencephaly and neuronal migration disorders page 156.

Early infantile epileptic encephalopathy with suppression burst (Ohtahara syndrome). There are characteristic EEG features. Exclude cortical malformations and respiratory chain disorders. See 'Epilepsy in infants and children', page 314.

Early myoclonic encephalopathy. There are characteristic clinical and EEG features. Exclude metabolic disease.

Benign neonatal convulsions and benign familial neonatal convulsions. See 'Epilepsy in infants and children', page 314.

In males: rare severe presentation of X-linked disorders. Consider mutation in *ARX, NEMO*, and *MeCP2*.

With dysmorphic features

Peroxisomal disorders (e.g. Zellweger). AR condition characterized by dysmorphic features with large fontanelle, high forehead, stippling at knees on X-ray, and raised VLCFAs. See 'Floppy infant', page 118.

Cholesterol biosynthetic defects (e.g. SLO syndrome, desmosterolosis). Prenatal growth deficiency, cleft palate (37–52%), cardiac defects (36–38%), hypospadias, and/or cryptorchidism (90–100%) in affected males. Y-shaped 2, 3 toe syndactyly (95%) and postaxial polydactyly (~50%). See 'Hypospadias', page 142.

Chromosomal disorders. Consider FISH for Miller–Deiker microdeletion 17p13.3.

Genetic advice

Recurrence risk

As for given diagnosis. If the cause remains undiagnosed, the possibility of a genetic condition needs to be considered with a risk of up to 25% for recurrence. Thorough testing usually gives a clue to the aetiological group even if a precise diagnosis is not possible.

If due to HIE, recurrence risk should be low, as long as the diagnosis is secure. Refer to fetal medicine specialist for expert supervision of future pregnancy and delivery.

Prenatal diagnosis

May be possible if known diagnosis; otherwise not possible.

Lay group contact: CLIMB (Children Living With Inherited Metabolic Diseases) <www.climb.org.uk>.

Expert adviser: Derek Applegarth, Emeritus Professor of Pediatrics, University of British Columbia, Vancouver, British Columbia, Canada.

References

Baxter P. Epidemiology of pyridoxine dependent and pyridoxine responsive seizures in the UK. *Arch Dis Child* 1999; **81**: 431–3.

Blankenberg FG, Loh NN, *et al.* Sonography, CT, and MR imaging: a prospective comparison of neonates with suspected intracranial ischaemia and haemorrhage. *Am J Neurol* 2000; **21**: 213–18.

Cowan F, Rutherford M, *et al.* Origin and timing of brain lesions in term infants with neonatal encephalopathy. *Lancet* 2003; **361**: 736–42.

Johnson JL. Prenatal diagnosis of molybdenum cofactor deficiency and isolated sulfite oxidase deficiency. *Prenat Diagn* 2003; **23** (1): 6–8.

Ment LR, Bada HS, *et al.* Practice parameter: neuroimaging of the neonate: report of the Quality Standards Subcommittee of the American Academy of Neurology and the Practice Committee of the Child Neurology Society. *Neurology* 2002; **58** (12): 1726–38.

Morrone A, Malvagia S, *et al.* Clinical findings and biochemical and molecular analysis of four patients with holocarboxylase synthetase deficiency. *Am J Med Genet* 2002; **111** (1): 10–18.

Saudubray JM, Nassogne MC, de Lonlay P, Touati G. Clinical approach to inherited metabolic disorders in neonates: an overview. *Semin Neonatol* 2002; **7**: 3–15.

Torres OA, Miller VS, *et al.* Folinic acid-responsive neonatal seizures. *J Child Neurol* 1999; **14**: 529–32.

Nystagmus

Nystagmus is an involuntary continuous oscillatory disorder of eye movement. It is commonly described by parents as 'wobbly eyes'. It is a symptom of disordered oculomotor control. In infancy it may be an indicator of bilateral visual impairment; adult onset nystagmus is more likely to be secondary to neurological disease. Nystagmus is usually horizontal, but can be vertical or rotatory.

Clinical approach

History: key points

- Three-generation family history, or more if a suggestion of X-linkage.
- Age of onset.
- Photophobia (achromatopsia, aniridia, albinism).
- Developmental milestones.
- Central nervous system (CNS) symptoms (especially cerebellar in adults).
- Seizures.
- Ensure adequate documentation of ophthalmic and neurological assessment from hospital notes.

Examination: key points

- Detailed eye examination by an ophthalmologist to include slit-lamp examination for iris translucency (albinism) and fundal examination.
- Neurological examination. Assess hypotonia or dystonia in infants; cerebellar and long tract signs in an adult.
- Dysmorphic features as a marker for possible intracerebral malformation.
- Skin (albinism).

Special investigations

- Ophthalmic assessment of eye structure, retina, and disc.
- Electrophysiology of visual system (electroretinography (ERG) and visual evoked potentials (VEPs)) to rule out retinal dystrophies and albinism.
- All children with acquired nystagmus of onset >6 months of age need a magnetic resonance imaging (MRI) brain scan to rule out chiasmal disease.
- Chromosome analysis if dysmorphic features or significant unexplained developmental delay.
- Metabolic and/or endocrine screen if there are signs of a progressive condition.
- DNA sample. Specific genetic testing may be available. If not, store DNA for possible future diagnostic use.
- Consider video of nystagmus if unusual.

Some diagnoses to consider

In infants

Optic nerve hypoplasia

Commonly presents with nystagmus, if bilateral. See 'Optic nerve hypoplasia', page 204.

Infantile retinal dystrophies

These include the following.

Rod monochromatism or achromatopsia. Total colour blindness is rare autosomal recessive (AR) disease characterized by early onset of photophobia, poor visual acuity, and total colour blindness that involves complete absence of all cone function. A number of mutations in the genes encoding the cone-specific α- and β-subunits of the cation channel (CNGA3 and CNGB3) and the α-subunit of transducin (GNAT2) have been implicated in this disorder.

X-linked blue cone monochromatism. A rare disorder that involves absence of red and green cone function. It is caused either by deletion of a critical region that regulates expression of the red/green gene array, or by mutations that inactivate the red and green pigment genes.

Congenital stationary night blindness. Normal fundus. Inheritance AR or X-linked (two X-linked genes have been identified). The autosomal dominant (AD) form of congenital stationary night blindess does *not* have nystagmus.

Leber congenital amaurosis. Leber congenital amaurosis (LCA) is one of the most common inherited cause of blindness in childhood and is characterized by a severe infantile rod–cone dystrophy that presents in the first few months of life with poor vision and nystagmus or roving eye movements. Eight genes have been identified that together account for ~50% of all LCA patients. These genes are expressed preferentially in the retina or the retinal pigment epithelium. Their putative functions are quite diverse and include retinal embryonic development (*CRX*), photoreceptor cell structure (*CRB1*), phototransduction (*GUCY2D*), protein trafficking (*AIPL1, RPGRIP1*), and vitamin A metabolism (*RPE65*) (Cremers *et al.* 2002). The fundus often appears normal in infancy but the ERG is very subnormal or, more usually, non-recordable. Later there may be signs of retinal degeneration. Variable neurological involvement and seizures may be present. Mostly AR. Retinal dystrophy similar to that in LCA is also seen in a number of syndromes including the following three.

Joubert syndrome. See 'Cerebellar anomalies', page 66.

Peroxisomal disorders. Check plasma very long chain fatty acids (VLCFAs) and phytanic acid.

Alstrom syndrome. Rare AR syndrome caused by mutations in *ALMS1* on 2p13. Alstrom syndrome is characterized by childhood obesity with type 2 diabetes mellitus (hyperinsulinism and chronic hyperglycaemia) and neurosensory defects, e.g.cone–rod retinal dystrophy. A subset of individuals have dilated cardiomyopathy, hepatic dysfunction, hypothyroidism, male hypogonadism, short stature, and mild/moderate developmental delay.

Ocular and oculocutaneous albinism

Ocular albinism is X-linked. Oculocutaneous albinism is AR.

X-linked ocular albinism (XLOA; Nettleship-Falls) affects ~1/50 000 males in the population and is due to mutations in *OA1* at Xp22.32. It results in hypopigmentation of the iris and retina, nystagmus, strabismus, foveal hypoplasia, abnormal decussation of the optic nerve fibres, and reduced visual acuity. Female carriers of XLOA have a classic pattern of mosaic retinal pigmentation and patchy iris translucency. Carriers also have macromelanosomes on skin biopsy. Approximately 50% of reported mutations in *OA1* are intragenic deletions and the rest are point mutations.

Oculocutaneous albinism (OCA). See 'Generalized disorders of pigmentation (including albinism)', page 126.

Other

Congenital idiopathic motor nystagmus. This is the most common form of childhood nystagmus and is usually non-genetic, but X-linked and AD forms are reported.

Pelizaeus–Merzbacher disease. Absent myelination on brain MRI scan. X-linked recessive. Mutations and duplications in the *PLP* gene.

Adult onset

Mostly caused by neurological diseases. It is important for a neurologist to evaluate the patient to exclude tumours and other non-genetic causes.

AD cerebellar ataxia. Test for *SCA* genes. Assess if retinopathy is a feature (ADCA type 7). See 'Ataxic adult', page 50.

Genetic advice

Recurrence risk

When no other disorder has been identified, and the nystagmus is an isolated feature, consider the possibility of **idiopathic** or **motor nystagmus**. This condition may be sporadic, but careful evaluation of the family may reveal a family history. AD, AR, and, most commonly, X-linked (XL) inheritance have been described. It is possible that the XL type may be allelic to other XL ophthalmic conditions such as: congenital stationary night blindness; ocular albinism; Åland island disease; X-linked optic atrophy.

Carrier detection

Possible by molecular genetic analysis in those families where the diagnosis is known and in whom a causative mutation has been identified.

Examination of the eye including fundal examination and electrophysiology in other family members may help, particularly in XL conditions.

Prenatal diagnosis

Available to those families where there is molecular confirmation of diagnosis.

Natural history and further management (preventative measures)

Long-term follow-up with an ophthalmologist or neurologist, or both, depending on the diagnosis.

Lay group contact: Nystagmus network <www.nystagmus.org>, Tel. 01392 627004; Albinism fellowship <www.albinism.org.uk>, Tel. 01282 771900.

Expert adviser: Anonymous.

References

Cremers FP, van den Hurk JA, *et al.* Molecular genetics of Leber congenital amaurosis. *Hum Mol Genet* 2002; **11**: 1169–76.

Deeb SS, Kohl S. Genetics of color vision deficiencies. *Dev Ophthalmol* 2003; **37**: 170–87.

Hearn T, Renforth GL. Mutation of ALMS1, a large gene with a tandem repeat encoding 47 amino acids, causes Alstrom syndrome. *Nat Genet* 2002; **31** (1): 79–83.

Hodgkins P, Harris CM. Paediatric eye movement disorders. In *Paediatric ophthalmology*, Fundamentals of Clinical Ophthalmology series (ed. A. Moore), Chapter 15, pp. 191–9. BMJ Books, London, 2000.

Kerrison JB. New genetic, pathophysiologic and therapeutic issues in nystagmus. *Curr Opin Ophthalmol* 1999; **10**: 411–19.

Oetting WS. New insights into ocular albinism type 1 (OA1): mutations and polymorphisms of the *OA1* gene. *Hum Mutat* 2002; **19**: 85–92.

Obesity with and without developmental delay

Obesity that prompts referral to the genetic clinic is usually severe (i.e. weight >99.6th centile, or major discrepancy between height and weight, e.g. height on 2nd centile, weight on 90th), and often there are accompanying learning difficulties. With currently available investigations the diagnostic yield is low. See 'Overgrowth', page 206, if all growth parameters are increased.

Body mass index (BMI). BMI = weight (kg)/height^2 (m^2). This formula is based on the assumption that most variation in weight for persons of the same height is due to fat mass. It provides some objective measure of the degree of obesity. The table shows the classification of BMI in adults.

The classification of obesity according to BMI in adults

BMI	WHO (1995) classification	Popular description
<18.5	Underweight	Thin
18.5–24.9	Normal	
25–29.9	Grade 1 overweight	Overweight
30.0–39.9	Grade 2 overweight	Obese
40.0 or greater	Grade 3 overweight	Morbid obesity

Distribution of fat mass. Truncal obesity is characteristic of some syndromes and the extremities can appear normal or even thin. In contrast, when obesity is secondary to excessive calorie intake, fat distribution is usually more generalized.

Clinical approach

History: key points

- Three-generation family tree noting height/weight of parents and siblings and birthweight of siblings and consanguinity.
- Pregnancy and perinatal history with close attention to growth parameters at birth (weight, length, occipital-frontal circumference (OFC)).
- Detailed feeding history in infancy. Were there feeding difficulties and hypotonia in the first year of life (Prader–Willi syndrome (PWS))?
- When did abnormal weight gain begin or was it present from birth (Bardet–Biedl syndrome (BBS), onset obesity within 1st year of life; PWS, onset after 1st year)
- What is the child's appetite like; is there food searching/stealing?
- Detailed developmental and behavioural profile.
- Is there any indication of visual deficit/night blindness (BBS/Cohen syndrome/Alstrom syndrome)?
- Deafness (Alstrom syndrome)

Examination: key points

- Growth parameters (height, weight, OFC).
- Distribution of obesity. Truncal obesity is typical of PWS, BBS, Alstrom syndrome, and Cohen syndrome.
- Are there dysmorphic features? Difficult to assess if there is facial obesity, but children with Albright hereditary osteodystrophy (AHO) have a flattened facial profile and those with Cohen syndrome typically have large prominent upper incisors. Red hair (POMC)
- Are the hands generally small (PWS/Smith–Magenis syndrome (SMS)); is there brachydactyly (BBS); are the 4th/5th metacarpals short (ask child to make a fist and

look at knuckle profile); AHO); is there syndactyly (usually 2,3 toes) or polydactyly (BBS/Carpenter syndrome)?
- Discrete foci of calcification in skin (AHO).
- Small genitalia are commonly seen in males with PWS and BBS. Female genital tract anomalies common in BBS.
- Is there acanthosis nigrigans (thickened hyperpigmentation of axillae and skin folds indicative of insulin resistance; AS)?
- Cardiovascular system. Hypertension, murmurs (aortic stenosis/left ventricular hypertrophy (LVH); BBS).
- Eyes should be examined for visual field defects, strabismus, myopia, photophobia, and retinal pigmentation (BBS, Alstrom syndrome, Cohen syndrome).

Special investigations

- Thyroxine (T4)/thryoid-stimulating hormone (TSH). Hypothyroidism can present with obesity in childhood; also high incidence of hypothyroidism in AHO.
- Consider random urine cortisol (to exclude Cushing syndrome).
- Consider measuring levels of testosterone, gonadotrophins, growth hormone, fasting glucose; consider glucose tolerance test (PWS, BBS, Alstrom syndrome).

If associated developmental delay also include the following.
- Chromosome analysis and telomere screen.
- DNA for fragile X syndrome (FRAXA) studies.
- PWS methylation studies if history of hypotonia with poor suck.
- Full blood count (FBC) with differential white blood cell (WBC) count. Neutropenia is seen in Cohen syndrome.
- Ophthalmology for retinitis pigmentosa (RP) plus electroretinogram (ERG) if considering BBS or Cohen syndrome (ERG not feasible in very young infants).
- Plasma Ca and parathyroid hormone (PTH; low Ca and high/normal PTH suggestive of AHO, but levels can be normal).
- Renal ultrasound scan (USS) if considering BBS.
- Hand X-ray to assess metacarpal length if clinically suspect (AHO).

Some diagnoses to consider

Prader–Willi syndrome (PWS). The most common recognized genetic form of obesity affecting 1/10 000–15 000 individuals. Babies have central hypotonia and feeding difficulties with failure to thrive in infancy. There is rapid weight gain between the ages of 1 and 6 years (usually 2–4 years), characterized by truncal obesity with small hands and feet, strikingly fat limbs, small genitalia in males, and short stature. Typically, there is insatiable appetite and food-seeking/hoarding. Most patients have intelligent quotients (IQs) in the 60s–low 70s, approximately 40% have borderline retardation or low normal intelligence, and 20% have moderate retardation. Overall, the IQ of a population-based sample of PWS patients is normally distributed with a mean IQ of 60, with parental and social factors accounting for the distribution as they do in the general population. Individuals with PWS are often good at jigsaws and word-find puzzles. Behavioural problems can be a major issue and 80% have some ritualistic behaviours (Holland *et al.* 2003). Most adults with PWS will require support/supervision in adult life and few will live independently. Both males and females have hypogonadotrophic hypogonadism. Sexual activity is uncommon and fertility is rare (but note if deletion; girls are at 50% risk for a child with Angelman syndrome (AS)—birth of an AS child to a PWS mother has been reported by Schulze *et al.* (2001)).

Due to imprinting, the maternally inherited genes on 15q11 (in the Prader–Willi/Angelman syndrome critical region (PWACR)) are usually inactivated and normal development is dependent upon paternally inherited genes. 75% of patients with PWS have del 15q11–13, 24% have maternal uniparental disomy (UPD)15, and only 1% have an imprinting defect (abnormal methylation but normal fluorescent *in situ* hybridization (FISH) and UPD studies). Small nuclear ribonuclear protein-associated polypeptide N (SNRPN) methylation analysis detects PWS in 99%.

Bardet–Biedl syndrome (BBS). Eight genes have been cloned (*BBS1-8*). One locus is allelic to McKusick–Kaufman syndrome (*BBS6*). The gene loci identified so far account for only 50% of cases suggesting the existence of further loci.

BBS is characterized by a pigmentary retinal dystrophy, postaxial polydactyly, obesity, cognitive impairment, and renal defects. For the majority of cases, BBS follows a Mendelian autosomal recessive (AR) pattern of inheritance; however, a few families exhibit 'triallelic inheritance'. In these families three mutations in at least two loci appear to be necessary to manifest the disorder, but occasionally the third mutant allele may modify the severity of the phenotype. The incidence in the UK is <1/100 000, but this is higher in some ethnic groups. Individuals with BBS are at risk for progressive renal insufficiency and creatinine and blood pressure should be monitored at 6 month intervals.

BBS has recently been shown to be caused by dysfunction of primary cilia as defined by photoreceptor degeneration, renal tubular disease and very occasional situs inversus (Snell).

Cohen syndrome. AR disorder consisting of characteristic craniofacial appearance with prominent upper incisors, global developmental delay, truncal obesity in mid-childhood with relatively short stature, severe myopia with visual impairment and choroidal–retinal dystrophy (mottled pigmentation of retina with ERG changes), and benign neutropenia. The myopia usually starts at <5 years and progresses to >–7 SD by the second decade. Young children have a 'bull's eye' maculopathy and, by the age of 10 years, patients have a generalized symptomatic retinopathy with attenuated or extinguished ERG. Visual handicap is progressive and significant with 35% registered partially sighted or blind. The neutropenia does not predispose to infection and does not generally require treatment. The gene for Cohen syndrome (*COH1*) was cloned recently and maps to 8q22–23. The incidence in the UK is probably <1/100 000.

Diagnostic criteria for Cohen syndrome (after Chandler *et al.* 2003) are as follows.
- Significant learning difficulties (children with Cohen syndrome have moderate to severe learning difficulties).
- At least two of the following three criteria:
  - facial gestalt, characterized by thick hair, eyebrows, and eyelashes, wave-shaped, downward slanting palpebral fissures, prominent beaked-shaped nose, upturned philtrum with grimacing expression on smiling;
  - pigmentary retinopathy;
  - neutropenia (defined as $<2 \times 10^9/\text{mm}^3$).

In addition there are a number of less specific but supportive criteria that are very common in Cohen syndrome: (1) early onset, progressive myopia; (2) microcephaly; (3) truncal obesity with slender extremities; and (4) joint hyperextensibility.

Albright hereditary osteodystrophy (AHO). This term describes a phenotype characterized by short adult stature with generalized obesity and relative microcephaly, brachydactyly particularly involving the distal phalanges (especially of the thumbs) and metacarpals/metatarsals, mild to moderate learning disability, and cutaneous ossifications (subcutaneous or intradermal lumps or flakes) in around 60%. The facial features are subtle but usually patients have a round face with a short neck, short nose, and mild mid-face hypoplasia. The obesity is not usually associated with hyperphagia. The brachydactyly is associated with cone-epiphyses and disharmonic bone age. Stature may be normal or above average in childhood but there is reduced longitudinal growth and early epiphyseal closure. The condition tends to be overdiagnosed largely because, with the exception of the cutaneous ossifications, the physical findings are non-specific.

The basis of the AHO phenotype is a 50% reduction in bioactivity of Gsα, a subunit of the heterotrimeric G-protein that transduces signals between various cell-surface hormone receptors and intracellular adenyl cyclase. It results from heterozygous deactivating mutations in the *GNAS* gene. *GNAS* is subject to tissue-specific imprinting. Mutations on the maternally derived allele are associated with **pseudohypoparathyroidism** (PHP type Ia) where individuals have variable hypocalcaemia due to end-organ resistance to PTH, and abnormal thyroid function due to resistance to TSH and thyroid-releasing hormone (TRH). Mutations of the paternally derived allele are not associated with endocrine abnormalities and these patients with AHO are said to have **pseudo-pseudohypoparathyroidism** (PPHP).

- **Diagnosis of AHO.** Where subcutaneous ossifications and/or PHP type Ia (including raised PTH and abnormal thyroid function) are present in association with other features of AHO, the diagnosis is very likely. Currently measurement of Gsα bioactivity is not routinely available. Screening *GNAS* for sequence changes in the exons and adjacent splice sites detected mutations in around 75% of a cohort with confirmed reductions in Gsα bioactivity. Most mutations are family-specific.
- **Diagnosis of PHP.** PTH stimulation testing is no longer performed owing to difficulties in obtaining PTH for human injection. Random PTH levels are usually very high in association with normal or low calcium and normal or raised inorganic phosphate. TSH levels are often high with triiodothyronine (T3)/T4 levels that may be normal or reduced. Note that PHP can occur in isolation (i.e. with a normal thyroid axis and no features of AHO) when it is known as PHP type Ib. Abnormal methylation of exon 1A, upstream of *GNAS* has been reported in at least some patients.

Uniparental disomy (UPD)14. The incidence is unknown, but it is worth considering if PWS investigations are negative and there are no other clues.

Smith–Magenis syndrome (SMS). Some patients are short and obese with small hands and feet, as well as square, rather heavy facies. They may have a history of hypotonia in infancy, developmental delay, behaviour disturbance (especially sleep), and sometimes food-searching behaviour. If PWS testing is negative, consider FISH for SMS (17p) if there is a history of sleep disturbance. Some individuals with SMS have mutations in *RAI1* a gene encompassed by the common 17p11.2 microdeletion (Slager *et al.* 2003).

Monosomy 1p36. Some patients with monosomy 1p36 develop childhood obesity. The clinical picture includes neonatal hypotonia, feeding problems in infancy and developmental delay often with seizures. See 'Submicroscopic chromosomal rearrangments', page 546.

Alstrom syndrome. Rare AR syndrome caused by mutations in *ALMS1* on 2p13. Alstrom syndrome is characterized by childhood obesity with type 2 diabetes mellitus (hyperinsulinism and chronic hyperglycaemia) and neurosensory defecits, e.g. cone–rod retinal dystrophy. A subset of individuals have dilated cardiomyopathy, hepatic dysfunction, hypothyroidism, male hypogonadism, short stature, and mild/moderate developmental delay.

Congenital leptin deficiency. Very rare AR disorder causing extreme obesity from early childhood. Children are born with a normal birthweight, but marked hyperphagia accompanied by weight acceleration begins after weaning. No cognitive impairment. The disorder is treatable with recombinant human leptin with dramatic effects on appetite and normalization of weight.

Leptin receptor deficiency. AR disorder characterized by hypogonadism, short stature, and hypothyroidism.

Pro-opiomelanocortin (POMC). AR disorder characterized by red hair, pale skin with isolated adrenocorticotrophic hormone (ACTH) deficiency presenting as adrenal crisis or features of cortisol deficiency in neonatal life, and hyperphagia.

Melanocortin 4 receptor (*MC4R*). Disorder characterized by increased growth velocity in childhood, hyperphagia, and severe hyperinsulinaemia. Usually autosomal dominant (AD) inheritance, but homozygotes with *MC4R* mutations have been identified in consanguineous families where heterozygotes have an intermediate phenotype suggesting co-dominant inheritance. This is the most common monogenic form of human obesity. Mutations in *MC4R* are found in 1–7% of patients with BMI >40 who become severely obese before the age of 10 years (Farooqi).

TrkB. Specific pattern of impaired short term memory, hyperactivity, impaired nociception and generalized developmental delay as well as hyperphagia and severe obesity. Caused by 'de novo' heterozygous mutations in *NTRK2*, which encodes TrkB which plays a crucial role of in the human nervous system (Yeo).

Hypothalamic disorder. Acquired hypothalamic injury from head injury, tumours, etc. can cause hyperphagia and behavioural disorders closely mimicking PWS. Consider paediatric neurology referral/magnetic resonance imaging (MRI) brain scan if problems are of recent onset with a short history to exclude a tumour.

Genetic advice

Recurrence risk

If you are able to make a syndromic diagnosis, counsel appropriately. In the majority of children it will not prove possible to make a diagnosis with currently available investigations.

Carrier detection

Not possible unless a molecular genetic diagnosis has been possible in the proband and the familial mutations are known.

Prenatal diagnosis

Not possible unless a specific diagnosis has been made with laboratory confirmation. Could look for polydactyly on USS for BBS, but this is not a universal feature.

Natural history and further management (preventative measures)

- Consider referral to paediatric endocrinologist.
- Refer to dietician.

Support group contacts: Prader–Willi Syndrome Association (UK) <www.pwsa.co.uk>, Tel. 01332 365676; Prader–Willi Syndrome Association (USA) Tel. 1 800 926 4797, <www.pwsausa.org>; LMBB (Lawrence–Moon–Bardet–Biedl) Society <www.lmbbs.org.uk>, Tel. 01892 682680; Cohen Syndrome Support Group Tel. 0161 653 0867.

Expert advisers: Philip Beales, Wellcome Trust Senior Research Fellow and Honorary Consultant, Institute of Child Health, London, Louise Wilson, Consultant Clinical Geneticist, Great Ormond Street Hospital, London, and Sadaf Farooqi, Wellcome Clinician Scientist Fellow, Department of Clinical Biochemistry, University of Cambridge, Cambridge, England.

References

Barshn GS, Farooqi IS, O'Rahilly S. Genetics of body weight regulation: applications and opportunities. *Nature* 2000; **404**: 644–51.

Beales PL, Elcioglu N, et al. New criteria for improved diagnosis of Bardet–Biedl syndrome: results of a population survey. *J Med Genet* 1999; **36**: 437–46.

Cassidy SB. Prader–Willi syndrome. In *Management of genetic syndromes* (ed. S.B. Cassidy and J.E. Allanson), Chapter 18, pp. 301–22. Wiley-Liss, New York, 2001.

Chandler KE, Kidd A, et al. Diagnostic criteria, clinical characteristics, and natural history of Cohen syndrome. *J Med Genet* 2003; **40**: 233–41.

Farooqi IS, Yeo GS, et al. Binge eating as a phenotype of melanocortin 4 receptor gene mutations. *N Engl J Med* 2003; **349**: 606–09.

Farooqi IS, Keogh JM, et al. Clinical spectrum of obesity and mutations in the melanocortin 4 receptor gene. *New Engl J Med* 2003; **348**: 1085–95.

Hearn T, Renforth GL, et al. Mutations of *ALMS1*, a large gene with a tandem repeat encoding 47 amino acids, causes Alstrom syndrome. *Nat Genet* 2002; **31**: 79–83.

Holland AJ, Whittington JE, et al. Behavioural phenotypes associated with specific genetic disorders: evidence from a population-based study of people with Prader–Willi syndrome. *Psychol Med* 2003; **33**: 141–53.

Juppner H. The genetic basis of progressive osseous heteroplasia. *New Engl J Med* 2002; **346**: 128–30.

Kolehmainen J, Black GCM, et al. Cohen syndrome is caused by mutations in a novel gene, *COH1*, encoding a transmembrane protein with a presumed roled in vesicle-mediated sorting and intracellular protein transport. *Am J Hum Genet* 2003; **72**: 1359–69.

Korner J, Leibel RL. To eat or not to eat—how the gut talks to the brain. *New Engl J Med* 2003; **349**: 926–8.

Schulze A, Mogensen H, et al. Fertility in Prader–Willi syndrome: a case report with Angelman syndrome in the offspring. *Acta Paediatr* 2001; **90**: 455–59.

Slager RE, Newton TL, et al. Mutations in *RAI1* associated with Smith–Magenis syndrome. *Nat Genet* 2003; **33**: 466–8.

Snell WJ, Pan J, et al. Cilia and flagella revealed: from flagellar assembly in Chlamydomonas to human obesity disorders. *Cell* 2004; **117**: 693–97.

World Health Organization (WHO). *Physical status: the use and interpretation of anthropometry. Report of a WHO Expert Committee*, WHO Technical Report Series, no. 854. WHO, Geneva, 1995.

Yeo GS, Connie Hung CC, et al. A de novo mutation affecting human TrkB associated with severe obesity and developmental delay. *Nat Neurosci* 2004; **7**: 1187–89.

Ocular hypertelorism

Ocular hypertelorism is otherwise known as widely spaced eyes. In clinical practice measurements are made of the inner and outer canthal distances and the interpupillary distance. In ocular hypertelorism the interpupillary distance is increased. Orbital measurements from X-rays can also be used.

It is important to distinguish true ocular hypertelorism from telecanthus (lateral displacement of the inner canthi and lacrimal puncta as seen in Waardenburg syndrome type 1) and epicanthic folds (see figure).

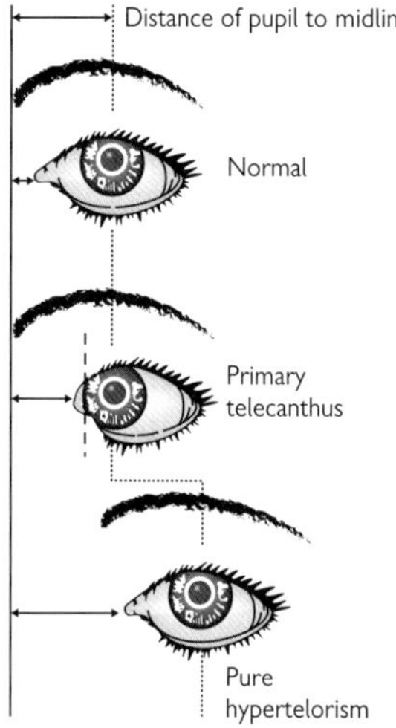

Comparison of telecanthus and ocular hypertelorism.

There is no single mechanism that gives rise to this feature. Isolated hypertelorism is rare; thus it is usually found as part of a syndrome. Chromosomal disorders, single gene disorders, and environmental factors can all give this phenotype. In this section we will concentrate on those syndromes where ocular hypertelorism is a major diagnostic feature.

Clinical approach

History: key points

- Family history. Note that some of the conditions are X-linked.
- Twin. Frontonasal dysplasia is more common in twins.
- Neurological problems/developmental delay.
- Laryngeal abnormalities and swallowing difficulties in Opitz syndrome.
- Environmental factors such as teratogen exposure.

Examination: key points

- Stature and proportions (short in Robinow and Aarskog syndromes).
- Cranial shape and size, any asymmetry, or plagiocephaly.
- Frontal encephalocele (frontonasal dysplasia).
- Hairline, widow's peak (Opitz syndrome).
- Bifid nose/nasal tip—grooved when viewed from above.
- Cleft lip/palate. Hypertelorism can occur secondary to major facial clefts.
- Gum hypertrophy (Robinow syndrome).

- Sloping shoulders (craniofrontonasal dysplasia (CFNS)).
- Cardiac murmur. Sometimes children with Noonan or LEOPARD (lentigines–ECG abnormalities–ocular hypertelorism–pulmonary stenosis–abnormal genitalia–retardation of growth–deafness) syndromes have hypertelorism but it is usually mild.
- Genitalia (shawl scrotum in Aarskog, small penis in Robinow, hypospadias in Opitz syndrome).
- Polysyndactyly (Greig syndrome).
- Longitudinal nail ridges/splits (CFNS)

Special investigations

- Careful eye measurements and ophthalmological assessment (eye measurements taken in clinic are difficult to do with accuracy especially interpupillary distance (IPD)). Beware of parallax errors. Eye measurements should be related to occipital-frontal circumference (OFC).
- Skull X-ray (craniosynostosis, small defects in frontal area).
- Brain imaging may be appropriate, especially to determine if there are any midline abnormalities, e.g. agenesis of the corpus callosum.
- Skeletal survey (Robinow syndrome).
- Consider referral for laryngoscopy in infants with Opitz syndrome.
- Chromosome analysis.
- DNA for storage or specific molecular genetic testing.

Syndromic diagnoses to consider

Frontonasal dysplasia is a malformation. It is usually sporadic and more common in twins. Severely affected infants have a midline facial cleft with encephalocele; those mildly affected have hypertelorism and bifid nasal tip.

Craniofrontonasal dysplasia (CFNS). The presence of coronal synostosis and facial asymmetry help distinguish this condition. Ridged nails, syndactyly, sloping shoulders, and cleft lip are other features. X-linked disorder mapping to Xp22 and caused by mutation in the ephrin-B1 gene (*EFNB1*) (Twigg). Females are more severely affected than males.

Opitz syndrome. Previously known as Opitz G/BBB and named after the initials of the original families. A gene *MID1*, on the X chromosome at Xp22 does not account for all cases and there is a second locus on 22q with autosomal dominant (AD) inheritance. In addition to ocular hypertelorism, affected individuals may have hypospadias and cleft lip and/or palate, and some have a laryngeal cleft that may cause feeding/respiratory problems.

Greig cephalopolysyndactyly. AD condition characterized by a high forehead with frontal bossing, macrocephaly, hypertelorism, and a broad base to the nose. Both pre- and postaxial polydactyly can occur but postaxial polydactyly is more common and is usually type B. The thumbs are often broad. Caused by mutations in *GLI3* on 7p13.

Aarskog syndrome (faciogenital dysplasia). Aarskog syndrome is a genetically heterogeneous developmental disorder characterized by short stature (rhizomelic), ptosis in some, hypertelorism, hypermetropia, shawl scrotum, and brachydactyly with hyperextendable proximal interphalangeal (PIP) joints. Facial features tend to normalize with age. Mental retardation is present in only a minority of affected males and is seldom severe. The X-linked form is caused by mutations in the *FGD1* gene. Behavioural and learning problems in childhood occur in ~50% of males with the X-linked form (Orrico *et al.* 2004). Some families appear to show AD inheritance.

Robinow syndrome. Both AD and autosomal recessive (AR) types. Skeletal survey to assess mesomelia, costovertebral abnormalities, and distinctive phalangeal changes. There is brachydactyly with abnormal orientation of the thumbs and occasional bifid thumbs. Large mouth and tongue, gingival hypertrophy, micropenis, and congenital heart defects. The AR type is due to homozygous abnormality in the *ROR2* gene. Different heterozygous mutations in *ROR2* cause brachydactyly type B.

Teebi syndrome. Teebi (1987) has reported, separately, patients with features similar to those of craniofrontonasal syndrome and Aarskog syndrome.

Genetic advice

Carefully examine parents and note ocular measurements before counselling an apparently sporadic case.

Recurrence risk

This is low in cases of frontonasal dysplasia and those syndromes where a *de novo* mutation has been established by DNA testing. Counsel for individual syndrome as appropriate.

Carrier detection

May be possible by molecular testing (see above) or by clinical examination.

Prenatal diagnosis

Although ultrasound scans (USS) can provide details of the phenotype from the second trimester onwards, and there are normal ranges for eye spacing at different gestations, only very significant hypertelorism could be confidently predicted from prenatal scans.

Natural history and further management (preventative measures)

Children with significant hypertelorism need multidisciplinary assessment by a specialist craniofacial team, including careful ophthalmological assessment (strabismus).

Support group contact: Many of the individual syndromes have their own support groups. See Contact a Family (UK) <www.cafamily.org.uk> and National Organisation for Rare Disorders (US) <www.rarediseases.org>.

Expert adviser: A.O.M. Wilkie, Nuffield Professor of Pathology and Honorary Consultant in Clinical Genetics, University of Oxford, Oxford, England.

References

Gorlin RJ, Cohen MM, Hennekam RCM. (ed.). *Syndromes of the head and neck*, 4th edn. Oxford University Press, Oxford, 2001.

Orrico A, Galli L, *et al.* Phenotypic and molecular characterisation of the Aarskog–Scott syndrome: a survey of the clinical variability in light of FGD1 mutation analysis in 46 patients. *Eur J Hum Genet* 2004; **12** (1): 16–23.

Patton M. Robinow syndrome. *J Med Genet* 2002; **39**: 305–10.

Teebi AS. A new autosomal dominant syndrome resembling craniofrontonasal dysplasia. *Am J Med Genet* 1987; **28**: 581–91.

Trockenbacher A, Suckow V, *et al.* MID1, mutated in Opitz syndrome, encodes an ubiquitin ligase that targets phosphatase 2A for degradation. *Nat Genet* 2001; **29**: 287–94.

Twigg SR, Kan R, *et al.* Mutations of ephrin-B1 (*EFNB1*), a marker of tissue boundary formation, cause craniofrontonasal syndrome. *PNAS* 2004; **101**: 8652–57.

Oedema—generalized or puffy extremities

Generalized oedema may occur in any very sick neonate, particularly if there has been inadequate nutritional support. It does not usually have a genetic basis. The causes of generalized oedema in the very preterm infant merge with the causes of fetal hydrops, some of which are genetic (see 'Oedema—nuchal translucency, cystic hygroma, and hydrops' page 618). If the infant is sick, severe anaemia and hypoalbuminaemia will usually have been excluded by the neonatologists before you are asked to review the baby.

Hereditary or primary lymphoedema, first described by Milroy in 1892, is a developmental disorder of the lymphatic system that leads to a disabling and disfiguring swelling of the extremities. Hereditary lymphoedema generally shows autosomal dominant (AD) inheritance with reduced penetrance, variable expression, and variable age at onset. Swelling may appear in one or all limbs. Swelling varies in degree and distribution and, if untreated, worsens over time. In rare instances, angiosarcoma may develop in affected tissues. Genetic analysis of families with Milroy disease led to the identification of mutations in *VEGFR3* as a cause of congenital lymphoedema, confirming the importance of VEGFR3 signalling in lymphatic development (Karkkainen *et al.* 2000). *FOXC2* appears to be the primary cause of the rare lymphoedema–distichiasis syndrome and is also a cause of lymphoedema in some families with phenotypes attributed to other lymphoedema syndromes (Finegold *et al.* 2001).

Clinical approach
History: key points
- Three-generation family history with specific enquiry for consanguinity, oedema, lymphoedema.
- Detailed pregnancy history. Enquire about polydramnios, fetal movements.

Examination: key points
- Are the facial features coarse?
- Are there medial epicanthic folds? A marker of intrauterine oedema, these are seen in a number of congenital lymphoedema syndromes.
- Are the ears low-set?
- Is the neck broad/webbed; are there redundant nuchal folds?
- Are the nipples wide-spaced?

Special investigations
- Karyotype (to exclude 45, X and other rare chromosome rearrangements). If clinical features are suggestive of Turner syndrome ask for mosaicism screen if routine karyotype normal.
- Echocardiogram (to assess for possible Noonan syndrome (NS)—pulmonary stenosis, cardiomyopathy).
- Urinalysis for protein to exclude nephrotic syndrome.
- White-cell enzymes if GM1 gangliosidosis or other lysosomal disorders are a possibility.
- Consider ophthalmological assessment.

Some diagnoses to consider
Presenting in infancy
Turner syndrome (45,X) or mosaic Turner syndrome. Lymphoedema that resolves *in utero* may present in the newborn as residual puffiness of the hands and feet and redundant nuchal folds. See 'Turner syndrome, 45, X and variants', page 558.

Noonan syndrome (NS). Lymphoedema that resolves *in utero* is thought to account for many of the dysmorphic features. Babies with NS have a tall forehead, thick eyelids with mild ptosis, epicanthic folds, small upturned nose, small chin, and short neck. See 'Noonan syndrome (NS)', page 402.

Milroy primary congenital lymphoedema (Milroy disease). Milroy disease is present at birth, when it mostly affects the dorsal aspects of the feet with chronic swelling due to dysfunction of lymphatic vessels. Inheritance is AD with reduced penetrance (80%) and it is caused by mutations in *VEGFR3* on 5q.

GM1 Gangliosidosis (β-galactosidase deficiency). A lysosomal disorder following autosomal recessive (AR) inheritance that presents from birth. Coarse features, facial oedema, pitting oedema of the hands and feet, large tongue, thick gums, floppy, poor feeding.

Progressive encephalopathy with (o)edema, hypsarrhythmia, and optic atrophy (PEHO syndrome). An AR neurodegenerative disorder first noted in Finnish patients and characterized by generalized hypotonia and oedema of face and extremities (hands and feet), profound psychomotor retardation, progressive cerebellar atrophy, and severe epilepsy (initially presenting with infantile spasms).

Hennekam syndrome. An AR condition comprising congenital lymphoedema, facial anomalies (flat face, flat and broad nasal bridge, and hypertelorism), intestinal lympangiectasia, and developmental delay. The lymphoedema is usually congenital; it can be markedly asymmetrical and is often gradually progressive.

Cholestasis–lymphoedema syndrome (CLS; Aagenaes syndrome). Patients with CLS suffer severe neonatal cholestasis that usually lessens during early childhood and becomes episodic; they also develop chronic severe lymphoedema. The condition maps to 15q.

Klippel–Trenaunay–Weber syndrome (KTW) can present with limb swelling at birth with associated cutaneous vascular naevus over the trunk or limbs, varicosities, and asymmetrical hypertrophy of all or part of a limb.

Microcephaly–lymphoedema syndrome. A rare AD condition characterized by microcephaly, lymphoedema, and chorioretinopathy with variable visual deficit and variable expression.

Presenting after puberty
Lymphoedema–distichiasis syndrome. Unusual AD syndrome characterized by primary lymphoedema with a double row of eyelashes (distichiasis is penetrant in ~95%) and caused by mutations in the forkhead transcription factor *FOXC2* on 16q24. As with most hereditary lymphoedema syndromes, the lymphoedema is delayed in onset until after puberty. Associated findings included ptosis (31%), congenital heart disease (6.8%), and cleft palate (4%) (Brice *et al.* 2002). Other than distichiasis, the most commonly occurring anomaly is varicose veins of early onset (49%).

Genetic advice
Counsel for specific diagnosis.

Recurrence risk
As for specific diagnosis.

Prenatal diagnosis
Possible only if a chromosomal abnormality or mutation has been defined in the proband.

Natural history and further management (preventative measures)
Refer to a dermatologist for management of the lymphoedema.

Lay group contact: Lymphoedema support network <www.lymphoedema.org>.

Expert advisers: Peter Mortimer, Professor of Dermatological Medicine, St George's Hospital, London and Dian Donnai, Professor of Medical Genetics, University of Manchester, Manchester, England.

References
Brice G, Mansour S, *et al.* Analysis of the phenotypic abnormalities in lymphoedema–distichiasis syndrome in 74 patients with FOXC2 mutations or linkage to 16q24. *J Med Genet.* 2002; **39** (7): 478–83.

Bull LN, Roche E, *et al.* Mapping of the locus for cholestasis–lymphedema syndrome (Aagenaes syndrome) to a 6.6 cm interval on chromosome 15q. *Am J Hum Genet* 2000; **67**: 994–9.

Ferrell RE, Levinson KL, *et al.* Hereditary lymphoedema: evidence for linkage and genetic heterogeneity. *Hum Mol Genet.* 1998; **7** (13): 2073–8.

Finegold DN, Kimak MA, *et al.* Truncating mutations in FOXC2 cause multiple lymphedema syndromes. *Hum Mol Genet.* 2001; **10** (11): 1185–9.

Karkkainen MJ, Ferrell RE, *et al.* Missense mutations interfere with VEGFR-3 signalling in primary lymphoedema. *Nat Genet* 2000; **25** (2): 153–9.

Limwongse C, Wyszynski RE, *et al.* Microcephaly–lymphedema–chorioretinal dysplasia a unique genetic syndrome with variable expression and possible characteristic facial appearance. *Am J Med Genet* 1999; **86**: 215–18.

Vanhatalo S, Somer M, *et al.* Dutch patients with progressive encephalopathy with edema, hypsarrhythmia, and optic atrophy (PEHO) syndrome *Neuropaediatrics* 2002; **33**: 100–4.

Oesophageal and intestinal atresia (including tracheo-oesophageal fistula)

For all types of gastrointestinal obstruction, the birth frequency is around 1 in 2000. A tracheo-oesophageal fistula (TOF) occurs in ~1/3000 livebirths (see figure); there is a small male preponderance. In >85% the fistula is associated with oesophageal atresia (OA). Approximately 50% have a major associated malformation. (David and O'Callaghan 1975). TOF results from incomplete division of the cranial part of the foregut into respiratory and oesophageal parts during 23–28 days post-conception.

The intestine develops as a hollow tube. The middle of the enteric tube is tethered to the umbilical cord by the vitelline duct. In the embryo this middle portion of the enteric system grows and rotates within the umbilical cord. By week 10 the intestines are situated within the abdominal cavity.

Atresias are thought to occur due to:

- problems with the vascular supply, e.g. vascular disruption (see Reid et al. 1986);
- occlusion;
- obstruction, e.g. pressure from malrotation or volvulus, annular pancreas.

Duodenal atresia is the most common form of intestinal atresia.

The role of the geneticist is to distinguish the syndromic causes of gut atresia.

Clinical approach

History: key points

- Family history: previous affected sib or parent, consanguinity.
- Maternal age (Down syndrome).
- Maternal diabetes, teratogen exposure.

- Prenatal features: polyhydramnios, premature delivery.
- Postnatal presenting features: abdominal distension, excessive gastric aspirates (bile-stained), vomiting.

Examination: key points

- If seen pre-operatively, features of atresia as described above.
- Features of Down syndrome: hypotonia, cardiac murmur, facial dysmorphic features.
- Omphalocele *or*
- Anorectal anomalies.
- Radial or thumb hypoplasia (VATER (vertebral defects–anal atresia–TOF–OA–renal anomalies)).
- Digital: short 5th fingers, syndactyly of toes (Feingold syndrome).
- Ear anomalies, pre-auricular skin tags (Goldenhar syndrome) and dysplastic external ears CHARGE (coloboma–heart defects–atresia choanae–retardation of growth and/or development–genital defect–ear anomalies and/or deafness syndrome).
- Eyes: corneal clouding (Fryns syndrome), colobomata (CHARGE), structural ocular abnormalities in several syndromes discussed below.
- Epidermolysis bullosa (associated with pyloric atresia).

Special investigations

- Operation. Note the surgical findings (site of atresia, single or multiple, malrotation, volvulus, 'apple peel atresia', vascular anatomy, structural abnormality of the pancreas).
- X-ray of spine (structural vertebral anomalies) in children with TOF and OA.
- X-ray lower spine and sacrum in infants of diabetic mothers.

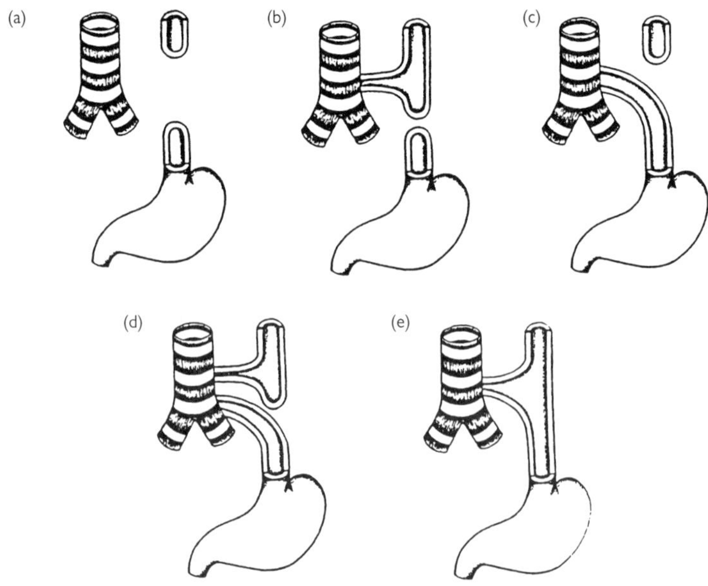

Schematics of various types of oesophageal atresnia (OA) and for tracheo-oesophageal fistula (TOF)
(a) OA without TOF   (b) OA with proximal TOF   (c) OA with distal TOF
(d) OA with proximal and distal TOF   (e) TOF without oesophageal atresia.
Reprinted from Stevenson. R. E. and Hall J. G. *Human malformation and related anomalies* (1993) with permission from Oxford University Press.

- Chromosome analysis (trisomy 21, trisomy 18, and possibly 22q11 fluorescent *in situ* hybridization (FISH)). Consider Fanconi testing in infants with bilateral upper limb anomalies.
- Consider DNA for storage.
- Mutation analysis for cystic fibrosis (CF) where indicated, e.g. jejuno-ileal atresia.
- Consider ophthalmology referral (for fundal exam for colobomata, e.g. CHARGE).
- Renal ultrasound scan (USS; for VATER/CHARGE).

Syndromic diagnoses to consider

Tracheo-oesophageal fistula (TOF) or oesophageal atresia (OA)

Isolated TOF presents with a characteristic triad of symptoms: choking and cyanosis on feeding; recurrent lower respiratory tract infection; and abdominal distension. Babies are invariably symptomatic from birth, although the symptoms may be intermittent and may vary in severity. A high index of suspicion is required because the symptoms are not specific. Establishing the diagnosis can be difficult and neither radiology nor bronchoscopy is infallible. Surgical division of the fistula is curative. Only ~45% of TOFs are isolated anomalies, so search carefully for other malformations.

Chromosomal anomalies. A wide variety of chromosomal conditions have been reported with TOF including trisomy 21, trisomy 18, del 22q11, and, rarely, 17q interstitial deletion.

Developmental malformation syndromes (usually sporadic).
- **VATER/VACTERL association.** Incidence 1.6/ 10 000. Hall suggests at least 1 anomaly from limb, thorax, and pelvis/lower abdomen for a secure opinion, and at least two anomalies in each of two of those regions for a probable one. The individual letters in VATER/ VACTERL have the following significance:
  - V, vertebral defects, usually upper to midthoracic and lumbar regions. Usually hemivertebrae, but dysseg- mented and fused vertebrae may occur—may be accompanying rib anomalies;
  - A, anal atresia—may be associated genital defects (hypospadias, bifid scrotum) or fistulae;
  - C, cardiac anomalies—present in ~80%; any type, any severity;
  - T, TOF;
  - E, (o)esophageal atresia—80% have an associated TOF;
  - R, renal; renal anomalies in 80%, e.g. renal agenesis/ dysplasia;
  - L, limb (radial defects)—preaxial with underdevelop- ment or agenesis of thumbs and radial bones; usually bilateral defects, but may be asymmetric. Reduced thenar muscle mass is mildest end of spectrum. The lower limbs are not affected.
- **Goldenhar (facio-auriculo-vertebral) syndrome.** TOF is a recognized but not common feature of this syndrome. See 'Ear anomalies', page 108 for additional details.
- **CHARGE syndrome.** TOF is present in ~10% of indi- viduals with CHARGE syndromes which is caused by mutations in the *CHD7* gene. There are some babies with features that overlap between CHARGE and VATER. See 'Ear anomalies', page 108.
- **OEIS.** OEIS complex refers to a combination of defects consisting of omphalocele, extrophy of the cloaca,

imperforate anus, and spinal defect. Mostly sporadic. See 'Anal anomalies (atresia, stenosis)', page 42.
- **Teratogens.**

Genetic syndromes.
- **Feingold syndrome.** AD. Also known as MODED (microcephaly–oculo–digito–(o)esophageal–duodenal) syndrome. A clinically variable disorder comprising hand and foot abnormalities (brachydactyly with clinodactyly of 5th fingers and bilateral syndactyly of toes 2,3 and 4,5: microcephaly: short palpebral fissures: learning dis- abilities; and oesophageal atresia (25%) and/or duodenal atresia (20%). The gene is 2p24–p25. MYCN (von Bokhoven)
- **Opitz syndrome.** Opitz (or G/BBB) syndrome is a pleiotropic genetic disorder characterized by hyper- telorism, hypospadias, laryngeal cleft, and additional midline defects. This syndrome is heterogeneous with an X-linked (XLOS) form caused by mutations in *MID1* on Xp22 and an autosomal dominant (ADOS) form. De Falco *et al.* (2003) found that laryngo-tracheo-(o)esophageal (LTE) defects are also common anomalies in males carrying a *MID1* mutation.
- **AEG syndrome.** Anophthalmia with oesphageal atresia and genital abnormalities (cryptorchidism and hypospadias in males). Neuronal migration defects in the central ner- vous system (CNS) are probably part of the syndrome. Caused by new dominant mutations of the *SOX2* gene .
- **Martinez–Frias syndrome.** AR. Low birthweight, TOF, duodenal atresia, intra- and extrahepatic biliary atresia, and hypospadias.
- **Epidermolysis bullosa-pyloric atresia.** AR. Pyloric atresia associated with junctional epidermolysis bullosa (PA-JEB) is a rare inherited disorder characterized by pyloric stenosis and blistering of the skin as primary manifestations. Mutations are reported in the integrin beta 4 gene in some families.
- **Hydrocephalus with features of VATER.** AR. Children have been reported with the cytogenetic features of Fanconi anaemia.

Duodenal atresia

NB. Duodenal stenosis may be associated with an annular pancreas.

Chromosomal anomalies. Down syndrome (trisomy 21) is the main condition to exclude in babies with duodenal atresia; it accounts for 30–50% of duodenal atresia.

Developmental malformation syndromes (usually sporadic).
- **Maternal diabetes and caudal regression.** See 'Maternal diabetes mellitus and diabetic embryopathy' page 612.
- **OEIS.** See above.
- **Vascular disruption.** See Reid *et al.* (1986).

Genetic syndromes.
- **Fryns syndrome.** A rare lethal AR condition with nail/ digital hypoplasia, corneal clouding, and diaphragmatic hernia as the main features.
- **Feingold syndrome.** See above.
- **Martinez–Frias syndrome.** See above.

Jejuno-ileal atresia

Developmental malformation syndromes. As for duodenal atresia. NB. Apple-peel atresia may also occur as a consequence of disruption.

Genetic associations/syndromes.

- **Cystic fibrosis (CF).** Roberts *et al.* (1998) calculated that the presence of jejuno-ileal atresia gave a 210 times increased risk for CF as 4 out of 38 Caucasian babies with jejuno-ileal atresia had CF.
- **Jejunal atresia (apple peel syndrome).** Familial AR inheritance has been reported.
- **Jejunal atresia (apple peel atresia), microcephaly, and ocular anomalies.** AR syndrome.

Colonic atresia

Accounts for 10% of bowel atresia and has a similar aetiology to that of jejuno-ileal atresia and multiple atresia.

Developmental malformation syndromes. As for duodenal atresia.

Multiple intestinal atresia

Developmental malformation syndromes. As for duodenal atresia.

Genetic associations/syndromes. May be an AR condition and has been reported more frequently found in French Canadian families.

Anal atresia

See 'Anal anomalies (atresia, stenosis)', page 42.

Genetic advice

Recurrence risk

Identify those infants with a syndromic cause and counsel appropriately.

- **Isolated TOF.** The recurrence risk for siblings of a child with an isolated TOF is very small at ~1%. The risk to offspring of an individual with an isolated TOF is very small and estimated at ~1% (Warren *et al.* 1979).
- **Isolated intestinal atresia.** As described above, there have been a small number of reports of familial occurrence of isolated bowel atresia, but the proportion that are recessive remains uncertain. The majority of isolated single-site bowel atresias are usually attributed to vascular disruption and are associated with a low recurrence risk. In a 10-year survey by the American Academy of Pediatricians the recurrence risk for sibs of infants with duodenal atresia was approximately 1 in 50. The recurrence risk may be higher than this in infants with multiple atresia or jejuno-ileal atresia.

Carrier detection

Not possible unless associated with CF or other genetic conditions with a known mutation or chromosomal rearrangement.

Prenatal diagnosis

USS in the second and third trimesters. USS findings suggesting TOF/OA include polyhydramnios and small or absent stomach. Approximately one-third of babies with gut atresias were prenatally detected (40% of these before 24 weeks) in the Haeusler *et al.* (2002) series.

Natural history and further management (preventative measures)

The primary management is surgical. Delivery should be planned at a hospital with full neonatal intensive care facilities and good links with a specialist paediatric surgical team. For suspected TOF/OA a senior paediatrician should be present at delivery since expert management of the neonate from the moment of delivery is necessary to minimize the risk of aspiration pneumonia.

Lay group contact: TOFS (Tracheo-oesophageal Fistula Support) <www.tofs.org.uk>, Tel. 0115 961 3092.

Expert adviser: Han G. Brunner, Professor, Department of Human Genetics, University of Nijmegen, Nijmegen, The Netherlands.

References

Boyd PA, Chamberlain P, Gould S, *et al.* Hereditary multiple intestinal atresia—ultrasound findings and outcome of pregnancy in an affected case. *Prenat Diagn* 1994; **14**: 61–4.

Buttiker V, Wojtulewicz, Wilson M. Imperforate anus in Feingold syndrome. *Am J Med Genet* 2000; **92**: 166–9.

Celli J, van Beusekom E, *et al.* Familial syndromic esophageal atresia maps to 2p23–p24. *Am J Hum Genet* 2000; **66**: 436–44.

David TJ, O'Callaghan SE. Oesophageal atresia in the South west of England. *J Med Genet* 1975; **12**: 1–11.

De Falco F, Cainarca S, *et al.* X-linked Opitz syndrome: novel mutations in the MID1 gene and redefinition of the clinical spectrum. *Am J Med Genet.* 2003; **120A** (2): 222–8.

Fonkalsrud EW, *et al.* Congenital atresia and stenosis of the duodenum: a review compiled from the members of the surgical section of the American Academy of Pediatrics. *Pediatrics* 1969; **43**: 79–83.

Haeusler MC, Berghold A, Stoll C, *et al.* Prenatal ultrasound detection of gastrointestinal obstruction: results from 18 congenital anomaly registers. *Prenat Diagn* 2002; **22**: 616–23.

Reid CO, Hall JG, *et al.* Association of amyoplasia with gastroschisis, bowel atresia and defects of the muscular layer of the trunk. *Am J Med Genet* 1986; **24**: 701–10.

Roberts HE, *et al.* Increased frequency of CF among infants with jejunoileal atresia. *Am J Med Genet* 1998; **78**: 446–9.

Warren J, Evans K, Carter CO. Offspring of patients with tracheo-oesophageal fistula. *J Med Genet* 1979; **16**: 338–40.

von Bokhoven H, Celli J et al. MYCN haploinsufficiency is associated with reduced brain size and intestinal atresias in Feingold syndrome. Nat Genet. 2005 May; **37**: 465–7.

Optic nerve hypoplasia

This is a non-progressive congenital anomaly that may be unilateral or bilateral and affect all, or part, of the optic nerve. The optic disc is small and pale and may show a peripapillary ring of pigmentation. The presenting feature is often nystagmus in bilateral cases, and strabismus in unilateral cases. Visual function varies from near normal to complete loss of vision. The prognosis is difficult to predict in small infants. The most important association to exclude is endocrine abnormalities due to a developmental disorder of the midline brain structures, e.g. septo-optic dysplasia or other midline anomalies. For this reason all infants with unilateral or bilateral ONH should see a paediatric endocrinologist. *PAX6* is involved in ocular morphogenesis and is expressed in the central nervous system (CNS) and numerous ocular tissues during development. Recently, *PAX6* mutations have been identified in some families with optic-nerve malformations including colobomata, morning glory disc anomaly, optic-nerve hypoplasia/aplasia, and persistent hyperplastic primary vitreous (Azuma *et al.* 2003).

Optic nerve hypoplasia is associated not only with other anomalies of the CNS (see above) and with teratogenic exposure (alcohol, anticonvulsants, maternal diabetes) but also with signs of general disturbance in fetal development. Risk factors include young maternal age, first parity, maternal smoking, preterm birth, and factors associated with preterm birth (Tornqvist *et al.* 2002).

Clinical approach

History: key points

- Three-generation family tree with specific enquiry regarding visual problems (*PAX6*).
- Pregnancy: alcohol exposure, anticonvulsant use.
- Maternal diabetes mellitus.
- Developmental milestones.
- Visual function.

Examination: key points

- Short stature (pituitary dysfunction, septo-optic dysplasia).
- Micropenis (pituitary dysfunction).
- Facial dysmorphic features.

Special investigations

- Ophthalmological assessment to differentiate optic nerve hypoplasia from optic atrophy and the crowded disc of hypermetropia.
- Refraction.
- Electrophysiology. Electroretinogram (ERG) normal, visual evoked responses (VER) abnormal.
- Brain and optic nerve magnetic resonance imaging (MRI; midline structural lesions).

- Endocrine investigations, particularly pituitary hormones. Refer to paediatric endocrinologist.
- Chromosome analysis if part of a malformation syndrome (trisomy 18, del 13q).
- DNA storage/specific mutational analysis.

Syndromic diagnoses to consider

Septo-optic dysplasia. Optic nerve hypoplasia with absent septum pellucidum and pituitary endocrine abnormalities. Mutations in *HESX1* (heterozygous and homozygous) have been found in a few individuals. See 'Structural intracranial anomalies (agenesis of the corpus callosum, septo-optic dysplasia, and arachnoid cysts)', page 248.

Environmental aetiology. Maternal diabetes, alcohol, or anticonvulsant use (see 'Maternal diabetes mellitus and diabetic embryopathy', 'Fetal alcohol syndrome (FAS)', and 'Fetal anticonvulsant syndrome' pages 612, 588 and 590).

Genetic advice

Recurrence risk

For isolated optic nerve hypoplasia the recurrence risk is low but there are rare reports of dominant inheritance. A recurrence may have more than just optic nerve hypoplasia; for example, there may be features of septo-optic dysplasia.

Carrier detection

May be available in families for conditions with a known mutation.

Prenatal diagnosis

Genetic testing may be available in families with a known mutation.

Natural history and further management (preventative measures)

A non-progressive developmental disorder. Visual function is difficult to predict in small infants.

Lay group contact: SOD/ONH Support Network <www.focusfamilies.org>.

Expert adviser: Anonymous.

References

Azuma N, Yamaguchi Y, *et al.* Mutations of the *PAX6* gene detected in patients with a variety of optic-nerve malformations. *Am J Hum Genet* 2003; **72**: 1565–70.

Golnik K.C. Congenital optic nerve abnormalities. *Curr Opin Ophthalmol* 1998; **9** (6): 18–26.

Tornqvist K, Ericsson A, Kallen B. Optic nerve hypoplasia: risk factors and epidemiology. *Acta Ophthalmol Scand* 2002; **80** (3): 300–4.

Overgrowth

Overgrowth can be defined as growth parameters (height and weight) in excess of the 99.6th centile. Insulin-like growth factors (IGF) and their receptors (IGFR) regulate embryonic and postnatal growth. In the embryonic phase, growth is largely IGF-2-dependent through IGF1R and the insulin receptor (IR), whilst later in fetal life and postnatally IGF-1 is dominant in growth regulation. Many of the overgrowth disorders are characterized by excessive growth in fetal life and infancy with subsequent decline in growth rate such that adults often have growth parameters within the normal range. Neonates with overgrowth require careful monitoring for hypoglycaemia.

Some of the overgrowth disorders, notably Beckwith–Wiedemann syndrome (BWS), but also Simpson–Golabi–Behmel (SGB) syndrome, have an increased risk for embryonal tumours with the risk maximal in early childhood. Others such as Bannayan–Riley–Ruvalcaba/Cowden syndrome (BRR-CS) have an increased risk for tumours in adult life

Diagnosis is often difficult because, apart from overgrowth, there are few other discriminatory features. The current development of molecular testing for BWS and Sotos syndrome should increase the proportion of children in whom a specific diagnosis is possible.

Clinical approach

History: key points

- Three-generation family tree.
- Parental birthweights, birth history, e.g. anterior abdominal wall defect, hypoglycaemia, and current height.
- Pregnancy history. Maternal diabetes? Gestation at earliest ultrasound scan (USS)? Were dates subsequently altered? Any abnormal USS findings?
- Birth history. Birthweight and occipital-frontal circumference (OFC; and length if available). Neonatal hypoglycaemia? Omphalocele or other congenital anomaly?
- Growth parameters to date.
- Developmental milestones.

Examination: key points

- Careful documentation of OFC, weight, and length/height.
- Ears for anterior linear lobe creases and posterior helical pits (BWS), ear creases (SGB).
- Face for frontal bossing and high forehead (Sotos), prominent mandible (Sotos) after first year, slow hair growth in frontoparietal regions (Sotos), and coarse facies (SGB).
- Tongue. Macroglossia in BWS; large tongue with exaggerated midline groove in SGB.
- Nipple line for polythelia (SGB).
- Hemihypertrophy.
- Skin. Thickened doughy skin in SGB, freckling (BRR-CS).
- Cardiac auscultation (Sotos, SGB).
- Spine for scoliosis (Sotos).

Special investigations

- Karyotype. Various chromosome anomalies, e.g. dup 4p, dup 11p15 (BWS), dup 12p, dup15qter, del15q35 (Sotos), and del 22q13, are characterized by overgrowth.
- DNA for *FRAXA* (fragile X syndrome) if developmental delay.
- DNA for molecular genetic analysis if features of BWS (UPD 11p15 and loss of methylation of KvDMR1) or Sotos (*NDS1*), or SGB (*glypican 3*). Note that Baujet found 11p15 anomalies in ~10% of patients with a clinical diagnosis of Sotos, and *NSD1* mutations in ~5% of patients with a clinical diagnosis of BWS
- Bone age. X-ray left wrist.
- Renal, USS (BWS, SGB as screening for Wilms tumour; Sotos for investigation of renal anomalies).
- Consider HbA1c in mother of newborn with overgrowth (unless recent glucose tolerance test (GTT) in pregnancy has been normal).

Some diagnoses to consider

Infant of diabetic mother. Fetal macrosomia with risk of neonatal hypoglycaemia and increased risk for congenital malformation, especially congenital heart disease, neural tube defects, and skeletal defects. See 'Maternal diabetes mellitus and diabetic embryopathy' page 612.

Beckwith–Wiedemann syndrome (BWS). Prevalence of ~1/15,000 Macrosomia, anterior abdominal wall defects, macroglossia, anterior ear lobe creases, and posterior helical pits. Risk of embryonal tumours. Complex genetics. See 'Beckwith–Wiedemann syndrome (BWS)' page 278.

Simpson–Golabi–Behmel (SGB) syndrome. X-linked recessive (XLR) disorder due to mutations in *glypican 3* (Xq26). Overgrowth is of prenatal onset and continues postnatally. Birthweight and birth OFC of affected males are usually both >97th centile. Other findings include hypertelorism, macroglossia, central groove of lower lip, supernumerary nipples, advanced bone age, vertebral segmentation defects, coarse facies in adults; most have normal intelligence quotient but some are mildly delayed (IQ). They may have cardiac/gastrointestinal malformations; refer for echo/electrocardiogram (ECG). Diagnostic overlap with BWS, but combination of minor facial anomalies, skeletal/ hand anomalies, and supernumerary nipples only occurs in SGB. Small risk of Wilms tumour. Consider periodic renal USS as for BWS, i.e. USS of kidneys, liver, and adrenals at 3–4 monthly intervals until 7–8 years.

Sotos syndrome. Prevalence ~1/15 000. Autosomal dominant (AD) disorder due to mutations or deletions of *NSD1* (5q35). Most are isolated cases due to *de novo* mutations, but familial cases do occur. Overgrowth from the prenatal stage, through childhood (especially first 4 years). Birthweight averages 4200 g in males and 4000 g in females. Final adult heights are often in the upper normal range. Characterized dysmorphic facies with long, thin face, broad forehead, fronto-temporal hair sparsity, down-slanting palpebral fissures and malar flushing. Developmental delay is almost always present, but varies from very mild to very severe. Associated features include cardiac and renal anomalies, neonatal jaundice and hypotonia, scoliosis, seizures and advanced bone age. Tumours are rare and no screening is recommended.

Weaver syndrome. Rare condition with overgrowth usually present at birth, but sometimes not apparent until a few months of age. Dysmorphic facies with broad forehead, hypertelorism, small chin which looks 'stuck on', and long philtrum. Some overlap with Sotos syndrome, but classic Weaver cases have much more prominent hypertelorism. Camptodactyly, fetal finger pads and flaring of metaphyses may be present. Developmental delay is usual but very variable in extent. Cases with clinical overlap with Sotos have *NSD1* mutations, but classic Weaver cases are due to unknown cause. Most are isolated cases, but some AD families reported.

Macrocephaly–cutis marmorata telangiectatica congenital (M-CMTC). Macrocephaly (often with hydrocephalus that may require shunting), macrosomia, philtral haemangioma, cutis marmorata (vascular mottling of skin), syndactyly toes 2,3 and/or fingers 3,4; may have postaxial polydactyly. Developmental delay. All cases reported to date are sporadic. See 'Macrocephaly', page 162.

PTEN (Bannayan–Ruvalcaba–Riley (BRR)/ Cowden syndrome (BRR-CS)). AD disorder due to mutations in *PTEN* (10q23). Birthweight usually >4000 g. Subsequent growth decelerates such that adults usually fall within normal centiles. Macrocephaly is a prominent feature, which is frequently progressive from birth, with OFC often increased to +4.5 standard deviations (SD) or more. Hypotonia with delayed gross motor skills is a common finding, and ~60% have a mild proximal myopathy with lipid deposition. Some patients have learning disability, which can vary from mild to severe. 25% have seizures. Most affected males with BRR have genital (penile or vulval) freckling. Lipomas and other hamartomas (e.g. haemangiomata) may occur in the skin. May have mild hypertelorism. Mutation carriers have an increased risk of thyroid tumours, gut hamartomas, breast fibroadenomas, and breast cancer.

Perlman syndrome. Rare autosomal recessive (AR) condition with macrosomia and a high incidence of Wilms tumour. Distinctive facial features and high neonatal mortality; learning disability is common.

Costello syndrome. Macrosomia, coarse facial features, and cardiac defects usually presenting in the neonatal period or early infancy. With time, failure to thrive may supervene and papillomata develop around the nose and periorally.

Proteus syndrome. Characterized by disproportionate overgrowth, vascular and lymphatic malformations, etc. Rarely presents as uniform overgrowth. Birthweight often normal, but can be increased or occasionally reduced. Features can be relatively unimpressive at birth and progress rapidly in infancy. See 'Hemihypertrophy and limb asymmetry', page 128.

Chromosomal disorders with overgrowth. Pallister–Killian (mosaic tetrasomy 12p) is associated with severe delay. Consider a 22q13 telomeric deletion if severe delay/autistic features, absent speech, and hypotonia are present (can be detected using telomeric control probe for routine 22q11 fluorescent *in situ* hybridization (FISH)).

Genetic advice
Recurrence risk
As for the specific disorder.

Carrier detection
As for the specific disorder.

Prenatal diagnosis
Usually only possible early in pregnancy if a specific mutation or chromosome anomaly has been identified. In an affected pregnancy, growth parameters are rarely significantly above the normal range until after ~20 weeks gestation.

Natural history and further management (preventative measures)
Referral to a paediatric growth clinic for monitoring is often appropriate.

Support group: Child Growth Foundation Tel: 020 8995 0257 <www.childgrowthfoundation.org> Sotos Syndrome Support Association (SSSA) <www.well.com/ user/sssa>.

Expert advisers: Trevor Cole, Consultant Clinical Geneticist, Birmingham and Nazneen Rahman, Senior Lecturer and Honorary Consultant in Clinical Genetics, Institute of Cancer Research, Sutton, Surrey, England.

References
Baujet G, Rio M, *et al*. Paradoxical *NSD1* mutations in Beckwith–Wiedemann syndrome and 11p15 anomalies in Sotos syndrome. *Am J Hum Genet* 1004; **74**: 715–20.

Biesecker LG, Happle R, *et al*. Proteus syndrome: diagnostic criteria, differential diagnosis, and patient evaluation. *Am J Med Genet* 1999; **84**: 389–95.

Cohen MM Jr, Neri G, Weksberg R. *Overgrowth syndromes*, Oxford Monographs on Medical Genetics. Oxford University Press, New York, 2002.

Tatton-Brown K, Rahman N. Clinical features of *NSD1*-positive Sotos syndrome. Clinical Dysmorphology 2004; **13**: 199–204.

Wilson HL, Wong AC, *et al*. Molecular characterisation of the 22q13 deletion syndrome supports the role of haploinsufficiency of *SHANK3/PROSAP2* in the major neurological symptoms. *J Med Genet* 2003; **40**: 575–84.

Patchy hypomelanotic skin lesions

As with the disorders of patchy hyperpigmentation, the differential diagnosis of these conditions depends on the distribution, shape of the lesions, and the presence of other features. The skin pigments (eumelanin and pheomelanin) are produced in melanosomes by melanocytes, which are large cells found among the basal cells of the epidermis. The melanosomes are then transferred to keratinocytes. Melanocytes are of neural crest origin.

Depigmentation ('amelanosis') describes the situation where melanocytes are absent; **hypopigmentation** describes a reduction in colour, where melanocytes are not entirely absent. Hypopigmented macules are present in <1% of white neonates and ~2% of black neonates (Alper and Holmes 1983). In older children and adults hypopigmented lesions attributable to chickenpox scars, trauma, and various dermatological conditions are a common finding.

Common causes of patchy hypomelanosis without significant genetic implications are the following.

- **Single hypopigmented macule.** Single lesions resembling the hypopigmented macules seen in tuberous sclerosis (TS) are found in 6–7% of normal children and 4% of adults <45 years of age with <1% having multiple lesions and no non-TS individual having more than three (Vanderhooft et al. 1996).
- **Vitiligo.** Autoimmune disorder in which the melanosomes are selectively destroyed.
- **Naevus anaemicus.** If the lesion is rubbed and intensifies and doesn't redden, this is the likely diagnosis. Benign.
- **Tinea versicolor.** Common fungal infection of the skin. Skin scrapes mounted on microscope slide in KOH and sent for microscopy or, if clinically typical, trial of treatment with appropriate antifungal agent.

Clinical approach

History: key points
- Three-generation family tree with specific enquiry regarding family members with similar lesions.
- Presence, or not, from birth.
- Increasing in number, or size?
- Deafness (Waardenburg syndrome (WS)).
- Neurological features, developmental delay, seizures.
- Hirschsprung disease or chronic constipation (WS).

Examination: key points
- Make a careful clinical and photographic record of the skin.
- Are the margins of the lesions sharply defined or irregular?
- Does the pattern of distribution follow Blaschko's lines?
- Document the number of lesions/areas of hypopigmentation.
- Do they cross the midline of the body?
- Other skin lesions, e.g. facial angiofibromas, shagreen patches, and ungual fibromas in TS.
- Areas/streaks of 'atrophic' hypopigmented skin with absence of appendages, e.g. hair in the involved areas (last stage of incontinentia pigmenti (IP) and Goltz syndrome).
- Any areas of hyperpigmentation?

- Hair. White forelock (piebaldism, WS); early greying (premature canities).
- Nervous system. Hypomelanosis of Ito, TS.
- Eye. Retinal hamartoma in TS; heterochromia (WS).

Special investigations
- Clinical photography.
- Examination under ultraviolet (UV; Woods) lamp.
- Karyotype of blood *and skin* in presence of developmental delay (unless the cause is thought to be a single gene disorder) or other structural malformations.
- Molecular genetic analysis is available for some conditions.

NB. In conditions with a mosaic aetiology, either of a single gene or chromosomal origin, blood testing has limited use and skin biopsies have an important role (although very occasionally they may miss the mosaic cell line).

Some diagnoses to consider

Tuberous sclerosis (TS). The hypopigmented lesion is described as a congenital hypomelanotic macule or ash leaf patch. However, even careful examination at birth may not reveal the lesions though they become apparent in the first few months of life. They are usually on the trunk, and are 1–5 cm in size. The number varies but most affected individuals have fewer than six. (See 'Tuberous sclerosis (TSC)' page 420.)

Piebaldism. A striking congenital disorder of depigmentation that most frequently involves the skin of the forehead, the anterior part of the scalp, and the hair growing from the depigmented area of scalp. There is a sharp margin to the area(s) of depigmentation.

Waardenburg syndrome (WS). Auditory–pigmentary syndromes are caused by physical absence of melanocytes from the skin, hair, eyes, and the stria vascularis of the cochlea. WS manifests with a white forelock, sometimes with more extensive depigmentation of the skin, sensorineural deafness, dystopia canthorum (an increased distance between the inner canthi), heterochromia of the irides, synophrys, and a high nasal bridge. Some patients have premature greying of the hair, WS typically follows autosomal dominant (AD) inheritance, but see 'Deafness', page 90, for exceptions and further details about the four types of WS. All forms of WS show marked variability from minor pigmentary changes to profound deafness even within families, and at present it is not possible to predict the severity, even when a mutation is detected.

Hypomelanosis of Ito. Large areas of the skin may be affected by hypopigmented streaks or whorls distributed along the lines of Blaschko. It may be particularly striking over the trunk. The streaks are mainly present on the limbs and the whorls on the trunk. The lesions are much easier to see under UV light. Swirly hyperpigmentation may also be seen. Seizures and developmental delay are often found. Brain imaging may reveal a migrational abnormality. A mosaic chromosomal aetiology has been found to be the cause in ~60% of reported individuals. The myriad of associated features reflects the extensive variety of aneuploid conditions seen. This pigment pattern can also be seen in otherwise apparently normal individuals. Its cause in them is unknown, but it is presumed to be due to mosaicism for single genes controlling pigment production.

Incontinentia pigmenti (IP) type 2 (NEMO). X-linked dominant (XLD) disorder caused by mutations in the *NEMO* gene on Xq28. 80% carry a common deletion. Skin features occur in four stages.

Stage 1 First few days or weeks of life: blistering lesions cropping in distribution of Blaschko's lines (vesicular fluid is highly eosinophilic) accompanied by marked peripheral blood eosinophilia. Linear distribution along limbs, circumferential on trunk, usually spares face (birth–4 months; there are rare reports of onset as late as 18 months).

Stage 2 Verrucous lesions (less widespread, often confined to lower legs; <6 months).

Stage 3 Streaky lines of hyperpigmentation especially in axilla and groin (childhood and teens).

Stage 4 Pale atrophic streaks particularly noticeable on back of calves (childhood–adult). 40% have nail dystrophy, 80% have dental abnormalities affecting deciduous and/or permanent dentition, e.g. missing teeth, small teeth, delayed eruption, conical teeth, accessory cusps. Hair is often sparse in childhood and later is wiry/coarse; there may be patchy alopecia. 30% have eye findings, but most have normal vision. Seizures in 14%, which are persistent in 6%. Learning disability in 10% of affected females (severe in 3%). Affected male pregnancies are usually lost spontaneously in first or early 2nd trimester, hydrops may be seen on ultrasound scan (USS) at 8–13 weeks gestation.

'Microphthalmia with linear skin defects' (MLS). Girls with MLS syndrome have microphthalmia with linear skin defects of face and neck, sclerocornea, corpus callosum agenesis, and other brain anomalies. This XLD, male-lethal condition is associated with heterozygous deletions of a critical region in Xp22.31. The *HCCS* gene, encoding human holocytochrome c-type synthetase, is the only gene located entirely inside the critical region (Prakash *et al.* 2002).

(Goltz syndrome) X-linked dominant (due to mutations in, or deletions encompassing, the *PORCN* gene at Xp11.23). Areas of focal dermal hypoplasia may be found on the trunk and limbs and there may fat herniation through the skin deficiency. (See 'Coloboma' page 82).

Rothmund–Thomson syndrome is characterized by poikiloderma congenita, with growth deficiency, alopecia, photosensitivity, dystrophic nails, abnormal teeth, cataracts, and hypogonadism. The skin abnormalities appear before 6 months of age with reticular or diffuse erythema on the face, hands, and extensor surfaces of the limbs. The trunk is relatively spared. It is caused by mutations in the helicase gene *RECQL4* on 8q24.

Lay group contacts: Tuberous Sclerosis Association <www.tuberous-sclerosis.org>; International Incontinentia Pigmenti International Foundation <http://imgen.bcm.tmc.edu/IPIF>; Unique—The Rare chromosome disorder support group <www.rarechromo.org>.

Expert adviser: Anonymous.

References

Alper JC, Holmes LB. The incidence and significance of birthmarks in a cohort of 4,641 newborns. *Pediatr Dermatol* 1983; **1**: 58–68.

Flannery DB. Pigmentary dysplasia, hypomelanosis of Ito and genetic mosaicism [editorial]. *Am J Med Genet* 1990; **35**: 18–21.

Flannery DB. Skin: pigmentary disorders. In *Human malformations and related anomalies*, (ed. R.E. Stevenson, J.G. Hall, and R.M. Goodman), Chapter 31, Vol. II, Oxford Monographs on Medical Genetics no. 27. Oxford University Press, New York, 1993.

Happle R. Incontinentia pigmenti versus hypomelanosis of Ito: the whys and wherefores of a confusing issue [letter]. *Am J Med Genet* 1998; **79**: 64–5.

Prakash SK, Cormier TA, *et al.* Loss of holocytochrome c-type synthetase causes the male lethality of X-linked dominant microphthalmia with linear skin defects (MLS) syndrome. *Hum Mol Genet* 2002; **11** (25): 3237–48.

Spritz R. Piebaldism, Waardenburg syndrome and related disorders of melanocyte development. *Semin Cutan Med Surg* 1997; **16**: 15–23.

Sybert VP. *Genetic skin disorders*, Oxford Monographs in Medical Genetics. Oxford University Press, New York, 1997.

Vanderhooft SL, Francis JS, *et al.* Prevalence of hypopigmented macules in a healthy population. *J Pediatr* 1996; **129**: 355–61.

Patchy pigmented skin lesions (including café-au-lait spots)

The skin pigments (eumelanin and pheomelanin) are produced in melanosomes by melanocytes, which are large cells found among the basal cells of the epidermis. The melanosomes are then transferred to keratinocytes. Melanocytes are of neural crest origin.

The differential diagnosis of these conditions depends on the distribution and shape of the lesions and the presence of other features.

Clinical approach

History: key points

- Presence, or not, from birth. Have they changed in character?
- Increasing in number, or size?
- Other skin lesions, e.g. plexiform neurofibroma in neurofibromatosis type 1 (NF1), or lipomas with *PTEN* mutations.
- Blistering in the neonatal period (incontinentia pigmenti (IP)).
- Family history of similar lesions.
- Neurological features, developmental delay, seizures.

Examination: key points

- Make a careful clinical and photographic record of the skin.
- Are the margins of the lesions sharply defined or irregular?
- Does the pattern of distribution follow Blaschko's lines?
- Are the lesions flat (macular) or raised (papular, verrucous)?
- Document the number of lesions/areas of hyperpigment-ation.
- Do they cross the midline of the body?
- How dark is the pigment and are there any darker areas within the area of hyperpigmentation?
- Areas of skin atrophy with loss of pigment and hair (last stage of IP).
- Any areas of hypopigmentation.
- 'Lumps and bumps', e.g. neurofibromas, lipomas.
- Eye and nervous system. These organs are particularly associated with skin disorders (neurocutaneous syndromes).

Special investigations

Some conditions have a presumed, or known, mosaic aetiology, either of a single gene or chromosomal origin.

- Clinical photography
- Examination under ultraviolet (UV; Woods) lamp.
- Chromosomal investigations including blood and skin in the presence of developmental delay, or structural malformations, unless a single gene condition is thought to be the cause. In NF1 about 5% have a deletion containing the NF1 gene.
- Molecular genetic analysis is available for some conditions.
- Skin biopsy for histology may sometimes be helpful. Consider referral to a dermatologist.

Some diagnoses to consider

Considering specific patterns of pigmentation narrows the differential diagnosis.

Irregular 'mosaic patterned' pigmentation

There are areas of macular hyperpigmentation that may either affect either whole blocks of skin, or may show a whorled pattern, or follow Blaschko's lines. Conditions in this group are thought to have a mosaic aetiology and either a single gene or chromosomal disorder.

Incontinentia pigmenti (IP). The familial form (IP2) is inherited as an X-linked dominant (XLD) condition that is usually lethal in affected males. IP is caused by mutations in the *NEMO* gene at Xp28. X-inactivation in females means that not all cell lines express the mutation—hence the mosaic patterning. Indeed X-inactivation is often very skewed in females with IP. Blistering skin eruptions develop shortly after birth to be followed by a verrucous phase that eventually fades to areas of skin atrophy. The hyperpig-mented phase begins between 3 and 6 months and the distribution follows Blaschko's lines (whorled on trunk and linear on limbs). See 'Patchy hypomelanotic skin lesions', page 208, for further details. The sporadic disorder IP1 has now been reclassified as hypomelanosis of Ito and is asso-ciated with rearrangements at Xp11 (see below).

McCune–Albright syndrome. The components of the condition are precocious puberty and polyostotic fibrous dysplasia. The pigment changes are sometimes described as giant café-au-lait patches (CALs) but they may be clinically distinct from typical CALs. They are more irregu-lar ('coast of Maine'), generally larger, and are more commonly found on the trunk. However, this is not always the case. The condition is caused by mosaicism for muta-tions in GNAS1α. The diagnosis is usually a clinical one, as molecular testing for mosaicism for mutations in GNAS1α is not routinely available (but may be available via a research lab). Referral to an endocrinologist is suggested.

Chromosomal mosaicism (see also hypomelanosis of Ito). A skin biopsy for chromosomal analysis is indicated when the skin pigmentary abnormalities are not typical for a known condition, and where there are dysmorphic features, epilepsy, congenital malformations, or develop-mental delay. Before proceeding to the biopsy check with your cytogenetic laboratory that they have already carefully examined at least 30 cells from a blood sample to exclude mosaicism. Take the biopsy at the margin of the pigmented skin. Two biopsies may increase the yield.

Café au lait spots (CALs)

CALs are the colour of milky coffee, though they are darker in individuals who are naturally dark-skinned. They have a sharply defined margin and are usually round or oval with a size between 0.5 and 20 cm. 10–20% of people have at least one CAL and up to three is within normal limits.

Neurofibromatosis type 1 (NF1). This is the most common cause of multiple CALs. Affected individuals typically have six or more CALs, 1.5 cm or larger in postpubertal individuals or 0.5 cm or larger in prepubertal individuals. See 'Neurofibromatosis type 1 (NF1)' page 396.

Neurofibromatosis type 2 (NF2). Typically 1–6 CALs. Only 4% of affected individuals in Evans *et al.*'s (19920 study had more than 3 spots; none had more than 6. See 'Neurofibromatosis type 2 (NF2)' page 470.

Ring chromosome phenotype. CALs indistinguishable from those of NF1 are found in association with ring chromosomal abnormalities. See 'Ring chromosomes' page 538.

Bannayan–Riley–Ruvalcaba (BRR; PTEN hamartomatous syndrome). A highly variable autosomal dominant (AD) disorder consisting of macrocephaly, vascular malformations, lipomas, and pigmented macules on the shaft of the penis. See 'Cowden syndrome (CS)' page 442.

Schimke immuno-osseous dysplasia. A rare autosomal recessive (AR) spondylo-epiphyseal dysplasia. The characteristic features include short stature with hyperpigmented macules and an unusual facies, proteinuria with progressive renal failure, lymphopenia with recurrent infections, and cerebral ischaemia (Boerkoel *et al.* 2000).

Urticaria pigmentosa (UP). UP is sometimes confused with NF1 because the mast cell infiltrates can resemble CALs. In this condition rubbing the brown spot initiates histamine release from the mast cells leading to localized oedema.

Recessive mutations in mismatch-repair (MMR) genes. Recessive mutations in the mismatch-repair genes *PMS2* and *MLH1* can cause a phenotype of CALs, axillary freckling, subtle generalized increase in skin pigmentation, primitive neuroectodermal tumours (PNETs), and non-Hodgkins lymphoma (NHL). This NF1-like condition has a highly malignant phenotype and follows AR inheritance (Sheridan *et al.* 2003).

Patchy pigmentation (not café au lait)

Areas of pigmented skin that are macular but are not typical CALs can be found in a number of rare genetic syndromes, including syndromes with associated malignancies. Consider the possibility of Fanconi syndrome, ataxia telangiectasia, Nijmegen breakage syndrome, and syndromes with PTEN mutations (Bannayan–Zonana, Cowden), and Turcot syndrome. See 'DNA repair defects' page 304.

Lentigines

These are brown to black in colour, with even pigmentation and a sharply defined border. They are darker than freckles. They are common and normal when seen on the skin, but are unusual on mucous membranes where they may be a hallmark of a single-gene disorder such as Peutz–Jeghers syndrome. They usually become apparent in early childhood. Lentigines are the cutaneous markers of several genetic disorders (Bauer) which include:

- **Peutz–Jeghers syndrome (PJS).** In PJS lentigines of the lips, buccal mucosa, and genital skin are found in association with polyps characteristically in the small intestine. See 'Peutz–Jeghers syndrome (PJS)' page 474.
- **LEOPARD syndrome.** An association of lentigines–electrocardiograph (ECG) abnormalities–ocular hypertelorism–pulmonary stenosis–abnormal genitalia–retardation of growth–deafness. LEOPARD syndrome is caused by mutations in the Noonan gene, *PTPN11*.

- **Carney complex (CNC).** An AD condition characterized by skin pigmentary abnormalities, cardiac and cutaneous myxomas, endocrine tumors, and schwannomas. See 'Multiple endocrine neoplasia' page 466.

Pigmented naevi (moles)

Moles are common and the average adult has 15–30. These common naevi should be distinguished from dysplastic naevi, which have the potential to develop into a malignant melanoma. Children with **Turner syndrome** may have an increased number of pigmented naevi.

Acanthosis nigricans

Raised, thickened areas of darkly pigmented skin more often seen in the axillae, groin, and neck areas. As the disorder progresses, the skin gets rougher and the affected areas enlarge. Acanthosis nigricans is believed to result from insulin resistance and can be associated with diabetes, obesity, or malignancy.

Syndromic causes of acanthosis nigricans include insulin resistance syndromes such as Donohue syndrome, Beradinelli syndrome, Crouzon syndrome, and Beare–Stevenson syndrome.

Poikiloderma

This condition is usually widespread, but is particularly found in sun-exposed areas. Although there is hyperpigmentation, this is accompanied by areas of hypopigmentation, atrophy, and telangiectasia and is dissimilar to CALs and other forms of hyperpigmentation. It is found in Rothmund–Thompson syndrome, xeroderma pigmentosum (XP; see 'DNA repair defects' page 304), progeria, and Majewski osteodysplastic primordial dwarfism (MOPD). There are non-genetic conditions with poikiloderma as well.

Genetic advice

Recurrence risk

Seek a specific diagnosis on which to base genetic advice.

Support group contact: International Incontinentia Pigmenti International Foundation <http://imgen. bcm.tmc.edu/IPIF>; Unique—The Rare chromosome disorder support group <www.rarechromo.org>.

Expert adviser: Anonymous.

References

Bauer AJ, Stratakis CA. The lentiginoses: cutaneous markers of systemic disease and a window to new aspects of tumourigenesis. *J Med Genet* 2005; **42**: 801–10.

Boerkoel CF, O'Neill S, *et al.* Manifestations and treatment of Schimke immuno-osseous dysplasia: 14 new cases and a review of the literature. *Eur J Pediatr*. 2000; **159**: 1–7.

Evans DGR, Huson SM, *et al.* A clinical study of type 2 neurofibromatosis. *Q J Med* 1992; **304**: 603–18.

Legius E, Schrander-Stumpel C, *et al.* PTPN11 mutations in LEOPARD syndrome. *J Med Genet.* 2002; **39** (8): 571–4.

Sheridan E, De Vos M, *et al.* Recessive mutations in MMR genes are a cause of an NF-1 like phenotype with a highly malignant phenotype and a high recurrence risk. *J Med Genet* 2003; **40** (Suppl. 1): SP28.

Sybert VP. *Genetic skin disorders*, Oxford Monographs in Medical Genetics. Oxford University Press, New York, 1997.

Plagiocephaly and abnormalities of skull shape

When asked to see a baby or infant who has an abnormality of the shape of the cranium, the aim is to distinguish a postural, deformational cause, which usually resolves with time, from syndromic or non-syndromic craniosynostosis.

Craniosynostosis, or craniostenosis, is premature fusion of one or more of the skull sutures. This fusion prevents or restricts growth perpendicular to the synostosis but not in the parallel direction. Characteristic skull shapes arise depending on the suture involved.

Descriptive terms for abnormalities of skull shape: These can be confusing. The skull shape can be described in terms of length, width, and the prominence of parts of the skull.

- **Dolicocephaly and scaphocephaly.** Increased length compared to width of skull. This can be a postural deformation associated with prematurity and breech presentation but is also a feature of sagittal synostosis.
- **Brachycephaly.** Flattening of the occiput with increased width compared to length of the skull. This is a common postural deformity but also occurs when there is excessive growth in the sagittal suture due to bilateral coronal synostosis.
- **Plagiocephaly.** Asymmetry of the head shape. Postural deformation needs to be distinguished from unilateral coronal or lambdoid synostosis.
- **Trigonocephaly.** The forehead assumes a triangular shape and is a feature of metopic synostosis.

- **Turricephaly, oxycephaly**, and **acrocephaly** all refer to a high, narrow 'tower'-shaped skull. This is found in association with severe coronal or multisuture synostosis.
- **Kleeblettschaedel, or clover leaf skull.** Premature fusion of all the cranial sutures. This is a serious life-threatening condition with considerable morbidity and mortality that requires urgent surgical management.

See figure in 'Craniosynostosis' in Chapter 3, 'Common consultations', page 288.

Deformation. Deformational plagiocephaly may occur if external forces are applied to a skull with normal sutures. Many babies are born with mild asymmetry of the skull due to one of the factors listed below.

- Immediately after a difficult vaginal delivery the baby's skull shape may have been 'moulded' due to cephalopelvic disproportion. Reassess the baby's skull shape at the 6 week baby check.
- Commonly, there is flattening of the frontal region due to mild compression in the later part of pregnancy. In most babies this resolves, but babies with hypotonia and developmental delay are at risk of gravitational forces accentuating the asymmetry if the child is unable to hold his/her head unsupported.
- The 'Back to sleep' campaign, to encourage parents to place babies in a supine sleeping position to reduce the risk of sudden infant death has led to increasing referrals

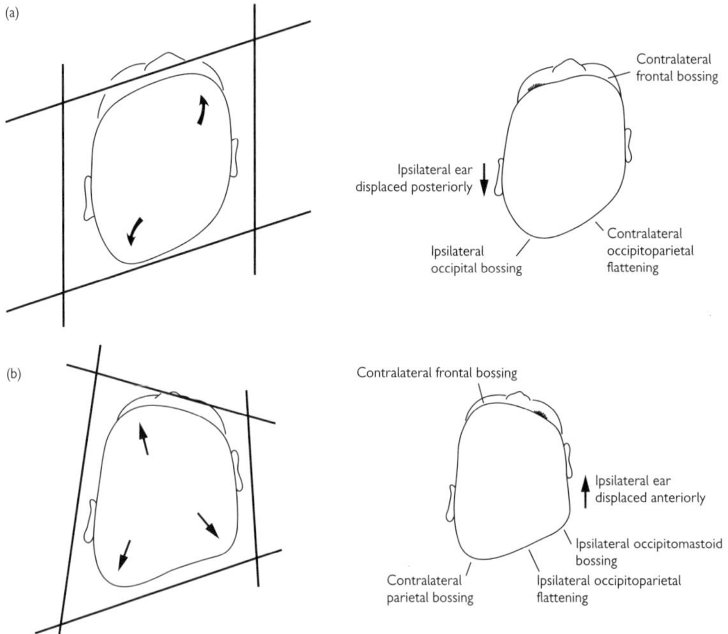

a) positional moulding of the L fronto-orbital region (the entire face and cranium are turning around a central axis) and (b) unilateral R-sided craniosynostosis.

Note that positional moulding results in a parallelogram-shaped head with the forehead flattening on the opposite side to the forward ear; whereas unilateral coronal craniosynostosis results in a trapezium-shaped head with the ear further forward on the side of the synostosis.

of infants with an unusually shaped skull (mainly brachycephaly) due to postural deformation.

In an infant with a postural deformation, the entire face and cranium appear to have turned around a central axis, with the forehead, brow, cheek, and ear all moving back and slightly down on the 'affected side' whilst reciprocal flattening is seen on the opposite side posteriorly. This point is very helpful when trying to distinguish between a postural cause and true craniosynostosis. In a postural deformity of the frontoparietal region the ear is pushed back on the side of the deformation, whereas in unilateral synostosis of the coronal suture the ear on the affected side is further forward (see figure).

If unable to determine if the asymmetry is due to a postural cause or, if the deformity is progressing refer to a craniofacial centre for evaluation.

Craniosynostosis. Premature fusion of one or more cranial sutures is found in 1 in 2500 livebirths. It is a heterogeneous condition and about 15–20% have a recognizable syndromic cause. Molecular testing is indicated in children with syndromic and non-syndromic synostosis. 30% of children with non-syndromic coronal craniosynostosis have mutations in FGFR3 (749C>G, Pro250Arg). The shape of the skull depends on which suture(s) are involved. An early referral to a specialist craniofacial unit should be arranged to assess whether there is raised intracranial pressure and to discuss timing of operative treatment. Untreated craniosynostosis may lead to increasing intracranial pressure and asymmetry of the midface and, if craniosynostosis is suspected, expert assessment is mandatory.

See 'Craniosynostosis' page 288.

Clinical approach

History: key points

- Three-generation family tree. Enquire for family history of craniosynostosis.
- Pregnancy. Decreased liquor, abnormal fetal presentation, persistent discomfort and sensation of 'head being stuck', twin pregnancy (deformation).
- Uterine abnormalities such as bicornuate uterus (deformation).
- Precipitate delivery (deformation). Relevant when assessing a neonate, but not for older infants.
- Obstructed labour (pre-existing synostosis).
- Skull shape unusual at birth.
- Progression of deformity.
- Sleeping position (deformation).
- Delayed motor milestones or prematurity may mean that an infant spends a longer period on his/her back rather than holding the head unsupported (deformation). Some craniosynostosis syndromes have associated delay and untreated synostosis may lead to developmental problems.
- Seizures (raised intracranial pressure from craniosynostosis).

Examination: key points

- Occipital-frontal circumference (OFC) and other growth parameters.
- Fontanelle. Position, size, and tension.
- Sutures. Palpate for sutural ridging (craniosynostosis).
- Skull shape. Examine the head from both sides, from above, and from the front. Describe the skull shape. Photographs of the head from the front, in profile, and from above (babies and young infants) can be very helpful and are also useful in documenting objectively whether there is progression or improvement in the skull shape over time. Look carefully for compensatory bulging/bossing (craniosynostosis).
- Ear position. Used in conjunction with the skull shape to assess if deformation is likely.
- Shape of face and supraorbital area, asymmetry.
- Eye spacing (measure) and/or exorbitism.
- Hands and feet for evidence of syndactyly. Fusion of digits in Apert syndrome; minor degrees of syndactyly in Pfeiffer and Saethre–Chotzen syndromes.
- Cleft palate (Apert syndrome).
- Broad thumbs and halluces (Pfeiffer syndrome), brachydactyly.
- Assessment of parental head shape.

Special investigations

- Skull X-ray. Posteroanterior (PA), lateral. Interpretation is difficult in infants and requires good quality films and expert reporting. The signs of synostosis are partial or total absence of the suture, indistinct zones along the suture, and perisutural sclerosis. Assess for evidence of a harlequin sign (elevation of the lesser wing of sphenoid) in coronal synostosis. If your clinical impression is that the child has craniosynostosis, seek expert advice even if a routinely reported skull X-ray is normal. Expert assessment and computerized tomographic (CT) scanning may be required to resolve matters.
- Chromosome analysis. Routine cytogenetic analysis in the normally developing infant with no features other than plagiocephaly is not indicated. The presence of developmental delay would be sufficient to warrant investigation. Consider fluorescent *in situ* hybridization (FISH) tests for *TWIST* and del 22q11.
- EDTA sample for molecular genetic analysis in infants with syndromic craniosynostosis or non-syndromic coronal synostosis.

Genetic advice

Recurrence risk

- In infants with developmental delay and hypotonia, investigate and counsel appropriately.
- If there is an identifiable uterine anomaly, the recurrence risk for future pregnancies will be high without treatment of the anomaly.
- For infants with craniosynostosis see 'Craniosynostosis' page 288.

Carrier detection

For infants with craniosynostosis see 'Craniosynostosis' page 288.

Prenatal diagnosis

For infants with craniosynostosis see 'Craniosynostosis' page 288.

Natural history and further management

In plagiocephaly or brachycephaly due to deformation the prognosis for normal skull shape is good.

Support group contact: For craniosynostosis: Headlines Craniofacial Support <info@headlines.org.uk>.

Expert adviser: A.O.M. Wilkie, Nuffield Professor of Pathology and Honorary Consultant in Clinical Genetics, University of Oxford, Oxford, England.

Reference

Wall S.A. Diagnostic features of the major non-syndromic craniosyostoses and the common deformational conditions which may be confused with them. *Curr Paediatr* 1997; **7**: 8–17.

Postaxial polydactyly

Postaxial polydactyly (PAP) is defined as an extra digit on the postaxial (radial or fibular) side of the hand or foot. Much is now known about the genes that control and initiate fetal limb development. The digits of the hand and feet are separated by 55 days postfertilization. The prevalence is between 1 in 1000 and 1 in 2000 newborns and PAP is particularly common in Africans. PAP is classified into two types (see figure).

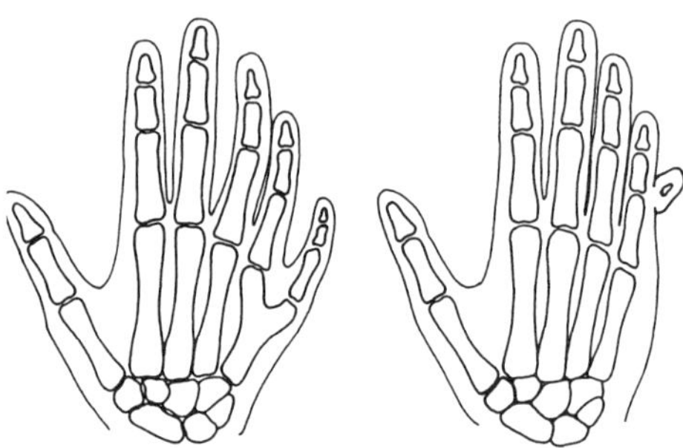

Postaxial polydactyly. Schematic shows type A postaxial polydactyly on left and type B on right. In type B, the extra digit is usually only a pedunculated tag attached to the fifth digit between the first and second flexion creases. (Taken from Stevenson *et al.* (1993), fig. 28.12, p. 822, by permission of Oxford University Press.)

- **Type A (PAP-A).** The digit is well formed and articulates with a metacarpal.
- **Type B (PAP-B).** The digit may be as small as a skin tag and is attached to the medial border of the 5th finger (pedunculated postminimus).

Postaxial polydactyly can be inherited as an isolated feature, (autosomal dominant (AD) with incomplete penetrance and variable expression) or can be a useful marker for a number of relatively common syndromes.

NB. Isolated dominant PAP-A and PAP-A/B are genetically heterogeneous. Some families have heterozygous mutations in the *GLI-3* gene on 7p13, but others are linked to 7q, 13q, or 19p.

Clinical approach

History: key points

- Three-generation family history with enquiry about presence in other family members and consanguinity.
- Maternal age (trisomy 13).
- Failure to thrive (marked in Smith–Lemli–Opitz (SLO) syndrome).
- Developmental delay.

Examination: key points

- Other types of polydactyly, syndactyly, and limb defects.
- Short stature (Ellis–van Creveld (EVC) syndrome).
- Overgrowth (Simpson–Golabi–Behmel (SGB) syndrome).
- Obesity (Bardet–Biedl syndrome (BBS)).
- Cranial shape (for craniosynostosis), size (macrocephaly and microcephaly), and skull defects/scalp aplasia.
- Irregular breathing (Joubert syndrome).
- Eyes (microphthalmia, trisomy 13), pigmentary retinopathy (BBS).
- Oral frenulae (EVC and Mohr–Majewski syndrome).

- Tongue hamartomas (Joubert and Mohr–Majewski syndromes).
- Cleft lip and/or cleft palate.
- Bell-shaped chest (Jeune and EVC syndromes).
- Cardiac defects.
- Renal anomalies, especially cysts (Joubert and Meckel syndromes).
- Genital anomalies (Kaufman–McKusick, BBS, and SLO syndromes).

Special investigations

- Photographs
- Chromosome analysis: trisomy 13, del 22q11, and many other abnormalities.
- Brain imaging for structural abnormalities of the central nervous system (CNS); may start with ultrasound scan (USS) in the neonatal period.
- Skeletal survey and skull X-rays if indicated from the examination.
- Renal USS if there are other features of a syndrome with known renal anomalies.
- Cardiac echo in the presence of a murmur or the presence of other features of a syndrome with known cardiac defects.
- 7-dehydrocholesterol analysis (SLO syndrome).
- DNA storage/gene analysis.

Some diagnoses to consider

When there is pre- or mesoaxial polydactyly and/or syndactyly the differential diagnosis has a bias towards syndromes with these features.

Chromosomal disorders

An example is trisomy 13 (see 'Patau syndrome (trisomy 13)' page 534.)

Syndromes that are usually lethal in the neonatal period

Meckel–Gruber syndrome. Lethal autosomal recessive (AR) syndrome with occipital encephalocele, bilaterally large kidneys with multicystic dysplasia and fibrotic changes of the liver, postaxial polydactyly. The kidneys are typically filled with thin-walled cysts of various sizes. In Fraser and Lytwyn's (1981) study of 38 secondarily ascertained cases of Meckel syndrome, 100% had cystic dysplasia of the kidney, 63% had an occipital meningocele, 55% had polydactyly, and 18% had no brain malformation. At least three loci are implicated, with Finnish Meckel syndrome linked to 17q22.

Hydrolethalus syndrome. AR condition similar to Meckel–Gruber syndrome but without cystic dysplasia of the kidneys. A rare disorder, but more common in Finland. Postaxial polydactyly occurs in 80%. See 'Short limbs' page 630.

Short-rib–polydactyly syndromes. A group of lethal skeletal dysplasias with AR inheritance characterized by markedly short ribs, short limbs, usually polydactyly, and multiple anomalies of major organs. See 'Short limbs' page 630.

Syndromes with craniosynostosis

Greig cephalopolysyndactyly. AD condition characterized by a high forehead with frontal bossing, macrocephaly, hypertelorism, and a broad base to the nose. Both pre- and postaxial polydactyly can occur but postaxial polydactyly is more common and is usually type B. The thumbs are often broad. Caused by mutations in *GLI3* on 7p13.

Syndromes with skeletal dysplasia

Ellis–van Creveld syndrome (EVC). AR condition characterized by PAP of the hands and occasionally of the feet. Shortening of the limbs, small deepset nails, multiple oral frenulae, and sometimes natal teeth. There is often congenital heart disease, usually an atrial septal defect (ASD). The ribs are short and the thorax is long and narrow. Radiologically, the features are indistinguishable from those of Jeune syndrome. The condition is caused by biallelic mutations in either *EVC* or *EVC2*—two non-homologous genes arranged in a head-to-head configuration on 4p16.

Jeune syndrome (asphyxiating thoracic dystrophy). AR condition characterized by a long narrow thorax with short ribs. There is also rhizomelic limb shortening. The face looks normal. Approximately 50% have PAP. Can be fatal in infancy due to respiratory insufficiency often exacerbated by a viral illness, e.g. bronchiolitis. Survivors may develop chronic renal failure with cystic changes in the kidney and also hepatic and pancreatic fibrosis and retinal degeneration. Genetically heterogeneous—one locus mapped to 15q13.

Mohr–Majewski syndrome. AR condition that is sometimes classified as oro-facial-digital (OFD) syndrome type IV and also as one of the short-rib–polydactyly syndromes, although the rib shortening is mild allowing survival. Typically there is a midline cleft or notch in the upper lip, a high-arched or cleft palate, oral frenulae, and fleshy hamartomas on the tongue. PAP of the hands is common, with pre-or postaxial polydactyly of the feet. Complex congenital heart disease, e.g. tetralogy of Fallot and transposition of the great arteries (TGA) may occur.

Kaufman–McKusick syndrome (hydrometacolpos–polydactyly syndrome). AR condition characterized by PAP sometimes with syndactyly. Female infants have hydrometacolpos with an imperforate hymen or vaginal atresia. Cyanotic congenital heart disease is common. Caused by mutations in the *MKKS* gene on 20p12 (allelic to *BBS6*—see below).

Other syndromes

Acrocallosal syndrome. AR condition characterized by mental retardation, agenesis of the corpus callosum, and preaxial polydactyly of the feet. PAP of the hands and/or feet may also occur

Bardet–Biedl syndrome (BBS). Characterized by pigmentary retinal dystrophy, PAP, obesity, cognitive impairment, and renal defects. AR condition that is genetically heterogeneous with seven loci mapped and five genes currently identified. *BBS6* and Kaufman–McKusick syndrome are allelic and caused by mutations in *MKKS* on 20p12. See 'Obesity with and without developmental delay', page 192.

Joubert syndrome. AR condition usually diagnosed in infancy with hypotonia and cerebellar vermis hypoplasia and a characteristic episodic respiratory pattern. Polydactyly is an occasional feature. Genetically heterogeneous. See 'Cerebellar anomalies', page 66.

Oro-facial-digital (OFD) syndromes especially OFD type 1. OFD type 1 is an X-linked dominant (XLD) malformation syndrome caused by mutation in *CXORF5*. The features in the hands are syndactyly, usually skin syndactyly affecting variable digits, brachydactyly, and PAP. Craniofacial anomalies are midline cleft lip, tongue cysts, and excess oral frenulae.

Otopalatodigital syndrome type 2 (OPD-2). An X-linked recessive (XLR) condition characterized by micrognathia and small mouth with cleft palate. Dislocated hips, flexed overlapping fingers, PAP, and syndactyly. There may be disharmonious growth of the toes, which may have bulbous tips ('tree-frog' feet). Radiographs may show curved or wavy long bones. Caused by specific localized mutations in the *FLNA* gene on Xq28.

Pallister–Hall syndrome (anocerebrodigital syndrome). Characterized by imperforate anus, postaxial (or often *mesoaxial*) polydactyly, hypopituitarism, and hypothalamic hamartoblastoma. Approximately 50% have a cleft larynx or bifid epiglottis. AD condition with very variable expression caused by mutations in *GLI3* on 7p13 (allelic to, Greig).

Simpson–Golabi–Behmel (SGB) syndrome. XLR condition characterized by overgrowth and caused by mutations in *glypican 3*. Some have PAP. See 'Overgrowth', page 206.

Smith–Lemli–Opitz (SLO) syndrome. Approximately 50% have PAP. Other features are pre- and postnatal growth deficiency and developmental delay (almost all), cleft palate (37–52%), cardiac defects (36–38%), hypospadias and/or cryptorchidism (90–100%) in affected males, Y-shaped 2,3 toe syndactyly (>95%). See 'Hypospadias', page 142.

Ulnar–mammary syndrome. AD with variable penetrance. Ulnar ray defects varying from hypoplasia of the 5th digit to absence of the ulna and ulnar ray (occasionally may have PAP). In addition, females have small/absent breast with hypoplastic nipples; males have small penises and delayed puberty and reduced fertility. Due to mutations in *TBX3* on 12q23.

Genetic advice

Recurrence risk

- **Syndromic PAP.** Counsel as appropriate for the underlying syndrome.
- **Isolated PAP** usually follows AD inheritance but the condition is not always fully penetrant and recessive pedigrees have been described.

Carrier detection

Possible if the familial mutations are known. Carriers of recessive syndromes such as BBS and SLO may occasionally have apparently isolated PAP, but most do not.

Prenatal diagnosis

- Genetic or chromosomal testing may be available.
- Biochemical testing (SLO).
- USS. A well-formed postaxial digit can be visualized from the second trimester. Other USS markers should be used to confirm a diagnosis.

Natural history and further management (preventative measures)

Consider referral to a plastic surgeon with special expertise in hand surgery.

Support group contact: Many of the syndromes have their own support groups. See <www.cafamily.org.uk>.

Expert adviser: Frances R. Goodman, Former Honorary Clinical Lecturer, Molecular Medicine Unit, Institute of Child Health, London, England.

References

Fraser FC, Lytwyn A. Spectrum of anomalies in the Meckel syndrome, or: 'Maybe there is a malformation syndrome with at least one constant anomaly'. *Am J Med Genet* 1981; **9** (1): 67–73.

Stevenson RE, Hall JG, Goodman RM. (ed.). *Human malformations and related anomalies*, Vol. II, Oxford Monographs on Medical Genetics no. 27. Oxford University Press, New York, 1993.

Temtamy SA, McKusick VA. *The genetics of hand malformations.* Alan R. Liss, New York, 1978.

Visapaa I, Salonen R, *et al.* Assignment of the locus for hydrolethalus syndrome to the highly restricted region on 11q23–25. *Am J Hum Genet* 1999; **65**: 1086–95.

Winth RM, Baraitser M (eds) London Dysmorphology Database. 2003.

Preaxial polydactyly

In preaxial polydactyly (PPD), the extra digit or duplicated digit is on the radial/tibial side of the hand/foot. The thumb and hallux are most commonly affected.

There is great variability from broad distal phalanges to complete duplication. It is less common than postaxial polydactyly (PAP) and, in isolated PPD, males are more frequently affected.

The aim is to establish if the polydactyly is an isolated event or part of a syndrome. Correct classification will aid syndrome diagnosis (see table and figure).

Classification of preaxial polydactyly (Temtamy and McKusick 1978)

Type of preaxial polydactyly	Description
Type I	Duplication of the thumb/hallux
Type II	Triphalangeal thumbs/duplication of the hallux
Type III	Absent thumbs: one or two extra preaxial digits
Type IV	Broad thumbs, preaxial polysyndactyly, postaxial polydactyly

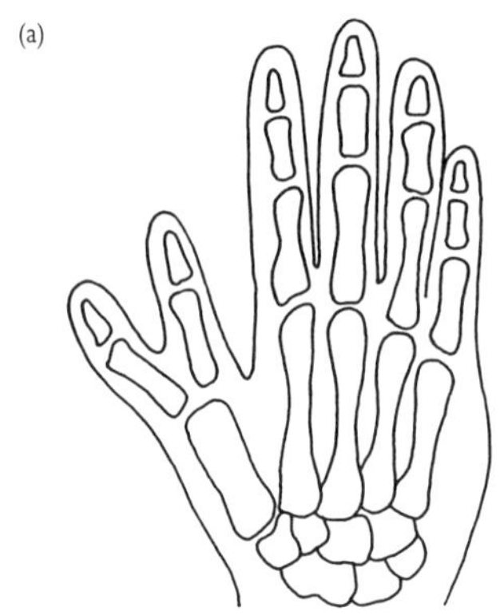

(a)

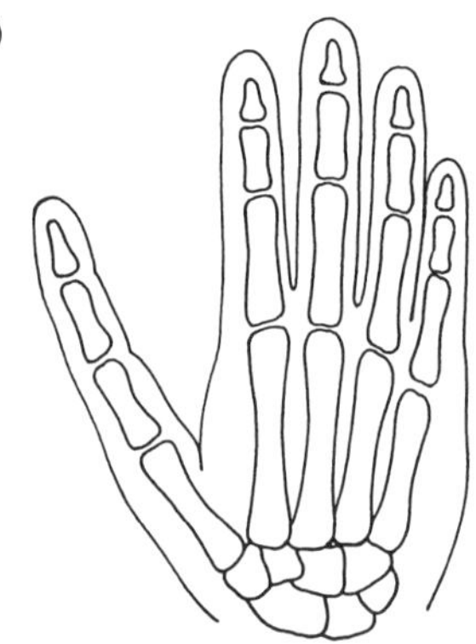

(b)

(a) Preaxial polydactyly type I, showing partial duplication of a biphalangeal thumb. (b) Preaxial polydactyly type II (triphalangeal thumb), showing three phalanges in thumb that is opposable. (Taken from Stevenson *et al.* (1993), figs 28.13 and 28.14, p. 822, by permission of Oxford University Press.)

NB. Numerous families with isolated dominant PPD-II, PPD-III, and triphalangeal thumb–polysyndactyly syndrome (MIM 190605) show linkage to 7q36; the underlying mutations are now thought to affect a regulatory element for the sonic hedgehog (*SHH*) gene.

Clinical approach

History: key points

- At least three-generation pedigree; explain to parents about the minimal signs that could indicate a gene carrier.
- Consanguinity (DOOR (deafness–onychodystrophy–onycholysis–retardation) syndrome, Carpenter syndrome, acrocallosal syndrome (ACS)).
- Neurological/developmental problems.
- Early pregnancy events/teratogen exposure, maternal diabetes.

Examination: key points

- Hands and feet. Describe shape and count the total number of digits. A good way to document this in the clinic is to put the hand/foot directly on the paper and draw around it.
- Thumb. Document structure and function:
  1 number of phalanges; three phalanges known as 'triphalangeal';
  2 if duplicated;
  3 if broad;
  4 opposition.
- Hallux (great or big toe) Document structure as above.
- Head and skull shape; macrocephaly (Greig syndrome), craniosynostosis (Pfeiffer and Carpenter syndromes).
- Features suggestive of any other skeletal abnormalities or limb shortening.
- Broad forehead (Greig syndrome).
- Face: clefts, hemifacial microsomia.
- Oral region: cleft palate, oral frenulae, tongue cysts (oral-facial-digital (OFD) syndromes).
- Cardiac murmurs (Holt–Oram and Townes–Brock (TBS) syndromes).
- Genital and renal anomalies (TBS).
- *Remember to examine the parents.*

Special investigations

- Photographs
- X-rays of the hands and feet are essential to assess the skeletal elements and to detect minor features not seen on clinical examination. The X-ray will assist in the process of definition.
- Skull X-rays and further skeletal films, if indicated from clinical assessment.
- Brain imaging:
  - agenesis of the corpus callosum in ACS;
  - cystic lesions in OFD2 syndrome;
  - cerebellar hypoplasia in Varadi–Papp (OFD6) syndrome.
- Full blood count and platelets (Aase syndrome).
- Hearing test (DOOR syndrome).
- Renal scans, if indicated.
- Urine organic acids (DOOR syndrome).
- Blood for DNA storage or genetic analysis if available.

Syndromic diagnoses to consider

PPD is a very good diagnostic marker for a number of rare syndromes. Although rare, many have very distinctive features, which will help when using a database such as the London Dysmorphology Database (LDDB). It is extremely important to use your information to classify the type of PPD in your patient. Many of the syndromes with this feature are noted above.

Acrocallosal syndrome (ACS; Schinzel syndrome). ACS is an autosomal recessive (AR) condition, characterized by agenesis of the corpus callosum, pre- and postaxial polydactyly, mild hypertelorism, and a spectrum of psychomotor retardation from mild to severe. Cranial cysts (including arachnoid cysts) were seen in 10/34 published cases of ACS (Koenig *et al.* 2002). There is some diagnostic overlap with Greig cephalopolysyndactyly syndrome, which is caused by mutations in *GLI3*.

Carpenter syndrome (acrocephalopolysyndactyly type II). A rare AR syndrome with PPD and brachydactyly in conjunction with craniosynostosis. The thumbs are often radially deviated. There is often hypoplasia of the middle phalanges.

Fanconi anaemia. A variety of radial ray anomalies are found in Fanconi anaemia including absent, hypoplastic, supernumerary or bifid thumbs and hypoplastic or absent radii. 20% have other skeletal problems (e.g. vertebral and rib anomalies). See 'DNA repair defects' page 304.

Greig cephalopolysyndactyly. Autosomal dominant (AD) condition characterized by a high forehead with frontal bossing, macrocephaly, hypertelorism, and a broad base to the nose. In the hands both PAP-B and, less commonly, PPD (broad thumbs with bifid nails and distal phalanges) can occur; also often central syndactyly. In the feet usually PPD (duplicated hallux) with syndactyly toes 1–3 occurs. Caused by mutations in *GLI3* on 7p13. The facial features of Greig can be subtle, especially in infancy. It is generally considered that PPD type IV is part of the spectrum of Greig syndrome and is caused by mutations in *GLI3*. Mutation analysis will help to determine if the cause is a new mutation in situations where there is clinical doubt.

Hydrolethalus. AR (*236680*). Usually the polydactyly is postaxial. Lethal in the neonatal period. See 'Postaxial polydactyly', page 214.

Lacrimo-auriculo-dental-digital (LADD) syndrome. AD condition characterized by absence or atresia of the lacrimal punctae causing overflow of tears (epiphora) and recurrent infection, simple, cup-shaped ears with sensorineural or conductive deafness, hypoplastic teeth, and bifid or triphalangeal thumbs with clinodactyly.

Pfeiffer syndrome. AD condition with coronal craniosynostosis, broad thumbs and halluces, and soft-tissue syndactyly. The halluces are usually in the varus position and a variety of anomalies are found including broad halluces, bifid halluces, and PPD. The face is similar to that in Crouzon syndrome but clover-leaf skull is a more frequent complication. Sometimes the thumbs and halluces are be broad and there may be a degree of skin syndactyly. Mutations are found in either *FGFR1* or *FGFR2*. *FGFR2* mutations may lead to a more severe craniofacial phenotype.

Syndromes in which triphalangeal thumbs (PPD type II) may occur

Paradoxically there is considerable overlap with syndromes causing hypoplastic or absent thumbs.

Diamond–Blackfan anaemia. Characteristically presents with hypoplastic macrocytic anaemia in the first year of life; 75% by 3 months of age. There is a 20-fold increased risk of leukaemia. Only ~20% of patients have thumb anomalies

(e.g. triphalangeal thumb). Most cases are sporadic but, when familial, kindreds usually show AD inheritance with variable expressivity (although AR inheritance is reported). Approximately 20% of patients have heterozygous mutations in the ribosomal subunit gene *RPS19* on 19q13.

DOOR (deafness–onychodystrophy–onycholysis–retardation) syndrome. A rare AR syndrome in which the nails can be absent with hypoplasia of the distal phalanges. There is congenital deafness and there may be triphalangeal thumbs.

Fanconi anaemia. See above.

Holt–Oram syndrome. AD heart–hand syndrome caused by mutations in *TBX5*. Penetrance is 100%. Skeletal defects affect the upper limbs exclusively and are invariably bilateral and usually asymmetrical. They range from clinodactyly, limited supination, and narrow, sloping shoulders to absent, hypoplastic, or triphalangeal thumb and severe reduction deformities of the upper arm (4.5%).

LADD syndrome. See above.

Townes-Brock syndrome (TBS) is an AD condition with imperforate anus, hand anomalies (triphalangeal thumb, hypoplastic thumb), and ear malformations (dysplastic ears and ear tags) with sensorineural hearing loss. Within and between families the phenotype displays striking variability. *SALL1*, a zinc finger transcription factor, is the disease-causing gene. High incidence of new mutations. Cardiac anomalies have been reported.

Genetic advice

A unilateral PPD without other features may be a sporadic event but bilateral changes affecting the hands and feet are likely to be genetic and most commonly dominantly inherited. Carefully examine parents and exclude features of syndromes.

Recurrence risk

Counsel as appropriate for the underlying syndrome. If use of anticonvulsant or other teratogen was the cause try to eliminate/reduce fetal exposure.

Prenatal diagnosis

- Genetic testing for some of these syndromes may be available.
- Ultrasound scans. A well-formed preaxial digit can be visualized from the second trimester. Other ultrasound markers should be used to confirm a diagnosis.

Lay group contact: Many of the syndromes have their own support groups. See <www.cafamily.org.uk>. and National Organization for Rare Disorders (US) www.raredisorders.org

Expert adviser: Frances R. Goodman, Former Honorary Clinical Lecturer, Molecular Medicine Unit, Institute of Child Health, London, England.

References

Draptchinskaia N, Gustavsson P, Andersson B, *et al.* The gene encoding ribosomal protein S19 is mutated in Diamond–Blackfan anaemia. *Nat Genet* 1999; **21**: 169–76.

Koenig R, Bach A, Woelki U, Grzeschik K-H, Fuchs S. Spectrum of the acrocallosal syndrome. *Am J Med Genet* 2002; **108**: 7–11.

London Dysmorphology Database. Winth RM, Baraitser M (eds) 2003.

Qazi Q, Kassner EG. Triphalangeal thumbs. *J Med Genet* 1988; **25**: 505–20.

Stevenson RE, Hall JG, Goodman RM. (ed.). *Human malformations and related anomalies*, Vol. II, Oxford Monographs on Medical Genetics no. 27. Oxford University Press, New York, 1993.

Temtamy SA, McKusick VA. *The genetics of hand malformations.* Alan R. Liss, New York, 1978.

Prolonged neonatal jaundice and jaundice in infants below 6 months

Jaundice manifests as yellow discoloration of the skin and the sclera of the eye. It is caused by deposition of bile pigments in the deep layers of the skin.

Jaundice (indirect hyperbilirubinaemia) is very common in newborn babies and many normal babies develop jaundice on the second or third day (physiological jaundice). Jaundice requires further investigation when it persists for more than 2–4 weeks.

Bilirubin comes from the breakdown of haemoglobin. This form of bilirubin is indirect bilirubin and is toxic to the brain (kernicterus and deafness) and cannot be excreted by the kidneys. Bilirubin is attached to albumin for transport and in the liver is conjugated with glucuronic acid by the action of the enzyme glucuronyl transferase. Bilirubin can then be excreted in the bile and through the kidneys.

Geneticists may be asked to see children with prolonged jaundice to determine if there is a genetic cause or contribution to the problem.

Clinical approach

History: key points

- Three-generation family history with specific enquiry regarding:
  - consanguinity (metabolic conditions);
  - ethnic origin (glucose-6-phosphate dehydrogenase (G6PD) deficiency, Niemann–Pick);
  - prolonged neonatal jaundice in sibling or parent;
  - drug/food reactions (G6PD);
  - other structural anomalies, i.e. congenital heart disease (Alagille syndrome).
- Intrahepatic cholestasis of pregnancy (found in some carriers of progressive familial intrahepatic cholestasis (PFIC)).
- Onset of jaundice, pruritus, scratching.
- Any fluctuation in the level of jaundice?
- Treatment given, eg. phototherapy or exchange transfusion.
- Failure to thrive, steatorrhoea.

Examination: key points

- Confirm jaundice clinically.
- Neurological abnormalities (Zellweger syndrome, Niemann–Pick disease).
- Large fontanelle.
- Facial dysmorphism (consider metabolic syndromes and Alagille syndrome).
- Cataract (galactokinase deficiency).
- Hepatospenomegaly (congenital infections, Zellweger syndrome, Niemann–Pick disease, cirrhosis).
- Heart murmur (Alagille syndrome).
- Bruising and bleeding (vitamin K deficiency).
- Contractures (ARC syndrome).
- Colour of urine and stool.

Special investigations

The geneticist is usually involved after the common paediatric causes of jaundice have been excluded. Note the following results.

- Bilirubin conjugated/unconjugated. Document levels and trends of conjugated and unconjugated bilirubin.
- Gamma glutamyl transpeptidase (gamma GT; low to normal in PFIC, elevated in most other causes of cholestasis).
- Other liver function tests and ammonia.
- Cholesterol.
- Urine reducing substances.
- Haematological investigations for evidence of haemolysis (Coombs test, rhesus and ABO incompatibility, abnormal red cells, e.g. spherocytes).
- Congenital infection screen. IgM (herpes, cytomegalovirus (CMV), rubella, coxsackie); TORCH (toxoplasmosis–other (including syphilis, varicella zoster, parvovirus)–rubella–cytomegalovirus–herpes simplex virus) screen.
- Thyroid function tests.
- Liver ultrasound scan (USS; structural lesions, choledochal cysts, biliary atresia) hepatobiliary scintigraphy (to evaluate biliary excretion) and/or liver biopsy.

Next consider the need for more specialized testing for genetic conditions.

- Bile acids (defects in bile synthesis).
- Alpha-1 antitrypsin level/phenotype.
- Very long chain fatty acids (VLCFAs; Zellweger syndrome).
- 7-Dehydrocholesterol if there are features of Smith–Lemli–Opitz (SLO) syndrome.
- Urine. Mass spectroscopy of bile acids, organic acids.
- Chest and vertebral X-rays (Alagille syndrome).
- Echocardiogram (Alagille syndrome).
- Ophthalmological exam (choriretinitis seen in intrauterine infections, anterior chamber defects seen in Alagille syndrome).
- DNA analysis or storage.

Some diagnoses to consider

Non-dysmorphic babies

Developmental anomalies affecting the biliary system.

- **Biliary atresia.** Jaundice gradually develops and is often not apparent for the first 2–3 weeks. It is important to detect the condition prior to irreversible liver damage occurring. The anatomy of the atresia must be defined and this is usually done radiologically. Extrahepatic atresia is the most amenable to surgical correction. Consider Alagille syndrome when there is paucity of the intrahepatic bile ducts. Once genetic causes of bile duct atresia have been excluded, the recurrence risk is low.
- **Choledochal cysts.** The typical presenting triad is pain, mass, and jaundice. However, they are sometimes detected prenatally on USS and may be an incidental finding later in infancy. Surgery is the treatment of choice. There is an association between congenital anomalies of the biliary tree and pancreatic duct and biliary tract malignancy later in life.

Alpha$_1$ antitrypsin deficiency. Alpha$_1$ antitrypsin deficiency is a common autosomal recessive (AR) disorder (1/1600–1/1800) characterized by predisposition to emphysema and cirrhosis. In Sveger's (1984) survey of 127 neonates with ZZ phenotype, virtually all had raised liver enzymes, and 14 (11%) had prolonged neonatal jaundice. Most of the infants with neonatal jaundice recovered but, overall, three (2.4%) of the ZZ cohort developed cirrhosis in infancy or childhood. It is important to diagnose this condition because cerebral haemorrhage can occur (vitamin K deficiency). See 'Alpha$_1$ antitrypsin deficiency' page 266.

Gilbert syndrome. Gilbert syndrome is one of the most common genetic disorders and is characterized by mild fluctuating unconjugated hyperbilirubinaemia (normal = 85 μmol/l) often precipitated by intercurrent illness. It is found in 4–7% of the general population. Penetrance is governed by other factors, e.g. gender (much less common in adult women possibly due to lower daily bilirubin production) and environmental factors. It is caused by homozygosity for the Gilbert-type promotor insertion (A(TA)$_7$TAA) in the UGT1A1 gene. Approximately 50% of the European and North American population is heterozygote for this promoter insertion and 9% are homozygous.

Prolonged neonatal jaundice is found in babies who are heterozygous or homozygous for Gilbert syndrome but in addition have G6PD, Coombs-negative ABO disease, spherocytosis, or prolonged breastfeeding.

Glucose-6-phosphate dehydrogenase deficiency (G6PD). G6PD is a red cell enzyme. Deficiency of G6PD is found more commonly in populations from Africa, South-east Asia and the Mediterranean. There are several subtypes. Haemolysis occurs after exposure to certain drugs and food (favism). It may contribute to prolonged neonatal jaundice if the child is also affected with Gilbert syndrome.

Galactosaemia is an AR condition caused by a deficiency of galactose-1-phosphate uridyl-transferase (which converts galactose to glucose) encoded by the *GALT* gene. Incidence in the UK is ~1/45 000 live births (estimated carrier frequency ~1/105); most patients are either homozygous or heterozygous for the Q188R mutation. Babies with galactosaemia usually present in the first days and weeks of life with feeding difficulties, vomiting, jaundice, failure to thrive, and liver and kidney disease. Untreated, the disorder can be fatal. Once galactose is removed from the diet, there is rapid improvement in the clinical symptoms. Babies may have cataracts, although many of these are minor and resolve with dietary treatment. Dietary treatment must be lifelong to stop recurrence of acute toxicity (Walter *et al.* 1999), but this does *not* prevent the long-term complications, which occur in the majority of patients (Schweitzer *et al.* 1993; Waggoner *et al.* 1990). These include ovarian failure in most females, speech problems, developmental delay, and specific learning difficulties. Growth may be delayed but the final height is normal. Girls may require induction of puberty and counselling about fertility. The life expectancy of treated individuals appears normal. However, there are reports of neurological complications such as movement disorders and intention tremor with increasing age. Cognitive function may worsen with age, and recent evidence suggests that there is endogenous production of galactose, which may be responsible for the emergence of these long-term effects despite early diagnosis and appropriate dietary treatment.

Crigler–Najjar types 1 and 2 (CN1 and CN2). These conditions are caused by mutations in the *UGT1A1* gene on 2q37. They are characterized by non-haemolytic unconjugated hyperbilirubinaemia; other hepatic functions are unaffected and the liver is morphologically normal.

- **CN1** is an AR condition that is rare in the Western hemisphere (prevalence <1/10^6; carrier frequency ~1/1000). It is caused by inactivating mutations in UGT1A1 resulting in a virtual absence of hepatic UGT1A1 enzyme activity and severe hyperbilirubinaemia (serum bilirubin, 340–685 μmol/l). Before the institution of phototherapy CN1 was uniformly lethal due to kernicterus.
- **CN2** is associated with intermediate levels of hyperbilirubinaemia (serum bilirubin, 120–340 μmol/l) as a result of incomplete deficiency of hepatic UGT1A1 activity caused either by compound heterozygosity for partial loss of function mutations or compound heterozygosity for a CN mutation together with a Gilbert-type promoter insertion (in *trans*).

Intermediate levels of hyperbilirubinaemia are observed commonly in families of patients with Crigler–Najjar.

Familial progressive intrahepatic cholestasis (PFIC). Babies present in the first few months. There is failure to thrive due to malabsorption. Loose stools are noted from birth. Liver biopsy is usually required to confirm the diagnosis. PFIC1 is due to mutation in *ATP8B1* and PFIC2 to mutation in *ABCB11*. Both are AR.

Neonatal haemochromatosis. This is a genetically heterogeneous and ill-defined entity.

Mitochondrial respiratory chain disorders. These may present with prolonged neonatal jaundice. See 'Mitochondrial DNA diseases' page 384.

With dysmorphic features

Alagille syndrome. An autosomal dominant (AD) multisystem condition characterized by bile duct paucity, cholestasis (abnormal liver function tests (LFTs) and raised cholesterol), congenital heart disease (especially tetralogy of Fallot and peripheral pulmonary artery stenosis (90%)), vertebral anomalies (e.g. butterfly vertebrae), opthalmological changes (posterior embryotoxon), and subtle facial dysmorphism (prominent forehead, deep-set eyes, straight nose with flattened tip, and a prominent and in some cases pointed chin). Alagille is caused by mutations in human *Jagged1* (JAG1), which is a ligand in the Notch signalling pathway and plays a role in early cell fate determination. 5–7% have a 20p12 deletion detectable by fluorescent *in situ* hybridization (FISH) with a *JAG1* probe. JAG1 mutations in Alagille syndrome include gene deletions and protein truncating, splicing, and missense mutations, suggesting that haploinsufficiency is the mechanism of disease causation. There is no clear genotype–phenotype correlation There is wide variation in expressivity. Investigate parents of an apparently sporadic case very carefully by:

- LFTs and cholesterol (typically cholestasis with raised cholesterol);
- vertebral Xray (e.g. butterfly vertebrae);
- echocardiogram;
- slit-lamp exam for posterior embryotoxon;
- assessment of facial features;
- molecular genetic studies if possible.

The new mutation rate is ~60%; a small proportion of parents with mild features may be gonosomal mosaics, however there is a great deal of clinical variability, even within families, amongst individuals with *JAG1* mutations.

The frequency of cardiac and liver disease is notably lower in secondarily ascertained mutation-positive relatives (Kamath).

Zellweger syndrome. An AR persoxisomal disorder often presenting in the neonatal period with central hypotonia ± seizures. The fontanelle is large and the forehead high. There may be stippled epiphyses (especially knees). See 'Floppy infant', page 118.

Niemann–Pick disease type A. An AR condition that is particularly prevalent in the Jewish population. Features are hepatomegaly, cholestatic jaundice, and neurological deterioration. There is deficiency of spingomyelinase and the causative gene is acid spingomyelinase (*SMPD1*) on 11p15.4. The prognosis is poor for those with type A. Niemann–Pick types B and C have an older age of onset.

Smith–Lemli–Opitz (SLO) syndrome. Failure to thrive, microcephaly, hypospadias in males, and 2,3 toe syndactyly are important features. Neonatal jaundice is not usually a significant problem. See 'Hypospadias', page 142.

ARC syndrome (Arthrogryposis, renal dysfunction, Cholestasis). AR syndrome characterised by arthrogryposis, neonatal cholestasis with bile duct hypoplasia and renal dysfunction. Affected infants fail to thrive and usually die in the first year of life. Caused by mutations in the *VPS33B* gene on 15q26.1 involved in regulation and fusion of membrane-bound organelles (Gissen).

Genetic advice

Recurrence risk
As appropriate for the cause of the jaundice.

Carrier detection
- Is possible in families where a causative mutation has been identified.
- May be possible for some biochemical abnormalities.

Prenatal diagnosis
Available to those families where there is molecular or biochemical confirmation of the diagnosis.

Natural history and further management (preventative measures)
Children with chronic liver disease should be under the care of a paediatric hepatologist. After biliary atresia, alpha-1 antitrypsin deficiency is the most frequent reason for liver transplantation in childhood.

Support group contact: Children's Liver Disease Foundation <www.childliverdisease.org>, Tel. 0121 212 3839.

Expert adviser: Ian D. Krantz, The Children's Hospital of Philadelphia, The University of Pennsylvania School of Medicine, Philadelphia, Pennsylvania, USA.

References
Gissen P, Johnson CA, *et al.* Mutations in VPS33B, encoding a regulator of SNARE-dependent membrane fusion, cause arthrogryposis-renal dysfunction-cholestasis (ARC) syndrome. *Nat Genet* 2004; **36**: 400–4.

Kadakol A, Sappal BS, *et al.* Interaction of coding region mutations and the Gilbert-type pomoter abnormality of the UGT1A1 gene causes moderate degrees of unconjugated hyperbilirubinaemia and may lead to neonatal kernicterus. *J Med Genet* 2001; **38**: 244–9.

Kamath BM, Bason L, *et al.* Consequnces of *JAG1* mutations. *J Med Genet* 2003; **40**: 891–95.

Kaplan M. Genetic interactions in the pathogenesis of neonatal hyperbilirubinaemia: Gilbert's syndrome and glucose-6-phosphate dehydrogenase deficiency. *J Perinatol* 2001; **21** (Suppl. 1): S30–4.

Krantz ID. Alagille syndrome; chipping away at the tip of the iceberg. *Am J Med Genet* 2002; **112**: 160–2.

Krantz ID, *et al.* Spectrum and frequency of JAGGED1 (JAG1) mutations in Alagille syndrome patients and their families. *Am J Hum Genet* 1998; **62**: 1361–9.

Schweitzer S, Shin Y, *et al.* Long term outcome in 134 patients with galactosaemia. *Eur J Paediatr* 1993; **152**: 36–43.

Shimotake T, Aoi S, *et al.* DPC-4 (Smad-4) and Kras gene mutations in biliary tract epithelium in children with anomalous pancreaticobiliary ductal union. *J Pediatr Surg* 2003; **38**: 694–7.

Sveger T. Prospective study of children with alpha 1-antitrypsin deficiency: eight-year-old follow-up. *J Pediatr* 1984; **104**: 91–4.

Waggoner DD, Buist NRM, *et al.* Long-term prognosis in galactosaemia: results of survey of 350 cases. *J Inherit Metab Dis* 1990; **13**: 802–18.

Walter JH, Collins JE, Leonard JV. Recommendations for the management of galactosaemia. UK galactosaemia steering group. *Arch Dis Child* 1999; **80**; 93–6.

Ptosis, blepharophimosis, and other eyelid anomalies

Ptosis (drooping of the eyelids) is an abnormality of eyelid elevation caused by poor function of the levator palpebrae superioris (LPS) muscle. This muscle has unique fibre types and is rich in mitochondria that make it fatigue-resistant. Ptosis is a feature of many neuromuscular conditions and may be due to a primary abnormality of the muscle or due to a disorder of its innervation. Despite the relatively long list of conditions of which ptosis is a featue, simple or congenital ptosis is the most common cause and results from a dysplasia of the levator muscle. It occurs sporadically and is non-progressive and usually unilateral.

Amblyopia may coexist with ptosis as a result of coexisiting squint or refractive error, but is only caused by the ptosis if the visual axis is obstructed (rare). The amblyopia is corrected before the ptosis, unless the pupil is obstructed.

Blepharophimosis is a decrease in palpebral fissure aperture. The distance between the internal and external canthi of each eye is reduced.

Cryptophthalmos is the covering of the globe of the eye by skin. The skin is adherent to the anterior structures of the eye. The main syndromal association is Fraser syndrome.

Clinical approach

History: key points

- Three-generation family tree with specific enquiry about ptosis and neurological problems.
- Congenital/acquired.
- Progressive, fatigability (congenital ptosis is non-progressive).
- Muscle weakness and dysphagia (mytotonic dystrophy, oculopharyngeal myopathy).
- Surgery to head and neck and other trauma.
- Central nervous system (CNS) disease.
- Developmental delay/mental retardation.

Examination: key points

- Eye movement, pupil size, and length of palpebral fissures (distance between the inner and outer canthus).
- Fundus. Pigmentary retinopathy in mitochondrial diseases.
- Muscle strength and myotonia (neurological disorders).
- Non-ocular dysmorphic features.
- Cardiac murmur (Noonan syndrome, Kabuki syndrome).
- Eczema (Dubowitz syndrome).
- 6% of ptosis is associated with a **Marcus Gunn phenomenon**. This is a unilateral ptosis that is reduced or overcompensated when chewing or sucking.

Special investigations

- DNA testing for mitochondrial conditions, myotonic dystrophy, blepharophimosis–ptosis–epicanthus inversus syndrome (BPES), and oculopharyngeal dystrophy is possible.
- Anticholinesterase antibodies and Tensilon test for myasthaenia (usually conducted by a neurologist).
- Blood creatine kinase (CK) to exclude muscle disease.
- Ophthalmological testing as necessary.
- Chromosome analysis if associated developmental delay or dysmorphic features. Consider fluorescent *in situ* hybridization (FISH) 22q11.

Ptosis: some diagnoses to consider

Non-genetic causes

- Congenital ptosis (simple ptosis). The most common cause of ptosis in children. Often unilateral and non-progressive.
- Trauma, Horner's syndrome, third nerve palsy. Often unilateral and non-progressive.

Muscle disorders associated with ptosis

Mitochondrial disorders.

- Chronic progressive external ophthalmoplegia (CPEO). Large-scale mitochondrial deletion.
- MELAS (mitochondrial myopathy–encephalopathy–lactic acidosis–stroke-like episodes). Point mutation.
- Kearns–Sayre. Large-scale mitochondrial deletion.
- Autosomal dominant (AD) CPEO.

Myotonic dystrophy. Myotonia, cataract, frontal balding in males. AD inheritance with anticipation through maternal inheritance. See 'Myotonic dystrophy (DM)' page 388.

Myasthenia gravis. Maternal transmission of antibodies to the fetus can cause arthrogryposis.

Oculopharyngeal myopathy (OPMD) is an AD disorder of late onset that commonly presents with ptosis and dysphagia. The genetic basis of the condition is a stable trinucleotide repeat expansion in exon 1 of the poly(A) binding protein 2 gene (*PABP2*), in which (GCG) (6) is the normal repeat length. The prevalence of OPMD is greatest in patients of French-Canadian origin (Hill *et al.* 2001).

Congenital fibrosis of the extraocular muscles. AD and autosomal recessive (AR) forms. One gene is *ARIX* (*PHOX2A*) encoding a homeodomain transcription factor protein that has an important role in the formation of the IIIrd and IVth cranial nerve nuclei (Nakano *et al.* 2001).

Dysmorphic syndromes

Aarskog syndrome (faciogenital dysplasia) is a genetically heterogeneous developmental disorder characterized by short stature (rhizomelic), ptosis in some, hypertelorism, hypermetropia, shawl scrotum, brachydactyly with hyperextendable proximal interphalangeal (PIP) joints. Facial features tend to normalize with age. Mental retardation is present in only a minority of affected males and is seldom severe. The X-linked form is caused by mutations in the *FGD1* gene. Behavioural and learning problems in childhood occur in ~50% of males with the X-linked form (Orrico *et al.* 2004). Some families appear to show AD inheritance.

Multiple pterygium syndrome. AD or AR inheritance. May be evidence of myopathy.

Neurofibromatosis type 1 (NF1). See 'Neurofibromatosis type 1 (NF1)' page 396.

Noonan syndrome. See 'Noonan syndrome' page 402.

Saethre–Chotzen syndrome. A disorder characterized by craniosynostosis caused by mutations in *TWIST* on 7p21. Asymmetric coronal suture involvement gives facial asymmetry. A low frontal hairline, ptosis, and small ears with a prominent crus are other helpful facial features. Examine for evidence of skin syndactyly and broad halluces.

Smith–Lemli–Opitz (SLO) syndrome. AR syndrome characterized by microcephaly, prenatal onset growth deficiency, cleft palate, 2–3 syndactyly of toes, small proximally placed thumbs, and sometimes postaxial polydactyly. Males have ambiguous genitalia or hypospadias with hypoplastic scrotum. 7-Dehydrocholesterol levels are elevated. Mutations in the *DHCR7* gene on 11q13 lead to deficient activity of 7-dehydrocholesterol reductase (DHCR7), the final enzyme of the cholesterol biosynthetic pathway (Jira *et al.* 2003).

Blepharophimosis (short palpebral fissures) with/without ptosis: some diagnoses to consider

Blepharophimosis, ptosis, epicanthus inversus syndrome (BPES). In this condition there is a reduced horizontal diameter of the palpebral fissures, droopy eyelids, and a fold of skin that runs from the lower lids inwards and upwards (epicanthus inversus). Mutations in *FOXL2*, a forkhead transcription factor on 3q, are found in ~67% of patients. Intelligence is mostly normal except where there is microdeletion encompassing the gene. In type I BPES eyelid abnormalities are associated with premature ovarian failure. Type II has eyelid defects only. For proteins with a truncation before the poly-Ala tract, the risk for development of premature ovarian failure is high (BPES type I). For mutations leading to a truncated or extended protein containing an intact forkhead and poly-Ala tract, no predictions are possible since some of these mutations lead to both type of BPES even within the same family. Poly-Ala expansions may lead to BPES type II.

Dubowitz syndrome. AR condition characterized by pre- and postnatal growth retardation, microcephaly, developmental delay/intellectual disability, sparse hair, telecanthus, ptosis, blepharophimosis, and prominent epicanthic folds.

Fetal alcohol syndrome (FAS). See 'Fetal alcohol syndrome (FAS)' page 588.

Ohdo syndrome. Blepharophimosis is the key feature in the recognition of this syndrome, which is also characterized by ptosis, very small teeth, and mild–moderate learning disability. Affected children are often very floppy at birth and have major feeding problems requiring tube feeding. They have generally decreased movements, particularly facial movements. Congenital heart disease is common and can be severe. Some have agenesis of the corpus callosum. All reports to date, except the original report by Ohdo *et al.* (1986) of two affected siblings and the report by Mhanni *et al.* (1998) of an affected mother and son, are of sporadic cases. A chromosomal aetiology has been suggested. Some children fit more closely with a similar phenotype described by Young and Simpson (1987) with severe mental retardation, a bulbous nose, and hypothyroidism.

Cryptophthalmos: some diagnoses to consider

Fraser syndrome. A rare AR syndrome with a birth incidence of approximately 1 in 250 000. Part of the skin of the forehead may be continuous with the cheek but the degree of cryptophthalmos is variable. In addition to crytophthalmos the features are:

- 50–60% of cases, cutaneous syndactyly;
- 40–60% of cases, malformed ears with degrees of conductive deafness;
- 40% of cases, renal agenesis;
- 25% of cases, laryngeal stenosis;
- 20% of cases have abnormal genitalia (ambiguous/vaginal atresia/cryptorchid testes).

There are several proposed loci. Two genes have been identified; the FRAS1 at *4q21* in Pakistani and Lebanese patients and the *FRAS 2* at 13q13 in 2 Spanish gypsy families. It is not known whether the variability of the condition is caused by mechanical effects or other genetic factors.

Long palpebral fissures: some diagnoses to consider

Kabuki syndrome. Characterized by facial dysmorphism with long palpebral fissures, eversion of the lateral one-third of the lower lid, and arched eyebrows that are more sparse laterally. Postnatal growth retardation, skeletal anomalies with joint laxity, mild to moderate mental retardation, and persistent fetal finger pads are present in most individuals with Kabuki syndrome. A highly arched palate or cleft palate, congenital heart defects, dental anomalies, and recurrent otitis media are very common. Breast development (premature thelarche) in female infants is frequently found. The genetic basis is currently unknown.

Eyelid coloboma: some diagnoses to consider

See 'Coloboma', page 82.

Genetic advice

Recurrence risk

- Most forms of ptosis are non-genetic, especially if unilateral and non-progressive.
- Isolated hereditary ptosis is usually AD and non-progressive.
- Counsel as appropriate for the specific syndrome.

Carrier detection

May be possible if the molecular or biochemical basis of a specific condition is identified.

Prenatal diagnosis

If the molecular or biochemical basis of a specific condition is identified, prenatal diagnosis may be possible.

Natural history and further management (preventative measures)

If there is severe ptosis, regular ophthalmological review is appropriate to ensure that the eyelids are not obstructing the visual axis. Eyelid surgery may be considered for cosmetic reasons in older children.

Support group contact: Many of the individual syndromes have their own support groups. See Contact a Family (UK) <www.cafamily.org.uk> and National Organisation for Rare Disorders (US) <www.rarediseases.org>.

Expert adviser: Anonymous.

References

De Baere E, Beysen D, *et al.* FOXL2 and BPES: mutational hotspots, phenotypic variability, and revision of the genotype–phenotype correlation. *Am J Hum Genet* 2003; **72**: 478–87.

Hill ME, Creed GA, *et al.* Oculopharyngeal muscular dystrophy: phenotypic and genotypic studies in a UK population. *Brain* 2001; **124** (Pt. 3): 522–6.

Hughes D. Eyelid disorders. In *Paediatric ophthalmology*, Fundamentals of Clinical Ophthalmology series (ed. A. Moore), Chapter 12, pp. 154–61. BMJ Books, London, 2000.

Jira PE, Waterham HR, *et al*. Smith–Lemli–Opitz syndrome and the DHCR7 gene. *Ann Hum Genet* 2003; **67** (Pt. 3): 269–80.

Mhanni AA, Dawson AJ, Chudley AE. Vertical transmission of the Ohdo blepharophimosis syndrome. *Am J Med Genet* 1998; **77** (2): 144–8.

Nakano M, Yamada K, *et al*. Homozygous mutations in ARIX (PHOX2A) result in congenital fibrosis of the extraocular muscles type 2. *Nat Genet* 2001 Nov; **29** (3): 315–20.

Ohdo S, Madokoro H, Sonoda T, Hayakawa K. Mental retardation associated with congenital heart disease, blepharophimosis, blepharoptosis, and hypoplastic teeth. *J Med Genet* 1986; **23**: 242–4.

Orrico A, Galli L, *et al*. Phenotypic and molecular characterisation of the Aarskog–Scott syndrome: a survey of the clinical variability in light of FGD1 mutation analysis in 46 patients. *Eur J Hum Genet* 2004; **12** (1): 16–23.

Young ID, Simpson K. Unknown syndrome: abnormal facies, congenital heart defects, hypothyroidism, and severe retardation. *J Med Genet* 1987; **24**: 715–16.

Radial ray defects and thumb hypoplasia

The most severe presentation is that of a radial club hand with a single often rudimentary forearm bone and absent thumb. Milder phenotypes involve only minimal disturbance of thumb development. Non-articulating thumbs attached by a small tissue band (floating thumbs) are also seen. Radial and thumb hypoplasia may be unilateral or bilateral, and about 50% of affected children will have other anomalies that aid diagnosis and understanding of the aetiology. The upper limb bud is formed on day 26–27 after fertilization and limb development is complete by day 55. Environmental factors within this time can lead to varying degrees of limb defects. Some genetic syndromes can affect predominantly radial ray development and these are more likely to lead to bilateral features with less variability between the left and right sides. There is a strong association with haematological and cardiac disorders.

Clinical approach

History: key points

- Three-generation family tree. Ask about mild features that may indicate an affected individual. Note consanguinity.
- Pregnancy. Medication, bleeding or threatened miscarriage, maternal diabetes, drug exposure (e.g. vitamin A, retinoids).
- Birthweight (much reduced in trisomy 18, de Lange syndrome).
- Anaemia or other haematological problem.
- Cardiac murmur or surgery.
- Developmental delay.

Examination: key points

- Carefully describe and photograph the upper limbs and hands.
- Growth parameters. Stature and head circumference and cranial shape.
- Cleft lip/palate (Diamond–Blackfan syndrome, Roberts syndrome, de Lange syndrome).
- Malar hypoplasia and micrognathia (Nager syndrome).
- Duane anomaly, which is a complex type of strabismus (Okihiro syndrome).
- Examine the feet and lower limbs, especially the tibial ray, and exclude terminal transverse defects.
- Examine for evidence of scoliosis and vertebral anomalies (VATER (vertebral defects–anal atresia–tracheo-oesophageal fistula–(o)esophageal atresia–renal anomalies) association).
- Cardiac murmur (Holt–Oram syndrome).
- Pigmented skin lesions (café-au-lait spots (CALs) develop with time in Fanconi anaemia), haemangiomata.

Special investigations

- Chromosome analysis. Basic G-banding to exclude trisomy 18, triploidy (in fetuses with extreme growth retardation), del 13q, and other visible abnormalities.
- Additional cytogenetic analysis. Please consult first with your laboratory as these are not routinely performed by all.
  - **Fanconi anaemia.** Increased chromosome breaks on exposure to mitomycin C and diepoxybutane (DEB).
  - **Roberts syndrome.** Chromosome 'puffing'. Should be seen on careful observation of a routine preparation.

- **Baller–Gerold syndrome.** This is a heterogeneous condition with reports of some patients having the same cytogenetic findings as those of Roberts syndrome and occasional reports of *TWIST* mutations (the gene for Saethre–Chotzen syndrome) in affected individuals.
- Haematological investigation. Full blood count (FBC) and platelet analysis. Referral to haematologist if abnormalities detected.
- X-ray of the affected limb(s). Consider chest and vertebral X-rays: vertebral abnormalities (VACTERL (vertebral defects–anal atresia–cardiac anomalies–tracheo-oesophageal fistula–(o)esophageal atresia–renal anomalies–limb defects)), cardiac enlargement, shoulder girdle (Holt–Oram).
- Cardiac echo and electrocardiogram (ECG; especially in the presence of a murmur or if there is a possibility of Holt–Oram syndrome or if there is a tracheo-oesophageal fistula (TOF)).
- Renal ultrasound scan (USS; VATER and Fanconi anaemia).

Some diagnoses to consider

Fetal/neonatal death

Consider triploidy (see 'Triploidy (69,XXX, 69,XXY, or 69,XYY)' page 556), trisomy 18 (see 'Edwards syndrome (trisomy 18)' page 526), and de Lange syndrome (see 'Limb reduction defects', page 152.

Haematological abnormalities

Fanconi anaemia. A variety of radial ray anomalies are found in Fanconi anaemia including absent, hypoplastic, supernumerary, or bifid thumbs and hypoplastic or absent radii. 20% have other skeletal problems (e.g. vertebral and rib anomalies). Prenatal diagnosis is not straightforward; consult your laboratory prior to counselling. See 'DNA repair defects' page 304.

Thrombocytopenia, absent radius (TAR) syndrome. Unlike many conditions that feature radial hypoplasia, *the thumb is present*. TAR syndrome is characterized by bilateral absence of the radii and a thrombocytopenia. The lower limbs and gastrointestinal, cardiovascular, and other systems may also be involved. In a survey of 34 cases, Greenhalgh *et al.* (2002) found that all cases had a documented thrombocytopenia and bilateral radial aplasia, 47% had lower limb anomalies, 47% cow's milk intolerance, 23% renal anomalies, and 15% cardiac anomalies. The inheritance is unclear. Autosomal recessive (AR) inheritance is possible but there have been fewer affected siblings than expected and a rarity of consanguinity.

Diamond–Blackfan anaemia. In this condition red cell anaemia develops and may be treated with corticosteroids. Short stature is almost always found and other features have been well documented by Alter *et al.* It is likely to be the same condition as Aase or Aase–Smith II syndrome. It is genetically heterogeneous. 20–25% of individuals have mutations in the ribosomal protein *RPS19*.

With dominant inheritance

Holt–Oram syndrome. See below.

Okihiro syndrome is the association of forearm malformation with Duane syndrome of eye retraction due to *SALL4* mutations on 20q13.13–q13.2 (Kolhase *et al.* 2002).

Nager syndrome (acrofacial dysostosis). Autosomal dominant (AD) condition with Treacher–Collins-like facies combined with radial ray limb defects, e.g. absent/hypoplastic thumbs and radial hypoplasia.

With recessive inheritance
Roberts syndrome (Pseudothalidomide syndrome)

AR disorder with symmetrical limb defects (severe shortening of the limbs, with radial defects and oligodactyly or syndactyly) together with craniofacial abnormalities. Caused by mutations in ESCO2 (Vega). See 'Limb reduction defects' page 152.

With cardiac anomalies
VATER/VACTERL association. Incidence, 1.6/10 000. Usually 3–4 features present. Hall (2001) suggests at least one anomaly from limb, thorax, and pelvis/lower abdomen for a secure diagnosis and at least two anomalies in each of two of those regions for a probable diagnosis. Normal cognitive development expected. Usually sporadic with low recurrence risk. The significance of the letters is as follows.

V   Vertebral defects. Usually upper to mid thoracic and lumbar regions. Usually hemivertebrae, but dyssegmented and fused vertebrae may occur. There may be accompanying rib anomalies.

A   Anal atresia. There may be associated genital defects (hypospadias, bifid scrotum) or fistulae.

C   Cardiac anomalies are present in ~80%—any type, any severity.

T   Tracheo-oesophageal fistula (TOF).

E   (O)esophageal atresia. 80% have an associated TOF.

R   Renal anomalies in 80%, e.g. renal agenesis/dysplasia.

L   Limb (radial defects). Preaxial with underdevelopment or agenesis of thumbs and radial bones, usually bilateral defects, but may be asymmetric. Reduced thenar muscle mass is mildest end of spectrum. Limb anomalies are restricted to the upper limbs.

Holt–Oram syndrome. AD heart–hand syndrome caused by mutations in *TBX5*. Penetrance is 100%.

• **Skeletal defects** affect the upper limbs exclusively and are invariably bilateral and usually asymmetrical. They range from clinodactyly, limited supination, and narrow, sloping shoulders to absent, hypoplastic, or triphalangeal thumb and severe reduction deformities of the upper arm (4.5%). Hypoplasia of the thenar eminence accompanies thumb hypoplasia. The radial ray is predominantly affected and the left side is usually more severely affected than the right.

• **Cardiac defects** include atrial septal defect (ASD; 34%), ventricular septal defect (VSD; 25%), mitral valve prolapse (MVP; 7%), with ECG changes only in 39% (long PR interval, bradycardia, and left or right axis deviation being the most frequent). Pectus deformity occurs in 40%. Cardiac defects (including minimal ECG changes) occur in 95%.

The offspring of a parent with Holt–Oram syndrome who inherits a *TBX5* mutation has a 1 in 3 chance of having a severe reduction defect of the upper limb, e.g. absent thumb, and a 5% risk of phocomelia. Prenatal USS may be helpful in identifying the more severe skeletal and cardiac defects. Sequence analysis of *TBX5* detects mutations in ~25% of sporadic cases and 53% of familial cases of HOS (Brassington).

Environmental and teratogenic effects
Thalidomide embryopathy is the most well known. Other drugs and agents that have a vasodilatory action can cause radial hypoplasia, e.g. carbamazepine, alcohol. Vitamin A teratogenicity can cause limb defects especially radial defects. Radial aplasia/hypoplasia is sometimes seen in diabetic embryopathy.

Genetic advice (for apparently isolated radial hypoplasia)
Examine carefully to exclude other features. Document if unilateral or bilateral. Examine lower limbs. Listen for cardiac murmur.

Recurrence risk
• **Apparently isolated and unilateral cases** with no family history of limb abnormality. Most are non-genetic. Recurrence risk low and offspring risk low. Explain that there is a small residual risk due to the variability of this feature in dominant conditions.

• **Apparently isolated and bilateral cases** with no family history. All Mendelian modes of inheritance have been described, but X-linkage is rare. Bilateral features increase the possibility of a genetic aetiology. Carefully exclude syndromic and environmental causes.

Prenatal diagnosis
The radius and ulna can be identified from the beginning of the second trimester. Hypoplasia of the thumb would not be detected unless there are absent bones.

Natural history and further management (preventative measures)
Consider the need for occasional blood counts.

Lay group contact: REACH (for upper limb defects) <www.reach.org.uk>, Tel. 08451 306225; Fanconi anaemia <www.fanconi-anaemia.co.uk>.

Expert adviser: Ruth Newbury-Ecob, Consultant in Clinical Genetics, St. Michael's Hospital, Bristol, England.

References
Brassington AM, Sung SS, *et al.* Expressivity of Holt–Oram syndrome is not predicted by TBX5 genotype. *Am J Hum Genet* 2003; **73**: 74–85.

Da Costa L, *et al.* Diamond–Blackfan anemia. *Curr Opin Pediatr* 2001; **13**: 10–15.

Greenhalgh KL, Howell RT, *et al.* Thrombocytopenia–absent radius syndrome: a clinical genetic study. *J Med Genet.* 2002; **39** (12): 876–81.

Gromp M, D'Andrea A. Fanconi anemia and DNA repair. *Hum Mol Genet* 2001; **10**: 2253–9.

Hall BD. VATER association. In *Management of genetic syndromes* (ed. S.B. Cassidy and J.E. Allanson), Chapter 28. Wiley-Liss, New York, 2001.

Joenje H, Patel KJ. The emerging genetic and molecular basis of Fanconi anemia. *Nat Rev Genet* 2001; **2** (6): 446–57.

Kohlase J, Heinrich M, *et al.* Okihiro syndrome is caused by *SALL4* mutations. *Hum Mol Genet* 2002; **11**: 2979–87.

Newbury-Ecob RA, Leanage R, Raeburn JA, Young ID. Holt–Oram syndrome: a clinical genetic study. *J Med Genet* 1996; **33**: 300–7.

Vega H, Waisfisz Q et al. Roberts syndrome is caused by mutations in ESCO2, a human homolog of yeast ECO1 that is essential for the establishment of sister chromatid cohesim. *Nat Genet* 2005; May **37**: 468–70.

Retinal dysplasia

Retinal dysplasia is a bilateral congenital structural abnormality of the retina. It is often associated with malformations of the central nervous system (CNS). Sometimes the description 'retinal folds' is used. In retinal dysplasia there is failure of retinal and vitreous development resulting in bilateral retinal detachment that is present at birth. Most cases are seen in males (Norrie disease is the most common cause of retinal dysplasia). The main conditions to exclude are retinoblastoma, severe forms of familial exudative retinopathy (FEVR) and, in premature infants, retinopathy of prematurity (ROP).

Clinical approach

History: key points

- Three-generation family history; consider X-linkage and consanguinity.
- Prenatal exposure to teratogens, trauma, or other adverse events.
- Gestation (ROP can give a similar picture).
- Neurological abnormality.
- Seizures.
- Bone fracture (osteoporosis pseudoglioma).
- Other eye pathology.

Examination: key points

- Microphthalmos and other structural eye abnormalities.
- Occipital-frontal circumference (OFC; either microcephaly or hydrocephalus may be found with muscle–eye–brain disease (MEB)).
- Encephalocele (MEB/Walker–Warburg syndrome (WWS)).
- Other growth parameters.
- Lymphoedema.
- Polydactyly (trisomy 13, Joubert syndrome).
- Congenital heart defect (trisomy 13).
- Neurological exam, particularly hypotonia and weakness (WWS).

Special investigations

- Full eye examination.
- Brain magnetic resonance imaging (MRI; migrational abnormalities, hydrocephalus).
- Creatinine kinase (CK; elevated in WWS and cerebroocular dysplasia–muscular dystrophy (COD-MD)).
- Muscle biopsy in children with an elevated CK.
- Karyotype.
- DNA for storage or specific genetic testing (e.g. mutation analysis of *NDP* in Norrie disease).

Syndromes to consider

The most common cause of retinal dysplasia by far is Norrie disease (see below), which can be confirmed by molecular genetic diagnosis (mutations in the *NDP* gene); other forms are rare.

Isolated ophthalmic disorders

Retinoblastoma. See 'Retinoblastoma' in Chapter 4, 'Cancer'.

Retinopathy of prematurity (ROP). A vasoproliferative retinopathy that may develop in very premature infants. In most infants, the disease is mild and undergoes spontaneous regression, but in a small minority the disorder progresses to total retinal detachment and blindness. The incidence and severity of ROP is inversely related to birthweight and gestational age. High levels of inspired oxygen are an important risk factor. Severe cicatricial disease is seen almost exclusively in infants weighing <1000 g at birth.

Persistent hyperplastic primary vitreous. This is always unilateral.

Autosomal dominant conditions

Familial exudative vitreoretinopathy (FEVR). Rare AD condition characterized by abnormal development of the retinal vasculature that may lead to vitreous hemorrhage and traction retinal detachment necessitating surgical intervention. Genetically heterogeneous with 4 loci (EVR1-4) (Toomes *et al.* 2005).

Autosomal recessive (AR) conditions

Walker–Warburg syndrome (WWS) and muscle–eye–brain disease (MEB) are disorders that share the combination of cerebral neuronal migration defects, ocular abnormalities, and a congenital muscular dystrophy. The features of WWS are hydrocephalus, agyria, retinal dystrophy, and sometimes an encephalocele. Thus its alternate name of HARD ± E. WWS is caused by mutations in the *O*-mannosyltransferase 1 gene (*POMT1*).

Osteoporosis pseudoglioma. Rare AR disorder characterized by severe juvenile-onset osteoporosis and congenital or early-onset blindness. Other features include muscular hypotonia, ligamentous laxity, mild mental retardation, and seizures. Mutation in the *LRP5* gene on 11q11–12.

Fryns syndrome. A rare lethal AR condition with nail/digital hypoplasia and diaphragmatic hernia. Retinal dysplasia is a feature but is rarely reported. Corneal clouding is more commonly documented.

AR retinal dysplasia. A rare recessive form of isolated retinal dysplasia.

X-linked disorders

Norrie disease. Affected infants are blind and have roving eye movements. Ophthalmological examination shows bilateral retrolental masses and ultrasound scan (USS) shows evidence of bilateral retinal detachment without evidence of intraocular calcification. Shallowing of the anterior chamber may cause pupil-block glaucoma, which is treated surgically. About 50% of males with Norrie have learning difficulties and may show poorly characterized behavioural abnormalities or psychotic-like features. At least 40% and probably the majority of affected males develop a progressive sensorineural hearing loss starting in early childhood. Some boys also develop epilepsy. The diagnosis of Norrie disease is often difficult. The ability to test for specific mutations permits clarification of diagnosis in atypical presentations.

Norrie disease follows X-linked recessive (XLR) inheritance and is caused by mutations in the NDP gene at Xp11 that encodes 'norrin'. The majority of mutations are unique point mutations, but intragenic and submicroscopic deletions, including NDP and adjacent regions, have been identified in about 15% of patients. There is no genotype–phenotype correlation. Mutations in *NDP* are associated with a spectrum of retinal disorders ranging from Norrie disease to X-linked familial exudative vitreoretinopathy (FEVR), including some cases of persistent hyperplastic primary vitreous (PHPV), Coats disease, and advanced ROP. A clinical phenotype in carrier females is rare.

Incontinentia pigmenti (IP) is an ectodermal multisystem disorder that can affect dental, ocular, cardiac, and neurological structures. The ocular changes of IP can have a very similar appearance to the retinal detachment of X-linked FEVR, which has been shown to be caused by the mutations in the Norrie disease gene. See 'Unusual hair, teeth, nails, and skin', page 256.

Juvenile X-linked retinoschisis is an XLR disorder resulting in visual loss in affected males in early life with splitting within the inner retinal membrane. A rare infantile form of juvenile X-linked retinoschisis may present with large bullous retinoschisi resembling retinal detachment. It is caused by mutations in the *RS1* gene on Xp22.1–22.1, which encodes a soluble secretory protein. There is no obvious genotype–phenotype correlation.

Chromosomal abnormalities
Trisomy 13. See 'Patau syndrome (trisomy 13)' in page 534.

Other

Microcephaly, lymphoedema, and choreoretinal dysplasia/retinal folds. This association has been noted in several families. Autosomal dominant (AD) inheritance is thought likely but there is reduced penetrance and variability.

Genetic advice
Recurrence risk
As appropriate for the diagnosis. For an isolated retinal dysplasia the geneticist should consult with ophthalmological colleagues over the likely aetiology.

Norrie disease. The majority of mothers of an apparently isolated male proband are carriers of an *NDP* disease-causing mutation, even when the family history is negative. Only rarely do affected males have a *de novo* mutation. Intrafamilial and interfamilial variability in the appearance and expression of the cognitive and behavioural difficulties is common.

Carrier detection
Available in families where there is a known mutation.

Prenatal diagnosis
* Available by genetic testing in families where there is a known mutation.
* If genetic testing is unavailable, USS for signs of the associated features such as hydrocephalus may be performed.

Natural history and further management (preventative measures)
Dependent on the diagnosis and associated features.

Lay group contact: Visual Impairment Scotland <www.ssc.mhie.ac.uk/eyeconds/norr.htm>, Tel. 0131 651 6078.

Expert adviser: Anonymous.

References
<www.geneclinics.org>.

Beltran-Valero Be Bernabe D, Currier S, *et al.* Mutations in the O-mannosyltransferase gene POMT1 give rise to the severe neuronal migration disorder Walker–Warburg syndrome. *Am J Hum Genet* 2002; **71**: 1033–43.

Cormand B, Pihko H, Bayes M, *et al.* Clinical and genetic distinction between WWS and MEB. *Neurology* 2001; **56**: 1059–69.

Limvongse C, Wyszynski RE, Dickerman LH, Robin NH. Microcephaly, lymphoedema and chorioretinal dysplasia: a unique genetic syndrome with variable expression and a possible characteristic facial appearance. *Am J Med Genet* 1999; **86**: 215–18.

Meindl A, Berger W, *et al.* Norrie disease is caused by mutations in an extracellular protein resembling C-terminal globular domain of mucins. *Nat Genet* 1992; **2**: 139–43.

Sabatelli P, Columbaro M, *et al.* Extracellular matrix and nuclear abnormalities in skeletal muscle of a patient with Walker–Warburg syndrome caused by *POMT1* mutations. *Biochem Biophys Acta* 2003; **1638**: 57–62.

Toomes C, Downey LM, *et al.* Further evidence of genetic heterogeneity in familial exudative vitreoretinopathy; exclusion of EVR1, EVR3, and EVR4 in a large autosomal dominant pedigree. *Br J Ophthalmol* 2005; **89**: 194–197.

Wang T, Waters CT, *et al.* Intracellular retention of mutant retinoschisin is the pathological mechanism underlying X-linked retinoschisis. *Hum Mol Genet* 2002; **11**: 3097–105.

Retinal receptor dystrophies

The outer receptor cell layer of the retina is comprised of rods and cones, the light-sensitive photoreceptors. Cones work best in good illumination and are important for detailed visual acuity and colour discrimination. Rods work best at low illumination and unlike cones can function at very low light levels. Most inherited retinal disorders affect cone as well as rod receptors. The age of onset of symptoms vary from early infancy to adult life depending on the causative genetic mutations. Most, but not all, of these disorders are progressive.

- **Rod dysfunction.** Patients with impaired rod function have poor vision in dim illumination (nyctalopia).
- **Cone dysfunction.** Symptoms of cone dysfunction include reduced central vision, sensitivity to light, and reduced colour vision. Those affected by cone disorders will often function better in dim illumination but be uncomfortable and severely dazzled in normal lighting.
- **Retinitis pigmentosa** (RP) is a heterogeneous group of disorders in which there is early loss of rod function followed by impaired peripheral cone function (causing field loss); foveal cones are affected late in the disease. In RP the loss of rods leads to early symptoms of night blindness and later there is loss of the peripheral visual fields, often starting in the mid-periphery. Examination of the fundus shows pigmentary changes in the mid-peripheral retina. RP may be isolated or occur as part of systemic disease or syndrome.
- Central degeneration with predominantly cone loss is known as either **macular degeneration** or **cone dystrophy**. Cone dystrophies can be distinguished from macular dystrophies by the finding of full-field electroretinography (ERG) abnormalities in the former. A progressive cone dystrophy leads to degeneration of the macular photoreceptors with morphological changes in the central fundus (bull's eye maculopathy) and early loss of colour vision and acuity.

In reality, there is a spectrum from pure rod dystrophies through rod/cone to cone/rod to pure cone dystrophy.

Stationary congenital cone dystrophies are discussed in 'Nystagmus', page 190.

The aim of this section is to determine if the retinal dystrophy is part of syndrome. If isolated please refer to 'Retinitis pigmentosa (RP)' page 406.

Clinical approach

History: key points

- Three generation family tree. Note if consanguinity is present.
- Age of onset.
- Neurological symptoms (mitochondrial disorders, autosomal dominant cerebellar ataxia (ADCA), Refsum disease).
- Developmental delay (Bardet–Biedl syndrome (BBS), peroxisomal disorders).
- Obesity (BBS, Cohen syndrome, Alstrom syndrome).
- Diabetes mellitus (obesity syndromes).
- Deafness (Usher syndrome, Refsum disease, Alstrom syndrome).
- Malabsorption (abetalipoproteinaemia).
- Renal disease (BBS).
- Cardiomyopathy (Alstrom syndrome, mitochondrial disorders).

Examination: key points

- Verify eye signs.
- Weight (obesity index), height, and occipital-frontal circumference (OFC).
- Blood pressure (renal disease).
- Facial dysmorphism (peroxisomal disorders).
- Prominent incisors (Cohen syndrome).
- Muscle weakness.
- Spasticity.
- Ataxia.
- Cardiac murmur/enlargement (structural defects and cardiomyopathy).
- Postaxial polydactyly (BBS).
- Acanthosis nigricans (Alstrom and insulin resistance).

Special investigations

- Ophthalmology assessment, including electrophysiology (ERG).
- Examine other family members (especially mother in affected males to exclude X-linked carrier state).
- Biochemistry. Basic biochemical screen of electrolyes, renal and liver function, fasting blood sugar to exclude diabetes.
- Phytanic acid (Refsum syndrome).
- DNA sample.

Further investigation is not required in AD or X-linked disease, but may be needed in the investigation of possible autosomal recessive (AR) disease.

- Metabolic investigations, if indicated, for neuronal ceroid lipofuscinosis (NCL), very long chain fatty acids (VLCFAs) and phytanic acid (Refsum), and abetalipoprotein B (abetalipoproteinaemia).
- Plasma amino acids (raised plasma ornithine in gyrate atrophy).
- Haematology. Neutrophil count (low in Cohen syndrome), acanthocytosis (abetalipoptroteinaemia), vacuolated lymphocytes (Batten).
- Renal ultrasound scan (USS; BBS).
- Electrocardiogram (ECG) and cardiac echo (Alstrom, BBS, mitochondrial disorders).
- Muscle biopsy (mitochondrial disorders).
- DNA sample. Mitochondrial DNA studies, *SCA7*. ADCA with RP, NCL (Batten), BBS, Usher syndrome. Store for future diagnostic purposes.
- Skin biopsy, ultraviolet (UV) irradiation (Cockayne syndrome).

Some diagnoses to consider

Autosomal recesssive (AR) syndromes

Usher syndrome. Sensorineural deafness (see 'Deafness', page 90).

Bardet–Biedl syndrome (BBS). Rod/cone dystrophy, mental retardation, postaxial polydactyly, obesity, renal abnormality (persistent fetal lobulation, dilatation of the collecting system with blind-ending cysts), vaginal atresia. At least five loci. McKusick–Kaufman syndrome is allelic. (See 'Obesity with and without developmental delay', page 192.)

Peroxisomal disorders.
- **Refsum syndrome***. A peroxisomal disorder that leads to very high phytanic acid levels with ataxia, deafness, and polyneuropathy.
- **Infantile Refsum syndrome.**
- **Neonatal adrenoleukodystrophy.**
- **Zellweger syndrome.** Presents in the neonatal period with hypotonia and seizures and dysmorphic features, e.g. large fontanelle, high forehead, stippled epiphyses. See 'Floppy infant', page 118.

Gyrate atrophy of the choroid and retina.* Rare, but treatable AR disorder caused by deficiency of the mitochondrial enzyme ornithine aminotransferase encoded by the *OAT* gene. Presents with night blindness and myopia. The ERG becomes abnormal as the disease progresses. Plasma ornithine levels are elevated, and treatment with pyridoxine may, in a small subset of patients, lead to reduced plasma ornithine levels and slowing of the progression of the retinal dystrophy. Most affected individuals need to follow an arginine-restricted diet in order to minimize progressive deterioration of vision.

Abetalipoproteinaemia.* Failure to thrive with fat malabsorption, acanthosis, ataxia, and absence of low-density lipoproteins (LDLs). Progressive pigmentary retinal degeneration accompanied by subnormal ERG changes are seen in patients with abetalipoproteinaemia caused by mutations in the microsomal triglyceride transfer protein (*MTP*) gene. Combined oral vitamin A and E supplementation that is initiated prior to 2 years of age can markedly attenuate the severe retinal degeneration.

Cockayne syndrome. AR neurodegenerative disorder characterized by low to normal birthweight, postnatal growth failure, brain dysmyelination with calcium deposits, cutaneous photosensitivity, pigmentary retinopathy and/or cataracts and/or optic atrophy, and sensorineural hearing loss. See 'DNA Repair defects' page 304.

Joubert syndrome (JS) is an AR developmental brain condition characterized by hypoplasia/dysplasia of the cerebellar vermis and by ataxia, hypotonia, oculomotor apraxia, and neonatal breathing dysregulation. A form of JS that includes retinal dysplasia and cystic dysplastic kidneys has been differentiated from other forms of JS, and is designated 'cerebello-oculo-renal syndrome' (CORS), and shows linkage to 11p12–q13.3 (Keeler *et al.* 2003). See page 66.

Neuronal ceroid lipofuscinoses (NCLs; Batten disease) are lysosomal storage disorders characterized by mental and motor deterioration, seizures, and visual loss. The juvenile form is Batten disease. Until recently confirmation of these diagnoses depended on electron microscopy detection of specific lysosomal storage material in tissue, a rectal or skin biopsy, or conjunctival tissue. It is now possible for most neurologists and geneticists to have access to molecular testing for the genes *CLCN 1, 2,* and *3* and enzyme analysis of palmitoyl-protein thioesterase (PPT)-1 and tripeptidyl-peptidase (TPP)-1. See also 'Developmental regression', page 96.

Carbohydrate deficient glycoprotein syndrome. Congenital disorders of glycosylation (CDG) are a group of AR metabolic disorders that are characterized biochemically by defective glycosylation of proteins (abnormal transferrin isoelectrophoresis). The most common type is

CDG-Ia, which is a multisytem disorder affecting the nervous system (cerebellar atrophy and encephalopathy), liver, kidney, heart, adipose tissue (lipodystrophy and abnormal fat pads), bone, and genitalia. It is caused by phosphomannomutase (PMM) deficiency, and mutations have been identified in the gene *PMM2*.

Cohen syndrome. Mental retardation, obesity, prominent incisors, neutropenia—due to mutations in *COH1* on 8q22–23. Most affected children are myopic. (See 'Obesity with and without developmental delay', page 192.)

Alstrom syndrome. Progressive deafness, obesity, small external genitalia in males, acanthosis nigricans, dilated cardiomyopathy, renal failure (glomerulosclerosis). Due to mutations in *ALMS1* on 2p13. See 'Obesity with and without developmental delay', page 192. The retinal dystrophy is an early onset cone–rod dystrophy and photophobia is a prominent early symptom.

Autosomal dominant (AD) conditions
Autosomal dominant cerebellar ataxia (ADCA) with retinal pigmentation, *SCA7*. (See 'Ataxic adult', page 50.)

X-linked conditions
- **Choroideraemia.** A diffuse progressive condition that presents in childhood with night blindness. Later there is development of peripheral field loss and ultimately in later adult life loss of central vision. In the early stages the fundal appearance may be confused with RP (although it is not primarily a photoreceptor dystrophy) but later in the disease there is a characteristic fundal appearance with extensive atrophy of the choriocapillaris and retinal pigment epithelium. Gene *REP-1* at Xq21. The visual prognosis is better than in X-linked RP, and most affected males keep good central vision until their fifth decade.
- **X-linked retinitis pigmentosa (XLRP).**
- **XLRP associated with deafness.**

Mitochondrial disorders
May be sporadic, maternal, or autosomal inheritance. (See 'Mitochondrial DNA diseases' page 384.)

Kearns–Sayre syndrome (KSS) is a subtype of chronic progressive external ophthalmoplegia (CPEO) with a poorer prognosis. Onset is <20 years and, in addition to the CPEO and pigmentary retinopathy, there is often a cardiac conduction defect and ataxia. Unlike CPEO the condition is usually life-limiting. See 'Mitochondrial DNA diseases' page 384.

Isolated macular degeneration
- Types include Stargardt disease, Best disease, Bietti crystalline dystrophy, and Sorsby fundus dystrophy.
- These diseases are genetically determined disorders that lead to macular atrophy.
- Diagnosis is based on clinical picture, electrophysiology, and pedigree.

Genetic advice
Recurrence risk
- For sporadic individuals with RP, cone–rod dystrophy, or macular dystrophy in whom a definitive diagnosis has not been made after thorough investigation, the presence of these eye changes suggests a genetic aetiology and a high recurrence risk. AR inheritance is the most likely mode of inheritance.
- X-linked conditions should be considered if there have been two or more affected boys and/or there is a family

history compatible with X-linkage, or if the ophthalmological findings are typical of an X-linked dystrophy. The mothers of isolated males with RP should have a careful fundus examination and ERG to see whether they have the typical carrier signs of the heterozygote. See 'Retinitis pigmentosa (RP)' page 406.

- Some families with AD RP may show incomplete penetrance. Some of the causative genes have been identified and molecular genetic diagnosis may be helpful in counselling (see splicing factor genes on 1q, 7p, and 19q). See 'Retinitis pigmentosa (RP)' page 406.
- Mitochondrial conditions pose difficult counselling problems; see 'Mitochondrial DNA diseases' page 384.
- Store DNA and/or fibroblast cell line for future diagnostic use. Check the literature for the availability of genetic testing.

Carrier detection

- Possible in those families in whom a causative mutation has been identified.
- May be possible for some biochemical abnormalities.
- Fundal examination and electrophysiology of other family members may help, particularly in choroideraemia and XLRP.

Prenatal diagnosis

Available to those families in where there is molecular or biochemical confirmation of diagnosis.

Natural history and further management (preventative measures)

The visual loss is usually progressive. Children should remain under the care of an ophthalmologist and have appropriate educational support.

Support group contacts: SPECS (Specific Eye Conditions) <www.eyeconditions.org.uk>, Tel. 01803 524238.; British Retinitis Pigmentosa Society <www.brps.demon.co.uk>, Tel. 01280 860363; Foundation Fighting Blindness (US) <www.blindness.org>; Macular disease society <www.maculardisease.org>, Tel. 0845 241 2041.

Expert adviser: Anonymous.

References

Chowers I, Banin E, *et al*. Long-term assessment of combined vitamin A and E treatment for the prevention of retinal degeneration in abetalipoproteinaemia and hypobetalipoproteinaemia patients. *Eye* 2001; **15**: 525–30.

Keeler LC, Marsh SE, *et al*. Linkage analysis in families with Joubert syndrome plus oculo-renal involvement identifies the CORS2 locus on chromosome 11p12–q13.3. *Am J Hum Genet* 2003; **73**: 656–62.

Michaelides M, Hunt DM, Moore AT. The genetics of inherited macular dystrophies [review]. *J Med Genet* 2003; **40**: 641–50.

Moore AT. Disorders of the vitreous and retina. In *Paediatric ophthalmology*, Fundamentals of Clinical Ophthalmology series (ed. A. Moore), Chapter 10. BMJ Books, London, 2000.

Rivolta C, Sharon D, De Angelis MM, Dryja TP. Retinitis pigmentosa and allied diseases, genes and inheritance patterns. *Hum Mol Genet* 2002; **11**: 1219–27.

Simunovic MP, Moore AT. The cone dystrophies. *Eye* 1998; **12**: 553–65.

Scalp defects

Aplasia cutis congenita.
Rare congenital malformation characterized by a local defect of epidermis, dermis, and subcutaneous tissue occurring predominantly over the vertex of the scalp. The underlying bone growth is abnormal. There may be a single area with a 'raw' appearance—the skin is a thin transparent membrane—or several small defects. It may occur as an isolated defect (when it may be familial) or occur as a feature of a chromosome disorder, genetic syndrome, or teratogen exposure. The defects often heal under conservative management. With time the defect may change into a raised area of scarred granulation tissue.

Clinical approach

History: key points

- Three-generation family history with special note of scalp defects, cardiac abnormalities, and limb defects (including neonatal deaths).
- Pyloric atresia in an affected individual (epidermylosis bullosa with pyloric atresia or Carmi syndrome).
- Pregnancy history with specific enquiry about drug exposure (e.g. methimazole, carbimazole, an anti-thyroid drug, or misoprostol) or infection (intrauterine varicella or herpes).
- History of delivery (was there a difficult instrumental delivery or any possibility that the defects are traumatic?). Often the lesions are thought to be traumatic when they are in fact congenital.
- Visual difficulties (cone–rod dysfuction and myopia).
- Deafness (Johanson-Blizzard syndrome (JBS)).
- Developmental delay (chromosomal anomalies).

Examination: key points

- Position and number of skin defects (bitemporal aplasia in Setleis syndrome and focal facial dermal dysplasia, random distribution in Goltz syndrome).
- Hair growth. Hair does not grow over the affected areas. Unruly hair with cow-licks in JBS; poor hair growth over the temples in Pallister–Killian syndrome.
- Examine very carefully for transverse limb deficiency (looking at all finger- and toe-nails is a convenient way to do this).
- Facies. Look carefully at alae nasae for features of JBS.
- Eyes. Structural malformations and epibulbar dermoids.
- Examine for other malformations, e.g. cardiac murmurs, hypospadias.
- Skin abnormalities at other sites, e.g deficiency, blisters, scarring, pigmentary abnormality.

Special investigations

- Clinical photography.
- Chromosome analysis if other malformations are present, or if there is developmental delay. Consider 4p– fluorescent *in situ* hybridization (FISH; scalp defects may occur in +13 and 4p– and a variety of rare unbalanced chromosome rearrangements).
- Fibroblast culture for chromosomal mosaicism (Pallister–Killian syndrome).
- Faecal elastase 1 (a screen for pancreatic exocrine sufficiency) and thyroid function if facies suggestive of JBS.

- Consider skull X-ray if the defect is very large (occasionally there are bony defects of the skull underlying cutis aplasia) to check for parietal foramina.
- Cranial ultrasound scan (USS) in infants.

Some diagnoses to consider

Adams–Oliver syndrome
Autosomal dominant (AD) condition featuring a combination of scalp defects and terminal transverse limb defects (usually minor reduction defects of fingers/toes and brachydactyly, although severe transverse deficiency can occur). Penetrance is incomplete and expression is highly variable making this a difficult disorder to counsel. Congenital heart disease (CHD) may occur. Examine the parents of affected children.

Johanson–Blizzard syndrome (JBS)
An autosomal recessive (AR) condition with intrauterine growth restriction (IUGR), scalp defects, and exocrine pancreatic insufficiency combined with dysmorphic features, notably a 'pinched' nose and notching of the alae nasi. CHD and deafness may occur. Faecal elastase is a useful test of pancreatic exocrine function.

Setleis syndrome
An AD condition in which the scalp defects are bitemporal and resemble 'forceps marks'. There may also be a coarse facial appearance, anomalies of the eyelashes and eyebrows, and periorbital puffiness. The mouth has a typical appearance with large lips, inverted 'V' contour, and downturned overly defined corners (McGaughran and Aftimos 2002). Patients usually have normal intelligence, but some have developmental delay. It is likely that Setleis syndrome is the same condition as Brauer syndrome and focal facial dermal dysplasia.

Microphthalmia with linear skin defects (MLS)
Girls with MLS syndrome have microphthalmia with linear skin defects of face and neck, sclerocornea, corpus callosum agenesis and other brain anomalies. This X-linked dominant male lethal condition is associated with heterozygous deletions of a critical region in Xp22.31. The *HCCS* gene, encoding human holocytochrome c-type synthetase, is the only gene located inside the critical region (Prakash *et al.* 2002).

(Goltz syndrome) X-linked dominant (due to mutations in, or deletions encompassing, the *PORCN* gene at Xp11.23). Areas of focal dermal hypoplasia may be found on the trunk and limbs and there may fat herniation through the skin deficiency. (See 'Coloboma' page 82).

Delleman syndrome (oculocerebrocutaneous syndrome)
Delleman syndrome is a rare disorder characterized by orbital cysts, micro/anophthalmia, malformations of the central nervous system (CNS), focal aplasia cutis, and multiple skin appendages (skin tags). The inheritance pattern is uncertain.

Parietal foramina
If the scalp defect is in the parietal area it may be associated with parietal foramina but *MSX2* mutation/deletion is not a frequent cause of scalp defects.

Epidermolysis bullosa with pyloric atresia or Carmi syndrome
A lethal AR condition. Mutations have been found in *ITGB2* and *ITGA6*. Prenatal diagnosis also described by USS and skin biopsy.

Epidermolysis bullosa dystrophica (EBD)
Consider if a skin disorder such as EBD could be the cause of the scalp lesions.

Genetic advice

Recurrence risk

- As for specific diagnosis.
- Isolated aplasia cutis congenita can follow AD inheritance. It is possible that apparent isolated aplasia cutis congenita could be part of the Adams–Oliver spectrum. Arrange detailed scans of the digits and heart in pregnancy.

Carrier detection
By careful clinical examination.

Prenatal diagnosis
Is possible for some of these conditions by fetal USS for structural abnormalities or by chromosomal or mutation analysis.

Natural history and further management (preventative measures)

Surgical management in a specialist centre because of the risk of associated vascular malformation and bleeding.

Support group contact: Many of the individual syndromes have their own support groups. See Contact a Family (UK) <www.cafamily.org.uk>; National Organisation for Rare Disorders (US) <www.rarediseases.org>.

Expert adviser: Dian Donnai, Professor of Medical Genetics, University of Manchester, Manchester, England.

References

Cambiaghi S, Levet PS, *et al.* Delleman syndrome: report of a case with a mild phenotype. *Eur J Dermatol.* 2000; **10** (8): 623–6.

Casanova D, Amar E, *et al.* Aplasia cutis congenita. Report on 5 family cases involving the scalp. *Eur J Pediatr Surg* 2001; **11**: 280–4.

Evers MEJW, Steijlen PM, Hamel BCJ. Aplasia cutis congenital and associated disorders: an update. *Clin Genet* 1995; **47**: 295–301.

McGaughran J, Aftimos S. Setleis syndrome: three new cases and a review of the literature. *Am J Med Genet* 2002; **111** (4): 376–80.

Prager W, Scholz S, *et al.* Aplasia cutis congenita in two siblings. *Eur J Dermatol* 2002; **12**: 228–30.

Prakash SK, Cormier TA, *et al.* Loss of holocytochrome c-type synthetase causes the male lethality of X-linked dominant microphthalmia with linear skin defects (MLS) syndrome. *Hum Mol Genet* 2002; **11**: 3237–48.

Verdyck P, Holder-Espinasse M. Hul VW, Wuyts W. Clinical and molecular study of 9 families with Adams–Oliver syndrome. *Eur J Hum Genet* 2003; **11**: 457–63.

Walkowiak J. Faecal elastase-1: clinical value in the assessment of exocrine pancreatic function in children. *Eur J Pediatr* 2000; **159**: 869–70.

Seizures with developmental delay/mental retardation

This section discusses the approach to the differential diagnosis in children with a seizure disorder and delayed development. For the child with isolated seizures please refer to 'Epilepsy in infants and children' page 314.

The average annual rate of new cases (incidence) of epilepsy in children is 5–7 cases per 100 000; about 5 in every 1000 children will have epilepsy. Epilepsy may occur as the endpoint of an acute or acquired process affecting the central nervous system (CNS), but genetic factors and genetically determined syndromes contribute in about 40% of patients.

There are several types of epilepsy syndromes that are unique to children, including infantile spasms (West syndrome), Lennox–Gastaut syndrome, and absence seizures.

Isolated epilepsy is managed by the paediatrician or paediatric neurologist. The geneticist is involved when there are features that may indicate a syndromic cause or when there is a strong family history that suggests a genetic basis. Genetic counselling for families of children with a severe seizure disorder and mental retardation, in whom no diagnosis has been made, is a common but difficult situation where the possibility of an underlying genetic cause has to be considered. The approach here is to high-light which of the features may indicate a condition with a genetic or chromosomal basis.

Clinical approach

History: key points

- Three-generation family tree with specific enquiry regarding family history of seizures, learning difficulties, skin signs of neurocutaneous disorders. Enquire about consanguinity.
- Onset of the seizures; frequency and type of seizure. Medication.
- Developmental progress before and since the onset of seizures. Try and establish if there is any evidence of developmental regression. This assessment is problematic in children with poorly controlled seizures on high doses of anti-epileptic drugs (pseudoregression).
- Parental consanguinity, previous affected sibling, other family history of epilepsy or developmental delay.
- Pregnancy (evidence of disturbance of brain develop-ment by congenital infections, severe bleeding, hypoxia, teratogenic drugs and alcohol, etc.).
- Perinatal period. Birth trauma, neonatal seizures, blistering rash, neonatal complications, e.g. prematurity.
- Occipital-frontal circumference (OFC) at birth and subsequent brain growth.
- Head injury (including non-accidental injury).

Examination: key points

- Growth parameters, particularly OFC.
- Dysmorphic features (chromosomal abnormalities and syndromic causes).
- Coarse facial features (metabolic problems) though features can coarsen on anti-epileptic medication.
- Hair sparse and brittle in Menkes syndrome. Sparse hair and alopecia have been reported with other genetic forms of epilepsy.

- Eyes. Retinal phakoma (tuberous sclerosis (TS)), pigment-ary retinopathy (mitochondrial disease, neuronal ceroid lipofuscinoses (NCLs) such as Batten disease), cataracts, and corneal clouding.
- Skin signs of neurocutaneous disorders: TS, neurofibro-matosis, biotinidase deficiency, Sturge–Weber syndrome.
- Neurological examination.
- Abnormal movements, behaviour, or gait (Angelman syndrome (AS), Rett syndrome).
- Signs of other organ involvement, e.g. hepatosplenomegaly.

Special investigations

- **Brain imaging**, preferably magnetic resonance imaging (MRI). An MRI carried out early in life, e.g. <15 months of age, may need to be repeated when the child is older.
- **Electroencephalography (EEG).** To look for specific diagnostic patterns or associated with known conditions, e.g. hypsarrythmia, burst suppression of Ohtahara, AS, ring chromosome 20. If the EEG has the features of AS, full molecular analysis including UBEA3 mutation testing is indicated (see 'Angelman syndrome' page 272).
- **Biochemical screening.** Basic biochemical screening has usually already been performed but should include plasma electrolytes (sodium, calcium, magnesium, and phosphate), liver function tests, acid/base status, fasting glucose, pyruvate and lactate, ammonia, amino acids, and congenital infection screen. Urine screen for glucose, ketones reducing sugars, amino and organic acids, mucopolysaccharides.
- Further biochemical testing to consider: biotinidase, white cell enzymes, long chain fatty acids.
- **Ultraviolet (UV) Woods light** to check for abnormalities of skin pigmentation (TS, incontinentia pigmenti and hypomelanosis of ITO).
- **Chromosome analysis** (routine analysis may reveal a variety of unexpected findings, e.g. ring chromosome 14, supernumerary marker 15 (inversion duplication 15 syndrome). Eight chromosomal disorders have a high association with epilepsy: the Wolf–Hirschhorn (4p–) syndrome, Miller–Dieker syndrome (del 17p13.3), AS (del 15q11–q13), the inversion duplication 15 syndrome, terminal deletions of chromosome 1q and 1p, and ring chromosomes 14 and 20 (Singh *et al.* 2002). Consider the following:
  - telomere or microarray analysis in children with mental retardation and malformations; if not avail-able, fluorescent *in situ* hybridization (FISH) for Wolf–Hirschhorn (del)4p, (del)1p36, (del)1q;
  - skin biopsy for fibroblast culture if streaky skin pigmentation suggestive of mosaicism (hypomel-anosis of Ito).
- Consider methylation analysis for AS (*SNRPN*) if there is associated developmental delay with minimal or absent speech, jerky movement disorder, and 2–3 Hz large-amplitude slow-wave bursts on EEG.
- **DNA.** Confirmatory or diagnostic testing, if available; otherwise storage for future testing. Diagnostic testing available for Rett syndrome, Batten disease (*CLN3*), Menkes syndrome, AS.

- Consider *UBEA3* in children who clinically have AS but with normal FISH and *SNRPN* methylation studies.
- Consider mitochondrial DNA analysis.
- Consider DNA storage in an undiagnosed child with severe epilepsy.

Some diagnoses to consider

One approach to diagnosing the symptomatic group of epilepsies is to consider the evidence for any of the following conditions.

Cytogenetic abnormalities

Seizures are found in a wide spectrum of chromosomal anomalies. Karyotype all children with non-isolated epilepsy and consider specific FISH analysis. Epilepsy in Down syndrome increases with age and is associated with diffuse abnormalities of the EEG consistent with dementia.

Brain malformations with epileptogenic potential

- Lissencephaly. Please refer to 'Lissencephaly and neuronal migration disorders', page 156, and the X-linked conditions noted below.
- Tuberous sclerosis (TS; see 'Tuberous sclerosis (TSC) page 420.
- Schizencephaly. Heterozygous mutation in EMX2 in some children.
- Focal areas of brain malformation often cause severe epilepsy, but these may have a mosaic genetic or a non-genetic aetiology.

Single gene disorders

Autosomal dominant (AD) disorders

- Tuberous sclerosis (TSC) is the most common dominant disorder and is caused by mutations in *TSC1* and *TSC2* (see 'Tuberous sclerosis (TSC)' page 420).
- Mowat–Wilson syndrome, due to mutation of *ZFHX1B* on chromosome 2q, often presents with microcephaly, seizures, developmental delay, and dysmorphic features. All cases to date appear to be *de novo* dominant mutations. See Clinical approach to 'Hypospasdias', page 142.

Autosomal recessive (AR) disorders

- Metabolic conditions, e.g. leukodystrophies, Batten disease, phenylketonuria (PKU), organic acidaemia (see 'Developmental regression', page 96).
- Genetically determined brain malformations, particularly disorders of neuronal migration.
- Significant microcephaly in association with seizures (see 'Microcephaly', page 172).
- Progressive myoclonic epilepsy (most are recessive; see below).
- PEHO (progressive encephalopathy–(o)edema–hypsarrhythmia–optic atrophy) syndrome. Originally described in Finland, there are reports from other parts of Europe. Progressive cerebellar atrophy is a key MRI feature.

X-linked disorders

- Menkes syndrome. Pili torti, abnormal skeletal survey, copper studies, and caeruloplasmin. Mutation analysis available.
- X-linked isolated lissencephaly sequence (XLIS; or DCX) mutations leading to subcortical band heterotopia in heterozygous females and predominantly anterior lissencephaly in hemizygous males.

- Bilateral periventricular nodular heterotopia (BPNH). Lethal in the perinatal period in males; focal epilepsy in carrier females who have BPNH on MRI scan. Filamin A (FLNA) gene at Xq28. See Clinical approach to 'Lissencephaly', page 156.
- ARX (Aristaless related homeobox) gene abnormalities. A spectrum of clinical phenotypes have been described with mutation in ARX.
- X-linked lissencephaly with abnormal genitalia in males and agenesis of the corpus callosum in females.
- X-linked infantile spasms (West syndrome).
- X-linked mental retardation.
- Partington syndrome (X-linked mental retardation with dystonia).
- Rett syndrome. See 'Rett syndrome' page 408.
- Seizures may occur with IP in heterozygous females but significant mental retardation is rare.

Mitochondrial disorders: MERFF, MELAS, NARP

MERFF, myoclonic epilepsy with ragged red fibres; MELAS, mitochondrial myopathy–encephalopathy–lactic acidosis–stroke-like episodes; NARP, neuropathy–ataxia–retinitis pigmentosa. See 'Mitochondrial DNA diseases', page 384.

Non-genetic causes

Moderate to severe trauma, infections, including congenital infections such as cytomegalovirus (CMV).

Genetic advice

Generalized symptomatic epilepsy, known cause

Symptomatic epilepsies are those where there is a known or suspected disorder of the CNS. Counsel as for the underlying condition.

Progressive myoclonic epilepsy (PME) is commonly referred to the geneticist whilst investigations are underway to find out the aetiology. PME is the triad of:

- stimulus-sensitive myoclonus;
- grand mal and absence epilepsy;
- progressive neurological deterioration/regression.

Most causes of PME are rare AR conditions. Exclude ceroid lipofuscinoses such as Batten disease (CLN genes), Unverricht–Lunborg disease (cystatin B), Lafora disease (laforin gene), sialodosis. Non-AR causes to exclude are MERFF and dentatorubro-pallidoluysian atrophy (DPRLA).

Generalized symptomatic epilepsy but no definite cause identified

In this group there will be some families with a high risk, and features such as true regression and progressive microcephaly are clues to a genetic aetiology with up to 25% recurrence. For more information on the counselling of specific epilepsy syndromes see 'Epilepsy in infants and children' and 'Epilepsy' pages 314 and 318.

Lay group contact: ⟨www.epilepsy.org.uk⟩; Epilepsy Foundation of America ⟨www.efa.org⟩.

Expert adviser: Jill Clayton-Smith, Consultant Clinical Geneticist, St Mary's Hospital, Manchester, England.

References

Cowan LD. The epidemiology of the epilepsies in children. *Ment Retard Dev Disabil Res Rev* 2002; **8**: 171–81.

Delgado-Escueta AV, Ganesh S, Yamakawa K. Advances in the genetics of progressive myoclonus epilepsy. *Am J Med Genet* 2001; **106**: 129–38.

Elmslie F, Gardiner M, Lehesjoki AE. The epilepsies. In *Emery and Rimoin's principles and practice of medical genetics*, 4th edn (ed. D.L. Rimoin, J.M. Conner, R.E. Pyeritz, and A.E.H. Emery). Churchill Livingstone, London, 2002.

Engel J Jr; International League Against Epilepsy (ILAE). A proposed diagnostic scheme for people with epileptic seizures and with epilepsy: report of the ILAE task force on classification and terminology. *Epilepsia* 2001; **42**: 769–803.

Guerrini R, Carrozzo R. Epileptogenic brain malformations: clinical presentation, malformative patterns and indications for genetic testing. *Seizure* 2001; **10**: 532–43.

Singh R, Gardner RJ, Crossland KM, Scheffer IE, Berkovic SF. Chromosomal abnormalities and epilepsy: a review for clinicians and gene hunters. *Epilepsia* 2002; **43** (2): 127–40.

Stromme P, *et al.* Mutations in the human ortholog of Aristaless cause X-linked mental retardation and epilepsy. *Nat Genet* 2002; **30**: 441–5.

Short stature

This is a common problem presenting to paediatricians and is also a feature of many syndromes. This section is a suggested approach to diagnosis in children whose weight and height/length are roughly proportionate (i.e. on similar centiles). If the child's weight is on a considerably lower centile than the height/length, use 'Failure to thrive', page 116.

A length/height of less than 0.4th centile is used to define short stature. Children with heights below the 0.4th centile, or who have sequential heights that cross successive centile bands merit further investigation. The two most common causes of short stature are:

- familial short stature;
- constitutional delay of growth and puberty.

These cause up to 75% of short stature. Other causes of short stature (with the approximate prevalence in children with short stature) are: chronic diseases (10%); syndromes (6%); chromosomal anomalies (5%); skeletal dysplasias (1%); growth hormone deficiency and receptor insensitivity (1–2%); others, including deprivation, psychological problems.

Clinical approach

History: key points

- Three-generation family tree including parental heights (mid-parental height) and consanguinity (rare skeletal dysplasias and inherited endocrine abnormalities).
- Enquire at what age the parents entered puberty and at what age they attained their final adult heights.
- Pregnancy. Maternal illness, medications, and ask about alcohol if appropriate. Did an ultrasound scan (USS) suggest limb shortening or small size?
- Birthweight/length/occipital-frontal circumference (OFC). Use to determine if the short stature was prenatal (most skeletal dysplasias). Correct for gestation.
- Postnatal growth chart.
- Medical history (chronic diseases).
- Surgical history, particularly orthopaedic procedures such as those to correct talipes, congenital dislocation of the hip (CDH).
- Developmental history.

Examination: key points

- The skeletal system.
  - Observe for disproportion and measure height/length, weight, OFC. If they appear disproportionate, measure arm span and upper and lower body segments (calculate ratio). See 'Skeletal dysplasia', page 246.
  - If the limbs are short, assess if this is predominantly affecting the proximal limb, e.g. humerus/femur (rhizomelic shortening) or forelimb, e.g. radius and ulna/tibia and fibula (mesomelic).
  - Deformity (bowing, talipes, Madelung deformity).
  - Asymmetry.
  - Hands and feet: brachydactyly, broad thumbs, short 4,5 metacarpals and metatarsals, clinodactyly.
- General systems.
  - Signs of poor nutrition.
  - Pubertal development (see 'Staging of puberty' in page 700).
  - Features of renal/cardiac disease.

- Features of hypothyroidism, growth hormone (GH) deficiency, and other endocrine disorders.
- Dysmorphic features and malformations.
- Note that overweight children tend to be tall not short in childhood, so short stature with obesity is an indication for investigation.

Special investigations

Parental heights

If the parents are phenotypically normal, measure their height and calculate the *mid-parental height* (MPH) and the *target centile range*. Children whose projected adult height falls outside the target centile range derived from their parents' heights merit further assessment. NB. This is misleading if one of the parents has a genetic cause of short stature.

- **Girls**
  - Mid-parental height (MPH) centile = [(Father's height − 13cm) + Mother's height (cm))]/2
  - Target centile range for girls = MPH centile ± 9 cm.
- **Boys**
  - Mid-parental height (MPH) centile = [(Mother's height + 13cm) + Father's height]/2
  - Target centile range for boys = MPH centile ± 10 cm.

[NB. 13cm is the average difference in height between adult males and females in the UK.]

Paediatric

- Baseline biochemistry (electrolytes, urea, thyroid function), haematology (full blood count (FBC) and erythrocyte sedimentation rate (ESR)), and urinalysis: to exclude chronic diseases.
- Antigliandin antibodies (coeliac disease).
- Bone age (left wrist).
- Additional endocrine investigations, particularly to exclude GH deficiency, are done under the supervision of a paediatric endocrinologist when the above results are normal but there are persistently subnormal growth rates. Cranial imaging of the pituitary gland may be performed.
- Karyotype on all girls (to exclude 45, X) and in presence of mental retardation/malformation/dysmorphic features in boys.

Genetic

- Consider if mosaicism screen (30 cells) is necessary— mainly applies to girls for investigation of Turner syndrome (45, X).
- Repeat cytogenetic analysis if previously done >5 years ago and if there is mental retardation or dysmorphic features. Chromosomal associations with short stature include:
  - Turner syndrome;
  - XX males, X-autosomal translocations;
  - deletions/mutations in the SHOX gene (see below);
  - most chromosomal imbalances have short stature as a feature but have additional dysmorphic features and mental retardation;
  - consider if the features are consistent with any known uniparental disomy (UPD) conditions;
  - consider microdeletion syndromes.
- Bone age. X-ray left wrist. Comparing the bone maturation (age) with the chronological age (CA) and height may help diagnostically, e.g. constitutional delay.

- Skeletal survey in children with disproportion, deformities, joint restrictions/dislocations. See 'Skeletal dysplasia', page 246 for details of which films to request.
- Molecular cytogenetic testing, e.g. fluorescent *in situ* hybridization (FISH) for SHOX gene on Xp 22.3.
- Consider molecular genetic analysis for maternal (mat)UPD7 in patients with Silver–Russell syndrome (SRS). Approximately 10% of patients with SRS have matUPD7 (maternal UPD in chromosome 7). Requires DNA from both parents, as well as child.
- DNA analysis for some endocrine disorders and some skeletal dysplasias. Molecular analysis can help provide carrier detection and prenatal diagnosis.

Some diagnoses to consider

Consider which of the following clinical groupings best fits the child you are assessing:

- short stature;
- short stature/history of low birthweight;
- disproportionate growth;
- short stature with dysmorphic features, mild or no mental retardation;
- short stature with moderate mental retardation.

Then use the headings below to assess suggested diagnoses.

Short stature

Familial short stature and constitutional delay. In familial short stature the bone maturation is consistent with the chronological age and final height may be estimated from the mid-parental target range. The bone maturation in the delayed puberty group is consistent with the height age and the prognosis for a normal adult height is good.

Mild Turner syndrome. Most of the short stature in Turner syndrome is due to SHOX haploinsufficiency. See 'Turner syndrome, 45,X and variants' page 558.

Noonan syndrome. See 'Noonan syndrome (NS)' page 402.

Leri–Weill dyschondrostosis (Leri–Weill syndrome). Madelung deformity of forearm (restricted pronation and supination). 2.4–7% of children with idiopathic short stature have a *SHOX* mutation, either a deletion or a point mutation (Morizio *et al.* 2003; Rappold *et al.* 2002). This prevalence is similar to that of GH deficiency and Turner syndrome in children with short stature.

Septo-optic dysplasia (SOD). SOD comprises two out of the three features of optic nerve hypoplasia (ONH), namely, unilateral or bilateral absence of the septum pellucidum and pituitary dysfunction. In one series 80% had GH deficiency. See 'Structural intracranial anomalies (agenesis of the corpus callosum, septo-optic dysplasia, and arachnoid cysts)', page 248.

Other midline intracranial defects may be associated with GH deficiency.

Short stature/history of low birthweight

88% of low-birthweight babies catch up over the first year of life. However, 'catch-up' may be delayed in preterm infants. Failure to catch up is more common if there has been early growth failure *in utero* and this may be detected by serial USS.

Silver–Russell syndrome (SRS). Failure to thrive, proportionately large head, but usually between 3rd and 25th centile, triangular face, and downturned mouth. Asymmetry is a key diagnostic feature. SRS is genetically heterogeneous. ~10% have maternal UPD7 and some others have an epimutation of the telomeric imprinting centre on 11p15 (Gicquel). See 'Failure to thrive', page 116.

Maternal uniparental disomy in chromosome 7 (MatUPD7). MatUPD7 has been reported in patients with only slight dysmorphic features and prenatal or postnatal growth retardation. Genetic screening for cases of matUPD7 among growth-retarded patients should be focused on patients with severe intrauterine growth retardation (IUGR) and features of SRS (Hannula *et al.* 2002). In addition, matUPD7 screening is advisable in individuals with cystic fibrosis and other recessive disorders mapped to chromosome 7 who have unusually short stature.

Mutations in IGF-1 receptor (IGF-1R). *IGF-1R* mutations are an uncommon cause of IUGR and postnatal growth failure (Abuzzahab *et al.* 2003). Typically patients who are haploinsufficient for *IGF-1R* have a height of (−2.5–3 SD) and delayed bone age.

Disproportionate growth

Hypochondroplasia. Disproportion and lumbar lordosis are key features. Arrange skeletal survey, consider DNA analysis of *FGFR3*. See 'Skeletal dysplasia', page 246.

Other skeletal dysplasias. Refer to 'Skeletal dysplasia', this chapter, page 246.

Short stature with dysmorphic features, mild or no mental retardation

Aarskog syndrome. Short stature (rhizomelic), ptosis in some, hypermetropia, shawl scrotum, brachydactyly with hyperextendable proximal interphalangeal (PIP) joints. Facial features tend to normalize with age. X-linked semi-dominant inheritance. Caused by mutations in the *FGD1* gene.

Noonan syndrome. Neck webbing, ptosis, and cardiac defects (especially pulmonary stenosis). See 'Noonan syndrome (NS)' page 402.

Pseudohypoparathyroidism (PHP). Albright hereditary osteodystrophy (AHO), GS alpha gene. See 'Obesity with and without developmental delay', page 192.

Floating-harbor syndrome. Predominantly postnatal short stature with growth − 4 to − 5 SD. The nose is broad, the mouth is large, and the ears are low-set and posteriorly rotated. The skull is long from front to back and affected children have had mild developmental delay, especially of expressive language. The eyes are deep-set. Bone age is markedly delayed.

Short stature with moderate mental retardation

There are many syndrome with short stature and mental retardation but particularly consider if the child has features of the following syndromes.

Rubinstein–Taybi syndrome. Normal birthweight, postnatal short stature and microcephaly, moderate–severe learning difficulties in most, broad thumbs and halluces, prominent fetal finger pads. See 'Broad thumbs', page 58.

Kabuki syndrome. Mild growth retardation, characteristic long palpebral fissures. See 'Ptosis, blepharophimosis, and other eyelid abnormalities', page 224.

Mild de Lange syndrome. Associated with the typical de Lange face but mild mental retardation and no radial defects.

Fetal alcohol syndrome (FAS). See 'Fetal alcohol syndrome (FAS)' page 588.

Genetic advice

Recurrence risk

- For children with apparently isolated constitutional delay with no mental retardation there may be familial factors that will increase the risk of short stature in other family members.
- For known diagnosis, as appropriate for the condition.

Carrier detection

SHOX testing can detect previously unknown carriers in large families. Complete deficiency of SHOX causes the severe Langer mesomelic dysplasia.

Prenatal diagnosis

See the 'Prenatal diagnosis' subsection of 'Skeletal dysplasia', this chapter on the pitfalls of predicting dysplasias at 20 weeks page 246.

Natural history and further management (preventative measures)

- Children with non-syndromic conditions require surveillance of their growth rate by a paediatrician or paediatric endocrinologist.
- GH treatment is beneficial in GH deficiency and in some girls with Turner syndrome and is licensed for the treatment of children who are small for gestational age and who fail to show catch-up growth by the age of 4 years. There is no clear-cut benefit in most syndromes or in skeletal dysplasias.
- Skeletal dysplasias require a plan of management to prevent complications, discuss prognosis, and to discuss procedures such as leg lengthening. See 'Skeletal dysplasias', page 246.

Support group contact: Child Growth Foundation 2 Mayfield Avenue, London W4 1PW; Restricted Growth Foundation, PO Box 4744, Dorchester DT2 9FA, UK <www.rgaonline.org.uk>; Little People of America <www.lpaonline.org>.

Expert adviser: David Dunger, Professor of Paediatrics, University of Cambridge, Cambridge, England.

References

Abuzzahab MJ, Schneider A, et al. IGF-1 Receptor mutations resulting in intrauterine and postnatal growth retardation. New Engl J Med 2003; **349**: 2211–22.

Dattani M, Preece M. Growth hormone deficiency and related disorders: insights into causation, diagnosis and treatment (Review). Lancet 2004; **363**: 1977–87.

Freeman JV, Cole TJ, Chinn S, Jones PRM, White EM, Preece MA. Cross sectional stature and weight reference curves for the U.K. 1990. Arch Dis Child 1995; **73**: 17–24.

Gicquel C, Rossignol S, et al. Epimutation of the telomeric imprinting center region on chromosome 11p15 in Silver-Russell syndrome. Nat Genet 2005; **37**: 1003–7.

Hannula K, Lipsanen-Nyman M, et al. Genetic screening for maternal uniparental disomy of chromosome 7 in prenatal and postnatal growth retardation of unknown cause. Pediatrics 2002; **109**: 441–8.

Morizio E, Stuppia L, et al. Deletion of the SHOX gene in patients with short stature of unknown cause. Am J Med Genet 2003; **119A**: 293–6.

Rappold GA, et al. Deletions in the homeobox gene SHOX (short stature homeobox) are an important cause of growth failure in children with short stature. J Clin Endocrinol Metab 2002; **87**: 1402–6.

Skeletal dysplasia

A skeletal dysplasia is a generalized structural abnormality of bone growth and modelling. The main structural protein of bone and cartilage is collagen. Bone modelling is a consequence of osteoblast and osteoclast activity and growth/morphogenetic factors are of importance in development. Mutations in these genes cause generalized dysplasia.

In clinical practice an infant or child may be referred with deformity, short stature, and/or disproportion to establish if he/she has an underlying skeletal dysplasia and, if so, to determine the diagnosis.

The terminology is as follows.

- **Epiphysis.** An area of secondary ossificiation, usually present at each end of long bones (the metacarpals and metatarsals only have one epiphysis each). Irregular bones such as the carpal bones each have a single ossification centre.
- **Metaphysis.** Immediately adjacent to the epiphysis, it is the growing area of the long bone.
- The **diaphysis** forms the central shaft of the bone. It is enclosed by the periosteum and in childhood some growth in thickness occurs here.
- **Spondylo,** pertaining to the spinal column or vertebrae.

Clinical approach

History: key points

- Three-generation family tree with enquiry about short stature (document estimated adult heights) and consanguinity.
- Family history of early osteoarthritis, hip replacement (Stickler syndrome, multiple epiphyseal dysplasia (MED), pseudoachondroplasia).
- History of the pregnancy. Were short limbs evident on antenatal ultrasound scan (USS)?
- Birth measurements of length and head circumference.
- At what age did the short stature become obvious?
- Joint pain, contractures and limitation of movement, e.g. pronation/supination of forearm in Lerri–Weill (*SHOX*).
- Pathological fractures (osteogenesis imperfecta (OI), osteopetrosis)—fractures resulting from trauma inadequate to fracture normal bone.
- Assess if evidence of developmental delay.

Examination: key points

- Measurementof height/length, arm span, upper to lower segment ratio:
  - arm span is the distance between middle finger tips when the arms are held out horizontally from the body;
  - upper to lower segment ratio (U/L) used to distinguish disproportionate growth. The bony landmark is the pubic bone. Sitting height using a 60 cm stool is an alternative;

$$\frac{\text{upper segment}}{\text{lower segment}} = \frac{(\text{height} - \text{lower segment})}{\text{lower segment}}$$

  U/L (for <10 years) >1.0; U/L (10 years) = 1.0; U/L (>10 years) <1.0.
- If limbs are short, measure using recognized bony landmarks and assess if this is proximal (rhizomelic shortening) or distal (mesomelic).

- Head circumference (macrocephaly in achondroplasia).
- Gait. Waddling gait due to hip disease; gait disturbance due to spinal stenosis in achondroplasia.
- Limbs:
  - talipes (diastrophic dysplasia, Kniest syndrome);
  - bowing of long bones;
  - Madelung deformity of the forearm (dyschondrosteosis);
  - asymmetry of limb length (X-linked dominant chrondrodysplasia punctata);
- Joints. Pain and limitation of movement, arthrogryposis, contractures, deformity, and swelling.
- Hands and feet:
  - brachydactyly, polydactyly (Ellis van Creveld and Jeune syndromes);
  - thumb abnormalities (hitchhiker thumb in diastrophic dysplasia, triphalangeal thumb with radial ray syndromes).
- Eyes. Cataract and myopia, detached retina.
- Palate. Cleft palate in Stickler syndrome, Kniest syndrome, and spondylo-epiphyseal dysplasia congenita (which are caused by *COL2 A1* mutations).
- Teeth (dentinogenesis imperfecta, Ellis van Creveld).
- Hair (thin in chondrodysplasia punctata, metaphyseal dysplasia type McKusick).
- Heart. Examine for signs of congenital heart disease (CHD).
- Neurological examination. Spinal stenosis, hydrocephalus.
- Exclude signs of a storage disorder (coarse features, hepatosplenomegaly).

Special investigations

- Radiological survey for skeletal dysplasia:
  - skull anteroposterior (AP) and lateral;
  - chest posteroanterior (PA);
  - spine AP with lateral;
  - pelvis with hips (most radiographers don't include hips if you just ask for 'pelvis');
  - humerus, radius, and ulna (unilateral);
  - hand, carpal bones, and phalanges (unilateral);
  - femur, tibia, and fibula (unilateral).

Good quality films and specialist interpretation of the radiographs are essential. Bone maturation in epiphyseal disorders is frequently delayed but can occasionally be advanced. Document changes over time. For some skeletal dysplasias radiological changes may not be obvious in infancy (e.g. hypochondroplasia). Children with a normal skeletal survey and delayed bone maturation require endocrine investigations.

- Magnetic resonance imaging (MRI) of the brain with cervical and lower spine scans may be indicated in conditions with suspected spinal stenosis.
- Scans or films in flexion or extension may be indicated to determine whether there is subluxation or absence of the odontoid in dysplasias where odontoid hypoplasia is a recognized complication. Arrange in conjunction with a neurologist/neuroradiologist. Particularly important prior to surgery/anaesthesia.
- Exclude metabolic bone disease in children with metaphyseal abnormalities and disorders of bone density.

- Molecular genetic analysis, e.g. *FGFR3* in achondroplasia and hypochondroplasia. Store DNA and investigate if testing available.
- Cytogenetic analysis if there are associated malformations and/or developmental delay. Certain disorders may have diagnostic cytogenetic changes (e.g. camptomelic dysplasia (*SOX9*), fluorescent *in situ* hybridization (FISH) analysis of *SHOX* on Xp dyschondreostosis/Leri–Weil).
- Metabolic screen for inborn errors of metabolism, e.g. mucopolysaccharidoses if a storage disorder is suspected (urine for glycosaminoglycans), and peroxisomal testing (very long chain fatty acids (VLCFAs)) and sterol analysis (sterol profile) with stippled epiphyses.
- Orthopaedic, rheumatology, and endocrine referrals as appropriate (particularly important in the growing child).

Some diagnoses to consider

- Differentiate between a skeletal dysplasia and other causes of short stature.
- Exclude the possibility of storage disorders and metabolic bone disease.
- Consider if other family members are affected and whether radiological investigation would help to establish this.
- If a skeletal dysplasia is present, aim to determine the broad diagnostic category even if the diagnosis is not certain. Enlist expert radiological assistance. The Skeletal Dysplasia Group in the UK have useful publications to help interpret the clinical and radiological features.

Clinical diagnostic groups (UK Skeletal Dysplasia Group)

Combine the radiological and clinical information and attempt to put into one of the following groups (Wynne-Davies 2004) page 698.

- **Short limbs/trunk less affected,** e.g. achondroplasia, hypochondroplasia, acromesomelic, pseudoachondroplasia.
- **Short limbs and trunk,** e.g. diastrophic dysplasia, Kniest dysplasia.
- **Epiphyseal disorders.** Delayed, small, irregular epiphyses in multiple epiphyseal dysplasia (MED), stippled epiphyses in the various types of chondrodysplasia punctata. The short stature in MED affects mainly the long bones.
- **Short trunk/limbs less affected,** e.g. spondyloepiphyseal and spondylometaphyseal dysplasias.
- **Metaphyseal disorders.** A difficult group to classify and differentiate from metabolic disorders such as rickets purely by radiographs.
- **Abnormal bone density.** Increased in osteopetrosis and pycnodysostosis; decreased in OI and hypophosphatasia. See 'The Non-lethal skeletal dysplasias', page 698.

Genetic advice

Recurrence risk

- **Known diagnosis.** Counsel as appropriate.
- **Unknown diagnosis.** If there is consanguinity, autosomal recessive (AR) is the likely mode of inheritance. An autosomal dominant (AD) or X-linked mode of inheritance may be established from the family history.

Carrier detection

Possible where there is a causative mutation, biochemical test, or radiological features.

Prenatal diagnosis

The two main techniques are ultrasound and chorionic villus sampling (CVS)/amniocentesis depending on the diagnosis and whether the causative mutation or biochemical defect has been identified. Early prenatal testing may be possible by CVS using molecular techniques but may not be appropriate for milder conditions or for conditions with a low recurrence risk. USS limb measurements may be normal at 20 weeks in conditions that cause marked short stature (e.g. achondroplasia). Milder conditions such as MED will not show prenatal limb shortening. See 'Short limbs' page 630.

Natural history and further management (preventative measures)

Long-term medical supervision is required for most children and adults, for example, to discuss the following:

- **Surgical management,** including limb lengthening.
- **Exercise.** The most beneficial forms of exercise to protect against joint damage, e.g. swimming. *Avoid* trampolining and baby bouncers/jumpers. *Avoid* contact sports, e.g. rugby, American football.
- **Medication,** e.g. bisphosphonates for children with OI.
- **Neurological complications,** e.g. spinal stenosis, nerve entrapment.
- **GH treatment.** Not shown to be of benefit in the majority of children.
- **Mobility aids.** Domiciliary assessment may also be helpful to determine whether kitchen/bathroom adaptations are needed.

Support group contact: Restricted Growth Association, PO Box 8919, Birmingham B27 6DQ, <www.restricted growth.co.uk>; United Kingdom Coalition of Short People, PO Box 18, Hereford, UK, email: <shortpeopleuk@aol.com>. Little People of America <www.lpaonline.org>.

Expert adviser: Ruth Wynne-Davies, Honorary Consultant in Orthopaedic Clinical Genetics, University of Oxford, Oxford, England.

References

European Skeletal Dysplasia Network <www.esdu.org>.

Horton WA. Skeletal development: insights from targeting the mouse genome. *Lancet* 2003; **362**: 560–9.

International Working Group on Constitutional Diseases of Bone. International nomenclature and classification of the osteochondrodysplasias. *Am J Med Genet* 1998; **79**: 376–82.

Seminars in Medical Genetics. Latest developments in skeletal dysplasias. *Am J Med Genet* 2001; **106C** (issue 4). <www.csmc.Pedu/genetics/skeldys>.

Wynne-Davies R, Hall CM, Hurst JA, UK Skeletal Dysplasia Group. *Skeletal dysplasias. A method of diagnosis of the non-lethal Skeletal dysplasias*. Skeletal dysplasia Group Occasional Publications No. 9a, 2004.

Structural intracranial anomalies (agenesis of the corpus callosum, septo-optic dysplasia, and arachnoid cysts)

Formation of the cerebral commissures begins as early as 6 weeks gestation gestation when axons destined to cross in the anterior commissure can be seen growing medially within the hemisphere. The most important fibre bundles cross in the lamina terminalis. At 10 weeks gestation the first fibres cross to form the anterior commissure. Fibres begin to cross in the corpus callosum from 11 gestation and over the next few weeks the corpus callosum grows enormously (see figure). The growth of the corpus callosum causes the lamina terminalis to become locally thinned and it forms the septum pellucidum. By 18–20 weeks gestation, the corpus callosum has assumed the adult form, although it continues to thicken and grow caudally for several months.

Agenesis of the corpus callosum (ACC)

ACC is one of the most common brain malformations with a prevalence of 3–7/1000. Its prevalence in children with developmental disabilities may be as high as 2%. It may occur as an isolated malformation, as one feature of a complex cranial malformation sequence, as part of a syndrome, or as a teratogenic consequence of an inborn error of metabolism.

The corpus callosum is relatively easy to visualize by cranial ultrasound scan (USS) in a neonate; it is also well seen on computerized tomography (CT) or magnetic resonance imaging (MRI) scans (see figure). As such, it is often identified fairly early in the investigations of a neonate with abnormal neurology or a child with developmental delay or seizures. Whilst it contributes to the

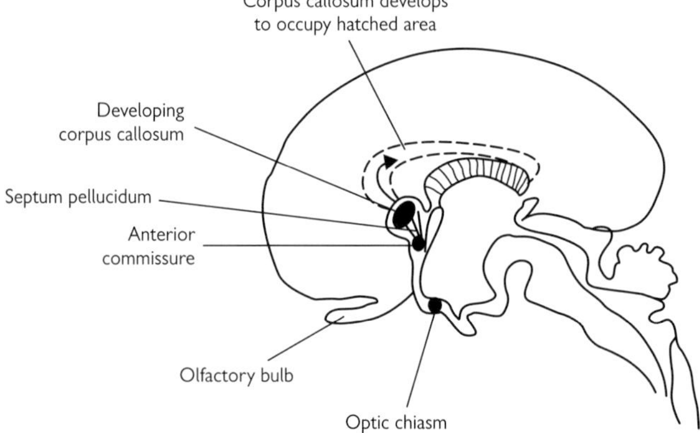

Line diagram to show sagittal view of brain of a 4-month-old fetus

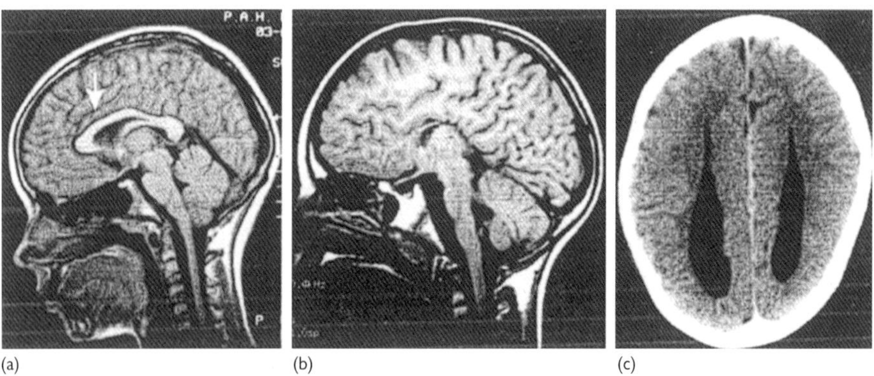

(a) Normal brain in a girl aged 2 years. A T_1-weighted sagittal MRI shows normal corpus callosum and cingulate gyrus (arrow). (b) Agenesis of the corpus callosum in a girl aged 6 years who has microcephaly and moderate learning difficulties. A T_1-weighted sagittal MRI shows absence of the corpus callosum and of the cingulate gyrus, which normally runs parallel to the corpus callosum. (c) Agenesis of the corpus callosum in the same girl as in (b). Axial CT shows typical appearance of parallel lateral cerebral ventricles, with divergence of the anterior horns of the ventricles and colpocephaly (dilated posterior part of the lateral ventricles). (Taken from Warrell (2003), figure 5, p. 1208 by permission of Oxford University Press.)

clinical picture it is a much less specific finding than is often thought. Occasionally it is an incidental finding in a child with otherwise normal development.

Clinical approach

History: key points

- Detailed three-generation family tree and enquire about consanguinity.
- Seizures.
- Developmental milestones.

Examination: key points

Look carefully for dysmorphic features and other congenital malformations.

Special investigations

- Chromosomes, include fluorescent *in situ* hybridization (FISH) for 4p–.
- Ophthalmology assessment. Optic nerve hypoplasia? Retinal lacunae (seen in Aicardi syndrome)?
- Review MRI for other midline anomaly, e.g. agenesis of septum pellucidum or evidence of more generalized migration defect, e.g. lissencephaly, or hydrocephalus (*L1CAM*).
- Urine for amino and organic acids.
- If seizures, cerebrospinal fluid (CSF) glycine (non-ketotic hyperglycinaemia) and lactate (pyruvate dehydrogenase deficiency). In a male infant consider neonatal adrenoleukodystrophy (very long chain fatty acids (VLCFAs)) and Menkes syndrome (caeruloplasmin).
- If optic nerve hypoplasia or absence of septum pellucidum, need to perform full investigation of hypothalamic pituitary axis (see below).

Some diagnoses to consider

Acrocallosal syndrome (ACS; Schinzel syndrome). ACS is an autosomal recessive (AR) condition that is likely to be genetically heterogeneous. It is characterized by agenesis of the corpus callosum, pre- and postaxial polydactyly, mild hypertelorism, and a spectrum of psychomotor retardation from mild to severe. Intracranial cysts (including arachnoid cysts) were seen in 10/34 published cases of ACS (Koenig *et al.* 2002). There is some diagnostic overlap with Greig cephalopolysyndactyly syndrome which is caused by mutations in *GLI3* and follows autosomal dominant (AD) inheritance with variable expressivity. In particular, large deletions involving *GLI3* may cause an overlap phenotype with ACS.

Mowat–Wilson syndrome. Characteristic facial appearance (hypertelorism, pointed chin, prominent columella, open-mouthed expression, broad, medial flared eyebrows and uplifted earlobes) together with severe mental retardation. Microcephaly, seizures, congenital heart defects, aplasia/hypoplasia of corpus callosum and urogenital anomalies (especially hypospadias in boys) are frequent findings. Caused by 'de novo' truncating mutations in *ZFHX1B*.

Genetic advice

Make every effort to make a specific diagnosis and to substantiate this by appropriate laboratory investigations and then counsel accordingly. If the ACC is isolated, this may be sporadic or follow AD, AR, or X-linked modes of inheritance.

Septo-optic dysplasia (SOD)

de Morsier's syndrome.

This is the association of optic nerve hypoplasia with agenesis of the septum pellucidum and disturbed hypothalamic/pituitary function. SOD comprises two out of the three features of optic nerve hypoplasia (ONH): unilateral or bilateral absence of the septum pellucidum and pituitary dysfunction. 50% of patients with this condition have a septum pellucidum present. In one series 80% had growth hormone (GH) deficiency, 60% had adrenocorticotrophic hormone (ACTH) deficiency, 40% had luteinizing hormone (LH)/follicle-stimulating hormone (FSH) deficiency, and 35% had diabetes insipidus. Visual impairment is extremely variable. Seizures in children with SOD are often secondary to hypoglycaemia (GH deficiency ± cortisol deficiency) rather than secondary to a primary brain abnormality. Overall, approximately half of cases have moderate or severe developmental delay. Children need specialist input from a paediatric endocrinologist and paediatric opthalmologist.

SOD is largely thought to be a sporadic disorder with a low recurrence risk. However, in the light of the recent identification of the *HESX1* gene, it is now clear that genetic mutations in this gene may account for some cases of SOD (Dattani *et al.* 1998; Tajima *et al.* 2003). Additionally, there is increasing evidence to suggest that SOD is a multigenic disorder, with other genes being involved, and possible interaction with environmental factors, ultimately leading to a phenotype.

Mutations in the homeobox gene *HESX1*, which is essential for pituitary and forebrain development, have been described in a handful of individuals with phenotypes ranging from severe SOD, relatively mild combined pituitary hormone deficiency (CPHD), to isolated GH deficiency (Dattani *et al.* 1998; Tajima *et al.* 2003). Very rarely the characteristic CNS and ocular abnormalities of SOD occur together with limb malformations (digital anomalies) as a distinct entity (Harrison).

Special investigations

- Full investigation of the hypothalamic pituitary axis (including post-pituitary).
- MRI scan, including imaging of optic chiasm and pituitary.
- Chromosomes, if associated developmental delay.
- DNA.

Arachnoid cysts

Arachnoid cysts are collections of CSF that develop within the arachnoid membrane because of splitting or duplication of the structure. They are developmental anomalies, which are often identified as an incidental finding during cranial imaging by USS, CT, or MRI. 40% are in the midline.

Arachnoid cysts are nearly always sporadic and single. The male to female ratio is greater than 2:1; they are more common on the left side. They are relatively rare, accounting for ~1% of intracranial space-occupying lesions. They cause concern when they are identified on a routine antenatal USS. They are usually asymptomatic, but can produce symptoms because of expansion or bleeding. Conservative management is usually indicated in the absence of symptoms or signs—but seek neurosurgical advice. Longstanding pressure effects may contribute to maldevelopment of the temporal lobe and may produce obstruction at the level of the IIIrd or IVth ventricle requiring shunting.

With widespread use of imaging, many arachnoid cysts are detected during the antenatal or neonatal period. Some may remain quiescent throughout life, some may resolve, and some may become symptomatic after several years of quiescence. Symptoms depend on size, location, and age. Seizure and headache are the most common symptoms of middle cranial fossa cysts (60%). 10–30% are found in the posterior fossa. There is a reported relationship between temporal lobe arachnoid cysts and attention deficit hyperactivity disorder (ADHD). Mental impairment and developmental delay have been associated with large arachnoid cysts.

Special investigations
Bilateral temporal arachnoid cysts occur in glutaric aciduria type 1. If present, do urine amino and organic acid screen.

Acrocallosal syndrome (Schinzel syndrome)
Intracranial cysts (including arachnoid cysts) were seen in 10/34 published cases of ACS (Koenig *et al.* 2002). See above.

Support group: SOD/ONH Support Network <www.focusfamilies.org>.

Expert adviser: Michael Baraitser, Emeritus Consultant Clinical Geneticist, Great Ormond Street Hospital, London, England.

References

Cameron FJ, Khadilkar VV, Stanhope R. Pituitary dysfunction and mortality with congenital midline malformation of the cerebrum. *Eur J Pediatr* 1999; **158**: 97–102.

Dattani MT, Martinez-Barbera JP, Thomas PQ, *et al.* Mutations in the homeobox gene HESX1/Hesx1 associated with septo-optic dysplasia in human and mouse. *Nat Genet* 1998; **19**: 125–33.

Dobyns WB. Absence makes the search grow longer [invited editorial]. *Am J Hum Genet* 1996; **58**: 7–16.

Gosalakkal JA. Intracranial arachnoid cysts in children: a review of pathogenesis, clinical features and management. *Pediatr Neurol* 2002; **26**: 93–8.

Gupta JK, Lilford RJ. Assessment and management of fetal agenesis of the corpus callosum [review]. *Prenatal Diagn* 1995; **15**: 301–12.

Harrison IM, Brosnahan D, *et al.* Septo-optic dysplasia with digital anomalies—a recurrent pattern syndrome. *Am J Med Genet* 2004; **131A**: 82–5.

Koenig R, Bach A, Woelki U, *et al.* Spectrum of the acrocallosal syndrome. *Am J Med Genet* 2002; **108**: 7–11.

Tajima T, Hattorri T, *et al.* Sporadic heterozygous frameshift mutation of HESX1 causing pituitary and optic nerve hypoplasia and combined pituitary hormone deficiency in a Japanese patient. *J Clin Endocrinol Metab* 2003; **88** (1): 45–50.

Warrell D. (ed.). *Oxford textbook of medicine*, 4th edn. Oxford University Press, Oxford, 2003.

Suspected non-accidental injury

Non-accidental injury (NAI) is suspected by the paediatric team when an infant presents with several fractures of varying ages with no clear history to account for them, or when an infant is found to have subdural haemorrhage (SDH) or when an infant/child presents with recurrent bruising. A genetic opinion may be sought if the diagnosis of NAI is uncertain or if there are clinical pointers suggesting a possible underlying genetic disorder. The paediatric team will usually have a protocol for managing suspected NAI and liase with appropriate agencies such as the child protection team, social services, and in some circumstances the police and the coroner.

In practice, for an infant or child presenting with fractures the most important differential diagnosis is osteogenesis imperfecta (OI); for an infant presenting with SDH it is important to exclude glutaric aciduria and, in males with developmental delay or seizures, Menkes syndrome. In SDH the paediatric team will investigate for coagulation disorders.

Recurrent fractures or fractures of different ages or occasions where the fracture seems disproportionate to the trauma sustained may all occur in OI. It is important to make a genetic diagnosis accurately and speedily in such circumstances to avoid inappropriate suspicion and investigation of child abuse.

Sadly, 'shaken baby syndrome' is a common cause of SDH in infants with an annual incidence of 2/10 000. SDH is commonly associated with other injuries (e.g. rib fractures from squeezing) and retinal haemorrhages. Isolated SDH or isolated retinal haemorrhages can both occur following intentional injury. Shaken baby syndrome is serious with a mortality of 12–30% and a high morbidity with 60–70% of survivors sustaining significant neurological handicap. SDH is not usually associated with an underlying genetic disorder.

Clinical approach

History: key points

- Three-generation family history including enquiry for fractures, dental problems, hearing loss, lax joints, short stature, or easy bruising.
- Detailed perinatal history. Was there any birth trauma? (SDH can follow traumatic delivery and be associated with retinal haemorrhage. SDH at birth may predispose to subsequent SDH in infancy.) Probable increased risk of fracture up to age 6 months in ex-premature infants born at less than 1000 g.
- Detailed developmental history. Was the child's development progressing normally prior to this episode?
- Is there any dietary deficiency (scurvy, rickets)?

Examination: key points

- Growth parameters. Height, weight, and occipital-frontal circumference (OFC).
- Record the size of the anterior fontanelle.
- Eyes. Are the sclerae blue (OI)? This is an age-dependent feature.
- Scalp. Sparse hair (Menkes)?
- Facial features (record with photographs).
- Documentation of bruising/fractures. Record briefly; full documentation will usually be completed by the paediatric team.

Special investigations

- Photographs.
- Full skeletal survey reviewed by a paediatric radiologist (look for wormian bones in OI and Menkes). Survey criteria can be found on the British Paediatric Radiololgy Society website http://www.bspr.org.uk/
- Consider a skin biopsy for fibroblast culture.
- Store DNA (EDTA (ethylenedinitrilotetraacetate) sample).
- Full blood count (FBC) with platelet count and coagulopathy screen (if SDH or bruising).
- Urine for organic and amino acids (to exclude glutaric aciduria).
- Samples for copper and caeruloplasmin in a male with subdurals (to exclude Menkes).
- Consider freezing urine, plasma, and serum samples to permit future analysis if the child is likely to die.
- Computerized tomography (CT) head scan is recommended whenever NAI is suspected.

Some diagnoses to consider

Osteogenesis imperfecta (OI). See 'Fractures', page 122. In Marlowe et al.'s (2002) study of biochemical analysis of fibroblasts in 262 children presenting with suspected NAI, 11 samples had alterations in the amount or structure of type I collagen synthesized, consistent with the diagnosis of OI. In 6/11, the diagnosis of OI was clinically suspected.

Glutaric aciduria. Associated with widening of the subdural space that can result in SDH due to stretching and rupture of subdural vessels. Case reports describe associated retinal haemorrhage.

Menkes syndrome. X-linked recessive disorder of copper metabolism. Main features are sparse, steely hair (with pili torti on microscopy) and progressive neurological impairment often with seizures and spasticity. Wormian bones on skull X-ray. Caused by mutations in *ATP7A* on Xq13.2–q13.3.

Deficiency disorders. Consider the possibility of scurvy or rickets.

Hypophosphatasia. Hypophosphatasia is a rare autosomal recessive (AR) inborn error of metabolism characterized by defective bone mineralization caused by a deficiency of liver-, bone-, or kidney-type alkaline phosphatase due to mutations in the tissue-non-specific alkaline phosphatase (*TNSALP*) gene. The clinical expression of the disease is highly variable, ranging from stillbirth with a poorly mineralized skeleton to pathological skeletal fractures that develop in late adulthood only. This clinical heterogeneity is due to the strong allelic heterogeneity in the *TNSALP* gene (Herasse et al. 2002).

Congenital insensitivity to pain with anhidrosis. Congenital insensitivity to pain with anhidrosis (CIPA) is a rare AR sensory autonomic neuropathy caused by mutations in the neurotrophic tyrosine kinase receptor type I (*NTRK1*). Skeletal findings include fractures, joint deformities, joint dislocations, osteomyelitis, avascular necrosis, and acroosteolysis. Mental retardation is common and cranial imaging may show mild loss of brain volume with some ventriculomegaly. Death from hyperpyrexia occurs in almost 20 % of patients in the first 3 years of life (Schulman et al. 2001).

Genetic advice

Recurrence risk

If a genetic disorder is diagnosed advise as appropriate. Social/environmental issues may generate a risk of recurrence even in the absence of a genetic risk. If a diagnosis of NAI is made, assessment and management of this risk is the responsibility of the paediatrician and child protection team.

Expert advisers: Christine Hall, Professor of Paediatric Radiology, Institute of Child Health, London and Nick Bishop, Professor of Paediatric Bone Disease, University of Sheffield, Sheffield, England.

References

Herasse M, Spentchian M, *et al.* Evidence of a founder effect for the tissue-nonspecific alkaline phosphatase (TNSALP) gene E174K mutation in hypophosphatasia patients. *Eur J Hum Genet* 2002; **10**: 666–8.

Kemp AM. Investigating subdural haemorrhage in infants. *Arch Dis Child* 2002; **86**: 98–102.

Marlowe A, Pepin MG, Byers PH. Testing for osteogenesis imperfecta in cases of suspected non-accidental injury. *J Med Genet* 2002; **39** (6): 382–6.

Nassogne MC, Sharrard M, *et al.* Massive subdural haematomas in Menkes disease mimicking shaken baby syndrome. *Childs Nerv Syst* 2002; **18**: 729–31.

Schulman H, Tsodikow V, *et al.* Congenital insensitivity to pain with anhidrosis (CIPA): the spectrum of radiological findings. *Pediatr Radiol* 2001; **31**: 701–5.

Syndactyly (other than 2,3 toe syndactyly)

For 2,3 toe syndactyly, see 'Minor congenital anomalies', page 180.

Syndactyly occurs when the digits fail to separate during days 52–55 (post-fertilization), or when an external disruptive event occurs during embryonic development. Failure to separate can have a genetic cause but environmental factors such as chorionic villus sampling (CVS) also need to be considered.

The aim is to distinguish whether the syndactyly is isolated or forms part of a syndrome or is secondary (see below). Correct description of the syndactyly is the first diagnostic step (see table).

Clinical approach

History: key points

- At least three-generation pedigree. Explain to parents the minimal signs that could indicate a gene carrier.
- Consanguinity (autosomal recessive (AR) syndromes).
- Increased paternal age (Apert syndrome).
- Early pregnancy events such as CVS, bleeding, teratogen exposure, fever.
- Neurological/developmental problems.

Examination: key points

- Hands and feet. Describe shape and count the total number of digits.
- Which fingers and toes are syndactylous?
- Does the syndactyly involve the whole length of the digits, i.e. complete or partial?
- Does the syndactyly appear to involve the bones or just soft tissues?
- Is there any skin webbing between the digits?
- Is there shortening of any of the digits, symbrachydactyly (Poland anomaly)?
- Bilateral or unilateral and symmetry.
- Thumbs and halluces. Are they involved? Document structure and function.
- Head and skull shape; craniosynostosis (Apert syndrome).
- Microphthalmia (oculodentodigital (ODD) syndrome).
- Hypoplastic alae nasi, 'pinched nose'(ODD).
- Oral region. Cleft palate, oral frenulae, tongue cysts (oral-facial-digital (OFD) syndromes).
- Other malformations (chromosomal disorders).
- Skin pigmentary abnormalities (chromosome mosaicism; especially consider diploid/triploid mosaicism).
- *Remember to examine the parents.*

Special investigations

- Clinical photographs.
- X-rays of the hands and feet are essential to assess the skeletal elements and to detect minor features not seen on clinical examination. The X-ray will assist in the process of definition.
- Skull X-rays and further skeletal films, if indicated from clinical assessment.
- Cytogenetic analysis if there are additional malformations or developmental delay.
- Skin fibroblast if chromosome mosaicism is likely.
- DNA storage and analysis if available.

Some diagnoses to consider

With asymmetric involvement

Moebius syndrome. Congenital cranial nerve palsies affecting VI (abduction of the eye) and VII (facial movement) in conjunction with terminal transverse defects. See 'Facial asymmetry', this chapter. Moebius syndrome may also be a feature of **oromandibular–limb–hypogenesis syndrome** (OMLH) and occur with **Poland anomaly**. See 'Limb reduction defects', page 152.

Be aware of the AR phenocopy, **Carey–Fineman–Ziter syndrome**, if talipes and muscle problems are features.

Amniotic bands. Early rupture of the amnion may lead to the production of fibrous mesodermal cords that constrict or cleave parts of the fetus, causing disruption of otherwise normal development. Another possible causal mechanism is the modification of fetal blood flow—the bands being a secondary phenomenon. Sometimes amniotic bands can be visualized by ultrasound scan (USS). There may be a clear history that, at delivery, fibrous cords were wrapped tightly round the affected digit(s). Sometimes the syndactyly is terminal and it is possible to pass a probe between the fingers proximally. Recurrence risk is very small, <2%.

Malformation syndromes

Synpolydactyly. Rare autosomal dominant (AD) disorder characterized by syndactyly between 3rd and 4th fingers and between 4th and 5th toes with a partly or completely duplicated digit in the syndactylous web. Penetrance incomplete and expressivity very variable. Severely affected males may also have hypospadias. Most patients have an expansion of a polyalanine tract in *HOXD13* on 2q31.

Apert syndrome (FGFR2**).** Severe syndactyly, often called a mitten hand. The feet are also affected and there is

Classification of the syndactylies (based on Temtamy and McKusick 1978)

Syndactyly type	Fingers	Toes	Comments
Type I (2q34–36)	3–4	2–3	Bilateral in 50%. Syndactyly of toes is 4 times as common as that of fingers
Type II (also known as synpolydactyly) (*HOXD13*)	3–4	4–5	Mesoaxial polydactyly frequently present (partial or complete duplication of a digit in the syndactylous web)
Type III (connexin 43, *GJA1*)	4–5		Found in oculodentodigital (ODD) dysplasia
Type IV	1–5		Rare, polydactyly common, hypoplastic or triphalangeal thumb
Type V	4–5 metacarpals	2–3: 4–5	
Complete syndactyly	2–5	2–5	Thumb may be involved. Mainly seen in Apert syndrome

coronal suture synostosis (see 'Craniosynostosis' page 288). Developmental delay is found even when there has been no evidence of raised intracranial pressure. Two recurrent mutations account for the majority of cases.

Cenani–Lenz syndrome. An AR syndrome where the hands and feet are similar to those in Apert syndrome but there is hypoplasia of the radius and ulna and fusion of the metacarpals.

Oculodentodigital (ODD) dysplasia. An AD syndrome with a characteristic nose, type III syndactyly, and dental anomalies. Approximately 50% of patients develop neurological features e.g. dysarthria, spastic bladder or gait disturbance, and cranial MRI may show white matter changes. Caused by mutations in connexin 43, *GJA1*, at 6q22–23 (Paznekas). There is a high new mutation rate.

Oro-facial-digital (OFD) syndromes especially OFD1
OFD1 is an X-linked dominant (XLD) malformation syndrome caused by mutation in *CXORF5*. The features in the hands are syndactyly (usually skin syndactyly affecting variable digits), brachydactyly, and postaxial polydactyly. Craniofacial anomalies are midline cleft lip, tongue cysts, and excess oral frenulae (Thauvin-Robinet).

Filippi syndrome. Type I syndacyly with microcephaly, mental retardation, and a distinctive nose. The inheritance is AR.

Chromosomal disorders

Triploidy. Consider this diagnosis in very growth-retarded fetuses with syndactyly. See 'Triploidy (69,XXX, 69,XXY, or 69,XYY)' page 556.

Diploid triploid mosaic. Arises from partial 'rescue' of a triploid conception, so the morula is mosaic ($3n/2n$). The affected fetus may not survive pregnancy or may continue to term and survive. Characteristic findings are syndactyly especially of fingers 3–4 and toes 2–3, with bulbous ends of the toes and clinodactyly. There may be body asymmetry and streaky skin with hyper- or hypopigmentation. Skin chromosomes are required to make the diagnosis. Genetic counselling is as for full triploidy. See 'Triploidy (69,XXX, 69,XXY, or 69,XYY)' page 556.

Deletion of 2q37. Some patients with syndactyly and brachydactyly type E and developmental delay have a 2q37 deletion.

Genetic advice

Recurrence risk

- Bilateral changes affecting the hands and feet, and fitting into one of the classification groups, are likely to be genetic and dominantly inherited. Carefully examine parents and exclude features of syndromes in affected individuals.
- In type II (see table) the penetrance is 96% in the upper limbs and 70% in the lower limbs. The expression is variable.
- Counsel as appropriate if there is an underlying syndrome.

Prenatal diagnosis

- Genetic testing for some of these syndromes may be available.
- USS. The digits can be visualized from the second trimester. Other USS markers should be used to confirm a diagnosis.

Support group contact: Many of the individual syndromes have their own support groups. See Contact a Family (UK) <www.cafamily.org.uk>; National Organisation for Rare Disorders (US) <www.rarediseases.org>.

Expert advisor: Dian Donnai, Professor of Medical Genetics, University of Manchester, Manchester, England.

References

Goodman FR. Congenital abnormalities of body patterning: embryology revisited. *Lancet* 2003; **362**: 651–62.

Paznekas WA, et al. Connexin 43 (GJA1) mutations cause the pleiotropic phenotype of oculo-dento-digital dysplasia. *Am J Hum Genet* 2003; **72**: 408–18.

Paznekas WA, Boyadjier SA, et al. Connexin 43 (GJA1) mutations cause the pleiotropic phenotype of oculodentodigital dysplasia. *Am J Hum Genet* 2003; **72**: 408–18.

Sharif S, Donnai D. Filippi syndrome: two cases with ectodermal features, expanding the phenotype. *Clin Dysmorpholo* 2004; **13**: 221–26.

Stevenson RE, Hall JG, Goodman RM. (ed.). *Human malformations and related anomalies*, Oxford Monographs on Medical Genetics no. 27. Oxford University Press, New York, 1993.

Temtamy SA, McKusick VA. *The genetics of hand malformations.* Alan R. Liss, New York, 1978.

Thauvin-Robinet C, Cossee M, et al. Clinical, molecular, and genotype-phenotype correlation studies from 25 cases of oral-facial-digital syndrome type 1: a French and Belgian collaborative study. *J Med Genet* 2006; **43**: 54–61.

Unusual hair, teeth, nails, and skin

The hair, teeth, nails, and epidermis are all tissues of ectodermal origin (the dermis of the skin is a mesodermal derivative). Hair follicles and sweat glands, two of the ectodermal appendages, are derivatives of both ectoderm and mesoderm. They arise from an interaction between the two germ layers when the overlying ectoderm extends into the underlying dermis. If an abnormality is noted in one ectodermal appendage, detailed enquiry and examination of the others is appropriate.

There are many ectodermal dysplasia syndromes, all sharing in common anomalies of some of these structures—the hair, teeth, nails, and sweat (and other homologous) glands. They are distinguished by the specific pattern of ectodermal structures involved and by associated anomalies, e.g. eyelid adhesion in AEC (ankyloblepharon–ectodermal dysplasia–clefting) syndrome, ectrodactyly in EEC (ectrodactyly–ectodermal dysplasia–clefting) syndrome. It is often not possible to make a specific diagnosis. However, detailed clinical assessment with accurate documentation and good photographs may help to establish a specific diagnosis. Sybert's (1997) excellent monograph is an invaluable tool.

The ectodermal dysplasias (EDs) are highly genetically heterogeneous and classification is in a state of transition as molecular genetic studies lead to a better understanding of the molecular basis of these disorders. Genes causing ED can be divided into four major functional subgroups, those with products involved in: cell–cell communication and signalling; adhesion; transcription regulation; and development (Lamartine 2003).

Clinical approach

History: key points

- Detailed three-generation family tree with specific enquiry about hair, teeth, nails, skin, infant death.
- Hair. Description of hair as a neonate. Has it ever been cut? Does it break easily? What is the colour?
- Teeth. When did the deciduous and permanent teeth erupt? Are they normally shaped? Are there a normal number and are they normally spaced?
- Nails. Description of nails as a neonate. Have they ever been cut? Do they seem to grow at a normal rate?
- Skin. Is the skin unusually dry? Has 'eczema' been diagnosed? Are any treatments used?
- Sweating. Does the individual sweat normally? Is there a history of heat intolerance/hyperpyrexia?
- Ankyloblepharon. Any history of eyelid fusion or strands of tissue between the lids at birth?
- Developmental delay/seizures (Coffin–Siris syndrome, sparse hair epilepsy syndromes).

Examination: key points

- Hair. Colour, texture (coarse, thin, unruly), sparse, short with broken ends?
- Teeth. Careful inspection of incisors and canines. Count upper and lower teeth (full complement of deciduous teeth is 20 and of permanent teeth is 32). Are the teeth normal in shape or conical or otherwise misshapen? Effacement of gum ridges in a neonate may indicate absence of teeth.
- Nails:
  - look carefully at each fingernail and each toenail. Nails may be thin, short, thickened, discoloured, and flattened or spoon-shaped (koilonychia);
  - absent nails, hypoplasia of the distal phalanges (DOOR (deafness–onychodystrophy–onycholysis–retardation) syndrome);
  - greatly thickened nails (pachonychia congenita);
  - defect down middle of nail (Ellis–van Creveld (EVC) syndrome, popliteal pterygium, nail patella syndrome).
- Finger deformities in trichorhinophalangeal syndrome (TRPS) develop from mid-childhood.
- Skin. If there is dry skin, what is its distribution?
- Clefts (EEC and other *p63* mutation syndromes).
- Nose (prominent nose in TRPS).
- Coarse facial features (Coffin–Siris syndrome).
- If nail patella syndrome (NPS) is a possibility (severe nail dysplasia; normal teeth, skin, and hair), palpate the patellae and examine extension and pronation/supination of elbow.

Special investigations

- Karyotype is not usually indicated if development is normal and there are no additional malformations, but may be appropriate for an isolated female case with a severe hypohidrotic ED phenotype. If Langer–Gideon (*TRPS2*) is suspected, fluorescent *in situ* hybridization (FISH) for the microdeletion on 8q24 is possible.
- If a specific diagnosis is made, e.g. hypohidrotic ectodermal dysplasia (HED), incontinentia pigmenti (IP), NPS, mutation analysis may be possible—5 ml EDTA (ethylenedinitrilotetraacetate) sample for DNA.
- If NPS is a possibility, radiographs of hands, elbows, pelvis, and knees and urine dipstick for proteinuria and measurement of plasma creatinine. Iliac horns (exostoses of the iliac crests) occur in 70% and are pathognomonic for NPS, but show age-dependent penetrance (see below).
- Consider referral for expert dermatological/dental opinion.

Some diagnoses to consider

Skin, hair, and nail abnormalities

X-linked hypohidrotic ectodermal dysplasia (HED). The most common ED. Males have reduced or absent sweating, dry skin, sparse hair, and missing and abnormally shaped teeth (conical or 'peg'-shaped).If the diagnosis is not recognized, there is a significant infant mortality risk in affected males due to hyperpyrexia with intercurrent infections. Females show very variable expressivity. The gene is cloned and known as *EDA-1*. There are autosomal dominant (AD) and autosomal recessive (AR) phenocopies; these are rarer. Even rarer are the very few males affected with X-linked HED and immunodeficiency due to mutations in *NEMO*, the gene mutated in IP (see below).

AD ectodermal dysplasia. There are many families with AD transmission of a relatively mild ED. The classification of some of these disorders is tricky due to overlapping phenotypes and genetic heterogeneity.

- **Witkop syndrome.** Hidrotic ectodermal dysplasia of hair, teeth, and nails. The hair may be fine, slow-growing, and sparse or may be normal. A variable degree of hypodontia of the permanent dentition is present. Teeth may be widely spaced and conical or peg-shaped. Deciduous teeth may also be conical. Nails are often slow-growing and toe-nails more severely affected. Many have small dysplastic nails that are spoon-shaped or concave. Most have normal skin but some have dry skin. Sweating is normal and heat intolerance is not a feature. AD with variable expression. The nail and hair signs are less noticeable in adults and may normalize. Affected individuals may have minimal signs, e.g. tapering crowns and widely spaced teeth.

- **Clouston syndrome.** An AD hidrotic ectodermal dysplasia with fine, sparse hair. The nails are dystrophic and there is often dyskeratotic skin that cracks easily and is rough to the touch on the palms and soles. The skin over the knuckles, elbows, knees, and axillae shows hyperpigmentation. Caused by mutations in the Connexin 30 gene, *GJB6* on 13q12 (Fraser).

Ectrodactyly-ectodermal dysplasia-clefting (EEC) syndrome (also ADULT (acro-dermato-ungual-lacrimal-tooth) and ankyloblepharon–ectodermal dysplasia–clefting (AEC or Hay–Wells) syndromes). EEC is an AD condition caused by mutations in *p63* on 7q21–22. Cleft lip and/or palate is common. Dry skin with variable hypohidrosis. Sparse fair dry hair often with absent eyebrows and eyelashes. Tear duct anomalies are common. Patients often have hypodontia. Nails are thin, brittle, and ridged. Mental development is usually normal. The middle rays of the limbs are affected to a variable degree ranging from no obvious defect to absence of the middle three rays.

p63 mutations are also found in ADULT, AEC, and limb–mammary syndromes and others.

Predominantly skin abnormalities

Incontinenti pigmenti type 2 (IP; NEMO). X-linked dominant disorder caused by mutations in the *NEMO* gene on Xq28. 80% carry a common deletion. Skin features occur in four stages:

1 first few days or weeks of life: blistering lesions cropping in distribution of Blaschko's lines (vesicular fluid is highly eosinophilic) accompanied by marked peripheral blood eosinophilia. Linear distribution along limbs, circumferential on trunk, usually spares face (birth–4 months, there are rare reports of onset as late as 18 months);

2 verrucous lesions (less widespread, often confined to lower legs; <6 months);

3 streaky lines of hyperpigmentation especially in axilla and groin (childhood and teens);

4 pale atrophic streaks particularly noticeable on back of calves (childhood–adults).

40% have nail dystrophy; 80% have dental abnormalities affecting deciduous and/or permanent dentition, e.g. missing teeth, small teeth, delayed eruption, conical teeth, accessory cusps. Hair is often sparse in childhood and later wiry/coarse—there may be patchy alopecia. 30% have eye findings, but most have normal vision. Seizures in 14%, which are persistent in 6%. Learning disability in 10% of affected females (severe in 3%). Affected male pregnancies are usually lost spontaneously in first or early second trimester. Hydrops may be seen on ultrasound scan (USS) at 8–13 weeks gestation.

Hypomelanosis of Ito. Large areas of the skin may be affected by hypopigmented streaks or whorls distributed along the lines of Blaschko. It may be particularly striking over the trunk. The streaks are mainly present on the limbs and the whorls on the trunk. The lesions are much easier to see under ultraviolet (UV) light. Swirly hyperpigmentation may also be seen. Seizures and developmental delay are often found. Brain imaging may reveal a migrational

abnormality. A mosaic chromosomal aetiology has been found to be the cause in ~60% of reported individuals. The myriad of associated features reflects the extensive variety of aneuploid conditions seen. This pigment pattern can also be seen in otherwise apparently normal individuals. Its cause in them is unknown, but presumed to be due to mosaicism for single genes controlling pigment production.

Predominantly nail abnormalities

Nail patella syndrome (NPS). AD disorder characterized by dysplasia of nails, patellae, and elbow joints, exostoses of iliac crest, and in some cases nephropathy. Fingernails are absent or abnormal (hypoplastic, fragile, split, and longitudinally ridged) from birth in 98%. Triangular or V-shaped lunules are characteristic. Nail abnormalities are most severe on the ulnar side of the thumb, decreasing to the little finger. Toenails are rarely involved. 40–60% may develop nephropathy. The first indication is chronic proteinuria, and 15% develop end-stage renal failure. The gene is *LMX1B* on 9q34, a transcription factor that regulates the *COL4A3* and *COL4A4* genes. Offer surveillance for nephropathy and glaucoma.

Pachyonychia congenita. Group of AD disorders characterized by symmetrical hypertrophic nail dystrophy affecting all nails and usually present from birth or developing in the neonatal period. The nails are greatly thickened and have a yellow–brown discolouration. Various subtypes are caused by mutations in keratin K6, K16, or K17.

DOOR syndrome (congenital deafness, onychodystrophy, onycholysis, retardation, and seizures) and **Yunis–Varon syndrome** (cleidocranial dysostosis with micrognathia, absent thumbs, and distal aphalangia) are rare AR syndromes in which the nails can be absent with hypoplasia of the distal phalanges. In DOOR there may be triphalangeal thumbs, whereas the thumbs are absent in Yunis–Varon.

Predominantly hair abnormalities

- **Coffin–Siris syndrome.** An AR malformation syndrome with sparse hair, coarse facial features, and nail hypoplasia, especially of the 5th finger. Carefully exclude chromosomal abnormalities.

- **Nicolaides–Baraitser syndrome.** Seizures, sparse hair. X-ray and clinical abnormalities of the phalanges with brachydactyly and swelling of the interphalangeal (IP) joints.

- **Trichorhinophalangeal syndrome (TRPS).** AD disorder characterized by fine, sparse growing scalp hair, dystrophic brittle nails, brachyphalangia with cone-shaped epiphyses on X-ray, and a pear-shaped bulbous nose. TRPS1 is in 8q24. It may be due to mutation in the gene or be part of a contiguous gene deletion syndrome. Specific molecular cytogenetic FISH analysis is available for the microdeletion.

- **Menkes syndrome.** X-linked recessive disorder of copper metabolism. Main features are sparse, steely hair (with pili torti on microscopy), progressive neurological impairment often with seizures and spasticity. Wormian bones on skull X-ray.

- **Other metabolic disorders.**

Predominantly dental abnormalities

Amelogenesis imperfecta. A defect of the enamel affecting both deciduous and permanent teeth. The teeth appear yellowed due to thinning of the enamel that allows the yellow colour of the dentine to show through the enamel layer. It is usually AD and due to mutations in the enamelin gene; it can also follow X-linked recessive (XLR) inheritance where it is caused by mutations in the amelogenin gene (female carriers show ridging of the teeth due to irregularity of the enamel covering). A few kindreds show AR inheritance.

Dentinogenesis imperfecta. Dentinogenesis imperfecta (DI), which is sometimes an accompanying symptom of osteogenesis imperfecta (OI), belongs to a group of genetically conditioned dentin dysplasias and is characterized clinically by an opalescent amber appearance of the dentin. Although the teeth of DI cases wear more easily and excessively compared to normal teeth, they do not appear to be more susceptible to dental caries than normal teeth. DI follows AD inheritance.

Genetic advice

Recurrence risk

- As for specific disorder.
- IP. New mutation rate is significant. 80% have a common deletion in NEMO. 70% of new mutations arise on the paternally inherited X. An adjacent pseudogene facilitates gene-conversion events. There is a small chance that parents may be asymptomatic mosaics so very careful examination of the parents, especially the mother, is important.

Carrier detection

If X-linked HED is a possibility careful physical examination of the mother including a starch-iodine sweat test is important, looking for mosaicism (lines of Blaschko) in carrier females. Molecular genetic testing for mutations in *EDA-1* may also be possible.

Prenatal diagnosis

May be possible if mutation is known.

Natural history and further management (preventative measures)

- Hyperpyrexia. Offer advice to prevent hyperpyrexia in infants who are unable to sweat (e.g. avoiding very hot environments, removal of items of clothing when the child feels hot, fans, and air conditioning). Precautions must be taken to limit upper respiratory infections. Tepid sponging and antipyretics for fever.
- Dental. Most people with ED have missing or malformed teeth. Dental treatment is necessary, beginning with dentures as early as age two, multiple replacements as the child grows, and perhaps dental implants thereafter. Orthodontic treatment may also be necessary. Refer to an orthodontist with specialist expertise.
- Skin. Care must be provided to prevent cracking, bleeding, and infection.
- Eyes may benefit from artificial tears if xerophthalmia is a problem, and review by a specialist is recommended.
- Other. Professional care may minimize the effects of vision or hearing deficits and surgical and/or cosmetic procedures may lessen facial and other deformities, thus reducing physical disfigurement.

Lay group contacts: Ectodermal Dysplasia Society (UK) <www.ectodermaldysplasia.org>; National Incontinentia Pigmenti International Foundation <http://imgen.bcm.tmc.edu/IPIF>; National Foundation for Ectodermal Dysplasias (NFED) <www.nfed.org>.

Expert adviser: Angus Clarke, Professor in Clinical Genetics, University of Wales College of Medicine, Cardiff, Wales.

References

Chitty LS, Dennis N, Baraitser M. Hidrotic ectodermal dysplasia of hair, teeth and nails: case reports and review. *J Med Genet* 1996; **33**: 707–10.

Donnai D. Incontinentia pigmenti. In *Management of genetic syndromes* (ed. S.B. Cassidy and J.E. Allanson), Chapter 11, pp. 185–93. Wiley-Liss, New York, 2001.

Fraser FC, Der Kaloustian VM. A man, a syndrome, a gene: Clouston's hidrotic ectodermal dysplasia (HED). *Am J Med Genet* 2001; **100**: 164–8.

Lamartine J. Towards a new classification of ectodermal dysplasias. *Clin Exp Dermatol* 2003; **28** (4): 351–5.

Sybert VP. *Genetic skin disorders*, Oxford Monographs in Medical Genetics. Oxford University Press, New York, 1997.

Common consultations

Chapter contents

Achondroplasia 260
Autosomal dominant polycystic kidney disease (ADPKD) 262
X-linked adrenoleukodystrophy (X-ALD) 264
Alpha₁-antitrypsin deficiency 266
Alport syndrome 268
Androgen insensitivity syndrome (AIS) 270
Angelman syndrome 272
Autism and austism spectrum disorders 274
Beckwith–Wiedemann syndrome (BWS) 278
Congenital adrenal hyperplasia (CAH) 282
Consanguinity 284
Craniosynostosis 288
Cystic fibrosis (CF) 292
Dementia 296
Diabetes mellitus 298
Dilated cardiomyopathy (DCM) 302
DNA repair defects 304
Duchenne and Becker muscular dystrophy (DMD and BMD) 308
Ehlers–Danlos syndrome (EDS) 312
Epilepsy in infants and children 314
Epilepsy 318
Facioscapulohumeral muscular dystrophy (FSHD) 322
Fragile X syndrome (FRAX) 324
Glaucoma 328
Haemochromatosis 330
Haemoglobinopathies 334
Haemophilia and other inherited coagulation disorders 338
Hereditary haemorrhagic telangiectasia (HHT) 342
Hereditary motor and sensory neuropathy (HMSN) 344
Hereditary spastic paraplegias (HSP) 348
Hirschsprung disease 352
Huntington disease (HD) 354
Hyperlipidaemia 358
Hypertrophic cardiomyopathy (HCM) 360
Immunodeficiency and recurrent infection 364
Incest 370
Leigh encephalopathy 372
Limb girdle muscular dystrophies 374
Long QT and Brugada syndromes 378
Marfan syndrome 380
Mitochondrial DNA diseases 384
Myotonic dystrophy (DM) 388
Neural tube defects 392
Neurofibromatosis type 1 (NF1) 396
Noonan syndrome (NS) 402
Parkinson disease 404
Retinitis pigmentosa (RP) 406
Rett syndrome 408
Sensitivity to anaesthetic agents 410
Spinal muscular atrophy (SMA) 412
Stickler syndrome 414
Thrombophilia 416
Tuberous sclerosis (TSC) 420

Achondroplasia

Achondroplasia is the most common cause of disproportionate short stature in children and adults. The prevalence at birth is estimated to be ~1/27 000. Individuals with achondroplasia have disproportionate short stature with shortening primarily of the limbs, a relatively normal-sized trunk, and contraction of the base of the skull, giving a large appearing head. There is considerable variation in severity, which is particularly apparent in the neonate and early infancy. Severity may range from so mild that there is uncertainty as to whether the clinical impression of rhizomelic limb shortening in a neonate is a real finding to a picture sufficiently severe that a differential diagnosis of thanatophoric dysplasia is considered. Final adult height in males is 120–145 cm and in females 115–137 cm. The Committee on Genetics, American Academy of Pediatrics (1995) have produced guidelines for the management of achondroplasia from birth to adult life. Medical care aims to prevent known complications, especially cervicomedullary compression, sleep apnoea, and spinal stenosis. The mortality in children with achondroplasia is twice normal with an excess of sudden death under the age of 4 years, of which 50% is due to brainstem compression. Hecht *et al.* (1987) found a 7.5% risk for death in the first year of life.

Achondroplasia is an autosomal dominant (AD) disorder caused by mutations in the *FGFR3* gene on chromosome 4p that potentiate the activity of FGFR3. 80% of affected individuals have *de novo* mutations. Mutations are almost invariably on the paternal chromosome and there is a marked paternal age effect. Two common mutations, G1138A and G1138C, account for 98% of mutations in affected individuals. When *FGFR3* is mutated at this site its normal inhibitory function is constitutively activated (i.e. activated even in the absence of bound fibroblast growth factor (FGF)), resulting in increased inhibition of growth of cartilage cells.

Clinical approach

History: key points
- Brief family tree unless you suspect that one of the parents is affected.
- Document parental heights and assess whether both parents are normal, or whether one of them may be affected. Document paternal age if *de novo*.
- Prenatal measurement of femur length. Often within normal range until after 22 weeks gestation.
- Respiratory difficulties and snoring.
- Hypotonia in infants (foramen magnum compression).
- Ability to walk more than 100 metres in older children and adults.

Examination: key points
- Clinical measurement. Height, weight, occipital-frontal circumference (OFC)—plot on achondroplasia-specific charts.
- Limb shortening predominantly rhizomelic with tibial bowing.
- Wedge-shaped gap between the 3rd and 4th fingers ('trident hand').
- Midface hypoplasia with depressed nasal bridge in infancy, relatively large jaw, and prominent forehead.
- Spine: thoracolumbar gibbus in infancy then lordosis when ambulant.
- Chest shape, respiratory rate, intercostal and subcostal recession (in infants).

- Limitation of elbow extension.
- Evidence of tonsillar or adenoid enlargement and glue ear.
- Dental malocclusion.
- Neurological examination: hypotonia in infants, hyperreflexia and ankle clonus, bowel and bladder disturbance.
- Gait abnormalities due to shape of pelvis and spinal cord claudication.

Special investigations
- Skeletal X-rays. To confirm the diagnosis.
  - Skull. The vault is large in comparison to the facial bones. The skull base is short.
  - Spine. Short pedicles. Scalloping of the posterior border of the vertebral bodies. Narrowing of the interpedicular distance between L1 and L5.
  - Chest. Short ribs.
  - Pelvis and hips. Horizontal acetabular roof, squared iliac wings, spur at the medial edge of the triradiate cartilage, splaying of the upper femoral metaphysis.
  - Limbs. Rhizomelic shortening, normal epiphyses, splayed metaphyses.
  - Hands. Metacarpals of equal length leading to trident appearence.
- Cranial ultrasound scan (USS) used in neonates and infancy to assess ventricular size.
- Magnetic resonance imaging (MRI) scans to assess the brain and cord. There is debate between experts as to whether these should be offered routinely or only if symptoms. Look for:
  - hydrocephalus, usually communicating;
  - cervicomedullary compression: foramen magnum size, displacement of the brainstem;
  - spinal compression due to stenosis or listhesis, often symptomatic.
- Sleep studies should be performed in all children to assess for central apnoea.

Alternative diagnoses/conditions to consider

There is an apparent clinical continuum from thanatophoric dysplasia, achondroplasia, hypochondroplasia through to short normal individuals. Skeletal radiographs together with mutation detection can be helpful in establishing a secure diagnosis in borderline cases. Many other rarer skeletal dysplasias are often misdiagnosed as 'achondroplasia' in the prenatal or neonatal period until the skeletal surveys have been reported by an expert, or until the molecular testing for achondroplasia is normal, prompting a review of the diagnosis.

Thanatophoric dysplasia is caused by *de novo* mutations in *FGFR3*. Thanatophoric dysplasia is a lethal disorder with profound limb shortening, macrocephaly, and a small chest. Infants are stillborn or die in the early neonatal period from respiratory insufficiency or central apnoea. The diagnosis may be evident on USS at 20 weeks gestation.

Hypochondroplasia. Approximately 60% are heterozygous for the N540K C > A, or the N540K C > G mutations in FGFR3. Clinical features resemble achondroplasia, but are milder with less involvement of the face, skull, and spine. Diagnostic changes may not be seen on radiographs until 2 years of age. Neurological problems are rare.

Pseudoachondroplasia. Short stature is often not apparent at birth or in infancy but becomes apparent in a toddler. Craniofacial appearance is normal. Limbs are short (as for achondroplasia) and there is joint hypermobility with early arthritis. Mutations in *COMP* gene on 19p13.1 (allelic with multiple epiphyseal dysplasia (MED)).

Genetic advice

AD, but many cases are new mutations. If a parent is affected, there will be a 50% risk to the offspring of any pregnancy. If *de novo* the sibling recurrence risk is 0.02% (Mettler and Fraser 2000). Germline mutations are rare.

If both parents have achondroplasia there is a 25% chance of a child with normal stature, a 50% chance of a child with achondroplasia, and a 25% chance of a child with homozygous achondroplasia (most die in the neonatal period due to respiratory difficulties with features very similar to those of thanatophoric dysplasia).

Variability and penetrance

Penetrance is 100%. Final adult height varies considerably (males 120–145 cm; females 115–137 cm).

Prenatal diagnosis

Possible by chorionic villus sampling (CVS) at 11 weeks gestation if the mutation is known. USS is not particularly useful as the fall-off in the growth of the long bones is not observed until after 20 weeks gestation.

Other family members

Achondroplasia is usually clinically apparent, so testing of other family members is rarely indicated unless there is clinical suspicion that they are affected.

Natural history and management

Cognitive outcome is normal in the great majority. Motor milestones are usually delayed, with independent sitting achieved at 9–20 months and walking at 14–27 months.

Handling in infancy requires special care with support given to the baby's head. Avoid baby bouncers and swings (risk of cervicomedullary compression and worsening of kyphosis).

Potential long-term complications

- **Anaesthetic risks.** Expert care of the cervical spine is required to avoid cervical cord compromise during intubation, etc.; increased risk for obstructive apnoea and postsedation obstruction (Berkowitz *et al.* 1990).
- **Cervical spinal stenosis.** In infants compression of the cervicomedullary junction can cause apnoea and sudden death; in children there is a risk of high cervical myelopathy. Avoid contact sports, e.g. rugby, ice hockey, or other sports where there is a high risk of impact, e.g. skiing, trampolining, gymnastics.
- **Glue ear** occurs in the majority and may cause conductive deafness, impairing acquisition of speech and language. Parental vigilance is important, with a low threshold for audiometry and ear, nose, and throat (ENT) referral.
- **Growth.** Growth hormone (GH) administration does lead to a small increase in the final height. The vertebrae are thought to grow more than the limbs, slightly increasing the disproportion. Such treatment should only be considered after a full discussion about the uncertainties and the small gain in height achieved by such therapy. Limb lengthening may give up to 10 extra inches but is complicated and considered expensive.
- **Hydrocephalus.** Most infants with achondroplasia are macrocephalic. OFC should be plotted on achondroplasia-specific charts and monitored serially (every 1–2 months) during the first years of life.

- **Pregnancy.** Women with achondroplasia can have successful full-term pregnancies. Main risks are respiratory compromise in late pregnancy and the neurological complications of hyperlordosis. Baseline pulmonary function tests early in the 3rd trimester may be helpful. Women should be under specialist obstetric care. Delivery is usually by elective lower segment Caesarean section (LSCS). Spinal anaesthesia should be avoided in women with achondroplasia.
- **Musculoskeletal.** Hypermobility is common at all joints except the elbow where there is restriction of movement. Most infants have a mild lumbar kyphosis, which changes to a marked or severe lumbar lordosis once they are old enough to walk. Their trunks should be supported until sufficient strength is gained to support the trunk independently.
- **Respiratory insufficiency.** Infants with achondroplasia have smaller than average chests. The respiratory compromise may be sufficient to cause tachypnoea and sweating, particularly with feeding. Such infants are particularly at risk with intercurrent infections, e.g. bronchiolitis.
- **Snoring and sleep apnoea.** Most individuals with achondroplasia snore loudly. Some suffer with obstructive apnoea, which can be helped by continuous positive airway pressure (CPAP).
- **Spinal stenosis.** Exercise-induced spinal claudication is present to some extent in most adults with achondroplasia due to stenosis of the lumbar spine. Adults with achondroplasia are also are risk for nerve root or cord compression, which is not exercise-related and may require urgent neurological/neurosurgical assessment (decompressive laminectomy).

Indications for surgery

- Cervical myelopathy with MRI evidence of compression and neurogenic apnoea.
- Thoracolumbar stenosis (inability to walk >100 m, neurological deficits).
- Limb straightening, usually of tibia varum.
- Correction of asymmetry in tibia/fibula and radius/ulna.
- Limb-lengthening procedures are another area of controversy but the topic should be discussed with all parents. This needs to be performed in specialist centres.

Support group: Restricted growth association <www.rgaonline.org.uk>; Little People of America <www.lpaonline.org>.

Expert adviser: Judith G. Hall, Emeritus Professor of Pediatrics and Medical Genetics, University of British Columbia, Vancouver, British Columbia, Canada.

References

Berkowitz ID, Raja SN, *et al.* Dwarfs: pathophysiology and anesthetic implications. *Anesthesiology* 1990; **73**: 739–59.

Committee on Genetics. American Academy of Pediatrics. Health supervision for children with achondroplasia. *Pediatrics* 1995; **95**: 443–51.

Hecht JT, Francomano CA, *et al.* Mortality in achondroplasia. *Am J Hum Genet* 1987; **41**: 454–64.

Hunter AGW, Bankier A, *et al.* Medical complications of children with achondroplasia: a multicenter patient review. *J Med Genet* 1998; **35**: 705–12.

Mettler G, Fraser FC. Recurrence risk for sibs of children with 'sporadic' achondroplasia. *Am J Med Genet* 2000; **31**: 250–1.

Pauli RM. Achondroplasia. In *Management of genetic syndromes* (ed. S.B. Cassidy and J.E. Allanson), Chapter 2, pp. 9–32. Wiley-Liss, New York, 2001.

Autosomal dominant polycystic kidney disease (ADPKD)

ADPKD is a common autosomal dominant (AD) disorder with a prevalence of 1/800 across all ethnic groups. It is a systemic disorder characterized by:

- age-dependent cysts (see table): kidney, liver, pancreas, and spleen;
- cardiovascular abnormalities: hypertension, mitral valve prolapse, intracranial aneurysms and left ventricular hypertrophy;
- connective tissue abnormalities: hernias, colonic diverticulae;
- Age at presentation with renal failure is earlier in PKD1 than PKD2, 54 years vs 74 years. (Hateboer et al. 1999b).

Diagnostic criteria for ADPKD as a function of age

Age (years)	Minimum number of renal cysts for diagnosis
<30	2 cysts either uni- or bilateral
30–59	2 cysts in each kidney
>60	4 cysts in each kidney

ADPKD is genetically heterogeneous. Mutations in PKD1 on chromosome 16 are found in ~85%, while mutations in PKD2 on chromosome 4 are found in ~15%. PKD3 is very rare. PKD2 has a milder phenotype, with most individuals not developing ESRF until their 70s. PKD2 patients are less likely to have hypertension, urinary tract infections (UTIs), or haematuria (Hateboer et al. 1999b). Many patients with PKD2 will die of another cause. Death due to subarachnoid haemorrhage (SAH) occurs in ~6% of patients with ADPKD, with aneurysmal rupture on average at age 41 years, a decade earlier than in sporadic cases. Patients with PKD2 as well as PKD1 are at risk of intracranial aneurysm.

Each renal cyst appears to arise by clonal proliferation following a second hit somatic mutation. 40–70% have hepatic cysts, but they rarely cause serious problems. Liver cysts occur more frequently and at a younger age in women than in men. Hypertension is frequent and of early onset.

Clinical approach

History: key points

- Three-generation family tree with specific enquiry about affected relatives, age of diagnosis, reason for diagnosis, age of onset of ESRF, history of SAH, cause of death.
- History of loin pain, haematuria, or recurrent UTIs.

Examination: key points

- Blood pressure (BP).
- Abdominal examination. Palpable kidneys? Palpable liver?
- Examine the heart. Midsystolic murmur or mitral valve prolapse?

Investigation

- Consider renal ultrasound scan (USS) after thorough discussion and careful consideration of the optimum age for investigation. Often the first USS is done at 20–25 years (see 'Predictive testing' below).
- DNA sample if PKD mutation analysis is available.

Other diagnoses/conditions to consider

Tuberous sclerosis (TS). A few renal cysts are seen in ~17% of individuals with TS. They are present from early childhood and do not appear to increase in number with age. Cysts in conjunction with seizures or ash-leaf macules, or other features suggestive of TS, raise the possibility of a contiguous gene deletion on 16p involving PKD1 and TSC2. See 'Tuberous sclerosis (TS)', page 420.

Von Hippel–Lindau (VHL) disease. Renal cysts may be detected from the second decade. Renal cell carcinoma is often but not invariably associated with cysts. The kidneys are not usually enlarged and there may be associated pancreatic cysts. See 'Von Hippel–Lindau (VHL) syndrome', page 484.

Oral-facial-digital (OFD) syndrome type 1 (OFD1). A rare X-linked dominant (XLD) condition caused by mutations in OFD1 on Xp22, which is lethal in affected males. Characterized in females by highly variable expressivity of polycystic kidneys, midline cleft or notch of upper lip, multiple oral frenulae, cleft palate, and lobulated tongue. Limb problems include brachydactyly and skin syndactyly of hands with preaxial polydactyly or bifid halluces. Structural central nervous system (CNS) anomalies may occur and some affected females have intellectual disability.

Branchio-oto-renal (BOR). AD condition caused by mutations in EYA1 on 8q11–13. Characterized by preauricular pits/tags, hearing loss in >75% (often with cochlear hypoplasia on magnetic resonance imaging (MRI)). Renal anomalies are very variable and include renal agenesis, duplex kidneys, and renal cysts. Branchial cleft/sinus/cysts occur in some mutation carriers.

Renal cysts and diabetes (RCAD). AD disorder characterized by unexplained familial renal cystic disease (renal cysts may be detected in utero), early-onset type 2 diabetes, genital tract malformations, and hyperuricaemia and early-onset gout. Renal biopsy shows cystic renal dysplasia or glomerulocystic disease. Renal cysts may present before the diabetes. It is caused by mutations in HNF-1β (hepatocyte nuclear factor-1β).

Autosomal recessive polycystic kidney disease (ARPKD) A severe form of polycystic kidney disease that presents primarily in infancy and childhood and that is characterized by enlarged kidneys and congenital hepatic fibrosis. The clinical spectrum is widely variable. About 30 to 50% of affected individuals die in the neonatal period, while others survive into adulthood. See 'Renal tract anomalies', page 624.

Genetic advice

Inheritance and recurrence risk

AD with 50% risk to offspring of a mutation carrier. There is usually an extensive family history. *De novo* mutations do occur, but are uncommon.

Variability and penetrance

Marked inter- and intrafamilial phenotypic variability. ADPKD is usually regarded as a disease of adult life. However, a small minority may present in childhood with loin pain, etc. Rarely (~1%) multiple intrarenal cysts may be detected during detailed antenatal USS. The phenotype may overlap with infantile polycystic kidney disease, but is seen in the context of a family history of ADPKD. Approximately 30% will die in the first few months of life, and survivors are at high risk for early hypertension and ESRF (MacDermot *et al.* 1998). The cause of this severe *in utero* form of ADPKD is unknown, but there appears to be a substantial sibling recurrence risk.

Striking familial clustering of intracranial aneurysms is observed with the rate of aneurysm five times higher in patients with a family history of ruptures of intracranial aneurysms than in those without. The position of the mutation in *PKD1* is predictive for development of intracranial aneurysms—5′ mutations are more commonly associated with vascular disease (Rossetti *et al.* 2003).

Prenatal diagnosis
Technically feasible by chorionic villus sampling (CVS) if the mutation is known, or if the kindred is large enough that clear linkage to chromosome 16 or 4 can be established. In practice, prenatal diagnosis is rarely requested.

Predictive testing
Renal USS is the mainstay for predictive testing; mutation analysis is not commonly available. Residual risk of ADPKD following a normal renal USS at 25 years is <5%; by 30 years the residual risk has dropped to 2%. Computerized tomography (CT) and MRI are more sensitive than USS, and may be used following a normal USS if an individual is contemplating donating a kidney to a member of the family with ESRF (living-related transplant). Linkage may also be desirable in clarifying the status of a potential donor, if mutation analysis is not feasible.

Other family members
Cascade approach to diagnosis in adult relatives is appropriate because of the benefits of good control of hypertension and the high morbidity and mortality associated with undiagnosed chronic renal failure.

Natural history and management
Potential long-term complications
- **ESRF.** Treated by renal transplantation, haemodialysis, or peritoneal dialysis.
- **Intracranial aneurysm (ICA).** Aysmptomatic 'berry aneurysms' are found in 8% of individuals with ADPKD (population risk is 1–2%). Incidence rises to 16–25% in the presence of a positive family history. The risk of interval rupture in ADPKD is unknown. Management is based on outcome in *individuals* without ADPKD in whom conservative management is suggested for aneurysms <10 mm diameter, and surgery considered if aneurysms are >10 mm. (There is a 1% mortality and 3–7% morbidity from surgical intervention.)
- **UTI.** Prompt treatment of infection is important: if infection becomes established in cysts it can be very difficult to eradicate.

Surveillance
- **Hypertension.** Blood pressure should be monitored annually from teenage years. Aggressive treatment of hypertension is important in reducing the risk of accelerated cardiovascular and cerebrovascular disease seen in ADPKD and in prolonging renal function.
- **Creatinine.** Once a diagnosis of ADPKD is made, plasma creatinine should be monitored annually if normal and, if plasma creatinine is elevated, the patient should be referred to a nephrologist.
- **ICA** screening by magnetic resonance angiography (MRA) may be considered if there is a family history of ICA from adulthood. If scans are negative they may be repeated at 5 yearly intervals; if an aneurysm is present, or there has been a previous intracranial bleed, repeat MRA at 2 yearly intervals. Screening should be arranged in conjunction with neurosurgical colleagues so that an agreed management plan is in place before imaging is undertaken.
- **Pregnancy.** Women with ADPKD usually tolerate pregnancy well. They should be under specialist supervision for monitoring of hypertension (which may worsen in pregnancy) and they are at some increased risk for pre-eclampsia (PET). Renal function usually remains stable throughout pregnancy.
- **Drugs.** Avoid nonsteroidal anti-inflammatory drugs (NSAIDs), e.g. ibuprofen, if renal function is abnormal. Prescribe all drugs with care if renal function is impaired.

Support group: Polycystic Disease Charity <www.pkdcharity.co.uk>, Tel. 01388 665004.

Expert advisers: Richard Sandford, Wellcome Trust Senior Fellow in Clinical Research and Honorary Consultant in Medical Genetics, Cambridge and John Firth, Consultant Physician and Nephrologist, Addenbrookes Hospital, Cambridge, England.

References
Ferrante MI, Giorgio G, *et al.* Identification of the gene for oral-facial-digital type 1 syndrome. *Am J Hum Genet* 2001; **68**: 569–76.

Hateboer N, Lazarou LP, *et al.* Familial phenotype differences in PKD1. *Kidney Int* 1999*a*; **56**: 34–40.

Hateboer N, van Dijk MA, *et al.* Comparison of phenotypes of polycystic kidney disease types 1 and 2. European PKD1–PKD2 Study Group. *Lancet* 1999*b*; **353**: 103–7.

MacDermot KD, Saggar-Malik AK, *et al.* Prenatal diagnosis of autosomal dominant polycystic kidney disease (PKD1) presenting *in utero* and prognosis for very early onset disease. *J Med Genet* 1998; **35**: 13–16.

Magistroni R, He N, *et al.* Genotype–renal function correlation in type 2 autosomal dominant polycystic kidney disease. *J Am Soc Nephr* 2003; **14**: 1164–74.

Rossetti S, Chauveau D, *et al.* Association of mutation position in polycystic kidney disease 1 (*PKD1*) gene and development of a vascular phenotype. *Lancet* 2003; **361**: 2196–201.

X-linked adrenoleukodystrophy (X-ALD)

ALD, adrenomyeloneuropathy, Schilder disease, sudanophilic leukodystrophy.

X-ALD is an X-linked metabolic disorder that is associated with accumulations of very long-chain fatty acids (VLCFAs; see table) in the adrenal gland and in the central and peripheral nervous systems. It is caused by mutations in the ABCD1 gene on Xq28 that encodes a peroxisomal ABC half-transporter (ALDP) of unknown function. The clinical consequences of this are highly variable. ALD is a disease with mixed features of axonal degeneration, leading to myeloneuropathy and a severe inflammatory reaction in the cerebral white matter resulting in demyelination. At least six phenotypic variants of X-ALD are recognized (Moser et al. 2000), with childhood cerebral ALD and adrenomyeloneuropathy accounting for 80% of cases.

- **Childhood cerebral ALD (CCALD).** Onset 3–10 years often presenting with behaviour problems, poor concentration, and decline in school performance. Seizures, spasticity, and dementia occur due to rapidly progressive cerebral demyelination. Once established, the process appears irreversible and most boys die 3–5 years from the onset of symptoms.
- **Adolescent cerebral ALD (AdolCALD).** As above but with onset between 10 and 21 years.
- **Adult cerebral ALD (ACALD).** Rare (1–3%) and usually presenting with predominantly psychiatric symptoms and worsening memory.
- **Adrenomyeloneuropathy (AMN).** Onset usually in the 20s to 40s. This is the most common phenotype and presents with slowly progressive paraparesis.
- **Isolated adrenocortical dysfunction (Addison disease).** Some patients present with isolated adreno-cortical dysfunction. Most develop neurological deficits later. Ronghe et al. (2002) identified a man who presented with Addison at the age of 5 years, but was only diagnosed with X-ALD at the age of 34 years when his AMN was recognized.
- **Asymptomatic or presymptomatic.** Mutation carriers with no symptoms.

It is not possible to predict phenotype by mutation analysis or biochemical assays. There is no apparent genotype–phenotype correlation. Different phenotypes may develop in different family members carrying the same mutation. Some patients have a mixed phenotype, e.g. AMD and Addison disease. Sometimes the phenotype evolves with time. Van Geel et al. (2001) found that, of 68 patients with AMN initially without brain involvement, 13 (19%) later developed cerebral demyelination. Most families have private mutations.

See also Moser et al. (1999) for the largest published experience of plasma VLCFAs.

Clinical approach

History: key points

- Three-generation family history with specific enquiry about Addison disease, gait disturbance, unexplained deaths in males. Enquire also about other neurological diagnoses in males and females. AMN may be misdiagnosed as multiple sclerosis (MS) or hereditary spastic paraplegia (HSP).
- Detailed developmental history. Are there any recent changes in school performance, personality, concentration?

Examination: key points

Examine carefully for spasticity particularly affecting the lower limbs (abnormal gait, increased tone, increased reflexes, clonus).

Investigation

- Plasma VLCFAs (raised in almost all affected males and in some carrier females).
- DNA for mutation analysis of ABCD1.
- Consider testing adrenocortical function in at-risk or affected males by arranging a short synacthen test (usually done in early morning with baseline cortisol, followed by administration of synacthen and repeat cortisol at 30 minutes).
- Consider magnetic resonance imaging (MRI); this is indicated if symptomatic.

Other diagnoses/conditions to consider

- **Other leukodystrophies.** See 'Leukodystrophy', page 150.
- **HSP.** See 'Hereditary spastic paraplegia (HSP)', page 348.
- **AAA (achalasia–addisonianism–alacrima) syndrome** (Allgrove syndrome). Autosomal recessive (AR) condition caused by mutations in aladin (AAAS) on 12q13 with defective tear production, autonomic dysfunction, and adrenal insufficiency.

Genetic advice

Only 5% of male probands and 1.7% of X-ALD hemizygotes have new mutations (Bezman et al. 2001).

Inheritance and recurrence risk

X-linked recessive, with expression in some carrier females (see below).

Variability and penetrance

20–50% of female heterozygotes develop neurological sequelae, usually AMN. Onset is usually in the 30s to 40s with slow progression. Adrenocortical insufficiency is very rare in female heterozygotes and is not routinely tested.

Reference ranges for VLCFAs*

VLCFA	Concentration (µmol/l) at age			Ratio at age	
	<10 years	**>10 years**		**<10 years**	**>10 years**
C_{22}	29–117	33–134			
C_{24}	24–83	25–98	C_{24}/C_{22}	0.56–1.06	0.59–0.94
C_{26}	0.20–1.44	0.25–1.24	C_{26}/C_{22}	0.003–0.029	0.003–0.022
Phytanate	<15	<15			

*East Anglian Regional Biochemical Genetics Unit, Addenbrooke's Hospital, Cambridge UK.

Prenatal diagnosis

Possible by chorionic villus sampling (CVS) at 11 weeks gestation by mutation analysis if familial mutation identified, or by analysis of VLCFAs in cultured chorionic villus cells or amniocytes.

Predictive testing

The introduction of bone marrow transplantation (BMT) raises the issue of predictive testing in at-risk males. Since BMT is a high-risk therapy with a significant morbidity and mortality, it is not usually considered in the complete absence of symptoms/signs. Identification of presymptomatic boys permits serial and careful follow-up by neuropsychological profiles and MRI studies at 6–12 month intervals beginning from age 3 years with recourse to BMT if initiation of CCALD is identified. BMT should be strongly considered if progressive MRI change is identified, even if neuropsychological function is still intact. BMT is not indicated in boys with normal MRI findings.

Since CCALD does not have its onset before 3 years of age predictive testing can be considered at any time during the first 2 years of life, with a view to arranging serial MRI and possible work-up for BMT from the age of 2.5 years.

VLCFAs are raised even in cord blood in most affected males. However, there are exceptional cases of affected males where plasma levels are within normal limits and abnormalities are only found in fibroblast assay. Mutation analysis is therefore the gold standard for family screening.

- **Carrier testing.** 15–20% of female heterozygotes have VLCFA levels within normal limits. Mutation analysis is therefore highly preferable in the evaluation of maternal female relatives. Some labs will accept samples from at-risk female relatives for mutation analysis even when no sample is available from the proband.
- **Extended family.** Cascade screening of the extended family provides the opportunity for identifying heterozygous females and presymptomatic males.

Natural history and management

A 5–10 year follow-up of 12 patients with CCALD (Shapiro *et al.* 2000) showed the long-term beneficial effect of BMT when the procedure was undertaken at an early stage in the disease. This approach offers hope to families where other males are identified in the presymptomatic phase of X-ALD following diagnosis in the proband.

Lorenzo oil (oleic and erucic acids) can lead to improvement in plasma VLCFAs, but is of limited value in correcting the accumulation of saturated VLCFAs in the brains of patients with ALD. Aubourg *et al.* (1993) found no evidence of clinically relevant benefit in a trial of 24 patients, but an international study by Moser *et al.* (2004) suggested that Lorenzo oil may have a preventative effect.

Surveillance

- Identification of presymptomatic boys and serial and careful follow-up by serial (6 monthly) neuropsychological and MRI studies with recourse to BMT if initiation of CCALD is identified.
- Surveillance for adrenal insufficiency in presymptomatic and affected boys.

Support group: ALD Family Support Trust <www.aldfst. org.uk>.

Expert adviser: Hugo Moser, Professor of Neurology and Pediatrics, Johns Hopkins University, Baltimore, Maryland, USA.

References

Aubourg P, Adamsbaum C, *et al.* A two-year trial of oleic and erucic acids ('Lorenzo's oil') as treatment for adrenomyeloneuropathy. *New Engl J Med* 1993; **329**: 745–52.

Bezman L, Moser AB, *et al.* Adrenoleukodystrophy: incidence, new mutation rate, and results of extended family screening. *Ann Neurol* 2001; **49**: 512–17.

Kemp S, Pujol A, *et al.* ABCD1 mutations and the X-linked adrenoleukodystrophy mutation database: role in diagnosis and clinical correlations. *Hum Mutat* 2001; **18**: 499–515.

Moser AB, Kreiter N, *et al.* Plasma very long chain fatty acids in 3,000 peroxisome disease patients and 29,000 controls. *Ann Neurol* 1999; **45**: 100–10.

Moser HW, Loes DJ, *et al.* X-linked adrenoleukodystrophy: overview and prognosis as a function of age and brain magnetic resonance imaging abnormality. A study involving 372 patients. *Neuropediatrics* 2000; **31**: 227–39.

Moser H, Dubey P, Fatemi A. Progress in X-linked adrenoleukodystrophy. *Curr Opin Neurol* 2004; **17** (3): 263–9.

Peters C, Charnas LR *et al.* Cerebral X-linked adrenoleukodystrophy: the international haematopoietic cell transplantation experience from 1982 to 1999. *Blood* 2004; **104**: 881–8.

Ronghe MD, Barton J, *et al.* The importance of testing for adrenoleucodystrophy in males with idiopathic Addison's disease. *Arch Dis Child* 2002; **86**: 185–9.

Shapiro E, Krivit W, *et al.* Long-term effect of bone-marrow transplantation for childhood-onset cerebral X-linked adrenoleukodystrophy. *Lancet* 2000; **356**: 713–18.

Suzuki Y, Isogai K, *et al.* Bone marrow transplantation for the treatment of X-linked adrenoleukodystrophy. *J Inherit Metab Dis* 2000; **23**: 453–8.

van Geel BM, Bezman L, Loes DJ, Moser HW, Raymond GV. Evolution of phenotypes in adult male patients with X-linked adrenoleukodystrophy. *Ann Neurol* 2001; **49** (2): 186–94.

Alpha₁-antitrypsin deficiency

Alpha₁-antitrypsin is a serine proteinase inhibitor that protects the connective tissue of the lungs from the elastase released by leucocytes. Alpha₁-antitrypsin deficiency is a common autosomal recessive (AR) disorder (1/1600–1/1800) characterized by a predisposition to emphysema and cirrhosis. Liver damage arises not from the deficiency of the protease inhibitor, but from pathological polymerization of the variant alpha₁-antitrypsin before its secretion from hepatocytes. Alpha₁-antitrypsin is encoded by the gene *SERPINA1* on 14q32.1.

Mutations in alpha₁-antitrypsin affect the electrophoretic mobility of the protein. Wild-type alpha₁-antitrypsin deficiency is termed M; the S variant (Glu264Val) results in a 40% reduction in plasma alpha₁-antitrypsin levels in homozygotes and the Z variant (Glu342Lys) results in an 85% reduction in homozygotes. Synthesis of the S and Z variants is normal, but intracellular processing and secretion are impaired and the protein is retained in the endoplasmic reticulum. Plasma concentrations in ZZ homozygotes and Z-null and SZ heterozygotes are insufficient to ensure lifelong protection from proteolytic damage, especially in smokers. Resulting lung damage results in the clinical phenotype of predominantly panlobular, basal emphysema. There is also an association with asthma and Wegener granulomatosis and possibly bronchiectasis. Recent work shows that neutrophils are chemotactically attracted to the polymerized Z protein and so polymerization may also play an important role in lung damage.

In Sveger's (1984) survey of 127 neonates with the ZZ phenotype, virtually all had raised liver enzymes, and 14 (11%) had prolonged neonatal jaundice. Most of the infants with neonatal jaundice recovered but, overall, 3 (2.4%) of the ZZ cohort developed cirrhosis in infancy or childhood. The neonatal period is a vulnerable period. One can speculate that, when polymerization of variant alpha₁-antitrypsin occurs, the immature liver is less able to degrade polymerized protein and is more readily overwhelmed, resulting in liver damage. Other factors such as intercurrent infection and fever may facilitate polymerization. Genetic variation in polymer degradation may be another important factor in the enormous variability in hepatic phenotype.

PiM is the normal protein. 10% of the European population are carriers for the S or Z variant (4% (1/25) of North Europeans carry Z, and 6% (1/17) carry S). Common phenotypes are PiMM, PiMS, PiMZ, PiSS, PiSZ, and PiZZ. Null variants are only distinguishable from homozygotes with genotyping.

Clinical approach

History: key points

- Three-generation family tree, with specific enquiry regarding emphysema and liver disease.
- Smoking history.

Investigation

- Clotted sample (serum) for alpha₁-antitrypsin phenotyping. If interpretation of phenotyping is problematical proceed to genotyping (5 ml EDTA (ethylenedinitrilotetraacetate) sample).

NB. If attempting alpha₁-antitrypsin typing on an individual who has had a liver transplant, the electrophoretic mobility of alpha₁-antitrypsin will reflect the genotype of the donor liver, and you will need to resort to mutation analysis (of DNA from lymphocytes) to determine the genotype of the transplant recipient.

Genetic advice

Inheritance and recurrence risk

AR inheritance. The possibility that apparently healthy parents of a ZZ or SZ child may themselves be ZZ or SZ should be borne in mind when offering phenotyping.

Variability and penetrance

If MZ parents have had a child with a ZZ phenotype and severe neonatal liver disease, it is easy to advise on the 1 in 4 risk for a subsequent ZZ child, but less easy to advise on the probability that subsequent ZZ children will develop severe liver disease. Accurate estimates are very difficult to establish. The risk quoted by Psacharopoulos *et al.* (1983) of 78% is almost certainly an overestimate. Current estimates are closer to 20–30% for significant liver disease in a ZZ sibling (i.e. overall 5–7% risk to a future pregnancy).

Prenatal diagnosis

This is available using chorionic villus sampling (CVS). Parents must have been phenotyped first, and subsequently genotyped. Prenatal diagnosis is by genotyping of DNA from CVS. Consult a specialist lab.

Other family members

- Most important message for family members is not to smoke. Smoking greatly accelerates lung disease in alpha₁-antitrypsin deficiency and markedly reduces life expectancy.
- Because carrier status is so common in the general population (10% (1/10)) and because so few ZZ individuals experience severe neonatal liver disease, cascade screening of the entire family is rarely appropriate. 4% (1/25) of North Europeans carry Z and 6% (1/17) carry S.
- Subsequent affected siblings of an alpha₁-antitrypsin deficient proband should receive intramuscular vitamin K at birth. Aim to minimize pyrexia and acute-phase inflammation by active treatment of incidental infections in ZZ homozygotes especially in infancy.

Natural history and management

The frequency of abnormal liver function tests (LFTs) in PiZZ individuals with alpha₁-antitrypsin deficiency who do not develop jaundice or hepatomegaly in infancy falls from 60% at 6 months of age to a plateau of ~15% at 12–18 years. Abnormal LFTs may be transient. Most of those with abnormal tests at 16 years were normal at 18 years and vice versa. PiZZ children may be vulnerable to new or worsening liver dysfunction during intercurrent illness, e.g. appendicitis or pneumonia. PiSZ infants have a better prognosis with a lower frequency of abnormal LFTs throughout childhood. In Sveger's (1984) study, none of the PiSZ neonates developed prolonged jaundice.

Potential long-term complications

- **Emphysema**. In healthy non-smokers, forced expiratory volume in 1 second (FEV₁) decreases by 35 ml/year, in ZZ non-smokers the average decrease is 45 ml/year, but in ZZ smokers, the rate is doubled at 70 ml/year reflecting the development of panlobar basal emphysema.

- **Cirrhosis**. The risk of cirrhosis in adult life is difficult to quantify, but ZZ individuals are at increased risk for chronic liver disease. Many have subclinical liver disease at post mortem.
- **Surveillance**. Watch for deteriorating LFTs (bilirubin, enzymes, clotting) in an individual with known alpha$_1$-antitrypsin deficiency. This should prompt assessment for liver transplantation.

Support groups: US `<www.alph1.org.uk www. alpha1.org>`.

Expert adviser: David A Lomas, Professor, Respiratory Medicine Unit, Department of Medicine, University of Cambridge, Cambridge, England.

References

Carrell RW, Lomas DA. Mechanisms of disease: alpha 1-antitrypsin deficiency—a model for conformational diseases. *New Engl J Med* 2002; **346**: 45–53.

de Serres FJ. Worldwide racial and ethnic distribution of alpha1-antitrypsin deficiency: summary of an analysis of published genetic epidemiologic surveys. *Chest* 2002; **122**: 1818–29.

Eriksson S, Carlson J, Velez R. Risks of cirrhosis and primary liver cancer in alpha 1-antitrypsin deficiency. *New Engl J Med* 1986; **314**: 736–9.

Ibarguen E, Gross CR. Liver disease in alpha-1-antitrypsin deficiency: prognostic indicators. *J Pediatr* 1990; **117**: 864–70.

Miravitlles M, Vila S, *et al.* Influence of deficient alpha1-antitrypsin phenotypes on clinical characteristics and severity of asthma in adults. *Respir Med* 2002; **96**: 186–92.

Primhak RA, Tanner MS. Alpha-1 antitrypsin deficiency. *Arch Dis Child* 2001; **85**: 2–5.

Psacharopoulos HT, Mowat AP, *et al.* Outcome of liver disease associated with alpha 1 antitrypsin deficiency (PiZ). Implications for genetic counselling and antenatal diagnosis. *Arch Dis Child* 1983; **58**: 882–7.

Sveger T. Prospective study of children with alpha 1-antitrypsin deficiency: eight-year-old follow-up. *J Pediatr* 1984; **104**: 91–4.

Alport syndrome

Nephropathy and deafness.

Alport syndrome (AS) is characterized by haematuria, proteinuria (<1–2 g of protein/24 hours), progressive renal failure, and sensorineural deafness. It is caused by mutations in the genes that code for type IV collagen. Type IV collagen is a major component of the basement membranes of the kidney, eyes, and cochlear, interweaving with laminins, nidogen, and sulfated proteoglycans. The basement membranes form a complex surface on which epithelial cells reside, providing morphogenic cues that determine the fate of cells, the polarization of subcellular constituents, and the location of cell receptors and transporters (Hudson *et al.* 2003).

The most serious complication is progressive renal failure. The glomerular basement membrane retains the fetal isoforms of type IV collagen, which appear to be more susceptible to proteolytic attack, and glomerulosclerosis develops.

Histological confirmation of Alport syndrome on renal biopsy may be replaced by molecular testing in families with known mutations.

The condition is genetically heterogeneous (see table). Most, approximately 85%, is X-linked (XLAS) with mutations in *COL4A5* encoding the α5(IV) collagen chain on Xq22–23. The next most likely mode of inheritance is autosomal recessive (ARAS) with mutations in *COL4A3* or *COL4A4* encoding the α3(IV) or α4(IV) chains on 2q35–37. A few families show autosomal dominant (AD) inheritance with dominant negative mutations in *COL4A3* or *COL4A4*.

The role of the geneticist is usually to provide genetic advice to families with Alport syndrome, in particular to estimate the risk of females carrying an XLAS mutation.

XLAS.

- **Males.** 67% of males present with macroscopic haematuria, usually during an intercurrent infection at an average age of 3 years (Flinter 2004). Once the macroscopic haematuria clears, there is residual microscopic haematuria. A male who has consistently normal urinalysis at the age of 5 years is very unlikely to develop XLAS. All affected males subsequently develop proteinuria; indeed, some 30% later develop nephrotic syndrome. Proteinuria never precedes haematuria in XLAS. High-tone sensorineural deafness affects 83% of affected males and first becomes apparent at an average age of 11 years. It is progressive and hearing may deteriorate rapidly during the teens, but some residual hearing is retained. Hypertension usually develop in the teens and the average age of reaching end-stage renal failure (ESRF) for males with XLAS is 21 years.
- **Females.** The clinical course is very variable. One-third present with macroscopic haematuria at an average age of 9 years, or present later when microscopic haematuria is detected on routine urinalysis. At the most severe end of the spectrum a small minority (1–2%) have a similar course to that of affected males. At the other extreme, women may remain asymptomatic into their 80s despite having microscopic haematuria on careful investigation. One-third develop hypertension (usually in mid-life) and the lifetime risk of ESRF is 8–15%.

Clinical approach

History: key points

- Family history. At least three generations. Consider X-linked (XL), AR, and AD modes of inheritance.
- Renal failure. Age, treatment, transplantation.
- Obtain copies of renal biopsy findings.
- Hearing problems, hearing aid.
- Visual problems.

Examination: key points

- Features of impaired renal function, elevated blood pressure (BP).
- Eyes. Observe if there are any abnormalities and use fundoscopy for retinal abnormalities.
  - Dot and fleck retinopathy in 85% of affected adult males.
  - Anterior lenticonus 25% (conical protrusion of the central portion of the lens into the anterior chamber may cause progressive myopia, anterior capsular cataract, or spontaneous rupture of the anterior capsule).
  - Posterior polymorphous corneal dystrophy (rare).
  - The eye findings are the same in XLAS and ARAS.
- Leiomyomatosis (contiguous gene deletion syndrome with submicroscopic deletion of Xq22 and loss of a

Classification of Alport syndrome (adapted from Hudson *et al.* 2003)

Description*	Cause
X-linked Alport syndrome (XLAS)	
Renal failure (average age of ESRF in males is 21 years); deafness, usually progressive during later childhood; anterior lenticonus in teens and adults	Deletions, nonsense, missense, and splice variant mutations in *COL4A5*
X-linked Alport syndrome and leiomyomatosis	
Early onset of renal failure with oesophageal dysfunction, genital leiomyomas, and occasional posterior cataract	Deletions from *COL4A5* to the 2nd exon of *COL4A6*
Autosomal recessive AS (ARAS)	
Early onset of renal failure (<30 years) in both males and females	Homozygous or compound heterozygous haploinsufficiency or splicing mutations in *COL4A3* or *COL4A4*
Autosomal dominant AS	
Renal failure of varying severity	Dominant negative mutations in *COL4A3* or *COL4A4*

* ESRF, End-stage renal failure.

variable portion of *COL4A5* and the first two exons of *COL4A6*).

Investigations

- Urinalysis. Microscopy (microscopic haematuria) and proteinuria. Send urine to lab for microscopy for red cells if positive on dipstick.
- Renal function. Creatinine.
- Refer for specialist ophthalmological examination ('dot and fleck' retinopathy, anterior lenticonus, and, rarely, posterior polymorphous corneal dystrophy).
- Audiometry to detect sensorineural hearing loss.
- DNA mutation analysis. In XLAS there is an approximately 50% detection rate by single-strand conformational polymorphism (SSCP).
- Cytogenetic analysis in the presence of mental retardation or other features (submicroscopic deletion of *COL4A5* and *FACL4*).
- Renal biopsy:
  - may not be necessary if there is a family history of Alport syndrome in which case renal ultrasound scan (USS) suffices to exclude other causes of haematuria, but may be indicated in an apparently solitary case;
  - typically shows thickening and splitting of the glomerular basement membrane. Tubules drop out, segmental glomerulosclerosis progresses, and the kidneys eventually fail because of interstitial fibrosis.
  - in XLAS, $\alpha3(IV)$, $\alpha4(IV)$, and $\alpha5(IV)$, collagens are undetectable in most glomeruli, tubules, and Bowman's capsule by immunostaining. Females may show a mosaic staining pattern. In patients with ARAS, $\alpha5(IV)$ staining is detectable in Bowman's capsule, but there are no detectable $\alpha3(IV)$ or $\alpha4(IV)$ collagens in glomerular or tubular basement membranes.

Other diagnoses/conditions to consider

Benign familial haematuria. AD mild haematuria or proteinuria that is non-progressive. Progression to renal failure is rare. Findings on renal biopsy are relatively normal except for a thin basement membrane (also found as a normal variant in 5–10% of the population). In some kindreds the condition is caused by mutations in the *COL4A3* or *COL4A4* genes (2q35–37).

Genetic advice

Inheritance and recurrence risk

In large families the inheritance pattern may be inferred from the family history. If there is only a single affected member consider the following.

- 85% of AS is XL due to mutation in *COL4A5*.
- The new mutation rate in AS due to *COL4A5* is 15%.
- Germline and gonosomal mosaicism in XLAS has been reported (Bruttini *et al.* 2000).
- ARAS is the next most frequent type after XLAS. Parental consanguinity and/or affected females may increase the likelihood of this.
- In families with documented male to male transmission, the inheritance may be AD but check the validity of the information.

Variability and penetrance

- In XLAS, the rate of progression of renal disease tends to run true to some extent within families. There are, however, a few notable families where the age at chronic renal failure (CRF) in affected males has varied by up to 20 years.
- Families vary in the rapidity of onset of organ failure. In XLAS, penetrance is close to 99% if the urine is tested carefully in female carriers (who are heterozygous for *COL4A5* mutations), but expressivity is variable. The lifetime risk for end-stage renal failure (ESRF) in female patients with XLAS is 8–15%.

Prenatal diagnosis

Possible by chorionic villus sampling (CVS) if the disease-causing mutation is known.

Predictive testing

Possible if the disease-causing mutation is known, or by linkage in suitable pedigrees.

Other family members

It is important to identify carrier females in XLAS. Mutation analysis is the preferred strategy.

Natural history and management

Potential long-term complications

- **Renal failure.** Progression to renal failure. Renal transplantation is the treatment of choice. 1–5% of individuals with Alport syndrome develop anti-GBM (glomerular basement membrane) nephritis after renal transplantation. The risk is higher for those who carry a mutation resulting in the absence of the non-collagenous (NC) domain.
- **Visual problems.** Lenticonus can be treated with lens implant as for cataracts.
- **Deafness.** Audiometry at diagnosis and subsequently, with provision of hearing aids as required.

Surveillance

Known mutation carriers and at-risk individuals should be under periodic surveillance by a nephrologist.

Support group: <renux.dmed.ed.ac.uk/EdREN>.

Expert adviser: Frances Flinter, Consultant Clinical Geneticist, Guy's Hospital, London, England.

References

Bruttini M, Vitelli F, *et al.* Mosaicism in Alport syndrome with genetic counselling. *J Med Genet* 2000; **37**: 717–19.

Colville D, Savige J. Alport syndrome: a review of the ocular manifestations. *Ophthal Genet* 1997; **18**: 161–73.

Flinter F. Alport syndrome. In *Genetics of renal disease*, Oxford Monographs on Medical Genetics (ed. F. Flinter, E. Maher, and A. Saggar-Malik), Chapter 8. Oxford University Press, Oxford, 2004.

Hudson BG, Tryggvason K, *et al.* Alport's syndrome, Goodpasture's syndrome, and type IV collagen. *New Engl J Med* 2003; **348**: 2543–56.

Kashtan CE. Alport syndrome. An inherited disorder of renal, ocular, and cochlear basement membranes. *Medicine* 1999; **78**: 338–60.

Lemmink HH, *et al.* The clinical spectrum of type IV collagen mutations. *Hum Mut* 1997; **9**: 477–99.

Androgen insensitivity syndrome (AIS)

AIS, complete androgen insensitivity (CAIS), testicular feminization syndrome, XY female, partial androgen insensitivity (PAIS).

AIS (1/20 000 live births) is caused by mutations in the androgen receptor gene on Xq11. Primary female sexual differentiation of the human embryo and fetus occurs even if the ovaries are absent and is not apparently under the influence of fetal hormones. Primary male sexual diffentiation is dependent on androgens (testosterone and dihydrotestosterone (DHT)) produced by the fetal testis in response to human chorionic gonadotrophin (hCG). Thus an XY embryo carrying a mutation in the androgen receptor gene that prevents androgen binding will develop as a female. In addition to testosterone the fetal testes produce anti-Müllerian hormone (AMH), which causes regression of the structures destined to develop into the Fallopian tubes, uterus, and upper vagina. The female infant with CAIS therefore usually has normal female external genitalia, but a blind-ending vagina.

Girls with CAIS are phenotypically normal females at birth. They present either in infancy/early childhood with bilateral inguinal herniae often containing testes or in young adult life with primary amenorrhoea. The diagnosis is suggested when a karyotype reveals 46,XY.

Girls who do not present in early childhood are often not diagnosed until quite late in their teens. At puberty, the testes produce a large amount of testosterone, which is converted to oestrogen promoting normal breast development. However, usually there is no or scant pubic hair and menarche does not occur.

Clinical approach

Families with a recent diagnosis of AIS are often confused and distressed. Careful, sensitive explanation of the biological basis for AIS is important. Emphasize the basic female pattern of the developing embryo and the normal female development of girls with AIS.

History: key points

- Three-generation family tree. In a family with AIS, a history of maternal female relatives who have been unable to have children raises suspicion.
- Determine how and when the diagnosis was made and obtain confirmation of the karyotype.

Examination: key points

Examination may not be appropriate if the diagnosis is secure. Otherwise:

- in infants and young children examine for bilateral inguinal herniae;
- in teenagers and adults examine for lack of axillary and pubic hair;
- consider pelvic ultrasound scan (USS) to confirm absence of uterus.

Investigation

- Karyotype to support diagnosis (if not already done).
- DNA for mutation analysis of the androgen receptor gene.

Other diagnoses/conditions to consider

The combination of bilateral inguinal herniae and normal phenotypic female development with a 46,XY karyotype is characteristic of CAIS, but in a girl ascertained coincidentally also consider SRY gene mutations. In PAIS, with ambiguous genitalia, the differential diagnosis is much wider and diagnosis more difficult.

Partial androgen insensitivity (PAIS). In this condition mutations in the androgen receptor gene impair androgen binding and signalling, but do not prevent it as in CAIS. The condition usually presents at birth with ambiguous genitalia. Problems with gender identity are often much greater in this group than in patients with CAIS. This may in part be due to the impaired (rather than absent) activity of androgens on the developing brain. Only a minority of females with a PAIS phenotype have a mutation in the gene encoding the androgen receptor; other genes are yet to be identified.

46,XY female due to mutation in SRY. The SRY gene on Yp encodes a testis-determining factor that promotes the indifferent early embryonic gonads to differentiate into testes. Mutations or deletions of this gene will result in female development but, unlike in CAIS, the testes are dysgenetic or streak gonads and AMH will not be produced so that the uterus and vagina will persist.

Genetic advice

Inheritance and recurrence risk

X-linked recessive. For a woman who is a carrier, there are four possible outcomes to a pregnancy, each equally likely: a normal daughter; a carrier daughter; a daughter with AIS; and a normal boy (i.e. 25% recurrence risk).

De novo mutations occur at a high rate within the androgen receptor gene (27% observed by Hiort *et al.* 1998; actual risk possibly ~33%). Germline and gonosomal mosaicism have been observed in mothers of affected sporadic cases. Hence as for Duchenne dystrophy, offer carrier detection to sisters of affected individuals even if the mother is proven on molecular studies not to be a carrier. (Risk is probably small, possibly a few %). Mothers may also wish to consider prenatal diagnosis in a future pregnancy because of the small risk of gonadal mosaicism.

Variability and penetrance

For CAIS the condition is fully penetrant and, apart from variation in time of presentation, there is little variability.

Prenatal diagnosis

If a mutation is identified, prenatal diagnosis by chorionic villus sampling (CVS) at 11 weeks gestation is technically feasible. Less certain is the decision to undertake prenatal diagnosis for a condition whose main impact is infertility.

Carrier testing

Mutation analysis is the gold-standard for accurate carrier detection, but note comments above about risks associated with gonadal mosaicism. If no mutation is known in the family, analysis of the size of the triplet repeat within the androgen-receptor gene can be used for intragenic linkage analysis, and may enable modification of the risk when combined with pedigree analysis (e.g. a woman who has inherited a different triplet repeat allele to that carried by an affected member of the family will be at low risk of being a carrier). Inability to determine the level in the family at which the mutation originated limits the utility of this approach in confirming carrier status in families with single affected individuals. A proportion of CAIS carrier females have reduced body hair (axillary and pubic hair).

Other family members
Maternal male relatives are unaffected, with no implications for their offspring. Maternal female relatives may be at risk of being carriers.

Natural history and management

Potential long term complications
Testes should be removed because of the risk of gonadoblastoma (~30% risk by age 50 years is often quoted, but may be an overestimate). Hormone replacement therapy (HRT) should be offered from adolescence to induce puberty and minimize the risk of osteoporosis. During teenage years consider referral to a gynaecologist with special expertise to assess whether the vagina is of sufficient size for sexual intercourse or whether vaginal dilatation or vaginoplasty should be offered.

Many normal adolescent girls feel relatively insecure about their personal and sexual identity. It is perhaps not suprising, therefore, that diagnosis of AIS in adolescence or young adult life can precipitate severe psychological distress.

Referral for ongoing psychological support, psychiatric help, or psychosexual counselling may be appropriate.

Surveillance
Periodic bone mineral density scans may be appropriate in adult life.

Support group: Androgen Insensitivity Syndrome Support Group <www.medhelp.org/www/ais>.

Expert adviser: Ieuan Hughes, Professor of Paediatrics, University of Cambridge, Cambridge, England.

References

Boehmer AL, Brinkmann AO, *et al.* Germ-line and somatic mosaicism in the androgen insensitivity syndrome: implications for genetic counselling. *Am J Hum Genet* 1997; **60**: 1003–6.

Boehmer AL, Brinkmann O, *et al.* Genotype versus phenotype in families with androgen insensitivity syndrome. *J Clin Endocrinol Metab* 2001; **86** (9): 4151–60.

Hiort O, Sinnecker GH, *et al.* Inherited and *de novo* androgen receptor gene mutations: investigation of single-case families. *J Pediatr* 1998; **132**: 917–18.

Angelman syndrome

Angelman syndrome (AS) is a distinctive neurobehavioural disorder resulting from disruption to the function of the maternally derived imprinted domain on 15q11.13 (more specifically, *UBE3A*). It affects ~1/12 000–1/40 000 children. All patients with classical AS exhibit:

- severe developmental delay;
- profound speech impairment. Many do not acquire speech or at the very most 3–4 words. Receptive and nonverbal communication skills are significantly better than expressive skills. Most children with AS use gesture to communicate and some are able to use sign language (e.g. Makaton). The PECS (picture exchange system) may be helpful.
- a movement and balance disorder: ataxic wide-based gait.
- specific behaviour with excitable personality and inappropriately happy affect. Hand-flapping when excited. Sociable and inquisitive. Love of water and fascination with reflections. Sleep disorder.

Other features include microcephaly, hypopigmentation (in some deletion patients), and seizures.

AS is caused by defects in the maternally derived imprinted domain on 15q11.13 that can arise in a variety of ways:

- interstitial deletion of 15q11–13mat (may be cytogenetically visible or need fluorescent *in situ* hybridization (FISH); 70%);
- paternal uniparental disomy (UPD) on chromosome 15 (2–5%);
- an imprinting defect (2–5%);
- mutation in the E3 ubiquitin protein ligase gene (*UBE3A*; 20%);
- unidentified.

All patients with an interstitial deletion, UPD, or an imprinting defect, i.e. ~80% in total, will have an *SNRPN* (small nuclear ribonuclear protein-associated polypeptide N) methylation abnormality (only unmethylated alleles). Normal individuals will show one methylated (maternal) and one unmethylated (paternal) allele. Patients with *UBE3A* mutations, AS of unidentified cause, and those with a phenocopy of AS but a different disorder will all show normal results on the *SNRPN* methylation assay.

Clinical approach

History: key points

- Three-generation family tree. Are there any other affected individuals? Would this fit with a maternally imprinted phenomenon?
- Feeding difficulties in infancy due to inefficient suckling. Oropharyngeal incoordination may cause difficulty in sucking and swallowing.
- Developmental milestones.
- Early onset of seizure disorder.
- Characteristic behavioural profile with frequent and sometimes inappropriate laughter, a love of water, and sleep disorder.

Examination: key points

- Growth parameters including occipital-frontal circumference (OFC; most have OFC < 25th centile by 3 years; severe microcephaly is very unusual).
- Happy and sociable affect. Smiling and laughing behaviours do not occur totally inappropriately, but are found

to increase in social situations and decrease in non-social situations.
- Wide-based, stiff-legged posture. Increased muscle tone in limbs.
- Jerky gait with arms often held with elbows bent and hands uplifted to shoulder level.
- Excitability with characteristic hand flapping.
- Facial features are subtle and include a wide, smiling mouth, prominent chin, and deep-set eyes.

Investigations

- Molecular genetic analysis by SNPRN methylation. 80% have abnormal methylation.
- Cytogenetic analysis. Karyotype with FISH for AS/Prader–Willi syndrome (PWS) critical region.
- UPD studies (parental DNA) if methylation abnormal, but cytogenetics normal.
- Mutation analysis of *UBE3A* if clinically typical, but methylation studies normal (44% detection rate in one study of methylation-negative sporadic patients), or if family history of AS and no cytogenetic abnormality. *UBE3A* mutations identified in 80% of familial cases and 15% of sporadic cases. Intragenic deletions can occur.
- Electroencephalography (EEG). 2–3 Hz large-amplitude slow wave bursts are characteristic. The EEG may be abnormal even if there is no history of seizures. However, a normal EEG does not exclude the diagnosis.

Other diagnoses/conditions to consider

Rett syndrome (in females). A proportion of children with a clinical diagnosis of AS, but negative genetic analysis have mutations in *MECP2*. See 'Rett syndrome', page 408.

Mowat–Wilson syndrome. All patients have typical dysmorphic features with upturned ear lobules in association with severe intellectual disability, and nearly all have microcephaly and seizures. Congenital anomalies include Hirschsprung's disease, congenital heart disease (CHD), hypospadias and genitourinary anomalies, and agenesis of the corpus callosum, Short stature is common. Caused by heterozygous deletions or truncating mutations in the *ZFHX1B* (*SIP1*) gene on 2q22.

X-linked alpha-thalassaemia/mental retardation syndrome (ATR-X) in males. The key facial features are the characteristic tenting of the upper lip associated with a small triangular-shaped nose and a flat nasal bridge. Abnormalities of the genitalia in males ranging from hypoplasia of the external genitalia to ambiguous genitalia are found. There is severe intellectual disability; patients rarely develop speech. Seizures are common. Search carefully for haemoglobin H (HbH) inclusions in erythrocytes stained with brilliant cresyl blue. The facial features have been confused with those of Coffin–Lowry syndrome, but in ATR-X carrier females do not have physical or intellectual manifestations of the condition. Carrier women may have some HbH inclusions, but it is not a reliable method of carrier detection. It is caused by mutations in the *XNP* gene on Xq13.

22q13 deletion syndrome. This condition is characterised by moderate to profound mental retardation, delay/absence of expressive speech, hypotonia, normal to accelerated growth and mild dysmorphic features.

Deletions are variable in size and are often submicroscopic requiring molecular cytogenetic methods eg FISH to detect them.

Genetic advice
Inheritance and recurrence risk
- Interstitial deletion of PWS/AS critical region (15q11–q13) on maternal homologue, with normal parental karyotypes. Risks are very low, probably <1%. Maternal germline mosaicism has been reported (Kokkonen and Leisti, 2000).
- UPD 15 (pat) arises as a sporadic event, sometimes following rescue of a trisomic conceptus, and so recurrence risks are very low, probably <1/200.
- *UBE3A* mutation. Women carrying a *UBE3A* mutation have a 50% risk of AS in each pregnancy (when transmitted by a father, development is normal because the gene is silenced).
- AS without a FISH deletion or UPD. Risks may be high (50%) if there is a *UBE3A* or imprinting centre mutation.

Variability and penetrance
Patients with cytogenetic deletions are the most severely affected, whilst UPD and imprinting defect patients are the least affected.

Prenatal diagnosis
If the cytogenetic basis for AS in the proband has been defined using FISH, then this is the method of choice for prenatal diagnosis. If there is a known *UBE3A* mutation, prenatal diagnosis by chorionic villus sampling (CVS) is also possible. If there is no detectable deletion or *UBE3A* mutation, but a methylation abnormality exists in the proband, a small study by Glenn et al. (2000) showed that correct prenatal diagnoses were obtained in 24/24 samples from amniocentesis and CVS using the 5' *SNRPN* locus. The DNA methylation imprint of 5' *SNRPN* arises in the germline and maintains the imprint in tissues suitable for prenatal diagnosis of AS and PWS. (Caution is advised in view of the theoretical possibilities of instability of imprints in trophoblast in early embryogenesis. Seek specialist advice from a lab with experience in this area.)

Predictive testing
Not usually relevant.

Other family members
Especially important if a *UBE3A* mutation or imprinting mutation is defined as some relatives may be at high genetic risk.

Natural history and management
Early motor skills are compromised by ataxia as well as learning disability and walking is often delayed until 3–4 years. Less than 10% may never achieve independent walking. Portage and other pre-school learning programmes have an important role. All children with AS will have special educational needs. Life expectancy can be normal. As an adult are likely to need supervision perhaps in a group home.

Potential long-term complications
Up to 90% develop seizures. (90% with deletion, 20% with UPD) usual onset is 12-18/12, 40% of adults develop scoliosis. Loss of mobility and development of joint contractures over time.

Surveillance
The child should be under the care of a multidisciplinary child development team.

Support group: Angelman Syndrome Foundation (US) <www.angelman.org>, Tel. 800 432 6435; ASSERT (Angelman Syndrome Support Education and Research Trust) <www.angelmanuk.org>.

Expert adviser: Jill Clayton-Smith, Consultant Clinical Geneticist, St Mary's Hospital, Manchester, England.

References
Clayton-Smith J, Laan L. Angelman syndrome: a review of the clinical and genetic aspects. *J Med Genet* 2003; **40** (2): 87–95.

Glenn CC, Deng G, et al. DNA methylation analysis with respect to prenatal diagnosis of the Angelman and Prader–Willi syndromes and imprinting. *Prenat Diagn* 2000; **20**: 300–6.

Kokkonen H, Leisti J. An unexpected recurrence of Angelman syndrome suggestive of maternal germ-line mosaicism of del (15) (q11q13) in a Finnish family. *Hum Genet* 2000; **107**: 83–5.

Lossie AC, Whitney MM, et al. Distinct phenotypes distinguish the molecular classes of Angelman syndrome. *J Med Genet* 2001; **38**: 834–45.

Moncla A, Malzac P, et al. Angelman syndrome resulting from UBE3A mutations in 14 patients from eight families: clinical manifestations and genetic counselling. *J Med Genet* 1999; **36** (7): 554–60.

Moncla A, Malzac P, et al. Phenotype-genotype correlation in 20 deletion and 20 non-deletion Angelman syndrome patients. *Eur J Hum Genet* 1999; **7**: 131–9.

Williams CA. Angelman syndrome. In *Management of genetic syndromes* (ed. S.B. Cassidy and J.E. Allanson), Chapter 3. Wiley-Liss, New York, 2001.

Williams CA. Neurological aspects of the Angelman syndrome. *Brain Dev* 2005; **27**: 88–94.

Autism and austism spectrum disorders

Autism is characterized by qualitative impairments in reciprocal social interaction and communication coupled with restricted and stereotyped patterns of interests and activities. The recurrence risk of autism in siblings is many times higher than the rate of the disorder in the general population. The concordance rate in monozygotic (MZ) twins (60–91%) is much higher than in dizygotic (DZ) twins (0–6%) suggesting a strong genetic component to autism susceptibility. In addition, the genetic liability to autism confers a risk for a broader range of more subtle autistic-like impairments in social communication and play development. These variants may be described as atypical autism, Asperger syndrome, or pervasive developmental disorder not otherwise specified. Collectively, these conditions are referred to as **autism spectrum disorders**.

Classical autism

With a prevalence of 1–2/1000, it is much more common in males with a M:F ratio of approximately 4:1. The prevalence of autism spectrum disorders is approximately 6/1000 (Fombonne 2003).

Autistic children fail to use eye-contact to regulate social interchanges and are often delayed in their language development with little babble. Some autistic children do not acquire speech; traditionally about half were found to be nonverbal or to have grossly impaired speech. However, these figures may need to be revised in the light of the changing concepts regarding diagnosis.

Although described in terms of social and behavioural abnormalities, autism is also associated with an uneven pattern of cognitive defects (see table). Many autistic individuals have full-scale intelligence quotient (IQ) scores <70, but show greater visuospatial than verbal skills. A small minority have one or more outstanding skill, well above their overall low level of functioning. There is evidence for an underlying neurodevelopmental disorder as 25–30% develop epilepsy by adult life (often with onset in teenage years) and 25% have head size >97th centile. The macrocephaly probably develops postnatally.

Only a small percentage of children with autism have a specific genetic diagnosis. Specific identifiable aetiologies include fragile X syndrome (FRAX), tuberous sclerosis (TS), Rett syndrome, and a variety of chromosomal anomalies. Recently, a microduplication of 15q13 has been implicated in a very small number of cases of familial autism. *De novo* chromosomal deletions at Xp22.3 have been observed in three autistic females (Thomas *et al.* 1999). Xp22.3 incorporates the neuroligin 4 gene (*NLGN4*). Mutations have recently been reported in two X-linked genes encoding neuroligins 3 and 4 in siblings with autistic spectrum disorders (Jamain *et al.* 2003). These genes encode synaptic cell-adhesion molecules and suggest that a defect in synaptogenesis may predispose to autism. They appear to be a rare cause of autism (Vincent).

In 90% the cause is unknown. A complex genetic basis is proposed with at least 3–4 loci implicated. Genome scans have mapped putative susceptibility loci to 2q, 7q, 15q, and 16p, although the findings are not entirely consistent across studies. Congenital rubella was implicated before mass vaccination reduced the frequency of the disease, so

---

ICD-10 criteria for autism (reproduced by permission of the World Health Organization ©1992)

A Abnormal or impaired development is evident before the age of 3 years in at least *one* of the following areas:

  1 receptive or expressive language as used in social communication;

  2 the development of selective social attachments or of reciprocal social interaction;

  3 functional or symbolic play.

B A total of at least 6 symptoms from (1), (2), and (3) below must be present, with at least two from (1) and at least one from each of (2) and (3).

  1 Qualitative abnormalities in reciprocal social interaction are manifest in at least two of the following areas:

    (a) failure adequately to use eye-to-eye gaze, facial expression, body posture, and gesture to regulate social interaction;

    (b) failure to develop (in a manner appropriate to mental age and despite ample opportunities) peer relationships that involve a mutuality of interests, activities, and emotions;

    (c) Lack of socioemotional reciprocity as shown by an impaired or deviant response to other people's emotions; or lack of modulation of behaviour according to social context; or a weak integration of social, emotional and communicative behaviours;

    (d) lack of spontaneous seeking to share enjoyment, interests, or achievements with other people (e.g. lack of showing, bringing, pointing out to other people objects of interest to the individual).

  2 Qualitative abnormalities in communication are manifest in at least one of the following areas:

    (a) delay in, or total lack of, development of spoken language that is not accompanied by an attempt to compensate through the use of gesture or mime as an alternative mode of communication (often preceded by a lack of communicative babbling);

    (b) relative failure to initiate or sustain conversational interchange (at whatever level of language skills is present) in which there is reciprocal responsiveness to the communications of the other person;

    (c) stereotyped and repetitive use of language or idiosyncratic use of words or phrases;

    (d) lack of varied spontaneous make-believe or (when young) social imitative play.

  3 Restricted, repetitive, and stereotyped patterns of behaviour, interests, and activities are manifest in at least one of the following areas:

    (a) an encompassing preoccupation with one or more stereotyped, restricted patterns of interest that are abnormal in content or focus; or one or more interests that are abnormal in their intensity and circumscribed nature though not in their content or focus;

    (b) apparently compulsive adherence to specific, non-functional routines or rituals;

    (c) stereotyped and repetitive motor mannerisms that involve either hand or finger flapping or twisting or complex whole body movements;

    (d) preoccupations with part-objects or non-functional elements of play materials (such as their odour, the feel of their surface, or the noise or vibration that they generate).

Characteristics of pervasive developmental disorders (after Rapin 2002)

Asperger disorder

Troublesome social ineptness, lack of insight

Behavioural inflexibility with a narrow range of interests

IQ ≥70 (affected children may be normally intelligent or gifted)

No delay in the emergence of speech

Often clumsiness

Pervasive developmental disorder not specified

Applies to less severely affected children who do not meet criteria for either classic autism or Asperger disorder

Disintegrative disorder

Early development entirely normal, including speech

Severe regression between the ages of 2–10 yrs affecting language, sociability, cognition, and competence in skills of daily life

Rett syndrome

Severe global regression in infant girls (rarely in boys) classically resulting in lifelong severe mental retardation, lack of language and purposeful hand use, and other neurological deficits

---

it has been postulated that viral/infectious diseases may cause autism or trigger the condition in susceptible individuals. However, as yet there is no established environmental aetiology.

Miles and Hillman (2000) evaluated 88 consecutive individuals with idiopathic autism. 58% were phenotypically normal on physical examination, 22% were clearly abnormal, and 20% were equivocal. The male excess was strongest in those with a normal physical examination (M:F, 7.5:1) and weakest in those who were phenotypically abnormal (M:F, 1.7:1).

The clinical picture is not attributable to the other varieties of pervasive developmental disorders (see table): specific developmental disorder of receptive language with secondary socioemotional problems; reactive attachment disorder or disinhibition attachment disorder; mental retardation with some associated emotional or behavioural disorder; schizophrenia of unusually early onset; and Rett syndrome.

Clinical approach

History: key points

- Three-generation family tree with specific enquiry about schooling, career choice, hobbies, and sociability of parents and other close relatives.
- Pre-, peri-, and postnatal history.
- Detailed developmental history especially of language development.
- Specific enquiry regarding regression/loss of skills.
- Detailed assessment of behaviour including:
  - repetitive activites (e.g. twirling, spinning);
  - play (whether it is imaginative);
  - social interaction, e.g. eye contact, greeting, turn-taking;
  - peer relationships;
  - response to close family members and to strangers;
  - response to new situations.

Examination: key points

- Complete physical examination focused on minor anomalies, neurology, social interaction, and behaviour.
- Careful examination of skin with Wood's light for hypopigmented macules (TS) especially if there is a history of seizures.
- Growth parameters. Height, weight, and occipital-frontal circumference (OFC).
- Assessment by child psychiatrist/clinical psychologist.

Investigation

- Chromosome analysis.
- Consider 15q11–13 fluorescent *in situ* hybridization (FISH) studies.
- FRAX studies.
- Consider *MECP2* analysis in girls with a history of normal early development and subsequent regression. Consider *NLGN3* and *NLGN4* mutation analysis if family tree suggestive of X-linked inheritance.
- Neuroimaging is not part of routine clinical assessment but is indicated for specific neurological signs. Focus on electroencephalogram (EEG) or triad of severe learning disability, autism, and epilepsy (Baird *et al.* 2003).

Other diagnoses/conditions to consider

Asperger syndrome. Asperger syndrome is characterized by higher cognitive abilities and more normal language function. It is much more common in males than females (M:F, 8:1). In Cederlund's study, there was a high rate of close relatives with autism spectrum problems but also high rates of prenatal and perinatal problems. It has recently been shown that classical autism and Asperger syndrome can both arise due to the same familial mutation in Neuroligin 4 (Jamain *et al.* 2003).

Tuberous sclerosis (TS). Autosomal dominant (AD) neurocutaneous disorder due to mutations in *TSC1* and *TSC2*. TS is reported in 1% of children with autism. In TS, autism is seen in ~25% of individuals and more broadly defined pervasive developmental disorders are seen in ~50%. Children who present with seizures, particularly infantile spasms, in the first 2 years of life are more likely to have learning disability and autism or autism spectrum disorders than those who develop seizures later or remain seizure-free. See 'Tuberous sclerosis (TS)', page 420.

Fragile X syndrome. Autistic features are common in fragile X syndrome. See 'Fragile X syndrome', page 324.

Inverted duplicated chromosome 15 syndrome. In this condition in which there is a small marker chromosome derived from the inversion and duplication of the 15q11–q13 region, all patients present with pervasive developmental disorder.

Genetic advice

Inheritance and recurrence risk

The rate of autism and other forms of pervasive developmental disorder in siblings of autistic probands is 3–5%

(45-fold increase in risk) with an additional 5–7% risk that he/she will have some type of broader social communication disorder of a less seriously handicapping variety (i.e. able to manage in mainstream education with appropriate support). Offspring of sibs are at a low risk (see below).

Variability and penetrance
Variable even amongst close family members.

Prenatal diagnosis
Not possible unless there is a specific monogenic (e.g. TS, FRAX) or chromosomal disorder.

Other family members
- Rate of autism in 2nd degree relatives is 0.13% (Jorde).
- Rate of autism in 3rd degree relatives is 0.05% (Jorde).

Natural history and management
Traditionally autism has been considered to be a lifelong and seriously handicapping disorder but, now that subtler forms of autism spectrum disorder are being recognized, it is becoming appreciated that the outcome may not always be so limited. Educational and behavioural interventions are the mainstay of management. Risperidone shows some promise as a treatment for tantrums, agression, or self-injurious behaviour in children with these associated features. Depressive and psychotic disorders may develop and require psychopharmacological treatment.

Potential-long term complications
About 30% will develop seizures by adult life (often with onset in teenage years). Most individuals with classic autism will not be able to live independently as adults.

Support group: The National Autistic Society <www.nas.org.uk>.

Expert adviser: Patrick Bolton, Professor of Child and Adolescent Psychiatry, The Institute of Psychiatry, London, England.

References
Baird G, Cass H, *et al*. Diagnosis of autism [review]. *Br Med J* 2003; **327**: 488–93.

Borgatti R, Piccinelli P, *et al*. Pervasive developmental disorders and GABAergic system in patients with inverted duplicated chromosome 15. *J Child Neurol* 2001; **16**: 911–14.

Cederlund M, Gillberg C. One hundred males with Asperger syndrome: a clinical study of background and associated factors. *Dev Med Child Neurol* 2004; **46**: 652–60.

Fombonne E. The prevalence of autism. *J Am Med Assoc* 2003; **289**: 87–9.

Jamain S, Quach H, *et al*. Mutations of the X-linked genes encoding neuroligins NLGN3 and NLGN4 are associated with autism. *Nat Genet* 2003; **34**: 27–8.

Jorde LB, Hasstedt SJ, *et al*. Complex segregation analysis of autism. *Am J Hum Genet* 1991; **49**: 932–8.

Miles JH, Hillman RE. Value of a clinical morphology examination in autism. *Am J Med Genet* 2000; **91**: 245–53.

Rapin I. The autistic-spectrum disorders (perspective). *New Engl J Med* 2002; **347**: 302–3.

Simonoff E, Rutter M. Autism and other behavioural disorders. In *Emery and Rimoin's principles and practice of medical genetics*, 4th edn (ed. D.L. Rimoin, J.M. Connor, R.E. Pyeritz, and B.R. Korf), vol. 3, pp. 2873–93. Churchill Livingstone, London, 2002.

Thomas NS, *et al*. Xp deletions associated with autism in three females. *Hum Genet* 1999; **104**: 43–8.

Vincent JB, Kolozsvari D, *et al*. Mutation screening of X-chromosomal neuroligin genes: no mutations in 196 autism probands. *Am J Med Genetics* 2004; **129B**: 82–84.

Volkmar FR, Pauls D. Autism [review]. *Lancet* 2003; **362**: 1133–41.

World Health Organization (WHO). *The ICD-10 classification of mental and behavioural disorders*. World Health Organization, Geneva, 1992.

Beckwith–Wiedemann syndrome (BWS)

Wiedemann–Beckwith syndrome, EMG syndrome (exomphalos, macroglossia, and gigantism).

BWS is a somatic overgrowth and cancer-predisposition syndrome estimated to affect ~1/13 700 individuals (see table for suggested diagnostic criteria). 85% of cases are sporadic and 15% the result of vertical transmission. The overall risk for tumour development in children with BWS is 7.5%. Tumours are predominantly of embryonal origin, e.g. Wilms, hepatoblastoma, and most of the increased tumour risk is in the first 5–8 years of life.

The genetic basis of BWS is complex. 11p15 encodes a 1 Mb cluster of genes involved in growth regulation, many of which are imprinted. These include *IGF2* (a paternally expressed embryonic growth factor), *H19* (a maternally expressed growth supressor gene), *p57KIP2* (also known as *CDKN1C*), which negatively regulates cell proliferation and is preferentially expressed from the maternal allele, and *LIT1*, an antisense transcript (encoded within the *KCNQ1* gene and normally expressed from the paternal allele resulting in methylation of an upstream target region) amongst others. Disturbance to the balance of gene expression, finely tuned by both growth-promoting and growth-suppressing genes and imprinting (with some genes preferentially expressed from the maternal chromosome and others from the paternal homologue), can result in the BWS phenotype. Paternal uniparental disomy (UPD) 11p15 causes increased expression of paternally expressed growth promoter genes (e.g. *IGF2*) and absence of maternally expressed growth suppressor genes (e.g. *H19*) and is found in 10–20% of BWS cases. Mosaic paternal UPD 11p15 is thought to arise as a consequence of somatic recombination. Mutations in *p57KIP2* are found in 5–10% and are more commonly found in familial cases.

There appears to be a 4.2-fold increase in risk of BWS after assisted reproductive technology, e.g. *in vitro* fertilization (IVF) and intracytoplasmic sperm injection (ICSI) (Maher *et al.* 2003).

Clinical approach

History: key points

- Three-generation family tree with parental and sibling birthweights and family history of overgrowth, exomphalos/-omphalocele/umbilical hernia. Were the parents unusually large/tall as children? Document current parental height. Particular attention should be paid to the maternal family history.
- Pregnancy history including enquiry about IVF or assisted reproductive technology, details of USS growth parameters. Polyhydramnios, prematurity (~50%)? Placental size (often placental weight is 2× normal)?
- Birthweight and neonatal problems (e.g. hypoglycaemia).

Examination: key points

- Growth parameters (height, weight, and occipital-frontal circumference (OFC)).
- Ears for creases of the ear lobe and helical pits (look along rim of outer helix).
- Forehead for naevus flammeus.
- Tongue for macroglossia.

Suggested diagnostic criteria for Beckwith–Wiedemann syndrome (BWS)*

Presence of *at least* 3 of the following features (2 major and 1 minor)

Major

Positive family history (one or more family members with a clinical diagnosis of BWS, or suggestive history and features)

Macrosomia (height and weight >97th centile)

Anterior linear ear lobe creases/posterior helical ear pits

Macroglossia

Omphalocele (exomphalos)/umbilical hernia

Visceromegaly involving one or more of liver, spleen, kidneys, adrenal glands, and pancreas

Embryonal tumour (e.g. Wilms tumour, hepatoblastoma, rhabdomyosarcoma) in childhood

Hemihyperplasia (asymmetric overgrowth of region(s) of the body)

Adrenocortical cytomegaly

Renal abnormalities including structural abnormalities, nephromegaly, and nephrocalcinosis

Cleft palate (rare)

Minor

Polyhydramnios

Prematurity

Neonatal hypoglycaemia

Facial naevus flammeus

Haemangioma

Characteristic facies, including midface hypoplasia and infraorbital creases

Cardiomegaly/structural cardiac anomalies/rarely cardiomyopathy

Diastasis recti

Advanced bone age

Monozygotic (MZ) twinning discordance

* No consensus criteria have yet been agreed upon. NB. Since children with milder phenotypes have developed tumours, tumour surveillance should be considered in individuals presenting with fewer than three features, e.g. macroglossia and umbilical hernia or hemihyperplasia only.

- Face for dysmorphic features.
- Face and limbs for hemihyperplasia.
- Abdomen for omphalocele, umbilical hernia, diastasis recti.

Investigation
- Monitor neonates for hypoglycaemia (30–50%) due to hyperinsulinaemia and islet cell hyperplasia.
- Karyotype looking carefully for 11p15 duplication (<1%).
- DNA sample for UPD studies of 11p15. The microsatellite marker *TH* that maps to the tyrosine hydroxylase locus is used to detect evidence of mosaic paternal isodisomy seen in 10–20% of sporadic cases of BWS.
- Consider 11p15.5 methylation assays if BWS likely and no UPD, e.g. assess for maternal methylation at *KvDMR1* (positive in 30–40%).
- Consider *p57KIP2* (*CDKN1C*) mutation analysis (5–10%) if above are negative and clinical diagnosis of BWS is strong. Most likely to be positive if there is a family history and exomphalos.
- Consider abdominal ultrasound scan (USS). USS surveillance (renal, adrenal, and hepatic USS) for nephroblastoma (Wilms), hepatoblastoma, and adrenal cortical tumours.
- Consider echocardiogram and electrocardiogram (ECG). Cardiomegaly of early infancy usually resolves. Cardiomyopathy is very rare but can be severe. Other structural cardiac malformations occur in ~5–15%. May be important if surgery is planned.

Other diagnoses/conditions to consider
See 'Overgrowth', page 206.
- Infant of a diabetic mother.
- Simpson–Golabi–Behmel (SGB) syndrome.
- Perlman syndrome.
- Costello syndrome.

Genetic advice
Inheritance and recurrence risk
85% are sporadic and 15% due to autosomal dominant (AD) transmission (but risks may be modified by parent of origin).
- Paternal UPD (10–20%). Sporadic; very low recurrence risk.
- 11p15 chromosome rearrangements, e.g. translocation/inversion/duplication (rare). Individual assessment required. Consult with cytogeneticists. but recurrence risk could be substantial.
- *p57KIP2* mutation (5–10%). 50% risk if carried by mother.
- Affected parent (10–15%). Recurrence risk may be up to 50% with preferential maternal transmission.
- Karyotype and UPD analysis normal and negative family history. Recurrence risk ~5%.

Variability and penetrance
Expressivity ameliorates with age. Very obvious features in infancy, e.g. macroglossia and macrosomia, may resolve by late childhood/early adult life. This makes it particularly important, when assessing parents of an apparently sporadic case, to obtain detailed information regarding parental birthweights and any neonatal complications the parents may have suffered, e.g. umbilical hernia and hypoglycaemia, and to examine the parents for ear lobe creases and helical pits as the diagnosis may be easy to miss in an adult and has major implications for the assessment of recurrence.

Prenatal diagnosis
- In the uncommon situation that a familial mutation (e.g. *KIP2*) or chromosome rearrangement predisposing to BWS has been identified, prenatal diagnosis by chorionic villus sampling (CVS) may be considered.
- Serial USS and growth parameters beginning with dating USS at 8–10 weeks gestation and including detailed fetal anomaly USS at 19 weeks gestation and subsequently (looking for macrosomia, macroglossia, anterior abdominal wall defect, nephromegaly, enlarged placenta, and polyhydramnios). Macrosomia does not usually become evident until late in second trimester.
- Maternal serum alpha-fetoprotein (AFP) at 15 weeks gestation as a marker for exomphalos (AFP is raised in anterior abdominal wall defects).

Natural history and management
If BWS is suspected antenatally, referral to a specialist in fetomaternal medicine is indicated in view of the obstetric risks of prematurity, polyhydramnios, pre-eclampsia, and fetal macrosomia. Neonates require surveillance for hypoglycaemia for the first few days of life and, if an omphalocele is present, may require sugery in the immediate neonatal period. Macroglossia may make intubation difficult.

Birthweights of babies with BWS are usually ~97th centile and length and weight are also ~+2 SD, although overgrowth is not invariably present. This trend continues through early childhood (bone age typically at upper limit of normal) and then excessive size becomes less dramatic with increasing age. Growth rate typically decreases from mid-childhood through puberty. Adult heights cluster between the 50th and 97th centile (i.e. within the top half of the normal range).

Weng *et al.*'s (1995) longitudinal survey of 15 children showed normal mental and social development in comparison with unaffected siblings and cousins. (Only exception is 11p15 duplication, which is associated with developmental delay, or if there have been major neonatal complications, e.g. severe prematurity, prolonged symptomatic hypoglycaemia.)

Potential long-term complications
- **Tumours.** Overall risk for tumour development estimated at 7.5%. Risk is greatest in pre-school children and 96% of all tumours in Beckwith's series of 121 BWS cases presented by 8 years. In a recent analysis of a cohort of BWS patients, patients with UPD 11p15 were more likely to have hemihypertrophy, cancer, and hypoglycaemia (Debaun *et al.* 2002).
- **Tongue.** Macroglossia if present can cause difficulties in intubation for anaesthesia and occasionally cause serious feeding/respiratory problems and speech problems. Mild to moderate macroglossia tends to improve with time as the mandible grows to accommodate the tongue; severe macroglossia may require surgical intervention by a specialist team with surgery usually undertaken at age 2–4 years.

Surveillance
- USS kidneys, liver, and adrenals at 3–4 monthly intervals (triannually) until 7–8 years.
- Consider 3–4 monthly AFP up to the age of 3 years. Note normal neonates have very high AFP levels (often several thousand kU/l, this declines with a half-life of 5.5 days so that by 4 months of age the mean is 70 kU/l (SD 56).

Adult levels are reached by 7–9 months. Normal adult range is <10 kU/l.

Support group: The Beckwith Wiedemann Support Network <www.geocities.com/bwsn>.

Expert adviser: Eamonn Maher, Professor of Medical Genetics, University of Birmingham, Birmingham, England.

References

Choyke PL, Siegel MJ, *et al.* Screening for Wilms tumor in children with Beckwith–Wiedemann syndrome or idiopathic hemihypertrophy. *Med Pediatr Oncol* 1999; **32**: 196–200.

Cohen MM Jr, Neri G, Weksberg R. Beckwith–Wiedemann syndrome. *Overgrowth syndromes*, Chapter 2, pp. 11–31, Oxford Monographs on Medical Genetics no. 43. Oxford University Press, Oxford, 2002.

Debaun MR, Niemitz EL, *et al.* Epigenetic alterations of H19 and LIT1 distinguish patients with Beckwith–Wiedemann syndrome with cancer and birth defects. *Am J Hum Genet* 2002; **70**: 604–11.

Maher ER, Brueton LA, *et al.* Beckwith–Wiedemann syndrome and assisted reproduction technology (ART). *J Med Genet* 2003; **40**: 62–4.

McNeil DE, Brown M, *et al.* Screening for Wilms tumour and hepatoblastoma in children with Beckwith–Wiedemann syndrome: a cost-effective model. *Med Pediatr Oncol* 2001; **37**: 349–56.

Shuman C, Weksberg R. Beckwith–Wiedemann syndrome. <www.geneclinics.org>.

Weksberg R, Shuman C. Beckwith–Wiedemann syndrome. In *Management of genetic syndromes* (ed. S.B. Cassidy and J.E. Allanson), Chapter 49, pp. 49–69. Wiley-Liss, New York, 2001.

Weng EY, Moeschler JB, *et al.* Longitudinal observations on 15 children with Wiedemann–Beckwith syndrome. *Am J Med Genet* 1995; **56**: 366–73.

Congenital adrenal hyperplasia (CAH)

Autosomal recessive (AR) condition with a prevalence of 1/12 000–1/15 000 resulting from a deficiency of one of the five enzymes required for synthesis of cortisol in the adrenal cortex.

- 21-hydroxylase deficiency (21-OHase). Carrier frequency 1/50. *CYP21* on 6p accounts for >90% of cases.
- 11β-hydroxylase deficiency (11β-OHase). Uncommon.
- 3β-hydroxysteroid dehydrogenase deficiency (3β-HSD). Rare.

21-hydroxylase is involved in the conversion of 17-OH-progesterone (17-OHP) to 11-deoxycortisol; it is also required for aldosterone biosynthesis. Accumulation of 17-OHP leads to increased androstenedione which is converted in the liver to testosterone. Hence the affected female fetus is exposed to increased fetal androgens from as early as 8 weeks gestation.

The clinical presentation of CAH is summarized in the table.

- Girls with classic CAH may be virilized to a variable degree (usually enlarged clitoris; often with labial fusion) due to testosterone production by the adrenal in early pregnancy. The vaginal opening may be normally sited or may open more anteriorly towards the back of the urethra, or even into the back of the urethra at a higher level. Females with classic CAH are likely to be identified at birth due to virilization (ambiguous genitalia).
- Boys with classic CAH usually present in the neonatal period at around 7–10 days old with poor feeding, failure to regain birthweight, dehydration, and collapse (low plasma Na, high K, acidosis, and elevated OH-progesterone (OHP), sometimes with hypoglycaemia).
- If recognized at birth the disorder is treatable by steroid therapy (hydrocortisone ± fludrocortisone and salt), and the subsequent physical and mental development of an affected infant should be normal (with expert supervision).
- Non-classic CAH may be asymptomatic or associated with signs of postnatal androgen excess. It occurs in ~0.2% of the White population, but is more frequent (1–2%) in some ethnic groups, e.g. Jews of Eastern European origin.

Clinical approach

Review results of the biochemical investigations undertaken when the diagnosis of CAH was made to ensure the diagnosis is secure. In 21-OHase deficiency these should show raised 17-OHP, raised testosterone, and elevated renin (if salt-losing). Take expert advice regarding diagnosis of 11 β-OHase or 3 β-HSD deficiency.

History: key points

- Three-generation family tree with specific enquiry about consanguinity and neonatal and infant deaths.

Examination: key points

- Growth parameters.
- Depending on age, examine for features listed in the table giving the clinical presentation.

Investigation

- DNA sample (EDTA (ethylenedinitrilotetraacetate)) to check for *CYP21* mutation in affected child and parents (if 21-OHase deficiency).

Other diagnoses/conditions to consider

Congenital adrenal hypoplasia can present very similarly to CAH with salt-losing crisis (low Na, high K, acidosis, and elevated adrenocorticotrophic hormone (ACTH)) in a male in the first month of life. The presence of normal or low serum 17-OHP strongly suggests X-linked adrenal hypoplasia congenita. One-third have a contiguous gene defect involving *DAX1*, glycerol kinase, and Duchenne muscular dystrophy (may be loss of terminal 3' exons that are not in routine multiplex screen, or deletion may extend more proximally or encompass the whole gene). One-third have other affected male relatives (nearly all have mutations in *DAX1*). One-third have isolated congenital adrenal hypoplasia with no family history (50–70% likelihood of finding a mutation in *DAX1*). Occasionally may present with adrenal failure later in infancy, and rarely with delayed puberty associated with mild or subclinical adrenal insufficiency.

Check creatine kinase (CK).

Pseudohypoaldosteronism. Condition manifesting as a lack of response to aldosterone at the receptor level in the kidney. Presents very similarly to CAH with salt-wasting in the neonatal period (poor feeding, failure to regain birthweight, dehydration, and collapse) but there is no virilization in females and investigations show low Na, high K, normal glucose, and normal 17-OHP and normal testosterone levels. Affected individuals require salt replacement, but unlike in CAH do not require hydrocortisone. The AR form is caused by mutations in the α-subunit (*SCNN1A*), the β-subunit (*SCNN1B*), or the γ-subunit (*SCNN1C*) of the epithelial sodium channel (ENaC). The autosomal dominant (AD) renal form is caused by

Clinical presentation of congenital adrenal hyperplasias (after Hughes 1998)

Type	Female	Male
Classic CAH		
At birth	Ambiguous genitalia	
Neonatal to infancy	Salt loss in 70%	Salt loss in 70%, pigmented scrotum (occasionally)
Early childhood		Penile growth, pubic hair, rapid linear growth, increased musculature
Non-classic CAH		
Late infancy	Clitoromegaly	
Childhood	Pubic hair, increased growth rate	Pubic hair, tall stature
Adolescence	Abnormal menses, hirsutism, acne	Not known
Adult	Hirsutism, oligomenorrhoea, infertility	Not known

Classes of congenital adrenal hyperplasia mutations

Class of CAH mutations	Enzyme activity	Phenotype
Deletions or nonsense mutations	Total loss of enzyme activity	Salt-wasting disease
I172N (missense mutation)	Enzyme activity 1–2% of normal	Simple virilizing disease
	Permits adequate aldosterone synthesis	
V281L, P30L	Enzymes retain 20–60% of normal activity	Non-classic disorder

mutations in the mineralocorticoid receptor gene (*NRJC2*) and tends to show some improvement with age.

Other causes of ambiguous genitalia. See 'Ambiguous genitalia (including sex reversal)', page 38.

Genetic advice

About 10 mutations have been described in the vast majority of patients with CAH, both classic and non-classic (see table). Homozygosity for deletion of *CYP21* causes classic CAH. In classic CAH ~20–25% have a gene deletion and ~30% have an intron 2 splice-site mutation. The missense mutation V281L is the most common mutation in non-classic CAH. Compound heterozygosity is one of the factors underlying phenotypic variation. An individual with non-classic CAH may be at risk of having a child with classic CAH if their partner carries a *CYP21* deletion, and, vice versa, an individual with classic CAH could have a child with non-classic CAH if their partner carried a 'mild' mutation.

1–2% of mutations are spontaneous mutations not carried by either parent (Speiser and White 2003).

Inheritance and recurrence risk

- Following the diagnosis of an affected infant the parents have a 1 in 4 risk for an affected pregnancy (1 in 8 risk for a virilized female).
- For an individual with CAH due to 21-OHase deficiency with an unrelated unaffected partner with no family history, the risk to a pregnancy is $1 \times 1/50 \times 1/2 = 1/100$ for an affected infant (1 in 200 for a virilized female).
- For the sibling of an individual with CAH due to 21-OHase deficiency with an unrelated unaffected partner with no family history, the risk to a pregnancy is $2/3 \times 1/50 \times 1/4 = 1/300$ for an affected infant (1 in 600 for a virilized female).

Variability and penetrance

There is some phenotypic variability amongst relatives carrying the same mutations (modifier genes?).

Prenatal diagnosis

Possible by chorionic villus sampling (CVS) at 11 weeks gestation if the familial mutation is known or if there is certainty over the diagnosis of 21-OH deficiency, in which case markers linked to *CYP21* can be used.

Discuss management of a future pregnancy and the options of:

1 no investigations and accepting 1 in 4 risk of affected infant, in which case make careful arrangements for expert review of at-risk baby after delivery;

2 prenatal diagnosis by CVS, and termination of pregnancy (TOP) in the case of an affected female pregnancy;

3 post-conception maternal steroid therapy to minimize virilization in an affected female pregnancy (see below). There is no evidence of a harmful effect on a baby of maternal dexamethasone therapy during pregnancy, but long-term effects on the developing child are still being evaluated.

Management of a high-risk pregnancy electing for prenatal therapy

- Prior to pregnancy establish the causative *CYP21* mutations and confirm that these are present in the parents. Alternatively, consider possibility of linkage-based prenatal diagnosis, but possibly some genetic heterogeneity with not all 21-OHase families linked to *CYP21*.
- Pregnancy test as soon as possible after late period for very early confirmation of pregnancy.
- If pregnant, start dexamethasone immediately (20 µg/kg/day—tds (*ter die sumendus*, i.e. three times a day) regimen). This regimen should be started early, preferably by 6/40 gestation and certainly by 8/40. Treatment started later than 8 weeks is not likely to completely prevent virilisation of the external genitalia
- CVS at 11 weeks gestation.
- If unaffected pregnancy or affected male pregnancy, stop dexamethasone by tailing dose off over 2 weeks.
- If affected female pregnancy, continue dexamethasone until term (careful antenatal monitoring required).

Management of an at-risk neonate

- Careful assessment for signs of virilization in a female.
- Plasma 17-OHP on day 3 (after first 48 hours) for *urgent* analysis.
- Urea and electrolytes (U & E) and blood glucose also on day 3 (look for low Na and high K; may have hypoglycaemia due to cortisol deficiency).

Other family members

Consider whether apparently unaffected siblings should be investigated with U & E and plasma 17-OHP, possibly repeated following synacthen stimulation.

Natural history and management

Management of a woman with CAH during pregnancy. Women with CAH should be under the joint care of an obstetrician and endocrinologist during pregnancy. Careful endocrine monitoring is required particularly to advise about the endocrine management of the stress of labour and delivery. Maternal circulating androgens have a low risk of causing virilization of a female fetus as placental aromatase efficiently converts testosterone to oestrogens.

Support group: CAH Group (CLIMB) <www.cah.org.uk>.

Expert adviser: Ieuan Hughes, Professor of Paediatrics, University of Cambridge, Cambridge, England.

References

CYP21 working party of the British Society for Paediatric Endocrinology and Diabetes. Protocol for the antenatal adrenal hyperplasia (CYP21) and the subsequent monitoring of outcome parameters post delivery. 2001.

Hughes IA. Congenital adrenal hyperplasia—a continuum of disorders [commentary]. *Lancet* 1998; **352**: 752–4.

Speiser PW, White PC. Congenital adrenal hyperplasia [review]. *New Engl J Med* 2003; **349**: 776–88.

Consanguinity

See also 'Developmental delay in the child with consanguineous parents', page 94 and 'Incest', page 370.

Proportion of nuclear genes shared as a function of degree of relationship

Relationship	Proportion of nuclear genes shared
Monozygotic twins	1 (100%)
First-degree relatives (siblings, parent: child, dizygotic twins)	1/2 (50%)
Second-degree relatives ((half-sibs, double first cousins, uncle/aunt:nephew/niece)	1/4 (25%)
Third-degree relatives (first cousins, half-uncle/aunt:niece/nephew)	1/8 (12.5%)

A consanguineous relationship is one between individuals who are second cousins or closer. Consanguineous marriage is customary in the Middle East, parts of South Asia including Pakistan, in some Jewish communities, and amongst Irish travellers. Although the custom is often perceived to be associated with Islam, in fact, it is (usually) independent of religion. Consanguineous marriage increases the birth prevalence of individuals with recessive disorders. In the Birmingham birth study amongst Northern European children (0.4% of parents related), the prevalence of recessive disorders was 0.28%, compared with British Pakistani children (69% of parents related) in whom the prevalence of recessive disorders was 3.0–3.3%. The effect is particularly marked for rare recessive disorders. The proportion of nuclear genes shared for a given degree of relationship is given in the table.

There is no measurable increase in the rate of spontaneous abortion or infertility in populations with a high incidence of customary consanguineous marriage.

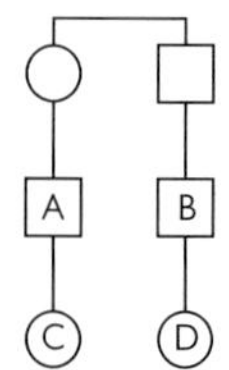 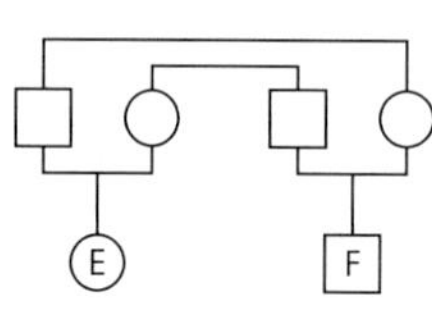

Diagram illustrating the terminology of relationships. A and B are first cousins. A and D and also B and C are first cousins once removed. E and F are double first cousins. C and D are second cousins.

The terminology for relationships is given here and illustrated in the figure.

- **First cousin.** Individuals are first cousins if one of each set of parents are siblings (A and B in figure).
- **Double first cousin.** Individuals are double first cousins if both of each set of parents, respectively, are siblings (E and F in figure).
- **First cousin once removed.** 'Removed' indicates a difference in generations, e.g. a first cousin once removed is the child of a first cousin (A and D in figure; also B and C).
- **Second cousins.** Individuals are second cousins if a paternal grandparent is sibling to a maternal grandparent, i.e. the offspring of first cousins are second cousins (C and D in figure).

Clinical approach

History: key points

- Detailed three-generation family tree including details of younger generations, i.e. cousins, nephews, and nieces. May be necessary to draw a more extensive family tree. Extend the family tree sufficiently far back that the common ancestors are shown.
- Where there is multiple consanguinity it may be helpful in clinic to document *in words* the stated relationships in the family, so that you can return to the family tree later (and if necessary redraw it!) to ensure that it accurately reflects the stated relationships in the family.
- If there is a family member with a known recessive disorder or a potentially recessive disorder (e.g. microcephaly), highlight that individual as the proband in the family tree.

Examination: key points

Usually not relevant.

Special investigations

These are determined by the ethnic origin of the family and the recessive disorders with known high carrier rates in that ethnic group.

- Northern European/Caucasian. Offer cystic fibrosis (CF) carrier testing.
- Mediterranean. Offer haemoglobinopathy screen (thalassaemia and sickle cell disorders) and CF carrier testing.
- Ashkenazi Jewish. Offer Tay–Sachs carrier testing (carrier risk ~1/30 in Ashkenazim) by plasma levels of hexosaminidase A and mutation analysis for the six common *HEXA* mutations (identifies ~98% of mutations in Jewish and 46% of mutations in non-Jewish carriers). Also offer CF carrier testing (including W1282X).
  - For Ashkenazim, DNA testing is the preferred method to ascertain Tay–Sachs carriers.
  - For Tay–Sachs carrier testing in non-Jewish individuals, enzyme assay should be done initially and positive or indeterminate results should be confirmed by DNA mutation analysis. If only one partner is descended from a high-risk group, that person should be tested first; only if he/she is a carrier should the other partner be tested. If the couple is pregnant at the time carrier testing is requested, both partners should have enzyme testing (leukocyte assay for the pregnant woman and serum assay for the father) and DNA testing sent concomitantly to expedite counselling (Sutton 2002).
- African-American/African-Caribbean/African. Offer haemoglobinopathy screen (sickle) and CF carrier testing. NB. Approximately 50% of the genes of African-Americans and African-Caribbeans are of Northern European origin.
- Indian/South-east Asian. Offer haemoglobinopathy screen (thalassaemia and sickle cell disorders) and CF carrier testing. The birth prevalence of children with CF is approximately the same amongst British Pakistanis as amongst northern Europeans (although the gene frequency is less) as a result of common consanguineous marriage.
- Other. Offer CF carrier testing.

Genetic advice—*no autosomal recessive (AR) disorder in extended family*

Two alternative approaches exist: the first is to rely on empiric (observed) data; the second to estimate the risk based on the assumption that each of the common grandparents carries one deleterious recessive gene.

First cousins
- *Empiric data.* Birth prevalence of serious congenital and genetic disorders diagnosed by 1 year for children of unrelated parents is 2.0–2.5%. For children of first-cousin parents the risk is doubled at 4.0–4.5%. Longer-term studies that include conditions diagnosed later in childhood (neurological disorders, thalassaemia, etc.) give an overall 4.0% risk for children of unrelated parents, with an approximate doubling of this risk to 8.0% in offspring of first cousins.
- *Estimated risk.* The probability that both first cousins will carry their grandfather's recessive gene is (1/4 × 1/4). The chance that they would have an affected child in each pregnancy is (1/4 × 1/4 × 1/4), i.e. 1/64. Similarly, the probability that both first cousins will carry their grandmother's recessive gene is (1/4 × 1/4). The combined probability for a pregancy homozygous for a recessive disorder is 1/64 + 1/64 = 1/32 (3%).

Second cousins
- *Empiric data.* The birth prevalence of serious congenital and genetic disorders diagnosed by 1 year for children of unrelated parents is 2.0–2.5%. For children of first cousins once removed, or second cousins the risk is increased by 1.0% to 3.0–3.5%.
- *Estimated risk.* The probability that both second cousins will carry their grandfather's recessive gene and that they would have an affected child is (1/8 × 1/8 × 1/4, i.e. 1/256). The probability that both second cousins will carry their grandmother's recessive gene is the same. The combined probability for a pregnancy homozygous for a recessive disorder is 1/128 (<1%).

Other relationships
See table.

Probability for a pregnancy homozygous by descent for an AR disorder in relationships other than first and second cousins

Relationship	Probability
Double first cousins (fathers are sibs, mothers are sibs))	1/16
Uncle/ aunt: niece/nephew	1/16
First cousins once removed	1/64
Double second cousins	1/64

Multiple consanguinity
The key step is to identify the common ancestors on the family tree. In the case of double first cousins this is the four grandparents or, with double second cousins, the four common great-grandparents. This can be tricky, especially if marriages have occurred between different generations. Once the common ancestors have been identified, then calculate the chance that a pregnancy will be homozygous by descent for each common ancestor, and sum them to obtain the overall risk.

Carrier detection
See above under special investigations.

Prenatal diagnosis
Detailed fetal anomaly ultrasound scanning (USS) will detect structural anomalies that occur in a small percentage of pregnancies affected by severe recessive disorders (e.g. polydactyly, cystic kidneys, congenital heart disease,

structural anomalies of the brain). Most severe recessive disorders will remain undetected as the great majority of metabolic disorders and neurodevelopmental disorders (leukodystrophies, etc.) will not be detectable by fetal USS. Detailed fetal anomaly USS should be offered to first-cousin relationships and closer, but the couple must recognize its limitations. Routine obstetric USS is appropriate for relationships less close than first cousins.

Genetic advice—known AR or possible AR disorder in extended family

If there is a known or possible recessive disorder in the family, other consanguineous relationships within the extended family are at *high* genetic risk for that disorder. The risks are summarized in the figures.

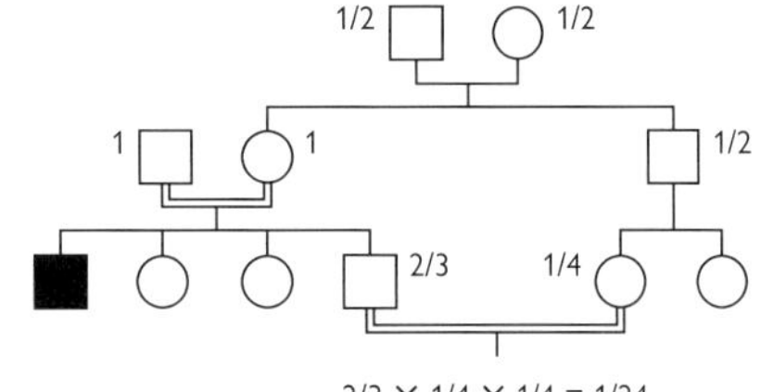

Risk to the offpring of an individual who has a sibling with an AR disorder who marries a first cousin.

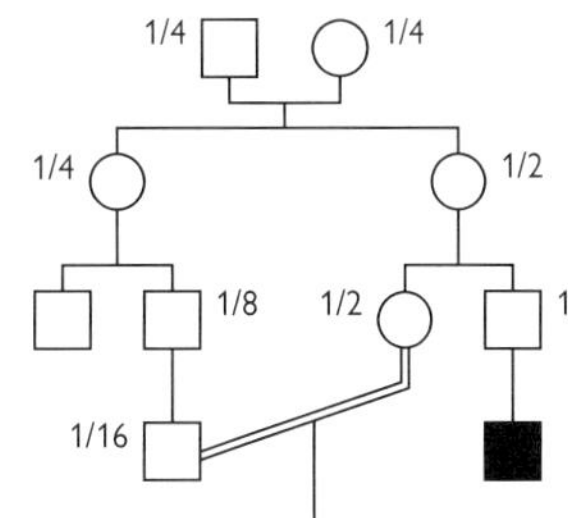

Risk to the offspring of an individual who has a nephew with an AR disorder who marries a first cousin once removed.

Method. Working from the nuclear family of the proband, assign the carrier status to the unaffected siblings (2/3) and the parents (1). Each parent will have inherited their carrier status from one or other of their parents, so assign carrier risk to each grandparent (1/2), and each of the parent's sibs will be at 50% risk (1/2). Continue in this manner until you reach each member of the couple seeking advice. The chance that they will have a child homozygous by descent for the disorder in any pregnancy is (carrier risk of father) × (carrier risk of mother) × 1/4.

Carrier detection
Carrier detection for many metabolic disorders by conventional biochemical methods is problematical due to an overlap in values between heterozygotes and normals. Where accurate carrier detection is not feasible by DNA mutation analysis or linkage studies, it may be preferable to rely on calculated risk from the pedigree combined with the offer of prenatal diagnosis.

Prenatal diagnosis
As for specific diagnosis in the family. Prenatal diagnosis is available for most metabolic disorders, but check with the lab providing the analysis re type of sample required (cultured/ uncultured CVS cells, amniotic fluid, amniocytes, DNA).

Expert adviser: Bernadette Modell, Emeritus Professor of Community Genetics, Royal Free and University College Medical School, London, England.

References

Bundey S, Aslam H. A five-year prospective study of the health of children in different ethnic groups, with particular reference to the effect of inbreeding. *Eur J Hum Genet* 1993; **1**: 206–19.

Harper P. *Practical genetic counselling*, 5th edn. Butterworth-Heinmann, London, 1998.

Kaback MM. Hexosaminidase A deficiency `<www.geneclinics.org>`.

Modell B, Darr A. Genetic counselling and customary consanguineous marriage. *Nat Rev Genet* 2002; **3**: 225–9.

Sutton VR. Tay–Sachs disease screening and counseling families at risk for metabolic disease. *Obstet Gynecol Clin N Am* 2002; **29**: 287–96.

Young ID. *Introduction to risk calculation in genetic couselling*, 2nd edn. Oxford University Press, Oxford, 1999.

Craniosynostosis

Craniosynostosis is defined as premature fusion of the cranial sutures. It has a prevalence of 1 in 2500 children and 15–20% of cases have a recognizable syndromic cause. The aetiology remains unknown in the majority of children with isolated craniosynostosis. Environmental factors are likely to be important determinants.

Craniosynostosis can be suspected clinically and confirmed by skull X-rays that show loss of the affected suture line(s). Computerized tomography (CT) scanning (with bone windows and three-dimensional reconstruction) gives greater precision in borderline cases. Copper beating is evidence of longstanding increased intracranial pressure, although normal markings on the inner vault are at their greatest at 3–4 years of age. Once diagnosed, the condition should be managed by a specialist surgical and medical team.

The sutures between the bones of the skull vault are the main sites of growth, which occurs at right angles to the line of the suture. Growth is controlled by a signalling system that includes ephrins which mark the suture boundaries, fibroblast growth factor receptors (FGFR) and the transcription factor *TWIST*. The five major sutures are coronal, lambdoid, and squamosal, all of which are paired, and the sagittal and metopic which are single. Fontanelles are found where sutures meet. (see fig p146).

Premature fusion leads to an abnormality in the shape of the vault and also affects the growth of the face. Brain growth may be restricted and increasing intracranial pressure can indicate that this is occurring.

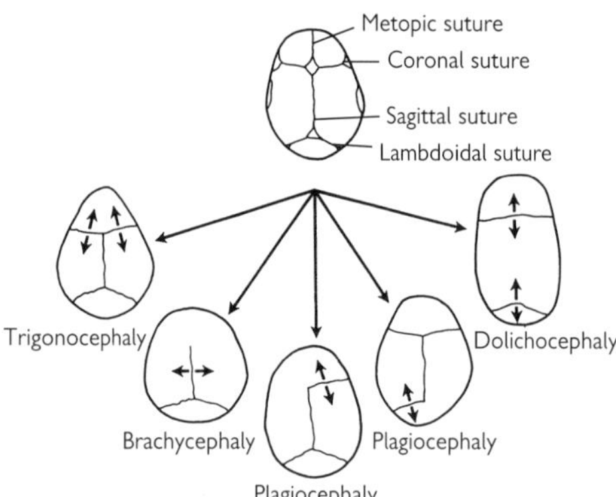

Skull shape resulting from abnormal patterns of suture fusion. (From Pruzansky (1973), by permission.)

The types of craniosynostosis and their effects on skull shape are as follows (see figure).

- **Unilateral coronal synostosis** (10–15%) causes a wide skull with orbital asymmetry.
- **Bicoronal synostosis** (5–10%). The skull is short with a compensatory increase in width and height. Most cases are syndromic. The two sutures may be variably involved so an asymmetric appearance is possible.
- **Lambdoid synostosis** (1%). Very rare.
- **Sagittal synostosis** (50–60%). Progressive elongation of the skull often with a palpable midline ridge.
- **Metopic synostosis** (5–10%). Triangular appearance of the frontal area.

- **Multiple suture involvement** can occur; many cases are syndromic.

Clinical approach

It is assumed that craniosynostosis has been proven. The aim is to determine whether the condition is isolated or part of a syndrome and to determine if there are any other affected family members.

History: key points

- Three-generation family history (consider variable penetrance of a dominant condition). Enquire about consanguinity.
- Pregnancy. Breech presentation, multiple pregnancy, reduced liquor volume, persistent discomfort, and history of head 'feeling stuck', uterine constraint. History of maternal hyperthyroidism. History of maternal drug ingestion eg. valproate (metopic synostosis), fluconazole (Antley-Bixler syndrome).
- Paternal age. Increased in association with *de novo* FGFR mutations.
- Age of presentation and progression of features.
- Neurodevelopmental abnormalities including seizures and delayed developmental milestones.

Examination: key points

- **Head.** Measure occipital-frontal circumference (OFC) and describe the shape of the head. Look for asymmetry. Palpate for ridging of the sutures; document presence and shape of the fontanelles.
- **Eyes.** Measure spacing and check for exorbitism and proptosis.
- **Face.** Midface hypoplasia and beaked nose in combination with exorbitism gives rise to the 'Crouzonoid' facies, which is important to recognize.
- Cleft palate.
- **Ears.** Small with prominent crus helices in Saethre–Chotzen syndrome.
- **Hands, feet, and limbs.** Mild cutaneous syndactyly in Saethre–Chotzen and Pfeiffer syndromes (occurs in less than 50%). Syndactylous bony fusion is diagnostic in Apert syndrome. Broad thumbs and/or halluces are diagnostic in Pfeiffer syndrome, with medial/radial deviation in more severe cases. The hallux may be broad in Saethre–Chotzen syndrome but the facial appearance is different. Muenke syndrome is associated with minor degrees of brachydactyly but this is not diagnostic. Polydactyly is present in Carpenter syndrome. Limited elbow movement is a feature of FGFR2 mutations.
- **Skin.** Acne, acanthosis nigricans, cutis gyratum (Beare–Stevenson syndrome).
- *Examine both parents* for the above features and review family photographs of the parents as children.

Special investigations

To be done in association with a specialist craniofacial team.

- Clinical photography.
- Molecular DNA analysis (EDTA sample). Not indicated for non-syndromic simple metopic and sagittal synostosis. Approximately 30% of children with non-syndromic

coronal craniosynostosis have mutations in *FGFR3* (749C >G, Pro250Arg). For syndromes see below.

- Cytogenetic analysis. Cytogenetic abnormalities are rarely found in a normally developing child with a single suture involved. Children with coronal synostosis, developmental delay, and other malformations require analysis. Consider fluorescent *in situ* hybridization (FISH) for the microdeletion at 7p21.1 involving the *TWIST* gene and for 22q11. Craniosynostosis occurs in ~1% of individuals with del 22q11.
- Further radiological investigations and intracranial pressure monitoring may be necessary.

Syndromic diagnoses to consider

Mutations in the genes for *FGFR1*, *2*, and *3*; *TWIST*; and *MSX2* have been identified in syndromic craniosynostosis. The *FGFR* and *MSX2* mutations act by gain of function, but *TWIST* by haploinsufficiency. Numbers in brackets are Online Mendelian Inheritance in Man (OMIM) database reference numbers.

The *FGFR* craniosynostosis syndromes. These all have autosomal dominant (AD) inheritance but new mutations are common.

- **Apert syndrome *FGFR2* (101200).** Severe syndactyly, often called a mitten hand, distinguishes this syndrome. Developmental delay is found even when there has been no evidence of raised intracranial pressure. Two recurrent mutations account for the majority of cases.
- **Beare–Stevenson syndrome *FGFR2* (123790).** Cutis gyrata are the key physical feature. AD. Often lethal in the newborn period.
- **Crouzon syndrome *FGFR2* (123500).** Shallow orbits leading to exorbitism and a hooked nose are characteristic features. Molecular testing can help to establish if there is a recurrence risk to parents as the clinical features in an affected parent can be mild.
- **Crouzon syndrome with acanthosis nigricans *FGFR3* (134934).** Coronal synostosis.
- **Muenke syndrome *FGFR3* (602849)** has a rather non-specific phenotype with coronal synostosis and occasionally brachydactyly and deafness. It is essential to exclude this diagnosis in every child with coronal synostosis (unilateral or bilateral). This can only be accomplished by molecular genetic testing.
- **Pfeiffer syndrome *FGFR1* and *FGFR2* (101600).** The face is similar to that in Crouzon syndrome but cloverleaf skull is a more frequent complication. Sometimes the thumbs and halluces are broad and there may be a degree of skin syndactyly. *FGFR2* mutations may lead to a more severe craniofacial phenotype.

Saethre–Chotzen syndrome *TWIST* (101400). Asymmetric coronal suture involvement gives facial asymmetry. A low frontal hairline, ptosis, and small ears with a prominent crus are other helpful features. Examine for evidence of skin syndactyly and broad halluces. The majority of patients with Saethre–Chotzen syndrome have mutations in the *TWIST* gene, which codes for a basic helix–loop–helix transcription factor. The presence of learning difficulties and developmental delay suggests a microdeletion of 7p21 rather than an intragenic *TWIST* mutation (approximately 10–20% of patients with Saethre–Chotzen have a large deletion involving *TWIST*). The clinical features show variability within families. Use molecular results to aid counselling.

Craniofrontonasal dysplasia (304110). An X-linked dominant (XLD) disorder that has paradoxically mild manifestations in males. The classical presentation is a female with gross hypertelorism, a midline nasal groove, coronal synostosis, sloping shoulders, characteristic longitudinal splits or ridges in the nails, and occasional syndactyly or polydactyly. Caused by diverse mutations in the *EFNB1* gene encoding ephrin-B1.

Boston craniosynostosis *MSX2* (604757). A rare cause of genetic craniosynostosis. AD inheritance.

Carpenter syndrome (acrocephalopolysyndactyly type II; 201000). A rare autosomal recessive (AR) syndrome with preaxial polysyndactyly. See 'Preaxial polydactyly', page 218.

Genetic advice—syndromic craniosynostosis

Recurrence risk

Test parents when a mutation is known. In the case of a *de novo FGFR* mutation, the recurrence risk is less than 1% and the majority of these mutations represent true sporadic events, often associated with increased paternal age. The recurrence risk in the case of a *de novo TWIST* mutation is unknown and the possibility of germline mosaicism should be considered.

Variability and penetrance

The Muenke and Saethre–Chotzen syndromes show marked variability. Very careful assessment of parents (supported by molecular genetic tesing) is needed.

Prenatal diagnosis

Theoretically possible by chorionic villus sampling (CVS) if a mutation is known. Severity is difficult to predict. Unless definitive prenatal diagnosis is possible and the fetus is known not to be affected, arrange for ultrasound scan (USS) at 36 weeks gestation to ensure that there is no cephalopelvic disproportion prior to delivery.

Other family members

In familial cases, evaluation of the extended family is indicated.

Genetic advice—isolated craniosynostosis

Sagittal synostosis is the most commonly found (approximately 50%). Bilateral involvement of the coronal sutures suggests a strong possibility of a genetic cause and careful examination to exclude syndromal causes and the presence of features in other members of the family as well. Molecular genetic testing for the Muenke syndrome mutation is advised. The observation of a significant environmental factor will help explain the aetiology. In many children the aetiology will be unknown.

Inheritance and recurrence risk

The majority will be sporadic events but sib recurrence risks of 5% for coronal synostosis and 2% for other synostoses, e.g. sagittal synostosis, cover the possibility of a genetic predisposition. Offspring risks for isolated Craniosynostosis have not been well documented in the literature.

Variability and penetrance

Carefully examine both parents and ask for early childhood photographs.

Prenatal diagnosis

Single suture involvement is unlikely to be detected on prenatal scans. The cranial sutures do not develop until after 16 weeks gestation. Arrange for fetal USS at 36 weeks gestation to ensure that there is no cephalopelvic disproportion prior to delivery.

Other family members

Risks to more distantly related individuals are very low.

Natural history and management of children with craniosynostosis

Potential long-term complications

Re-stenosis of a surgically opened suture, raised intracranial pressure, poor growth of the midface, sleep apnoea, exposure keratitis, hearing loss, dental malocclusion, and, rarely, syringomyelia.

Surveillance

Patients should remain under the care of a craniofacial team until facial and cranial growth is complete.

Support group contact. Headlines Craniofacial Support <info@headlines.org.uk>.

Expert adviser: A.O.M. Wilkie, Nuffield Professor of Pathology and Honorary Consultant in Clinical Genetics, University of Oxford, Oxford, England.

References

Cai J, Goodman BK. Increased risk for developmental delay in Saethre–Chotzen syndrome is associated with *TWIST* deletions: an improved strategy for *TWIST* mutation screening. *Hum Genet* 2003; **114**: 68–76.

Cohen MM, MacLean RE. *Craniosynostosis: diagnosis, evaluation and management*, 2nd edn. Oxford University Press, New York, 2000.

Fluck CE, Tajima T, *et al.* Mutant P450 oxidoreductase causes disordered steroidogenesis with and without Antley-Bixler syndrome. *Nat Genet* 2004; **36**: 228–30.

Muenke M, Wilkie AOM. Craniosynostosis syndromes. In *The metabolic and molecular bases of inherited disease*, 8th edn (ed. C.R. Scriver *et al.*), pp. 6117–46. Mc Graw Hill, New York, 2001.

Shackleton C, Marcos J, *et al.* Biochemical diagnosis of Antley-Bixler syndrome by steroid analysis. *Am J Med Genet* 2004; **128A(3)**: 223–31.

Wilkie AOM. Craniosynostosis: genes and mechanisms. *Hum Mol Genet* 1997; **6**: 1647–56.

Cystic fibrosis (CF)

CF is the most common life-limiting autosomal recessive (AR) disorder in the White population. Three clinical phenotypes are associated with mutations in the CF transmembrane conductance regulator gene (*CFTR*) on 7q31–32.

1 Classical CF. Obstructive lung disease, bronchiectasis, exocrine pancreatic insufficiency, elevation of sweat chloride concentration (>60 mM), and infertility in males due to congenital bilateral absence of the vas deferens (CBAVD).

2 Non-classical CF. Chronic pulmonary disease ± pancreatic exocrine disease ± elevated sweat chloride (>60 mM) ± CBAVD.

3 CBAVD. See 'Male infertility: genetic aspects' page 606.

The incidence of CF in Caucasians of European extraction is 1/2000–1/4000 newborns (1/2500 in the UK). CF is rare in native Africans and Asians. The mutation spectrum and frequency are highly dependent on ethnic background. See the first table for the diagnostic criteria for CF.

More than 1000 mutations in CFTR have been identified (see the second table), of which the most common by far is delta F508 (ΔF508). ΔF508 encodes a three-nucleotide deletion resulting in a CFTR protein lacking phenylalanine (F) at postion 508 in the protein. This causes misfolding of the newly synthesized mutant CFTR so that it does not integrate into the cell membrane, but remains in the cytoplasm where it is degraded by the ubiquitin–proteosome pathway. ΔF508 accounts for ~70% of CF alleles, but the exact proportion varies depending on ethnic origin. The next most common mutations are G542X, G551D, delta1507, W1282X, and N1303K, each accounting for only 1–2.5% of known CF alleles. W1282X is common in the Ashkenazi Jewish population. Standard commercial kits for DNA diagnosis usually identify ~29 mutations. In the English population this accounts for ~87% of CF alleles. Thus, using a standard screen, 76% of English patients with CF will have two identifiable CFTR mutations, 22% will have a single identifiable CF mutation, and 2% of patients with CF will have no identifiable mutation. Specialist labs may offer rare mutation screens.

Polythymidine (Poly-T) tracts in intron 8 affect the splicing efficiency of a CFTR allele. The most efficient polymorphism is 9T, 7T has reduced efficiency, and 5T has significantly reduced efficiency. R117H in *cis* with 5T, with ΔF508 as the other allele, usually results in non-classical CF (pancreatic sufficient), whereas R117H in *cis* with 9T with

Criteria for the diagnosis of CF (after Rosenstein and Cutting 1998)

Diagnosis requires at least one criterion from each group

Group 1
- One or more characteristic phenotypic features (see below), e.g. chronic sinopulmonary disease, gastrointestinal and nutritional abnormalities, salt loss syndromes, and male urogenital abnormalities, e.g. CBAVD
- Sibling with CF
- Positive neonatal IRT (immunoreactive trypsinogen test)

Group 2
- Sweat chloride >60 mM on 2 occasions (≥75 mg of sweat is critical to reliability). Some laboratories assay sweat osmolality which is increased in CF (normal range is 62–196 mOsm/kg)
- Identification of 2 CF mutations
- Abnormal nasal potential difference (measure of CFTR-mediated ion transport)

Phenotypic features consistent with diagnosis of CF (after Rosenstein and Zeitlin 1998)
- Chronic sinopulmonary disease. Persistent colonization with typical CF pathogen (*Staphylococcus aureus*, *Haemophilus influenzae*, *Pseudomonas aeruginosa*, *Burkholderia cepacia*), chronic cough and sputum production, persistent chest X-ray abnormalities (bronchiectasis, atelectasis, infiltrates, hyperinflation), airway obstruction (wheezing and air trapping), nasal polyps, X-ray or computerized tomography (CT) abnormalities of paranasal sinuses, clubbing
- Gastrointestinal and nutritional abnormalities. Meconium ileus (10–20%), rectal prolapse (20%), distal intestinal obstruction, pancreatic insufficiency, recurrent pancreatitis, focal biliary cirrhosis or multilobular cirrhosis, failure to thrive (protein–calorie malnutrition), hypoproteinaemia and oedema, complications secondary to lack of fat-soluble vitamins
- Salt loss syndromes. Acute salt depletion, chronic metabolic acidosis
- Male urogenital abnormalities resulting in obstructive azoospermia. CBAVD

Functional classification of CFTR alleles (after McKone et al. 2003)

Class	Functional effect of mutation	Allele
I	Defective protein production	G542X, R553X, W1282X, R11162X, 621–1G → T, 1717–1G → A, 1078ΔT, 3659ΔC
II	Defective protein processing	ΔF508, Δ1507, N1303K, S549N
III	Defective protein regulation	G551D, R560T
IV*	Defective protein conductance	R117H, R334W, G85E, R347P
V*	Reduced amounts of functioning CFTR protein	3849 + 10 kbC → T, 2789+5G → A, A455E
Unknown		711+1G → T, 2184DA, 1898+1G → A

* Compared with class II (including ΔF508 homozygotes). classes IV and V have a significantly lower mortality rate and milder clinical phenotype.

ΔF508 as the other allele typically causes the much milder phenotype of CBAVD without respiratory symptoms.

See <http://www.genet.sickkids.on.ca/cftr> for the Cystic Fibrosis Analysis Consortium CF mutation database.

Clinical approach

History: key points

- Three-generation family tree.
- Genotype of affected individual if known.

Examination: key points

Usually not relevant if affected individual is under the care of CF paediatrician/physician or you are seeing another family member.

Investigation

DNA sample for mutation analysis of *CFTR*.

Genetic advice

Inheritance and recurrence risk

- Autosomal recessive (AR) and so the recurrence risk to parents of an affected child = 1/4. The following recurrence risks are based on pedigree analysis and assuming no consanguinity, no family history of CF in a partner, and a CF carrier rate of 1/23 (see below for carrier rates in different ethnic groups). This risk estimate can be substantially modified by CF mutation analysis in the relative and his/her partner (see below).
- Risk to offspring of healthy sib of an affected child is $2/3 \times 1/23 \times 1/4 = 1/138$.
- Risk to offspring of aunt/uncle or half-sib of an affected child is $1/2 \times 1/23 \times 1/4 = 1/184$.
- Risk to offspring of an affected individual is $1 \times 1/23 \times 1/2 = 1/46$.

Variability and penetrance

Homozygosity for ΔF508 and compound heterozygosity or homozygosity for other non-functional alleles are associated with the classical form of CF. Even in classical CF the age of onset and rate and progression of pulmonary disease are very variable (influenced by modifier genes, infection, nutrition, therapy, smoking, etc.). ΔF508 homozygotes vary considerably in their manifestation of gastrointestinal, hepatobiliary, and pulmonary disease. Monozygotic CF twins are more concordant than dizygotic CF twins. The CF phenotype may be modified by loci in the partially imprinted region on 7q 3' of *CFTR* that determine stature, food intake, and energy homeostasis. All classical cases of CF (ΔF508 homozygotes) have pancreatic insufficiency but there is considerable variability in pulmonary disease. Decline in lung function in CF is associated with colonization by *Pseudomonas aeruginosa* and *Burkholderia cepacia*.

A partially functional allele in combination with a non-functional allele (e.g. ΔF508) is a typical picture in non-classical CF. However, since the standard screening panel comprises mainly non-functional alleles, many patients with non-classical CF will have only one identifiable CF allele, i.e. those patients in whom clinical diagnosis is most challenging are often those most difficult to diagnose genetically.

In comparison with ΔF508 homozygotes, ΔF508/R117H, ΔF508/A455E, ΔF508/3849 + 10 kb C → T and ΔF508/ 2789 + 5G → A are associated with mild clinical manifestations (McKone *et al.* 2003).

Prenatal diagnosis

Possible by chorionic villus sampling (CVS) at 11 weeks gestation if both mutations are known. If a single or neither mutation is known, diagnosis of CF is secure, and paternity is certain, it is possible to offer linkage studies to capture unidentified allele(s) and enable prenatal diagnosis. Pre-implantation genetic diagnosis (PGD) for ΔF508 homozygotes is available in some centres.

Predictive testing

This may be applicable in younger siblings of a child recently diagnosed with CF, in view of the benefits of treatment with prophylactic antibiotics and pancreatic and vitamin supplements.

Other family members

When an individual is diagnosed with CF, and mutation analysis is performed, it is routine practice to offer carrier testing to both parents. Cascade screening of the extended family for the mutation identified in their relative can then be offered. Where an individual is shown to be a CF carrier, population-based screening (see table) can be offered to his/her partner to determine the risk to their offspring. Carrier testing of children is usually deferred until 16 years when they are of an age to be involved in decision-making and old enough to understand the implications of the result.

Carrier rates and mutation detection rates in different ethnic populations

Population	Carrier frequency	Mutation detection rate with panel appropriate to ethnic group (%)
Ashkenazi Jewish	1 in 23	97
Northern European	1 in 23	90
Hispanic	1 in 46	57
African-American	1 in 65	75
Asian	1 in 90	30

Natural history and management

Potential long-term complications

- **Respiratory failure.** Pulmonary disease is the main cause of morbidity and mortality in patients with CF. Heart–lung transplantation may be considered for end-stage disease.
- **Diabetes.** 25–50% have an abnormal glucose tolerance test (GTT) by their 20s and 5% require insulin.
- **Liver disease.** 5% of adults have cirrhosis and portal hypertension.
- **Male infertility.** 97% of males with CF have CBAVD with obstructive azoospermia. Pregnancy may be possible with assisted reproductive technology (see 'Male infertility: genetic aspects' page 606), in which case offer mutation analysis to partner.

Surveillance

Evidence is emerging that management of CF in paediatric and adult CF centres results in a better clinical outcome. In the US median survival has reached 31.1 years for men and 28.3 years for women. Survival to the 30s and 40s is no longer rare. Median survival for patients with pancreatic sufficiency (non-classical CF) is 56 years.

Pregnancy in women with CF

Fertility in women with CF is impaired, but successful pregnancy is possible. In a retrospective study from France, of 75 pregnancies, 64 were liveborn (18% premature and 30% low-birthweight), there were 5 miscarriages, 5 therapeutic abortions, and one maternal death. Three women died in the year following a pregnancy, all of whom had a forced expiratory volume in 1 second (FEV_1) <50% before pregnancy (Gillet *et al.* 2002). A retrospective audit of 33 successful pregnancies from Scandinavia found that preterm delivery occurred in 24% (Odegaard *et al.* 2002). The lung function of women delivering preterm was significantly lower than that of those delivering at term, and they were most likely to have other CF complications including diabetes, asthma, or liver disease. Lung function did not deteriorate during pregnancy, but the need for intravenous (IV) antibiotics was doubled. Women with mild to moderate disease may safely go through pregnancy.

- Offer mutation analysis to partner (offer CVS if partner is a CF carrier).
- Refer to CF physician for assessment of likely impact of pregnancy on respiratory reserve.
- Increased risk of gestational diabetes due to pancreatic insufficiency in women with classical CF.
- Consider the drug regimen of your patient and whether any of the drugs have teratogenic potential.
- Pregnancy should be jointly managed by an obstetrician with special expertise in maternal and fetal medicine and a CF specialist.

Neonatal screening

Most neonatal screening programmes for CF combine assay of immunoreactive trypsinogen (IRT) on a dried blood spot (Guthrie card), with analysis for common CF mutations, e.g. ΔF508. An IRT of 60–70 μg/l is equivocal and >70 μg/l is positive. This approach has been well studied but misses some children with CF and detects more ΔF508 carriers than expected. The excess of ΔF508 heterozygotes is associated with the presence of a second mutation or the 5T allele in some infants. In one study of 57 subjects with positive IRT who were ΔF508 heterozygotes, three had clinical CF at 1 year.

Support group: Cystic Fibrosis Trust <www.cftrust.org.uk>.

Expert advisers: David A. Lomas, Professor, Respiratory Medicine Unit, Department of Medicine, University of Cambridge, Cambridge and Di Bilton, Consultant Respiratory Physician and Director of the Adult CF Unit, Papworth Hospital, Cambridge, England.

References

Dankert-Roelse JE, te Meerman GJ. Screening for cystic fibrosis—time to change our position? [editorial]. *New Engl J Med* 1997; **337**: 997–8.

Durie PR. Pancreatitis and mutations of the cystic fibrosis gene [editorial]. *New Engl J Med* 1998; **339**: 687–8.

Gillet D, de Braekeleer M, *et al.* Cystic fibrosis and pregnancy. Report from French data (1980–1999). *Br J Obstet Gynaecol* 2002; **109**: 912–18.

Mahadeva R, Webb K, *et al.* Clinical outcome in relation to care in centres specialising in cystic fibrosis: cross sectional study. *Br Med J* 1998; **316**: 1771–7.

Massie RJ, Wilcken B, *et al.* Pancreatic function and extended mutation analysis in DeltaF508 heterozygous infants with an elevated immunoreactive trypsinogen but normal sweat electrolyte levels. *J Pediatr* 2000; **137**: 214–20.

McKone EF, Emerson SE, *et al.* Effect of genotype on phenotype and mortality in cystic fibrosis: a retrospective cohort study. *Lancet* 2003; **361**: 1671–6.

Mekus F, Laabs U, *et al.* Genes in the vicinity of CFTR modulate the cystic fibrosis phenotype in highly concordant or discordant F508del homozygous sib pairs. *Hum Genet* 2003; **112**: 1–11.

Neill AM, Nelson-Piercy C. Hazards of assisted conception in women with severe medical disease. *Hum Fertil* 2001; **4**: 239–45.

Odegaard I, Stray-Pedersen B, *et al.* Maternal and fetal morbidity in pregnancies of Norwegian and Swedish women with cystic fibrosis. *Acta Obstet Gynecol Scand* 2002; **81**: 689–705.

Rosenstein BJ, Cutting GR. The diagnosis of cystic fibrosis: a consensus statement. *J Pediatr* 1998; **132**: 589–95.

Rosenstein BJ, Zeitlin PL. Cystic fibrosis. *Lancet* 1998; **351**: 277–82.

Dementia

The Royal College of Physicians Committee on Geriatrics (1981) defined dementia as 'The global impairment of higher cortical functions including learned perceptuomotor skills, the correct use of social skills, and the control of emotional reactions in the absence of gross clouding of consciousness. The condition is often irreversible and progressive'.

Clinically, dementia affects memory, speech, perception, and mood. The risk of developing dementia increases with age. Alzheimer disease is the most common neurodegenerative condition affecting older people. Alzheimer disease has a prevalence of 1–2% among those aged 65–69 years increasing to 40–50% among persons 95 years of age and over. Dementia is a feature of many progressive disorders affecting the central nervous system (CNS) but the most common dementia over the age of 40 years is Alzheimer disease. Other common causes include vascular dementia, Lewy body dementia, frontotemporal dementia, and Parkinson disease.

Pathologically, Alzheimer disease and many other neurodegenerative disorders are characterized by neuronal loss and intracellular and/or extracellular aggregates of proteinaceous fibrils. In Alzheimer disease these are intracytoplasmic neurofibrillary tangles (hyperphosphorylated forms of the microtubular protein tau) and extracellular amyloid or senile plaques. The amyloid in senile plaques is a cleavage product of β-amyloid precursor protein formed by the action of the β- and γ-secretases. Another group of dementing disorders are known as tauopathies (e.g. some fronto-temporal dementia) where the tangles are 'tau'-rich and another group are called synucleinopathies (e.g. Parkinson disease, Lewy body dementia, multisystem atrophy) where the filamentous lesions comprise α-synuclein. There is not, however, a simple relationship between disease, mutation, and pathology as, for example, there is accumulation of 'tau' protein in Alzheimer disease. The references address these complex issues in more detail.

Early-onset Alzheimer disease can be defined as onset at age <65 years. Campion *et al.* (1999) undertook a prevalence study based on the population of Rouen and (using a very strict definition of early-onset Alzheimer disease with age of onset <61 years) found a prevalence of early-onset Alzheimer disease of 41.2/100 000 persons at risk and of familial Alzheimer disease (defined as early-onset Alzheimer disease in three generations) of 5.3/100 000 persons at risk.

Clinical approach

Affected individuals need a full systems interview, examination, and diagnostic evaluation by an appropriate specialist (e.g. neurologist or old-age psychiatrist) in order to identify potentially treatable causes of cognitive impairment or dementia.

History: key points

- Three-generation family history with specific enquiry regarding affected relatives, age of onset, rate of progression, age at death. Is the progression of the memory loss gradual (Alzheimer disease) or step-wise (vascular dementia)?
- Past medical history and social history (association of dementia with trauma, infection, alcohol excess, seizures).
- Is there an associated movement disorder (Huntington disease (HD), Parkinson disease)?
- Is there a history of stroke or transient ischaemic attacks (cerebral autosomal dominant arteriopathy with

subcortical infarcts and leukoencephalopathy (CADASIL), multi-infarct dememtia)?

Examination: key points

- Not usually indicated if you are seeing an asymptomatic relative.
- If you are concerned that the consultand is affected then refer to a neurologist for specialist evaluation and diagnosis.
- There are no clinical differences between sporadic Alzheimer disease and early-onset autosomal dominant (AD) types other than the age of onset.

Investigation

- Affected individuals may require diagnostic evaluation before genetic counselling is given to related individuals.
- Consider DNA storage on affected individuals when a genetic aetiology is possible, after obtaining appropriate consent.
- Consider β*APP*, *PSEN1*, and *PSEN2* mutation analysis in an affected member of the family if they have early-onset disease (onset at <61 years) or a family history of the disease (e.g. affected relative in three generations with at least one having early-onset disease).

Other diagnoses/conditions to consider

Genetic dementia

- **Alzheimer disease** (see below).
- **AD frontotemporal dementia with parkinsonism (including Pick disease).** The second most common presenile dementia after Alzheimer disease. AD and caused by mutation in the tau gene (*MAPT*) on 17q21 which encodes the microtubule-associated protein tau, the primary component of neurofibrillary tangles found in Alzheimer disease and some other neurodegenerative disorders.
- **Lewy body dementia.** One of the three most common causes of dementia in older people (with Alzheimer disease and vascular dementia). Clinical presentation is typically with fluctuating cognitive impairment, visuospatial dysfunction, marked attentional deficits, psychiatric symptoms (especially complex visual hallucinations), and mild extrapyramidal features (Wilcock 2003).
- **CADASIL** (cerebral AD arteriopathy with subcortical infarcts and leukoencephalopathy). Associated with *NOTCH* gene mutation.
- **Huntington disease** (HD) is characterized by an involuntary movement disorder (chorea), psychiatric disturbance, and dementia. AD and caused by a triplet repeat expansion (CAG) in the huntingtin gene on 4p. (see 'Huntington disease', page 354).
- **Prion diseases** (Gerstmann–Straussler–Shencker syndrome and Creutzfeld–Jakob disease (CJD)). AD and caused by mutations in the *PRNP* gene on 20p. Prion diseases may also be sporadic or have infectious aetiologies (eg. new-variant CJD).
- **Late-onset metabolic disorders**, e.g. adrenoleukodystrophy (X-linked) and other rare, mainly autosomal recessive (AR) disorders.

Multifactorial dementia

- **Sporadic Alzheimer disease.**
- **Vascular dementia due to repeated infarcts (excluding CADASIL).**

Other causes
- Aids-related. The most prevalent dementing disease in the USA among those aged <40 years.
- Treatable conditions such as drug toxicity in the elderly, nutritional deficiency, hypothyroidism.
- Alcohol-related.
- Tumour.
- Vasculitis.
- Head injury.
- Transmitted CJD.

Genetic advice

Family history of Alzheimer disease

Alzheimer disease may be caused by monogenic, high penetrance mutations, but Alzheimer disease risk can also be influenced by complex predisposition alleles, e.g. apolipoprotein E (*APOE*). As stated above, there is no clinical or pathological way of distinguishing genetic from sporadic Alzheimer disease in an individual. Family history and age of onset are used to initially determine the likelihood of an inherited Alzheimer disease.

Linkage analysis of familial Alzheimer disease has identified three causative genes: β-amyloid precursor protein (β*APP*) on chromosome 21; presenilin 1 (*PSEN1*) on chromosome 14; and presenilin 2 (*PSEN2*) on chromosome 1. The presenilin and β*APP* mutations found in familial early-onset Alzheimer disease appear to result in the increased production of Aβ_{42}, which is probably the principal neurotoxin in these forms of Alzheimer disease.

The inheritance of different *APOE* genotypes affects the age of onset and apparent risk of Alzheimer disease. Three variants, *APOEε2*, *ε3*, and *ε4*, exist. Carrying one *APOEε4* allele doubles the lifetime risk of Alzheimer disease from 15% to 29%, whereas not carrying an *APOEε4* allele cuts the risk by 40% (Campion *et al.* 1999). Nevertheless, the rate of disease-free survival in individuals homozygous for *APOEε4* is high. The main effect of the *APOEε4* allele seems to be to shift the age of onset an average of 5–10 years earlier in the presence of one allele and 10–20 years earlier in homozygotes in persons with an underlying susceptibility to Alzheimer disease (Meyer *et al.* 1998). The usefulness of *APOE* testing is controversial—50% of those with a pathological diagnosis of Alzheimer made at post mortem do not carry an *APOEε4* allele. APOE testing is generally not indicated in a clinical setting, e.g. for clinical diagnosis/prediction. However, it may be useful in research contexts.

Mutation testing for the other three genes is offered by some centres, usually as part of a research facility. Using a very strict definition of AD Alzheimer disease (early-onset disease in three generations), Campion *et al.* (1999) found *PSEN1* mutations in ~50% and β*APP* mutations in 15%.

Inheritance and recurrence risk

Early-onset dementia For families with a known mutation, or clearly dominant FH, Mendelian risks may be used.

Later-onset dementia For most families empiric risks are all that can be given. These are discussed by Breitner (2002) who gives a three to four fold risk of developing Alzheimer disease in the first-degree relatives of individuals with Alzheimer disease compared to controls (19% against 5%).

Variability and penetrance

In the families with genetic Alzheimer disease there is age-dependent penetrance with variability caused by other genetic and environmental factors.

Prenatal diagnosis
Theoretically possible by chorionic villus sampling (CVS) in families with a known mutation.

Predictive testing
Has been reported in families with known Alzheimer disease mutations using a protocol similar to that used in HD.

Other family members
Later-onset disease See Breitner (1991). Risks for second-degree relatives are about twice that for controls (i.e. ~10%).

Natural history and management

Individuals affected by early-onset dementia should be referred to a neurologist or psychiatrist with special expertise in dementia for comprehensive evaluation, investigation, and care. Cholinesterase inhibitors, e.g. Arisept, may be of limited benefit. Drug therapy for vascular dementia is under development.

Potential long-term complications
Progressive loss of higher mental functions with loss of independence.

Surveillance
At-risk individuals are advised to avoid deleterious environmental factors such as alcohol excess. Folic acid supplementation may have some protective value.

Support group: <www.alzheimers.org.uk>.

Expert advisers: David Rubinsztein, Wellcome Senior Clinical Fellow, Cambridge Institute for Medical Research, Cambridge and Judy Rubinsztein, Clinical Lecturer in Old Age Psychiatry, University of Cambridge, Cambridge, England.

References

Baraitser M. *London Neurology database*. Oxford University Press, Oxford.

Breitner JC. Clinical genetics and genetic counselling in Alzheimer disease. *Ann Intern Med* 1991; **115**: 601–6.

Campion D, Dumanchin C, *et al.* Early-onset dominant Alzheimer disease: prevalence, genetic heterogeneity and mutation spectrum. *Am J Hum Genet* 1999; **65**: 664–70.

Meyer MR, Tschanz JT, *et al.* APOE genotype predicts when—not whether—one is predisposed to develop Alzheimer disease. *Nat Genet* 1998; **19**: 321–2.

Morishima-Kawashima M, Ihara Y. Alzheimer's disease: beta-amyloid protein and tau. *J Neurosci Res* 2002; **70**: 392–401.

Nussbaum RL, Ellis CE. Alzheimer's disease and Parkinson's disease. *New Engl J Med* 2003; **348**: 1356–64.

Roses AD, Pericak-Vance MA, Saunders A. Alzheimer disease and other dementias. *Rimoin's principles and practice of medical genetics*, 4th edn (ed. D.L. Rimoin, J.M. Connor, R.E. Pyeritz, and B.R. Korf). Churchill Livingstone, London, 2002.

Royal College of Physicians Committee on Geriatrics. Organic mental impairment in the elderly. *J R Coll Physicians London* 1981; **15**: 141–67.

Selkoe DJ, Podlisny MB. Deciphering the genetic basis of Alzheimer's disease. *Annu Rev Genomics Hum Genet* 2001; **3**: 67–99.

Tobin SL, *et al.* The genetics of Alzheimer disease and the application of molecular tests. *Genet Test* 1999; **3**: 37–45.

Trojanowski JQ. Tauists, Baptists, Syners, apostates, and new data. *Ann Neurol* 2002; **52**: 263–5.

Wilcock GK. Dementia with Lewy bodies [commentary]. *Lancet* 2003; **362**: 1689–90.

Yip AG, Brayne C, *et al.* Apolipoprotein E4 is only a weak predictor of dementia and cognitive decline in the general population. *J Med Genet* 2002; **39**: 639–43.

Diabetes mellitus

Diabetes mellitus is a common and rapidly growing medical problem arising from a combination of environmental and genetic risk factors. The condition is divided into two types.

- Type 1 diabetes mellitus (T1D) formerly known as insulin-dependent diabetes mellitus (IDDM).
- Type 2 diabetes (T2D) formerly known as non-insulin-dependent diabetes mellitus (NIDDM), although in fact ~50% of T2D subjects require insulin within 6 years of diagnosis.

Type 1 diabetes affects about 0.3% of Caucasians with the highest rates in northern Europe, (1–1.5% in Finland). The condition becomes less frequent moving south in Europe to Africa. It is 10 times less common in Japan than in the USA. The condition is caused by selective destruction of the pancreatic β-cells. Insulin deficiency leads to the presenting signs of polyuria and polydipsia as the glucose level in the blood rises and causes an osmotic diuresis. Treatment of T1D is insulin replacement therapy by percutaneous injection. The aetiology is complex and the condition arises from the action of many genes and environmental factors. There is rarely evidence for monogenic inheritance.

  Type 2 diabetes is becoming more common as the population becomes older and fatter. It is estimated that 1 in 10 of European and US individuals will develop T2D.

  T2D is pathologically heterogeneous, but is most commonly the result of defects in the action of insulin (insulin resistance) with a secondary failure of the β-cells to compensate with increased insulin production. Thus at diagnosis, the insulin levels may be high although insufficient to overcome the insulin resistance, but as the disease progresses the insulin levels fall as β-cells become exhausted, and so absolute, rather than just relative insulin deficiencies may be seen at later stages.

  Treatment is by dietary and lifestyle manipulation and oral hypoglycaemic medication in the early stages, with many progressing to insulin therapy within a few years.

  Although the environmental factors are more apparent than in T1D, there has been more success in identifying monogenic forms of T2D.

Neonatal diabetes

Transient neonatal diabetes (TND) is a rare but distinct type of diabetes. Classically, neonates present with growth retardation and diabetes in the first week of life. Apparent remission occurs by 3 months but there is a tendency for children to develop diabetes in later life. Evidence suggests it is the result of overexpression of an imprinted and paternally expressed gene/s within the TND critical region at 6q24 (Temple and Shield 2002). Three genetic mechanisms have been shown to result in TND: paternal uniparental isodisomy of chromosome 6; paternally inherited duplication of 6q24; and a methylation defect at a CpG island overlapping exon 1 of *ZAC/HYMAI* (two imprinted genes that have been identified as potential candidates).

Permanent neonatal diabetes One third of patients with permanent neonatal diabetes and 4% of those with transient neonatal diabetes have activating mutations in *KCNJ11* encoding the potassium channel Kir6.2 subunit. Five cases with a *KCNJ11* mutation have significant developmental delay, epilepsy, contractures and mild facial dysmorphic features (Gloyn).

Clinical approach

History: key points

- Three-generation family history. Any evidence of mitochondrial inheritance?
- Autoimmune diseases, e.g. hypo- or hyperthyroidism, vitiligo, Addison disease, systemic lupus erythematosus (SLE), rheumatoid arthritis.
- Deafness, muscle weakness, stroke-like episodes, ophthalmoplegia, pigmentary retinopathy (mitochondrial disorders).
- Growth failure in children and adolescents (due to insulin resistance).
- Weight gain (insulin resistance).

Examination: key points

- Height and weight. Body mass index. Blood pressure.
- Skin. Acanthosis nigricans (insulin resistance), vitiligo (autoimmune disease).
- Body fat distribution. Look carefully for features of lipodystrophy—Inherited lipodystrophy is usually either total or predominantly limb/gluteal, Acquired lipodystrophy has patchy areas of loss of subcutaneous fat, e.g. typically on the face, also on the shoulders and upper arms.
- Pseudoacromegaly in severe insulin resistance; large jaw and hands.
- Insulin resistance may be associated with hyperandrogenism (hirsutism, acne, polycystic ovary syndrome).
- Features of mitochondrial disease (e.g. ptosis).
- Evidence of diabetic complications in affected individuals.

Investigation

- Fasting insulin level if there are signs of insulin resistance.
- Autoantibodies are positive in 90% of northern Europeans at the time of diagnosis of T1D (most commonly anti-glutamic acid decarboxylase (GAD), anti-islet cell).
- Mitochondrial DNA testing. 3243 bp mitochondrial deletion commonly found in MELAS (mitochondrial myopathy–encephalopathy–lactic acidosis–stroke-like episodes) in families with a maternal mitochondrial mode of inheritance (consider if there is another affected family member in the matrilineal line or if associated with deafness or other features of MELAS).
- Mutation analysis may be available in monogenic causes of T2D including lipodystrophies.

If you are seeing an 'at-risk' family member consider:

- blood glucose. A fasting blood glucose >7 mmol/l on two occasions = diabetes mellitus (American Diabetic Association diagnostic criteria); a fasting blood glucose 5.6–6.9 mmol/l = impaired fasting glucose (i.e. needs follow-up by GP/physician). NB. Individuals with mutations in gluokinase (see 'Maturity-onset diabetes of the young (MODY)' below) have stable hyperglycaemia throughout life.

Diagnoses/conditions to consider

Type 1 diabetes

The HLA (human leukocyte antigen), or MHC (major histocompatibility complex), region and the insulin gene region are thought to contain the main susceptibility genes for IDDM, although at least 20 regions have been linked to IDDM.

- The IDDM1 locus contains several genes in the MHC complex on 6p21.3 and accounts for about 40% of the familial aggregation of IDDM.
- The IDDM2 locus is at 11p15.5. The insulin minisatellite, INS VNTR, is 596 bp upstream from the translation initiation site of the insulin gene. It is associated with increased susceptibility to IDDM and also NIDDM, polycystic ovarian syndrome, and variation in birth size.
- Most studies have been on European and US families and there may be ethnic differences. Risks follow a multifactorial mode. Genetic factors can be seen in the difference in concordance between monozygous twins and siblings.

Type 2 diabetes

There are major environmental risk factors for the development of T2D but as a geneticist it is important to recognize the monogenic types of T2D where there has been progress in identifying the susceptibility genes. Owen *et al.* (2003) studied 268 unselected Caucasians presenting with apparent T2D at ages 18–45 years. 10% were positive for a β-cell antibody, one had familial partial lipodystrophy with a lamin A/C mutation, two had the MELAS 3243 mitochondrial point mutation, two of a selected subset had HNF-1α mutations.

Maturity-onset diabetes of the young (MODY). MODY is a form of T2D with autosomal dominant (AD) inheritance, non-obese body habitus, and an age of onset before 25 years. It accounts for 1–2% of people with diabetes. Five genes account for 87% of UK MODY.

- ***HNF*-1α** (hepatocyte nuclear factor-1α gene). 70% of MODY cases have mutations in this gene. Two-thirds remain non-insulin-dependent throughout life, although one-third ultimately require insulin. Patients are extremely sensitive to sulfonylureas (Pearson *et al.* 2003).
- **Glucokinase gene.** A relatively benign form that does not progress to insulin requirement
- **Renal cysts and diabetes (RCAD).** *HNF*-1β (hepatocyte nuclear factor-1β). AD disorder characterized by unexplained familial renal cystic disease (renal cysts may be detected *in utero*), early-onset T2D, genital tract malformations, hyperuricaemia, and early-onset gout (Edgehill). Renal biopsy shows cystic renal dysplasia or glomerulocystic disease. Pancreas atrophy is common (Bellanne-Chantelot). ~50% of cases result from a large genomic deletion (>1Mb) encompassing the gene.
- ***HNF*-4α** (hepatocyte nuclear factor 4-α gene). Less common that *HNF*-1α, but with similar characteristics, although age of diagnosis may be later.
- ***IPF1*** (insulin promoter factor-1 gene).

Mitochondrial mutations. The most common symptom other than the diabetes is *deafness* and this usually precedes the diabetes. Other signs of mitochondrial disease may be present and should be considered in all affected members of the family. The most common mutation found is the 3243 bp deletion, which is also found in MELAS. For more details about genetic advice, see 'Mitochondrial DNA diseases', page 384.

Insulin receptor mutation.

1 When two mutations are present there is severe insulin resistance and extremely high insulin levels.
- **Donohue syndrome** (leprechaunism). This is the most severe form presenting in infancy with pre- and postnatal failure to thrive, hirsutism, aged face with thick lips and prominent ears, and enlargement of breasts and genitalia. Inheritance is autosomal recessive (AR).
- **Rabson–Mendenhall syndrome** (acanthosis nigricans, polycystic ovaries, virilization of females) is a less severe form presenting later. Inheritance is AR.

2 AD inheritance of a single dominant-negative mutation may cause type A Insulin resistance +/– diabetes mellitus.

Lipodystrophy

Lipodystrophy syndromes are characterized in broad terms by loss of subcutaneous adipose tissue and have similar metabolic attributes including insulin resistance, hyperlipidaemia, and diabetes.

Familial partial lipodystrophy (Dunnigan variety). AD disorder caused by missense mutations in lamin A/C gene (*LMNA*). It is characterized by loss of subcutaneous fat from the extremities and trunk and accumulation of fat in the head and neck region beginning at puberty.

'Diabetes plus'—diabetes as a component of a syndrome

See table 'Association between syndromes and diabetes' (below)

Wolfram syndrome (diabetes insipidus–diabetes mellitus–optic atrophy–deafness (DIDMOAD)). AR condition. It is caused by mutations in *WFS1* on 4p 16.1. Patients often have renal tract anomalies, e.g. hydronephrosis.

Genetic advice

Inheritance and recurrence risk

- **T1D**.
  - 30–50% concordance in monozygous twins.
  - Sibling risk 6% (up to 10% in some studies with a higher background rate) with HLA identical sibs having a greatly increased risk of developing T1D.
  - Offspring risks show some differences between affected fathers and mothers; a greater proportion of fathers (approximately 4%) than mothers (approximately 2%) of children with IDDM have the disease themselves.
- **MODY** follows AD inheritance.
- **Insulin receptor mutations.** Both Donohue and Rabson–Mendenhall syndrome follow AR inheritance.

Associations between syndromes and diabetes

Deafness	Eye signs*	Renal disease	Severe obesity	Severe insulin resistance
MELAS[†]	Prader—Willi (RP)	Renal cysts and diabetes	Prader—Willi[ø]	Donohue
Wolfram[ø]	Alstrom (RP)	Wolfram	Alstrom	Rabson—Mendenhall
	Bardet-Biedl (RP)	Bardet—Biedl[ø]	Bardet-Biedl	partial lipodystrophy
	Wolfram (OA)			

* RP, Retinitis pigmentosa; OA, optic atrophy.
[ø] See 'Mitochondrial disorders' in Common conditions
[†] See Clinical approach to 'Obesity with/without developmental delay

Type A Insulin Resistance (less severe) may also be AD

Variability and penetrance
- **T1D.** Although thought of as a disease of childhood, the onset is after 20 years in 50%.
- **MODY.** Penetrance is high, ~95%. Environmental factors influence the age of onset.

Prenatal diagnosis
- **T1D.** Not available.
- **MODY.** Not usually offered.
- **Donohue syndrome.** Available by chorionic villus sampling (CVS) if mutations are known.

Predictive testing
- **T1D.** HLA testing of sibs has been used but half of HLA-compatible sibs will never develop the condition. There is no presymptomatic treatment to alter the disease process. Consider the ethical position and issues of informed consent. Autoantibodies (anti-islet cell, anti-GAD, etc.) have been used predictively to assess risk in sibs in research, but not in routine clinical practice.
- **MODY.** Possible in those with a known mutation but issues of consent as above.

Other family members
- **T1D.** Individuals who are at high genetic risk should know the symptoms of diabetes mellitus and attend for prompt assessment if they develop these features.
- **MODY.** Mutation testing is recommended for other affected family members in order to confirm the aetiology of their diabetes. Asymptomatic individuals who are at high genetic risk require baseline biochemical investigation for diabetes, e.g. oral glucose tolerance test. Predictive molecular genetic testing is possible in families where the causative mutation has been defined. In MODY due to *HNF1α*, median age of onset of symptoms is 16 yrs (6–25). OGT usually becomes positive 1 yr before this. Commence monthly urine analysis from age of 6 yr and yearly blood glucose. Consider predictive testing in children (if familial mutation is known) since this may enable dietary modification ahead of the onset of symptoms.

Natural history and management
Potential long-term complications
The long-term complications of diabetes are well documented but it is important to remind patients and their doctors of the risks in pregnancy to the fetus if the diabetes is poorly controlled. (See 'Maternal diabetes mellitus and diabetic embryopathy' page 612.)

Surveillance
Individuals with all types of diabetes require regular medical and nursing supervision to ensure accurate control of the disease in order to help prevent long-term complications. Assessment of cardiovascular risk is probably the most important part of management of T2D in terms of prognosis due to the constellation of associated metabolic risk factors for atherosclerosis.

Support group: Diabetes UK <www.diabetes.org.uk>.

Expert advisers: Robert Semple, Wellcome Clinical Research Training Fellow, Department of Clinical Biochemistry, University of Cambridge, Cambridge and David Savage, Wellcome Trust Training Fellow, Department of Clinical Biochemistry, University of Cambridge, Cambridge, England.

References
<http://care.diabetesjournals.org/cgi/content/full/26/suppl 1/s5>. American Diabetes Association Consensus Document—detailed discussion of classification, terminology, and diagnostic criteria.

<www.ex.ac.uk/diabetesgenes/> Exeter website.

Bellanne-Chantelot C, Chavean D *et al.* Clinical spectrum associated with hepatocyte nuclear factor-1 beta mutations. *Am Intern Med* 2004; **140**: 510–17.

Edghill EL, Bingham C, *et al.* Mutations in hepatocyte nuclear factor-1beta and their related phenotypes. *J Med Genet* 2006; **43**: 84–90.

Fajans SS, Bell GI, Polanky KS. Molecular mechanisms and clinical pathophysiology of maturity-onset diabetes of the young. *New Engl J Med* 2001; **345**: 971–80.

Gloyn AL, Pearson ER, *et al.* Activating mutations in the gene encoding the ATP-sensitive potassium-channel subunit Kir6.2 and permanent neonatal diabetes. *NEJM* 2004; **350**: 1838–49.

Mein CA, Esposito L, Dunn MG, Johnson GCL, Timms AE, Goy JV, Smith AN, Sebag-Montefiore L, Merriman ME, Wilson AJ, Pritchard LE, Barnett AH, Bain SC, Todd, JA. A search for type 1 diabetes susceptibility genes in families from the United Kingdom. *Nat Genet* 1998; **19**: 297–300.

Onengut-Gumuscu S, Concannon P. Mapping genes for autoimmunity in humans: type 1diabetes as model. *Immunol Rev* 2002: **190**: 182–94.

Owen KR, Stride A, *et al.* Etiological investigation of diabetes in young adults presenting with apparent type 2 diabetes. *Diabetes Care* 2003; **26**: 2088–93.

Pearson ER, Starkely BJ, *et al.* Genetic causes of hyperglycaemia and response to treatment in diabetes. *Lancet* 2003; **362**: 1275–81.

Pociot F, McDermott MF. Genetics of type 1 diabetes mellitus. *Genes Immunol* 2002; **3**: 235–49.

Seminars in Medical Genetics. The genetics of diabetes mellitus. *Am J Med Genet* 2002; **115C** (Issue 1).

Temple IK, Shield JP. Transient neonatal diabetes, a disorder of imprinting. *J Med Genet* 2002; **39** (12): 872–5.

Dilated cardiomyopathy (DCM)

DCM is a disease of the myocardium characterized by dilatation and impaired contraction of the left ventricle (or both ventricles) causing progressive heart failure and ventricular arrhythmia. Impaired left ventricle (LV) function is most commonly due to coronary artery disease, and this must be excluded to make a diagnosis of DCM. DCM can be associated with alcohol excess, viral myocarditis, metabolic disorders (e.g. haemochromatosis), systemic disorders (hypothyroidism, hypocalcaemia), late pregnancy, and the puerperium. In an individual without a family history, take care to ensure that other causes have been adequately excluded before assuming a genetic basis as only about one-half of cases appear to be hereditary.

DCM is sometimes inherited as an isolated trait but familial DCM is often associated with other features (see below). Familial DCM has a prevalence of >2/10 000. Currently there are nine nuclear-encoded genes cloned for familial DCM, one mitochondrial gene, and a further seven chromosomal localizations. However, mutations in these genes appear to account for <20% of familial DCM. Clinically there are four broad categories of clinical presentation.

1 **DCM with rapid progression in young men.** Likely to be X-linked with mutation in dystrophin (Xp21). (Mutations in tafazzin (Xq28) usually cause a cardiomyopathy that is fatal in infancy (Barth syndrome), but patients can survive to adult life.)

2 **DCM without additional features.** Likely to follow autosomal dominant (AD) inheritance. Mutations have been identified in three cardiac sarcomere genes that are also critical genes in hypertrophic cardiomyopathy (HCM): troponin T; β-myosin heavy chain (MHC); and cardiac actin. Mutations in δ-sarcoglycan, which is implicated in one form of limb–girdle dystrophy, can also cause familial DCM with no/subclinical skeletal muscle involvement.

3 **DCM with early conduction disease.** Likely to follow AD inheritance. Mutations have been identified in lamin A/C (mutations in this gene also cause AD Emery–Dreifuss), and desmin (mutations in this gene usually cause a severe skeletal myopathy).

4 **DCM with sensorineural hearing loss.** One autosomal locus (6q23–24) and one mitochondrial-encoded gene (tRNA–Lys).

Clinical approach
History: key points
- Three-generation family history with specific enquiry about:
  - heart failure;
  - sudden death, conduction disorders (palpitations, dizzy spells, 'faints', pacemakers), atrial fibrillation;
  - stroke (embolic from thrombus forming in dilated cardiac chambers);
  - 'muscular dystrophy', muscle weakness (ability to climb stairs or get up from a chair), abnormal gait, wheelchair use, contractures;
  - sensorineural deafness.
- Fits, faints, or funny turns.
- Exercise tolerance and breathlessness.
- Enquire about muscle weakness. Difficulty rising from chairs implies hip girdle involvement; difficulty lifting arms above head, e.g. brushing hair, hanging out washing, implies shoulder girdle involvement.
- Current level of mobility. Rising from chairs, walking on flat, use of aids,

Examination: key points
- If not already seen by a cardiologist, basic cardiovascular assessment, e.g. pulse, blood pressure, jugular venous pressure (JVP), palpate apex, auscultation of heart.
- Muscle bulk (e.g. calf hypertrophy in Becker muscular dystrophy (BMD)), and limb-girdle muscle power (Gower's manoeuvre and lifting arms above head).
- Look for contractures especially at the elbows and ankles (Emery–Dreifuss).

Investigation
All first-degree relatives should be offered investigation with an electrocardiogram (ECG) and echocardiogram. Genetic investigations should be focused on a single clearly affected family member, unless a specific mutation is identified, in which case predictive testing and carrier testing may become possible.
- Echocardiogram.
- 12-lead ECG with rhythm strip.
- 24 hour tape.
- Creatine kinase (CK: total CK and isoenzyme CK-MB).
- Dystrophin deletion/duplication screen (if family history consistent with X-linked recessive (XLR) inheritance, i.e. no male–male transmission and CK elevated).
- If young males only affected, no accompanying muscle weakness, and family history compatible with XLR inheritance, check for promoter mutations in dystrophin and for exon 29 deletions (deletion of exon 29 from the midrod regions disrupts sarcoglycan assembly in cardiac muscle, but not in skeletal muscle).
- Consider lamin A/C mutation analysis if family tree consistent with AD Emery–Dreifuss or AD DCM, especially if there are early atrial fibrillation and conduction disease. (Mutations in lamin A (*LMNA*) are a rare cause of isolated DCM.)

Other diagnoses to consider
Becker muscular dystrophy (BMD)
BMD is caused by in-frame mutations in dystrophin on Xp21. Cardiac complications (DCM) are a major cause of morbidity and mortality in BMD. BMD patients should be under regular review by a cardiologist with regular surveillance from the teens onwards (annual ECG and echocardiogram in the first instance). See 'Duchenne and Becker muscular dystrophy (DMD and BMD)', page 308.

Emery–Dreifuss muscular dystrophy
Usually XLR due to mutations in *emerin* on Xq28 but some AD forms exist, e.g. lamin A/C (*LMNA*). Variable muscular dystrophy with development of contractures (especially elbows and knees) from teens. Cardiac conduction defects are a prominent feature. See 'Limb-girdle muscular dystrophies', page 374.

Genetic advice
Inheritance and recurrence risk
The great majority of familial DCM follows AD inheritance. Autosomal recessive (AR) inheritance is less common

Major and minor criteria for the diagnosis of DCM in adult members of affected families (after McKenna 2003)

Major criteria

- A reduced ejection fraction of the LV (<45% of normal) and/or fractional shortening (<25%) as assessed by echocardiography, radionuclide scanning, or angiography
- An increased LV end-diastolic diameter corresponding to >117% of the predicted value corrected for age and body surface area

Minor criteria

- Unexplained supraventricular or ventricular arrhythmia
- A low degree of dilatation (>112% of the predicted value)
- An intermediate impairment of LV dysfunction
- Conduction defects
- Segmental wall motion abnormalities in the absence of intraventricular conduction defect
- Ischaemic heart disease
- Unexplained sudden death of a first-degree relative or stroke at <50 years

Diagnosis of inherited DCM is fulfilled in a first-degree relative of an affected individual in the presence of:

- one major criterion *or*
- LV dilatation plus one minor criterion *or*
- three minor criteria

---

accounting for ~15% of affected families. Homozygous mutation in cardiac troponin 1 has been identified in one such family (Murphy *et al.* 2004). X-linked inheritance is particularly important for families presenting with rapidly progressive DCM affecting young males. DCM is a significant cause of death in men with BMD; female carriers for BMD and DMD may develop cardiomyopathy, but this is usually mild and subclinical. DCM is a feature of some mitochondrial disorders (both matrilineal and nuclear), usually with additional abnormalities.

Variability and penetrance
Clinical features can be quite variable even among family members carrying the same mutation. Penetrance is age-dependent and overall (for categories 2 and 3 above) is estimated at 10% in those <20 years, 34% in young adults of 20–30 years, 60% in adults of 30–40 years, and 90% in those >40 years.

Prenatal diagnosis
In a family with a known mutation (the minority) this is technically possible.

Predictive testing
In a family with a known mutation (the minority) this could be offered so that cardiac surveillance could be targeted more appropriately. Otherwise screening of at-risk relatives should be offered.

Other family members
See table.

Natural history and management
Beta-blockers have an important role in reducing overall mortality and hospitalization rates for heart failure. Angiotensin-converting enzyme (ACE) inhibitors have a role in the management of heart failure due to DCM. Pacemakers should be considered in families with conduction disorders. Amiodarone may be of value in patients with ventricular arrhythmia. Trials are in progress to assess the value of implantable defibrillators in patients with a high risk of sudden death from ventricular arrhythmia. Cardiac transplantation or left-ventricular assist devices have a role in the management of some individuals with end-stage heart failure due to DCM.

Potential long-term complications
Systemic and pulmonary emboli are common, and anticoagulation with warfarin may be advised for patients in atrial fibrillation, with intracardiac thrombus, a history of stroke, or severe ventricular dilatation and dysfunction.

Surveillance
Affected individuals should be under regular long-term surveillance by a cardiologist. It is difficult to know how long cardiac surveillance should be continued in an apparently unaffected individual, but infrequent surveillance is probably advisable at least until the age of 45 years (see 'Variability and penetrance' above).

Support group: Cardiomyopathy Association <www.cardiomyopathy.org>.

Expert adviser: Hugh Watkins, Professor of Cardiovascular Medicine, University of Oxford, John Radcliffe Hospital, Oxford, England.

References
Franz W-M, Muller OJ, Katus A. Cardiomyopathies: from genetics to the prospect of treatment [review article]. *Lancet* 2001; **358**: 1627–37.

McKenna WJ. The cardiomyopathies: hypertrophic, dilated, restrictive and right ventricular. In *The Oxford textbook of medicine*, 4th edn (ed. D.A. Warrell, T.M. Cox, and J.D. Firth). Oxford University Press, Oxford, 2003.

Murphy ET, Mogensen J, *et al.* Novel mutation in cardiac troponin 1 in recessive idiopathic dilated cardiomyopathy. *Lancet* 2004; **363**: 371–2.

Sebillon P, Bouchier C, *et al.* Expanding the phenotype of *LMNA* mutations in dilated cardiomyopathy and functional consequences of these mutations. *J Med Genet* 2003; **40**: 560–7.

DNA repair defects

These disorders all share defects in the DNA repair mechanisms of the cell. They are caused by mutations in 'caretaker genes' that encode the proteins that function to protect the genome against acquired alterations. Typically, DNA damage is generated by ultraviolet (UV) radiation, ionizing radiation, free radicals, and exogenous chemicals. The impaired capacity to maintain genomic integrity results in the accelerated accumulation of key genetic changes that promote cellular transformation and neoplasia. DNA repair proteins also have a role in joining the double-stranded breaks between the variable (V), diversity (D), and joining (J) gene segments of the lymphocyte immunoglobulin and antigen receptor genes to generate immunological diversity. Deficiency of this repair process may contribute to the immunodeficiency characteristic of these disorders. Some have distinctive features, e.g. radial hypoplasia in Fanconi anaemia (FA), but for others there is considerable phenotypic overlap. As a group they are probably significantly underdiagnosed.

- **Nucleotide excision repair (NER)** is a DNA repair pathway that removes DNA damage (such as UV-light-induced thymidine dimers) by excising the region of DNA that contains the damaged base(s). Defective in xeroderma pigmentosum (XP) and trichothiodystrophy (TTD).
- **Transcription-coupled repair** is a specialized pathway that facilitates the repair of damaged DNA during transcription. The transcribed strand of active genes is preferentially repaired. Defective in Cockayne syndrome (CS) and cerebro-oculo-facial-skeletal syndrome (COFS).
- **Cross-linking agent repair.** Agents such as mitomycin C (MMC) and diepoxybutane (DEB) and a variety of cytotoxic agents (e.g. cisplatin, cyclophosphamide) form covalent cross-links in double-stranded DNA (either between the two strands, or between adjacent bases) that obstruct DNA replication. Specific repair pathways are required to detect the DNA damage and facilitate its repair. Defective in FA.

Clinical approach

History: key points

- Three-generation family history with specific enquiry for consanguinity.
- Pregnancy history with birthweight.
- Developmental milestones and postnatal growth.
- Sun-sensitivity.

Examination: key points

- Growth parameters. Height, weight, occipital-frontal circumference (OFC); short stature is common.
- Face. Deep-set eyes, pinched nose, premature ageing (CS), microcephaly with prominent mid-face (Nijmegen breakage syndrome (NBS)), freckling (XP and NBS), solar keratoses and brown spots (XP), butterfly rash (Bloom syndrome).
- Skin. Café au lait spots (CALs) and areas of increased pigmentation (FA), excessive sunlight-induced skin injury (XP), especially pigmentation changes (XP) and sunburn (XP, CS, TTD).
- Eyes. Telangiectasiae (ataxia telangiectasia (AT)), cataract (CS).

- Neurology. Balance (AT), spasticity (CS).
- Brittle, sulphur-deficient hair (TTD).

Investigation

- **AT**
  - Serum alpha-fetoprotein (AFP). Usually unmeasurable levels in childhood, but high levels in AT.
  - Full blood count (FBC) for white cell counts.
  - EDTA (ethylenedinitrilotetraacetate) sample (3–5 ml) for Ig subclasses (IgA and IgG2 deficiency is common) and lymphocyte subsets.
  - 5 ml blood in LiHeparin (LiHep) for radiosensitivity assay (up to 10-fold increased chromosome breakage after irradiation in lab). Also present in peripheral T cells is a high frequency of chromosome translocations involving chromosomes 7 and 14. Lymphoblastoid cell line can be made from the heparin sample and tested for reduced level/absence of ATM protein by Western blotting (6 weeks). Identification of the *ATM* mutations can then follow using the same cell line.
- **Bloom syndrome.** Measurement of sister chromatid exchanges (SCEs) in blood sample.
- **CS and COFS.** Skin biopsy for fibroblast culture for study of RNA synthesis following exposure to UV light. Reduced RNA synthesis recovery is seen on exposure of cells to UV light. Unlike in XP, excision repair after UV damage is grossly normal, but there is a slow recovery of DNA and RNA synthesis.
- **FA**
  - FBC for haematological indices.
  - AFP is often elevated.
  - Spontaneous and DEB-induced chromosome breakage analysis in LiHep blood sample. In FA, both measures of chromosome breakage are increased. Exact levels are lab-dependent, but in the Guy's Hospital lab, spontaneous breaks/cell in control samples are 0.00–0.20 and in Fanconi samples 0.08–2.03, and DEB-induced breaks/cell in control samples are 0.00–0.23, and in Fanconi samples 0.48–18.40.
- **NBS**
  - FBC for white cell counts.
  - EDTA sample (3–5 ml) for Ig subclasses and lymphocyte subsets.
  - 5 ml blood in LiHep for radiosensitivity assay. Increased breakage of chromosomes, as for AT. In unirradiated peripheral T cells there is an increased frequency of chromosome translocations involving chromosomes 7 and 14, again as for AT. A lymphoblastoid cell line can be made from heparin sample and tested for absence of Nbs1 protein by Western blotting, 6 weeks. If suggestive, proceed to mutation analysis of *NBS1* (EDTA sample). A common 5 bp deletion is present in homozygous or compound heterozygous form in the majority of patients.
- **TTD**
  - Skin biopsy for fibroblast culture for study of NER following UV-irradiation (as for XP).
  - Blood sample for FBC and haemoglobin electrophoresis (TTD patients show β-thalassaemia triad: decreased mean corpuscular volume (MCV);

decreased mean corpuscular haemoglobin (MCH); increased HbA_2.

- **XP**
  - Skin biopsy for fibroblast culture for analysis of NER using unscheduled DNA synthesis (UDS) assay following UV-irradiation—defective in 80% of XP cases. Levels of UDS are 0–50% of normal.
  - In variant form (20%), UDS is normal. Assay involves UV irradiation, incubating for 2 days in caffeine, then measuring replicative DNA synthesis as measure of survival—defective in XP variants.

Diagnoses/conditions to consider

Ataxia telangiectasia (AT)

Prevalence ~1/300 000. Child with AT usually appears normal until he/she begins to walk and ataxia becomes evident. Characteristics include:

- neurological problems, e.g. unsteady (wobbly) gait, difficulty standing without swaying. Progressive difficulty with eye movements (oculomotor apraxia) and squint, slurred speech (dysarthria), and drooling may be evident from early years; involuntary movements (fidgety movement of hands) can make skilled movements difficult in late childhood; dysfunctional swallowing can be problematic in teens;
- telangiectasiae usually visible on sclerae by 4–8 years. Sun sensitivity and premature ageing of skin with dark spots and occasional grey hairs;
- immunodeficiency in 80%—variable, typically sinusitis and/or bronchitis/pneumonia;
- impaired growth and delayed/incomplete puberty;
- predisposition to cancer, especially lymphoma and leukaemia. 10–30% of AT patients including 15% <16 years;

AT is an autosomal recessive (AR) disorder caused by mutations in ATM (A-T mutated) on chromosome 11. Mutations occur throughout the gene (66 exons) and are usually truncating. The ATM protein activates cellular responses to DNA damage caused by radiation, certain chemicals, or normal cellular metabolism. Chromosome instability in lymphocytes from AT patients takes the form of non-random translocations and inversions that preferentially involve the T- and B-cell receptor gene involving chromosomes 7 and 14. Avoid therapeutic doses of ionizing radiation (seek advice); avoid diagnostic X-rays where possible. Life-limiting condition, but life expectancy varies.

Approximately 1/200 individuals are carriers for AT. Hence, there is low risk to extended family unless there is consanguinity, e.g. risk for sibling having an AT child is 2/3 × 1/200 × 1/4 = 1/1200 or aunt/uncle having an AT child is 1/2 × 1/200 × 1/4 = 1/1600. Determining AT carrier status for someone from general population not generally feasible. Prenatal diagnosis usually possible for parents of an affected child.

Heterozygous carriers for AT are at a 3.6-fold risk of breast cancer. Current advice is to avoid regular mammographic screening because of potential radiation risk and consider breast awareness or clinical evaluation from 50 years in lieu of mammographic screening. AT carriers should minimize exposure to diagnostic X-rays, e.g. restrict exposure to situations where X-ray would significantly alter management.

An AT-like disorder (ATLD) that is neurologically indistinguishable from AT has been described. At the cellular level there is also an increased sensitivity to ionizing radiation. The patients do not have mutations in the *ATM* gene, but in the *hMRE11* gene.

Bloom syndrome

Very rare AR disorder caused by mutations in *BLM* on 15q26.1, which encodes a RecQ DNA helicase involved in the maintenance of DNA integrity. Children with Bloom syndrome are small and usually have an erythematous 'butterfly rash' that is sensitive to sunlight, excessive hyper- and hypopigmented skin lesions located anywhere on the body, and a high rate of bacterial infections due to immunodeficiency. They are prone to cancer, chronic lung disease, and diabetes. Bloom syndrome is more common among Ashkenazi Jews.

Cerebro-oculo-facial-skeletal syndrome (COFS)

AR, rapidly progressive neurological disorder leading to brain atrophy with calcifications, cataracts, microcornea, optic atrophy, progressive joint contractures, and growth failure. Usually presents in fetal or neonatal life. COFS is part of the spectrum of NER disorders, which includes XP, CS, and TTD, and is probably a variant of CS.

Cockayne syndrome (CS)

AR neurodegenerative disorder characterized by low to normal birthweight, postnatal growth failure, brain dysmyelination with calcium deposits, cutaneous photosensitivity, pigmentary retinopathy and/or cataracts and/or optic atrophy, and sensorineural hearing loss. The facies are characteristic with a prematurely aged appearance with deep-set eyes and a pinched appearance to the nose (loss of subcutaneous fat). There is microcephaly with developmental delay, spasticity, and often ataxia. Patients usually have sun-sensitivity. More severe form (sometimes called type II) shows features from birth.

CS is caused by mutations in the genes *CSA* or *CSB*. Cultured CS cells are hypersensitive to UV radiation, because of impaired NER of UV-induced damage in actively transcribed DNA (global genome NER is unaffected).

Fanconi anaemia (FA)

AR disorder caused by mutations in six FA genes, *FANC A, C, D2, E, F,* and *G*, and also biallellic mutations in *BRCA2* (*FANCA* accounts for the majority, with *FANCC* most common amongst Ashkenazi Jews). An X-linked form of FA has recently been identified, encoded by the gene FANCB on Xp22.31 (Meetei). The clinical phenotype of all FA complementation groups is similar and is characterized by:

- pre- and postnatal growth retardation; 50% of FA patients are <3rd centile for height;
- radial ray anomalies: absent, hypoplastic, supernumerary, or bifid thumbs and hypoplastic or absent radii. 20% have other skeletal problems (e.g. vertebral and rib anomalies);
- structural renal malformations: 25% have unilateral renal agenesis, rotated, misshapen, or fused kidneys;
- pigmentary skin changes: many FA patients develop CALs. In some the entire body or large areas of the body may have a suntanned appearance (hyperpigmentation);
- other features may include: microcephaly; microphthalmos; congenital heart disease (e.g. atrial septal defect (ASD), ventricular septal defect (VSD)); and learning disability;
- aplastic anaemia: median age of onset of marrow failure is 7 years (usual range 3–12 year). Bone marrow transplantation is sometimes offered;
- increased risk for myelodysplasia, acute myeloid leukaemia (AML), and other cancers, especially squamous

carcinomas of head, neck, and oesophagus and cancers of female reproductive tract.

The chromosomal aberrations that occur spontaneously and randomly in dividing FA cells affect the newly replicated DNA. They are microscopically visible at metaphase as broken chromatids. Cells show increased sensitivity to cross-linking agents such as MMC and DEB. This forms the basis of diagnostic testing (see above). Misrepair leads to quadriradial formation. Overall life expectancy is reduced to an average of 20 years (range 0–50 years). Prenatal diagnosis is not straight-forward, but is usually possible by chorionic villus sampling (CVS)—consult your laboratory prior to counselling.

Nijmegen breakage syndrome (NBS)

NBS is extremely rare. Affected children have micro-cephaly, intrauterine growth restriction (IUGR), short stature, prominent midface, growth retardation, mild learning difficulties, susceptibility to infections with panhy-pogammaglobulinaemia, and susceptibility to lymphoma and other tumours. AR due to mutations in *NBS1* on 8q, which encodes 'nibrin', a novel protein involved in DNA double-strand break repair. Cells show increased sensitiv-ity to ionizing radiation. A common 5 bp deletion is present in homozygous or compound heterozygous form in the majority of patients.

Rothmund–Thomson syndrome

Rothmund–Thomson syndrome is characterized by poikiloderma congenita, with growth deficiency, alopecia, photosensitivity, dystrophic nails, abnormal teeth, cataracts, and hypogonadism. 20% have radial ray defects. The skin abnormalities appear before 6 months of age with reticular or diffuse erythema on the face, hands, and extensor sur-faces of the limbs. The trunk is relatively spared. It is caused by mutations in the helicase gene *RECQL4* on 8q24.

Trichothiodystrophy (TTD)

Rare condition characterized by brittle sulphur-deficient hair (trichorrhexis nodosa on microscopy), short stature, mental retardation, and sometimes icthyosis. Genetically heterogeneous and can be caused by mutations in *XPB*, *XPD*, (most common) and *TTDA*. Patients with *XPD* mutations have reduced expression of β-globin genes resulting in β-thalassaemia trait.

Werner syndrome

Werner syndrome is a progeroid syndrome characterized by premature greying and thinning of the hair, prematurely aged appearance, short stature, diabetes mellitus type 2, hypogonadism, osteoporosis, premature atherosclerosis, a weak or hoarse voice, and cataracts. It is caused by muta-tions in *WRN*, which is a member of the *RECQ* family of DNA helicases. The mean age of diagnosis is 39 years (SD 7.7 years), with the mean age of initial symptoms being 13 years. Some patients with atypical Werner syndrome have mutations in the lamin A/C gene *LMNA*.

Xeroderma pigmentosum (XP)

XP is a rare AR disorder characterized by extreme sensitivity of the skin to sunlight-induced changes. Many people with XP will get unusually severe sunburn after a short sun exposure. The sunburn will last much longer than expected —perhaps for several weeks—and usually occurs during a child's first sun exposure. Some people with XP will not get sunburnt more easily and the disease may go unrecognized until the occurrence of multiple skin cancers (basal cell carcinoma, squamous cell carcinoma, and melanoma) at an early age suggests the diagnosis. Individuals with XP have a 1000-fold increase in incidence of sunlight-induced skin cancers. Most patients with XP develop dense freckling at an early age. Other skin changes, such as irregular dark spots, thinning of the skin, excessive dryness, and solar keratoses typical of those usually seen in the elderly, begin in infancy and are almost always present by age 20 years. The eyes are often painfully sensitive to the sun. Corneal clouding and cancerous and non-cancerous growths on the eyes may occur. Approximately 20% develop neurological problems, e.g. deaf-ness, impaired coordination, spasticity, and developmental delay. Neurological problems are usually progressive. Note that early diagnosis followed by strict and complete protec-tion from sunlight with UV-resistant face-masks, gloves, and UV-resistant film on windows can completely prevent all skin symptoms.

Genetically, XP is complex with features in the majority of patients resulting from a defect in one of seven genes (*XPA*, *XPB* … *XPG*), controlling NER. Approximately 20% of XP patients have normal levels of NER and are known as XP variant (XP-V) and have mutations in the gene encod-ing DNA polymerase η causing a reduced ability to replic-ate DNA after irradiation. Even though some patients with XP-V have a high incidence of tumours, many of them sur-vive to a relatively old age compared with NER-defective patients with XP.

Genetic advice

Inheritance and recurrence risk

All are AR, except X-linked FA with 1 in 4 risk to future pregnancies.

Variability and penetrance

All are 100% penetrant in the homozygous or compound heterozygous state, but especially for XP and CS features are very variable.

Prenatal diagnosis

Usually possible by CVS at 11 weeks gestation, but liaise carefully with expert laboratory as these are highly special-ized investigations.

Other family members

In FA careful consideration should be given to testing apparently healthy siblings. Occasionally chromosome breakage tests demonstrate FA in an apparently healthy sibling with no congenital anomalies and normal FBC.

Natural history and management

Potential long-term complications

These are life-limiting disorders. See individual disease entries.

Surveillance

Refer to specialist centre for advice.

Support groups: Ataxia-Telangiectasia Society <www.atsociety.org.uk>; Fanconi anaemia <www.fanconi-anaemia.co.uk>; xeroderma pigmentosum <http://xpsupportgroup.org.uk/>;<www.xps.org/> (US).

Expert advisers: Malcolm Taylor, Professor of Cancer Genetics, University of Birmingham, Birmingham and Alan Lehmann, Professor and Chairman, Genome Damage and Stability Centre, University of Sussex, Brighton, England.

References

Broughton BC, Cordonnier A, *et al.* Molecular analysis of mutations in DNA polymerase η in xeroderma pigmentosum-variant patients. *Proc Natl Acad Sci USA* 2002; **99**: 815–20.

Graham JM Jr, Anyane-Yeboa K, *et al.* Cerebro-oculo-facio-skeletal syndrome with a nucleotide excision-repair defect and a mutated XPD gene, with prenatal diagnosis in a triplet pregnancy. *Am J Hum Genet* 2001; **69**: 291–300.

International Nijmegen Breakage Syndrome Study Group. Nijmegen breakage syndrome. *Arch Dis Child* 2000; **82**: 400–6.

Joenje H, Patel KJ. The emerging genetic and molecular basis of Fanconi anaemia. *Nat Rev Genet* 2001; **2**: 446–57.

Lederman HM, Crawford TO. *Ataxia-telangiectasia: a handbook for families and caregivers*, 1st edn. Ataxia-Telangiectasia Society, London, 2000.

Meetei AR, Levitus M *et al.* X-linked inheritance of Fanconi anaemia complementation group B. *Nat Genet* 2004; **36**: 1219–24.

Duchenne and Becker muscular dystrophy (DMD and BMD)

Meryon disease

Duchenne muscular dystrophy (DMD) affects ~1 in 3000–4000 male births. It is the most common and severe form of childhood muscular dystrophy. The natural history of the disease is that it results in early loss of ambulation between the ages of 7 and 13 years (mean age 9 years) and death in the late teens or early twenties. DMD is an X-linked recessive (XLR) disorder caused by mutations in the dystrophin gene (*DMD*) on Xp21. Dystrophin is a protein localized to the inner side of the plasma membrane that interacts with a group of proteins linking into the extracellular matrix and also on the intracellular surface with actin. Immunolabelling of a muscle biopsy from a boy with DMD using antibodies to dystrophin shows a complete or almost complete absence of the protein with secondary loss of the dystrophin-associated proteins in the muscle fibre membrane.

60–65% of DMD is caused by large out-of-frame deletions that remove one or more exons. At least a further 5% result from exon duplication. There are two hotspot regions for deletions: at the 5' end, affecting exons 3–8, and towards the 3' end, affecting exons 44–60, but deletions may occur anywhere in the gene. The remaining cases of DMD are mostly nonsense or frameshift mutations that cause chain termination. Loss of the 3' end of the gene, as in the contiguous gene deletion syndrome involving *DAX1* and glycerol kinase, also results in DMD.

Approximately 30% of boys with DMD have a mild learning disability that is not progressive. They may present with developmental delay, especially with speech delay and late walking.

Lifespan is markedly reduced in DMD. For boys receiving specialist care and nocturnal ventilation the mean age of death is 25.3 years (Eagle *et al.* 2002). Cardiomyopathy is almost universal and early detection may allow appropriate treatment; severe symptomatic cardiomyopathy is usually a poor prognostic indicator.

Becker muscular dystrophy(BMD) is clinically similar to DMD but milder, with a mean age of onset of 11 years. Loss of the ability to walk may occur late (e.g. 40s or 50s) and many individuals with BMD survive into middle age and beyond. Often cramps on exercise are the only problem initially, but some affected boys are late in learning to walk and are unable to run fast. Later in the teens and twenties, muscle weakness becomes evident causing difficulty in rapid walking, running, and climbing stairs. It may become difficult to lift objects above waist height. Cognitive impairment is not a major feature of BMD. BMD is caused by 'in-frame' mutations in dystrophin that result in reduced dystrophin being produced. Immunolabelling of muscle biopsy from a man with BMD shows a reduction in the intensity of staining which may vary within and between fibres.

Some patients present with an **intermediate dystrophin phenotype**, i.e. a clinical picture intermediate between those of DMD and BMD. See figure for an illustration of the predominant muscle weaknesses in DMD and BMD.

Manifesting female carriers. In Hoogerwaard *et al.*'s (1999a) survey of 129 carriers of muscular dystrophy, ~5% had myalgia/cramps and 17% had mild/moderate muscle weakness on testing (but only ~10% were aware of symptoms prior to testing). None had severe weakness, and

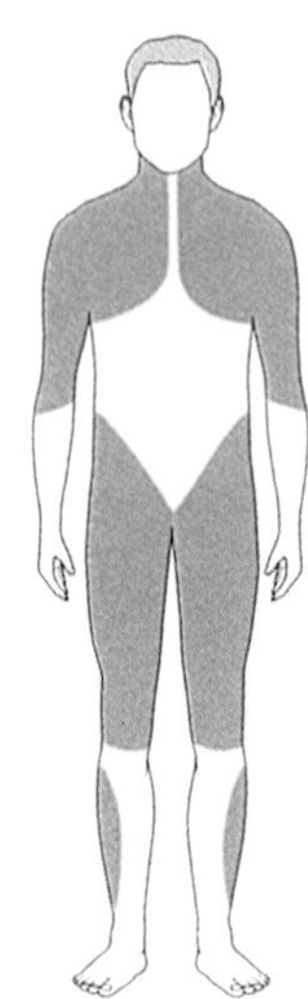

Distribution of predominant muscle weakness in Duchenne and Becker muscular dystrophy. (Reproduced from Emery (1998), fig. 1a, p. 992, by permission of the BMJ Publishing Group.)

severe disabling muscle weakness among carriers is probably rare. Onset of symptoms in this study did not occur at <16 years and the average age of onset was 33 years. 70% of women who complained of myalgia, cramps, or muscle weakness were weak on testing. Weakness was primarily proximal and asymmetric and in 40% only the shoulder-girdle or upper arm was affected. Severe disabling muscle weakness among carriers is probably rare, but can occur. Carriers of BMD are less frequently and less severely affected than carriers of DMD. Serum creatine kinase (CK) was raised in 53% of carriers of DMD and 30% of carriers of BMD. Mean serum CK was 306 u/l (range, 48–1860). Surprisingly, there was no significant difference in mean CK activity between carriers with, and carriers without, muscle weakness. Immunohistochemistry of muscle biopsy from a manifesting DMD carrier using labelled antibodies shows some reduction in the intensity of staining which varies both between and within fibres.

- Approximately 20% of carriers have evidence of cardiac involvement on investigation.
- Females with early onset or severe muscle weakness should have a karyotype (X-autosome translocations, androgen insensitivity syndrome (AIS), etc.).

Clinical approach

History: key points

- Detailed three-generation family tree, with careful enquiry for other affected males (e.g. maternal brother, uncles, and great-uncles). Extend the family tree as far as possible on the affected side of the family.
- Detailed developmental history. Boys with DMD usually have mild delay of motor-milestones, e.g. late-walking and tip-toe and unsteady gait.
- Difficulty rising from the floor (leading to Gower's manoeuvre where the child pushes up on his thighs with

his hands to get up off the floor) and difficulties going upstairs (e.g. needing to get both feet on to the step before tackling the next step). Ungainly and slow running are common in the first 2–3 years of life.

Examination: key points
- Observe the child's gait. You may need more space to observe this than is available in the consulting room. Abnormalities of gait become much more evident when a child tries to hurry.
- Boys with DMD never achieve a normal run; very few of them ever learn to jump with both feet together.
- Proximal limb weakness.
- Calf hypertrophy occurs in most children in the early phase of the disease.

Investigation
- CK: usually several thousand. Children with DMD invariably have *serum or plasma* levels >10 times normal. (See 'Predictive testing' below.)
- DNA for dystrophin deletion/duplication analysis and linkage studies if no mutation identified. Dystrophin sequencing will enable a higher proportion of DMD families to be offered direct testing avoiding the errors inherent in linkage-based approaches.
- Muscle biopsy if no dystrophin mutation identified and clinical picture indicative of a dystrophic process meriting invasive diagnostic investigations. Examination of dystrophin in the muscle biopsy gives a more quantitative idea of the effect of the mutations and can provide further prognostic information though it needs to be interpreted in the context of the clinical and genetic findings
- Echocardiogram and electrocardiogram (ECG) at diagnosis.

Other diagnoses/conditions to consider
See 'Limb girdle muscular dystrophies', page 374.

Genetic advice
Inheritance and recurrence risk
XLR. In any pregnancy of a carrier female there are four possible outcomes, each equally likely: normal male; normal female; affected male; carrier female. Carrier rate is similar across different ethnic groups.

Variability and penetrance
Penetrance is complete in males inheriting a pathogenic dystrophin mutation. A small percentage of women are manifesting carriers with raised CK and a variable degree of muscle weakness (see above).

Prenatal diagnosis
- Available to carriers of a known dystrophin mutation by chorionic villus sampling (CVS) at 11 weeks gestation.
- Available to mothers of an apparently *de novo* Duchenne mutation because of the significant risk arising from germline mosaicism (see below).
- Available in families where a mutation has not been found, but where a 'high risk X' can be identified by linkage studies. If the pregnancy is found to carry the high risk X, and a termination of pregnancy is requested, consider dystrophin staining of fetal muscle tissue to gain additional information for future pregnancies.
- First step is fetal sexing (e.g. amelogenin probe). Molecular genetic analysis is usually only pursued if the

pregnancy is male. Reliable, non-invasive methods of fetal sexing, e.g. using a combination of fetal ultrasound scan (USS) and free-fetal DNA in maternal serum late in the first trimester, may become available in the near future (L. Chitty, personal communication, 2003).
- Pre-implantation genetic diagnosis (PGD) with selection of female pregnancies is a theoretical possibility for women with a high carrier risk in a family where the causative mutation is unknown.

Predictive testing
- **Newborn males.** Women at risk of being carriers who decline prenatal testing, and who give birth to a son may wish their infant son to be tested before embarking on another pregnancy. CK is often elevated in cord blood or in blood samples taken within the first week after delivery. CK may also be elevated following intramuscular (IM) injections (e.g. infant immunizations). Affected males, even as neonates, will usually have a CK of several thousand. A value in the normal range excludes DMD. CK levels on cord blood are fine if they are very high or in the normal range; CK values in the hundreds or just outwith the normal range should be repeated at 6 weeks of age. If arranging CK estimation on cord blood, ensure that the family understand that if the result is equivocal they may need to wait until the boy is 6 weeks old for a repeat test; otherwise defer testing until the infant is 6 weeks old.
- **Becker muscular dystrophy.** CK levels in BMD can be as high as in DMD but usually are not. CK levels in BMD fall with disease progression, so you may get almost normal levels in very elderly people. It is difficult to be dogmatic about levels in early infancy (linkage may be an adjunct to assessment, if the familial mutation is unknown).

Other family members—carrier testing and assessment of risk of carrier status in female relatives
Assemble the maximum information available using:
- family tree—include accurate information about unaffected males, and symptomatic enquiry about muscle weakness, muscle cramps, cardiomyopathy, etc. in 'at risk' females;
- confirmation of diagnosis in proband (e.g. muscle biopsy result, dystrophin mutation analysis);
- serial CKs in consultand, if no mutation known in proband, see page 662.

Mutation known
If the mutation in the affected individual is known, determination of carrier status is straightforward by direct analysis of the consultand's DNA for the known dystrophin mutation in the family—but *note risks arising from germline mosaicism*. The precise incidence of germline mosaicism in DMD is not clear. The following is based on an estimated risk.
- For the mother of an affected boy with a known mutation that is not present in the mother's genomic DNA there is a suggested 1 in 5 (20%) risk to a future son who inherits the same X chromosome as his affected brother (i.e. there is an overall 5% risk to future pregnancies).
- In families with a single affected boy with a known mutation, not present in his mother's genomic DNA, *it is important that sisters of the affected boy are offered mutation-based carrier testing*. Sisters inheriting the same maternal X as the affected boy will have a 20% risk

of being carriers as a result of maternal germline mosaicism.

Mutation unknown

If the mutation in the affected individual is unknown, assessment of carrier status in female relatives is more complex.

- Families with a single affected male—unknown mutation.
  1 Identify the closest female relative from whom both the consultand and proband are descended—this is the 'dummy consultand'.
  2 Use Bayes's theorem to calculate the risk that the 'dummy consultand' is a carrier for DMD/BMD— include the mother of the affected boy in the risk calculation (see worked examples in the Appendix page 646)—include conditional information about unaffected sons of the 'dummy consultand', the mother of the affected boy, the mother of the consultand, and the consultand herself.
  3 Use linkage where possible to determine whether or not the consultand is carrying the 'high risk X'. Samples from maternal grandparents and from unaffected males may be helpful here
  4 Use serial CKs from the consultand as conditional information in the Bayes analysis.
- Families with more than one affected male—unknown mutation.
  1 If the affected males are in different generations, all intervening female relatives are obligate carriers (e.g. a woman with an affected maternal uncle and an affected son is an obligate carrier, as is her mother, and the maternal grandmother has a two-thirds chance of being a carrier).
  2 As above, identify the closest female relative from whom both the consultand and the nearest affected male relative are descended—the 'dummy consultand'.
  3 Use Bayes's theorem to derive the carrier risk, unless this is immediately apparent, i.e. the daughter of an obligate carrier will have a 50% carrier risk (unless she has had unaffected male pregnancies which can be included as conditional information and will lower her risk).
  4 Use linkage where possible to determine whether or not the consultand is carrying the 'high risk X'. Samples from maternal grandparents and from unaffected males may be helpful here.
  5 Use three serial CK's from the consultand as conditional information in the Bayes analysis.

Natural history and management

Gene therapy remains a hope for the future. Possibilities currently under development include upregulation of utrophin and targeted exon-skipping to restore the reading frame.

Potential long-term complications in DMD

- **Loss of ambulation.** Muscle weakness is progressive and children with DMD will lose ambulation between 7 and 13 years (mean age ~9 years) and become wheelchair-dependent. This is due to a combination of weakness and contractures affecting the ankles, knees, and hips. Ankle splints to prevent contracture of the tendo-achilles are important in maintaining ambulation for as long as possible. Some boys may also find long leg calipers beneficial for the prolongation of ambulation.

In large-scale randomized control trials, daily prednisolone has been shown to preserve ambulation and delay the development of other complications. Side-effects require careful monitoring and may necessitate the introduction of alternative regimes and careful dietary control. Prednisolone does not slow contracture development.

- **Scoliosis.** Affected children confined to a wheelchair are at high risk of developing a scoliosis. More than 90% of boys with DMD will eventually develop a significant scoliosis. Bracing may reduce the rate of progression of the scoliosis, but often major surgery is required to stop the progression. Surgery is high risk and should be undertaken in specialist centres that have the facility to undertake a comprehensive cardiac assessment prior to intervention.
- **Nocturnal hypoventilation.** Respiratory muscles are also affected and this becomes a clinical problem usually in the late teens. Respiratory failure causing nocturnal hypoventilation is common at this age and can be treated with night-time facial or nasal mask ventilation. Without treatment, death often ensues within a few months.
- **Cardiac problems.** Because of their immobility, patients with DMD rarely develop signs of cardiac failure; however, on investigation signs of cardiomyopathy are almost universal. Patients are at significantly increased risk of arrhythmia and other cardiac problems perioperatively. Guidelines exist for cardiovascular investigations and management, see below (Bushby et al. 2003).
- **Cognitive impairment** may be a significant part of the condition and may particularly have an effect on verbal rather than performance intelligence quotient (IQ).

Potential long-term complications in BMD

- **Impaired mobility.** Some men with BMD retain ambulation throughout their lives, but others will become dependent on aids (sticks/walking frames) and eventually become wheelchair-dependent.
- **Cardiac complications** (e.g. dilated cardiomyopathy (DCM)) are a major cause of morbidity and mortality in BMD. BMD patients should be under regular review by a cardiologist with regular surveillance from their teens onwards (annual ECG and echocardiogram in the first instance). As for DMD, BMD patients are at increased risk perioperatively and an anaesthetist should always be made aware of the diagnosis. Guidelines exist for cardiovascular investigations and management, see below (Bushby et al. 2003).

Potential long-term complications in carriers for DMD or BMD

There is unequivocal evidence that ~10% of female carriers of dystrophin mutations (DMD or BMD) develop overt cardiac failure even in the absence of skeletal muscle involvement (Hoogerwaard et al. 1999b; Bushby et al. 2003).

Surveillance

One model of care is for the local community paediatric team to share care with a specialist centre with expertise in paediatric neuromuscular disorders.

- **DMD.** Cardiac investigations (echo and ECG) every 2 years to age 10 years and annually thereafter. Echo and ECG should be repeated before any surgery.

- **BMD.** Cardiac investigations (echo and ECG) every 5 years.
- **Carriers.** All carriers of DMD or BMD should have an echo and ECG at diagnosis or after the age of 16 years and at least every 5 years thereafter. Carriers manifesting severe skeletal muscle symptoms or cardiac symptoms require more frequent investigation (Bushby *et al.* 2003).

Support group: Muscular Dystrophy Campaign <www.muscular-dystrophy.org>; Duchenne Family Support Group <www.dfsg.org.uk>. Parent Project UK–Muscular dystrophy www.ppuk.org.

Expert adviser: Kate Bushby, Action Research Professor in Neuromuscular Genetics, Institute of Human Genetics, University of Newcastle, Newcastle-upon-Tyne, England.

References

<cmgs.org/BPG/Guidelines/1st_ed/dmd.htm>.

Bundey S. Calculation of genetic risks in Duchenne muscular dystrophy by geneticists in the United Kingdom. *J Med Genet* 1978; **15** (4): 249–53.

Bushby K, Muntoni F, Bourke JP. 107th ENMC International Workshop: the management of cardiac involvement in muscular dystrophy and myotonic dystrophy. 7th–9th June 2002, Naarden, the Netherlands. *Neuromuscul Disord* 2003; **13**: 166–72.

Connolly AM, Schierbecker J, *et al.* High dose weekly oral prednisone improves strength in boys with Duchenne muscular dystrophy. *Neuromuscul Disord* 2002; **12**: 917–25.

Eagle M, Baudouin SV, *et al.* Survival in Duchenne muscular dystrophy: improvements in life expectancy since 1967 and the impact of home nocturnal ventilation. *Neuromuscul Disord* 2002; **12**: 926–9.

Emery AE. The muscular dystrophies. *Br Med J* 1998; **317**: 991–5.

Hoogerwaard EM, Bakker E, *et al.* Signs and symptoms of Duchenne muscular dystrophy and Becker muscular dystrophy among carriers in the Netherlands: a cohort study. *Lancet* 1999a; **353**: 2116–19.

Hoogerwaard EM, van der Wouw PA, *et al.* Cardiac involvement in carriers of Duchenne and Becker muscular dystrophy. *Neuromuscul Disord* 1999b; **9**: 347–51.

Wong BL, Christopher C. Corticosteroids in Duchenne muscular dystrophy: a reappraisal. *J Child Neurol* 2002; **17**: 183–90.

Young ID. *Introduction to risk calculation in genetic counselling*, 2nd edn. Oxford University Press, Oxford 1999.

Ehlers–Danlos syndrome (EDS)

All forms of EDS cause clinical problems such as skin fragility, unsightly bruising and scarring, musculoskeletal discomfort, and susceptibility to osteoarthritis (see table). However, only the vascular type is associated with an increased risk of death. Approximately 1/5000 people is affected by EDS.

Vascular EDS. Autosomal dominant (AD) due to mutations in *COL3A1*, encoding type III collagen. Affected individuals are prone to arterial rupture, intestinal perforation (usually colon), and uterine rupture. Complications are rare in infancy, but occur in up to 25% before 20 years, and 80% before 40 years. Median life expectancy is 48 years with arterial rupture accounting for most deaths. Arterial repairs are technically challenging because the vessels are extremely friable.

Diagnosis is based on specific facial features, thin translucent skin, propensity to bleeding, and rupture of vessels. There may be increased joint mobility of the hands. Diagnosis is confirmed by finding abnormalities in type III collagen and/or a mutation in *COL3A1*. Although arterial tears are the hallmarks of vascular EDS, ~25% of all complications affect the gastrointestinal tract.

In Pepin *et al.*'s (2000) study, most deaths resulted from arterial dissection or rupture. Approximately 80% of these deaths involved thoracic or abdominal vessels and <10% resulted from intracranial haemorrhage. Most of the bowel complications affected the colon, especially the sigmoid. Perforation of the small bowel and gastric perforation were uncommon. Vascular EDS should be suspected in any young person presenting with unexplained arterial rupture or visceral rupture, carotid dissection, or colonic perforation.

- **Molecular pathogenesis.** Mutations in *COL3A1* have a 'dominant negative' effect. Patients who are heterozygous for mutations in *COL3A1* that do not cause premature chain termination produce about equal amounts of normal and abnormal type III procollagen polypeptides. These interact to form the homotripolymer type III procollagen protein. However, only ($1/2 \times 1/2 \times 1/2$), i.e. 1/8 of the proteins, will contain three normal polypeptides, whereas the other 7/8 will contain at least one mutant polypeptide and will function abnormally.

Clinical approach

History: key points

- Three-generation family tree with specific enquiry regarding joint hypermobility, easy bruising, or abnormal scarring. (For vascular EDS enquire about arterial or intestinal rupture.)
- Enquire about dislocation/subluxation of joints (especially shoulders, patellae, temperomandibular joints, and digits).

Examination: key points

- Assess Beighton score (see 'Hypermobile joints' page 138.
- Ask the patient whether they have any 'party tricks' to demonstrate their joint hypermobility.
- Assess skin. Is it soft and velvety? Is it hyperextensible (pick up a small fold of skin over the upper arm and gently draw it away from the underlying muscle)?
- Examine skin over elbows and knees for abnormal scarring (e.g. thin atrophic ('cigarette paper' scars); also examine any scars from surgery for abnormal widening and thinning.
- Examine for bruising.

Investigation

- Consider skin biopsy for electron microscopy for ultrastructural analysis and for fibroblast culture for collagen studies—type V collagen in classical EDS, type III collagen in vascular EDS. Abnormal migration of type I collagen is seen in kyphoscoliosis and arthrochalasia types.
- Consider DNA for mutation analysis in one family member (not feasible in most families with hypermobile EDS). Molecular testing is available for vascular (IV), kyphoscoliosis (VI), and arthrochalasia (VII) types.
- Consider echocardiogram for mitral valve prolapse (MVP) and aortic root diameter in adults with classical EDS, hypermobile EDS, and kyphoscoliotic EDS.
- Consider magnetic resonance imaging (MRI) of thoracic and abdominal aorta and iliac arteries in symptomatic individuals with vascular EDS (whether there is a role for

Villefranche classification of EDS (1997; taken from Beighton et al. (1998))

Classical (types I and II). AD; up to 50% are due to mutations in *COL5A1* and *COL5A2*
Soft, hyperextensible skin with easy bruising and thin atrophic scars; joint hypermobility; varicose veins; risk of prematurity in affected fetuses

Hypermobility (type III). AD
Common and usually mild disorder. Soft skin with hypermobility of large and small joints (Beighton score 5/9 or greater)

Vascular (type IV). AD due to mutations in *COL3A1* encoding type III collagen
Uncommon but serious disorder. Characteristic facies with prominent eyes due to decreased adipose tissue below the eyes and thin, slightly 'pinched' nose, thin lips, and hollow cheeks. Thin translucent skin with visible veins, easy bruising. No significant large joint hypermobility (Beighton score <5/9). Risk of arterial rupture and rupture of bowel, bladder, and uterus leads to reduced life expectancy

Kyphoscoliosis (type VI). AR due to mutations in *PLOD1* (lysyl hydroxylase deficiency)
Soft hyperextensible skin, joint hypermobility, muscle hypotonia, scoliosis, and rupture of the optic globe

Arthrochalasia (type VIIA and B). AD due to exonic deletions in *COL1A1* or *COL1A2*
Soft skin with or without abnormal scarring, severe joint hypermobility, and congenital hip dislocation

Dermatosporaxis (type VIIC). AR due to mutations in type I collagen *N*-peptidase (ADAMTS2)
Severe skin fragility with sagging, redundant skin

Other variants
e.g. X-linked (type V) and AD Periodontal EDS (type VIII), AR Progeroid (XGPT1 mutation) and AR EDS without scaring (*tenascin-X* deficiency)

repair of unruptured aneurysms in patients with this syndrome is not clear).

Other diagnoses/conditions to consider
Benign joint hypermobility syndrome. This term is sometimes used synonymously with EDS—hypermobility type. See 'Hypermobile joints' page 138.

Cutis laxa. Inherited cutis laxa is a connective tissue disorder characterized by loose skin and variable internal organ involvement, resulting from paucity of elastic fibres. Mutations in the elastin gene have been reported in three families with AD inheritance, and a family with autosomal recessive (AR) cutis laxa was recently reported to have a homozygous missense mutation in the fibulin-5 (*FBLN5*) gene. Markova *et al.* (2003) reported a patient with a heterozygous tandem duplication within (*FBLN5*). There may be other genes in addition to *ELN* and *FBLN5*.

Marfan syndrome. See 'Marfan syndrome', page 380.

Genetic advice
Inheritance and recurrence risk
Most are AD—see table above.

Variability and penetrance
Some inter- and intrafamilial variability is seen. Significant variability is uncommon, but mild phenotypic variability is commonly seen.

Prenatal diagnosis
Technically possible if the familial mutation is known, but rarely indicated (with the possible exception of vascular EDS).

Predictive testing
Although no specific therapies delay the onset of complications in patients with vascular EDS, knowledge of the diagnosis may influence the management of surgery, pregnancy, and major complications. Patients should avoid any activity that leads to a sudden increase in blood pressure.

Natural history and management
Potential long-term complications
- **Pregnancy.** There is an increased risk for preterm delivery in fetuses affected by classical EDS. Overall, post-partum haemorrhage and complicated perineal wounds are more common in women with EDS than without (19% versus 7% and 8% versus <1%, respectively). Women with vascular EDS have a risk of uterine rupture (as well as arterial and bowel rupture). In Pepin *et al.*'s (2000) study the mortality rate amongst women with vascular EDS who became pregnant was 1 death per 23 pregnancies. Although several women died of uterine rupture at term, it is uncertain whether the use of elective lower segment Caesarean section (LSCS) would decrease mortality (uterine rupture may occur before the onset of labour).
- **Early arthritis.** Joint hypermobility can predispose to premature onset of osteoarthritis in early or mid adult life.
- **Aortic root dilatation.** In Wenstrup *et al.*'s (2002) study of 71 individuals with EDS, 14/42 (33%) individuals with classical EDS and 6/29 (20%) with hypermobile EDS had aortic root dilatation. The risk of aortic root rupture appears to be significantly less than in Marfan syndrome but, nevertheless, occasional cases have been reported in both classical and hypermobile types.

Support group: The Ehlers–Danlos National Foundation <www.ednf.org>; The EDS support group (UK) <www.ehlers-danlos.org>.

Expert adviser: Nigel Burrows, Consultant Dermatologist, Addenbrooke's Hospital, Cambridge, England.

References
Beighton P, De Paepe A, *et al.* Ehlers–Danlos syndromes: revised nosology, Villefranche 1997. Ehlers–Danlos National Foundation (USA) and Ehlers–Danlos Support Group (UK). *Am J Med Genet* 1998; **77**: 31–7.

Germain DP. Clinical and genetic features of vascular Ehlers–Danlos syndrome. *Ann Vasc Surg* 2002; **16**: 391–7.

Lind J, Wallenburg HC. Pregnancy and the Ehlers–Danlos syndrome: a retrospective study in a Dutch population. *Acta Obstet Gynecol Scand* 2002; **81**: 293–300.

Malfait F, Coucke P, *et al.* The molecular basis of classic Ehlers-Danlos syndrome: a comprehensive study of biochemical and molecular findings in 48 unrelated patients. *Hum Mutat* 2005; **25**: 28–37.

Markova D, Zou Y, *et al.* Genetic heterogeneity of cutis laxa: a heterozygous tandem duplication within the fibulin-5 (FBLN5) gene. *Am J Hum Genet* 2003; **72**: 998–1004.

Pepin M, Schwarze U, *et al.* Clinical and genetic features of Ehlers–Danlos syndrome type IV, the vascular type. *New Engl J Med* 2000; **342**: 673–80.

Pyeritz RE. Ehlers–Danlos syndrome [editorial]. *New Engl J Med* 2000; **342**: 730–2.

Schalkwijk J, Zweers MC, *et al.* A recessive form of the Ehlers-Danlos syndrome caused by teanscin-X deficiency. *NEJM* 2001; **345**: 1167–75.

Wenstrup RJ, Hoechstetter LB. The Ehlers–Danlos syndromes. In *Management of genetic syndromes* (ed. S.B. Cassidy and J.E. Allanson), Chapter 8, pp. 131–49. Wiley-Liss, New York, 2001.

Wenstrup RJ, Meyer RA, *et al.* Prevalence of aortic root dilation in the Ehlers–Danlos syndrome. *Genet Med* 2002; **4**: 112–17.

Epilepsy in infants and children

This section discusses epilepsies of infancy and childhood that have specific electroencephalographic (EEG) and clinical features. These conditions are often difficult to control and are associated with developmental delay, and families ask for genetic advice about recurrence risk and prenatal diagnosis.

Ion channels provide the basis for the regulation of excitability in the central nervous system (CNS), and most of the idiopathic epilepsies with a known molecular basis are channelopathies. Where the ion channel defects have been defined, however, they generally account for a minority of families and sporadic cases with the syndrome in question. The data suggest that ion channel mutations of large effect are a common cause of rare monogenic idiopathic epilepsies, but a rare cause of common epilepsies (Mulley et al. 2003).

As there is rapid progress on the molecular aetiology of these conditions, genetic risks may be more accurately determined in the future by molecular methods, but at present these are not usually available except through research centres and currently only a tiny proportion of cases have defined mutations (see table).

Clinical approach

History: key points

- Three-generation family history for epilepsy, including febrile convulsions (may indicate a dominant, recessive, or X-linked pattern of inheritance).
- Parental consanguinity and previous affected sibling increase the probability of a recessive disorder.
- Pregnancy (congenital infections, severe bleeding, hypoxia, teratogenic drugs, and alcohol by disturbance to brain development).
- Perinatal period: birth trauma, neonatal seizures, blistering rash (incontinentia pigmenti (IP)).
- Occipital-frontal circumference (OFC) at birth and subsequent brain growth.
- Onset of the seizures; frequency and type of seizure. Medication.
- Developmental progress before and since the onset of seizures. Try and establish if there is any evidence of developmental regression. This assessment is problematic in children with poorly controlled seizures on high doses of anti-epileptic drugs (pseudoregression).

Examination: key points

- OFC. Beware OFC falling down the centiles.
- Neurological signs (pyramidal features, ataxia).
- Eyes and fundus.
- Dysmorphic features/other system involvement indicate a possible syndromic cause (see 'Dysmorphic child' page 102).
- Neurocutaneous signs. Woods light examination.

Investigation

- Review biochemical and metabolic investigations (see 'Neonatal encephalopathy and intractable seizures in the neonate' and 'Seizures with developmental delay/mental retardation' page 238).
- Magnetic resonance imaging (MRI) brain scan to exclude structural malformation.
- EEG for specific diagnostic changes. Consider if repeats are required or if additional family members should have an EEG if they have features suggestive of a seizure disorder.
- Cytogenetic testing in children with complex seizure disorders or with developmental delay (see 'Seizures with developmental delay/mental retardation' page 238).
- DNA storage/ diagnostic testing. Consider mitochondrial DNA analysis.

Other diagnoses/conditions to consider

Symptomatic and syndromic causes of epilepsy (see 'Seizures with developmental delay/mental retardation' page 238).

Generalized cryptogenic epilepsies in infants and children
Early infantile epileptic encephalopathy with suppression burst (Ohtahara syndrome). This is the earliest type of age-dependent epileptic encephalopathy that has characteristic clinical and EEG features. It is a heterogeneous condition and, whilst it is mostly sporadic, there are familial cases. Migrational abnormalities in the brain and other structural abnormalities should be excluded by MRI and/or neuropathology. Cytochrome oxidase deficiency has been reported in one case. Defects in energy metabolism should be considered. There is a poor prognosis with severe handicap; early death is likely.

Epilepsy syndromes in infants and children associated with single-gene mutations

Epilepsy syndrome	Gene	Gene product
AD nocturnal frontal lobe epilepsy (ADNFLE)	*CHRNA4*	Subunit of nicotinic acetylcholine receptor
	CHRNB2	Subunit of nicotinic acetylcholine receptor
AD juvenile myoclonic epilepsy (ADJME)	*GABRA1*	GABA$_A$-receptor subunit
	EFHC1	Associates with calcium channel
Benign familial neonatal convulsions	*KCNQ2*	Potassium channel
	KCNQ3	Potassium channel
	ATP1A2	Na$^+$, K$^+$-ATPase pump
Childhood absence and febrile seizures	*GABRA1*	GABA$_A$-receptor subunit
Generalized epilepsy with febrile seizures plus (GEFS(+))	*SCN1A*	Sodium-channel subunit
	SCN2A	Sodium-channel subunit
	SCN1B	Sodium-channel subunit
	GABRG2	GABA$_A$-receptor subunit
Idiopathic generalized epilepsy (variable phenotype)	*CLCN2*	Voltage-gated chloride channel

Infantile spasms and West syndrome. West syndrome is the triad of infantile spasms, hypsarrhythmia, and developmental delay. An infantile spasm is a sudden bilateral and symmetrical contraction of the muscles. The prevalence is 0.4 per 100 000 and it is more common in boys.

The symptomatic group accounts for more than 85% of children with infantile spasms; in these children there is an underlying abnormality affecting brain development. All children with infantile spasms should have brain imaging.

Before counselling the family of a child with infantile spasms, check particularly that the following conditions have been excluded.

- Lissencephaly (see 'Lissencephaly and neuronal migration disorders' page 156).
- Tuberous sclerosis accounts for 25% of cases (see 'Tuberous sclerosis', page 420).
- Metabolic disorders, including untreated phenylketonuria (PKU).
- PEHO (progressive encephalopathy–(o)edema–hypsarrthymia–optic atrophy) syndrome. Autosomal recessive (AR) condition characterized by hypsarrhythmia, hypotonia, hyperreflexia, and oedema of the extremities.
- Mitochondrial or other defects of energy metabolism.
- X-linked infantile spasms in males (*ARX*).
- Early onset infantile spasma with severe neurodevelopmental retardation in females due to 'de novo' mutations in *STK9* (Tao)
- Non-genetic causes include trauma and infections.

The condition is described as cryptogenic when the aetiology is unknown and, prior to the spasms, the infant had normal development. The prognosis is better in the cryptogenic group. Prompt recognition and treatment also improve the outcome.

Epilepsy with myoclonic–astatic epilepsy (MAE), severe myoclonic epilepsy in infancy (SMEI or Dravet syndrome), and intractable childhood epilepsy with generalized tonic–clonic seizures (ICEGTC) are epileptic encephalopathies where multiple seizure types begin in the first year of life along with slowing of developmental progress and regression in the severe phenotypes.

Generalized epilepsy with febrile seizures (GEFS(+)) is a familial epilepsy where febrile convulsions persist past early childhood and/or afebrile fits occur. Genetically heterogeneous, mutations have been identified in three sodium channel subunit genes and a GABA_A subunit gene and (*SCN1A, SCN1B, SCN2A, GABRG2*).

Idiopathic generalized epilepsy
Mutations in 10 genes causing distinct forms of idiopathic epilepsy have been identified so far, but the genetic basis of many idiopathic generalized epilepsy subtypes is still unknown.

Juvenile myoclonic epilepsy (JME) accounts for 5–10% of seizures. It is the most frequent cause of hereditary grand mal seizures. The peak age of onset is in adolescence but it presents from childhood onwards. 90% have tonic clonic seizures and 30% have absence seizures in addition to myoclonic seizures. Autosomal dominant (AD) juvenile myoclonic epilepsy was recently demonstrated in some families, to be a channelopathy associated with mutations in the gene encoding a GABA(A) receptor alpha-1 subunit (*GABRA1*). Mutations in *EFHC1* on 6p11–12 have been found to segregate with epilepsy or EEG polyspike wave in some other families (Suzuki).

Benign childhood epilepsy with centrotemporal spikes (BCECTS) includes benign rolandic epilepsy and benign focal epilepsy.

Benign familial neonatal convulsions. AD disorder presenting in the first year of life caused by mutations in a potassium-channel gene (*KCNQ2/KCNQ3*). Seizures occur repeatedly in the first days of life and remit by approximately 4 months of age; a subset of families has onset of seizures in infancy (Singh *et al.* 2003).

Benign familial neonatal–infantile seizures. AD disorder presenting in the first year of life caused by mutations in the sodium channel subunit gene *SCN2A*. This is a benign familial epilepsy syndrome beginning in early infancy, an age at which seizure disorders frequently have a sombre prognosis (Heron *et al.* 2000).

Genetic advice
Those cryptogenic and idiopathic epilepsy syndromes that are commonly referred for counselling are discussed here.

Recurrence risk: generalized cryptogenic epilepsies in infants and children

Early infantile epileptic encephalopathy with suppression burst (Ohtahara syndrome) is a heterogeneous condition and, whilst it is mostly sporadic, there are familial cases. Consanguinity may indicate AR inheritance.

Infantile spasms and West syndrome (cryptogenic). When identifiable inherited diseases have been excluded, the recurrence risk is low, less than 2%. In a small subgroup this will underestimate the risk. Dulac *et al.* (1993) reported that clinical signs of a progressive encephalopathy such as postnatal microcephaly and myoclonus are features that may predict a recurrence. Of the 11 familial cases, four were due to 'non-genetic' factors (twin pregnancy, recurrent maternal toxaemia).

MAE, SMEI, and ICEGTC and GEFS(+). Consider the following when counselling.
- It has been shown that MAE, SMEI, and ICEGTC are part of the syndrome GEFS(+).
- Changes in three sodium channel subunit genes and a GABA_A subunit gene and (*SCN1A, SCN1B, SCN2A, GABRG2*) have been identified in all three epilepsy syndromes.
- MAE has occurred in individuals from large pedigrees with GEFS(+).
- 50% of children with SMEI have a family history of seizures.
- More severe *de novo* truncating mutations of *SCN1A* have been found in SMEI.

Recurrence risk: idiopathic generalized epilepsy
JME. There is often a family history but not following a Mendelian pattern. Both AR and AD modes of inheritance have been proposed. Apparently unaffected individuals in families have had abnormalities on EEG and subclinical seizures. With no family history, recurrence and offspring risks of around 5% for significant epilepsy will underestimate the risks for some families.

BCECTS. 15% risk of epilepsy in sibs and just over 50% show EEG abnormalities.

Benign familial neonatal convulsions. AD inheritance.

Benign familial neonatal–infantile seizures. AD inheritance.

Carrier detection
Not available unless a causative mutation has been identified in the proband.

Prenatal diagnosis
Not available unless a causative mutation or biochemical abnormality has been identified in the proband.

Natural history and further management
Patients require long-term management by a paediatric neurologist.

Support group: <www.epilepsy.org.uk>; Epilepsy Foundation of America <www.efa.org>.

Expert adviser: R.M. Gardiner, Professor, Department of Paediatrics and Child Health, Royal Free and University College Medical School, London, England.

References

Chang BS, Lowenstein DH. Mechanisms of disease; epilepsy [review]. *New Engl J Med* 2003; **349**: 1257–66.

Dulac O, *et al.* Genetic predispopsition to West syndrome. *Epilepsia* 1993; **34**: 732–7.

Engel J; International League against Epilepsy (ILAE). A proposed diagnostic scheme for people with epileptic seizures and with epilepsy: report of the ILAE task force on classification and terminology. *Epilepsia* 2001; **42**: 769–803.

Haug K, Warnstedt M, *et al.* Mutations in CLCN2 encoding a voltage-gated chloride channel are associated with idiopathic generalized epilepsies. *Nat Genet.* 2003; **33** (4): 527–32.

Heron SE, Crossland KM, *et al.* Sodium-channel defects in benign familial neonatal–infantile seizures. *Lancet* 2002; **360** (9336): 851–2.

Lerche H, Jurkat-Rott K, *et al.* Ion channels and epilepsy. *Am J Med Genet.* 2001; **106** (2): 146–59.

Mulley JC, Scheffer IE, Petrou S, Berkovic SF. Channelopathies as a genetic cause of epilepsy. *Curr Opin Neurol* 2003; **16**: 171–6.

Scheffer IE. Severe infantile epilepsies: molecular genetics challenge clinical classification. *Brain* 2003; **126**: 513–14.

Scheffer IE, Wallace R, *et al.* Clinical and molecular genetics of myoclonic–astatic epilepsy and severe myoclonic epilepsy in infancy (Dravet syndrome). *Brain Dev* 2001: **23**: 732–5.

Singh NA, Westenskow P, *et al.* KCNQ2 and KCNQ3 potassium channel genes in benign familial neonatal convulsions: expansion of the functional and mutation spectrum. *Brain* 2003; **126** (pt 12): 2726–37.

Singh R, Gardner RJ, Crossland KM, Scheffer IE, Berkovic SF. Chromosomal abnormalities and epilepsy: a review for clinicians and gene hunters. *Epilepsia* 2002; **43**(2): 127–40.

Suzuki T, Delgado-Escueta AV, *et al.* Mutations in *EFHC1* cause juvenile myoclonic epilepsy. *Nat Genet* 2004; **36**: 842–49.

Tao J, Van Esch H, *et al.* Mutations in the X-linked cyclin-dependent kinase-like 5 (*CDKL5/STK9*) gene are associated with severe neurodevelopmental retardation. *Am J Hum Genet* 2004; **75**: 1149–54.

Vanmolkot KR, Kors EE, *et al.* Novel mutations in the Na$^+$, K$^+$-ATPase pump gene *ATP1A2* associated with familial hemiplegic migraine and benign familial infantile convulsions. *Ann Neurol* 2003; **54**: 360–66.

Epilepsy

This chapter primarily considers the counselling of an individual with apparently idiopathic epilepsy, or someone who has a family history of this. See also 'Epilepsy in infants and children', page 314, and 'Seizures with developmental delay/mental retardation' page 238 and 'Neonatal encephalopathy and intractable seizures in the neonate' page 186, 'Clinical approach'.

Epilepsy is a disorder of the brain. It may occur as part of an acute or acquired process affecting the central nervous system (CNS). Genetic factors and genetically determined syndromes contribute in many patients. Epilepsy and seizures are common medical problems. In the general population the cumulative incidence for developing epilepsy to the age of 40 years is just under 2%.

Bianchi *et al.* (2003) in a huge epidemiological survey of >10 000 patients with epilepsy found that the prevalence of epilepsy in first-degree relatives of patients with idiopathic generalized epilepsies was 5.3%. Probands with idiopathic generalized epilepsies were highly concordant with respect to their relative's type of epilepsy. Risks to relatives were higher when the epilepsy in the proband began at <14 years of age. Berkovic *et al.* (2001) studied twin pairs with seizures and found that concordance was higher in monozygotic (MZ) twin pairs than in dizygotic (DZ) twin pairs (casewise concordance 0.62 and 0.18, respectively). In 94% of concordant MZ pairs and 71% of concordant DZ pairs, both twins had the same major epilepsy syndrome. This strongly suggests the presence of syndrome-specific genetic determinants rather than a broad genetic predisposition to seizures.

Most genetic epilepsies have a complex mode of inheritance and genes identified so far account only for a minority of families and sporadic cases (Gutierrez-Delicado). Genes associated with idiopathic generalised epilepsy are within the ion-channel family. Mutations in non-ion channel genes are implicated in AD lateral temporal lobe epilepsy, malformations of cortical development and X-linked mental retardation syndromes in which seizures are a component.

To understand the epilepsy literature it is helpful to review the current definitions and classification.

- **Epileptic seizure.** A transient episode of abnormal cortical neuronal activity (see first table). This may manifest as a motor, sensory, cognitive, or psychic disturbance.
- **Epilepsy.** A disorder of the brain characterized by recurrent (two or more) unprovoked seizures (see second table).

Neurologists manage and investigate the patient with epilepsy. Correct classification of the epilepsy is required prior to genetic counselling.

Clinical approach

History: key points

- Family history. Three-generation family tree with specific enquiry about seizures.

Simplified classification of epileptic seizures

1 **Partial seizures.*** The initial changes are caused by activation of neurons in part of one cerebral cortex
- Simple partial seizures. Consciousness retained. Motor (e.g. limb or adversive head turning), sensory (e.g. visual or pins and needles), autonomic, psychic presentation
- Complex partial seizures. Altered consciousness. A simple partial seizure may evolve into a complex partial seizure
2 **Generalized seizures**. The electroencephalographic (EEG) changes are bilateral from the onset. Consciousness may or may not be altered
- Absence seizures. Sudden onset of a brief impairment of consciousness
- Tonic–clonic seizures. Sudden loss of consciousness. Tonic muscle contraction is followed by clonic jerking
- Myoclonic seizure. Brief jerk, either in single muscle or generalized, of rapid onset and cessation. No loss of consciousness
- Atonic seizures

* Sometimes partial seizures progress and become generalized, the focal onset being followed by a generalized tonic–clonic seizure. This is termed a partial seizure with secondary generalization.

Classification of epilepsy

1 Partial epilepsy
- Idiopathic. No underlying cause other than a possible genetic component. Includes some Mendelian inherited epilepsy syndromes
- Symptomatic. Secondary to a known or suspected disorder of the brain
- Cryptogenic. Presumed to be symptomatic, but cause cannot be identified in the individual concerned
2 Generalized epilepsy
- Idiopathic. No underlying cause other than a possible genetic component. Includes some Mendelian inherited epilepsy syndromes
- Cryptogenic. Presumed to be symptomatic but cause cannot be identified in the individual concerned, e.g. infantile spasms
- Symptomatic. Secondary to a known or suspected disorder of the brain
3 Epilepsies and syndromes undetermined as to whether focal or generalized
4 Special syndromes
5 Situation-related seizures
- Febrile seizures
- Hypoglycaemic seizures
- Other acute metabolic or toxic factors

Genetic risks in idiopathic epilepsy (modified after Harper (2004))

Individual affected	Cumulative risk of clinical epilepsy to age 20 years (%)*
Monozygotic twins	~60
Dizygotic twins	~10
Sibling with onset <10 years	6
Sibling with onset >25 years	1–2
Overall sibling risk	2.5
Parent	4(1.5–7.5)
Parent and sibling	~10
Both parents	~15
General population	~1

* Excluding febrile convulsions.

- Perinatal history, past medical history. Is there evidence of an acquired cause for the epilepsy such as head injury, meningitis?
- Developmental milestones. Delay/mental retardation.
- Natural history of the seizures. Age of onset, e.g. neonatal, change in seizure type with age, seizure type, frequency, precipitating factors, medication. An eye witness account is often invaluable in determining the seizure type. Are there nocturnal seizures?

Examination: key points
Consider examination of affected individuals when the aetiology is unknown.
- Focal neurological signs.
- Skin examination for signs of a neurocutaneous syndrome. Consider Woods light to exclude depigmented lesions of tuberous sclerosis (TS), incontinentia pigmenti (IP), and hypomelanosis of Ito.
- Eye and fundal examination.
- Dysmorphic features: storage, metabolic, or chromosomal conditions.

Investigation
- Electroencephalogram (EEG). Note if specific diagnostic features have been seen.
- Brain imaging. If this has not already been performed, magnetic resonance imaging (MRI) may be required prior to counselling to exclude genetically determined structural malformations of the brain.
- Electrocardiogram (ECG). Arrhythmias, long QT interval leading to syncope and an erroneous diagnosis of epilepsy.
- Cytogenetic analysis if dysmorphic features and/or mental retardation. (See 'Seizures with developmental delay/mental retardation' page 238.)
- DNA analysis is available for some epilepsy syndromes, e.g. TSC, *SCN1A*. Consider if mitochondrial DNA analysis is necessary (MERFF (myoclonic epilepsy with ragged red fibres), MELAS (mitochondrial myopathy– encephalopathy–lactic acidosis–stroke-like episodes)).

Other diagnoses/conditions to consider
- **Long QT syndromes.** See 'Long QT and Brugada syndromes', page 378.

- **Non-epileptic causes**, e.g. syncope, pseudoseizures, Munchausen syndrome (by proxy in children). These diagnoses should be evaluated by a neurologist.

Genetic advice
Idiopathic epilepsy. Define the epileptic syndrome as far as possible. Analyse the family tree to determine evidence for a Mendelian pattern of inheritance. Ensure that a structural brain lesion has been excluded in the proband (by cranial imaging).

Known autosomal dominant (AD) syndromes:
- AD nocturnal frontal lobe epilepsy (mutations in neuronal nicotinic acetyl choline receptor genes *CHRNA4*, *CHRNB4*);
- benign familial neonatal convulsions (potassium channel genes *KCNQ2*, *KCNQ3*);
- generalized epilepsy with febrile seizures (GEFS(+); voltage-gated sodium channel genes *SCN1B*, *SCN1A* and the GABA(A) receptor *GABRG2*). In most families GEFS(+) is not AD.
- remember to exclude TSC.
- there are many other AD syndromes some with known genes, e.g. AD partial epilepsy with auditory features (*LG11*) and benign familial infantile seizures mapped to chromosomes 16 and 19 (genes unknown).

In practice genetic testing is rarely available. Locus and allelic heterogeneity make DNA analysis problematic in idiopathic AD epilepsies which are mainly caused by ion channel gene mutations.

Inheritance and recurrence risk
Where possible use figures that are specific for the type of epilepsy, these may be found by consulting the references listed below.

For isolated/idiopathic epilepsy with no clear familial inheritance, multifactorial inheritance is assumed and empiric risk figures used. The offspring risk for epilepsy is between 1.5% and 7.5%.

Variability and penetrance
Most of the familial epilepsy syndromes show intra- and interfamilial variability with some mutation carriers unaffected with epilepsy.

Prenatal diagnosis
Only available in conditions with a known mutation or cytogenetic abnormality. Be alert to the teratogenic effects of anti-epileptic medications (see 'Fetal anticonvulsant syndrome (FACS)' page 590).

Other family members
For AD families, pedigree analysis may refine carrier risks. Multifactorial inheritance for other idiopathic types means that risks for second-degree relatives are not much higher than population risks.

Natural history and management
Potential long-term complications
- Fetal anti-epileptic drug effects and increased risk of neural tube defects. See 'Fetal anticonvulsant syndrome' page 590. Possible neurodevelopmental consequences for fetus of frequent maternal tonic-clonic seizures in pregnancy (Adab).
- Increased risk of sudden death in patients with epilepsy (mainly attributable to the underlying disease, accidents, or suicide), especially in certain groups (e.g. young people and those with frequent generalized seizures and mental retardation).

- Restrictions on driving; possible discrimination; long-term effects of the epilepsy, seizures, and medication.

Surveillance
By a neurologist.

Support group: <www.epilepsy.org.uk; www.epilepsynse.org.uk>; Epilepsy Foundation of America <www.efa.org>.

Expert adviser: S.M. Sisodiya, Department of Clinical and Experimental Epilepsy, University College London Institute of Neurology, London, England.

References

Adab N, Kini U, *et al.* The longer term outcome of children born to mothers with epilepsy. *JNNP* 2004; **75**: 1575–83.

Berkovic SF, Howell RA, *et al.* Epilepsies in twins: genetics of the major epilepsy syndromes. *Ann Neurol* 1998; **43**: 435–45.

Bianchi A, Viaggi S, Chiossi E. Family study of epilepsy in first degree relatives: data from the Italian Episcreen Study. *Seizure* 2003; **12**: 203–10.

Callenbach PM, Geerts AT, *et al.* Familial occurrence of epilepsy in children with newly diagnosed multiple seizures; Dutch Study of Epilepsy in Childhood. *Epilepsia* 1998; **39**: 331–6.

Chang BS, Lowenstein DH. Mechanisms of disease; Epilepsy [review]. *New Engl J Med* 2003; **349**: 1257–66.

Elmslie F, Gardiner M, Lehesjoki AE. The epilepsies. In *Emery and Rimoin's principles and practice of medical genetics*, 4th edn (ed. D.L. Rimoin, J.M. Conner, R.E. Pyeritz, and A.E.H. Emery). Churchill Livingstone, London, 2002.

Engel J Jr; International League Against Epilepsy (ILAE). A proposed diagnostic scheme for people with epileptic seizures and with epilepsy: report of the ILAE task force on classification and terminology. *Epilepsia* 2001; **42**: 769–803.

Gutierrez-Delicado E, Serratosa JM. Genetics of the epilepsies (Review). *Curr Opin Neurol* 2004; **17**: 47–53

Harper PS. *Practical genetic counselling*, 6th edn. Arnold, London, 2004.

Kjeldsen MJ, Kyvik KO, *et al.* Genetic and environmental factors in epilepsy: a population-based study of 11900 Danish twin pairs. *Epilepsy Res* 2001; **44**: 167–78.

Lerche H, Jerkat-Rott K, Lehmann-Horn F. Ion channels and epilepsy. *Am J Med Genet* 2001; **106**: 146–59.

Seminars in Medical Genetics. The Genetics of Epilepsy. *Am J Med Genet* 2001; **106C** (Issue 2).

Sutierrez-Decicado E, Serratosa JM. Genetics of the epilepsies (Review). *Curr Opin Neurol* 2004; **17**: 147–53.

Facioscapulohumeral muscular dystrophy (FSHD)

Landouzy–Dejerine muscular dystrophy, facioscapuloperoneal muscular dystrophy.

FSHD is an autosomal dominant (AD) disorder caused by deletion of an integral number of tandem 3.3 kb repeats, termed *D4Z4*, on 4q35. Prevalence is estimated at ~1/20 000 in the UK (Lunt *et al.* 1995). Deletion of *D4Z4* may lead to the inappropriate transcriptional de-repression of genes on 4q35 in muscle, the overexpression of which leads to FSHD (Gabellini *et al.* 2002). Contraction in the polymorphic *D4Z4* repeat array is associated solely with the 4qA allele and not with the 4qB allele (Lemmers *et al.* 2002).

FSHD typically presents before the age of 20 years with weakness of the facial muscles and the stabilizers of the scapula (see figure). The legs are affected to some degree in ~50%, with weakness of the dorsiflexors of the foot often being an early feature. Hearing impairment may be associated (Brouwer *et al.* 1987; Rogers *et al.* 2002), as also may an asymptomatic retinal vasculopathy comprising telangiectasia and microaneurysms visible with fluorescein angiography (Fitzsimmons *et al.* 1987). Early childhood-onset cases are often 'de novo'.

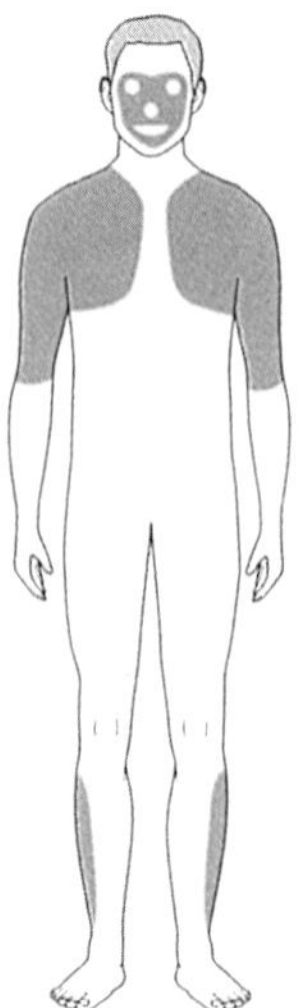

Distribution of predominant muscle weakness in facioscapulohumeral muscular dystrophy. (Reproduced from Emery (1998), fig. 1d, p. 992, by permission of the BMJ Publishing Group.)

Clinical approach

History: key points

- Three-generation family tree with specific enquiry regarding:
  - facial weakness (reduced facial expression, especially when smiling; sleeping with eyes slightly open; unable to whistle or blow up balloons);
  - weakness of shoulders (difficulty lifting arms above head, e.g. combing hair, pegging out washing);
  - weakness of the ankles ('foot drop').
- Developmental milestones and participation in sports and physical education at school.
- Document age at which weakness was first noted. A baby or child may show little facial expression. Later excessive aching around the shoulders with 'rounded' or 'dropped' shoulders may be noted. Shoulder symptoms often begin unilaterally, usually being noted first in the dominant arm in the second or third decade.

Examination: key points

- Facial weakness. More in the lower facial muscles than the upper (inability to bury the eyelashes, puff the cheeks, purse the lips, or whistle).
- Scapular winging (ask the patient to face the wall with their arms bent and hands at shoulder height and to place their palms on the wall and lean with their weight on their palms). Observe from behind to detect winging.
- Observe for stepping of the shoulders on elevation of the arms.
- Thin upper arms with wasting of biceps and triceps. Asymmetry is common.
- Examine for weakness of ankle dorsiflexors (may cause foot drop).
- Severely affected patients may have some hip girdle weakness—difficulty rising from a chair or from the floor.
- Reflexes are often reduced.

Investigations

- Creatine kinase (CK). Usually normal or mildly elevated. Rarely more than 3–5 times the upper limit of normal.
- DNA for analysis of deletion of the *D4Z4* motif. Disease alleles are typically 34 kb or smaller; normal alleles are usually >42 kb. In ~5% the typical deletion may be obscured in the testing method; whether 4q35 FSHD can occur without a typical deletion is not known. (Alleles between 34 and 42 kb represent an overlap region between normal and mild FSHD (usually presenting with mild scapulohumeral weakness), probably with an increasing likelihood of clinical symptoms with reducing fragment size.)
- Muscle biopsy. With the advent of molecular genetic diagnosis it is usually possible to avoid a muscle biopsy for diagnostic purposes. If performed, it typically shows non-specific chronic myopathic changes, often including small angular fibres, and sometimes with a mononuclear inflammatory reaction.

Other diagnoses/conditions to consider

Myotonic dystrophy. AD muscle disorder characterized by myotonia with facial weakness, weakness of sternomastoid muscles with weakness, and wasting of forearm and hand muscles in the early stages. See 'Myotonic dystrophy (DM)', page 388.

Limb girdle muscular dystrophies. Especially LGMD2A with shoulder girdle onset prior to pelvic girdle. See 'Limb girdle muscular dystrophies', page 374.

Nemaline myopathy is a diagnosis made by the identification of nemaline bodies ('rods') on histological analysis of a muscle biopsy. It is caused by mutations in one of at least six different genes. The clinical picture varies widely, in terms of the grade and the distribution of muscle weakness. Muscle weakness is usually most severe in the face, the neck flexors and the proximal limb muscles. In familial cases, autosomal recessive (AR) inheritance is more common than AD inheritance, and in some patients the disorder is caused by new dominant mutations. Because of the genetic heterogeneity and the large size of 'nebulin', one of the genes commonly involved, no routine molecular genetic testing is yet available, with the exception of the actin gene (*ACTA1*) which accounts for 15–25% of cases. Diagnosis often rests on clinical and histological criteria. Management of patients with nemaline myopathy requires regular monitoring of respiratory capacity to detect the onset of insidious hypoventilation (Wallgren-Pettersson 2002).

Mitochondrial myopathy. See 'Mitochondrial DNA diseases', page 384.

Becker muscular dystrophy (BMD) is clinically similar to Duchenne muscular dystrophy (DMD) but milder, with a mean age of onset of 11 years. Loss of the ability to walk may occur late (e.g. 40s or 50s) and many individuals with BMD survive into middle age and beyond. Often, cramps on exercise are the only problem initially, but some affected boys are late in learning to walk and are unable to run fast. Later in the teens and twenties, muscle weakness becomes evident, causing difficulty in rapid walking, running, and climbing stairs. It may become difficult to lift objects above waist height. See 'Duchenne and Becker muscular dystrophy (DMD and BMD)', page 308.

Emery–Dreifuss muscular dystrophy. See 'Limb girdle muscular dystrophies', page 374.

Genetic advice

The great majority of families are linked to 4q35, but a small group of families do not map to this locus.

Inheritance and recurrence risk

AD with 50% risk to offspring of an affected individual. In view of the wide variability and incomplete penetrance, testing of asymptomatic adult family members should be considered before giving advice about risks to their offspring. High *de novo* mutation rate of 10–30%. In general, patients with *de novo* disease have shorter 4q35 fragments than those with familial disease and tend to be symptomatic earlier with more severe disease. At least 40% of new mutations for FSHD arise in mitosis (presumably in the early blastocyst) giving somatic and germline mosaicism (van der Maarel *et al.* 2000). This should be checked for in parents of an apparently isolated case as the recurrence risk in sibs would be significant. Even in molecularly apparent *de novo* mutations, there is a small theoretical risk of sibling recurrence due to parental germline mosaicism.

Variability and penetrance

Penetrance is fairly high. Zatz *et al.* (1998) found a penetrance of 83% by 30 years that was higher in males than females. Signs of muscle weakness (particulary in the face) are evident by 12 years in at least 50% of mutation carriers. The disease shows high interfamilial variability—some patients with severe infantile FSHD have muscle weakness at birth, whereas other mutation carriers can remain asymptomatic throughout life. Non-penetrance may be more likely with larger alleles. Within a family the severity tends to follow a similar trend. It is unusual to find siblings who are affected to very different degrees. There is some genotype–phenotype correlation with earlier age of onset, earlier age of loss of ambulation, and muscle weakness all correlated with shorter 4q35 fragments.

Prenatal diagnosis

Possible by chorionic villus sampling (CVS), but tends to be requested only in the context of the more severe presentations because, otherwise, FSHD is usually a condition of adult life with normal cognition and fairly normal life expectancy.

Predictive testing

FSHD is usually penetrant by early adult life. For those adults wishing to clarify their status, perhaps before starting a family, this is feasible if the proband has a short 4q35 fragment.

Other family members

If 'at-risk' children are symptomatic, testing has an important role in diagnosis. Testing of unaffected 'at-risk' children is generally discouraged so that testing can be deferred until the individual is mature enough to give their own consent (usually as an adult).

Natural history and management

Potential long-term complications

- **Loss of mobility.** Up to 20% of sufferers eventually require a wheelchair. The earlier in life the weakness appears, the greater its eventual severity. Foot splints may be helpful for patients with 'foot drop'.
- **Impaired use of arms in severe disease.** The operation of scapula fixation (attaching the scapula to the ribs) may help some patients to regain useful arm function; however, if an individual has rapidly progressive disease, the benefits may be short-lived.
- **Hearing impairment.** High-tone sensorineural hearing loss can be a feature, although there is no good agreement between different studies on a figure for the proportion of FSHD patients who have an abnormal audiogram (Brouwer *et al.* 1991; Rogers *et al.* 2002).

Surveillance

No specific surveillance is currently advised. An increased incidence of atrial tachyarrhythmias has been noted (Laforet *et al.* 1998), but these are rarely symptomatic and cardiac surveillance is not routinely indicated.

Support group: Muscular Dystrophy Campaign <www.muscular-dystrophy.org>.

Expert adviser: Peter Lunt, Consultant Clinical Geneticist, St. Michael's Hospital, Bristol, England.

References

Brouwer OF, Padberg GW, *et al.* Hearing loss in facioscapulo-humeral muscular dystrophy. *Neurology* 1991; **41**: 1878–81.

Emery AE. The muscular dystrophies. *Br Med J* 1998; **317**: 991–5.

Fitzsimmons RB, Gurwin EB, Bird AC. Retinal vascular abnormalities in facioscapulohumeral muscular dystrophy. A general association with genetic and therapeutic implications. *Brain* 1987; **110** (Pt. 3): 631–48.

Gabellini D, Gren MR, Tupler R. Inappropriate gene activation in FSHS: a repressor complex binds a chromosomal repeat deleted in dystrophic muscle. *Cell* 2002; **110**: 339–48.

Laforet P, de Toma C, *et al.* Cardiac involvement in genetically confirmed facioscapulohumeral muscular dystrophy. *Neurology* 1998; **51**: 1454–6.

Lemmers RJ, de Kievit P, *et al.* Facioscapulohumeral muscular dystrophy is uniquely associated with one of the two variants of the 4q subtelomere. *Nat Genet* 2002; **32**: 235–6.

Lunt PW, Jardine PE, *et al.* Phenotypic–genotypic correlation will assist genetic counselling in 4q35-facioscapulohumeral muscular dystrophy. *Muscle Nerve* 1995; **2S**: 103–9.

Rogers MT, Zhao F, Harper PS, Stephens D. Absence of hearing impairment in adult onset facioscapulohumeral muscular dystrophy. *Neuromuscul Disord* 2002; **12**: 358–65.

Van der Maarel SM, Deidda G, *et al.* De novo facioscapulohumeral muscular dystrophy: frequent somatic mosaicism, sex-dependent phenotype, and the role of mitotic transchromosomal repeat interaction between chromosomes 4 and 10. *Am J Hum Genet* 2000; **66**: 26–35.

Wallgren-Pettersson C. Nemaline and myotubular myopathies. *Semin Pediatr Neurol.* 2002; **9** (2): 132–44.

Zatz M. Marie SK, *et al.* The facioscapulohumeral muscular dystrophy (*FSHD1*) gene affects males more severely and more frequently than females. *Am J Med Genet* 1998; **77**: 155–61.

Fragile X syndrome (FRAX)

FMR1, Martin–Bell syndrome

FRAXA is the most common inherited cause of mental retardation with approximately 1 in 5500 males carrying a full mutation. *FMR1*, at Xq27.3, contains a triplet repeat $(CGG)_n$ in the 5' untranslated region of the gene. Allele sizes outside the normal range are unstable in meiosis. The triplet repeat expansion in FRAXA is a dynamic mutation. Several studies have shown strong somatic stability of the expansion size after the initial period of expansion during which one or more different allele sizes may be generated (see table).

Full, premutation, intermediate, and normal allele sizes in FRAXA*

Normal individuals	<45 repeats
Intermediate allele	45–54 repeats
Premutation carrier females and normal-transmitting males	55–200 repeats
Affected individuals and full-mutation carrier females	>200 repeats

* In FRAXA as in the other repeat disorders there are no distinct boundaries separating the different repeat size categories. Individuals with intermediate-size alleles have ~45 to ~60 repeats, whereas males and females with premutation alleles have ~55 to ~200 repeats. The distinction between intermediate and premutation alleles is made by family history and repeat instability. Categories vary considerably in different publications.

In the presence of a full mutation the *FMR1* gene is methylated and, although mRNA may be produced, no FMR protein (FMRP) is produced. Polysomal association of *FMR1* mRNA, which is high in normal cells, becomes progressively lower with increasing (CGG) repeat expansion. Impairment of *FMR1* mRNA translation may be the cause of the lower FMRP levels that lead to clinical involvement. The level of FMRP correlates with the degree of cognitive involvement in both males and females (Tassone *et al.* 2000).

FRAXE is less common with ~1 in 23 000 males carrying a full mutation. It is caused by a triplet repeat $(GCC)_n$ in *FMR2* on Xq28. The phenotype tends to be milder and the disorder is considerably less common than FRAXA. Whereas FRAXA (*FMR1*) is tested for routinely in the evaluation of developmental delay, FRAXE (*FMR2*) is usually only tested if the family history is suggestive of X-linked mental retardation.

Full mutation in males (fragile X syndrome)

- **Developmental delay.** Hypotonia and mild motor delay is relatively common.
- **Speech and language.** Variable, ranging from no speech through to mild communication problems. Speech is often not very fluent. The speech of affected individuals tends to be characterized by the use of many incomplete sentences, repetition, and echolalia.
- **Intelligence quotient (IQ).** Males with a full mutation that is methylated have an average IQ of 41. Males mosaic for a full and premutation have an average IQ of 60. Males with a full mutation with >50% of cells unmethylated have an average IQ of 88.
- **Behaviour.** Overactivity and impulsiveness with marked concentration problems, fidgetiness, and distractability. Affected individuals are easily overwhelmed by a variety of sensory stimuli. Autistic features with gaze avoidance, stereotyped repetitive behaviours such as hand flapping, resistance to change of routines or environment, and strong preoccupations or fascinations are common. Perseveration with an affected individual becoming fixated on a particular activity or asking questions about the same issue over and over again is quite common. Most children with FRAXA are affectionate and have an interest in relating socially, but have notable difficulty in social interaction and tend to be shy and anxious in group situations.
- **Adult life.** Adults with full mutations often show strengths in skills of daily living, relative to their communication and socialization abilities. Nevertheless, a degree of supported living is needed by many.

Full mutation in females

Females are less affected by fragile X than males, because the nomal X produces variable amounts of FMRP. The level of FMRP correlates with the degree of cognitive involvement in both males and females (Tassone *et al.* 2000). Up to 50% of females with a full FRAX mutation demonstrate learning and behavioural difficulties that are similar to, but usually less severe than those seen in affected males. However, more subtle problems with learning, behavioural, and emotional difficulties are common even in females with a full mutation who have a normal IQ. As is the case for affected males, verbal abilities tend to be better than performance skills, and special needs in arithmetic, visuospatial abilities, and visual and auditory memory are common.

Premutation alleles

On rare occasions, individuals with a premutation may be clinically affected with learning disabilities or cognitive defects, although the vast majority of individuals with the premutation have an IQ in the normal range (Hagerman *et al.* 1996; Tassone *et al.* 2000). When a child with learning difficulties is found to have a premutation, this should not be assumed to be the cause and other investigations should be considered.

Pesso *et al.* (2000) offered preconception and antenatal screening for FRAXA to 8426 Israeli women without a family history of FRAX. They identified 58 women with a premutation (expansion size 55–199 repeats)—this gives an incidence of 0.68% for premutation carrier status for FRAXA in that population

Intermediate alleles

Youings *et al.* (2000) tested 2932 mother to boy transmissions and found only 8 changes in transmission in the common and intermediate range—5 at FRAXA and 3 at FRAXE. For FRAXA these were: 34–37, 43–42, 45–47, 47–48, and 53–54. Transmissions from females with common or intermediate repeats are remarkably stable (in the absence of a family history of FRAX), although instabilities are approximately 90 times more frequent for alleles in the size range 40–59 repeats than for alleles <40 repeats. In a much smaller series (136 transmissions from 92 mothers) Nolin *et al.* (2003) found that 19% of transmissions in the size range 49–54 repeats were unstable. Intermediate alleles are potential precursors of a full mutation in future generations. By definition, only premutation alleles have the potential to expand to full mutations in one generation and so any potential small risk is to more distant generations, with grandchildren being the closest possible generation at risk.

Some intermediate alleles are stably transmitted within families, whilst others show allele instability and may be the potential precursors of a premutation in a subsequent generation. The differences are likely due, at least in part, to differences in AGG interruptions within the FMR1 repeat. In the normal population, the CGG repeat is interrupted by AGG trinucleotides, most often at positions 10 and 20. In contrast, premutation alleles are distinguished by the absence of AGG or the presence of only one AGG interruption at the 5' end of the repeat and long tracts of uninterrupted CGG repeats at the 3' end.

Clinical approach

History: key points

- Three-generation family tree that may need to be extended to further generations in the maternal line to facilitate cascade carrier testing.
- Pregnancy and perinatal history.
- Developmental milestones including language development and schooling.
- Behaviour.

Examination: key points

- Height, weight, occipital-frontal circumference (OFC).
- Face and ears. Classically, individuals with FRAXA have a long face and mildly prominent ears with cupping of the upper pinnae, but this is rarely striking and usually only evident in older boys. Many young children look entirely normal.
- Joints. Joint hypermobility is common.
- Large testes in postpubertal individuals.
- Heart. Examine for mid-systolic click or murmur (mitral valve prolapse (MVP)).
- Behaviour. Eye contact, hyperactivity, motor incoordination.

Investigation

- DNA for FRAXA $(CGG)_n$ repeat size or FRAXE $(GCC)_n$ repeat size.
- Assessment of methylation status. Use of a methylation-sensitive enzyme (Eagl) that cuts non-methylated DNA at the CpG island, but leaves methylated DNA uncut, allows an analysis of the methylation status of *FMR1*.

Other diagnoses/conditions to consider

See 'Mental retardation with apparent X-linked inheritance' page 164.

Genetic advice

Inheritance and recurrence risk

Females. Expansion of a triplet repeat may not occur with every pregnancy in a woman carrying a premutation, but huge expansion into the full mutation range is a potential risk with all premutation alleles. Women with a FRAX premutation face four possible outcomes to each pregnancy: each equally likely. These are: a normal male; a normal female; a male with a FRAX premutation or full mutation; and a female with a FRAX premutation or full mutation.

In Nolin *et al.*'s (2003) study of the offspring of ~1500 premutation females (see table), the smallest size of premutation allele that expanded to a full mutation in one generation was 59 repeats and this was observed on only two occasions in the study.

Risk of maternal premutation expansion to full mutation (Nolin *et al.* 2003)

Maternal CGG premutation	Risk of expansion to >200 CGG repeats (%)
55–59	3.7
60–69	5.3
70–79	31.1
80–89	57.8
90–99	80.1
100–139	>94
>140	100

Males. Males with the premutation will pass this on to all of their daughters and none of their sons. The repeat size is likely to remain fairly stable (although small expansions and contractions are possible). Males with the full mutation are unlikely to form mature sexual relationships as adults. Several studies have found that adult FRAXA males who carry a full mutation in their somatic tissues have only premutation size repeats in their sperm/gonadal tissue.

Variability and penetrance

- Males with a full mutation that is methylated have an average IQ of 41.
- Males mosaic for a full and premutation have an average IQ of 60.
- Males with a full mutation with >50% of cells unmethylated have an average IQ of 88.
- Females. Approximately one-half of females with a full mutation have learning and behavioural difficulties that are similar to, but usually less severe than those seen in males with a full mutation. As for affected males, verbal abilities tend to be better than performance skills and special needs in arithmetic and difficulties with visuospatial skills and abstract concepts are common.

Prenatal diagnosis

Feasible by chorionic villus sampling (CVS; adequate sample size needed), but note difficulty of predicting phenotype in females carrying a full mutation. Direct genomic Southern blot analysis using a probe that flanks the CGG repeat region is the standard methodology (in addition to polymerase chain reaction (PCR)-based analysis). Exclude maternal cell contamination.

Daughters of mothers carrying a full or premutation

Testing of sisters of affected boys who have no schooling problems is generally deferred until 16 years of age or later when they may wish to discover their carrier status before planning a family. Sisters who experience mild difficulties at school should be offered a vision and hearing check and, for younger girls, a paediatric developmental assessment or, for older girls, an assessment by an educational psychologist. Once these are complete and if there is evidence for a learning difficulty and no obvious alternative cause (e.g. poor hearing due to glue ear), then it may be helpful to pursue diagnostic testing for FRAX.

Other family members

Cascade screening of adult family members is indicated. A premutation in a female may have been inherited from her mother or her father, but a full mutation can only be maternally inherited. Remember that, if the familial mutation is maternally inherited, normal brothers may be premutation carriers (normal transmitting males) and should be offered testing because of the potential risk to their daughters' offspring.

Natural history and management

Refer to a developmental paediatrician who will arrange pre-school learning support and liase with community paediatric services. Individuals with FRAX have special educational needs. Most can manage in mainstream primary school with appropriate support, but others may benefit from a special needs school. Children with FRAX are readily overwhelmed by noisy and busy environments, e.g. supermarkets, leading to tantrums, overactivity, withdrawal, repetitive behaviour, etc. Careful thought needs to be given to this in planning educational support. Children often learn best when auditory and visual distraction is minimized and work is packaged into short (maximum 15 minutes) blocks (see Fragile X Society for further information on educational needs).

Potential long-term complications in affected individuals

- **Recurrent otitis media** occurs in 60–80% causing conductive hearing loss. Consider grommets and/or prophylactic antibiotics if this is troublesome.
- **Seizures** occur in approximately 20%. They usually resolve by adolescence.
- **MVP** is rare in childhood but may occur in ~50% of adults.

Potential long-term complications in premutation carriers

- **Males.** Some adult males with FRAX premutations may develop a progressive neurological syndrome, fragile X tremor ataxia syndrome (FXTAS), with cerebellar tremor/ataxia, cognitive decline, and generalized brain atrophy characterized by intranuclear inclusions (Greco et al. 2002). The origin of the inclusions is unknown, although elevated FMR1 mRNA levels in these premutation carriers may lead to the neuropathological changes.

The prevalence of this disorder amongst males with premutations is not currently known.

- **Females.** Approximately 24% of female premutation carriers will undergo premature menopause (cessation of menses at <40 years). This information may be helpful to carrier women for reproductive planning. See 'Premature ovarian failure (POF)' page 620.

Support group: Fragile X Society, Tel. 01424 813147, <www.fragilex.org.uk>; National Fragile X Foundation (US) <www.fragileX.org>.

Expert adviser: Angela Barnicoat, Consultant in Clinical Genetics, Institute of Child Health, London, England.

References

de Graaf E, Willemsen R, et al. Instability of the CGG repeat and expression of the FMR1 protein in a male fragile X patient with a lung tumour. Am J Hum Genet 1995; **57**: 609–18.

Greco CM, Hagerman RJ, et al. Neuronal intranuclear inclusions in a new cerebellar tremor/ataxia syndrome among fragile X carriers. Brain 2002; **125**: 1760–71.

Hagerman RJ, Staley LW, et al. Learning disabled males with a fragile X CGG expansion in the upper premutation size range. Pediatrics 1996; **97**: 122–6.

Heitz D, Devys D, et al. Inheritance of the fragile X syndrome: size of the fragile X premutation is a major determinant of the transition to full mutation. J Med Genet 1992; **29**: 794–801.

Nolin SL, Lewis FA, Ye LL, et al. Familial transmission of the FMR1 CGG repeat. Am J Hum Genet 1996; **59**: 1252–61.

Nolin SL, Brown WT, et al. Expansion of the fragile X CGG repeat in females with premutation or intermediate alleles. Am J Hum Genet 2003; **72**: 454–64.

Pesso R, Berkenstadt M, et al. Screening for fragile X syndrome in women of reproductive age. Prenat Diagn 2000; **20**: 611–14.

Tassone F, Hagerman RJ, et al. Clinical involvement and protein expression in individuals with FMR1 premutation. Am J Med Genet 2000; **91**: 144–52.

Youings SA, Murray A, et al. FRAXA and FRAXE: the results of a five year survey. J Med Genet 2000; **37**: 415–21.

Glaucoma

Glaucoma is an optic neuropathy with characteristic field loss that may or may not be associated with increased intraocular pressure. It is classified according to the mechanism causing the glaucoma into the following.

1 Primary open angle glaucoma (POAG) is due to an intrinsic disorder of the trabecular meshwork.

2 Closed angle glaucoma (acute and chronic).

3 Secondary glaucomas arise as a consequence of disease or abnormality either elsewhere in the eye or in other systems.

Most adult-onset glaucoma is a complex disease showing multifactorial inheritance, and family history is an important risk factor (Tielsch *et al.* 1994).

Glaucoma in infancy and childhood may form part of a wider condition, but is usually an isolated occurrence. Primary congenital glaucoma is also known as **buphthalmos** and has a birth incidence of ~3/100 000 (Bermejo and Martinez-Frias 1998).

The aim is to determine whether the glaucoma is a purely ocular condition or if there are non-ocular features that suggest a syndrome diagnosis. 'Anterior segment eye malformations' page 46 may also be useful.

Clinical approach

History: key points

- Family history. At least three-generation family tree. Enquire for consanguinity.
- Growth. Most chromosomal condition show poor growth. Rieger syndrome is associated with pituitary abnormalities.
- Developmental progress, allowing for visual difficulties.
- Vision, photophobia.

Examination: key points

- Ophthalmology opinion to confirm diagnosis by measuring intraocular pressure (may require general anaesthesia in infants), examination of optic discs, and visual testing in adults and older children.
- Exclude other structural abnormalities of the eye such as iris hypoplasia, aniridia, sclerocornea, megalocornea, microphthalmia, lens abnormality.
- Uni- or bilateral?
- Growth parameters (short stature in Peter's plus syndrome, Rieger syndrome).
- Orofacial clefts (Peter's plus syndrome, Kivlin syndrome).
- Abnormal dentition (Rieger syndrome).
- Hypospadias (Rieger syndrome).
- Redundant per-umbilical skin (Rieger syndrome).
- Olfaction (abnormalities may be found with PAX6 mutations).

Special investigations

- *Examine parents* to exclude minor signs of anterior segment dysgenesis.
- Chromosome analysis in children with malformation syndromes and/or developmental delay. Exclude deletion 11p13 in children with aniridia (fluorescent *in situ* hybridization (FISH) 11p13).
- Save DNA for possible genetic testing.
- Echocardiogram if there is dislocation/subluxation of the ocular lens or if there are other features of Marfan syndrome.

Syndromic diagnoses to consider

Secondary causes of childhood glaucoma

Anterior segment disorders. See 'Anterior segment eye malformations' page 46 for more details.

- Aniridia (*PAX6* gene).
- Axenfeld–Rieger syndromes.
- Peter's anomaly.

Neurofibromatosis type 1 (NF1). Typically six or more café-au-lait spots (CALs). Glaucoma is really only seen in a rare form of NF1 with extensive ipsilateral plexiform neuroma. See 'Neurofibromatosis type 1 (NF1)', page 396.

Sturge–Weber syndrome. Association of facial capillary haemangioma (port-wine stain) involving the ophthalmic division of the Vth cranial nerve with meningeal angiomata. Seizures and mental retardation may be complications. Most cases are sporadic.

Secondary causes of juvenile and adult glaucoma

As above plus the following.

Nail patella syndrome. Autosomal dominant (AD) disorder characterized by dysplasia of nails, patellae, and elbow joints, exostoses of iliac crest, and in some cases nephropathy. Fingernails are absent or abnormal in 98%. Gene is *LMX1B* on 9q34, a transcription factor that regulates the *COL4A3* and *COL4A4* genes. Offer surveillance for nephropathy. See 'Unusual hair, teeth, nails, and skin' page 256.

Nanophthalmos or simple microphthalmia. The nanophthalmic eye has a proportionately thicker sclera but the lens is of normal size, which leads to a narrow anterior chamber, and glaucoma may develop. See 'Microphthalmia and anophthalmia' page 176.

Marfan syndrome and ectopia lentis. AD condition characterized by tall stature, long limbs, pectus deformity, and aortic root enlargement. Caused by mutations in fibrillin (FBN1) on 15q. Acute glaucoma secondary to lens dislocation may develop. See 'Marfan syndrome', page 380.

Homocystinuria. An autosomal recessive (AR) condition caused by deficiency of cystathionine synthetase encoded on 21q22 and characterized by lens-dislocation (typically downward displacement) and thrombophilia. Most thrombotic events are cerebrovascular. Acute glaucoma secondary to lens dislocation may develop.

Norrie disease. Secondary angle closure glaucoma may occur as a result of lens dislocation and may complicate retinal dysplasia in Norrie disease. See 'Retinal dysplasia' page 230.

Genetic advice

Inheritance and recurrence risk

Buphthalmos/primary congenital glaucoma. Corneal opacification, photophobia.

- Exclude other anterior segment anomalies.
- Exclude secondary causes of glaucoma (see above).

Recessive inheritance possible. Genetic heterogeneity with at least three loci. One is *CYP1B1* on 2p21. Another, the forkhead transcription factor gene FKHL7 on 6p25, is responsible for a spectrum of glaucoma phenotypes including primary congenital glaucoma, Rieger anomaly, Axenfeld anomaly, and iris hypoplasia (Nishimura *et al.* 1998). In the absence of consanguinity recurrence risks are about 5%.

Juvenile and adult primary glaucoma. AD inheritance; many loci. Mutations in myocilin gene (*MYOC*) are found in a proportion (~6–8%) of families with POAG and juvenile glaucoma (Bruttini *et al.* 2003; Williams-Lyn *et al.* 2000). The phenotype associated with mutation in *MYOC* is highly variable even within the same kindred, ranging from normal through ocular hypertension to severe open angle glaucoma (OAG; Cobb *et al.* 2002). Compared with adult-onset POAG, there is a higher incidence of affected family members in juvenile onset disease. Nevertheless, many cases of juvenile glaucoma do not have a family history. Most adult glaucoma is a complex (multifactorial) disease.

Tielsch *et al.* (1994) in a population-based study found age-adjusted associations of POAG with a history of glaucoma were higher in siblings (odds ratio (OR) = 3.69) than in parents (OR = 2.17) or children (OR = 1.12).

Secondary causes of glaucoma. Counsel for the specific syndrome diagnosed.

Prenatal diagnosis
Most glaucoma is treatable if appropriate surveillance is offered and it is identified early. Parents may desire prenatal diagnosis for congenital glaucoma where the visual results may be poor despite treatment, but this will only be feasible if the mutation(s) are known.

Predictive testing
Possible in the few families in which molecular genetic testing has been done which has identified the causative mutation. Note that mutations in MYOC may have variable expressivity and penetrance. Predictive testing could be used to target surveillance.

Other family members
Offer ophthalmological surveillance to first-degree relatives. The age at which to begin screening will depend on the family history. Seek guidance from your ophthalmological colleagues.

Natural history and management
Potential long-term complications
Untreated glaucoma can lead to irreversible constriction of the visual fields.

Surveillance
Ensure ophthalmological surveillance for affected individuals and arrange ophthalmological follow-up for 'at risk' family members.

Support group: International Glaucoma Association <www.iga.org.uk>, Tel. 020 7737 3265.

Expert adviser: Anonymous.

References
Alward WLM. Glaucoma genetics 1999. Presented at Ninth Robert J. Gorlin Conference on Dysmorphology, October 1999.

Bermejo E, Martinez-Frias ML. Congenital eye malformations: clinical–epidemiological analysis of 1,124,654 consecutive births in Spain. *Am J Med Genet* 1998; **75**: 497–504.

Bruttini M, Longo I, *et al.* Mutations in the myocilin gene in families with primary open-angle glaucoma and juvenile open-angle glaucoma. *Arch Ophthalmol* 2003; **121**: 1034–8.

Cobb CJ, Scott G, *et al.* Rapid mutation detection by the transgenomic wave analyser DHPLC identifies MYOC mutations in patients with ocular hypertension and/or open angle glaucoma. *Br J Ophthalmol* 2002; **86**: 191–5.

Nishimura DY, Swiderski RE, *et al.* The forkhead transcription factor gene FKHL7 is responsible for glaucoma phenotypes which map to 6p25. *Nat Genet* 1998; **19**: 140–7.

Tielsch JM, Katz J, *et al.* Family history and risk of primary open angle glaucoma. The Baltimore Eye Survey. *Arch Ophthalmol* 1994; **112**: 69–73.

Weinrab RN, Khaw PT. Primary open-angle glaucoma (Seminar). *Lancet* 2004; **363**: 1711–20.

Williams-Lyn D, Flanagan J, *et al.* The genetic aspects of adult-onset glaucoma: a perspective from the Greater Toronto area. *Can J Ophthalmol* 2000; **35**: 12–17.

Haemochromatosis

Hereditary haemochromatosis (HH), genetic haemochromatosis (HC).

HH type 1 is an autosomal recessive (AR) disorder of iron metabolism of low penetrance. It is characterized by progressive iron overload and caused by mutations in the *HFE* gene (HLA-H) on chromosome 6. *HFE* is expressed in the intestinal crypt cells, and is likely to play a key role in coupling the iron-sensing mechanism of the crypt cells to iron absorption by the mature enterocyte. The predominant feature of HH is excessive absorption of dietary iron. Eventually, deposition of iron in parenchymal tisuues results in cirrhosis of the liver, diabetes mellitus, skin pigmentation, and testicular failure. Genetically predisposed individuals occur with an estimated frequency ranging from 1/2000 (Finland) to 1/200 (Utah). In evolutionary terms, heterozygotes for mutations in *HFE* may have been at a selective advantage when diets were poor and infestation with gut parasites was common.

There are two common mutations C282Y and H63D. Approximately 90% of patients with HH are homozygous for C282Y; a further 4% are compound heterozygotes for C282Y/H63D. H63D homozygotes do not develop HH. HH due to C282Y is common in populations associated with Celtic migrations, e.g. the UK especially Northern Ireland, Brittany, and Australia. It is rare in Asia, the Middle East, and most of Africa. Penetrance of clinical haemochromatosis amongst individuals homozygous for C282Y is age-dependent and incomplete. In the UK the S65C mutation may be implicated in ~1% of cases of HC, but appears to be associated with a mild form of HH.

In *HFE* C282Y homozygotes, it is unusual to get tissue injury from iron overload before 20 years. If HH is diagnosed early, before irreversible liver damage, treatment by serial phlebotomy is both straightforward and effective and many of the non-specific symptoms are reversible (except arthralgia). It is presumed that iron depletion treatment that is initiated before cirrhosis develops results in a near normal life expectancy. If a late diagnosis is made and irreversible organ damage has resulted, life expectancy is reduced.

Haemochromatosis is genetically heterogeneous and, although *HFE* is much the most common cause amongst the Caucasian population, haemochromatosis can also occur due to mutations in transferrin receptor 2 gene on 7q22 (AR) (type 3) and in the ferroportin 1 gene (*SLC11A3*) on 2q32 (autosomal dominant (AD)) (type 4).

- **Juvenile haemochromatosis** (type 2) is an inherited condition of high penetrance in which there is clinical onset between 10 and 30 years of age. Most juvenile-onset cases are AR and caused by homozygous mutation in hemojuvelin (*HJV*) on 1q21. Rare cases of Juvenile haemochromatosis are caused by homozygous mutation in the *HAMP* gene on 19q13.1 which encodes hepcidin, a peptide which plays a key role in regulating intestinal iron absorption. Liver involvement is a constant feature; cardiomyopathy, diabetes and hypogonadotrophic hypogonadism are more prominent than in adult-onset HH. Digenic inheritance of mutations in *HFE* and *HAMP* can result in either juvenile haemochromatosis or hereditary haemochromatosis, depending upon the severity of the mutation in *HAMP* (Robson).
- **Neonatal haemochromatosis** is a condition of acute liver damage with iron accumulation. This encompasses severe iron overload in neonates of undefined pathogenesis (not all are genetic) and is not linked to HFE.

Clinical approach

Prior to the consultation, try to confirm the diagnosis in the affected relative and, if possible, determine whether genotyping has been done.

History: key points

- Family tree. Estimate the relationship to the proband and the genetic risk, based on a crude carrier rate of 10% (1 in 4 for siblings, 1 in 20 for offspring).
- For siblings enquire for symptoms of HH. Late features of the disease are well known, e.g. bronzed skin pigmentation, cirrhosis, and diabetes mellitus, but early features are characteristically non-specific:
  - weakness and lethargy;
  - arthralgia, especially interphalangeal (IP) and metacarpophalangeal (MCP) joints of hands (especially digits II and III);
  - abdominal pain;
  - impotence or amenorrhoea (endocrine failure secondary to Fe deposition in pituitary);
  - dyspnoea (cardiomyopathy).

Examination: key points

- Hands for arthropathy of small joints.
- Pigmentation (especially shins).
- Cardiac arryhthmia.
- Signs of hypogonadism.

Special investigations

- DNA sample for genotype for C282Y and H63D mutations in *HFE*, unless juvenile onset in which case consider mutation analysis of *HJV* and *HAMP*
- Iron studies including serum Fe, ferritin (reflects total body Fe stores) and transferrin saturation (best screening test).
  - **Ferritin.** In normal subjects, ferritin concentrations of >300 μg/l for men and postmenopausal women and >200 μg/l for premenopausal women indicate elevated iron stores (levels may vary between different labs). Serum ferritin is an acute phase reactant and so may be raised in intercurrent illness or inflammation.
  - **Transferrin saturation.** If transferrin saturation >50%, repeat on a fasting morning sample. Fasting transferrin saturation >55% (men) and >50% (women) is abnormal and indicates Fe accumulation. Normal values are 20–40%, carriers may have intermediate levels and genotyping may be helpful in determining significance. (In exceptional cases significant tissue iron storage can occur in the absence of an elevated serum ferritin, although in most cases the serum transferrin and iron saturation will be elevated.)
- If symptomatic include measurement of liver function tests (LFTs) and glucose, alpha-fetoprotein (AFP) for primary hepatoma, luteinizing hormone (LH)/follicle-stimulating hormone (FSH) if impotence/amenorrhoea, and electrocardiogram (ECG) and echocardiogram if dyspnoeic. Refer to appropriate physician.
- A liver biopsy may be considered for any patient with a raised transferrin saturation, a serum ferritin concentration of >1000 μg/l, and/or evidence of liver damage (hepatomegaly or raised aspartate transaminase (AST) activity). For patients with a raised transferrin saturation,

a ferritin of <1000 μg/l, no hepatomegaly, and normal AST activity, biopsy is usually not necessary because the risk of hepatic fibrosis or cirrhosis being present is low. Biopsy of the liver may assist in determining prognosis.

Genetic advice for type 1

Compound heterozygotes for C282Y/H63D may accumulate Fe, but the risk of clinical haemochromatosis is much less than that for C282Y homozygotes.

Inheritance and recurrence risk
AR. The general population allele frequencies for both mutations are high, e.g. 8% for C282Y and 15.7% for H63D in a survey in north-east Scotland. Frequency of heterozygosity for C282Y is 9.6% in Whites from the USA, 17.3% in Northern Ireland, 13.2% in New Zealand, 9.6% in northern Germany, and 13.3% in Denmark—overall an approximate 1/10 risk for carrier status in the general population.

Genetic risk to sibs is 1 in 4, to offspring is $(1 \times 1/10 \times 1/2) = 1/20$, to grandchildren is $(1 \times 1/10 \times 1/4) = 1/40$, and to nephews/nieces is $(2/3 \times 1/10 \times 1/4) = 1/60$.

Variability and penetrance
Although HH is often underdiagnosed, penetrance is incomplete and disease expression is variable, so many of those with genetic predisposition to HH will never manifest serious clinical features. Males are more often affected than females with ratio ~10M:1F. In Beutler et al.'s (2002) large population-based study, the penetrance of haemochromatosis in individuals (average age ~50 years) homozygous for C282Y was <1%. The validity of this study and the population base from which it is drawn is hotly debated; the real value in Caucasian populations is probably rather higher, say a few per cent. What the comparable penetrance figure is for family members who may share important genetic modifiers is unknown, but it is likely that homozygotes ascertained through cascade screening of families will have a higher penetrance than individuals in the general population. Nevertheless, the penetrance is likely to remain fairly low even amongst close family members. Mura et al. (2001) found a lack of correlation of the Fe marker status between pairs of sibs homozygous by descent for C282Y, indicating a variable phenotypic expression of Fe loading independent of *HFE* genotype.

Prenatal diagnosis
Technically feasible, but rarely requested since this is a treatable condition in which complications are largely preventable and lifespan should be normal with careful monitoring of Fe storage and venesection where indicated.

Predictive testing
Appropriate in adult life (see below) to identify which members of a family require regular monitoring of Fe status.

Other family members
Offer testing by *HFE* genotyping, transferrin saturation, and serum ferritin concentration to:
- siblings (1 in 4 risk for HH genotype; lower risk for symptomatic disease);
- parents.

In addition, testing should be offered in the following situations.
- If the proband has children, the partner should be offered testing to determine the risk to offspring. There is a 1/10 chance that the partner will carry C282Y and a 1/5 chance that the H63D mutation will be present. If the partner is not a carrier of C282Y or H63D, offspring can be reassured that they are obligate carriers, but not at risk of disease.
- If the proband's partner is not available or declines testing, offer testing to offspring from the age of 15 years (if in their teens or 20s they may choose to have iron studies only, rather than risk a 'genetic' diagnosis of HH with implications for life insurance, pensions, etc., or, since the risk of diagnosis is fairly low at 1/20, they may choose to have genetic testing in an attempt to avoid the need for future screening and evaluation). Some, but not all, insurance companies take the view that HH properly diagnosed and managed does not justify refusal of cover or increased premiums.

The low penetrance of *HFE* makes cascade screening of extended families inappropriate. Risks to second-degree relatives, e.g. grandchildren (1/40 × penetrance of say 5% = 1/800) and nephews/nieces (1/60 × penetrance of say 5%' ≤ 1/1000), and third-degree relatives, e.g. cousins, become sufficiently small that systematic iron studies and genetic testing are not indicated.

Natural history and management

For C282Y homozygotes diagnosed with haemochromatosis, the mean age of onset is 44.1 years in males and 49.8 years in females (Mura et al. 2001). In homozygotes, serum ferritin rises progressively with age. If patients are diagnosed in the pre-cirrhotic, pre-diabetic stage and treated with venesection to remove excess Fe, then life expectancy is normal.

Our practice is to advise all individuals with C282Y/C282Y or C282Y/H63D against taking over-the-counter preparations containing Fe, such as multivitamin and mineral supplements, and to avoid a very high dietary intake of Fe (red meat, red wine, etc.).

Potential long-term complications
- **Liver cirrhosis**—with increased risk for hepatocellular carcinoma—irreversible.
- **Hepatoma** is responsible for one-third of deaths from HH. The great majority of hepatomata occur in cirrhotic livers, but they have been reported in non-cirrhotic livers.
- **Arthritis** is irreversible.
- **Congestive cardiomyopathy.** Early cardiac changes on echocardiography may improve with venesection.
- **Diabetes mellitus.** Non-insulin-dependent diabetes or impaired glucose tolerance may be improved in a small proportion of patients by venesection; insulin-dependent diabetics will remain insulin-dependent.
- **Impotence.** Hypogonadotrophic hypogonadism may improve or resolve after iron depletion.

Surveillance
- Repeat normal Fe studies in homozygotes every 3 years in males, and every 5 years in females and compound heterozygotes (C282Y/H63D) with referral for specialist assessment if results indicate Fe overload.
- Proven heterozygotes do not require repeated measures of iron status if initial studies are normal.

Treatment
For individuals with HH who have already accumulated excess Fe, the usual treatment is weekly venesection. Once excess Fe has been removed, the transferrin

saturation should be maintained below 50% and the serum ferritin at <50 μg/l, which can often be achieved on a programme of venesection 2–4 times per year.

Support group: The Haemochromatosis Society <www.ghsoc.org>; Hemochromatosis Foundation <www.hemochromatosis.org>.

Expert adviser: T.M. Cox, Professor of Medicine, University of Cambridge, Cambridge, England.

References

Beutler E, Felitti VJ, et al. Penetrance of 845G→A (C282Y) HFE hereditary haemochromatosis mutation in the USA. *Lancet* 2002; **359**: 211–18.

British Committee on Standards in Haematology 2000. Guideline on Haemochromatosis. <www.bcshguidelines.com>.

Camaschella C, Roetto A, et al. Genetic haemochromatosis: genes and mutations associated with iron loading. *Best Pract Res Clin Haematol* 2002; **15**: 261–76.

Dooley J, Wowood M. *Genetic haemochromatosis. British Committee for Standards in Haematology. Guideline on diagnosis and therapy.* British Society for Haematology, London, 2000.

Haddow JE, Bradley LA. Hereditary haemochromatosis: to screen or not. Conditions for screening are not yet fulfilled. *Br Med J* 1999; **319**: 531–2.

Miedzybrodzka Z, Loughlin S, et al. Haemochromatosis mutation in North-East Scotland. *Br J Haematol* 1999; **106**: 385–7.

Mura C, Le Gac G, et al. Variation of iron loading expression in C282Y homozygous haemochromatosis probands and sib pairs. *J Med Genet* 2001; **38**: 632–6.

Pietrangelo A. Medical Progress: Hereditary Haemochromatosis— A new look at an old disease (Review). *NEJM* 2004; **350**: 2383–97.

Report of a meeting of physicians and scientists at the Royal Free Hospital School of Medicine. *Lancet* 1997; **347**: 1688–93.

Robson KJ, Merryweather-Clarke AT, et al. Recent advances in understanding haemochromatosis: a transition state. *J Med Genet* 2004; **41**: 721–30.

Worwood M. Inherited iron loading: genetic testing in diagnosis and management. *Blood Rev* 2005; **19**: 69–88.

Haemoglobinopathies

Haemoglobinopathies are the most common single-gene disorders in the world population, with ~7% of the population being carriers. The incidence of the various haemoglobinopathies varies enormously in different population groups so that detailed knowledge of your patient's ethnic background is often extremely helpful.

Haemoglobin (Hb) is a tetramer composed of two different pairs of globin chains. Adult haemoglobins are HbA ($A_2\beta_2$), HbA_2 ($\alpha_2\delta_2$), HbF ($\alpha_2\gamma_2$). The α-globin chains are present in both fetal and adult Hb, so severe homozygous forms of α-thalassaemia cause intrauterine death (IUD) or neonatal death. β-chain abnormalities do not become clinically significant until Hb synthesis switches from HbF to HbA in early infancy. There are two α-globin genes in tandem array on chromosome 16 (normal genotype: $\alpha\alpha/\alpha\alpha$). The β-like globin cluster is on chromosome 11 and contains one β-, two γ-, and one δ-globin gene (normal β-genotype: β/β). Therefore α-globin gene defects can be co-inherited with β-globin gene defects.

There are two main types of haemoglobinopathy: (1) disorders caused by structural variant haemoglobins, e.g. sickle cell anaemia; and (2) disorders in which there is a reduced rate of production of one or more of the globin chains, e.g. thalassaemia. Heterozygotes are often referred to as 'trait' and homozygotes as 'disease'. Several disorders result from the inheritance of the sickle cell gene together with different forms of thalassaemia (β- and δ β-) or other structural variants.

Structural variants. Structural variants are named after letters of the alphabet (e.g. S, C, D, E) or places where they were discovered (e.g. Zurich, Constant Spring). More than 750 abnormal Hbs have been characterized, the majority comprising α- and β-chain variants. The majority are clinically silent and do not cause any disease. However, a number have altered properties, either being unstable, having a higher oxygen affinity (resulting in polycythaemia), a lower oxygen affinity (resulting in cyanosis in some cases), reduced synthesis (resulting in thalassaemia), or altered solubility, e.g. HbS.

Most variants have a single amino acid replacement due to a point mutation. For example, HbS differs from HbA due to a missense mutation in the B-globin gene E6V (glutamic acid at amino acid 6 is changed to valine). This substitution alters the solubility of the Hb molecule in the deoxygenated state resulting in aggregation with consequent sickling of the red cell. Sickled red cells have increased fragility and shortened survival leading to chronic haemolytic anaemia. The sickled red cells can themselves aggregate in the microvasculature leading to a thrombotic crisis.

Hereditary Persistence of Fetal Hemoglobin (HPFH). In this AD condition, expression of the δ-globin gene of HbF persists at high levels in adult erythroid cells. Increased levels of fetal hemoglobin (HbF) ameliorate the clinical course of inherited disorders of β-globin gene expression, such as β-thalassemia and sickle cell anemia.

Hb electrophoresis. See the table for normal red cell indices and those for some haemoglobinopathies.

- In normal adults ~97% of Hb is HbA, 0–3.5% HbA_2, and 0–1% HbF.
- In α-thalassaemia, Hb electrophoresis is normal. DNA analysis is required to make the diagnosis.
- In β-thalassaemia trait, HbA_2 is >3.5% (usually 4–6%; but not in the presence of Fe deficiency), with a slight elevation of HbF to 1–3% in some. A few mutations are associated with borderline normal HbA_2 values of 3.3–3.8% (normal HbA_2 β-thalassaemia) and a few very rare ones with borderline normal HbA_2 values and normal red cell indices (silent β-thalassaemia). In homozygous β°-thalassaemia there is no HbA—only HbF and HbA_2. In homozygous β^+ thalassaemia, HbF ranges from 30% to 90% and HbA_2 is usually normal.

Normal red cell indices and red cell indices for some haemoglobinopathies*

	Hb (g/dl)	MCH (pg)	MCV (fl)	HbA₂ (%)	HbF (%)
Normal red cell indices					
Male	13–17	27–32	82–102	0–3.5	0–1
Female	12–16	27–32	82–102	0–3.5	0–1
Typical red cell indices for some haemoglobinopathies					
α^+-thalassaemia trait	11–16	24–28	75–90	1.5–3.0	0–1
Homozygous α^+-thalassaemia	11–16	21–24	68–76	1.5–3.0	0–1
α°-thalassaemia trait	11–15	20–23	65–75	1.5–3.0	0–1
HbH disease	8–11	17–21	55–70	1–2	0–1
β-thalassaemia trait	8–16	18–25	63–80	3.5–7	0–8
Normal $A_2\beta$-thalassaemia	12–16	23–26	67–79	3.3–3.8	0–2
Silent β-thalassaemia	12–16	27–29	80–90	3.3–3.8	0–2
Thalassaemia intermedia	5–13	14–22	50–85	1–7	5–100
Thalassaemia major	2–7	12–18	50–60	1–7	15–100
HbE/β-thalassaemia	5–10	16–23	61–75	3.5–8	5–85
AS	12–16	26–32	80–95	3.0–5.0	0.5–1.5
SS (African)	6–10	26–32	80–95	1.5–3.5	5–10
SS (Arab–Indian)	8–10	26–32	80–95	1.5–5	10–25
S/β°	7–11	18–25	60–80	3.5–6	5–15
S/β^+	9–11	20–25	65–80	3.5–6	5–15
S/$\delta\beta^\circ$	10–12	20–25	65–80	1.5–2.5	10–25
S/HPFH	12–16	24–30	68–88	1–2	20–35

* MCH, Mean corpuscular haemoglobin; MCV, mean corpuscular volume, HPFH, hereditary persistence of fetal haemoglobin.

- Most Hb variants have been detected by electrophoretic methods due to the variant having a change in electric charge. For example, HbS migrates differently from HbA and appears as a distinct band (heterozygotes have both HbA and HbS; those with sickle cell disease have HbS and no HbA and a variable amount of HbF).
- In HbSC disease, HbS and HbC are present in approximately equal proportions.
- In HbC disease, HbC is present with small amounts of HbF and no HbA.

Clinical approach

History: key points

- Three-generation family tree with specific enquiry about ethnic origin and consanguinity. Specific detail about the country of origin of relatives can be very helpful.
- Enquire about previous pregnancies, miscarriages.

Investigations

- Full blood count (FBC) with red cell indices.
- Hb electrophoresis.
- Sickle test if indicated by ethnic background.
- DNA for molecular studies where indicated, e.g. diagnosis of α-thalassaemia carrier status, or to permit future prenatal diagnosis for α- or β-thalassaemia or structural variants, e.g. HbS, C. In the UK samples may be referred to the National Haemoglobinopathy Reference Laboratory, Oxford Haemophilia Centre, Churchill Hospital, Oxford OX3 7LJ; Tel. 01865 225329 after prior discussion with the laboratory.

Specific diagnoses/conditions to consider

Sickling disorders

Frequent in African Black populations and, sporadically throughout the Mediterranean and Middle East. Occur in some parts of India, but *not* in South-east Asia. The heterozygous state for sickle cell may confer resistance to malaria. It should be noted that the term 'sickle-cell disease' is often used to describe a similar phenotype that is seen with any of several genotypes (SS, SC, S/β-thalassaemia, S/D Punjab, or S/O Arab).

Sickle cell anaemia (genotype β^S/β^S). The clinical course is extremely variable ranging from crippling haemolytic anaemia with frequent crises to mild disorder. It usually presents in infancy with jaundice and anaemia from about 3 months of age. Hb is typically 6–8 g/dl; transfusion is not usually required. Crises due to blockage of vessels by sickled erythrocytes may cause infarction of bone and bone marrow, abdominal pain, chest syndrome (shortness of breath, pleuritic chest pain, and fever), and neurological syndrome (transient ischaemic attacks (TIAs) and strokes). Crises may be precipitated by infection or dehydration but often no precipitant is identified. Repeated splenic infarction in early childhood makes children vulnerable to infection, and prophylactic penicillin reduces early mortality. In the long term, avascular necrosis of the hip, renal impairment, and ischaemia of the retinal vasculature may occur. A study based on survival of >3000 patients attending a Jamaican clinic estimated median survival for men at 53 years and for women at 58.5 years. Patients from the Eastern Province of Saudi Arabia and central India have higher HbF levels and a milder clinical course than patients of African origin.

Sickle cell trait (β^S/β). Normal FBC. Diagnose by positive sickling test and Hb electrophoresis demonstrating HbA and HbS (34–40%). NB. The co-inheritance of α-thalassaemia causes reduced red cell indices and lowers the %HbS to 29–34% for $\alpha\alpha/\alpha-$ and to 24–28% for $\alpha-/\alpha-$ genotypes. Asymptomatic, except in conditions of extreme anoxia. It is possible for heterozygotes to suffer vaso-occlusive episodes if they become unusually hypoxic during anaesthesia. Apart from advice about anaesthaesia and avoidance of unpressurized aircraft or deep-sea diving, individuals with sickle trait require no treatment.

Haemoglobin SC disease (β^S/β^C). Relatively common in west Africa, e.g. Ghana. Characterized by a milder anaemia than sickle cell anaemia (SS) and may be undiagnosed until adult life when patients present with one of the complications. Aseptic necrosis of the femoral head and unexplained haematuria are common complications. Widespread thrombosis may occur in pregnancy/puerperium or during intercurrent infection. Infarction of retinal vasculature may lead to retinitis proliferans with retinal detachment and loss of vision.

Haemoglobin C disease (β^C/β^C). Homozygous state for HbC is characterized by mild haemolytic anaemia with splenomegaly. Film shows 100% target cells. This is a mild disorder for which no treatment is required.

β-thalassaemias

These produce severe anaemia in their homozygous and compound heterozygous states. They occur widely in a broad belt stretching from the Mediterranean and parts of north and west Africa through the Middle East and India to South-east Asia including the Balkans and southern parts of Russia and southern China (see figure). Some mutations are inactivating (β°) and others cause reduced levels of β-globin synthesis (β^+).

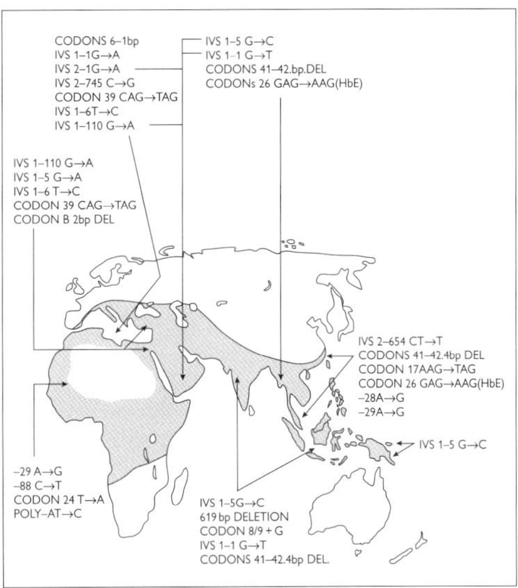

Map showing the distribution of the different β-thalassaemia mutations. (Figure 4, p. 679 from Weatherall (2003) by permission of Oxford University Press.)

Homozygous β-thalassaemia (β°/β°, β°/β^+, β^+/β^+). Most homozygous β°-thalassaemia presents in the 1st year with failure to thrive and intermittent bouts of fever. Hb at presentation ranges from 2 to 8 g/dl. If regular transfusion is instigated development progresses reasonably normally until puberty when side-effects of secondary haemochromatosis become apparent with lack of secondary sexual characteristics and short stature. In the absence of intensive iron chelation therapy, death usually occurs in the late teens or 20s due to progressive cardiac damage from iron overload. However, with regular transfusion and compliance with optimal iron chelation therapy, life expectancy improves considerably and patients can survive to their third or fourth decade with a good quality of life.

A few β^+-thalassaemia mutations have a milder phenotype than the majority of β^0 and β^+ mutations. Homozygotes for these mutations have a milder condition called *thalassaemia intermedia*. Patients have a Hb of 6–9 g/dl, splenomegaly, and some bone deformities, but are not dependent on regular transfusions for survival. Thalassaemia intermedia is caused by a wide range of different genotypes, e.g. homozygous $\delta\beta$-thalassaemia, and by the co-inheritance of ameliorating factors, e.g. homozygous β-thalassaemia with co-inherited α-thalassaemia.

Heterozygous β^0-thalassaemia (β/β^0) and heterozygous β^+thalassaemia (β/β^+). Carriers for β-thalassaemia are usually asymptomatic except in periods of stress such as pregnancy when they may become anaemic. Life expectancy is normal. Hb is 9–11 g/dl with hypochromia and microcytosis and low mean corpuscular volume (MCV) and mean corpuscular haemoglobin (MCH). *A heterozygous state for β-thalassaemia may mask a coexistent carrier state for α-thalassaemia (the latter is usually characterized by microcytosis and reduced MCH, which may be attributed to the β-thalassaemia trait).*

α-thalassaemias

These are more common than the β-thalassaemias but pose less of a health problem as the homozygous forms of the severe types (α^0-thalassaemias) are lethal. They occur widely throughout the Mediterranean, parts of west Africa, the Middle East, parts of India, and throughout South-east Asia. The most serious forms of α-thalassaemia are restricted to some of the Mediterranean island populations (e.g. Cyprus) and South-east Asia (see figure).

Heterozygotes are of two main types: α^0 in which both alpha genes on one chromosome 16 are deleted ($\alpha\alpha/- -$) and α^+ in which there is a deletion or mutation in only one of the two tandem alpha globin genes ($\alpha\alpha/\alpha-$ or $\alpha\alpha/\alpha^T\alpha$). (See figure for the genetics of α-thalassaemia.)

Homozygous α^0 thalassaemia (haemoglobin Bart's hydrops fetalis syndrome) (– –/– –)

Common cause of fetal loss throughout South-east Asia and also in Greece and Cyprus. Affected infants produce no alpha chains and so are unable to make HbA or HbF. Usually stillborn in third trimester (their fetal blood is 80% Hb Bart's, i.e. β-globin tetramers and 20% embryonic Hb). High risk of pre-eclampsia (PET) and other obstetric problems due to enlarged placenta.

HbH disease ($\alpha-/- -$). Usually compound heterozygotes for α^0 and α^+. Absence of 3 alpha genes leads to formation of β-globin tetramers. Microcytic anaemia with Hb 7–10 g/dl. Splenomegaly is common and haemolytic crises may occur in response to infection. Most patients survive to adulthood but life expectancy is shortened.

α-thalassaemia homozygote ($\alpha-/\alpha-$); α heterozygote ($\alpha\alpha/- -$); α^+-thalassaemia heterozygote ($\alpha\alpha/\alpha-$). α^+ homozygotes and α^0 heterozygotes are well, with a mild microcytic hypochromic anaemia; α^+ heterozygotes are well with a normal Hb level, but mild microcytosis and hypochromia.

Thalassaemias with variant haemoglobins

Sickle cell β^0-thalassaemia (β^S/β^0) or sickle cell β^+-thalassaemia (β^S/β^+). Variable phenotype. In Mediterranean populations where one parent may have β^0 and the other β^S, the picture is one of sickle cell disease. In African Blacks several mild forms of β^+ thalassaemia are commonly found that, when they interact with β^S, produce a condition with mild anaemia and few sickling crises and normal life expectancy. HbS also interacts with $\delta\beta$-thalassaemia to produce sickle cell disease, in contrast to the interaction of HbS with hereditary persistence of fetal haemoglobin (HPFH) where patients are clinically normal.

Haemoglobin C β-thalassaemia (β^C/β^0 or β^C/β^+). Found in west Africans and some north African and southern Mediterranean populations. Mild haemolytic anaemia

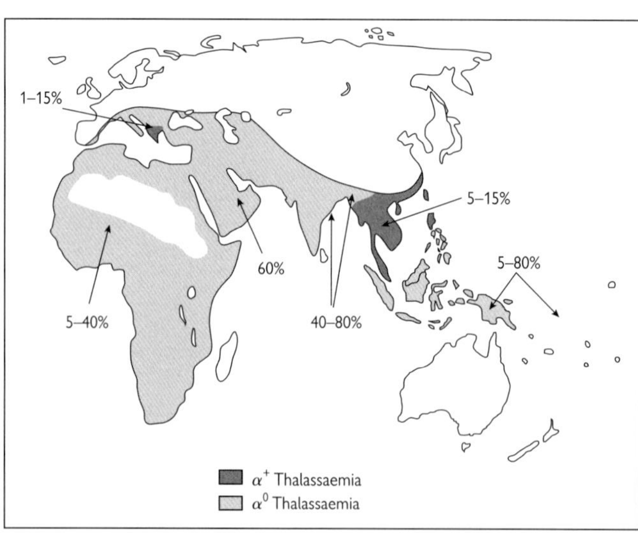

Map showing the distribution of the α-thalassaemias. (Figure 14, p. 684 from Weatherall (2003) by permission of Oxford University Press.)

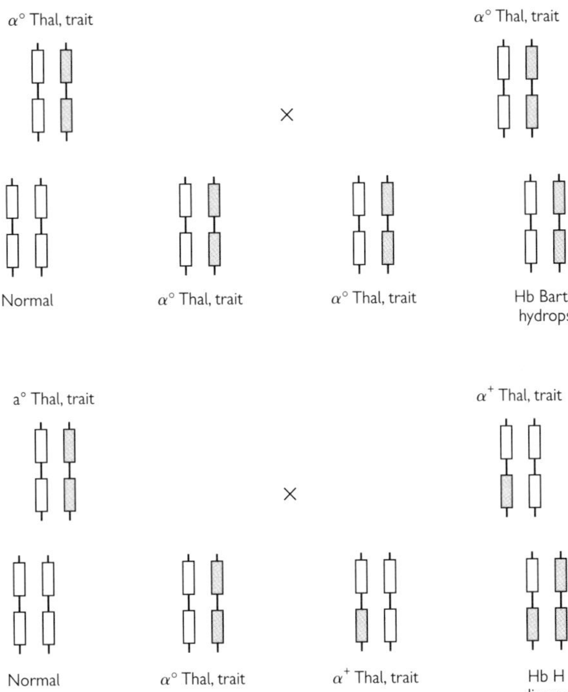

The genetics of α-thalassaemia. The black α genes represent gene deletions or otherwise inactivated genes. The open α genes represent normal genes. α° Thalassaemia and α⁺ thalassaemia are defined in the text. (Figure 16, p. 685 from Weatherall (2003) by permission of Oxford University Press.)

associated with splenomegaly. Hb electrophoresis shows mainly HbC.

Haemoglobin E β-thalassaemia (β^E/β° or β^E/β^+). The most common severe form of thalassaemia in Southeast Asia and India. The majority of the β-thalassaemia alleles commonly found with HbE are the β° or the severe β^+ type. HbE is inefficiently synthesized and, when co-inherited with a β°-thalassaemia allele, there is marked deficiency in β-chain production and a picture that can be similar to that of homozygous β°-thalassaemia.

Genetic advice

Inheritance and recurrence risk

- **Sickle cell disease and other structural variants.** Autosomal recessive (AR) with 25% sibling recurrence risk.
- **Thalassaemias.** AR with 25% sibling recurrence risk.
  - Beware the possibility of interaction of thalassaemia with variant haemoglobins.
  - Beware the possibility that β-thalassaemia trait may mask coexistent α-thalassaemia trait.

Variability and penetrance
See text concerning individual conditions.

Prenatal diagnosis
Always test both parents to define their genotype before embarking on prenatal diagnosis. Prenatal diagnosis by chorionic villus sampling (CVS) at 11 weeks gestation is available if mutations have been identified in both parents.

Carrier testing
Carrier testing is appropriate in the following circumstances.

- If there is a significant incidence of haemoglobinopathy in individuals of a given ethnic group.
- If a partner has a known haemoglobinopathy, the other partner should be tested even if they are from a low-risk group (since haemoglobinopathies can occur at very low incidence in most populations).

Other family members
Cascade testing of families and of partners should be offered.

Natural history and management

Potential long-term complications
See individual conditions.

Surveillance
Refer affected individuals to a haematologist.

Support group: UK Thalassaemia society <www.ukts.org>; The Sickle Cell Society <www.sicklecellsociety.org>. Advice for carriers: <www.chime.ucl.ac.uk/APoGI/menu.htm>

Expert adviser: John Old, National Haemoglobinopathy Reference Laboratory, Churchill Hospital, Oxford, England.

References

Forget BG. Molecular basis of hereditary persistence of fetal hemoglobin. *Ann N Y Acad Sci.* 1998; **850**: 38–44.

Stuart MJ, Nagel RL. Sickle-cell disease (Seminar) *Lancet* 2004; **364**: 1343–60.

Weatherall DJ. Disorders of the synthesis or function of haemoglobin. In *Oxford textbook of medicine*, 4th edn, (ed. D.A. Warrell, et al.), Chapter 22.05.07.00. Oxford University Press, Oxford, 2003.

Wierenga KJ, Hambleton IR, et al. Survival estimates for patients with homozygous sickle-cell disease in Jamaica: a clinic-based population study. *Lancet* 2001; **357**: 680–3.

Haemophilia and other inherited coagulation disorders

The geneticist's main role is to clarify the nature of the bleeding disorder in the family, to determine its severity, and to assess the level of risk to the consultand. Of the families we have encountered in clinic who were referred with a family history of 'haemophilia', only ~50% actually had a relative with factor VIII or factor IX deficiency. Other diagnoses that have emerged during further investigation included von Willebrand disease (VWD) and factor XI deficiency. Consultands or their families may have links with one or more haemophilia centres; it is important for geneticists to collaborate closely with haemophilia centre staff.

Haemophilia A (factor VIII deficiency) and haemophilia B (factor IX deficiency or Christmas disease) are clinically indistinguishable. The incidence of haemophilia A is 1 in 5000 male births and that of haemophilia B is 1 in 30 000 male births. Females with disadvantageous X-inactivation may have mild haemophilia, but severe disease is rare in females unless there is extreme skewing of X-inactivation or the girl has Turner syndrome or the child has a father who is a haemophiliac and a mother who is a carrier. Bleeding occurs in haemophilia owing to failure of secondary haemostasis. Primary haemostasis (formation of a platelet plug) occurs normally, but stabilization of the plug by fibrin is defective because inadequate amounts of thrombin are generated. The type and severity of haemophilia run true in families. There is no known family history in approximately one-third of haemophiliacs. The classification of haemophilia is outlined in the table.

Factor VIII—haemophilia A. The factor VIII gene is located on Xq28 and consists of 26 exons. 45% of patients with severe haemophilia A have an inversion in intron 22 that disrupts the factor VIII gene. This mutation arises almost exclusively in the male germline. Other mutations are predominantly point mutations (85% missense, 15% nonsense) with about 5% being large or small deletions and insertions. Approximately 2% of patients with severe haemophilia A do not have a detectable mutation on sequencing of the factor VIII gene.

A proportion of patients who make no, or virtually no, native factor VIII protein will produce antibodies in response to treatment with exogenous factor (inhibitors). This can significantly complicate treatment. Haemophilia A patients carrying the intron 22 inversion, large deletions, or nonsense mutations have an ~35% incidence of inhibitors (antibodies that inactivate factor VIII), whereas those with missense mutations and small deletions have an ~5% risk. Overall, ~10% of patients with haemophilia A develop inhibitors.

Factor IX—haemophilia B. The factor IX gene is located on Xq27 and consists of 8 exons. The vast majority of mutations are point mutations (~67% missense), with ~7% short insertions or deletions and 3% large-scale gene deletions or complex rearrangements. Mutations in the promoter region cause the unusual **factor IX Leiden** phenotype. Usually endogenous factor IX (and factor VIII) levels do not change significantly with age, but, in those with the factor IX Leiden mutation, the factor IX concentration rises with hormonal changes at puberty. Severe haemophiliacs become mild, and mild haemophiliacs may develop normal factor IX concentrations.

In haemophilia B, patients with gene deletions or rearrangements have a risk of inhibitor development (see above) of ~50%, whereas for frameshift, premature stop, or splice-site mutations the risk is ~20%. Those with missense mutations almost never develop inhibitors. In general, inhibitors are less common in haemophilia B than in haemophilia A.

Clinical approach

History: key points

- Three-generation family history with specific enquiry re bleeding disorders; ask about joint bleeding. For milder disorders it is particularly helpful to ask if anyone has bled after surgery, e.g. dental extractions or tonsillectomy. Extend family tree further if other affected relatives are known.
- Detailed history of proband. Try to clarify the type of bleeding disorder (factor VIII, factor IX, VWD, etc.). Try to assess level of severity. Factor VIII injections? Joint injury from haemarthroses, etc.? Try to establish which haemophilia centre the affected individual attends.

Examination: key points
Usually not relevant.

Investigation
When the diagnosis in proband is certain:

- specific factor level, e.g. factor VIII level if family history is of haemophilia A, factor IX level for family history of haemophilia B;
- DNA (EDTA (ethylenedinitrilotetraacetate) sample) for molecular diagnosis if familial mutation known or for linkage.

When the diagnosis in proband uncertain (involve a haematologist):

- full blood count (FBC) for platelet count;
- coagulation screen (prothrombin time (PT), activated partial thromboplastin time (APTT)). Note that a normal screen does not rule out VWD or some other disorders;
- Von Willebrand factor antigen (VWF: Ag);
- ristocetin cofactor (VWF:RiCof)—a functional assessment of VWF;

Classification of haemophilia

Severity of haemophilia	Concentration of factor VIIIC or IXC	Clinical features
Mild	5–40% (>0.05–0.40 IU/ml)	Spontaneous bleeding does not occur; excessive bleeding after surgery, dental extractions, and accidents
Moderate	1–5% (0.01–0.05 IU/ml)	Bleeding into joints and muscles after minor injuries; excessive bleeding after surgery and dental extractions
Severe	<1% (<0.01 IU/ml)	Spontaneous joint and muscle bleeding; bleeding after injuries, accidents, and surgery

- specific factor levels, e.g. factor VIII or IX;
- consider DNA storage (EDTA sample) for future studies.

Other diagnoses/conditions to consider

Von Willebrand disease (VWD). Deficiency or dysfunction of the adhesive glycoprotein von Willebrand factor (VWF). VWF protects factor VIII from premature proteolytic degradation and concentrates it at sites of vascular injury. VWD is common with incidence figures varying between 0.1% and 1%. There are several different subtypes of VWD, but the phenotype is usually relatively mild. Mucosal bleeding predominates but it is also an important cause of menorrhagia in affected families. VWD is not clearly autosomal dominant, the inheritance is more variable and there is a strong school of opinion that the common mild type 1 may be related to genetic or environmental influences independent of the von Willebrand factor (eg. blood group).

Factor VII deficiency. Autosomal recessive (AR) disorder affecting 1/500 000 located on chromosome 13.

Factor X deficiency. AR disorder affecting 1/100 000 located on chromosome 13.

Factor XI deficiency (previously called haemophilia C). Autosomally inherited disorder affecting 1/1 000 000. The gene for factor XI is located on chromosome 4. In most cases a mild bleeding disorder. Heterozygotes may have a bleeding tendency that is poorly related to the factor XI level. Factor XI deficiency is particularly common in Askenazim where 1/190 have severe deficiency and 8% (~1/12) of the population are carriers.

Other coagulation factor deficiencies. Congenital deficiencies can occur in any of the coagulation factors, but all are rare. Inheritance is autosomal with these disorders being more common in racial groups where cousin marriages occur. Such disorders should be discussed with a haemophilia specialist.

Genetic advice

Inheritance and recurrence risk
X-linked recessive.

Factor VIII deficiency. Mutations originate ~3 times more often in males than in females. This implies that 80% of mothers of an isolated patient are expected to be haemophilia carriers.

Variability and penetrance
Haemophilia is fully penetrant. It runs true in families, so if one relative has 'mild' disease, other affected relatives will also be likely to be mildly affected. Similarly for severe disease.

Prenatal diagnosis
This is usually only considered for severe haemophilia. Most patients with mild haemophilia enjoy a normal lifestyle, with appropriate advice about management of trauma or major surgery. Possible by chorionic villus sampling (CVS) at 11 weeks gestation if familial mutation known or by linkage. Pre-implantation genetic diagnosis (PGD) with selection of female embryos may be another option to consider.

Predictive testing
Testing of cord blood of 'at risk' males is indicated to guide future management.

Other family members
Carrier testing of female relatives is often problematic unless the familial mutation is known. Only a proportion of carriers have factor levels below the normal range.

A reproducibly normal result does not exclude carrier status. Linked markers may be helpful in excluding carrier status or in identifying the 'high-risk' X. Some carrier females have low concentrations of factor VIIIC or IXC that can predispose to excessive bleeding, with levels in the mild haemophilia range. Factor concentrations should therefore be measured in girls and women who are definite or possible carriers. Mutation testing to determine carrier status is usually deferred until the mid-teens when a girl is able to engage actively in the testing process.

Natural history and management

People with bleeding disorders should be referred to a Haemophilia Centre for registration, advice, and for management of bleeding episodes. Haemophilia care in the UK is provided by a network of specialist centres and coordinated by the UK Haemophilia centre Doctor's Organisation (UKHCDO) who provide relevant protocols and guidelines for management.

- **Factor concentrates** are the treatment of choice for people with severe and moderate haemophilia A or B.
- **Plasma-derived factors**. During the 1980s, production of factor concentrates from pooled plasma resulted in a large number of haemophiliacs acquiring one or more of hepatitis B, hepatitis C, and human immunodeficiency virus (HIV). Virus-inactivation procedures are currently used in product manufacture, but concerns remain about prions (e.g. new variant Creutzfeld–Jakob disease (CJD)). Hepatitis B can be prevented by immunization.
- **Recombinant products** are the treatment of choice. In the UK all patients will be transferred to recombinant products by 2005–6.
- **DDAVP (desamino-8-D-arginine vasopressin).** In mildly affected patients with haemophilia A and mild VWD (some subtypes) it is often possible to use DDAVP instead of factor VIII concentrate. Patients with severe VWD require factor concentrates containing VWF; these are plasma-derived.

Potential long-term complications
- **Complications of the disorder**. Recurrent joint bleeding with inadequate treatment in severe haemophilia leads to chronic arthropathy, pain, and loss of function which may lead to crippling. Death from bleeding (eg. intracranial haemorrhage) may occur.
- **Complications related to treatment**:
  - transfusion-transmitted infections, e.g. hepatitis B, hepatitis C, HIV (risk is very much reduced with virally inactivated concentrates; risk thought to be eliminated with recombinant products);
  - development of antibodies (inhibitors).

Surveillance
Guidelines for the management of pregnancy in carriers for haemophilia (from Giangrande 1998) are as follows.
- Baseline factor VIII or IX level should be checked at booking and at 34 weeks gestation.
- Fetal sex should be determined by ultrasound scan (USS) and the obstetrician informed prior to delivery.
- Routine lower segment Caesarean section (LSCS) is *not* indicated because of possible haemophilia, but would be performed if there were other obstetric reasons.
- If required for obstetric indications, LSCS may be carried out without haemostatic support if the maternal factor level is ≥0.5 IU/ml or 50% of normal.

- Epidural anaesthaesia is permitted if the factor level is >0.4 IU/ml or 40% of normal.
- The use of invasive fetal monitoring techniques such as fetal scalp electrodes or the collection of fetal scalp vein samples should be avoided during the delivery of affected males (or if the status of a male infant is unknown).
- Vacuum extraction (Ventouse delivery) *should be avoided*. Use of forceps is not contraindicated, but particular care is required, and if the child proves to be affected coagulation factor treatment will be required after delivery.
- A cord blood sample should be taken after delivery for testing for haemophilia.
- Vitamin K should *not* be given by im injection until the result is known (can be given orally).
- There is no need to administer coagulation factor concentrates to a haemophiliac neonate after a normal vaginal delivery, if there is no evidence of any bleeding (e.g. cephalhaematoma). Recombinant coagulation factor concentrate should be used for the treatment of neonates if treatment is needed after delivery for any reason (e.g. after forceps delivery).
- Special observations after delivery may be warranted. Risk of intracranial bleeding after a normal vaginal delivery is very low (~1–4% in severe haemophiliacs), but it is a recognized complication. It is most likely within the first week and some units routinely carry out USS of the brain to exclude this possibility.

Support group: Haemophilia Society (UK) <www.haemophilia.org.uk>; National Hemophilia Foundation (USA) <www.infonhf.org>.

Further information: The Haemophilia Alliance <www.haemophiliaalliance.org.uk> is a national partnership whose aim is to advance and promote high levels of care for people with haemophilia and related disorders.

Expert advisers: Paula Bolton-Maggs, Consultant Haematologist, Manchester Comprehensive Care Haemophilia Centre, Manchester Royal Infirmary, Manchester and Paul Giangrande, Consultant Haematologist, Oxford Haemophilia Centre and Thrombosis Unit, Churchill Hospital, Oxford, England.

References

Bolton-Maggs PHB, Pasi KJ. Haemophilias A and B [seminar]. *Lancet* 2003; **361**: 1801–9.

Giangrande PLF. Management of pregnancy in carriers of haemophilia. *Haemophilia* 1998; **4**: 779–84.

Mannucci PM, Tuddenham EGD. The haemophilias—from royal genes to gene therapy. *New Engl J Med* 2001; **344**: 1773–9.

Hereditary haemorrhagic telangiectasia (HHT)

Rendu–Osler–Weber syndrome.

HHT is an autosomal dominant (AD) vascular dysplasia, with a prevalence of approximately 1/10 000. There is locus heterogeneity with two loci, endoglin (*ENG*) on chromosome 9 and activin-like receptor kinase (*ALK-1*) on 12q13, responsible for almost all cases of HHT. Both endoglin and *ALK*-1 encode proteins involved in serine–threonine kinase signalling in the endothelial cell. The proteins form a homodimeric integral membrane glycoprotein that is the surface receptor for the transforming growth factor β (TGF-β) superfamily that mediates vascular remodelling through effects on extracellular matrix production (Fuchizaki *et al.* 2003).

The characteristic lesions of HHT are cutaneous and mucosal telangiectasia (that consist of focal dilatations of postcapillary venules) and visceral arteriovenous malformations (AVMs). Pulmonary arteriovenous malformations (PAVMs), found in 15–20%, create clinically significant right–left shunts and are much more common in families with endoglin mutations (Berg *et al.* 2003). Primary pulmonary hypertension is a rare complication in some families with *ALK-1* mutations (Trembath *et al.* 2001). Most patients with familial primary pulmonary hypertension have defects in the gene for bone morphogenetic protein receptor II (*BMPR2*), which like *ENG* and *ALK-1* is a member of the TGF-β superfamily of receptors. Criteria for the diagnosis of HHT are given in the table.

The Curaçao criteria for the diagnosis of HHT (Shovlin *et al.* 2000)

Criteria

1 **Epistaxis**: spontaneous, recurrent nosebleeds*

2 **Telangiectasia**: multiple, at characteristic sites: lips, oral cavity, fingers, nose

3 **Visceral lesions**: such as: gastrointestinal telangiectasia, pulmonary AVM, hepatic AVM, cerebral AVM, spinal AVM

4 **Family history**: a first-degree relative with HHT according to these criteria

The diagnosis of HHT is:

Definite if three criteria are present[†]

Possible or suspected if two criteria are present

Unlikely if fewer than two criteria are present

* Epistaxis should occur spontaneously on more than one occasion.

[†] Within HHT families a firm diagnosis can be made on the basis of two separate visceral manifestations.

Clinical approach

History: key points

- Detailed three-generation family tree with specific enquiry about nosebleeds, telangiectasia, stroke, etc.
- Nosebleeds. Do they occur spontaneously? Age of onset, frequency? Night-time bleeds are particularly suspicious.
- Previous unexplained anaemia or gastrointestinal bleeding.
- History of headache, epilepsy, intracranial haemorrhage due to cerebral AVMs (CAVMs) or transient ischaemic attack (TIA), stroke, or cerebral abscess as a complication of PAVMs (paradoxical embolization)
- History of exertional dyspnoea; rarely, haemoptysis or haemothorax due to PAVMs.

Examination: key points

- Look carefully at the lips, mouth, and tongue for telangiectasia. These may be very subtle and only apparent on close inspection.
- Look carefully at the finger pulps and nail beds for telangiectasia, which again may not be apparent without close inspection.
- Examine for clubbing, cyanosis.
- Listen for an hepatic or pulmonary vascular bruit.

Special investigation

If there is a clinical diagnosis or strong suspicion of HHT the following are appropriate.

- Posteroanterior (PA) and left lateral chest X-rays for evidence of PAVMs (rounded, circumscribed lesions, sometimes with shadows of feeding/draining vessels).
- Refer to a respiratory specialist or lung function lab for screening for PAVMs by pulse oximetry (SaO_2 after lying for 10 mins and standing for 10 mins) to detect resting desaturation and orthodeoxia—most PAVMs are in the lower lobes.
- Consider DNA for mutation analysis of endoglin (especially in families with PAVMs) and *ALK-1* if available.
- If PAVMs evident on chest X-ray or suspected from SaO_2 readings, the right–left shunt can be quantified using 100% oxygen method or renal imaging following intravenous (IV) injection of $^{99}Tc^m$-albumin-labelled microaggregates (Chilvers *et al.* 1988). Angiography allows detailed localization and embolization.

Genetic advice

Inheritance and recurrence risk

AD inheritance. 50% risk to offspring of affected individual.

Variability and penetrance

Age-dependent penetrance. 62% symptomatic by 16 years, 83% by 26 years, and 97% by 35 years. Fully penetrant by 40 years.

Epistaxis (from telangiectasia in nasal septum and inferior turbinate) is usually the first symptom with onset around puberty. Mucocutaneous telangiectasia appear 5–20 years after onset of epistaxis and increase in number with age.

Prenatal diagnosis and pregnancy

Prenatal diagnosis is technically feasible only if there is a known familial mutation. Pregnancy is a risk period for progression of PAVMs. *Women with PAVMs in association with HHT are at high risk in pregnancy* when ~50% experience complications (intrapulmonary bleeding, worsening shunt, etc.). Some women experience a reduction or cessation in nosebleeds during pregnancy, but for others the frequency of nosebleeds increases and they may develop new telangiectasia.

Other family members

Cascade screening of the extended family is important because of the potential for serious avoidable complications. PAVMs do not usually occur before mid–late teenage years and so screening (chest X-ray and lying/standing pulse oximetry) is usually offered from the teens onwards, and only to those with recurrent nosebleeds (or other bleeding site) or clinically evident telangiectasia (i.e. two or more diagnostic criteria—see the table above).

Natural history and management

Telangiectasia and AVMs tend to increase both in size and number with age.

- **Gastrointestinal AVMs** (11–40%) can result in Fe-deficient anaemia or gastrointestinal haemorrhage.
- **PAVMs** (14–30%) can cause hypoxaemia leading to respiratory failure and polycythaemia and paradoxical embolism causing stroke and cerebral abscesses. Embolization in a specialist centre is the preferred treatment for these lesions.
- **Hepatic AVMs** (8–31%) can rarely cause high-output cardiac failure or port–caval shunting and may cause an unusual appearance on hepatic imaging. Embolization is best avoided.
- **Central nervous system (CNS; brain, spinal cord) (5–11%).** CAVMs can bleed, although numerically more neurological events occur secondary to PAVMs than intracranial AVMs. Risk/benefit of screening for asymptomatic CAVMs is uncertain. Risk of haemorrhage of untreated CAVMs, estimated at approximately 2% per annum, needs to be balanced against risks of neurosurgical intervention. Some centres offer screening by digital subtraction angiography (DSA), but in the absence of symptoms most do not screen.
- **Skin telangiectasia** (13–89%) may occur on the oral mucosa, face, conjunctivas, trunk, extremities, nail beds, and finger pads.
- **Nasal telangiectasia (>90%).** Management of nosebleeds is difficult and there is no wholly satisfactory approach. Most nosebleeds are self-limiting and patients learn to manage them independently.
  - Routine treatment with packing and humidification. Fe and transfusion when necessary.
  - Laser treatment may be successful.
  - Surgery (septal dermoplasty) may be successful in expert hands—but vessels regrow.
  - Cautery has only a limited role.

Surveillance

- Five yearly screening investigations for PAVMs (chest X-ray and lying and standing pulse oximetry). Since pregnancy is a time when PAVMs may develop/ progress, arrange repeat screening between pregnancies.
- Low threshold for checking haemoglobin (Hb) in those with frequent nosebleeds (may need regular Fe supplementation).

Support group: Telangiectasia Self Help Group <www.telangiectasia.co.uk>; HHT Foundation International <www.hht.org> (useful site for clinicians too).

Expert advisers: Mary Porteous, Consultant Clinical Geneticist, Edinburgh, Scotland and Edwin Chilvers, Professor of Respiratory Medicine, University of Cambridge, Cambridge, England.

References

Berg J, Porteous M, *et al.* Hereditary haemorrhagic telangiectasia: a questionnaire based study to delineate the different phenotypes caused by endoglin and *ALK1* mutations. *J Med Genet* 2003; **40**: 585–90.

Chilvers ER, Peters AM, *et al.* Quantification of right to left shunt through pulmonary arteriovenous malformations using $^{99}Tc^{m}$-albumin microspheres. *Clin Radiol* 1988; **39**: 611–14.

Fuchizaki U, Miyamori H, *et al.* Hereditary haemorrhagic telangiectasia (Rendu–Osler–Weber disease)—eponym. *Lancet* 2003; **362**: 1490–4.

Shovlin CL, Guttmacher AE, *et al.* Diagnostic criteria for hereditary haemorrhagic telangiectasia (Rendu–Osler–Weber syndrome). *Am J Med Genet* 2000; **91**: 66–87.

Shovlin CL, Letarte M. Hereditary haemorrhagic telangiectasia and pulmonary arteriovenous malformations: issues in clinical management and review of pathogenic mechanisms. *Thorax* 1999; **54**: 714–29.

Trembath RC, *et al.* Clinical and molecular genetic features of pulmonary hypertension in patients with hereditary haemorrhagic telangiectasia. *New Engl J Med* 2001; **345**: 325–34.

Hereditary motor and sensory neuropathy (HMSN)

Charcot–Marie–Tooth disease (CMT), peroneal muscular atrophy.

Usually presents between the ages of 5 and 15 years with difficulty walking due to problems picking up the feet ('foot drop'), progressive foot deformity, high instep, and claw toes. Gradual loss of muscle bulk in lower calves leads to 'inverted champagne bottle' appearance with weakness of dorsiflexion and eversion of foot and high-arched feet (pes cavus). Weakness of hands may occur later and is rarely symptomatic before adult life. The weakness is very slowly progressive. Affected individuals may also have a loss of sensation in the hands and feet. Sometimes does not present until much later, even into middle age. Severe disease can also present in infancy and early childhood. A few people with HMSN1 have a tremor (Roussy–Levy syndrome).

There is a wide range of severity. A few gene carriers may be asymptomatic in adult life and a few may have severely impaired mobility and become wheelchair-dependent. For the majority, HMSN causes problems with sporting activities and footwear in childhood and adolescence and some impairment of mobility by middle life. HMSN is not uncommon with a prevalence of 1/3300.

Hereditary motor sensory neuropathy (HMSN/CMT) represents a clinically and genetically heterogeneous group of inherited neuropathies caused by aberration of the intimate relationship between the myelin sheath and the axon. Disorders causing demyelination are classified as HMSN1 (CMT1) and those causing axonal loss as HMSN2 (CMT2). The mechanisms by which mutations disturb the relationship of the myelin sheath and axon are not fully understood. Some mutations affect this relationship more profoundly than others, and thus account for the paradox that mutation of a 'myelin gene' can present with electrophysiological features of CMT2 and vice versa (Boerkoel et al. 2002). There are currently 37 genes implicated in CMT. Many of these genes play a role in axonal transport and protein trafficking (Shy).

The most common molecular defect in HMSN1 (CMT1) is a 1.5 Mb duplication at 17p11.2 arising from unequal crossing over of homologous chromosomes at regions of low copy repeats flanking the duplicated region. Deletion of the same region causes the milder phenotype, hereditary neuropathy with liability to pressure palsies (HNPP)—see below.

Classification of HMSN/CMT (see table) is in a transition state between classifications based on clinical presentation and neurophysiology and those based on - molecular genetics. No consensus is currently agreed. In the pre-molecular era HMSN was classified on the basis of the inheritance pattern (autosomal dominant (AD), autosomal recessive (AR), or X-linked) and whether the neuropathy was demyelinating or axonal. A median nerve conduction velocity (NCV) of 38 m/s was taken as the cut-off with slower velocities classified as demyelinating. It is now apparent that some individuals with NCVs >38 m/s have a mutation in a myelin protein gene, e.g. connexin 32.

Clinical approach

History: key points

- Three-generation family tree (or more if affected members are known in previous generations) with detailed enquiry for high arches, unusual gait, impaired mobility, e.g. use of sticks, wheelchair.
- Developmental milestones. Difficulty running, walking, participation in sport at school.
- Enquire about difficulty undoing buttons, clumsiness, or frequent falls.
- Document current level of disability.
- Enquire about vision and hearing.

Examination: key points

- Observe gait. Is there foot drop with slapping or high-stepping gait?
- Test walking on heels (usually difficult due to weakness of foot dorsiflexion) and abduction of fingers.
- Examine for wasting of calf muscles, high instep, clawing of toes, and enlargement of peripheral nerves. Examine for wasting of interossei muscles in hands.
- Test for loss of vibration sense in feet and hands.
- Test reflexes. Ankle jerks are usually lost early, with progressive loss of other reflexes. (NB. Sometimes the ankle jerks remain present even in some people with substantial weakness.)
- Palpate the greater auricular nerve (running behind the ear lobe near the mastoid bone) for enlargement. Often present in HMSN1, but not seen in HMSN2 or X-linked HMSN1 (HMSN1 X).
- If sporadic, look for retinitis pigmentosa (RP).
- If accompanying learning difficulty, consider karyotype with Smith–Magenis fluorescent in situ hybridization (FISH).

Special investigations

If there is a known family history, it may be appropriate to proceed directly to molecular genetic investigation. Even if not, if the clinical picture is of typical HMSN it may be reasonable to do DNA testing for a PMP22 duplication before proceeding to nerve conduction studies to clarify the diagnosis.

- Molecular genetic investigations (DNA):
  - if family history shows AD inheritance, look for duplication 17p11.2–12 (PMP22), or point mutation of PMP22 or MPZ (P0);
  - if no male–male transmission, i.e. family history consistent with X-linked inheritance, look for connexin 32 (GJB1) mutations. (NB. Females are often symptomatic, but usually later than males, so that the family history may appear to be 'AD' but closer scrutiny shows the absence of male–male transmission.)
- NCVs:
  - motor conduction velocities in full-term infants are approximately 50% of those in adults and approach adult values by ~3 years. HMSN1 motor NCVs are usually in range 10–38 m/s;
  - in adults normal NCV studies show a velocity of >40–45 m/s.
- Additional investigations to consider for sporadic case in early childhood:
  - NCVs in both parents to detect asymptomatic gene carrier for HMSN;
  - testing for Friedreich's ataxia (FRDA; triplet repeat expansion in Frataxin gene). It can be difficult to distinguish cases of HMSN2 with unsteadiness from early stages of FRDA;

Classification of HMSN/CMT

Inheritance and proportion of HMSN	Genetic basis*	Pathology	Clinical features†
HMSN1 (CMT1) AD, ~70–80%	*PMP22* in 70–80% (1A). Most are gene duplications. Some are point mutations (which tend to give a more severe phenotype) *MPZ* in 5–10% (1B) *LITAF* uncommon (1C) *EGR2* uncommon (1D)	Abnormal myelin. Slow NCVs typically 10–30 m/s	Distal muscle weakness and atrophy associated with mild/moderate glove and stocking sensory loss, depressed reflexes, and pes cavus. A few people with HMSN have a tremor (Roussy–Levy syndrome)
HMSN1 X (CMTX) X-linked semidominant, ~10–20%	*Connexin 32* (also known as *GJB1*) (1X)	Most have a predominantly demyelinating picture but some have a relatively axonal form that may be confused with HMSN2	Affected males are clinically very similar to HMSN1, but males are consistently more severely affected than females
HMSN2 (CMT2) AD, ~10%	*KIF1B-MFN2* (2A) *RAB-7* (2B) *6ARS* (2C) *Neurofilament triplet L protein* (2E)	Axonopathy. NCVs usually normal or mildly slowed (38–48 m/s), but amplitude is reduced	Clinically similar to HMSN1 but in general less disabling and with less sensory loss
HMSN3 (CMT3), congenital HMSN, 'Dejerine–Sottas'‡ AD for CMT1A, 1B, and 1D and AR for CMT4. Most are *de novo* AD mutations, i.e. reclassified as HMSN1	*PMP22* (CMT1A) *MPZ* (CMT1B) *EGR2* (CMT1D and CMT4)	Usually abnormal myelin with very slow NCVs	Severe demyelinating neuropathy of infancy and childhood with marked clinical weakness and hypertrophy of nerves
HMSN4 (CMT4) AR, rare	Genetically heterogeneous with 7 loci including: *EGR2* (CMT4E) *PRX* (CMT4F)·	Either abnormal myelin or axonopathy	Often early childhood onset
Complex forms of HMSN § Rare	Genetically heterogeneous. Some may possibly represent contiguous gene deletions		Neuropathy may be combined with other features, e.g. deafness, retinitis pigmentosa, vocal cord paralysis

* *PMP22*, Peripheral myelin protein 22; *MPZ*, myelin protein zero; *EGR2*, early growth response protein 2; *KIF1B*, kinesin-like protein KIF1B; *MFN2*, Mitochondrial GTPase mitofusin 2; *RAB7*, Ras-related protein Rab-7; *6ARS*, glycyl-tRNA synthetase; *NEFL*, neurofilament triplet L protein; *GJB1*, connexin 32. *LITAF*, lipopolysaccharide – induced TNF factor.

† Subtypes related to the different genes are clinically indistinguishable.

‡ This clinical category is genetically heterogeneous and has been reclassified on the basis of the genetic pathology, usually as HMSN1.

§ Consider the possibility of an alternative diagnosis especially in a sporadic case.

- ophthalmology assessment for pigmentary retinopathy or optic atrophy;
- phytanic acid (Refsum may resemble other demyelinating neuropathies, e.g. HMSN2 and HMSN3, but, in addition, children develop night blindness and pigmentary retinopathy);
- magnetic resonance imaging (MRI) scan if any hint of regression, history of seizures, or other central nervous system (CNS) abnormality;
- sural nerve biopsy if DNA studies are non-contributory.

Other diagnoses/conditions to consider

Hereditary neuropathy with liability to pressure palsies (HNPP). The history is of recurrent nerve palsies often with an AD history of similar problems. Caused by deletion of the *PMP22* gene (the same region that is duplicated in HMSNA 1A).

Hereditary neuralgic amyotrophy (familial brachial plexus neuropathy). AD disorder characterized by sudden onset of pain and weakness in the shoulder or upper arm associated with weakness. Typically asymmetric, recurring on the same or opposite side. Some recovery of function is usual, particularly early in the course of the disease.

Distal spinal muscular atrophy (SMA). A heterogeneous group of neuromuscular disorders caused by progressive anterior horn cell degeneration and characterized by progressive motor weakness and muscular atrophy, predominately in the distal parts of the limbs. One AR variety maps to 11q13. Mutations in *HSP22* and *HSP27* encoding small heat-shock proteins have been found in some families with AD distal hereditary motor neuropathy (Evgrafor, Irobi).

Friedreich's ataxia (FRDA). Mean onset 15.5 ± 8 years with range 2–51 years. The most common inherited ataxia. AR and caused by mutations in frataxin on 9q. Frataxin is a nuclear-encoded mitochondrial protein. It is characterized by a dying back from the periphery of the longest and largest myelinated fibres (e.g. large fibres arising in dorsal root ganglia). Carrier frequency in Caucasian population is ~1:85 with a disease prevalence of 1/29 000; it is rare in Africans and Asians. 98% of mutations are triplet repeat expansions of $(GAA)_n$ in intron 1 and 2% are point mutations or deletions. Normal triplet repeat allele size is 6–34, mutations have 67–1700 repeats. Repeat size is unstable with a tendency to decrease in size when paternally transmitted and increase or decrease when maternally transmitted. The disease is slowly but relentlessly progressive with loss of walking ~15 years after onset and mean age of death at ~37.5 years (usual cause is cardiomyopathy). Late-onset FRDA (onset >25 years) has been recognized since the onset of molecular testing. See 'Ataxic child' page 50 for more details.

Genetic advice

Inheritance and recurrence risk

Discuss AD inheritance or X-linked or AR as appropriate.

Variability and penetrance

Variability is often displayed within the extended family and gives parents an idea of the range of possible severity. Approximately 10% of affected individuals are asymptomatic

and detected either by careful clinical assessmement or NCVs.

Prenatal diagnosis

Technically possible by chorionic villus sampling (CVS) if the familial mutation is known, but not usually requested.

Predictive testing

Possible for at-risk adult members of the family if the familial mutation has been defined. Genetic testing is usually undertaken in children if they are symptomatic.

Other family members

Prenatal diagnosis is theoretically possible if a mutation has been identified, but is seldom requested or desired.

Natural history and management

Management

- Ankle–foot orthosis (AFO) if foot drop.
- Referral to orthopaedic surgeon if severe foot deformity.
- Care of feet if sensory deficit to prevent development of ulcers, etc.
- Monitor adolescents for development of scoliosis.
- Mobility aids, e.g. walking sticks, handrails; wheelchairs, may be required by some over time.
- If adults are drivers, they should inform the Driver and Vehicle Licensing Agency (DVLA).
- Avoid neurotoxic drugs, e.g. vincristine, taxol, cisplatin (chemotherapy), isoniazid (tuberculosis), and nitrofurantoin (antimicrobial used in treatment of urinary tract infections (UTIs)).

Potential long-term complications

- **Pes cavus.** Daily stretching exercises to prevent Achilles tendon shortening may be helpful. Careful choice of footwear which has good ankle support. Severe cases may benefit from orthopaedic surgery.
- **Loss of mobility.** With time, some patients may need aids such as walking sticks, but <5% need wheelchairs.
- **Scoliosis** is more common in those with early onset of symptoms. It is rarely severe.

Support group: CMT UK <www.cmt.org.uk>.

Expert adviser: David Hilton–Jones, Consultant Neurologist, Oxford Radcliffe Hospitals NHS Trust, Oxford, UK.

References

Boerkoel CF, Takashima H, Lupski JR. The genetic convergence of Charcot–Marie–Tooth disease types 1 and 2 and the role of genetics in sporadic neuropathy. *Curr Neurol Neurosci Rep* 2002; **2** (1): 70–7.

Evgrafor OV, Mersiyanova I *et al*. Mutant small heat-shock protien 27 causes axonal Charcot-Marie-Tooth disease and distal hereditary motor neuropathy. *Nat Genet* 2004; **36**: 602–06.

Irobi J, Van Impe K *et al*. Hot-spot residue in small heat-shock protien 22 causes distal motor neuropathy. *Nat Genet* 2004; **36**: 597–61.

Kijima K, Numakura C, *et al*. Mitochondrial GTPase mitofusin 2 mutation in Charcot-Marie-Tooth neuropathy type 2A. *Hum Genet* 2005, **116**: 23–27.

Ouvrier RA, McLeod JG, Pollard JD. *Peripheral neuropathy in childhood*, 2nd edn. MacKeith Press, London, 1999.

Shy ME. Charcot-Marie-Tooth disease: an update (Review) *Curr Opin Neurol* 2004; **17**: 579–85.

Wilmshurst JM, Pollard JD, *et al*. Peripheral neuropathies of infancy. *Dev Med Child Neurol* 2003; **45**: 408–14.

Hereditary spastic paraplegias (HSP)

Hereditary spastic paraparesis.

The HSPs are single-gene disorders in which the axons of the corticospinal tract either fail to develop normally or show progressive degeneration after initially normal development. The principal clinical feature in all HSPs is the presence of a bilaterally symmetrical, slowly progressive lower limb spastic paralysis. This occurs in relative isolation in the pure HSPs (PHSPs), or with other neurological or extra-neurological features in the complicated HSPs (CHSPs). Autosomal dominant (AD), autosomal recessive (AR), and X-linked recessive (XLR) inheritance patterns have been described for both pure and complicated HSPs, with AD PHSP the most common form (70–80% of families) in northern Europe and North America. XLR inheritance is rare. Most HSPs, including probably all of the AD PHSPs, are associated with neurodegeneration rather than abnormal neurodevelopment. Histopathological studies in PHSP have characterized this neurodegeneration as a length-dependent 'dying back' of the terminal ends of the corticospinal tract and dorsal column axons.

At least 20 HSP loci are recognized and 11 associated genes have been cloned (see table). Mutations in spastin (SPG4) on chromosome 2p21–22 are found in approximately 40% of families with AD PHSP, while mutations in atlastin (SPG3A; 14q12–21) are responsible in approximately 10% of families. Mutations in these genes are much less frequent in sporadic cases or in cases with an uncertain family history. The functions of the spastin and atlastin proteins are not yet known, though spastin may have a role in regulation of the microtubule cytoskeleton. Paraplegin mutations are a rare cause of AR pure or complicated (by optic, cortical, or cerebellar atrophy) HSP. They are associated with defects in mitochondrial oxidative phosphorylation, with characteristic structural and functional abnormalities on muscle biopsy.

Diagnosis in a family with AD PHSP is often known, and the role of the geneticist lies in advising about inheritance and assessing 'at risk' family members. Beware misdiagnosis in other family members, e.g. 'multiple sclerosis'. Penetrance is age-dependent and this together with the striking disease variability within families makes giving accurate genetic advice a considerable challenge in the absence of an identified mutation.

Clinical approach

History: key points

- Three-generation family history with special attention to gait disturbance, mobility.
- Age of onset. Paraplegia may begin in early childhood, presenting with delayed motor milestones and clumsiness

Genetic loci for HSP*

Gene symbol	MIM number	Chromosomal location	Gene product	Phenotype [†]
Autosomal dominant				
SPG3A	**182600**	**14q12–q21**	**Atlastin**	**PHSP**
SPG4	**182601**	**2p21–p24**	**Spastin**	**PHSP; ?CHSP (subtle cognitive impairment)**
SPG6	600363	15q11.2–q12	NIPA1	PHSP
SPG8	603563	8q24	—	PHSP
SPG9	601162	10q23.3–q24.2	—	CHSP (HSP with cataracts, motor neuropathy, short stature, skeletal abnormalities, gastro-oesophageal reflux)
SPG10	604187	12q13	KIF5A	PHSP
SPG12	604805	19q13	—	PHSP
SPG13	605280	2q24–q34	HSP60	PHSP
SPG17	270685	11q12–q14	Seipin	CHSP (Silver Syndrome—HSP with severe distal amyotrophy)
SPG19	607152	9q33–q34	—	PHSP
Autosomal recessive				
SPG5	270800	8q11–q13	—	PHSP
SPG7	602783	16q24.3	Paraplegin	PHSP; CHSP (HSP complicated by optic, cerebellar, or cerebral atrophy)
SPG11	604360	15q13–q15	—	PHSP; CHSP (HSP with thin corpus callosum)
SPG14	605229	3q27–q28	—	CHSP (HSP complicated by mild mental retardation and motor neuropathy)
SPG15	606859	14q22–q24	—	CHSP (Kjellin syndrome—HSP complicated by retinal degeneration)
SPG20	275900	13q12.3	Spartin	CHSP (Troyer syndrome—HSP complicated by dysarthria and distal muscle wasting)
SPG21	248900	15q22.31	Maspardin	CHSP (Mast syndrome—HSP with dementia and cerebellar and extrapyramidal signs)
SPG23	—	1q24–q32	—	CHSP (HSP with skin pigmentary abnormalities)
X-linked recessive				
SPG1	312900	Xq28	L1-CAM	CHSP; XLH
SPG2	312920	Xq22	PLP; DM20	PHSP; CHSP; PMD
SPG16	300266	Xq11.2	—	PHSP; CHSP

* **Common genes** denoted in **bold** type. MIM, Mendelian Inheritance in Man (database).

[†] CHSP, Complicated HSP; PHSP, pure HSP; XLH, X-linked hydrocephalus; PMD, Pelizaeus–Merzbacher disease.

(25% of cases in AD families are symptomatic by 5 years). Difficulty with physical education at school.
- Gait disturbance (shoe scuffing), history of trips and falls. Enquire about the maximum distance walking on flat ground, and whether aids, e.g. walking stick(s), are used.
- Spasticity affects lower limbs, and symptomatic involvement of upper limbs is rare.
- Severity. Spectrum varies from asymptomatic (10–20%) to chairbound (10–20%) and very rarely bed-ridden. Insidiously progressive.
- Aggravating features. Tiredness, cold, alcohol.
- Associated features. Bladder or bowel dysfunction.
- Complicating features, e.g. muscle wasting (e.g. Silver syndrome), cerebellar signs, dystonia, dementia, epilepsy, sensory neuropathy, optic atrophy, central retinal degeneration (Kjellin syndrome), ichthyosis (Sjögren–Larsson syndrome), disordered skin pigmentation, adducted thumbs + mental retardation (MASA (mental retardation–aphasia– shuffling gait–adducted thumbs) syndrome).

Examination: key points
- Observe gait and examine footwear for toe scuffing.
- Examine for foot deformity (65%). Pes cavus.
- Increased tone is disproportionately severe in comparison to weakness.
- Deep tendon reflex (DTRs) increased especially in lower limbs (99%). 7% have decreased power and increased reflexes in upper limbs.
- Clonus. Examine for sustained clonus (>4 beats; 45%).
- Extensor plantar reflexes (80%).

Signs in HSP are predominantly confined to the motor system. However, abnormal vibration sense is found in 40% of patients and other sensory modalities may be involved less frequently (involvement of dorsal columns). Mild distal muscle wasting may be found in longstanding cases.

Special investigations
In the absence of a causative mutation in a family, HSP is a diagnosis of exclusion. Investigations to be considered are the following.
- DNA for spastin or atlastin mutational analysis. Paraplegin mutation analysis can be considered in recessive families, but the pick-up rate appears low.
- Very long chain fatty acids (VLCFAs) for adrenoleukodystrophy, if inheritance is compatible with XLR, i.e. no male–male transmission.
- In cases lacking sensory symptoms, consider a trial of L-dopa, to exclude dopa-responsive dystonia.
- Magnetic resonance imaging (MRI) of the brain and spinal cord in one member of an affected family, and particularly in sporadic cases. In AD PHSP this may show spinal cord atrophy, especially in the cervical and thoracic regions, while some recessive HSPs are associated with thinning of the corpus callosum.
- Consider white cell enzymes if atypical features present eg, significant peripheral neuropathy.

A firm diagnosis of HSP should only be made where at least two family members have a progressive spastic gait disturbance with frank corticospinal tract signs in the lower limbs, i.e. hyperreflexia with either bilaterally extensor plantar reflexes or bilateral sustained (5+ beats) clonus.

Other diagnoses/conditions to consider
Pure HSP is a distinctive clinical entity, and diagnosis is usually straightforward. Occasional confusion may occur with the following.

Hereditary motor and sensory neuropathy (HMSN). Reflexes usually depressed in this condition (rather than increased). Peripheral nerve conduction velocities (NCVs) are almost always normal in HSP, and abnormal in HMSN. See 'Hereditary motor and sensory neuropathy (HMSN)', page 344.

Freidreich's ataxia (FRDA). Consider atypical FRDA (with preservation of reflexes) if inheritance compatible with AR (DNA for frataxin mutation analysis). See 'Ataxic child' page 52.

Dopa-responsive dystonia (Segawa syndrome). This may rarely present with a spastic paraplegia. Response to a trial of L-dopa is dramatic and sustained and should be considered in any case where sensory signs are not present. See 'Dystonia' page 106.

X-linked adrenoleukodystrophy. The adrenomyeloneuropathy phenotype may mimic HSP and should be considered in families lacking male to male transmission. A normal brain MRI does not exclude this condition. See 'X-linked adrenoleukodystrophy (X-ALD)', page 264.

Genetic advice
Inheritance and recurrence risk
Most PHSP follows AD inheritance (70–80%; see table), but AR inheritance (10–20%) and XLR inheritance (<5%) both occur. Most CHSPs are inherited in an AR pattern, although AD and XLR (notably the *L1-CAM* associated disorders) forms exist.

Risk of having inherited disease gene for clinically normal offspring of affected individuals (for families with AD disease and age of onset predominantly <35 years)

Age (years)	Residual risk of having disease gene (%)
20	24
25	22
30	19
35	13
40	11
45	9

The frequency of asymptomatic gene carriers means that every effort should be made to examine parents of apparently sporadic or recessive PHSP cases. If parents are both normal, recessive inheritance is most likely. If both parents of affected siblings cannot be examined, empiric figures indicate a 1/6 chance that one parent was affected, giving a risk to offspring of affected siblings of 1/12. No empiric figures are available for risks to offspring of apparently sporadic cases, where the possibility of AR inheritance, a non-penetrant AD parent, and a *de novo* mutation must all be considered.

Variability and penetrance
For AD families, because 10–20% of gene carriers are asymptomatic, risk of symptomatic disease in offspring of a gene carrier is 40–45%.

Prenatal diagnosis
Technically possible by chorionic villus sampling (CVS) if familial mutation is known or if family is large enough for linkage analysis.

Predictive testing

Theoretically possible if familial mutation is known or if family is large enough for linkage analysis, but restrict to adults who are able to engage fully in the decision-making process and approach as for other adult-onset neurodegenerative conditions.

Other family members

Anxiety may complicate assessment of 'at-risk' family members by causing mildly increased tone, hyperreflexia, and non-sustained clonus. (Don't overinterpret soft physical signs.)

Natural history and management

Surveillance

Because the disorder progresses so insidiously, it may be several years since diagnosis and the patient's disability may have progressed substantially since last reviewed. It may be appropriate to arrange for evaluation of the following.

- **Driving**. HSP may impair ability to use pedals in the car. Patients should notify the Driver and Vehicle Licensing Agency (DVLA) of their diagnosis and may need conversion of car to hand controls.
- **Home** may need bathroom alterations (e.g. walk-in-shower, rails), stair-lift, or downstairs bedroom.

- **Urinary symptoms**. <50% of patients with HSP have urinary frequency, urgency, or hesitancy. If symptomatic or recurrent infections, consider referral to urologist. Males may suffer erectile impotence.
- **Physiotherapy**. No therapy is currently available that slows disease progression. Treatment is aimed at maximizing functional ability and preventing contractures.
- **Antispasmodic medication** may benefit some patients and should be prescribed under the supervision of a neurologist.

Support group: Familial Spastic Paraplegia Group, Tel. 01702 218184.

Expert adviser: Evan Reid, University Lecturer and Honorary Consultant in Medical Genetics, University of Cambridge, Cambridge, England.

References

Errico A, Ballabio A, et al. Spastin, the protein mutated in autosomal dominant hereditary spastic paraplegia, is involved in microtubule dynamics. *Hum Mol Genet* 2002; **11**: 153–63.

Harding AE. Hereditary 'pure' spastic paraplegia: a clinical and genetic study of 22 families. *J Neurol Neurosurg Psychiatry* 1981; **44**: 871–83.

Reid E. The hereditary spastic paraplegias. *J Neurol* 1999; **246**: 995–1003.

Hirschsprung disease

Congenital intestinal aganglionosis, HSCR, aganglionic megacolon.

Hirschsprung disease is an important genetic cause of functional intestinal obstruction. It is characterized by the absence of neural-crest-derived enteric neural ganglia along a variable length of the intestine. The critical period in embryonic life for cranial–caudal migration of vagal neural crest cells and invasion of the neural-crest-derived ganglion cells into the intestinal wall is 5–12 weeks gestation. Ultrashort segment Hirschsprung disease (uncommon and even questionable) involves only the very distal rectum. Short-segment Hirschsprung disease (60–85%) is characterized by absence of intestinal ganglion cells from the wall of the rectum through to the upper sigmoid colon. Long-segment Hirschsprung disease (15–25%) involves the rectum through to a short section of the ascending colon. Total colonic aganglionosis (3–5%) involves the rectum and entire colon and variable parts of the ileum. Different degrees of Hirschsprung disease may occur within the same family.

Hirschsprung disease affects 1/5000 neonates. Males are more susceptible than females (4.5M:1F for short-segment and 1.75M:1F for long-segment Hirschsprung disease). Most present in neonatal period with failure to pass meconium in first 48 hours and/or abdominal distension and vomiting. Rectal biopsy is needed to confirm the diagnosis. Treatment is surgical with excision of the aganglionic bowel.

70% occur as an isolated finding, 20% are syndromic or have another congenital anomaly, and 10% are chromosomal (especially Down syndrome). Isolated Hirschsprung disease appears to be a multigenic malformation.

Hirschsprung disease is genetically heterogeneous, with eight genes known to be involved (mainly in the *RET* and endothelin signalling pathways). *RET* is regarded as the major locus in multigenic Hirschsprung disease.

Clinical approach

History: key points

- Careful three-generation family tree with particular attention to Hirschsprung disease or unexplained neonatal or early infant deaths, deafness and pigmentary anomalies, neurological features, thyroid cancer, phaeochromocytoma, or parathyroid hyperplasia.
- Determine the extent of gut inolved, e.g. short-segment/long-segment.
- Confirm diagnosis from histology report (if available).

Examination: key points

- Examine for pigmentary anomalies (white forelock, heterochromia, skin streaking).
- Examine for dysmorphic features.
- Careful cardiac assessment (5% of patients with Hirschsprung disease have a cardiac lesion, mostly atrial or ventricular septal defects (ASD or VSD, respectively)).
- Examine for distal limb anomalies. There are a series of rare syndromes with Hirschsprung disease and polydactyly, brachdactyly, or hypoplasia of distal phalanges and nails.

Investigation

- Karyotype if any anomaly in addition to Hirschsprung disease.
- Consider echocardiogram and renal ultrasound scan (USS) in view of significant incidence of additional anomalies.
- Consider *RET* mutation analysis. 40–50% of familial cases and 15–20% of sporadic cases have RET mutations with a penetrance of 50–70% in familial cases. Because of poor genotype–phenotype correlation as well as low and gender-dependent pentrance, the benefit of mutation screening for non-syndromic Hirschsprung appears very low. In addition, mutations are scattered all along the gene-coding sequence with no hot spot.
- Consider *ZFHX1B* (*SMADIP1*) mutation analysis in patients with Hirschsprung disease, microcephaly, and mental retardation and typical dysmorphic features with upturned ear lobules.
- Consider 7-dehydrocholesterol for Smith–Lemli–Opitz (SLO) if associated features are involved such as intrauterine growth restriction (IUGR), microcephaly, distal limb anomalies, etc.

Other diagnoses/conditions to consider

Waardenburg (WS) and related pigmentary anomalies. WS causes pigmentary anomalies and sensorineural deafness due to absence of melanocytes of the skin and the stria vascularis of the cochlea. The combination of Waardenburg plus Hirschsprung disease is termed Shah–Waardenburg or WS4 and is genetically heterogeneous, including homozygous endothelin pathway mutations and heterozygous *SOX10* mutations. In the latter case, various neurological symptoms with demyelinization might occur. See 'Deafness' page 90.

MEN2A (multiple endocrine neoplasia type 2A) and familial medullary thyroid cancer (MTC). Both MEN2A (age-related predisposition to MTC, phaeochromocytoma, and parathyroid hyperplasia) and familial MTC can be associated with Hirschsprung disease in some families. Screen for mutations in *RET* exon 10 and 11. See 'Multiple endocrine neoplasia (MEN)' page 466.

Mowat–Wilson syndrome. All patients have typical dysmorphic features with upturned ear lobules in association with severe intellectual disability, and nearly all have microcephaly and seizures. Congenital anomalies include Hirschsprung disease, congenital heart disease, hypospadias and genitourinary anomalies, agenesis of the corpus callosum. Short stature is common. Caused by heterozygous deletions or truncating mutations in the *ZFHX1B* (*SMAD1P1*) gene on 2q22.

Haddad syndrome. Both congenital central hypoventilation syndrome (CCHS, Ondine's curse) and Hirschprung disease can occur and nearly all patients have a heterozygous polyalanine expansion mutation in the *PHOX2B* gene.

Additional isolated congenital anomaly. A variety of additional anomalies are described: cardiac defects (5%); renal dysplasia/agnesis (4%); genital anomalies, e.g. hypospadias (2–3%).

Genetic advice

Inheritance and recurrence risk

Assess the family tree. If there are several affected family members and the inheritance pattern is suggestive of autosomal dominant (AD) or autosomal recessive (AR) inheritance, counsel for that, incorporating advice about very low penetrance. Use the table if the Hirschsprung disease is non-syndromic and there is no discernible Mendelian inheritance pattern or you are dealing with a sporadic case. Overall recurrence risk in sibs of a proband is 4%.

Empiric risk for non-syndromic Hirschsprung disease (Badner et al. 1990)

Sex of proband	Risk (%) to	
	Male sib	Female sib
Male short segment	5	1
Male long segment	17	13
Female short segment	5	3
Female long segment	33	9

Variability and penetrance

For Mendelian forms, penetrance is variable and gene-specific. In families carrying a mutation in RET, penetrance is 50–72% in gene carriers, mostly depending on the gender of the carrier individual.

Prenatal diagnosis

Prenatal diagnosis for Hirschsprung disease *per se* is not possible. If the mutation is known it would be theoretically possible, but may not be desired in view of the low penetrance of most mutations and the availability of surgical treatment.

Natural history and management

Potential long-term complications
Chronic constipation and soiling (10–15%).

Support group: American Hirschsprung's Disease Society <www.tiac.net/users/aphs>.

Expert adviser: Stanislas Lyonnet, Professor of Genetics, Hôpital Necker–Enfants Malades, Paris, France.

References

Amiel J, Lyonnet S. Hirschsprung disease, associated syndromes, and genetics: a review. *J Med Genet* 2001; **38**: 729–39.

Amiel J, Epinosa-Parilla Y, *et al*. Large-scale deletions and SMADIP1 truncating mutations in syndromic Hirschsprung disease with involvement of midline structures. *Am J Hum Genet* 2001; **69**: 1370–7.

Badner JA, Sieber WK, Garver KL, *et al*. A genetic study of Hirschsprung disease. *Am J Hum Genet* 1990; **46**: 568–80.

Huntington disease (HD)

Previously known as Huntington's chorea.

HD is a progressive neurological disorder. Macroscopic examination of the brain at autopsy in advanced disease shows striking degeneration of the basal ganglia structures. The caudate nucleus is particularly atrophied, although the putamen and globus pallidus are also affected. The brain is generally smaller, especially the frontal lobes.

The features are an involuntary movement disorder, psychiatric disturbance, and dementia. In the early stages of the condition, chorea may be prominent (especially with onset >40 years) but, as the disorder progresses, dystonia, bradykinesia, and decreased voluntary movements are the predominant motor features. Rigidity rather than chorea is found in juvenile HD; psychiatric problems and behavioural problems are common presenting features in young adults. Death occurs 15–20 years after the first signs. The clinical diagnosis is made after recognition of the symptoms described in the history, physical signs on examination, and family history. HD is confirmed by specific molecular testing.

The prevalence of the HD in the UK is 4–10 per 100 000. The birth incidence is about 2.5 times the prevalence or, to express it differently, there are several asymptomatic gene carriers for every affected individual. The peak age of onset is between 40 and 45 years. The South Wales study showed 4.5% with onset under 20 years (juvenile HD) and 8% over 60 years (HD in the elderly).

HD is caused by an increased (CAG) trinucleotide repeat number within the huntingtin gene (*HD*) on 4p16. The expanded (CAG) repeat is the underlying mutation in all populations studied. The trinucleotide repeat is unstable during meiosis, which gives rise to the term 'dynamic mutation'. Epidemiological studies had shown evidence for an earlier age of onset through the generations (anticipation) and this was shown to be due to expansion of the (CAG) repeat (see table). Large increases of >70 repeats are almost exclusively seen in the children of affected fathers. The relationship between an increased number of (CAG) repeats and a younger age of onset shows strongest correlation for juvenile onset; however caution is advised in using the number of repeats to predict age of onset.

Intermediate alleles are rare in the general population. They may be found in the parent (usually the father) of an apparently new mutation for HD. Intermediate alleles are not likely to cause clinical features of HD.

Juvenile HD is uncommon. It is almost invariably paternally inherited and associated with repeat sizes usually in excess of ~60. Presentation is different to the adult disorder, with schooling difficulties and paucity of facial movement. Diagnosis and progression of HD in a parent can itself account for schooling difficulties amongst younger members of the family. Assessment by a paediatric neurologist and formal psychometric testing repeated at an interval of 4–6 months may be helpful in determining whether there is progression and an organic basis to the difficulties. Magnetic resonance imaging (MRI) should also be performed (looking for basal ganglia changes) to establish a clinical diagnosis before embarking on diagnostic testing to determine the HD repeat size. (Otherwise, if the young person does not have juvenile HD, there is a 50% risk that an inadvertent predictive test is performed.)

Clinical approach

History: key points

- Three-generation family tree; extend further if possible to include all known affected family members. Note maiden names of females, addresses of long-term care institutions.
- Age of onset of affected family members and age of death.
- Psychiatric disease, suicide, or dementia in apparently unaffected family members (may actually have been HD).

Examination: key points

- Many individuals with early HD have few, if any, signs on examination. Observation during the consultation may be more informative. Many genetic centres have an examination check-list for individuals at risk of HD.
- Clinical examination is not usually performed on the first meeting with an apparently unaffected individual at risk of HD unless specifically requested. This meeting is to give information about the HD and an explanation of the role of the geneticist in such issues as predictive testing.
- Fidgety movements of the legs or facial grimacing may increase suspicion. Many patients consulting about HD are very anxious, which may manifest as restlessness or facial twitching, so be wary of overinterpretation.

Investigation

In the case of a clinically unaffected 'at risk' individual, accurate confirmation of diagnosis (preferably with molecular confirmation) is required from at least one affected member of the family. *Written informed consent will be required before predictive testing is undertaken* (see below).

In an individual with suspected HD but no, or unavailable family history, the following investigations might be undertaken.

- Diagnostic molecular testing for HD.
- Thick wet blood film for acanthocytes (neuroacanthosis).
- Diagnostic molecular testing for dentatorubropallidoluysian atrophy (DRPLA).
- Diagnostic molecular testing for hereditary spinocerebellar ataxias.
- Copper studies for Wilson disease with a juvenile or rigid presentation.
- DNA storage for future diagnostic studies.

In children the issues surrounding genetic testing need special consideration.

Other diagnoses/conditions to consider

Conditions associated with chorea

Benign familial chorea. Autosomal dominant (AD). Onset in early childhood with no progression, dementia, or psychiatric features.

Dentatorubropallidoluysian atrophy (DRPLA). AD. This is very rare but is the closest clinically to HD. Ataxia, choreoathetosis, dementia, myoclonus, and epilepsy are features. The neuropathology is diagnostic. DRPLA is also a triple repeat condition with an expansion of CAG in the gene, found on chromosome 12. It is more common in Japan but is increasingly recognized throughout the world since the advent of diagnostic molecular testing.

Neuroacanthosis. Autosomal recessive (AR). Mostly described in the Japanese. Onset in early adult life with a movement disorder involving the muscles of the face and mouth. Chorea and dystonic movements develop but dementia is not a prominent feature.

Disorders of the basal ganglia
Parkinson disease. Diagnostically there is not usually any confusion except in the juvenile rigid form of HD. Some affected individuals with HD have an erroneous diagnosis of Parkinson disease.

Tardive dyskinesia. Problems arise when an at-risk individual is treated with phenothiazines for a psychosis.

Wilson disease. AR. Is in the differential diagnosis for the juvenile and rigid forms of HD.

Spinocerebellar ataxia (SCA). SCA 3, in particular, has a pronounced movement disorder. See 'Ataxic adult' page 50.

Conditions associated with dementia
Chorea rather than dementia is the presenting feature in early HD. See 'Dementia', page 296.

Psychiatric conditions
HD has often been misdiagnosed as schizophrenia or paranoid psychosis, but it is also important to note that both conditions are more common in patients with HD.

Genetic advice—unaffected individual at risk of HD
Inheritance and recurrence risk.
AD. As HD is due to an unstable triplet repeat, both anticipation and the parental origin may influence the age of onset and presentation.

Families appreciate help and advice in how to talk about the condition in the family and how and when to go about telling the children about HD. This and other issues may be helped by contact with HD support groups.

Variability and penetrance
The main considerations are the age of the person concerned, the age of onset in other family members, the presence of juvenile HD in the family, and whether the mutation is maternally or paternally inherited. Age of onset curves and risks of an unaffected individual at 50% risk of HD carrying the HD gene at a particular age are indicated in the tables.

Prenatal diagnosis
Both direct gene analysis and prenatal exclusion testing are available. Prenatal exclusion is the procedure whereby an at-risk individual can avoid the birth of a child carrying the HD gene but without themselves having a diagnostic test. Linked markers are used to define a haplotype around the HD gene. The 'at risk' parent will have inherited one chromosome 4 from the affected grandparent and one from the unaffected grandparent. The haplotype from the affected grandparent carries a 50% risk. The fetus is at 50% risk if it inherits this grandparental haplotype, but at population risk if it inherits the haplotype from the unaffected grandparent. Couples choosing an exclusion test need to weigh the benefits of ensuring that their offspring will not inherit HD (whilst choosing not to disclose their own status) against the prospect in the event of a 'high risk' result of terminating a pregnancy that has a 50% chance of being unaffected.

Allele classification

	$(CAG)_n$ repeat range
Normal allele	<30 repeats
Intermediate allele	30–35 repeats
HD allele—reduced penetrance	36–39 repeats
HD allele	>39 repeats

Risk for a healthy individual at 50% prior risk of HD carrying a pathological HD gene expansion at different ages (after Harper and Newcombe 1992)*

Age (years)	Risk (%)	Age (years)	Risk (%)	Age (years)	Risk (%)
20	49.6	40	42.5	60	18.7
25	49	45	37.8	65	12.8
30	47.6	50	31.5	70	6.2
35	45.5	55	24.8	72.5	4.6

* This table is *not* intended for use in advising individual patients because the risks for an individual are heavily governed by: (1) the age of onset in the family; (2) whether the mutation is maternally or paternally inherited; and (3) the expansion size. These figures are included here simply to remind the clinician that the risks for an apparently healthy individual remain quite high even into later life.

Influence of expansion size on age at onset (from Brinkman and Mezel 1997)*

CAG repeat size	Median age at onset (years)[†]	95% CI for median age at onset (years)[‡]
39	66	72–59
40	59	61–56
41	54	56–52
42	49	50–48
43	44	45–42
44	42	43–40
45	37	39–36
46	36	37–35
47	33	35–31
48	32	34–30
49	28	32–25
50	27	30–24

* This table is *not* intended for use in advising individual patients. These figures reflect the median onset for a group of individuals with a known expansion size. Hence the age of onset for an *individual* cannot be estimated with the precision that this table implies. Nevertheless, this data gives the clinician a useful 'feel' for the importance influence of expansion size in determining age of onset.

[†] Age by which 50% of individuals will be affected.

[‡] CI, Confidence interval.

Predictive testing
Predictive testing for HD has been the model upon which much of the predictive testing for other genetic conditions have been based. There is usually a series of three or more meetings between the at-risk individual and a genetic counsellor to explore the reasons why they wish to have the test and to discuss possible outcomes and future management.

About 15–25% of first-degree relatives opt for predictive testing. Follow-up is offered to at-risk relatives to keep them informed of new developments and, if they wish, for a clinical assessment for signs of HD. See 'Testing for genetic status' page 28.

Other family members

Predictive testing for those at less than 50% risk has a number of difficulties, particularly ethical, that require thought and discussion before testing and results are offered. A predictive test for the intervening relative has effectively been performed if an individual at 25% genetic risk is found to carry the (CAG) expansion.

Natural history and management (of at-risk individuals and known gene carriers)

Potential long-term complications

Onset of signs and symptoms of HD. Psychological, social, and family problems that can arise from this knowledge.

Surveillance

Follow-up is offered to all gene carriers and those at risk who have declined testing. They may wish to be informed if there are any signs of HD. There is also an obligation for the counsellor to disclose such information to the individual if they are considered unsafe to drive a car or to be a danger to themselves or other people as a result of HD.

Close liaison with HD workers in the community helps ensure that appropriate supportive help is given.

Treatment

For presymptomatic individuals new research into treatment offers real hope.

- There is experimental work on animals to investigate whether histone deacetylase inhibitors prevent the neuronal damage found in HD.
- Stem cell and fetal striatal transplantation is another area of research.
- Symptomatic treatment of HD is available for the movement disorder and psychiatric complications.

Support group: Huntington's Disease Society of America <http://hdsa.mgh.harvard.edu>; Huntington Disease Association, UK <http://www.hda.org.uk>.

Expert adviser: Peter S. Harper, Emeritus Professor of Genetics, University of Wales College of Medicine, Cardiff, Wales.

References

Bates G, Harper PS, Jones A (2002) (eds). Huntington's Disease. 3rd edition OUP. Oxford.

Brinkman RR, Mezel MM. The likelihood of being affected with Huntington disease by a particular age, for a specific CAG size. *Am J Hum Genet* 1997; **60**: 1202–10.

Clinical Genetics Society (1994) Report of a working party on the genetic testing of children. *J Med Genet* 1994; **31**: 785–97.

Craufurd D, Tyler A. Predictive testing for Huntington's disease: protocol of the UK Huntington's Predictive Consortium. *J Med Genet* 1992; **29**: 915–18.

Harper PS, Newcombe RG. Age at onset and life table risks in genetic counselling for Huntington's disease. *J Med Genet* 1992; **29** (4): 239–42.

Huntington's Disease Collaborative Research Group. A novel gene containing a trinucleotide repeat that is expanded and unstable on Huntington's disease chromosomes. *Cell* 1993; **72**: 971–83.

Karpuj MV, *et al.* Prolonged survival and decreased abnormal movement in transgeneic model of HD with administration of the transglutaminase inhibitor cystamine. *Nat Med* 2002; **8**: 143–9.

Hyperlipidaemia

The level of serum cholesterol increases in an individual with advancing age, and is the result of the interplay between a number of genetic and environmental factors; hypercholesterolaemia in the population has a multifactorial basis. Hydroxymethyl glutaryl coenzyme (HMG-CoA) reductase inhibitors ('statins') have revolutionized the treatment of hypercholesterolaemia. This section deals primarily with some of the most common monogenic forms of hyperlipidaemia.

Clinical approach

History: key points

- Three-generation family tree, with enquiry about relatives with hypercholesterolaemia, heart attacks (document age), angina (document age of onset), and cause of death (document age).
- History of Achilles 'tenosynovitis'.

Examination: key points

- Examine carefully for tendon xanthomata over the Achilles tendons (often there is fibrous swelling overlying cholesterol accumulation deep within the tendon, so the xanthoma may feel hard) and over the tendons overlying the knuckles with the fingers outstretched.
- Look for an arcus senilis.

Investigation

- Lipid profile.
- DNA for molecular genetic testing in an affected member of the family.

Diagnoses/conditions to consider

Familial hypercholesterolaemia (FH). Approximately 1/500 of the population in Europe and North America are heterozygous for mutations in the low-density lipoprotein (LDL) receptor (*LDLR*). There is a much higher incidence of FH in certain populations, such as the Afrikaaners (1/80), Christian Lebanese, Finns, and French-Canadians, due to founder effects. Serum cholesterol concentrations are elevated from birth and generally approximately twice normal values. By adult life serum cholesterol in heterozygotes is typically 9.0–14.0 mmol/l. Heterozygotes develop xanthomata over tendons, especially the Achilles tendons and the tendons overlying the knuckles of the hand. Corneal arcus and xanthelasma also tend to develop at a younger age than in the generally population. Heterozygotes are at high risk of coronary heart disease, and without treatment the elevated serum cholesterol concentrations lead to a more than 50% risk of fatal or nonfatal coronary heart disease by age 50 years in men and at least 30% in women aged 60 years (Marks *et al.* 2003). The clinical diagnosis of FH is based on a family history of hypercholesterolaemia and premature coronary atherosclerosis, the lipid profile, and the presence of xanthomata (Betteridge *et al.* 1999). Treatment is with statins, which are usually started in the late teens in men and later, perhaps after completion of child-bearing, in women. Lifestyle modifications such as a healthy diet and especially avoidance of smoking are important adjuncts to drug therapy.

Homozygotes and compound heterozygotes have very severe hypercholesterolaemia, and develop xanthomata in childhood over tendons, the skin of the popliteal and antecubital fossae, buttocks, and in the webs between the fingers. Statins have only a minor effect on cholesterol levels, and the LDL apheresis is the mainstay of treatment. Life expectancy is severely curtailed and most die by the age of 20 years due to supravalvular aortic stenosis and coronary heart disease.

Familial defective apoB-100 (FDB). Approximately 1/1000 of the European population are heterozygous for a mutation in apolipoprotein B (*APOB*) on 2p23–24. There is a common mutation, Arg3500Gln, that occurs in the LDLR-binding domain of apoB-100 (Rader *et al.* 2003). In ~25% of heterozygotes, plasma levels of LDL-cholesterol overlap with the upper end of the normal range. Clinically, FDB is indistinguishable from FH, although there are fewer tendon xanthomata. Treatment is with statins and lifestyle modification.

FDB homozygotes have levels of plasma LDL-C comparable to those in FH heterozygotes rather than those in FH homozygotes.

Autosomal recessive (AR) hypercholesterolaemia (ARH). AR hypercholesterolaemia is caused by mutations in the *ARH* gene that encodes an novel adaptor protein involved in the intracellular trafficking of the LDLR (Rader *et al.* 2003). Plasma levels of LDL-cholesterol in ARH patients tend to be intermediate between those in FH heterozygotes and homozygotes. The onset of coronary heart disease is later in ARH patients than in patients with homozygous FH. Despite having lower plasma levels of cholesterol than FH homozygotes, patients with ARH often have large, bulky xanthomata (Rader *et al.* 2003). Treatment is with statins, but LDL apheresis is necessary to maintain optimal cholesterol levels in most affected patients.

Sitosterolaemia. Sitosterolaemia (also known as phytosterolaemia) is a rare AR disorder characterized by the presence of tendon and tuberous xanthomata, accelerated atherosclerosis, and premature coronary artery disease. In normal individuals, cholesterol constitutes more than 99% of circulating sterols; non-cholesterol sterols, such as sitosterol, are present in only trace amounts. In sitosterolaemia, plasma levels of cholesterol are normal, but sitosterol levels are elevated more than 50-fold. The disorder is caused by mutations in either the *ABCG8* or *ABCA5* genes, which encode ABC half transporters expressed in the intestine (Rader *et al.* 2003).

Genetic advice

Mutations are currently only detected in 30–50% of patients with a clinical diagnosis of FH (Heath *et al.* 2001).

Inheritance and recurrence risk

As for individual condition.

Variability and penetrance

Some families with FH are more susceptible to coronary heart disease than others and, in a few, coronary heart disease occurs at a strikingly young age, e.g. affecting men in their 20s.

Prenatal diagnosis

May be considered for the homozygous form of FH, but is not generally indicated for the heterozygous form for which treatment is available.

Predictive testing

Is possible by analysis of lipid profiles or more definitively by molecular genetic analysis if the familial mutation has been defined.

Other family members

Cascade screening of family members is indicated, but in FH, since treatment is not usually initiated until the late teens, it may be appropriate to defer genetic testing until individuals are in their mid-teens and able to participate in the testing process.

Guidelines for a diagnosis of FH (Scientific Steering Committee on behalf of the Simon Broome Register Group 1999) are a serum cholesterol >6.7 mmol/l in children <16 years, or >7.5 mmol/l in adults plus tendon xanthomata in the patient or a first- or second-degree relative of the patient.

Natural history and management

The prognosis for patients with heterozygous FH has improved with the introduction of more effective treatment, with recent studies showing a decline in the relative risk of coronary mortality in patients aged 20–59 years from an 8-fold risk prior to 1992 and the introduction of statin therapy to 3.7-fold thereafter.

Surveillance

Affected patients should be under the care of a lipid clinic.

Support group: Heart UK, Tel. 01628 628638 <www.heartuk.org.uk>.

Expert adviser: Steve E. Humphries, Professor of Cardiovascular Genetics, British Heart Foundation Laboratories, Royal Free and University College Medical School, London, England.

References

Betteridge DT, Broome K *et al.* Mortality in treated heterozygous familial hypercholesterolaemia: implications for clinical management. *Atherosclerosis* 1999; **142**: 105–12.

Durrington P. Dyslipidaemia [seminar]. *Lancet* 2003; **362**: 717–31.

Heath KE, Humphries SE, Middleton-Price H, Boxer M. A molecular genetic service for diagnosing individuals with familial hypercholesterolaemia (FH). *Eur J Hum Genet* 2001; **9**: 244–52.

Lee MH, Gordon D, *et al.* Fine mapping of a gene responsible for regulating dietary cholesterol absorption; founder effects underlie cases of phytosterolaemia in multiple communities. *Eur J Hum Genet* 2001; **9**: 375–84.

Marks D, Thorogood M, *et al.* A review on the diagnosis, natural history, and treatment of familial hypercholesterolaemia. *Atherosclerosis* 2003; **168** (1): 1–14.

Rader DJ, Cohen J, Hobbs HH. Monogenic hypercholesterolemia: new insights in pathogenesis and treatment. *J Clin Invest* 2003; **111**: 1795–803.

Hypertrophic cardiomyopathy (HCM)

Hypertrophic obstructive cardiomyopathy (HOCM).
HCM is a disease of the myocardium characterized by ventricular hypertrophy (usually asymmetric left ventricular hypertrophy (LVH) with preferential hypertrophy of the septum and anterior left ventricle (LV) wall). Individuals with HCM are at risk for arrhythmia (which may cause sudden death), myocardial ischaemia, and heart failure. Cardiac hypertrophy can also be secondary to hypertension and valvular or supravalvular aortic stenosis; in the absence of a family history, these need to be excluded before a diagnosis of HCM is made. It can also occur in Noonan syndrome, Friedreich's ataxia (FRDA), and some mitochondrial disorders.

Familial HCM affects up to 1/500 young adults. It follows an autosomal dominant (AD) mode of inheritance and currently there are nine identified genes (see table). Eight of these encode cardiac sarcomere proteins. About 30% of familial HCM can be attributed to mutations in beta-myosin heavy chain, 20% to myosin binding protein C, 5% to troponin T, and 5% to troponin I. Overall, mutations in one of these eight genes are found in 60–70% of families with HCM. *De novo* mutations do occur, but account for <10% of cases. Most mutations are 'private' missense mutations. LVH develops during childhood and adolescence, but is not progressive in adults (except myosin binding protein C which is characterized by late-onset disease). Hypertrophy is variable in pattern and extent and only a minority of patients have obstruction.

Clinical approach

History: key points

Three-generation family history with specific enquiry about the following.

- Deaths attributed to heart problems.
- Sudden unexplained deaths.
- Shortness of breath, chest pain/discomfort, palpitation, light-headedness, and black-outs.
- Try to obtain death certificate/post-mortem report/copy of echocardiogram report to verify diagnosis in an affected family member and to establish whether hypertrophy was obvious or subtle.

Examination: key points

- If not already seen by a cardiologist, basic cardiovascular assessment, e.g. pulse (jerky?), blood pressure, jugular venous pressure (JVP), palpate apex (forceful?), auscultation of heart (ejection systolic murmur due to LV outflow tract obstruction?).

- Are there any features of Noonan (may be subtle in adult)? Coexisting pulmonary stenosis or short stature would make this a likely diagnosis.

Investigation

- 12-lead electrocardiogram (ECG).
- Echocardiogram. Assess thickness of ventricular wall and interventricular septum; observe for systolic anterior motion (SAM) of the mitral valve.
- If abnormalities on echo/ECG, consider 24 hour tape and exercise test for risk stratification.
- Mutation analysis in one member of family (samples from other affected members may be helpful for linkage studies or to confirm segregation of a potential mutation with disease in the family).
- If late-onset disease, consider mutation analysis for myosin binding protein C.
- If multiple sudden deaths in children and adolescents, or if deceased had only mild hypertrophy, prioritize mutation analysis for cardiac troponin T.
- If mutation analysis is not available, consider storing DNA from an affected family member.
- If no antecedent family history in a young patient, consider *de novo* mutation (~10%), but also consider possibility of Friedreich's ataxia (FRDA; frataxin triplet repeat disorder) as cardiac manifestations may precede neurological symptoms in some.
- If fatigue and exercise limitation is disproportionate to the echo findings, and the family history is consistent with maternal inheritance, or sporadic, consider a mitochondrial disorder (see 'Mitochondrial DNA diseases', page 384).

Other diagnoses/conditions to consider

Noonan syndrome. Typically, pulmonary valve stenosis, peripheral pulmonary artery stenosis, or HCM with short stature and characteristic facies (*PTPN11* mutations are found in ~40%). A stenotic and often dysplastic pulmonary valve is found in 20–50% of affected individuals. See 'Noonan syndrome (NS)', page 402.

LEOPARD (lentigines–ECG abnormalities–ocular hypertelorism–pulmonary stenosis–abnormal genitalia–retardation of growth–deafness). AD condition. The lentigines are small (<5 mm) numerous dark brown spots mainly over the face and trunk. Deafness (sensorineural) is variable ranging from normal to severe.

Gene defects associated with HCM (after Franz)

Gene product	Chromosome	% of familial HCM	Comment
β-myosin heavy chain	14q11.2–12	~30	Degree of hypertrophy and risk of sudden death variable. Some mutations (L908V, G256E, & V606M) associated with benign course, others (R403Q, R453C, & R719W) with high risk of sudden death
Myosin binding protein C	11p11.2	~20	More benign clinical course, progressive hypertrophy with rather late onset
Troponin T	1q3	~5	High risk of sudden death, mild or absent hypertrophy (except R92L which is benign)
Troponin I, cardiac	19q13.4	~5	

Friedreich's ataxia (FRDA). Mean onset 15.5 ± 8 years with range 2–51 years. The most common inherited ataxia. Autosomal recessive (AR) and caused by mutations in frataxin on 9q. Frataxin is a nuclear-encoded mitochondrial protein. It is characterized by a dying-back from the periphery of the longest and largest myelinated fibres (e.g. large fibres arising in dorsal root ganglia). The disease is slowly but relentlessly progressive with loss of walking ~15 years after onset and mean age of death ~37.5 years (usual cause is cardiomyopathy). See 'Ataxic child' page 50 for more details.

Fabry disease. X-linked semi-dominant disorder caused by deficiency of α-galactosidase on Xq. Characterized by angiokeratoma (small raised red vascular lesions around the buttocks and genital region), episodes of neuropathic pain (burning sensation in the extremities worsened by exercise and extremes of temperature), and cardiac hypertrophy (especially LV) with conduction defects leading to a shortened PR interval and prolonged QRS complex. Stroke and renal failure are the most common causes of death. Median age of death in untreated males is 48–49 years; life expectancy in heterozygous women is also shortened. See 'Corneal clouding' page 88.

Arrhythmogenic right ventricular dysplasia (ARVD) or cardiomyopathy (ARVC) is an AD heart muscle disorder that causes arrhythmia, heart failure, and sudden death. It is characterized by replacement of the right ventricular (RV) myocardium by adipose and fibrous tissue. A total of 14.5% of cases have cardiac hypertrophy, assessed by an increase in heart weight and/or left ventricular wall thickness. See 'Long QT and Brugada syndromes', page 378.

Genetic advice

Inheritance and recurrence risk
AD with 50% risk to offspring of affected individuals.

Variability and penetrance
Variable expression of disease is common even amongst family members carrying the same mutation. Penetrance is age-dependent and incomplete. Finding of a normal ECG and echo in a child or adolescent reduces the probability of developing HCM, but does not exclude it (see 'Surveillance' below).

Prenatal diagnosis
In a family with a known mutation this is technically possible. It is usually only considered by families with mutations carrying a high risk of sudden death.

Predictive testing
In a family with a known mutation this could be offered so that cardiac surveillance could be targeted more appropriately. Otherwise, screening of at-risk relatives should be offered. See 'Testing for genetic status' page 28 for a discussion of the issues relating to genetic testing in children.

Other family members
See table.

Natural history and management
Progression of symptoms due to LV dysfunction is usually slow, but about 10% develop a dilated end-stage cardiomyopathy. Beta-blockers, calcium channel antagonists, and disopyramide may improve symptoms. Surgery or catheter intervention is an option for patients with obstruction that has not responded to medical therapy. LV outflow tract

---

Major and minor criteria for the diagnosis of HCM in adult members of affected families (after McKenna et al. 1997)*

Major criteria
Echocardiographic features
    LV wall thickness ≥ 13 mm in the anterior septum or posterior wall or ≥15 mm in the post septum or free wall
    Severe systolic anterior motion of the mitral valve (septal–leaflet contact)
Electrocardiographic (ECG) features
    LVH + repolarization changes
    T wave inversion in leads I and aVL (≥3 mm; with QRS–T wave axis difference ≥30°), V3–V6 (≥3 mm) or II and III and aVF (≥5 mm)
    Abnormal Q (>40 ms or >25% R wave) in at least 2 leads from II, III, aVF (in absence of left anterior
      hemiblock), V1–V4; or I, aVL, V5–V6

Minor criteria
Echocardiographic features
    LV wall thickness of 12 mm in the anterior septum or posterior wall or 14 mm in the posterior septum or free wall
    Moderate systolic anterior motion (SAM) of the mitral valve (no leaflet–septal contact)
    Redundant mitral valve leaflets
Electrocardiographic (ECG) features
    Complete bundle branch block (BBB) or (minor) interventricular conduction defect (in LV leads)
    Minor repolarization changes in LV leads
    Deep S V2 (>25 mm)
Clinical features
    Unexplained chest pain, dyspnoea, or syncope

Diagnosis of HCM in a first-degree relative of a patient with HCM is fulfilled by:
• One major criterion *or*
• Two minor echocardiographic criteria *or*
• One minor echocardiographic plus two minor ECG criteria

* NB. Diagnosis of HCM in the presence of other potential causes of LVH (athletic training, hypertension, obesity) is problematical. Diagnostic criteria in those <10 years old requires a body surface area corrected LV wall thickness of >10 mm. HCM may not be expressed until after adolescent growth is complete.

obstruction at rest is a predictor of progression to severe symptoms of heart failure and of death.

Potential long-term complications

- **Sudden death**. Some genetic defects, e.g. cardiac troponin T, may cause sudden death in the absence of symptoms or hypertrophy. Most patients who die from HCM have only mild (15–20 mm) or moderate (20–25 mm) LVH. Annual cardiovascular mortality is 0.7–1.4%. The greatest risk is in young patients with recurrent syncope or with strong family history of sudden death. Intense physical exertion may trigger sudden death and should be avoided in high-risk patients. Amiodarone reduces risk of sudden death and implantable cardioverter-defibrillators have a role in some high-risk patients.
- **Arrhythmia**. Ventricular arrhythmias during 48 hour ambulatory ECG monitoring are a predictor of risk in adults. Atrial fibrillation poses a risk of embolism and anticoagulation is advised.
- **Subacute bacterial endocarditis (SBE)**. Patients with outflow obstruction and/or mitral regurgitation need antibiotic prophylaxis, e.g. for dental work.

Surveillance

Affected individuals should be under regular long-term surveillance by a cardiologist. In 'at risk' relatives it is difficult to know how early cardiac surveillance should be started, or for how long it should be continued. The family history is a very important factor in informing these decisions. Presentation in pre-school children is rare (and raises suspicion of a disorder such as NS) and presentation is unusual in children of primary school age.

In most circumstances children should be screened clinically every 2 years from around 8–10 years of age and then annually through puberty. Except in families where affected adults have minimal hypertrophy or clearly late-onset hypertrophy (as distinct from late presentation), an entirely normal ECG and echo by late teens is sufficient to discontinue surveillance. Where the familial mutation is known, definitive genetic testing may be possible to determine who needs surveillance.

Family support group: Cardiomyopathy Association <www.cardiomyopathy.org>.

Expert adviser: Hugh Watkins, Professor of Cardiovascular Medicine, University of Oxford, John Radcliffe Hospital, Oxford, England.

References

Cannon III RO. Assessing risks in hypertrophic cardiomyopathy. *New Engl J Med* 2003; **349**: 1016–18.

Elliott P, McKenna WJ. Hypertrophic cardiomyopathy (Seminar). *Lancet* 2004; **363**: 1881–91.

Maron BJ, et al. Epidemiology of hypertrophic cardiomyopathy-related death: revisited in a large non-referral based patient population. *Circulation* 2000a; **102**: 858–64.

Maron BJ, Shen WK, Link MS, et al. Efficacy of implantable defibrillators for the prevention of sudden death in patients with hypertrophic cardiomyopathy. *New Engl J Med* 2000b; **342**: 365–73.

Martin MS, Olivotto I, et al. Effect of left ventricular outflow tract obstruction on clinical outcome in hypertrophic cardiomyopathy. *New Engl J Med* 2003; **248**: 295–303.

McKenna WJ, Spirito P, et al. Experience from clinical genetics in hypertrophic cardiomyopathy: proposal for new diagnostic criteria in adult members of affected families. *Heart* 1997; **77**: 130–2.

Watkins H, McKenna WJ, Thierfelder L, et al. Mutations in the genes for cardiac troponin T and alpha-tropomyosin in hypertrophic cardiomyopathy. *New Engl J Med* 1995; **332**: 1058–64.

Immunodeficiency and recurrent infection

Congenital immunodeficiency disorders are genetically heterogeneous and result from mutations in the many genes involved in the development of the immune system and the immune response. Broadly speaking, most primary immunodeficiencies fall within the classification of B-cell (antibody) deficiencies, T-cell (cell-mediated) defects, combined (T and B cell) deficiencies, or phagocytic disorders.

Most families will come to the genetic clinic with a clinical diagnosis already established by an immunologist or haematologist. In some families the molecular diagnosis may have been established but, despite recent advances, some familial disorders remain uncharacterized. Immunodeficiency can also be acquired, e.g. in critically ill children with overwhelming infection. Discussion with an immunologist will usually enable you to determine whether the immunodeficiency was a component of the underlying condition (i.e. a useful diagnostic handle) or an acquired feature.

Most primary immunodeficiency disorders are caused by single-gene defects and present in infancy or preschool years.

Lymphocyte phenotyping. B lymphocytes, $CD19^+$ cells; T lymphocytes, $CD3^+$, $CD4^+$, and $CD8^+$ cells.

Clinical approach

History: key points

- Three-generation family tree, extended further on the maternal side if possible, with specific enquiry about immunodeficiency, infant or childhood death either unexplained or due to infection, malignancy, and haematological disorders.
- Document the postnatal history of the proband including the types of infections they have experienced, the ages at which they occurred, and the nature of the pathogens. Is the child prone to bacterial or viral infections or both? Have there been any opportunistic or fungal infections?

Examination: key points

- Growth parameters. Height, weight, occipital-frontal circumference (OFC). Failure to thrive is common.
- Examine the skin (eczema, erythroderma).
- Examine for lymphadenopathy, presence or absence of tonsils, hepatosplenomegaly.

Investigation

- Blood for molecular genetic analysis for the specific disorder (if available); otherwise store a DNA sample for future use.
- For certain disorders specific protein analysis is appropriate before embarking on mutation screening.

In addition, if the child has not been diagnosed or comprehensively evaluated by a clinical immunologist and the process of investigation is just beginning, it is important to discuss appropriate tests with an immunologist. In most cases the following investigations should be included.

- Full blood count (FBC; in EDTA (ethylenedinitrilotetraacetate)) for white cell count and differential count.
- Immunoglobulins: clotted sample.
- T-cell subsets (EDTA). This will need to be discussed beforehand with the immunology laboratory.
- Antibody response to prior immunization, e.g. tetanus diphtheria: clotted sample.
- Neutrophil function tests in some cases.

Specific diagnoses/conditions to consider

Severe combined immunodeficiencies (SCID)

SCID affects ~1/30 000 livebirths and is genetically heterogeneous, being caused by mutations that influence the maturation of lymphocytes, particularly T-cells. Symptoms usually start at <7 months with failure to thrive and diarrhoea, oral candidiasis, and opportunistic infections such as *Pneumocystis carinii* pneumonia (PCP). Other infections include viral infections, systemic aspergillosis, and systemic candidiasis. Most patients die within 2 years if they do not receive a successful bone marrow transplant. The tonsils are usually absent, as is the thymic shadow on chest X-ray. Most affected infants are lymphopenic, with absent or low T cells. Subtypes of SCID are defined by lymphocyte phenotyping for CD3, CD4, CD8, CD19, and CD16/56. Inheritance is either X-linked or autosomal recessive (AR). The underlying genetic defect can be defined in approximately 70% of cases. Most cases are treated by bone marrow transplantation (BMT).

X-linked SCID (T^-, B^+, natural killer (NK)$^-$). Caused by mutations in the common γ-chain (γ_c) gene (also known as interleukin-2 receptor γ-chain). The γ_c chain is an essential component of five cytokine receptors, all of which are necessary for the development of T cells and natural killer cells. The causative mutation is identifiable in most families. Affected males become unwell in the first few months and fail to thrive because of frequent infections. Most infants are treated by BMT, although some recent successes with gene therapy have been reported. Female carriers show unilateral X-inactivation in purified T cells.

AR SCIDs.

- **Defects in VDJ recombination (T^-, B^-, NK^+).** Molecular defects in the recombinase-activating genes (*RAG1* or *RAG2*) lead to a variable phenotype depending on the amount of residual protein activity. In complete *RAG1* or *RAG2* deficiency, severe SCID results from the failure to express functional T- and B-cell receptors. Partial RAG deficiency may result in a SCID variant known as Ommen syndrome, characterized by severe failure to thrive, erythrodermic skin rash, lymphadenopathy, hepatosplenomegaly, and severe infections. Complete SCID and Ommen syndrome may occur within the same pedigree.
- **Adenosine deaminase (ADA) deficiency (T^-, B^-, NK^-).** A defect in purine metabolism that leads to accumulation of metabolites that are toxic to lymphocytes. ADA has an important role in the intermediate pathways of purine metabolism in all tissues, and deficiency may also cause a variety of other abnormalities including skeletal, renal, and neurodevelopmental abnormalities. This condition was the first disorder to be treated by enzyme replacement therapy in clinical medicine and also the first disease to be treated by gene therapy (with only partial success). Many cases are still treated by BMT.
- **Purine nucleoside phosphorylase (PNP) deficiency (T^{low}, B^{low}, NK^{low}).** Another defect in purine metabolism, but much rarer than ADA deficiency, with only a few cases reported worldwide. The immunodeficiency in PNP deficiency often presents later, and neurodevelopmental problems are frequent.
- **Interleukin 7 receptor α (IL-7Rα) deficiency (T^-, B^+, NK^+).** A rare form of SCID caused by defects

in the IL-7Rα gene, which is essential for normal development of T cells.

- **Janus-associated kinase 3 (Jak-3) deficiency (T⁻, B⁺, NK⁻)**. An AR form of SCID, immunologically indistinguishable from the X-linked form. Jak-3 is part of the same T-cell signalling pathway as common γc.

Other combined immunodeficiencies

MHC (major histocompatibility complex) class 2 deficiency (bare lymphocyte syndrome). Defects in several regulatory genes essential for expression of MHC class 2 (DR) molecules cause a severe immunodeficiency characterized by a clinical syndrome similar to SCID, with low CD4⁺ T cells, hypogammaglobulinaemia, and absence of DR expression. Survival beyond the first decade is unusual without BMT.

CD40 ligand deficiency (X-linked hyper-IgM syndrome). Mutations in the CD40 ligand gene cause absence or defective function of CD40 ligand on the surface of activated T cells, resulting in failure of the T cell/B cell interaction required for immunoglobulin isotype switching, as well as a functional T-cell defect. Affected boys usually present with recurrent bacterial infections or PCP. There is a high incidence of liver disease. Supportive treatment is with immunoglobulin replacement and anti-infective prophylaxis but, increasingly, BMT is performed because of the poor long-term survival.

Wiskott–Aldrich syndrome. An X-linked disorder characterized by thrombocytopenia (with small platelets), atypical eczema, and immunodeficiency, with susceptibility to opportunistic and pyogenic infections and lymphoproliferative disease or lymphoid malignancy, often associated with Epstein–Barr virus (EBV). Supportive treatment is with immunoglobulin, anti-infectives, platelet transfusions, and sometimes splenectomy, but BMT is usually recommended. Caused by mutations in *WASP*, which is involved in the regulation of the actin cytoskeleton and is found only in blood cells. Female carriers have non-random X chromosome inactivation in whole blood.

X-linked lymphoproliferative (XLP) syndrome (Duncan syndrome). A rare disorder characterized by inability to effectively handle EBV infection. Manifestations include severe (often fatal) infectious mononucleosis, acquired hypogammaglobulinaemia, lymphoproliferative disease or lymphoma, haemophagocytic lymphohistiocytosis-like syndromes, and aplastic anaemia. Caused by defects in the *SH2D1A* gene, encoding the SAP (SLAM-associated protein). However, although almost all affected males lack SAP expression by Western blotting, mutations in the SAP gene can only be found in 55–60% of cases.

Primary antibody deficiency

X-linked agammaglobulinaemia (XLA; Bruton disease). XLA is characterized by early-onset bacterial infections (recurrent otitis media, pneumonitis, sinusitis, and conjunctivitis), marked reduction in all classes of serum immunoglobulins, and very low or absent B cells (CD19⁺ cells). Babies are usually well in the first few months of life (until transplacentally acquired maternal immunoglobulins wane.) Treatment is with lifelong immunoglobulin replacement and early intervention with antibiotics for infection. The long-term outlook is good, although there is a risk of chronic lung disease and enteroviral meningoencephalitis. XLA is caused by mutations in *BTK* on Xq21.3–22. 50% of males with newly diagnosed XLA have no family history.

In this instance, 15–20% have *de novo BTK* mutations, and in 80–85% the mother is a carrier (with the mutation usually arising in her father).

AR immunoglobulin deficiencies. Clinically and immunologically indistinguishable from XLA, resulting from mutations in other genes that are required for normal B-cell development including μ heavy chain, Igα, λ5, or *BLNK*.

Common variable immunodeficiency (CVID). The most common form of antibody deficiency. CVID most frequently presents in young adulthood but can present at any age. It is characterized by low immunoglobulin levels, variable abnormalities of T and B cell numbers and function, and an increased incidence of autoimmunity, granulomatous disease, and malignancy. There is often a family history of IgA deficiency. Variable patterns of inheritance, with some families showing an autosomal dominant (AD) pattern. Exclusion of molecularly defined forms of immunodeficiency is required. In most individuals with CVID the molecular defect is not known, although rare families have been described with a defect in the *ICOS* gene.

Phagocytic disorders

Chronic granulomatous disease (CGD) is characterized by recurrent severe catalase-positive bacterial and fungal infections, e.g. pneumonia, lymphadenitis, cutaneous infections, hepatic abscesses, osteomyelitis. It is a genetically heterogeneous disorder characterized by defective production of superoxide (O₂⁻) by neutrophils, monocytes, and eosinophils, as a result of defects in components of the membrane-linked NADPH (reduced nicotinamide–adenine dinucleotide) oxidase. One X-linked and three autosomal genes encode protein components of the respiratory burst oxidase. The X-linked form of CGD accounts for the majority of cases; the other forms are AR. The diagnosis is confirmed by the nitroblue tetrazolium (NBT) slide test confirming abnormal neutrophil superoxide or peroxide production. Treatment includes antibiotic and antifungal prophylaxis, and interferon γ (IFNγ) may be helpful during severe infective episodes. BMT may be recommended. Female carriers of the X-linked type show intermediate levels of NBT reduction as a result of Lyonization. The molecular type can be confirmed by Western blotting prior to mutation screening.

Leukocyte adhesion deficiency. AR disorder caused by genes that encode components of the three integrin complexes on the neutrophil cell surface causing impaired adhesion of leukocytes to the endothelium, impaired chemotaxis, and impaired phagocytosis. The condition is very genetically heterogeneous with at least five genes defined. Typically presents in infancy with delayed separation of the umbilical cord. Foci of infection show a lack of neutrophils. Severely affected patients often die in infancy or early childhood without BMT.

Chediak–Higashi syndrome. AR disorder characterized by partial albinism, abnormal leukocytes containing giant granules, easy bruising, and neurological abnormalities. Most affected individuals progress to an 'accelerated' lymphoproliferative or haemophagocytic lymphohistiocytosis-like phase that is fatal without BMT. Caused by defects in *LYST* (*CHS1*), which plays an important role in lysosomal protein trafficking.

Congenital neutropenia

Congenital agranulocytosis (Kostmann syndrome). Rare AD disorder characterized by severe persistent neutropenia. Bone marrow aspirate shows arrest of neutrophil maturation in the promyelocyte stage. Caused by mutations in the gene encoding neutrophil elastase. Treatment with G-CSF (granulocyte colony-stimulating factor) prolongs life by increasing absolute neutrophil counts and reducing vulnerability to overwhelming infection. However, patients are at increased risk of developing acute myeloid leukaemia (AML) and myelodysplastic syndromes. BMT may be recommended.

Cyclic neutropenia. Rare AD disorder of haematopoiesis also caused by mutations in the gene encoding neutrophil elastase. Cyclic dips in neutrophil counts approximately every 21 days and lasting 3–7 days. Along with neutropenia there are also cyclic drops in the reticulocyte and monocyte counts. Episodes of neutropenia may be severe, e.g. $<200 \times 10^6/\mu l$ sometimes with fever, pharyngitis, and bacterial infections. Can be treated with G-CSF.

Cytokine/cytokine receptor deficiencies
IFNγ receptor/interleukin 12 (IL-12) pathway defects. AR defects in various componenets of this pathway (IFNγ receptor, IL-12, IL-12 receptor) lead to susceptibility to infection with intracellular organisms including mycobacterial infection and salmonella. The severity varies, and some patients can be managed with antimicrobial prophylaxis and/or IFNγ replacement. BMT has been performed in a few patients with variable results.

Other disorders
DiGeorge syndrome/velocardiofacial (del 22q11 syndrome). There is a wide spectrum of immunological abnormalities in 22q11 microdeletion syndrome. A small percentage (<2%) of infants have complete DiGeorge syndrome with absent T cells and may require corrective therapy (thymic transplant or BMT), but most have only a moderate T-cell lymphopenia, mainly affecting CD8 T cells, that improves over the first few years of life. Some affected individuals have a variable degree of humoral immunodeficiency. See '22q11 deletion syndrome' page 490.

DNA repair defects. Immunodeficiency is a feature of many of these, especially ataxia telangiectasia (AT) and Nijmegen breakage syndrome (NBS) and, occasionally, Fanconi syndrome. See 'DNA repair defects', page 304.

Other defects
An increasing number of molecular defects are being defined, and more will emerge. The tables provide a summary of the current major known defects. There are many other complex syndromes that include immunodeficiency as a component.

Genetic advice
Inheritance and recurrence risk
Counsel for the specific diagnosis in question.

XLA. X-linked recessive. 80–85% of mothers of isolated cases are carriers. Most *de novo* mutations arise in the maternal grandfather; maternal grandmothers are carriers in <20% of isolated cases. The risk of carrier status in a woman whose sister has a son with XLA where there is no other family history is therefore <10%. More than 90% of affected boys have detectable mutations in *BTK*. The causative mutation provides a cornerstone for advising family members about their carrier status. Even if the mother is not a carrier there is a small possibility (<5%) of recurrence due to germline mosaicism.

Prenatal diagnosis
- **Mutation analysis**. Usually possible by chorionic villus samling (CVS) if the causative mutation in the proband has been identified. Prenatal testing by mutation screening is routinely available in the UK for:
  - XLA;
  - SCID;
    - X-linked SCID (common γ-chain ($γ_c$) deficiency);
    - Jak-3 deficiency;
    - RAG 1 and 2 deficiency;
  - X-linked hyper-IgM syndrome (CD40 ligand deficiency);
  - Wiskott–Aldrich syndrome;
  - XLP syndrome (Duncan syndrome).

  For other defined molecular defects mutation screening and prenatal diagnosis may be available in research or other laboratories worldwide.
- **Linkage analysis**. If the diagnosis is secure but the mutation cannot be defined prenatal diagnosis may be possible by linkage analysis.
- **Enzyme analysis**. Prenatal testing for ADA and PNP deficiency is reliably performed by enzyme analysis of CVS tissue.
- **Fetal blood sampling**. For families affected by SCID where the molecular defect cannot be defined, but the phenotype is clear-cut, second trimester prenatal diagnosis by lymphocyte subpopulation analysis of fetal blood can be offered.

X-linked immunodeficiencies

Disorder	Gene	Chromosome
X-linked chronic granulomatous disease (CGD)	gp91*phox*	Xp21
X-linked agammaglobulinaemia (XLA)	Bruton tyrosine kinase (Btk)	Xq22
X-linked severe combined immunodeficiency (SCID)	Common γ chain ($γ_c$)	Xq13
X-linked hyper-IgM syndrome (CD40 ligand deficiency)	CD40 ligand (CD154)	Xq26
Wiskott–Aldrich syndrome	WASP	Xp11
X-linked lymphoproliferative (XLP; Duncan) syndrome	SAP	Xq25
Properdin deficiency	Properdin	Xp21
Dyskeratosis congenita (variable immunodeficiency) Hoyeraal–Hreidarsson syndrome severe combined immunodeficiency (T^+, B^-, NK^- SCID)	Dyskerin (*DKC1*)	Xq28
IPEX (immunodysregulation, polyendocrinopathy, enteropathy, X-linked)	FoxP3	Xp11

Autosomal recessive immunodeficiencies

Disorder	Gene	Chromosome
I Severe combined immunodeficiency (SCID)		
Adenosine deaminase (ADA) deficiency	Adenosine deaminase	20q12–13
Purine nucleoside phosphorylase (PNP) deficiency	Purine nucleoside phosphorylase	14q11
Recombinase-activating gene (RAG 1 & 2) deficiency Ommen syndrome	RAG1/RAG2	11p13
T-cell receptor deficiencies	CD3γ/CD3 ε	11q23
Zap70 deficiency	ZAP70	2q12
JAK3 deficiency (T⁻, B⁺,NK⁻ SCID)	JAK3	19p13
IL-7 receptor deficiency	IL-7 receptor α	5p13
DNA repair defects	DNA ligase IV	13q22
	Artemis	10p
II Non-SCID		
Leucocyte adhesion deficiency type 1	CD11/CD18	21q22
Chronic granulomatous disease (CGD)	p47phox	7q11
	p67phox	1q25
	p22phox	16p24
Chediak–Higashi syndrome	LYST	1q42
Congenital neutropenia Cyclical neutropenia	Elastase	19p13.3
MHC class II deficiency	CIITA (MHC2TA)	16p13
	RFXANK	19p12
	RFX5	1q21
	RFXAP	13q13
MHC class I	TAP2	6p21
	TAP1	6p21
Autoimmune lymphoproliferative (ALP) syndrome	APT1 (Fas)	10q24
Ataxia telangiectasia (AT)	ATM	11q22
Inherited mycobacterial susceptibility	Interferon γ receptor	6q23
	IL-12 p40	5q31
	IL-12 receptor β1	19p13
Autosomal recessive agammaglobulinaemia	μ heavy chain	14q32.33
	Igα	
	λ5	22q11.2
	BLNK	10q23
Common variable immunodeficiency (CVID)*	ICOS	2q33
	CD19	
	BAFF-R	22q13
	TACI	

* Only two families reported.

Other family members

- **Carrier testing** for X-linked disorders where the causative mutation has been defined is feasible. Carrier testing is also possible by biochemical methods for AR SCID due to ADA or PNP deficiency.
- **Cord blood analysis and storage**. For all severe immunodeficiencies where stem cell transplantation may be required it is appropriate to consider umbilical cord-blood stem-cell banking at the time of delivery of new siblings. Cord blood from unaffected infants is a potential source of stem cells for affected siblings, while cord blood from infants who are affected by the disorder may be used for future gene therapy. For pregnancies where prenatal diagnosis has not been possible, or families have chosen not to have predictive testing, umbilical cord blood should be sent for lymphocyte phenotyping or other testing as appropriate to the disorder. Ideally, this should be arranged in advance with the obstetric unit and the immunology laboratory.

Natural history and management

The natural history in primary immunodeficiency disorders is highly variable, and the severity of individual disorders can also vary within families. For primarily antibody deficiency syndromes the long-term outlook should be good, provided that the diagnosis is made without delay and that treatment and monitoring are optimal. The mainstay of management is long-term immunoglobulin replacement therapy.

Infants affected by SCID are unlikely to survive beyond the first 2 years of life in the absence of corrective treatment. For many of the other disorders the long-term outlook is also less favourable, and BMT, other forms of stem cell transplantation, or gene therapy are increasingly recommended.

Bone marrow transplantation (BMT) and gene therapy. For infants affected by all forms of SCID, BMT from an HLA (human leucocyte antigen)-identical sibling is the best treatment, with a >90% chance of success. Transplantation from an HLA-matched unrelated donor, phenotypically identical family member, or haplo-identical parent has a variable success rate of between 60% and 80%, depending on the nature of the underlying disorder, complications at the time of transplant, and the closeness of the match. Early successes with gene therapy have been reported in X-SCID and ADA deficiency, and this may be an appropriate approach in the absence of a matched sibling donor. Gene therapy is likely to be developed for other severe forms of immunodeficiency.

Potential long-term complications

Complications of primary immunodeficiency may arise either as a result of damage caused by infection or as a result of the immune dysregulation that occurs in many immune disorders.

- **Organ damage caused by infection** is most frequently chronic lung disease—bronchiectasis—which still occurs in patients with primary antibody deficiency, particularly if immunoglobulin replacement is inadequate or intercurrent infection is not treated aggressively.
- **Enteroviral meningoencephalitis** also occurs with increased frequency in XLA and CVID. **Autoimmunity** and **granulomatous disease** are common in CVID and other undefined combined immunodeficiencies.
- **Liver disease** is a particular risk in CD40 ligand deficiency, but liver disease also occurs in other combined immunodeficiencies.

- **Lymphoproliferative disease and malignancy** are risks in many immunodeficiency disorders, the latter most particularly in the chromosome breakage disorders.

Surveillance

Affected individuals should be under the care of a clinical immunologist.

Support groups: Primary Immunodeficiency Association <www.pia.org.uk>, Tel. 020 7976 7641; Chronic Granulomatous Disease Trust <www.cgd.org.uk>, Tel. 01725 517977.

Expert adviser: Alison Jones, Consultant Paediatric Immunologist/Honorary Senior Lecturer, Great Ormond Street Hospital/Institute of Child Health, University College, London, England.

References

Conley ME, Mathias D, et al. Mutations in btk in patients with presumed X-linked agammaglobulinaemia. Am J Hum Genet 1998; **62**: 1034–43.

Ochs HD, Smith CIE, Puck JM (eds.). Primary immunodeficiency diseases: a molecular and genetic approach. Oxford University Press, Oxford, 1999.

Sinning J, Berliner N. Leucocytes in health and disease. In Oxford textbook of medicine, 4th edn (ed. D.A. Warrell, T.M. Cox, J.D. Firth, and E.J. Benz), Chapter 22.4.1. Oxford University Press, Oxford, 2003.

Webster ADB. Immunodeficiency. In Oxford textbook of medicine, 4th edn (ed. D.A. Warrell, T.M. Cox, J.D. Firth, and E.J. Benz), Chapter 5.6. Oxford University Press, Oxford, 2003.

Incest

Incest is defined as sexual intercourse between close relatives. In English law it is the crime of sexual intercourse between parent and child or grandchild, or between siblings or half-siblings (*Shorter Oxford English dictionary*). Incest has major genetic implications because of the greatly increased risk of autosomal recessive (AR) disorders or multiple recessive disorders occurring in the offspring. Incest also has major social implications because it is illegal in many communities, and the offspring (if they survive) may be offered for adoption/fostering.

There is a high chance that the offspring will be homozygous for a recessive disorder, or possibly multiple recessive disorders. There is also an increased risk for disorders that follow multifactorial inheritance.

Clinical approach

History: key points

- Detailed family tree documenting the precise relationship between the parents of the pregnancy/child in question. Include full three-generation family tree taking particular care to identify if there are any known/possible recessive disorders in the extended family.
- Routine history of pregnancy, birth, and development.

Examination: key points

- Measurement of weight, length, and occipital-frontal circumference (OFC).
- Detailed assessment for dysmorphic features and congenital anomalies.
- Detailed neurological examination with particular emphasis on hearing and vision.

Special investigations

- DNA from parents and child (after suitable consent).
- Urine amino and organic acids.
- Plasma amino acids.
- Consider testing for common recessive disorders depending on ethnic background, e.g. cystic fibrosis (CF) in northern Europeans. See 'Consanguinity', page 284.

Genetic advice

For offspring of first-degree relationships (parent:child, sib:sib)

- **Empiric risk.** There is an observed increase of 30% in severe abnormalities and mortality, giving an overall risk of ~1/3 for death in childhood or severe abnormality. In addition, there is an increased risk for mental retardation without physical anomaly bringing overall risk close to 1/2 (50%).
- **Estimated risk.** The probability that a pregnancy will be homozygous by descent in a relationship between parent:child, or siblings is 1/8 (12.5%); this

is considerably less than the observed excess, and so empiric data is preferable over estimated data.

For offspring of second-degree relationships (half-sibs, uncle/aunt:niece/nephew)

See table.

Probability that a pregnancy will be homozygous by descent for a recessive disorder for second-degree relationships

Relationship	Probability
Half-siblings	1/16 (6%)
Uncle/aunt:niece/nephew	1/16 (6%)

- **Empiric risk.** The excess risk for mental retardation without physical anomaly recognized for offspring of first-degree relationships is less frequently noted in offspring of first-cousin relationships, but an intermediate risk may exist for offspring of second-degree relationships.
- **Estimated risk.** The calculations for half-sibs, and uncle/aunt:niece/nephew relationships probably considerably underestimate the risk (see above).

Adults who themselves are the product of an incestuous relationship

Children born as the product of an incestuous relationship who develop normally are not at increased genetic risk when they have children of their own.

Prenatal diagnosis

Detailed fetal anomaly ultrasound scan (USS), but note limitations as only a small minority of recessive diseases have structural anomalies.

Adoption

Harper (2001) estimates that around 75% of severe recessive disorders will manifest in the first 6 months of life.

Natural history and management

Surveillance

- Children who are born as the product of an incestuous relationship require careful neurological and developmental follow-up.
- The mother who has been involved in an incestuous relationship may require support and protection from social services.

Expert adviser: Ian D. Young, Consultant Clinical Geneticist, Leicester, England.

References

Harper PS. *Practical genetic counselling*, 5th edn, revised reprint. Arnold, London, 2001.

Young ID. *Introduction to risk calculation in genetic counselling*, 2nd edn. Oxford University Press, Oxford, 1999.

Leigh encephalopathy

Subacute necrotizing encephalomyelpathy, Leigh's disease, Leigh's syndrome.

Leigh encephalopathy presents one of the most challenging clinical problems encountered in the genetics clinic. The diagnosis is often rather vague, the affected members of the family may have died, and the recurrence risks are potentially high. The varied inheritance patterns (autosomal recessive (AR), mitochondrial, and X-linked (XL)) encountered in Leigh encephalopathy add to the difficulty. The extreme genetic heterogeneity in AR Leigh complicates matters even further. The first priority is to try to establish a clear clinical diagnosis and determine whether the proband really did have features consistent with a diagnosis of Leigh encephalopathy.

Leigh encephalopathy is a neurodegenerative disorder. The prevalence is ~1/32 000–1/40 000 with a slight male preponderance. The condition presents in infancy with non-specific features such as feeding difficulties, vomiting, regurgitation, hypotonia, seizures, and developmental delay. Later, psychomotor regression, spasticity, ataxia, optic atrophy, and chronic progressive external ophthalmoplegia (CPEO) may develop. Blood lactate is often elevated, and cerebrospinal fluid (CSF) lactate is usually significantly elevated. Cranial magnetic resonance imaging (MRI) shows bilateral, usually symmetrical changes in the basal ganglia, (especially the putamen), brainstem, and thalami. The prognosis for patients presenting in infancy is poor—they usually die within months or a few years.

Despite genetic heterogeneity all of the known defects affect intracellular energy production. A subset of patients carry the mitochondrial (mt)DNA point mutations T8993G or T8993C (also seen in neuropathy–ataxia–retinitis pigmentosa (NARP)). Mutations in the nuclear-encoded *SURF1* gene underlie 75% of cytochrome-oxidase-deficient Leigh encephalopathy (i.e. 10–20% of all Leigh syndrome) and follow AR inheritance.

Clinical approach

History: key points

- Three-generation family tree with specific enquiry about consanguinity. Extend on the maternal line as far as possible.
- Details of affected family members. Age of onset, clinical features, progression, whether tissue or DNA is stored.
- Age of onset of signs and symptoms. Regression? Seizures?
- Careful documentation of development and loss of skills.

Examination: key points

- Growth parameters; height, weight, and occipital-frontal circumference (OFC). Note if any deceleration in head growth.
- Neurological features. Hypotonia, spasticity, ataxia.
- Neuromuscular features. Muscle wasting and weakness.
- External ophthalmoplegia.
- Cardiac examination (cardiomyopathy).

Investigation

- Blood and CSF lactate.
- DNA for investigation and storage.
- MtDNA investigations; point mutations, and depletion.
- Skin biopsy for fibroblast culture for investigation and storage.
- Consider the need for a muscle biopsy.

- MRI brain scan. The key feature of Leigh encephalopathy is the presence of symmetrical necrotic lesions in the basal ganglia. It rarely affects the cortex of the brain.
- Ophthalmological assessment of the retina and optic disc.

Other diagnoses/conditions to consider

Other neurogenerative conditions. See 'Developmental regression' page 96.

Genetic advice

The following are the most common causes of Leigh encephalopathy.

- Pyruvate dehydrogenase deficiency (PDH). X-linked.
- Cytochrome oxidase (COX) deficiency (itself very heterogeneous—many nuclear genes including *SURF1* are involved in COX assembly).
- NADH (reduced nicotinamide–adenine dinucleotide) dehydrogenase (complex I) deficiency (both nuclear and mitochondrial genes).
- T8993G mitochondrial mutation.

Other causes include:

- other mtDNA mutations, e.g. the T10158C mutation (McFarland et al. 2004);
- complex II deficiency;
- mtDNA depletion.

Inheritance and recurrence risk

Even where there is good clinical and MRI evidence of Leigh disease, it is currently possible to make a genetic diagnosis in <40% of patients despite thorough investigation in a specialist research laboratory.

An *empiric risk* of 33% was estimated by van Erven *et al.* (1987)—this may be an overestimate since the calculation was not corrected for unascertained sibships. See White *et al.* (1999a) for estimate of risk for patients carrying T8993G or T8993C. Recurrence risk for Leigh disease due to *SURF1* mutations is 25%. Recurrence risk for PDH deficiency is very low, when occurring as a new mutation.

Variability and penetrance

Variation in presentation is very great overall, but may be more consistent in siblings with *SURF1* mutations or other AR nuclear gene defects.

Prenatal diagnosis

Once a genetic diagnosis is established, this should be relatively straightforward by chorionic villus sampling (CVS) in families with *SURF1* and *PDH* mutations, also with nuclear gene causes of complex I deficiency (but not as widely available). Prenatal diagnosis of mitochondrial 8993 mutations appears relatively robust.

Predictive testing

Technically feasible once the genetic defect in the proband has been identified.

Other family members

Straightforward once the genetic defect in the proband has been identified.

Natural history and management

Potential long-term complications

Progressive accumulation of neurological damage, especially following intercurrent illnesses. Common outcome is respiratory failure.

Support group: CLIMB (Children Living with Inherited Metabolic Diseases) <www.climb.org.uk>, Tel. 0870 770 0326; NORD (National Organisation for Rare Disorders) <www.rarediseases.org>.

Expert adviser: Garry Brown, University Lecturer, Genetics Unit, Department of Biochemistry, University of Oxford, Oxford, England.

References

Darin N, Oldfors A, et al. The incidence of mitochondrial encephalomyopathies in childhood: clinical features and morphological, biochemical, and DNA anbormalities. *Ann Neurol* 2001; **49** (3): 377–83.

McFarland R, Kirby DM, et al. De novo mutations in the mitochondrial ND3 gene as a cause of infantile mitochondrial encephalopathy and complex I deficiency. *Ann Neurol* 2004; **55** (1): 58–64.

Montpetit VJA, Andermann F, et al. Subacute necrotising encephalomyelopathy: a review and study of two families. *Brain* 1971; **94**; 1–30.

Rahman S, Blok RB, et al. Leigh syndrome: clinical features and biochemical and DNA abnormalities. *Ann Neurol* 1996; **39**; 343–51.

Van Erven PMMM, Cillessen JPM, et al. Leigh syndrome, a mitochondrial encephalo(myo)pathy. A review of the literature. *Clin Neurol Neurosurg* 1987; **89**: 217–30.

White S, Collins V, et al. Genetic counselling and prenatal diagnosis for the mitochondrial DNA mutations at nucleotide 8993. *Am J Hum Genet* 1999a; **65**: 474–82.

White SL, Shanske S, et al. Two cases of prenatal analysis for the pathogenic T to G substitution at nucleotide 8993 in mitochondrial DNA. *Prenat Diagn* 1999b; **19**: 1165–8.

Zhu Z, Yao J, et al. SURF1, encoding a factor involved in the biogenesis of cytochrome c oxidase, is mutated in Leigh syndrome. *Nat Genet* 1998; **20**: 337–43.

Limb girdle muscular dystrophies

The limb girdle muscular dystrophies (LGMD) are a heterogeneous group of genetically determined progressive muscular dystrophies that are defined by predominant involvement of the pelvic girdle and shoulder girdle musculatures (see figure). LGMD used to be very much a diagnosis of exclusion but, as the molecular basis of many types of LGMD can now be delineated, an attempt should be made in all patients to achieve a precise diagnosis. This may necessitate specialized referral and investigation. The different types of LGMD put together probably still only represent in most populations about one-third the frequency of Becker muscular dystrophy (BMD) and, within the LGMD classification, some of the subgroups are extremely rare indeed. It is important to recognize therefore that, on empirical grounds, in a patient presenting with a 'limb girdle' pattern of muscular dystrophy, dystrophinopathy is a more likely diagnosis than LGMD and should be excluded by gene and protein analysis. This is particularly important from a genetic counselling perspective because of the risk to female relatives in the dystrophinopathies.

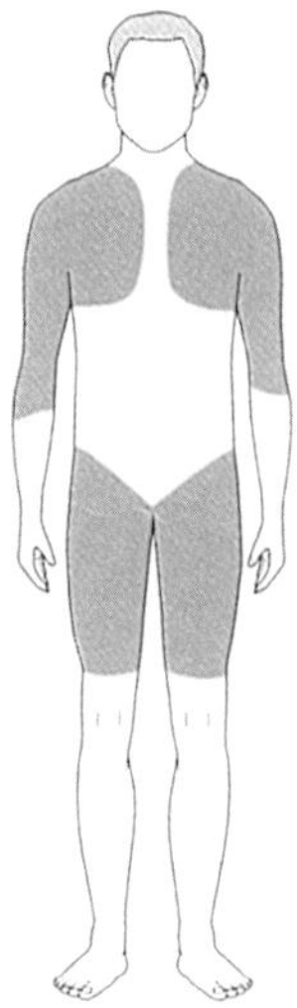

Distribution of predominant muscle weakness in limb girdle muscular dystrophy. (Reproduced from Emery (1998), fig. 1a, p. 992, by permission of the BMJ Publishing Group.)

In addition to the genetic counselling implications for patients with LGMD, there may be significant management points in the various subtypes, e.g. in terms of cardiac and respiratory surveillance.

The number of genetically distinct types of LGMD continues to grow (see table). Sixteen forms of limb-girdle muscular dystrophies (6 autosomal dominant (AD) and 10 autosomal recessive (AR)) have already been identified. The protein product of the 10 genes responsible for the AR forms, which account for more than 90% of the cases, has been identified (Zatz *et al.* 2003). Diagnosis and management of patients with limb girdle dystrophies is a highly specialized area and the patient should be under the care of a neurologist with expertise in muscle disease.

Clinical approach

History: key points

- Three-generation (or more) family tree with specific enquiry regarding muscle weakness, premature cardiac death, cardiac failure.
- Onset of muscle weakness. Obtain a history of early motor milestones, participation in physical education at school, etc.
- Muscle groups affected. Difficulty rising from chairs implies hip girdle involvement, difficulty lifting arms above head, e.g. brushing hair, hanging out washing, implies shoulder girdle involvement.
- Current level of mobility. Rising from chairs, walking on flat, use of aids.
- Fits, faints, or funny turns.
- Exercise tolerance and breathlessness.
- Sleep history. Difficulty breathing when lying flat may indicate diaphragmatic weakness; difficulty rising in the morning may indicate nocturnal hypoventilation.

Examination: key points

It is often necessary to seek advice from an expert to facilitate diagnosis in LGMD. Photography may be a useful adjunct to clinical assessment for this purpose and also to document progression.

- Is there evidence of muscle wasting?
- Which muscle groups are weak? (Humero-peroneal weakness is suggestive of Emery–Dreifuss.) Involvement of distal muscle groups, facial muscles (suggests facioscapulohumeral muscular dystrophy (FSHD)), or extraocular muscles (suggests mitochondrial disorder) is not a feature of LGMD.
- Is there facial involvement? (Consider FSHD.)
- Are deep tendon reflexes present?
- Are there any contractures, e.g. at elbows (inability to fully extend elbows), Achilles tendons (inability to plantar flex the foot), and spine (restricted neck flexion)? These would indicate a need to consider laminopathy or X-linked Emery–Dreifuss, or Bethlem myopathy.

Special investigations

- Creatine kinase (CK). Usually elevated <10× normal in dominant disease, though LGMD1C may be higher than this; often elevated >10× normal or up to 100× normal in recessive disease.
- DNA for mutation analysis or storage. A dystrophin deletion/duplication screen is appropriate in patients without contractures, unless a muscle biopsy excludes a dystrophinopathy.
- Cardiac assessment. Electrocardiogram (ECG) and echocardiogram.
- Muscle biopsy with multiple stains if diagnosis remains unknown (biopsy may need to be sent to a specialist centre since LGMD is such a genetically heterogeneous condition).
- If LGMD refer to a neurologist with expertise in muscle disorders (if not already involved).

Other diagnoses/conditions to consider

Becker muscular dystrophy (BMD). BMD is clinically similar to Duchenne muscular dystrophy (DMD) but

Classification and genetic basis of some of the more common types of limb-girdle muscular dystrophies (after Bushby 1999*a*)

Nomenclature	Locus	Gene product	Muscle biopsy	Clinical features
LGMD1B	1q21	Lamin A/C*	Absent/reduced lamin A/C	Invariable cardiac conduction defects and in some patients also DCM
LGMD1C	3	Calveolin 3	Absent/reduced caveolin 3	Variable, may also present with hyperCKaemia or rippling muscle disease
LGMD2A	15q	Calpain 3	Nomal sarcoglycan; absent/ reduced calpain 3	Onset 8–15 years. Progression variable
LGMD2B	2p	Dysferlin	Normal sarcoglycans and calpain 3	Onset 16–25 years. Progression often slow. Some variability—may present with proximal or distal disease
LGMD2C	13q	γ-sarcoglycan	Absent/reduced γ-sarcoglycan; reduced α-, β-sarcoglycan	Extremely variable severity with onset from childhood to adult life. All sarcoglycanopathies are at risk of cardiac and respiratory complications
LGMD2D	17q	α-sarcoglycan	Absent/reduced α-sarcoglycan; reduced β-, γ-sarcoglycan	
LGMD2E	4q	β-sarcoglycan	Absent/reduced β-sarcoglycan; reduced α-, γ-sarcoglycan	
LGMD2I	19	Fukutin-related protein (FKRP)	May be secondary reduction in in laminin α2, variable reduction of α-dystroglycan expression	Very variable severity, cardiac and respiratory disease common

*Laminopathies. Several diseases share mutations at the Lamin A/C gene, *LMNA*. These include AD Emery–Dreifuss muscular dystrophy, dilated cardiomyopathy type 1A, limb girdle muscular dystrophy type 1B, familial partial lipodystrophy, Charcot–Marie–Tooth disease type 2, mandibuloacral dysplasia, atypical Werner syndrome, and a rare childhood syndrome of premature ageing, Hutchinson–Gilford syndrome. Overlapping phenotypes may exist. In all patients with muscle disease due to laminopathy there is a major risk of cardiac conduction defects and sudden death.

milder, with a mean age of onset of 11 years. Loss of the ability to walk may occur late (e.g. 40s or 50s) and many individuals with BMD survive into middle age and beyond. Often cramps on exercise are the only problem initially, but some affected boys are late in learning to walk and are unable to run fast. Later in the teens and twenties, muscle weakness becomes evident causing difficulty in rapid walking, running, and climbing stairs. It may become difficult to lift objects above waist height. Cognitive impairment is not a major feature of BMD. BMD is caused by 'in-frame' mutations in dystrophin that result in reduced dystrophin being produced. Immunolabelling of muscle biopsy from a man with BMD shows a reduction in the intensity of staining, which may vary within and between fibres. See 'Duchenne and Becker muscular dystrophy (DMD and BMD)', page 308.

X-linked Emery–Dreifuss muscular dystrophy (XLEDMD).
Emery–Dreifuss muscular dystrophy is characterized by early contractures of the Achilles tendons, elbows, and spine, slowly progressive muscle wasting and weakness with a distinctive humeroperoneal distribution (upper arms and lower legs; see figure), and cardiac conduction defects leading to dilated cardiomyopathy (DCM). Onset is usually in childhood; onset after 20 years is rare. Contractures usually develop *before* there is significant weakness. These involve the elbows (arms carried in a flexed position), Achilles tendon (toe-walking), and the spine (limitation of flexion, especially neck flexion). There may be extensor contractures of the wrist and/or flexion contractures of the fingers. Caused by mutations in *STA* on Xq28. The gene product, emerin, associates with the nuclear envelope.

AD Emery–Dreifuss muscular dystrophy.
There is a broad phenotypic spectrum from those with predominant features of dilated DCM and little or no apparent

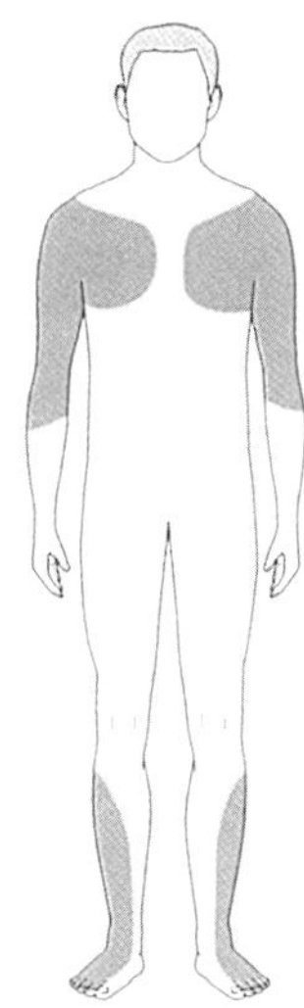

Distribution of predominant muscle weakness in Emery–Dreifuss muscular dystrophy. (Reproduced from Emery (1998), fig. 1a, p. 992, by permission of the BMJ Publishing Group.)

involvement of skeletal muscle to those in whom a progressive limb girdle muscular dystrophy, very similar to that seen in XLEDMD, dominates the clinical picture. There is marked intrafamilial variability, often with different family members exhibiting different aspects of the phenotype. Early-onset conduction disease is an important clinical prompt to this diagnosis. It is caused by mutations in the lamin A/C gene (*LMNA*) on 1q21. As for XLEDMD, the gene product is known to associate with the nuclear envelope.

Facioscapulohumeral muscular dystrophy (FSHD). FSHD is often clinically easily recognizable, and the diagnosis can be confirmed in 95% of cases by molecular genetic analysis for the disease-associated deletion on chromosome 4q35. However, there are some patients in whom facial weakness may be very minor and in these patients LGMD may be suggested as the diagnosis. Careful examination for the other characteristic signs of FSHD (prominent scapular winging, stepping of the shoulders on elevation of the arms, foot drop, frequent asymmetry) should suggest the diagnosis. FSHD is important to diagnose as it is an AD condition, though with a high rate of new mutations and germline mosaicism. See 'Facioscapulohumeral muscular dystrophy (FSHD)', page 322.

Bethlem myopathy. Bethlem myopathy is an AD disease that causes proximal muscle weakness associated with frequent contractures, typically of the elbows, finger flexors, and Achilles tendons, but, as these contractures may be relatively subtle, patients may be misdiagnosed as LGMD. An additional clinical clue may be the presence of keloid scarring and follicular hyperkeratosis. Bethlem myopathy is caused by mutations in one of the genes encoding collagen 6A1, 6A2, or 6A3 (the same genes as those implicated in Ullrich congenital muscular dystrophy).

Clinical diagnostic clues to the different forms of LGMD
Genotype–phenotype correlations in this highly heterogeneous group may be difficult (Zatz *et al.* 2003), but there are some useful clinical correlates.
- LGMD2I, which is probably the most common type of LGMD in the European population, is phenotypically the most similar to dystrophinopathy, with frequent calf hypertrophy and cardiomyopathy.
- The sarcoglycanopathies also share these clinical similarities to dystrophinopathy.
- LGMD2A or calpainopathy is relatively rarely associated with muscle hypertrophy and is usually a very atrophic disease with predominant weakness and wasting of the posterior musculature of the lower limbs and frequent scapular winging.
- LGMD2B or dysferlinopathy can present with either predominantly proximal or distal disease and the first clinical problem may be standing on the toes. These patients often present with a very clear onset at the end of the second decade.
- Contractures, cardiac conduction disease, and lipodystrophy may be a clue to the diagnosis of laminopathy.
- LGMD1C may be suggested by calf and other hypertrophy and a history of rippling muscle disease.
- For AR LGMD, unlike most AR disorders, a discordant phenotype, ranging from a relatively severe course to mildly affected or asymptomatic carriers, may be seen in patients carrying the same mutation even within the same family. Careful clinical assessment is used in combination with pedigree analysis and immunohistochemical staining of the muscle biopsy to obtain a precise genetic diagnosis.

Molecular analysis for the disease-causing mutations may then be possible.

Genetic advice
Recurrence risk
This is dependent on the specific diagnosis. After excluding BMD and XLEDMD, undiagnosed LGMD may follow an AR or AD pattern of inheritance. If both parents are normal the mode of inheritance is most likely to be AR, but ~10% of individuals probably have a *de novo* AD mutation.

Carrier detection
Possible if the familial mutation is known.

Prenatal diagnosis
Possible by chorionic villus sampling (CVS) if the familial mutation is known.

Natural history and further management (preventative measures)
Cardiac surveillance
- **XLEDMD.** Annual ECG with interpretation by a cardiologist (ECG changes may be subtle and difficult to interpret). Annual 24-hour ECG (Holter monitor). Periodic echocardiogram. Consider permanent pacemaker in asymptomatic patients when ECG begins to show signs of sinus node or atrial ventricular (AV)-node disease. Carrier females should be offered periodic ECG surveillance (Bushby *et al.* 2003).
- **Laminopathy.** Except for the partial lipodystrophy and Charcot–Marie–Tooth (CMT) phenotypes there is strong evidence for cardiac involvement that is progressive with age. DCM may develop as well as conduction defects. Management should be in a specialist centre with expertise in cardiac electrophysiology and may include consideration of an implantable defibrillator. If atrial fibrillation/flutter or atrial standstill occur frequently, consider anticoagulation with warfarin (Bushby *et al.* 2002).
- **Sarcoglycanopathy (LGMD2C–F).** Screen for the development of cardiomyopathy (echo and ECG) every 5 years. Routine surveillance is not needed in LGMD2A, 2B, 2G, 2H, 1A, 1C (Bushby *et al.* 2002).
- **LGMD2I.** Screen for the development of cardiomyopathy by annual echo and ECG. There is a high risk of cardiomyopathy especially in patients who are not homozygous for the common CA26A mutation (Poppe).

Respiratory surveillance
All of these groups are at risk of respiratory failure with increasing disease. Diaphragmatic weakness may be an additional feature in LGMD2I especially. All patients should be followed with regular forced vital capacity (FVC) in sitting and lying positions and additional investigations (e.g. overnight pulse oximetry) as indicated.

Support group: Muscular Dystrophy Campaign <www.muscular-dystrophy.org>.

Expert adviser: Kate Bushby, Action Research Professor in Neuromuscular Genetics, Institute of Human Genetics, Newcastle upon Tyne, England.

References

Bione, S, Maestrini, E, *et al.* Identification of a novel X-linked gene responsible for Emery–Dreifuss muscular dystrophy. *Nat Genet* 1994; **8**: 323–7.

Brockington M, Yuva Y, *et al.* Mutations in the fukutin-related protein gene (FKRP) identify limb girdle muscular dystrophy 2I as a milder allelic variant of congenital muscular dystrophy MDC1C. *Hum Mol Genet.* 2001; **10** (25): 2851–9.

Bushby KMD. The limb-girdle muscular dystrophies—multiple genes, multiple mechanisms. *Hum Mol Genet* 1999a; **8**: 1875–82.

Bushby KM. Making sense of the limb-girdle muscular dystrophies. *Brain* 1999b; **122** (pt. 8): 1403–20.

Bushby K, Muntoni F, Bourke JP. 107th ENMC International Workshop: the management of cardiac involvement in muscular dystrophy and myotonic dystrophy. 7th–9th June 2002, Naarden, the Netherlands. *Neuromuscul Disord* 2003; **13**: 166–72.

Emery AE. The muscular dystrophies. *Br Med J* 1998; **317**: 991–5.

Helbling-Leclerc A, Bonne G, Schwartz K. Emery–Dreifuss muscular dystrophy. *Eur J Hum Genet* 2002; **10** (3): 157–61.

Poppe M, Bourke J, *et al.* Cardiac and respiratory failure in limb-girdle muscular dystrophy 2I. *Annals of Neurology* 2004; **56**: 738–41.

Poppe M, Cree L, *et al.* The phenotype of limb-girdle muscular dystrophy type 2I. *Neurology* 2003; **60** (8): 1246–51.

Zatz M, de Paula F, Starling A, Vainzof M. The 10 autosomal recessive limb-girdle muscular dystrophies. *Neuromuscul Disord* 2003; **13** (7–8): 532–44.

Long QT and Brugada syndromes

Romano–Ward syndrome (autosomal dominant (AD)), Jervell and Lange–Nielsen syndrome (autosomal recessive (AR)).

Long QT syndromes are usually AD and characterized by prolonged ventricular repolarization that predisposes carriers to life-threatening arrhythmia, most characteristically torsade de pointes, a type of ventricular tachycardia that causes syncope but may degenerate to ventricular fibrillation and cause cardiac arrest. Mutations in the potassium-channel genes, *KCNQ1* (LQT1) and *KCNH2* (LQT2), and gain-of-function mutations in the sodium-channel gene, *SCN5A* (LQT3), are the most common causes of long QT syndrome, being responsible for ~60%, 35%, and 5% of families with identifiable mutations, respectively. Mutations in other potassium channels, *KCNE1*(LQT5), *KCNE2* (LQT6), and *KCNJ2* (LQT7), account for some of the remaining families, but about 30% of families do not have detectable mutations in any of these genes with other genes clearly still to be identified.

Birth incidence is unknown but has been estimated at 1/5000–1/7000. Typically, syncope occurring during physical activity or emotional upset begins in pre-teen to teenage years and usually continues into the 20s, but may present at any age. First cardiac events are uncommon after 30–40 years. Importantly, it is estimated that in excess of 30–50% of carriers of mutations associated with this syndrome never have symptoms. Most others have one or many episodes of syncope but do not die suddenly. Sudden cardiac death occurs in only about 4% of affected individuals (International LQTS Registry). Syncope typically occurs without warning as distinct from, e.g. vasovagal syncope in which patients feel dizzy or faint prior to collapse. Long QT syndrome is often misdiagnosed as epilepsy especially in children and this needs careful attention.

Approximately one-third of carriers have a QT interval corrected for heart rate (QT_c) of 400–460 ms on the electrocardiogram (ECG), which overlaps with the normal range. ($QT_c = QT/\sqrt{RR}$ (ventricular response rate)). The QT interval is influenced by the genetic locus and, in general, those patients with QT_c >500 ms are at substantially increased risk for cardiac events compared to those with a shorter QT_c (Priori *et al.* 2003).

Diagnosis of long QT syndrome. This is often a difficult diagnosis relying on careful evaluation of the patient's history, his/her non-invasive test results especially the 12-lead ECG, his/her family history, and, ideally, genetic analysis. Criteria for diagnosis are:

- a prolonged QT_c on the ECG (>470 ms in men or >480 ms in women). If there is a definite diagnosis of long QT in the family then $QT_c \geq 450$ ms in men or $QT_c \geq 460$ ms in women is highly suggestive of affected status with the following qualifications:
  - ensure that QT_c has been used to determine the diagnosis (QT interval is longer at slower heart rates), and that the proband was not hypokalaemic or taking drugs known to prolong the QT interval at the time the diagnosis was made;
  - if $QT_c < 400$ ms, long QT is highly unlikely as << 1% of gene carriers have a QT_c in this range, but ~30% of gene carriers have QT_c intervals in the range 400–460 ms, which overlaps with the normal range, and 'at risk' family members with a QT_c in this range have uncertain status.

- *or* presence of a pathogenic mutation in *KCNQ1, KCNH2, SCN5A, KCNE1,* or *KCNE2*.

Known triggers for long-QT-related arrhythmias include:

- swimming, running;
- startle: alarm clock, loud horn, ringing phone;
- emotions: anger, crying, test taking, or other stressful situations.

NB. Sudden death may also occur during sleep.

Clinical approach

History: key points
Three-generation family tree with specific enquiry for history of fainting, 'epilepsy', sudden death, and congenital deafness.

Investigation
- ECG with calculation of QT_c.
- DNA sample for molecular genetic analysis.

Other diagnoses/conditions to consider

Jervell and Lange–Nielsen syndrome. Homozygous form of long QT characterized by profound congenital deafness and long QT. AR with 1 in 4 sibling recurrence risk. Parents will both be carriers for long QT and sibs will be at two-thirds carrier risk for long QT.

Timothy syndrome. A rare condition characterised by long-QT syndrome and syndactyly due to mutations in $Ca_v1.2$, the L-type calcium channel (Splawski). Additional features which may be present include mild facial dysmorphism, congenital heart disease, intermittent hypoglycaemia, cognitive abnormalities and autism.

Brugada syndrome. A rare AD condition caused in ~15% by loss-of-function mutations in the cardiac sodium channel gene *SCN5A* (LQT3) that predispose to a variety of arrhythmias including bradycardia, atrioventricular conduction delay, and ventricular fibrillation (VF). The genetic basis in the remaining 85% is currently unknown.

Hypertrophic cardiomyopathy (HCM). HCM may predispose affected individuals to life-threatening arrhythmia. The post-mortem examination should indicate if this is the cause of sudden death in a family. See 'Hypertrophic cardiomyopathy (HCM)', page 360.

Arrhythmogenic right ventricular dysplasia (ARVD) or cardiomyopathy (ARVC) is an AD heart muscle disorder that causes arrhythmia, heart failure, and sudden death. It is characterized by replacement of the right ventricular myocardium by adipose and fibrous tissue. This disorder may be as prevalent as 6 in 10 000. In a large French population-based analysis, ARVC/D accounted for ~10% of cases of unexpected sudden cardiac death (Tabib *et al.* 2003). Males and females were equally affected and nearly one-third of all deaths occurred during the fourth decade, usually during everyday circumstances at home. Death was not precipitated by exercise, and 10% of cases occurred perioperatively. Adipose infiltration of the right ventricle was either isolated (20%) or associated with fibrosis (74.5%) and lymphocytes (5.5%). A total of 14.5% of cases had cardiac hypertrophy, assessed by an increase in heart weight and/or left ventricular wall thickness. In most cases, the His bundle and its branches were abnormal either because of infiltration of adipose tissue, fibrosis, or both.

Nine genetic loci associated with this disease have been identifed, and mutations in genes at three loci have been discovered. Heterozygous mutations in genes encoding desmoplakin (*DSP*) and plakoglobin (*JUP*) suggest that altered integrity at cardiac myocyte cell–cell junctions may promote myocyte degeneration and death, with the repair process consisting of replacement of myocardium by adipose and fibrous tissue. Mutations in the gene encoding plakophilin-2 (*PKP2*) may account for 25–30% of cases (Gerull).

Catecholaminergic polymorphic ventricular tachycardia (CPVT). CPVT is a severe arrhythmic disease characterised by salvoes of exercise-induced bidirectional and polymorphic tachycardias. It usually follows AD inheritance. Laitinen identified mutations in the ryanodine receptor 2 (*RYR2*) in some individuals. The resting ECG can look entirely normal in affected individuals—an exercise ECG may be needed to demonstrate the condition.

Naxos disease is the triad of AR ARVC with biventricular dilated cardiomyopathy, palmoplantar keratoderma, and woolly hair caused by mutations in the junction plakoglobin gene (*JUP*) on chromosome 17q21.

Genetic advice

Inheritance and recurrence risk
AD with low *de novo* mutation rate.

Variability and penetrance
The disease exhibits both inter- and intrafamilial variability. Penetrance is incomplete with approximately 50% of gene carriers remaining asymptomatic.

Prenatal diagnosis
Technically feasible by chorionic villus sampling (CVS) if the familial mutation is known.

Predictive testing
Cascade screening of family members can be used to clarify status if the familial mutation is known. In asymptomatic 'at risk' family members with QT_c in the equivocal range, molecular genetic analysis may be the only way to definitively assign status.

Natural history and management

- **Lifestyle modification.** Patients should be advised to avoid activities associated with intense physical activity and/or emotional stress, e.g. competitive sports, amusement park rides, scary movies, jumping into cold water, etc.
- **Avoidance of drugs that prolong the QT interval.** See <www.qtdrugs.org> for list.

- **β-blockers**. The first-choice therapy in patients with long QT. Effective in ~70% of patients; cardiac events continue in the remaining 30%.
- **Implantable cardioverter defibrillator (ICD)**. May be necessary for those with symptoms despite β-blockade or for those with a history of cardiac arrest.

Potential long-term complications
Sudden death occurs in ~4% of mutation carriers.

Surveillance
At-risk family members should be reviewed by a specialist cardiologist.

Support group: SADS UK (The Sudden Arrhythmic Death Syndrome Foundation UK) <www.sadsuk.org>; The Cardiac Arrhythmia Research and Education Foundation <www.longqt.org>.

Expert adviser: Andrew Grace, Consultant Cardiologist, Papworth Hospital, Cambridge, England.

References

Ahmad F. The molecular genetics of arrhythmogenic right ventricular dysplasia–cardiomyopathy. *Clin Invest Med* 2003; **26**: 167–78.

Gerull B, Heuser A, *et al.* Mutations in the desmosomal protein plakophilin-2 are common in arrhythmogenic right ventricular cardiomyopathy. *Nature Genetics* 2004; **36**: 1162–64.

Jervell FLN. Congenital deaf-mutism, functional heart disease with prolongation of the Q–Y interval and sudden death. *Am Heart J* 1957; **54**: 59–68.

Laitinen PJ, Swan H, *et al.* Molecular genetics of exercise-induced polymorphic ventricular tachycardia: identification of three novel cardiac ryanodine receptor mutations and two common calsequestrin 2 amino-acid polymorphisms. *Eur J Hum Genet* 2003; **11**: 888–91.

Moss AJ. Long QT syndrome. *J Am Med Assoc* 2003; **289**: 2041–4.

Papadatos GA, Wallerstein PMR, *et al. Proc Natl Acad Sci, USA* 2002; **99**: 6210–15.

Priori SG, Napolitano C. Genetics of cardiac arrhythmias and sudden cardiac death (Review). *Ann N Y Acad Sci* 2004; **1015**: 96–110.

Priori SG, Schwartz PJ, *et al.* Risk stratification in the long-QT syndrome. *New Engl J Med* 2003; **348**: 1866–74.

Splawski I, Timothy KW, *et al.* $Ca_v1.2$ Calcium channel dysfunction causes a multisystem disorder including arrhythmia and autism. *Cell* 2004; **119**: 19–31.

Tabib A, Loire R, *et al.* Circumstances of death and gross and microscopic observations in a series of 200 cases of sudden death associated with arrhythmogenic right ventricular cardiomyopathy and/or dysplasia. *Circulation* 2003; **108**: 3000–5.

Vincent GM. The long-QT syndrome—bedside to bench to bedside [perspective]. *New Engl J Med* 2003; **348**: 1837–8.

Marfan syndrome

Marfan syndrome (MFS) is a multisystem disorder caused in the majority of classically affected individuals by mutations in the fibrillin gene (*FBN1*) on 15q21 (Loeys). Recently a second gene for Marfan syndrome, *TGFBR2* on 3p24.1, has been identified (Mizuguchi). MFS has an estimated prevalence of 1/3000–1/5000. Fibrillin is a component of microfibrils. The microfibrillar meshwork in the extracellular matrix is important in the integrity of the connective tissue. Various components of the extracellular matrix such as collagens, elastin, and fibrillin are present in varying proportions in different tissues and contribute to the elasticity, tensile strength, and durability of various types of connective tissue. Fibrillin is particularly rich in the wall of the proximal aorta and the zonule of the ocular lens.

Cardiovascular involvement is the main cause of major morbidity and mortality in MFS. In untreated MFS, life expectancy is reduced by 30–40%. Death is typically due to rupture or dissection of an aneurysm of the aortic root, or severe aortic regurgitation.

In practical terms, there appears to be a continuum between patients at the extreme end of the normal population, through patients with mild connective tissue phenotypes, to Marfan syndrome. In many centres, fibrillin mutation analysis is not routinely available, and diagnosis relies on careful clinical evaluation (see table).

Classification of aortic dissection. Aortic dissection may be classified into type A, proximal or ascending aorta, and type B, distal or descending aorta.

Clinical approach

History: key points

- Three-generation family tree with specific enquiry about parental heights, abnormal chest shape or scoliosis, eye problems (lens dislocation, myopia, retinal detachment), heart problems (aortic aneurysm/dissection, mitral valve replacement (MVR), aortic valve replacement (AVR), sudden cardiac death). Carefully document whether aortic rupture was thoracic or abdominal.
- Joint problems. Hypermobility, subluxation, disclocation, discomfort, 'clicky' joints.
- Dental overcrowding and orthodontic treatment.
- Hernias.
- Easy bruising/abnormal scarring.
- Past medical history, e.g. spontaneous pneumothoraces.

Examination: key points

- Height, weight, span, and lower segment (LS).
- Face shape, palate, dental overcrowding.
- Hands for arachnodactyly with wrist and thumb signs, and contractures.
- Joint hypermobility (Beighton score).
- Chest shape and back for scoliosis.
- Skin for striae (lumbar region and over shoulders) and unusual scarring.
- Feet for pes planus and medial rotation of medial malleoli on standing.

Investigation

- Height and weight. Plot height on centile chart; calculate body surface area for normograms of aortic root diameter.
- Echocardiogram.

- Slit-lamp examination of the eyes.
- DNA for *FBN1* mutation analysis.
- Urine for homocystinuria if sporadic case with lens dislocation or family history consistent with autosomal recessive (AR) inheritance.
- If aortic root enlargement is present, consider magnetic resonance imaging (MRI) scan of thoracic aorta—a more objective measure of aortic root size and shape.
- MRI scan of lumbosacral spine for dural ectasia if the finding of one additional major criterion (see table) would secure diagnosis and clarify management (age-dependent penetrance so probably best deferred until late teens or adult life).

Other diagnoses/conditions to consider

Marfan syndrome Type II (MFS2). A newly described condition caused by mutation in the transforming growth factor β genes (*TGFBR1* and *TGFBR2*) and characterized by hypertelorism, bifid uvula/cleft palate and generalised arterial tortuosity with aneurysm and dissection of the ascending aorta. AD inheritance with variable expressivity. Other findings in some affected individuals include: craniosynostosis, structural brain abnormalities, mental retardation, congenital heart disease and aneurysms with dissection throughout the arterial tree (Loeys 2005). From the limited data currently available, ectopia lentis does not seem to be feature.

MASS phenotype (mitral valve prolapse, mild aortic involvement (<2 SD), skeletal, and skin anomalies).

Congenital contractural arachnodactyly CCA (FBN2). Beal syndrome. Typically there is a history of neonatal contractures that improve during infancy. Ears may appear crumpled at birth. Scoliosis may be severe and cardiovascular involvement is generally mild. Autosomal dominant (AD) inheritance, caused by mutations in *FBN2* on 5q.

Ehlers–Danlos syndrome, hypermobility type (previously type III). Common and usually mild AD disorder. Soft skin with hypermobility of large and small joints (Beighton score 5/9 or greater). There can be considerable diagnostic overlap with MFS. See 'Ehlers–Danlos syndrome (EDS)', page 312.

Ehlers–Danlos syndrome, vascular type (previously type IV). This is an uncommon but serious AD disorder caused by mutations in *COL3A1* encoding type III collagen. The facial features are subtle and include prominent eyes due to decreased adipose tissue below the eyes and thin, slightly 'pinched' nose, thin lips, and hollow cheeks. Thin translucent skin with visible veins and easy bruising. No significant large joint hypermobility (Beighton score <5/9). Risk of arterial rupture and rupture of bowel, bladder, and uterus leads to reduced life expectancy. See 'Ehlers–Danlos syndrome (EDS)', page 312.

Stickler syndrome. A dominantly inherited disorder of collagen, resulting in a congenital vitreous gel anomaly, myopia, variable orofacial features including cleft palate in some, sensorineural deafness, and arthropathy. Joint hypermobility and a habitus characterized by slender extremities with long fingers may cause diagnostic overlap with MFS (although height is normal). Characteristic vitreoretinal changes observed during ophthalmological diagnosis

Ghent diagnostic criteria for Marfan syndrome (De Paepe et al. 1996)

Requirements for diagnosis for the index case

- If family/genetic history is not contributory, major criteria in at least 2 different organ systems and involvement of a third organ system
- If mutation known to cause MFS in others is detected, one major criterion in an organsystem and involvement of a second organ system

Requirements for diagnosis for a relative of the index case

- Presence of a major criterion in the family history and one major criterion in an organ system and involvement of a second organ system

Skeletal system (1 major criterion requires presence of 4 or more of criteria listed under 'Major' below)

Major	**Minor**
• Pectus carinatum	• Pectus excavatum of minor severity
• Pectus excavatum requiring surgery	• Joint hypermobility
• US:LS ratio <0.86* *or* arm span/height ratio >1.05	• Highly arched palate with crowding of teeth
• Wrist *and* thumb signs[†]	• Facial appearance (dolicocephaly, malar hypoplasia,
• Scoliosis of >20° or spondylolisthesis	enophthalmos, retrognathia,
• Reduced extension of elbows (<170°)	down-slanting palpebral fissures)
• Medial displacement of the medial malleoli causing pes planus	
• Protusio acetabulae of any degree (X-ray)	

Ocular system (for this to be involved, at least 2 minor criteria must be present)

Major	**Minor**
• Ectopia lentis	• Abnormally flat cornea (keratometry)
	• Increased axial length of globe (>23.5 mm in adult)
	• Hypoplastic iris or hypoplastic ciliary muscle

Cardiovascular system (for this to be involved either 1 major or 1 minor criterion must be present)

Major	**Minor**
• Dilatation of the ascending aorta[§] with or without aortic regurgitation and involving at least the sinuses of Valsalva	• Mitral valve prolapse ± mitral valve regurgitation
• Dissection of the ascending aorta	• Dilatation of the main pulmonary artery <40 years
• Calcification of the mitral annulus <40 years	
• Dilatation or dissection of the descending thoracic or abdominal aorta <50 years	

Pulmonary system (for this to be involved 1 of the minor criteria must be present)

Minor

- Spontaneous pneumothorax
- Apical blebs (on chest X-ray)

Skin (for this to be involved 1 of the minor criteria must be present)

Minor

- Striae atrophicae (stretch marks) not associated with weight changes, pregnancy, or repetitive stress
- Recurrent or incisional herniae

Dura (for this to be involved the major criterion must be present)

Major

- Lumbosacral dural ectasia by computerized tomography (CT) or magnetic resonance imaging (MRI)

Family/genetic history

Major

- Having a parent, child, or sib who meets these diagnostic criteria independently
- Presence of a mutation in *FBN1* known to cause MFS
- Presence of a haplotype around *FBN1* inherited by descent, known to be associated with unequivocally diagnosed MFS in the family (linkage)

---

* Upper segment (US)/lower segment (LS) ratio = (height−LS)/LS. Need chart for children <16 years (see Hall p. 272–73).

[†] Wrist sign, thumb overlaps terminal phalanx of 5th digit when grasping contralateral wrist; thumb sign, entire nail of thumb projects beyond ulnar border of hand when hand is clenched without assistance.

[‡] Increased axial length causes myopia. If ultrasound scan (USS) measurement of axial length is not available consider substituting high–moderate or high myopia.

[§] See charts of normal range or aortic root dimensions (Roman *et al.* 1989).

should alert the clinical team to this diagnosis, but sensorineural deafness and cleft palate are other important diagnostic prompts. See 'Stickler syndrome', this chapter.

Homocystinuria. An AR condition caused by deficiency of cystathionine synthetase encoded on 21q22 and characterized by lens dislocation (typically downward displacement) and thrombophilia. Most thrombotic events are cerebrovascular. The course is variable and often unpredictable. Lens dislocation is rarely present before 3 years; glaucoma, cataracts, myopia, and retinal detachment may also occur. Patients are usually tall and thin and deformity of the chest wall is common. Learning disability can occur, but this is not always the case. If the diagnosis is strongly suspected despite normal urine amino acids, do plasma amino acids and consult a metabolic specialist (a methionine load may be needed to demonstrate the biochemical defect).

Sex chromosome anomalies (e.g. XXX, XXY, XYY). Tall stature may sometimes cause diagnostic overlap, but major features of MFS are not present on careful scrutiny.

Myotonic dystrophy. See 'Myotonic dystrophy (DM)', page 388.

Marfanoid habitus with learning difficulties. MFS itself does not cause cognitive impairment. Consider X-linked Fryns syndrome in males, or mosaic trisomy 8, or 15q21 interstitial deletion.

Neonatal Marfan syndrome. Babies presenting with MFS in the neonatal period have a severe phenotype with extreme arachnodactyly, contractures and cardiac/aortic disease. They are unusually long and are often floppy due to ligamentous laxity and may develop a scoliosis. Neonatal MFS is usually caused by a 'de novo' mutation in the *FBN1* gene, usually in exons 24–32 (the central portion of the gene).

Genetic advice

Inheritance and recurrence risk
AD condition with 50% risk to offspring. High new mutation rate ~30%. If sporadic case and both parents are normal on full clinical assessment (including echocardiogram and slit-lamp), recurrence risk for future pregnancies is low. If it is possible to identify an *FBN1* mutation in the proband, this greatly facilitates risk assessment.

Variability and penetrance
The phenotype can be very variable. Ectopia lentis can be discordant between affected related individuals. In general cardiovascular involvement tends to be more severe in men than women. Some families show fairly consistent severe cardiovascular involvement, but others do not. Penetrance is age-dependent and this is crucial when determining whether 'at risk' family members are affected or not.

Prenatal diagnosis
If an *FBN1* mutation has been identified in the parent, this is possible by chorionic villus sampling (CVS), but in practice is not often requested unless there is an adverse family history.

Predictive testing
If a pathological *FBN1* mutation has been identified in an affected member, predictive testing is possible and may be offered so that surveillance can be targeted more effectively.

Other family members
Parents of an individual with MFS should be offered comprehensive evaluation with clinical assessment, echocardiogram, and slit-lamp examination. If parents are not available, or results are not known, offer evaluation to siblings too. All children of an affected individual are at 50% risk and should be offered periodic review. If the proband has an identifiable, pathological *FBN1* mutation, this greatly facilitates assessment of other family members.

Natural history and management

- **Progressive dilatation of the aortic root.** Beta-blockade slows progression of aortic root dilatation by decreasing the stress on the aortic wall (Shores *et al.* 1994).
- **Scoliosis** is usually non-progressive once growth has ceased. If a fixed (i.e. non-postural) spinal deformity is noted in a child or adolescent, refer on for specialist assessment.
- **Pneumothorax.** Pleurodesis is recommended after recurrent pneumothorax.
- **Retinal detachment.** Patients with high myopia and increased axial globe length are at increased risk. Contact sports and diving from a board should be avoided.
- **Glaucoma.** Increased risk particularly in individuals with ectopia lentis.

Surveillance
- All individuals with MFS should be offered annual echocardiography. Individuals with marked aortic root dilatation (>4.5 cm) should be reviewed more frequently, as should women in pregnancy and those with a rapidly changing aortic root diameter.
- Instigate beta-blockade if aortic root diameter >2 SD from mean (consider earlier intervention if child clearly affected and severe cardiovascular phenotype in family). NB. asthma is a relative contraindication to beta-blockade.
- Patients with an aortic root diameter at the sinuses of Valsalva of >5.0 cm should be referred for consideration of elective replacement of the aortic root with a composite graft.
- Periodic ophthalmic review is appropriate in childhood and early adolescence. If ectopia lentis is going to develop, it most often becomes evident in preschool years and is slowly progressive, particularly in childhood and early teens. If there is no ocular involvement, adult patients can probably be safely managed by regular review by an optometrist/dispensing optician.
- Growth should be monitored in childhood and adolescence. Interventions to reduce growth potential such as hormonal treatment and epiphyseal stapling are rarely used.
- Spine. Monitor children and adolescents for scoliosis.

Lifestyle issues
- Sports. Enquire specifically about leisure pursuits, and assess individually. In general isometric exercise, e.g. weight-lifting, rowing, press-ups, should be avoided (severe cardiovascular stress). Contact sports such as football, basketball, hockey, volleyball, boxing, and wrestling are contraindicated (risk of retinal detachment and deceleration injury to aorta). Regular rhythmic activity such as walking, swimming, and non-competitive cycling is fine.

- The Marfan Association produces a range of booklets for children, teenagers, and adults and also for teachers and can provide help with outlets for clothing and shoes.

Pregnancy

Pregnancy increases the risk of dissection of an aneurysm, the risk increasing with gestational age. Women need to be aware that the increased risk for dissection associated with pregnancy persists until 6–8 weeks post-partum.

- If there is evidence of cardiovascular compromise, e.g. moderate or more severe aortic regurgitation or aortic root diameter >40 mm, and/or a family history of early dissection, the risk of dissection in pregnancy is greatly increased.
- If cardiovascular involvement is minor and aortic root diameter <40 mm, pregnancy is usually tolerated well with favourable maternal and fetal outcomes, and no evidence of aggravation of aortic root dilatation with time (Meijboom).
- Periodic echocardiographic surveillance is recommended during pregnancy and the puerperium. It is our practice to offer an echocardiogram in each trimester and a fourth scan 4–8 weeks post-partum.
- There do not seem to be specific contraindications to the use of atenolol in pregnant patients with MFS, throughout pregnancy.
- Delivery should be by the least haemodynamically stressful method. Ideally, MFS patients should have a vaginal delivery in the lateral decubitus position with minimal maternal expulsive efforts and a low threshold for forceps or vacuum extraction to shorten the second stage (Rossiter *et al.* 1995).

Support group contact: Marfan Association UK <www.marfan.org.uk>; National Marfan Foundation (US) <www.marfan.org>.

Expert adviser: Sally J. Davies, Consultant in Medical Genetics, University Hospital of Wales, Cardiff, Wales.

References

De Paepe A, Devereux RB, *et al.* Revised diagnostic criteria for the Marfan syndrome. *Am J Med Genet* 1996; **62**: 417–26.

Hall JG, Froster–Iskenius UG, Allanson JE. Handbook of normal physical measurement. OUP Oxford 1995.

Loeys B, De Backer J, *et al.* Comprehensive molecular screening of the FBN1 gene favors locus homogeneity of classical Marfan syndrome. *Hum Mutat* 2004; **24**: 140–6.

Loeys BL, Chen J *et al.* A syndrome of altered cardiovascular, craniofacial, neurocognitive and skeletal development caused by mutations in *TGFBR1* or *TGFBR2*. *Nat Genet.* 2005; **37**: 275–81.

Meijboom LJ, Vos FE *et al.* Pregnancy and aortic root growth in the Marfan syndrome: a prospective study. *Eur Heart J.* 2005; **26**: 914–20.

Mizuguchi T, Collod–Beroud G, *et al.* Heterozygous *TGFBR2* mutations in Marfan syndrome. *Nat Genet* 2004; **36(8)**: 790–2.

Roman MJ, Devereux RB, *et al.* Two-dimensional aortic root dimensions in normal children and adults. *Am J Cardiol* 1989; **64**: 507–12.

Rossiter JP, Repke JT, *et al.* A prospective longitudinal evaluation of pregnancy in the Marfan syndrome. *Am J Obstet Gynecol* 1995; **173**: 1599–606.

Shores J, Berger KR, *et al.* Progression of aortic root dilatation and the benefit of long-term beta-adrenergic blockade in Marfan's syndrome. *New Engl J Med* 1994; **330**: 1335–41.

Mitochondrial DNA diseases

Disorders following mitochondrial inheritance present some of the most challenging situations in genetic counselling and precise advice may not always be possible at the current time. Prenatal diagnosis for mitochondrial disorders is highly problematical and expert advice should always be sought where this is considered. An accurate diagnosis enables appropriate screening for other systems that may be affected, e.g. conduction defects and diabetes in Kearns–Sayre syndrome (KSS). Mitochondrial disorders encoded by nuclear DNA, e.g. Friedreich ataxia (FRDA), are discussed elsewhere.

Figures from Sweden (Darin *et al.* 2001) have shown an incidence of mitochondrial respiratory chain (MRC) dysfunction in children under 6 years of age of 1/11 000. The same study showed prevalence figures of 1/21 000 in the paediatric population (<16 years). Studies from the UK looking at adults gave a potential prevalence of 1/8000 and combining the figures for children and adults suggests that MRC disease is far from rare, and may occur as frequently as 1/8500.

Mitochondrial DNA (mtDNA) is exclusively maternally inherited with very rare exceptions (Schwartz and Vissing 2002). It is a circular double-stranded molecule of 16 569 bp. The genome encodes two ribosomal RNAs, 22 tRNAs involved in translation of mRNA into protein, and 13 polypeptide components of the oxidative phosphorylation (OXPHOS) system. Thousands of copies of mtDNA are present in each nucleated somatic cell. Changes in mtDNA sequence can be inherited or somatic. Human mtDNA has a mutation rate 10–20 times that of nuclear DNA, probably due to failure of proof-reading by mtDNA polymerase. In normal individuals all the copies of mtDNA have the same sequence (homoplasmy); in many patients with mitochondrial disease there is a mixture of normal and mutant sequence within the same cell (heteroplasmy). A variety of mutations occur in mitochondrial disease including deletions, duplications, and point mutations. *Point mutations are commonly maternally inherited whilst deletions and duplications are most often sporadic.* The percentage of mutant DNA may vary between different tissues and also change with time. Blood levels are a very poor reflection of mutant load in A3243G (MELAS (mitochondrial myopathy–encephalopathy–lactic acidosis–stroke-like episodes)) and rearrangements. Preferential accumulation of mutant mtDNAs in affected tissues appears to explain the progressive nature of mitochondrial disorders.

Individual oocytes from a woman at risk of transmitting mitochondrial disease may contain markedly different levels of mutant mtDNA. There is increasing evidence for a 'bottleneck' early in embryological development so that all mtDNA in an individual is derived from a small number of progenitors (Brown 1997). The degree of heteroplasmy in the progenitors probably governs the subsequent mutant load in the individual.

Some useful nomenclature follows.

- **Homoplasmy.** All of an individual's mtDNA is identical.
- **Heteroplasmy.** The existence of more than one mitochondrial DNA (mtDNA) type in the same individual, e.g. mitochondria containing a mixture of mtDNA carrying the MELAS 3243 point mutation and mtDNA with the wild-type sequence. In mitochondrial disorders because of the thousands of mitochondria in each cell the percentage of mutant and wild-type mtDNAs often varies between different cells and especially between different tissues.

- **OXPHOS.** Oxidative phosphorylation, the core of the energy-producing pathway in the mitochondrion, is a system of five multisubunit complexes located on the inner mitochondrial membrane. Adenosine triphosphate (ATP) is generated by complex V (ATPase). 70 of the 83 polypeptide components of the system are encoded by nuclear genes; the other 13 by mtDNA. Some tissues, e.g. brain and muscle, are highly dependent on the OXPHOS system for energy.
- **COX.** Cytochrome oxidase, complex IV of the OXPHOS system.
- **SDH.** Succinate dehydrogenase, complex II of the OXPHOS system.

Mitochondrial diseases are often late in being diagnosed, either because they present insidiously or because the clinical features (see table) are so heterogeneous that the diagnosis is missed. The organs most often affected in mitochondrial disorders are highly energy-demanding tissues, such as the central nervous system (CNS), skeletal and cardiac muscle, pancreatic islets, liver, and kidney. Features that should particularly alert suspicion are highlighted in bold in the table. Several features together increase the likelihood of an underlying mitochondrial disorder.

Clinical clues to mitochondrial disorders (after Leonard and Schapiro 2000)

CNS	Developmental delay/regression
	Generalized seizures
	Ataxia
	Myoclonus
	Stroke-like episodes
	Encephalopathy
Muscle	Myopathy—weakness/fatigue/hypotonia
Eyes	**Ptosis**
	External ophthalmoplegia
	Optic atrophy
	Pigmentary retinopathy
	Cataract
	Sudden loss of vision (LHON)
Ears	**Sensorineural deafness** (including aminoglycoside deafness)
Heart	Cardiomyopathy
	Conduction defects
Pancreas	**Diabetes mellitus**
Kidney	Renal tubular dysfunction (Fanconi syndrome) with generalized amino aciduria and glycosuria
Bone marrow	Sideroblastic anaemia/pancytopenia

* Features highlighted in bold should particularly arouse suspicion of a mitochondrial disorder. NB. *Any of the above features in combination with lactic acidosis* is highly suggestive of a mitochondrial disorder. Particular combinations, e.g. *diabetes and sensorineural deafness*, are very suggestive of an underlying mitochondrial disorder.

Clinical approach

History: key points

Three-generation family tree with specific enquiry about muscle weakness, vision, hearing, and neurological problems. Extend the family tree as far as possible through the maternal line. If there are other potentially affected members in the family take a careful history noting the scope of their problems and the age of onset and progress of their symptoms. Mitochondrial disorders often display extraordinary intrafamilial variability.

Examination: key points

- Growth parameters. Height, weight, occipital-frontal circumference (OFC).
- Examine eyes, looking for ptosis and nystagmus and testing for external ophthalmoplegia.
- Neurological examination for hypotonia, myoclonus, and ataxia.
- Ophthalmological examination for pigmentary retinopathy, cataract.

Investigation

- DNA for mutation analysis of mitochondrial genome or nuclear-encoded mitochondrial genes. Note that mtDNA rearrangements are not usually found in blood, whilst the common point mutations frequently are; both types are seen in muscle.
- Electrocardiogram (ECG) for conduction disorder.
- Urinalysis for tubular dysfunction (generalized amino-aciduria and glycosuria), which may occur in Pearson syndrome, KSS, and MELAS.
- Blood lactate.
- Blood glucose.
- Creatine kinase (CK) is usually normal or only mildly elevated.
- Consider cerebrospinal fluid (CSF) lactate (important in the investigation of possible Leigh disease).
- Consider muscle biopsy with Gomori trichrome staining for 'ragged red fibres' and staining for COX (complex IV) and SDH (complex II). Occasional COX-negative fibres may be found as a normal variant in individuals >40 years of age, but these never exceed 5%. In order to gain maximum information, the biopsy should be processed and examined in a specialist facility that can undertake light microscopy, electron microscopy, immunostaining, storage of muscle for subsequent assay of individual complex activity, and DNA extraction from muscle for mutation analysis. Muscle biopsy is the single most useful test in the diagnosis of mitochondrial disorders, although occasional patients with Leber hereditary optic neuropathy (LHON) and with mitochondrial myopathy due to mtDNA mutations may have normal biopsies.
- Consider magnetic resonance imaging (MRI) if there are symptoms of encephalopathy, e.g. seizures, regression, ataxia, myoclonus, stroke-like episodes.
- Audiometry.

Specific mitochondrial disorders and genetic advice

Most patients with mtDNA mutations present as apparently sporadic cases.

Chronic progressive external ophthalmoplegia (CPEO) with or without retinitis pigmentosa (RP) or limb weakness and fatigue is usually caused by a single deletion in mtDNA, although ~30% of cases may be due to nuclear genes (following AD or AR inheritance) involved in mtDNA nucleotide metabolism or replication which cause multiple deletions. It typically presents in teenage or young adult life and usually runs a benign course with little involvement of other organs. Most patients with CPEO do not have a family history and presumably develop from ova in which mutations have arisen *de novo*.

- **Recurrence risks.** Females with a single mtDNA deletion have a very low (<1–5%) chance of transmitting the disease to their offspring. If mtDNA duplications are present the recurrence risk is higher.

Kearns–Sayre syndrome (KSS). KSS is a subtype of CPEO with a poorer prognosis. Onset is at <20 years and, in addition to the CPEO and pigmentary retinopathy, there is often a cardiac conduction defect and ataxia. Unlike CPEO the condition is usually life-limiting. Patients with KSS usually have a single mtDNA deletion, but duplications may be found in patients with diabetes and deafness. Most patients with KSS and a single mtDNA deletion do not have a family history and presumably develop from ova in which mutations have arisen *de novo*.

- **Recurrence risks.** Females with a single mtDNA deletion have a very low (<1–5%) chance of transmitting the disease to their offspring. If mtDNA duplications are present the recurrence risk is higher.

Leber hereditary optic neuropathy (LHON). Leber hereditary optic neuritis. NB. Leber has several eponymous conditions, e.g. Leber congenital amaurosis (autosomal recessive (AR)), a congenital retinal dystrophy causing blindness, so ensure that the diagnosis really is LHON before giving genetic advice.

The most common mutation in LHON is 11778 (70%); 3460 accounts for 15% and 14484 for a further 5%. LHON causes a fairly rapid and irreversible loss of vision. It is more penetrant in males than females. 40% of patients with G11778A have no family history of the disease. Visual loss is usually irreversible except with the T14484C mutation where some visual recovery is seen in up to 70% of patients; some visual recovery is also occasionally seen in 3460. The relative risk to women is higher in 3460 families as the sex ratio is less skewed to males.

Currently there are no effective interventions to prevent visual loss. Advise at-risk family members to avoid known retinal toxins such as smoking and excess alcohol. Age of onset of visual loss is very variable: 5% by age 10 years; 45% by age 20 years; 70% by age 30 years; 80% by age 40 years; 95% by age 50 years; 100% by age 70 years. The risk diminishes with age. Males who have reached 20 years without problems have halved their lifetime risk; for females this occurs at 27 years (Harding *et al.* 1995).

Measuring blood levels is not very helpful in predicting outcome in LHON. The symptom-free maternal relatives may carry identical mutant loads. Some individuals with the G11778A mutation present with a multiple-sclerosis like illness. The G11778 mutation is commonly homoplasmic.

The offspring risks for LHON are summarized in the table on page 386.

Leigh syndrome (subacute necrotizing encephalomyopathy). See also 'Leigh encephalitis' page 372. Usually presents in infancy with non-specific features such as hypotonia, seizures, and developmental delay. Prevalence ~1/32 000–1/40 000. Spasticity, RP, ataxia, and CPEO may develop later. Blood lactate is often elevated, and CSF lactate is usually significantly elevated. MRI shows bilateral, usually symmetrical changes in the

Remaining lifetime risk for LHON at age* (Mackay)

	Birth	14 yr	26 yr	37 yr	50 yr	61 yr
European[†] male	50%	42%	25%	8%	1%	0.07%
European female	No data					
Australian[†] male	20%	17%	10%	3%	0.4%	0.02%
Australian female	4%	3.3%	2%	0.7%	0.1%	0.01%

*A mother with 100% mutant has a 99% chance that the child will be the same so these risks apply to the offspring of these maternal members of the family. Ie. most families stay the same.

[†] The difference between Australian and European risks is thought to be due to environmental factors but could be due to better ascertainment in Australia of all family members.

upper brainstem and thalami. The prognosis for patients presenting in infancy is poor—they usually die within months or a few years. Leigh syndrome is a genetically heterogeneous condition caused by several biochemical defects including pyruvate dehydrogenase (PDH) deficiency and OXPHOS defects. A subset of patients carry the mtDNA point mutations T8993G and T8993C (also seen in NARP (neuropathy–ataxia–retinitis pigmentosa)). Mutations in the nuclear-encoded *Surf1* gene underlie 75% of COX-deficient Leigh syndrome (i.e. 10–20% of all Leigh syndrome) and follow AR inheritance.

- **Recurrence risks.** An empiric risk of 33% was estimated by van Erven *et al.* (1987); this may be an overestimate since the calculation was not corrected for unascertained sibships. See White *et al.* (1999*a*) for estimate of risk for patients carrying T8993G or T8993C. The recurrence risk for Leigh syndrome due to *Surf1* mutations is 25%.

MELAS (mitochondrial encephalomyopathy–lactic acidosis–strokes).

One of the most common of the mitochondrial disorders (1/10 000), and one of the most *variable*. 90% of cases are caused by the A3243G point mutation in the tRNA[leu] gene. Despite the acronym, the most common presenting features are diabetes and progressive deafness and some patients do not develop other symptoms. Approximately 10% develop a cardiomyopathy. Blood levels in A3243G are a very poor reflection of mutant load, and may diminish with age.

- **Recurrence risks.** Everyone in the A3423G maternal line is at increased risk for diabetes (usual onset in early adult life, initially diet-controlled, but patients usually become insulin-dependent fairly rapidly), deafness (progressive sensorineural), and (cardiomyopathy).
  - Low load (<30% in muscle, <10% in blood) or asymptomatic or diabetes only: likely lowish offspring risk ~15–25%.
  - Moderate load (>50% in muscle) or symptomatic other than diabetes and/or deafness: likely offspring risk >60%.

MERRF (myoclonic epilepsy with ragged red fibres).

In addition to myoclonic epilepsy, the clinical spectrum includes cerebellar ataxia, deafness, and dementia. Caused by mtDNA point mutations, typically A8344G in the tRNA[lys] gene

- **Recurrence risks.** In a small analysis of 47 women carrying the A8344G mutation (Chinnery *et al.* 1997), <5% of the offspring were affected when the mutant load in maternal blood was <35%, 15% were affected when the mutant load was 40–59%, 20% when the mutant load was 60–79%, and 80% when the mutant load was 80–100%.

NARP (neurogenic weakness, ataxia, retinitis pigmentosa).

Caused by the T8992G and T8993C mutations (which can also cause a subset of Leigh syndrome).

- **Recurrence risks.** Risks depend on the base change, the T8993G being more severe than T8993A. See White *et al.* (1999*a*) for further details.

Pearson syndrome

usually presents in infancy with transfusion-dependent sideroblastic anaemia or pancytopenia often with malabsorption (exocrine pancreatic failure). May develop villous atrophy, diabetes mellitus, renal tubular dysfunction, etc. Caused by mtDNA deletions. Morbidity and mortality are high. If infants survive, the clinical picture evolves into KSS because the red and white blood cells with higher mutant loads are selected against and gradually lost from the blood, but tissues such as brain and heart where cells do not turn over rapidly gradually acquire more deletions.

- **Recurrence risks.** The recurrence risk for pure mtDNA deletions is likely to be very low (<1–5%). If mtDNA duplications are present the recurrence risk is higher.

Respiratory chain defects where the precise molecular basis is unknown.

- **Recurrence risks.** Genetic counselling of this group is extremely difficult as they embrace such a wide group of disorders. In the largest study of Leigh disease recurrence risks were between 1 in 8 and 1 in 4. If, however, a mother carries a mtDNA mutation (which may be unrecognized), then the recurrence risk can be much higher.

Sensorineural deafness.

A1555G is the most common mutation, but usually only causes hearing impairment in early life if there has been exposure to aminoglycosides (e.g. gentamicin). Hearing loss is progressive. A74445G is the second most common mitochondrial mutation (sometimes associated with palmoplantar keratoderma). 7472insC can cause isolated progressive deafness or deafness with ataxia/dysarthria/myoclonus. Overall, mitochondrial mutations are found in up to 30% of families with members affected by sensorineural deafness in two or more generations related through the maternal line, but only 1% of sporadic early-onset non-syndromic deafness. Age of onset of deafness can be very variable (Estivill *et al.* 1998).

- **Recurrence risks.** A1555G is homoplasmic in nearly all pedigrees.

Genetic advice

A major problem for genetic counselling is that the correlation between phenotypic severity and level of mutant mtDNA is poor in many mitochondrial diseases.

Inheritance and recurrence risk
See individual conditions. Offspring of affected males are not at risk.

Variability and penetrance
Mitochondrial disorders often display extraordinary intrafamilial variability, with different family members inheriting different mutant loads.

Prenatal diagnosis
Prenatal diagnosis for mitochondrially encoded disorders should be undertaken only in conjunction with a centre with specialist expertise in mitochondrial genetics. Each mtDNA mutation needs to be considered separately. The available data from studies of human fetal tissues with

mtDNA mutations (White *et al.* 1999*a*) suggest that there is little or no tissue-variation or selection operating on mtDNA mutations *in utero*. Current data therefore suggest that mutant load in a prenatal sample (chorionic villus sampling (CVS)/amniocentesis) does appear to predict the mutant load in most tissues at birth (Thorburn and Dahl 2001). However, the main difficulty lies in accurately predicting the phenotype from the mutant load and, even with expert advice, there may be a high degree of uncertainty.

CVS/amniocentesis may be suitable for women with a low recurrence risk (this approach relies on a woman having a sufficient proportion of oocytes with low mutant loads to have a reasonable chance of a successful outcome). Donor oocyte *in vitro* fertilization (IVF) may be a suitable option for women with moderate to high mutant loads. Pre-implantation genetic diagnosis (PGD) and nuclear or cytoplasmic transfer may become available in the future but are not in routine use currently.

Predictive testing

This can be offered to maternal relatives; however, as noted above, the main difficulty lies in accurately predicting the phenotype from the mutant load. Even with expert advice there may be a high degree of uncertainty.

Natural history and management

No curative treatment is available. Patients should be under the care of a paediatric neurologist or neurologist and/or metabolic paediatrician/physician.

Surveillance

Check ECG and blood glucose periodically.

Drugs to avoid in mitochondrial disorders

- Sodium valproate inhibits several pathways of intermediate metabolism so use with caution.
- Barbiturates (used in general anaesthetics). Avoid since they are inhibitors of OXPHOS.
- Gentamicin may cause sensorineural deafness.
- Ciprofloxacin is an mtDNA inhibitor.
- Chloramphenicol is a mitochondrial translation inhibitor.
- Tetracycline is a mitochondrial translation inhibitor.
- Zidovudine (antiviral agent) causes mitochondrial depletion.

Treatment

There are no specific treatments for disorders due to mitochondrial respiratory chain dysfunction. Early diagnosis and supportive treatment of complications such as diabetes, cardiomyopathy, epilepsy, and undernutrition are, therefore, extremely important. Rare cases of primary coenzyme Q (ubiquinone) deficiency may respond to oral replacement using ubiquinone or idebenone that crosses the blood–brain barrier. Anecdotal reports suggest that patients with complex I deficiency and lipid storage benefit from carnitine treatment and that riboflavin may help some patients with

MELAS and the A3243G. Other forms of supplementation therapy have been tried without apparent benefit. See <www.enmc.org/workshops/reports.cfm?p=122>.

Support group: European Mitochondrial Disease Network <www.netcentral.co.uk/emdn>.

Expert adviser: Joanna Poulton, Professor of Mitochondrial Genetics, University of Oxford, Oxford, England.

References

Brown GK. Bottlenecks and beyond: mitochondrial DNA segregation in health and disease. *J Inherit Metab Dis* 1997; **20**: 2–8.

Chinnery PG, Howell N, *et al.* Molecular pathology of MELAS and MERFF: the relationship between mutation load and clinical phenotype. *Brain* 1997; **120**: 1713–21.

Darin N, Oldfors A, *et al.* The incidence of mitochondrial encephalomyopathies in childhood: clinical features and morphological, biochemical, and DNA anbormalities. *Ann Neurol* 2001; **49** (3): 377–83.

Estivill X, Govea N, *et al.* Familial progressive sensorineural deafness is mainly due to the mtDNA A1555G mutation and is enhanced by treatment of aminoglycosides. *Am J Hum Genet.* 1998; **62** (1): 27–35.

Harding A, Sweeney M, *et al.* Pedigree analysis in Leber hereditary optic neuropathy in families with a pathogenic mtDNA mutation. *Am J Hum Genet* 1995; **57**: 77–86.

Leonard JV, Schapiro AHV. Mitochondrial respiratory chain disorders I: mitochondrial DNA defects [seminar]. *Lancet* 2000; **355**: 299–304.

Mackey D, Howell N. A variant of Leber hereditary optic neuropathy characterised by recovery of vision and by an unusual mitochondrial genetic etiology. *Am J Hum Genet* 1992; **51**: 1218–28.

Mackey DA. Mitochondrial Diseases. In: Traboulsi EI, editor.Genetic Diseases of the Eye. New York: OUP 1998: p 729.

Poulton J, Macaulay V, Marchington DR. Transmission, genetic counselling and prenatal diagnosis of mitochondrial DNA disease. In *Genetics of mitochondrial disease* (ed. I. Holt), Oxford Monographs in Medical Genetics no. 47, Chapter 16, pp. 309–26. Oxford University Press, Oxford, 2003.

Schwartz M, Vissing J. Paternal inheritance of mitochondrial DNA. *New Engl J Med* 2002; **347**: 576–80.

Seminars in Medical Genetics. Mitochondrial diseases *Am J Med Genet* 2001; **106C** (Issue 1).

Thorburn DR, Dahl HH. Mitochondrial disorders: genetics, counseling, prenatal diagnosis and reproductive options. *Am J Med Genet* 2001; **106C**: 102–14.

Van Erven PMMM, Cillessen JPM, *et al.* Leigh syndrome, a mitochondrial encephalo (myo)pathy. A review of the literature. *Clin Neurol Neurosurg* 1987; **89**: 217–30.

White S, Collins V, *et al.* Genetic counselling and prenatal diagnosis for the mitochondrial DNA mutations at nucleotide 8993. *Am J Hum Genet* 1999*a*; **65**: 474–82.

White SL, Shanske S, *et al.* Two cases of prenatal analysis for the pathogenic T to G substitution at nucleotide 8993 in mitochondrial DNA. *Prenat Diagn* 1999*b*; **19**: 1165–68.

Myotonic dystrophy (DM)

Dystrophica myotonica, Steinert disease.

DM is the most common heritable neuromuscular disorder with a prevalence of 1/8000. It is caused by a triplet repeat expansion (CTG) in the non-coding region of the myotonin gene at 19q13.3. The condition is characterized by extreme variability, anticipation, and differential expansion in the maternal and paternal germline.

The normal number of repeats is 4–37 (most common allele is 5 triplets (34%); 11, 12, 13, and 14 are also quite common). Alleles of >30 repeats are uncommon (<2%). Affected individuals with DM have an increased number of repeats from 50 to many thousand. Less than 100 repeats is usually visible as a clear band, but greater than 100 repeats is usually seen as a smear on Southern analysis due to mitotic instability in triplet repeat number. Pathogenic expansions are liable to expand during both paternal and maternal transmission (but contraction noted in ±6%). There is potential for much greater expansion if maternally inherited. Women carrying a DM expansion who are symptomatic or who have clinical signs are at risk for a congenitally affected infant.

Paradoxically 'protomutations' (50–80 repeats) can be inherited stably through females for several generations, but often (70%) result in a large increase into the full disease range >100 repeats if transmitted by males.

The table demonstrates overlaps between the clinical presentation and the repeat size and the uncertainty of predicting the phenotype on the basis of the molecular results.

Congenital myotonic dystrophy (CMD)

The pregnancy is often complicated by polyhydramnios. At delivery severely affected infants are floppy and often have respiratory problems with diaphragmatic hypoplasia and may require ventilatory support. Some severely affected infants may die; the neonatal mortality is 20%. Severe feeding problems may necessitate nasogastric feeding. Infants and young children do not show myotonia. Bilateral facial diplegia and a 'tented mouth' and inability to smile are characteristic features.

Babies who receive ventilatory support through the early weeks/months may subsequently improve and breathe independently and become less floppy. Most will

Overlap between clinical presentation, CTG repeat size, and phenotype

Number of CTG repeats	Designation	Clinical features
4–37	Normal allele	None
38–49	Premutation	None
50–80	Protomutation	Usually asymptomatic or associated with mild late-onset disease, e.g. cataracts without neuromuscular disease
200–500	Mutation	Usually associated with onset in third and fourth decade
230–1800 (mean 830)	Mutation	Childhood onset but not usually congenital
>1000	Mutation	May cause congenital myotonic dystrophy

later have significant learning disability requiring specialist educational support and usually ongoing support in adult life, with few living independently. The South Wales survey reported few deaths between the age of 1 and 20 years, but only half survived to the mid-30s and none beyond 40 years (not many studied at this age).

Some individuals with CMD do not have severe neonatal respiratory problems (although usually a history of slow or difficult feeding is elicited) and present later with developmental delay and the characteristic facial appearance. Myotonia usually has its onset in adolescence and other features of classical myotonic dystrophy are then gradually superimposed.

Clinical approach

History: key points

- Three-generation family tree with specific enquiry for cataracts, diabetes, myotonia, muscle weakness, etc.
- Hands 'locking up', e.g. using can-opener, turning key in lock, holding steering wheel, peeling potatoes. Tends to be exacerbated by cold weather.
- Fatigue (tire easily); may have reduced exercise tolerance.
- Chest infections?
- Palpitations?
- Choking on food/ difficulty swallowing lumps?
- Sleep/sleep pattern. Fall asleep during daytime? Sleep with eyes open? Snoring?
- Gastrointestinal symptoms similar to those of irritable bowel syndrome.

Examination: key points

- Facies. Ptosis; long face with reduced ability to wrinkle forehead, bury eyelashes, or clench masseter muscles; frontal balding.
- Sternomastoids. Test muscle power against hand placed on side of chin. Note sternomastoid muscle bulk and power (both often reduced in DM).
- Test power of wrist extension (weakness and wasting of forearm muscles is characteristic).
- Tap thenar eminence to elicit myotonic contraction.
- Ask patient to clench hands into a tight fist, hold, and then quickly release (may elicit myotonia). Alternatively, ask them to grip hold of your index and middle finger and then quickly release (may take many seconds to gradually unfurl hand).
- Deep tendon reflexes may be normal if mildly affected case, but become difficult to elicit and may be absent in more severely affected individuals.
- Pilomatrixoma. Benign tumour of the hair matrix.

Investigation

- Mutation analysis for $(CTG)_n$ triplet repeat expansion in myotonin gene.
- Electrocardiogram (ECG) looking for heart block.
- Blood glucose (diabetes mellitus).
- Ophthalmology referral if suspected cataract. Otherwise recommend regular surveillance by optometrist/optician.

Other diagnoses/conditions to consider

Proximal myotonic myopathy (PROMM/DM2). An autosomal dominant (AD) condition only distinguished from DM after cloning of the myotonin gene. The weakness is predominantly proximal, myotonia is mild, and muscle pain is a notable feature. PROMM is also known as DM2 and a (CCTG) expansion in the *ZNF9* gne has been found. This mutation should be checked in cases of suspected DM where the expected (CTG) expansion proves negative. Muscle biopsies show preferential type 2 fibre atrophy in contrast to type 1 fibre atrophy seen in DM1 (Vihola *et al.* 2003).

Congenital non-progressive myotonias.

- **Thomsen disease (AD) and Becker disease (AR).** Characterized by impaired muscle relaxation after forceful contraction (myotonia), which is more pronounced after inactivity and improves with exercise. These diseases are similar except that transient weakness is seen in Becker disease, but not in Thomsen disease. Mutations in the *CLCN1* chloride channel gene have been found in both types.

- **Schwartz–Jampel syndrome.** Blepharospasm and skeletal dysplasia. Inheritance is AR with mutation in the perlecan gene *HSPG2*.

Moebius syndrome. The facial weakness in Moebius syndrome is due to cranial nerve palsy (usually VI and VII), but the facial appearance can be confused with that of DM.

Genetic advice

Inheritance and recurrence risk
Inheritance is AD. The risk of having a child with CMD depends on the sex of the transmitting parent and the clinical features in the parent, and CMD only occurs if the fetus inherits a myotonin expansion. See Cobo *et al.* for an analysis of CTG repeat sizes in 124 affected mother–child pairs.

- Risk for CMD in offspring of mothers carrying (CTG) expansion.
  - Mothers with minimal disease and a small expansion size (<80 repeats). In such women the chance of expansion into the CMD range is minimal and the mutation is likely to remain relatively stable.
  - Mothers with neuromuscular involvement and moderate expansion size (200–500 repeats) with no previous children: 10–30% risk of a child with CMD.
  - Mothers with neuromuscular involvement and moderate expansion size (200–500 repeats) with previous child with CMD: 40–50% risk
- Risk for CMD in offspring of fathers carrying (CTG) expansion. The risk of transmission of congenital disease from an affected father is extremely small with only a few reported cases in the world literature.
- Other offspring risks for males.
  - Males with minimal disease and a small expansion size (<80 repeats). There may be a considerable expansion with offspring at risk for earlier and more severe disease (but not for CMD).
  - Males with neuromuscular involvement and moderate expansion size (200–500 repeats). There is a variable outlook for offspring of affected male as mutation could contract, stay stable, or expand.

Variability and penetrance
Affected families exhibit anticipation in their offspring with a tendency to increasing severity in successive generation. Older generations may be minimally affected, e.g. by cataract alone with no neuromuscular symptoms.

Prenatal diagnosis
Possible by chorionic villus sampling (CVS) using triplet repeat (CTG) expansion. This will determine whether or not the fetus has inherited the expansion. Predicting prognosis is more difficult. Most (but not all) infants with CMD have expansions of greater than 1000 repeats, though some at this size will have childhood onset. It is usually possible to distinguish whether a fetus is carrying an expansion consistent with minimal or adult-onset disease or an expansion consistent with a risk of CMD. Polymerase chain reaction (PCR)-based assay to determine size and presence of normal alleles is quick but, if only one normal allele is seen, Southern blotting to determine size of expansion may take 2–3 weeks.

Predictive testing
Chance that a sibling/offspring aged 21–40 years with a normal clinical examination carries a (CTG) expansion is 10% (of which only one-half will have significant neuromuscular involvement). When considering predictive testing in a healthy younger person, due consideration needs to be given to potential implications for children, insurance, and financial arrangements.

Other family members
Cascade approach to family screening is appropriate. Even mildly affected women may be at risk of having offspring with CMD. The risk of CMD in offspring of women (21–40 years old) who are entirely clinical normal on examination is low.

Natural history and management

The age of onset of symptoms is between 20 and 30 years, though the diagnosis may be delayed when there is no clear family history. The impact of the disease can be obtained from a large study of an affected family in Canada where 20% of affected males and 50% of affected females never worked. The disease does not follow a clear pattern and the rate of progress is difficult to predict. In a large Dutch registry study the mean age of death in females was 59 years and in males 60 years. The observed survival to the ages of 25, 45, and 65 years was 99%, 88%, and 18%, respectively, compared with an expected survival of 99%, 95%, and 78%, respectively. Pneumonia and cardiac arrhythmias were the most frequent primary causes of death, each occurring in approximately 30% (de Die- Smulders *et al.* 1998).

In young adults the potential problems to discuss are the following.

- Reproductive issues and fertility. Fertility is reduced in males and females and women have a higher miscarriage rate. There are particular obstetric problems:
  - failure to progress in labour;
  - polyhydramnios, 15%;
  - prematurity, <38/40 13%;
  - retained placenta, 10%;
  - post-partum haemorrhage, 5%;
  - anaesthetic risks (see below).
- Mobility and muscle weakness.
- Gastrointestinal tract; irritable bowel syndrome.
- Consider whether the patient's symptoms could affect driving.

Potential long-term complications
Discuss the benefits of carrying a Medic-alert card with details of the patient's diagnosis.

- **Anaesthetics.** There is an increased sensitivity to sedatives and opiates given as premedication. There is an increased risk for adverse reaction to commonly used anaesthetic agents (e.g. suxamethonium), cardiac dysrhythmias, aspiration pneumonia, and prolonged recovery. Consider regional blocks or spinal or epidural anaesthaesia. If a general anaesthetic is required, it should be given in a hospital with high dependency unit or intensive care unit facilities for postoperative support and monitoring. Postoperatively, patients with DM are at increased risk for chest infections (weak respiratory muscles + sensitivity to opiate analgesia). A preoperative ECG is advised.

- **Diabetes mellitus** due to insulin resistance.
- **Cataract.** Posterior subcapsular cataract.
- **Cardiac involvement.** There is clear evidence of an increased risk of conduction disease, but not of ischaemic heart disease or of impaired myocardial function (Bushby *et al.* 2003). Ventricular arrhythmias are likely to explain some cases of sudden death. Additional investigations should include Holter monitoring (24-hour tape) if annual ECGs show increasing PR interval or other evidence of increased risk of bradycardia. Treatment with a pacemaker is indicated when a progressive arrhythmia is detected even prior to symptoms (Bushby *et al.* 2003).
- **Endocrine** disorder with gondadal atrophy in males, premature menopause in females.
- **Cholelithiasis**.
- **Somnolence.** Excessive daytime sleepiness is typical in advanced disease but may also be a consequence of nocturnal sleep apnoea. Consider referral for sleep studies.
- **Apathy** and impaired cognitive processing are features of advanced disease.

Surveillance

Arrange annual follow-up for all affected individuals, usually with a neurologist or GP. A standardized pattern of assessment is recommended that includes:

- annual ECG with careful assessment of PR interval (30–80% of patients with DM have some abnormality);
- specific enquiry for symptoms suggestive of diabetes and investigation if indicated.

Support group: Myotonic dystrophy support group <www.mdsuk.org>.

Expert adviser: Peter S. Harper, Emeritus Professor of Genetics, University of Wales College of Medicine, Cardiff, Wales.

References

Bennun M, Goldstein B. Continuous propofol anaesthesia for patients with myotonic dystrophy. *Br J Anaesth* 2000; **85** (3): 407–9.

Brunner HG, Nillesen W, *et al.* Presymptomatic diagnosis of myotonic dystrophy. *J Med Genet* 1992; **29**: 780–4.

Bushby K, Muntoni F, Bourke JP. 107th ENMC International Workshop: the management of cardiac involvement in muscular dystrophy and myotonic dystrophy, 7th–9th June 2002, Naarden, the Netherlands. *Neuromuscul Disord* 2003; **13**: 166–72.

Buxton J, Shelbourne P, *et al.* Detection of an unstable fragment of DNA specific to individuals with myotonic dystrophy. *Nature* 1992; **355**: 547–8.

Cobo AM, Poza JJ *et al.* Contribution of molecular analysis to the estimation of the risk of congenital myotonic dystrophy. *J Med Genet* 1995; **32**: 105–8.

de Die-Smulders CE, Howeler CJ. Age and causes of death in adult-onset myotonic dystrophy. *Brain* 1998; **121** (8): 1557–63.

Gennarelli M, Novelli G, *et al.* Prediction of myotonic dystrophy clinical severity based on the number of intragenic $(CTG)_n$ trinucleotide repeats. *Am J Med Genet* 1996; **65**: 342–7.

Harley HG, Rundle SA, *et al.* Unstable DNA sequence in myotonic dytrophy. *Lancet* 1992; **339**: 1125–8.

Harper PS. *Myotonic dystrophy*, 3rd edn, Major problems in Neurology, no 37. W.B. Saunders, Philadelphia, 2001.

Harper PS. *Myotonic dystrophy—the facts.* Oxford University Press, Oxford, 2002.

Martorell L, Monckton DG, *et al.* Frequency and stability of the myotonic dystrophy type 1 premutation. *Neurology* 2001; **56**: 328–35.

Vihola A, Bassez G, *et al.* Histopathological differences of myotonic dystrophy type 1 9DM1) and PROMM/DM2. *Neurology* 2003; **60**: 1854–57.

Zhang J, George AL Jr, *et al.* Mutations in the human skeletal muscle chloride channel gene (*CLCN1*) associated with dominant and recessive mytonia congenital. *Neurology* 1996; **47**: 993–98.

Neural tube defects

Includes anencephaly, encephalocele, myelocele or rachischisis, iniencephaly, meningomyelocele, spina bifida, and spina bifida occulta.

Neural tube defects (NTDs) arise from failure of closure of the neural tube, which normally occurs 18–28 days post-fertilization. The prevalence of NTDs varies considerably from 1/300 (0.003) in Northern Ireland to <1/1000 (0.001) in parts of the USA. The birth prevalence of NTDs was declining substantially even before the introduction of peri-conceptual folate supplementation and prenatal screening, perhaps due to improved maternal nutrition. Infants of diabetic mothers have an increased risk for NTDs with a relative risk of 11.5 (Greene 1999). Folic acid antagonists, e.g. valproate, are teratogenic early in the first trimester of pregnancy (see below). Several studies have shown an increased risk for NTDs associated with pre-pregnancy maternal obesity. In a population-based case-control study, Watkins et al. (1996) found obese women were more likely than average-weight women to have an infant with spina bifida (unadjusted odds ratio (OR) 3.5).

The figures indicate the normal development of the neural tubes.

Of all cases with NTDs, approximately 50% have spina bifida, 40% have anencephaly, 8.5% have encephalocele, and 1.5% have iniencephaly. More females are affected than males (1M:1.3F).

- **Anencephaly** results from failure of fusion of the caudal folds of the neural tube 18–28 days after ovulation (4.5–6 gestational weeks). The forebrain fails to develop and the defect is lethal.
- **Chiari II malformation.** Downward protrusion of the medulla below the foramen magnum to overlap the spinal cord (can cause lower cranial nerve palsies and central apnoea). It is present in >70% of cases with meningomyelocele. Increasing symptoms with age. See 'Cerebellar anomalies' in Chapter 2, 'Clinical approach'.
- **Diastematomyelia.** The presence of a sagittal cleft that divides the spinal cord into two halves, each surrounded by its own pia mater. A bony or cartilaginous spur may transfix the cord, fixing it in a low position as the child grows. The cleft is usually in the low thoracic or lumbar region, but cervical clefts have been reported. In 75% of cases with diastematomyelia an overlying midline skin abnormality is present, and plain radiographs show abnormalities in most cases. These include abnormal vertebral segmentation, spina bifida, and scoliosis.

- **Dysraphism.** Continuity between posterior neuro-ectoderm and skin.
- **Encephalocele.** Outpouching of the brain through a bony defect. Sometimes anterior or lateral, but most are occipital. Occipital defects usually project through an apical defect of the occipital bone or enlarged posterior fontanelle.
- **Iniencephaly/Craniorachischisis.** Developmental abnormality of the skull and upper spine in which the brain and spinal cord protrude through an opening in the occiput and upper spinal canal.
- **Spina bifida.** See figure.
  - **Spina bifida cystica** results from failure of fusion of the rostral folds of the neural tube between days 18 and 28 of embryonic development (4.5–6 gestational weeks). Lesions may occur anywhere along the length of the spine, but most commonly in the lumbosacral region. In a **meningocele** there is no neural tissue present in the cystic lesion; in a **myelomeningocele** the spinal cord is a component of the cyst wall. Hydrocephalus complicates ~90% of cases with lumbosacral meningomyelocele. When an extensive length of the spine is open—the defect is sometimes termed **rachischisis**—there is also usually fusion of vertebrae.
  - **Spina bifida occulta** may include a hairy patch of pigmented or abnormal skin, subcutaneous mass, dimple, or sinus over the lumbosacral spine associated with failure of fusion of the dorsal vertebral arches (usually at L5/S1). As a radiological finding only, in the absence of cutaneous or neurological findings, it is fairly common (~5% of the population) and not thought to confer an increased risk of NTD to offspring.

Isolated NTDs usually have a multifactorial basis, with contribution from environment (dietary folate) and genetic

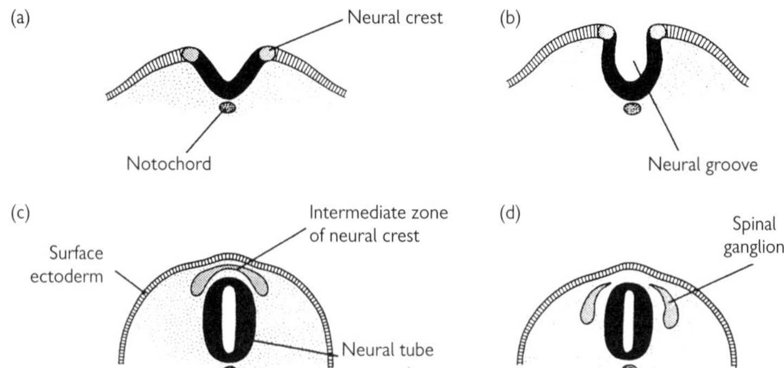

Schematic drawing of a number of transverse sections through successively older embryos, showing the formation of the neural folds, neural groove, neutral tube and neural chest. The cells of the neural crest, initially forming an intermediate zone between the neural tube and surface ectoderm (c), develop into the spinal and cranial sensory ganglia (d).

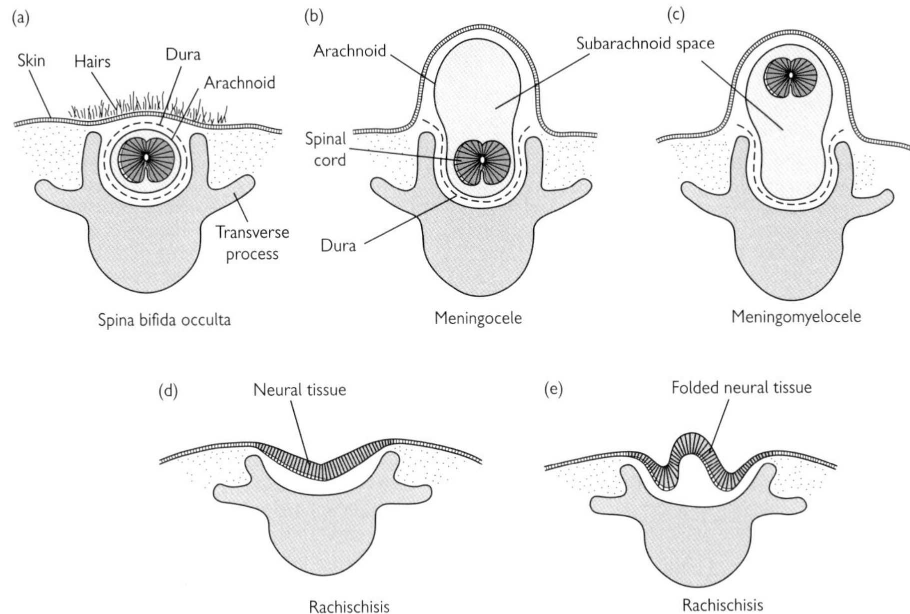

Schematic drawings to show the various types of spina bifida

factors. Several genes are implicated in the elevation of the neural folds. There is considerable variation in the ethnic prevalence for NTD, with rates generally being high in Celtic populations and Canadian Sikhs. Polymorphisms in the 5,10-methylenetetrahydrofolate reductase (*MTHFR*) gene are associated with increased risk of NTD in population studies, but the relative risks are low (e.g. twofold) and mutation analysis is currently not routinely used in the clinical setting.

Clinical approach

Most cases are straightforward and involve an isolated NTD, either anencephaly or spina bifida, or both. Care is needed to ensure that you are dealing with a primary NTD and not one that is occurring as a feature of a syndrome, a chromosome anomaly, or teratogenic exposure. Vertebral anomalies and hydronephrosis are commonly seen in 'isolated' NTDs.

History: key points
- Three-generation family tree with enquiry about still-births and neonatal deaths.
- Enquiry about pre-conceptual folic acid ingestion.
- Detailed pregnancy history including enquiry about drug exposure, e.g. folic acid antagonists, and maternal diabetes.

Examination: key points
- **Affected individual** Try to examine the affected individual or obtain a post-mortem report to confirm that the NTD is an isolated anomaly. Additional anomalies are present in ~20% but, if additional anomalies are found, the possibility of a syndrome or chromosomal anomaly should be revisited. NB. There is an increased incidence of NTD in association with congenital heart disease, diaphragmatic aplasia, and oesophageal atresia.

- **Parents or intervening relative.** Examine for **spina bifida occulta** (hairy patch or pigmented or abnormal skin, subcutaneous mass, dimple, or sinus over the lumbosacral spine associated with failure of fusion of the dorsal vertebral arches (usually at L5/S1)) and enquire about bladder control. A spinal cord abnormality may cause asymmetrical lower motor neuron weakness with wasting, and diminished reflexes in the lower limb, or spasticity with hyperreflexia. Magnetic resonance imaging (MRI) of spinal cord indicates if any of these features are present and counsel as if affected by NTD.

Investigation
- If NTD is the only anomaly, karyotyping is not routinely indicated.
- Karyotype if other anomalies are present.
- X-ray/MRI if NTD is not adequately defined or if any suspicion of occult NTD in parent.

Other diagnoses/conditions to consider

Meckel syndrome. Lethal autosomal recessive (AR) syndrome with occipital encephalocele, bilaterally large kidneys with multicystic dysplasia and fibrotic changes of the liver, and postaxial polydactyly. The kidneys are typically filled with thin-walled cysts of various sizes. In Fraser and Lytwyn's study of 38 secondarily ascertained cases of Meckel syndrome, 100% had cystic dysplasia of the kidney, 63% had an occipital meningocele, 55% had polydactyly, and 18% had no brain malformation. Several loci are implicated, and two genes have now been cloned. These are *MKS1* which has a role in ciliary function (Kyttala) and *MKS3* which encodes the transmembrane protein meckelin (Smith).

Triploidy. Severe intrauterine growth retardation (IUGR), syndactyly. See 'Triploidy (69,XXX, 69,XXY, or 69,XYY)' page 556.

e.g. anticonvulsants (sodium valproate, carbamazepine, phenytoin, phenobarbitone or primidone) or sulfasalazine, triamterene, or trimethoprim. Valproate-induced NTDs predominantly affect the lower lumbar and sacral region.

Genetic advice

Inheritance and recurrence risk

- **Anencephaly and spina bifida.** See table.
- **Spina bifida occulta.** As a radiological finding only, in the absence of cutaneous or neurological findings, it is fairly common (~5% of the population) and not thought to confer an increased risk of NTD to offspring (see above).

Variability and penetrance

In non-syndromal NTD there is *no* tendency for the site of the NTD, e.g. high or low spina bifida, to breed true in subsequent affected pregnancies.

Prenatal diagnosis

- **Ultrasound scanning (USS).** Anencephaly is detectable on USS from 11–12 weeks gestation; spina bifida is detectable with fetal anomaly scanning from 19 weeks gestation; large defects may be visible earlier, e.g. from 13 weeks gestation. Boyd *et al.* (2000) found the sensitivity of prenatal diagnosis by USS in an unselected population to be 98% for anencephaly and 75% for spina bifida. A sensitivity higher than this may be possible when USS is specifically targeted because of an increased risk.
- **Maternal serum screening for alpha fetoprotein (AFP).** Serum screening using a cut-off of 2.5 MoM (multiple of the median) at 16 weeks gestation is a reliable method of screening with a detection rate for spina bifida of 82% for a false-positive rate of 1.9%. It does not detect closed defects (i.e. those covered by intact skin); hence it is wise to use it in conjunction with detailed anomaly USS if monitoring a subsequent pregnancy. It is less sensitive in women taking valproate, which is unfortunate since the risk of NTDs is increased in valproate-exposed pregnancies.
- **Amniocentesis.** Due to the efficacy of detailed USS in combination with maternal serum screening, amniocentesis is nowadays rarely used for the sole indication of prenatal diagnosis of NTD.

Natural history and further management (preventative measures)

If diagnosed prenatally, Caesarean section gives a better outcome than vaginal delivery.

- **To prevent first occurrence of NTD**, women who are planning a pregnancy should take 400 μg daily of folic acid from at least 1 month before conception and continue until the 12th week of pregnancy.
- **To prevent recurrence of NTD**, women who are planning a pregnancy should take 5 mg daily of folic acid from at least 1 month before conception and continue until the 12th week of pregnancy. High-dose folate prevents approximately 70% of recurrences. No known or suspected adverse effects of folic acid at the proposed 5 mg daily dose have been recorded, and it has no contraindications, though women with epilepsy should have their anticonvulsant treatment reviewed.

Where a recurrence occurs on high-dose folate, reconsider whether there is a syndromal association. It is our practice to continue with high-dose folate supplementation in a subsequent pregnancy, but with little expectation of benefit and, therefore, a 10% recurrence risk is appropriate.

Other situations where **high-dose folate** (5 mg per day) may be appropriate include the following.

- One or other parent has spina bifida occulta with a hairy patch or abnormal skin over the lumbosacral spine.
- The mother needs to continue with anticonvulsant therapy during pregnancy.
- Affected second-degree relatives, e.g. mother's sib, may be advised to take high-dose folate (5 mg per day) since this should result in an 85% reduction in their absolute risk which is somewhat increased (1–2% versus 0.1–0.5%), compared with the ~36% risk reduction resulting from the standard 400 μg dose.

Long-term outcome

Hunt and Oakeshott (2003) reviewed the outcome of 117 unselected consecutive babies with open spina bifida who had their backs surgically closed in the immediate neonatal period. Morbidity and mortality were strongly correlated with the level of the sensory deficit; with the best outcome in those with the lowest defects. On review 35 years later, 54 were still alive of the survivors with a sensory level in infancy below L3, 71% had a cerebrospinal fluid (CSF) shunt, 88% had an intelligence quotient (IQ) = 80, 67% were able to walk ≥50 m with aids if required, 33% were continent, 58% were living independently and able to drive, and 38% were in open employment.

Support group: Association for Spina Bifida and Hydrocephalus (ASBAH) <www.asbah.org>, Tel. 01733 555988.

Expert adviser: Jill Clayton-Smith, Consultant Clinical Geneticist, St Mary's Hospital, Manchester, England.

Anencephaly and spina bifida: approximate recurrence risks (%) without folate supplementation in relation to population incidence

Relationship of affected individual to 'at risk' pregnancy	Recurrence risk (%) for population incidence of		
	0.005	0.002	0.001
One sibling	5	3	2
Two siblings	12	10	10
One 2nd-degree relative	2	1	1
One 3rd-degree relative	1	0.75	0.5
One parent	4	4	4

Normal

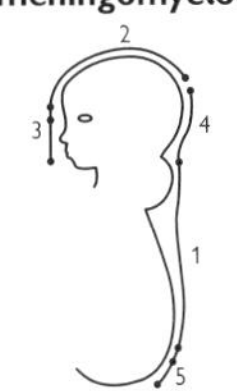

**Lumbar meningocoele
or meningomyelocoele**

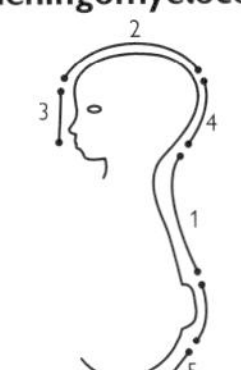

Failure of caudal closure 1

Anencephaly

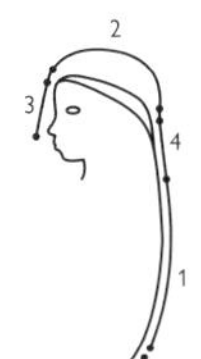

Merocranium. Failure of
closure 2 Holoacranium.
Failure of closure 2 and 4

**Cervical meningocoele
or meningomyelocoele**

Failure of rostral closure 1

Occipital encephalocoele

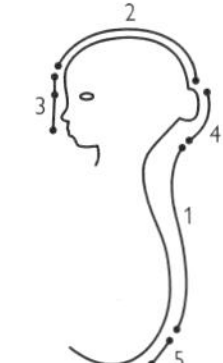

Failure of closure 4

Craniorachischisis

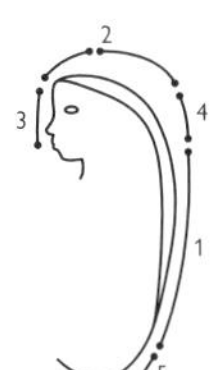

Failure of closure 2, 4, 1

Neural tube defects arising from errors in the multisite closure of the neural tube (modified from Van Allen MI, Kalovsek DF *et al. Am J Med Genet* 1993; **47**: 723–43).

Expert adviser: Jill Clayton-Smith, Consultant Clinical Geneticist, St Mary's Hospital, Manchester, England.

References

American Academy of Pediatrics—Committee on Genetics. Folic acid for the prevention of neural tube defects. *Pediatrics* 1999; **104**: 325–7.

Boyd PA, Wellesley DG, *et al.* Evaluation of the prenatal diagnosis of neural tube defects by fetal ultrasonographic examination in different centres across Europe. *J Med Screen.* 2000; **7** (4): 169–74.

British National Formulary. Department of Health, London, 2003.

Drainer E, May HM, Tolmie JL. Do familial neural tube defects breed true? *J Med Genet* 1991; **28**: 605–8.

Feuchtbaum LB, Curruer RJ. Neural tube defect prevalence in California (1990–1994): eliciting patterns by type of defect and maternal race/ethnicity. *Genet Test* 1999; **3**: 265–72.

Fraser FC, Lytwyn A. Spectrum of anomalies in the Meckel syndrome, or: 'Maybe there is a malformation syndrome with at least one constant anomaly'. *Am J Med Genet* 1981; **9**: 67–73.

Greene MF. Spontaneous abortions and major malformations in women with diabetes mellitus. *Semin Reprod Endocrinol* 1999; **17**: 127–36.

Harris MJ, Juriloff DM. Mini-review: toward understanding mechanisms of genetic neural tube defects in mice. *Teratology* 1999; **60**: 292–305.

Hernandez-Diaz S, Werler MM, *et al.* Neural tube defects in relation to use of folic acid antagonists during pregnancy. *Am J Epidemiol* 2001; **153**: 961–8.

Hunt GM, Oakeshott P. Outcome in people with open spina bifida at age 35: prospective community based cohort study. *Br Med J* 2003; **326**: 1365–6.

Kyttala M, Tallila J, *et al.* MKS1, encoding a component of the flagellar apparatus basal body proteome, is mutated in Meckel syndrome. *Nat Genet.* 2006; **38**: 155–7.

McDonnell RJ, Johnson Z, Delaney V, Dack P. East Ireland 1980–1994: epidemiology of neural tube defects. *J Epidemiol Community Health* 1999; **12**: 782–8.

Mitchell LE, Adzick NS, *et al.* Spina bifida (Seminar). *Lancet* 2004; **364**: 1885–95.

Salonen R, Paavola. Syndrome of the month—Meckel syndrome. *J Med Genet* 1998; **35**: 497–501.

Smith UM, Consugar M, *et al.* The transmembrane protein meckelin (MKS3) is mutated in Meckel-Gruber syndrome and the wpk rat. *Nat Genet.* 2006; **38**: 191–6.

Wald NJ, Law MR, *et al.* Quantifying the effect of folic acid. *Lancet* 2001; **358**: 2069–73.

Watkins ML, Scanlon KS, Mulinare J, Khoury MJ. Is maternal obesity a risk factor for anencephaly and spina bifida? *Epidemiology* 1996; **7**: 507–12.

Neurofibromatosis type 1 (NF1)

von Recklinghausen disease, MIM (Mendelian Inheritance in Man (database)) number, 162200.

NF1 is an autosomal dominant (AD) disorder with a birth incidence of 1 in 2500 and a prevalence of 1 in 4000. The cardinal features are café-au-lait spots (CALs), neurofibromata, and Lisch nodules in the iris (see table). NF1 shows hugely variable expressivity and many of the features of NF1 show age-dependent penetrance.

NF1 is caused by mutations in the *NF1* gene on 17q11.2 that encodes the protein neurofibromin. The *NF1* gene is large, spanning 350 kb of DNA with an mRNA of 11–13 kb and 59 exons. There are three alternatively spliced exons, 9a, 23a, and 48a. The mutational spectrum includes nonsense, frameshift, splice mutations, missense and/or small in-frame deletions, and deletions of the entire *NF1* gene. About 30% of NF1 patients may carry a splice mutation resulting in the production of one or several shortened transcripts (Messiaen *et al.* 2000). For new mutations there is a predominance of paternal mutations but no paternal age effect. About 70% of germline mutations cause trunctation of the neurofibromin protein. One of the main functions of the gene is as a guanosine triphosphate (GTP)ase-activating protein (GAP) regulating 'ras' in the cell cycle.

There is a risk of serious complications arising throughout life and regular surveillance is required to try and detect these at an early time when they are potentially treatable.

Clinical approach

History: key points

- Detailed family history enquiring specifically for other relatives with CALs, lumps, or bumps on their skin, other tumours.
- Previous medical and surgical history (may reveal complications not previously considered to be due to NF1).

- Developmental progress, including schooling difficulties, which are extremely common. Language, reading, visuospatial, neuromotor, and concentration problems are particularly found in NF1.
- Seizures and other neurological symptoms.
- Pain or rapid growth of any soft tissue lesions (indicating possible malignancy).

Examination: key points

- **Growth parameters**. Height (13% have a height <2 SD), weight, occipital-frontal circumference (OFC; 24% have an OFC >2 SD).
- **Skin.**
  - CALs. Examine with a Woods light if fair-skinned;
  - axillary, neck, or groin **freckling** (usually appears at 3–5 years of age);
  - most diffuse disfiguring **plexiform neurofibromata** are apparent within the first 2 years of life, or at least evident by a patch of skin with increased pigmentation;
  - **dermal neurofibromata** appear from late childhood onwards. They are raised and red purplish in colour and may increase in number and size at puberty and during pregnancy;
  - **xanthogranulomata**, small raised yellow lesions often on the forehead that completely disappear in late childhood;
  - some patients with NF1 show a subtle generalized increase in skin pigmentation in comparison with unaffected family members.
- **Facial features.** Some coarsening of the features, or Noonan-like features, may be seen (particularly in those with gene deletions).
- **Spine.** Scoliosis found in 11% and spinal tumours (arrange neurology/neurosurgery opinion and magnetic resonance imaging (MRI) if there are gait abnormalities,

Diagnostic criteria for NF1 (National Institutes of Health Consensus Development Conference 1988)

Criteria	NF1 patients with this feature (%)*
The patient should have two or more of the following features	
1 6 or more café-au-lait spots • 1.5 cm or larger in postpubertal individuals • 0.5 cm or larger in prepubertal individuals	86.7%
2 2 or more neurofibromata of any type or 1 or more plexiform neurofibromata	59.4% (cutaneous neurofibroma), 45.5% (subcutaneous neurofibroma), 15.3% (plexiform neurofibroma)
3 Freckling in the axilla, neck, or groin	83.8% (axillary) 42.3% (groin)
4 Optic glioma (tumour in the optic pathway)	
5 2 or more Lisch nodules (benign iris hamartomas)	63%
6 A distinctive bony lesion • Dysplasia of the sphenoid bone • Dysplasia or thinning of the long bone cortex	
7 A first-degree relative with NF1	71.2%

*Data from north-west England register-based study (McGaughran *et al.* 1999).

spasticity, increased reflexes). If there are no neurological symptoms/signs consider orthopaedic referral for management of scoliosis.

- If patient <2 years old, check for tibial bowing (pseudarthrosis of the tibia is found in 2%).
- **Blood pressure.** Renal artery stenosis especially in those under 20 years; at risk for phaeochromocytoma throughout life.
- **Heart.** Pulmonary stenosis is a feature of Watson syndrome.
- Check visual acuity (VA) in each eye separately and check visual fields (optic pathway gliomas are seen in pre-school years, peak incidence is at 4–6 years).
- Precocious puberty (which if present is usually found in association with a chiasmal optic glioma).
- Document existing soft tissue lesions carefully, and enquire whether any recent change has been noted.
- **Examine parents for NF1.** Don't rely on patient's own assessment; whereas most adults with full blown NF1 are aware of this, segmental NF1 is easily missed.

Investigation

- **Ophthalmology referral** to examine for Lisch nodules (requires slit lamp). Some authorities recommend annual ophthalmic surveillance for optic glioma in children <6 years old (King *et al.* 2003). Lisch nodules are not usually present in preschool children.
- **Cytogenetic analysis.** Dysmorphic facial features, especially hypertelorism, cardiac anomalies, and learning disability, are signs that should lead to the suspicion of a microdeletion at 17q11.2 found in 5–20% of patients with NF1 (Venturin *et al.* 2004). However, Kehrer-Sawatski *et al.* found a significant frequency of mosaic deletions in sporadic NF1 patients without dysmorphic features or MR and suggest that deletion-sensitive analysis e.g. FISH or MLPA should be undertaken in all subjects with NF1 [in whom a mutation is not identified]. The common 1.4Mb deletion incorporates the NF1 gene and is caused by unequal homologous recombination of NF1 repeats, ~30% of deletion patients have a 1.2Mb deletion mediated by recombination between *JJAZ1* and its pseudogene. Recognition is important because of the increased risk of malignant peripheral nerve sheath tumour (MPNST) (de Raedt).
- **Molecular DNA analysis.** Mutation analysis of neurofibromin may be available, and may be especially helpful in establishing the diagnosis in a borderline patient within a family with a known mutation, or in cases with an atypical presentation. Limited availability of testing means that generally NF1 remains a clinical diagnosis.
- **Brain imaging.** Some authorities do not advocate routine imaging because of the high frequency of changes of doubtful clinical significance. The main cause of difficulty is the presence of high signal intensity changes, which are predominantly found in the basal ganglia, thalamus, brainstem, and cerebellum. These are called unidentified bright objects (UBOs). Imaging, e.g. MRI, is strongly indicated in the presence of:
  - a rapidly expanding head circumference in a baby to exclude aqueduct stenosis;
  - focal neurological signs (brain and spinal cord need to be considered);
  - epilepsy;
  - visual problems;
  - precocious puberty or failing growth velocity.

Other diagnoses/conditions to consider

In most affected individuals over the age of 5 years the diagnosis can be made according to the criteria in the table above and is not in doubt. Atypical skin pigmentary changes and unusual disorders of growth can cause diagnostic problems. See 'Patchy pigmented skin lesions (including café au lait spots)' page 210 and also 'Lumps and bumps', page 160.

Segmental NF1. Typical skin changes are only found in one segment of the body. A postzygotic mutation is the cause.

Watson syndrome. CALs, Noonan-like facies, and pulmonary stenosis. Also due to mutations in neurofibromin but these usually cause a mutant protein rather the truncated protein of NF1.

Neurofibromatosis type 2 (NF2). This is less common than NF1 but can cause diagnostic confusion. Approximately 43% have a few CALs (with only 4% having >3 spots and none having >6 in Evans's series). NF1-like cutaneous neurofibromas occur in 27%. There is a high incidence of central nervous system (CNS) tumours. Spinal neurofibromata seen in NF1 can appear identical to the spinal Schwannomas seen in NF2, both radiologically and at surgery. They are distinct histologically, but may need expert review by a neuropathologist for definitive diagnosis. Deafness is a common feature of NF2 due to vestibular Schwannomas, but is rare in NF1. See 'Neurofibromatosis type 2 (NF2)' page 470.

Proteus syndrome. Thickening of the skin on the soles of the feet, macrodactyly, and pigmented skin lesions that look like a linear sebaceous naevus. The lesions are usually asymmetric and may grow rapidly. Germline and mosaic mutations in *PTEN* have been reported, though there is some controversy as to whether these patients have typical Proteus syndrome.

Recessive mutations in mismatch-repair (MMR) genes. Recessive mutations in the mismatch-repair genes *PMS2* and *MLH1* can cause a phenotype of CALs, axillary freckling, subtle generalized increase in skin pigmentation, primitive neuroectodermal tumours (PNETs), non-Hodgkins lymphoma (NHL), and bowel polyps predisposing to bowel cancer. This NF1-like condition has a highly malignant phenotype and follows autosomal recessive (AR) inheritance (Sheridan *et al.* 2003).

Genetic advice

Counselling the parents of a newly diagnosed child, who is fit and well, but nevertheless is affected with NF1, is challenging. It is necessary to balance the possibility of complications and disfigurement with the equal possibility of a lifetime with few difficulties. Parent support groups with their specialist staff can be a great help to families at this time.

Inheritance and recurrence risk

- **Parent affected**. The inheritance is autosomal dominant (AD) with a 50% risk to offspring. The new mutation rate is approximately 50%, although McGaughran *et al.* (1999) found a lower rate of 28.8% in her register-based study.
- **Parents unaffected**. If the parents are unaffected (after careful clinical assessment and eye examination) or the proband is known to have a *de novo* mutation, the

recurrence risk is less than 1%. (Germline mosaicism has been reported by Lazaro *et al.* (1994) in a clinically normal father who had two affected children and was found to carry an NF1 mutation in 10% of his sperm). Note the importance of examining the parents for segmental NF1 as a small but significant proportion of parents are gonosomal mosaics (see below).

- **Parent with segmental NF1.** In individuals with mosaic or localized manifestations of NF1 (segmental neurofibromatosis type 1), disease features are limited to the affected area, which varies from a narrow strip to one quadrant and occasionally to one-half of the body. Distribution is usually unilateral but can be bilateral, either in a symmetrical or asymmetrical arrangement (Ruggieri and Huson 2001). Risks to offspring are generally lower than for parents with non-mosaic NF1 but the exact risk is not definable, varying from <1%–50% depending on the degree of gonadal involvement. Animal studies suggest that the risk is proportional to the percentage of body area involved (Ruggieri and Huson 2001). Overall, a figure of ~5% may be reasonable.

Variability and penetrance

NF1 is fully penetrant. The frequencies of the most common complications are given in the table. Many of the features show age-dependent expression (see table). NF1 shows highly variable expressivity and it is unwise to predict the manifestations of the condition based on the presence or absence of complications in other family members.

Prenatal diagnosis

Possible by chorionic villus sampling (CVS) and mutation analysis if the familial mutation is known, or by linkage in a family with two or more affected individuals if the markers have been worked up in advance and are informative. Within current UK practice it is not often requested.

Predictive testing

Clinical examination of at-risk individuals. The children of affected individuals are seen annually, if there are no signs, to 2 years and then checked once more at 5 years. Genetic testing is possible if the familial mutation is known.

Other family members

Clinical evaluation should be offered, together with mutation testing if the familial mutation is known.

Natural history and management

Potential long-term complications

The lifespan is reduced with a mean age of death of 54 years ($n = 70$) and median of 59 years ($n = 74$). This reduction is almost entirely due to malignant soft tissue tumours. Some complications present at different ages and this can be useful for reassurance.

- **Optic nerve pathway tumours** tend to arise in the toddler or early childhood years. Approximately 15% of individuals with NF1 have thickening of the optic nerve tracts visible on MRI scan. A much smaller proportion of these become symptomatic, but all merit careful surveillance. Clinical progression following presentation occurs in < one-third of patients. Symptoms include loss of visual acuity, decreased field of vision, proptosis, agitation, and behavioural changes with signs including optic nerve pallor, sometimes with fullness of the optic disc. Most follow a benign course, even when symptomatic. However, a small number impinge on the optic nerves causing irreversible blindness and, if involving the optic chiasm, can lead to precocious puberty. Tubular

Frequency of NF1 complications for counselling purposes (data from population-based study of Huson et al. (1989) and (in italics) from register-based study of McGaughran et al. (1999))

Complication	Frequency in NF1 (%)	Risk in NF1	Overall risk in pregnancy of NF1 parent
Intellectual handicap*	33.0	1 in 3	1 in 6
Moderate–severe retardation	3.2		
Mild–moderate learning difficulties	29.8		
Developing in childhood with lifelong morbidity	8.5	1 in 12	1 in 24
Severe plexiform neurofibromata of head and neck	1.2		
Scoliosis requiring surgery	5.2		
Severe pseudoarthrosis	2.1 *(1.9)*		
Treatable complications that can develop	15.7	1 in 6	1 in 12
Aqueduct stenosis	2.1		
Epilepsy	4.2 *(4.3)*		
Spinal neurofibromata	2.1 *(2.1)*		
Visceral neurofibromata	2.1		
Endocrine tumours (e.g. phaeochromocytoma)	3.1		
Renal artery stenosis	2.1		
CNS and malignant tumours	4.4–5.2 *(9.4)*	1 in 20	1 in 40
Optic gliomas			
Symptomatic	0.7		
Asymptomatic	4.5		
Other CNS tumours	0.7–1.5		
Rhabdomyosarcoma	1.5		
Peripheral nerve malignancy	1.5[†] *(8–13)*		

*McGaughran *et al.* (1999) found that learning difficulties of varying severity occurred in 62%.

[†]The median age at diagnosis for malignant peripheral nerve sheath tumours is 26 years.

Features and complications of NF1 showing age-dependent expression

Café-au-lait patches	Infancy through childhood; most have 6 or more patches by 2 years
Sphenoid wing dysplasia	Infancy <2 years
Pseudoarthrosis	Infancy <2 years
Plexiform neurofibroma	Most disfiguring plexiform neurofibromata are evident by 2 years of age
Lisch nodules	Not usually present at birth, 50% by 5 years, 75% by 15 years, 90% by 25 years
Optic glioma	Usually arise in toddler and early childhood years <6 years
Axillary and groin freckling	Childhood
Dermal neurofibromata	Adolescence through adulthood especially during puberty and pregnancy
Nerve sheath tumours	Adolescence through adulthood

expansion of the optic nerves, often with lengthening and kinking, and extension to include the chiasm are highly characteristic of NF1 optic pathway gliomas (OPG). The period for highest risk for the development of OPG in NF1 is the first 6 years of life.

- **Xanthogranuloma and chronic myelogenous leukaemia (CML).** An association has been noted between juvenile xanthogranuloma and CML and >25 cases are recorded in the literature (Morier et al. 1990). Consider haematological surveillance, e.g. 6-monthly full blood count (FBC).
- **Malignant peripheral nerve sheath tumours (MPNST).** Median age at diagnosis in NF1 patients is 26 yrs compared with 62 yrs in sporadic tumours (Evans). Some originate in existing plexiform tumours, but most arise in deep-seated locations e.g. brachial plexus or sciatic nerve. Almost all MPNSTs present with pain or rapid growth. Any NF1 patient with these symptoms should have rapid access to specialist advice and imaging. Risk may be increased after radiotherapy, so radiation treatment should only be used in NF1 patients when absolutely necessary.

Surveillance

Arrange follow-up according to needs of your patient and their family. Options include the following.

- Routine annual follow-up for children with no ongoing problems with a paediatrician:
  - general symptom enquiry;
  - development and schooling;
  - growth parameters (height, weight, OFC) and blood pressure;
  - skin;
  - spine (check for scoliosis);
  - vision (check VA in each eye and check visual fields.)
- Routine annual follow-up for adults with no ongoing problems with a general practitioner:
  - general symptom enquiry;
  - blood pressure;
  - review of skin;
  - reinforce genetic advice as appropriate.
- Surveillance by a Clinical Geneticist for patients with ongoing genetic investigations, e.g. work-up for possible prenatal testing or features that require surveillance by a doctor with experience of NF1.

- Specialist NF clinic for patients with ongoing surgical or complex medical management or diagnostic issues.

NB. In addition, *all* children with NF1 should have annual ophthalmological examinations during the first 6 years of life (King et al. 2003).

Support group: The Neurofibromatosis Association <www.nfa.zetnet.co.uk>; National Neurofibromatosis Foundation (US) <www.nf.org>.

Expert advisers: Susan M. Huson, Hon Consultant in Clinical Genetics, Regional Genetics Service, Manchester, England and Charles ffrench-Constant, Professor of Neurogenetics, University of Cambridge, Cambridge, England.

References

De Raedt T, Brems H, et al. Elevated risk for MPNST in NFI microdeletion patients. *Am J Hum Genet* 2003; **72**: 1288–92.

Evans DGR, Baser ME, et al. Malignant peripheral nerve sheath tumours in neurofibromatosis 1. *J Med Genet* 2002; **39**: 311–14.

Friedman JM, Gutmann DH, MacCollin M, Riccardi VM. *NF phenotype, natural history and pathogenesis*, 3rd edn. Johns Hopkins University Press, Baltimore, 1998.

Huson SM, Compston DAS, Harper PS. A genetic study of von Recklinghausen neurofibromatosis in south east Wales II. Guidelines for genetic counselling. *J Med Genet* 1989; **26**: 712–21.

Kehrer – Sawatski H, Kluwe L, et al. High frequency of mosaicism among patients with neurofibromatosis type 1 (NF1) microdeletions caused by somatic recombination of the JJAZ1 gene. *Am J Hum Genet* 2004; **75**: 410–23.

King A, Listernick R, et al. Optic pathway gliomas in neurofibromatosis type 1: the effect of presenting symptoms on outcome. *Am J Med Genet* 2003; **122A**: 95–9.

Lazaro C, Ravella A, et al. Neurofibromatosis type 1 due to germline mosaicism in a clinically normal father. *New Engl J Med* 1994; **331** (21): 1403–7.

Mc Gaughran JM, Harris DI, Donnai D. Teare D, Macleod R, Westerbeek R, Kingston H, Super M, Harris R, Evans DGR. A clinical study of neurofibromatosis 1 in north west England. *J Med Genet* 1999; **36**: 192–6.

Messiaen LM, Callens T, et al. Exhaustive mutation analysis of the NF1 gene allows identification of 95% of mutations and reveals a high frequency of unusual splicing defects. *Hum Mutat* 2000; **15** (6): 541–55.

Morier P, Merot Y, et al. Juvenile chronic granulocytic leukemia, juvenile xanthogranulomas, and neurofibromatosis. Case report and review of the literature. *J Am Acad Dermatol* 1990; **22** (5, pt. 2): 962–5.

National Institutes of Health Consensus Development Conference. Neurofibromatosis Conference statement. *Arch Neurol* 1988; **45**: 575–8.

Rasmussen SA, Colman SD, Ho VT, Abernathy CR, Arn PH, Weiss L, Schwartz C, Saul RA, Wallace MR. Constitutional and mosaic large NF1 gene deletions in neurofibromatosis type 1. *J Med Genet* 1998; **35** (6): 468–71.

Rassmussen SA, Yang Q, Friedman JM. Mortality in NF1: an analysis using US death certificates. *Am J Med Genet* 2001; **68**: 1110–18.

Ruggieri M, Huson SM. The clinical and diagnostic implications of mosaicism in the neurofibromatosis. *Neurology* 2001; **56** (11): 1433–43.

Seminars in Medical Genetics. Neurofibromatosis 1. *Am J Med Genet* 1999; **89C** (Issue 1).

Sheridan E, De Vos M, *et al*. Recessive mutations in MMR genes are a cause of an NF-1 like phenotype with a highly malignant phenotype and a high recurrence risk. *J Med Genet* 2003; **40** (suppl. 1): SP28.

Szudek J, Birch P. Growth in North American white children with NF1. *J Med Genet* 200; **37**: 933–5.

Vandenbroucke I, Callens T, De Paepe A, Messiaen L. Complex splicing pattern generates great diversity in human NF1 transcripts. *BMC Genomics* 2002; **3** (1): 13.

Venturin M, Guarnieri P, *et al*. Mental retardation and cardiovascular malformations in *NF1* microdeleted patients point to candidate genes in 17q11.2 *J Med Genet* 2004; **41**: 35–41.

Noonan syndrome (NS)

Noonan syndrome (NS) is a relatively common autosomal dominant (AD) disorder affecting ~1/2500 people. It may also occur *de novo* as a new mutation, but caution is necessary in ascribing unaffected status to a parent as the typical facial features in childhood become more subtle with time. A family history is reported in 50% of cases. Many individuals with NS probably remain undiagnosed; it is not uncommon to diagnose several members of a family with the condition once a diagnosis is made in the proband. One gene for NS was identified in 2001 as *PTPN11* on 12q, a gene encoding the non-receptor protein tyrosine phosphatase SHP-2, which is involved in multiple intracellular cascades. The vast majority of *PTPN11* mutations are located in 5 of the 15 exons. All are missense.

Clinical approach

History: key points

- Three-generation family tree with specific enquiry regarding short stature, congenital heart disease, learning difficulty.
- Detailed pregnancy history with specific enquiry for exposure to alcohol and to anticonvulsants (phenotypic overlap with some of the dysmorphic features) and for nuchal thickening/cystic hygroma or polyhydramnios. Birthweight usually normal or increased because of oedema.
- Was there failure to thrive or poor feeding in infancy?
- Detailed developmental history (developmental milestones may be delayed, e.g. sitting at 10 months, walking at 21 months, simple two-word phrases at 31 months; Allanson 2001).
- Schooling.
- History of easy bruising or prolonged bleeding after venepuncture, tooth extraction, surgery.

Examination: key points

- **Growth parameters.** Height (mean height follows 3rd centile until puberty), weight, occipital-frontal circumference (OFC).
- **Face.** Tall forehead, hypertelorism, low-set posteriorly rotated ears with thickened helix, short up-turned nose, deeply grooved philtrum with high, wide peaks to the vermilion border of the upper lip, small pointed chin. Overall the features may appear coarse, particularly in infancy and childhood.
- **Eyes.** Heavy eyelids or ptosis, epicanthic folds, irides often pale.
- **Low posterior hairline and short neck** with redundant skin/webbing.
- **Chest.** Wide-spaced nipples, prominence of sternum superiorly and depression inferiorly.
- **Heart.** 50–80% have a cardiac defect. Most common defect is pulmonary stenosis, but may have atrial or ventricular septal defect (ASD or VSD, respectively), branch pulmonary artery stenosis, tetralogy of Fallot, coarctation of aorta. Hypertrophic cardiomyopathy (HCM) may occur in 20% and may present at birth, in infancy, or in childhood.
- In males examine for **cryptorchidism** (60%).
- **Hypotonia** and **joint hyperextensibility** are common in infancy and childhood.
- **Skin**. Check carefully for café-au-lait spots (CALs). There is some phenotypic overlap with NF1 (Watson

syndrome) and it is important not to miss this diagnosis. Check for lentigines; there is considerable phenotypic overlap with LEOPARD (lentigines–ECG abnormalities–ocular hypertelorism–pulmonary stenosis–abnormal genitalia–retardation of growth–deafness) syndrome.

Investigation

- Karyotype in all sporadic females (phenotypic overlap with 45, X) and all patients with developmental delay.
- Echocardiogram and electrocardiogram (ECG), if not already done.
- Prothrombin time (PT), activated partial thromboplastin time (APTT), platelet count. Thrombocytopenia, platelet dysfunction, and varied coagulation factor defects (factors V, VIII, XI, and XII and protein C) may occur alone or in combination in ~50% of patients with NS.
- Eye examination.

Other diagnoses/conditions to consider

LEOPARD (lentigines–ECG abnormalities–ocular hypertelorism–pulmonary stenosis–abnormal genitalia–retardation of growth–deafness). AD condition. The lentigines are small (<5 mm) numerous dark brown spots mainly over the face and trunk. Deafness (sensorineural) is variable ranging from normal to severe. Allelic to Noonan syndrome and also caused by mutations in *PTPN11*.

Williams syndrome. Microdeletion on 7q11.23, which encompasses the elastin gene (*ELN*). Coronary heart disease occurs in 80%, 75% have supravalvular aortic stenosis (SVAS), and ~25% have a discrete supravalvular pulmonary stenosis. Peripheral pulmonic stenosis is found in 50–75% of infants, but improves with time. The elastin anomaly is generalized and almost any artery can be narrowed, e.g. renal artery stenosis (40%). Aortic insufficiency (20%) and mitral valve prolapse (MVP; 15%) may occur in some adults. Characteristic facial features: infants and young children have periorbital fullness, bulbous nasal tip, long philtrum, wide mouth, full lips, full cheeks, and small widely spaced teeth; older children and adults have a more gaunt appearance with coarser facial features. Developmental delay with very variable mental retardation ranging from severe to low-average with most having mild mental retardation, strengths in language but poor visuospatial skills, overfriendly personality, short attention span, and anxiety. Approximately 15% of infants have hypercalcaemia.

Watson syndrome (NF1). CALs, short stature, mental retardation, and pulmonary stenosis. Due to specific mutations in neurofibromin. These usually cause a mutant protein rather the truncated protein of NF1. Lisch nodules are not seen.

Cardiofaciocutaneous (CFC) syndrome. CFC is characterized by congenital heart defects, a Noonan-like facial appearance, short stature, ectodermal and gastrointestinal abnormalities, and mental retardation. All reported cases are sporadic. Caused by *de novo* missense mutations in three genes within the mitogen-activated protein kinase (MAPK) pathway (Rodriguez-Viciana).

Costello syndrome. Feeding difficulties in infancy and Noonan-like features. Patients with Costello syndrome have a high birthweight and develop papillomas around the nose and mouth. 20% have HCM, and others may have a structural defect and chaotic rhythms. Developmental delay and an increased risk of malignancy are other features (Kerr). Caused by mutations in the *HRAS* gene on 11p13.1 (Aoki).

Genetic advice

Inheritance and recurrence risk

AD. If one of the parents is affected a 50% offspring risk is appropriate. If the NS appears *de novo* and both parents have only possible or no signs of Noonan syndrome an empiric recurrence risk of 5% is appropriate (Sharland *et al.* 1993). If a *PTPN11* mutation is identified and this is not present in either parent, the sibling recurrence risk will be lower (small theoretical risk of gonadal mosaicism).

Parental evaluation should include:

- clinical examination;
- assessment of childhood photographs;
- echocardiogram and ECG.

Variability and penetrance

Features change with age.

Prenatal diagnosis

Monitor for nuchal oedema and polyhydramnios. Pulmonary stenosis is difficult to detect by fetal echocardiography. Lymphatic abnormality with increased nuchal oedema is more common in *PTPN11*. Mutation analysis possible by chorionic villus sampling (CVS) if the familial mutation has been defined.

Natural history and management

Surveillance

- **Heart.** Specialist cardiological follow-up if a heart defect is identified.
- **Growth.** Short stature is a very common manifestation of NS and is accompanied by a variable delay in bone age. Bone age is often delayed by ~2 years. If height is <0.4th–2nd centile refer to a paediatric growth specialist for further management. Mild delay of puberty is common in both males and females, with mean age of menarche 14.5 years. Mean final adult height for males is 162.5 cm (2nd centile) and for females 151 cm (2nd centile). Noonan found over half of the females and nearly 40% of males had an adult height below the 3rd percentile. Some centres may consider growth hormone therapy in children with NS.
- **Fertility.** Normal in females, but may be reduced in males who have had cryptorchidism.

- **Hearing.** Approximately 30% have chronic serous otitis media in infancy and childhood. Increased parental awareness for hearing impairment and low threshold for referral to ear, nose, and throat department are appropriate.
- **Vision.** More than 50% have strabismus and/or a refractive error so orthoptic referral is appropriate in children at the time of diagnosis.
- **Bleeding.** Two-thirds of individuals with NS give a history of abnormal bleeding or mild to severe bruising. The coagulopathy is variable and may be subclinical, cause easy bruising, or cause severe surgical haemorrhage.
- **Development and education.** Early milestones may be delayed (see above). Intelligence quotient (IQ) usually falls in normal range and most are educated in normal school, but 10–15% require special education. Mild mental retardation is seen in <one-third (Allanson 2001). Verbal IQ is frequently lower than non-verbal IQ.

Support groups: UK <www.noonan.co.uk>; US <wandar@bellatlantic.net>.

Expert adviser: Judith Allanson, Professor of Pediatrics, University of Ottawa, Ottawa, Ontario, Canada.

References

Allanson JE. Noonan syndrome. In *Management of genetic syndromes* (ed. S.B. Cassidy and J.E. Allanson), Chapter 32, 2nd edition. Wiley-Liss, New York, 2004.

Allanson JE, Hall JG, Van Allen MI. Noonan syndrome: the changing phenoype. *Am J Med Genet* 1985; **21**: 507–14.

Aoki Y, Niihori T, *et al.* Germline mutations in HRAS proto-oncogene cause Costello syndrome. *Nat Genet*. 2005; **10**: 1038–40.

Kavamura MI, Pomponi MG, *et al.* PTPN11 mutations are not responsible for the cardiofaciocutaneous (CFC) syndrome. *Eur J Hum Genet* 2003; **11**: 64–8.

Kelnar CJ. Growth hormone therapy in Noonan syndrome. *Horm Res*. 2000; **53** (suppl. 1): 77–81.

Kerr B, Delrue MA, *et al.* Genotype-phenotype correlation in Costello syndrome; HRAS mutation analysis in 43 cases. *J Med Genet*. 2006 Jan 27.

Noonan JA, Raaijmakers R, Hall B. Adult height in Noonan syndrome. *Am J Med Genet*. 2003; **123A** (1): 68–71.

Rodriguez-Viciana P, *et al.* Germline Mutations in Genes within the MAPK Pathway Cause Cardio-facio-cutaneous Syndrome. *Science*. 2006 Jan 26.

Sharland M, Morgan M, *et al.* Genetic counselling in Noonan syndrome. *Am J Med Genet* 1993; **45**: 437–40.

Tartaglia M, Mehler EL, *et al.* Mutations in PTPN11 encoding the protein tyrosine phosphatase SHP-2 cause Noonan syndrome. *Nat Genet* 2001; **29**: 465–8.

Parkinson disease

Parkinson disease is a neurodegerative disease characterized by tremor, slowness of movement and difficulty initiating movement, rigidity, and poor postural reflexes. This disturbance of motor function is due to the loss of neurons in the substantia nigra and elsewhere in association with the presence of Lewy bodies (ubiquitinated cytoplasmic protein deposits containing aggregates of α-synuclein) and thread-like proteinaceous inclusions within neurites, also containing α-synuclein (Lewy neurites). It is the second most common neurodegenerative condition after Alzheimer disease with a prevalence of 0.5–1% at age 65–69 years and 1–3% amongst persons of 80 years and older.

Most cases are sporadic, but there are occasional families with dominant or recessive inheritance. There are few patients with clear Mendelian inheritance compared with the number of sporadic cases.

Late-onset Parkinson disease, the most usual form of the disease, does appear to have a familial component. Monozygotic (MZ) twins with early-onset disease have a very high rate of concordance (much higher than for dizygotic (DZ) twins) suggesting a significant genetic component, at least in early-onset disease. Payami et al. (2002) investigated familial aggregation of early- and late-onset Parkinson disease and found that, compared with controls, the age-specific risk of Parkinson disease was increased 7.75-fold in the relatives of patients with early-onset disease and nearly threefold in the relatives of those with late-onset disease. Kurz et al. (2003) in a Norwegian community-based study found a 3- to 4-fold increased risk for Parkinson disease in the families of patients with the disease. Current models favour a rare major Mendelian gene with incomplete and age-dependent penetrance (Maher and Currie 2002).

Nine genetic loci have been reported in the Mendelian forms (*PARK1–8* and *PARK-10*). Rare genetic mutations in α-Synuclein Gene (*SNCA*) result in the aberrant accumulation of this protein, causing toxic gain of function leading to the development of Parkinson disease. Singleton et al. (2003) reported a kindred with a triplication of the α-synuclein gene and showed that elevation in wild-type α-synuclein protein is sufficient to develop the early-onset form of the disorder.

The very rare condition autosomal recessive (AR) juvenile Parkinson disease may be caused by mutations in *parkin* (Lucking et al. 2000). Subsequently, heterozygous mutations in *parkin* have been reported in some apparently sporadic cases of Parkinson disease with onset under 60 years (Lucking et al. 2000) and in autosomal dominant (AD) familial Parkinson disease (Kobayashi et al. 2003). See the table for some monogenic causes of Parkinson disease.

Clinical approach

History: key points

- Three-generation family tree with careful enquiry about who in the family is/was affected and the age at onset of symptoms, treatment given, and age and cause of death.
- Does the consultand have any symptoms of Parkinson disease? If so, refer to a neurologist for evaluation.
- Other neurological features in the affected individual or other family members: especially dementia but also dystonia, ataxia, non-specific tremor, and response to L-dopa (dopa-responsive dystonia (DRD) can present as AD parkinsonism).

Examination: key points

Observe for resting tremor and bradykinesia and other neurological features. If present refer to a neurologist for evaluation.

Investigation

- Consider storing a DNA-sample from an affected member of the family. Mutations in α-synuclein appear to be very rare. Mutation analysis for *parkin* and *α-synuclein* is usually only available as part of a research programme.
- Post-mortem reports are very helpful as the diagnosis is not always accurate in life.

Other diagnoses/conditions to consider

Parkinsonism may be postencephalitic, drug-induced (antipsychotic agents), or arteriosclerotic and these may all cause confusion with the idiopathic or familial forms of Parkinson disease. Huntington Disease in previous generations is not infrequently mistaken for PD.

AD Parkinson disease. See below.

Tauopathies, e.g. frontotemporal dementia with parkinsonism (including Pick disease). The second most common presenile dementia after Alzheimer disease. Mutation in tau gene, AD. See 'Dementia', page 296.

Lewy body dementia. One of the three most common causes of dementia in older people (with Alzheimer disease and vascular dementia). Clinical presentation is

Some monogenic causes of parkinsonism occurring worldwide (after Hardy et al. 2003)

Gene	Inheritance	Disease*	Clinical description				Other	Pathology
			Dementia	Asymmetry	Resting tremor	Response to L-dopa		
PARK1 (*SNCA*)	AD	PD plus DLB* (A53T)	++ (+/no)	+++	+++	+++	Onset typically <45 years	PD plus for DLB A53T
PARK2 (*parkin*)	Mainly AR, some pseudo-dominant	PD, dystonia	No	+/no	+/no	+++	Foot dystonia, sleep benefit. insidious course	Nigral cell loss, no Lewy bodies
FTDP17 (*tau*)	AD	Frontotemporal dementia with parkinsonism)	+++	No	No	No	Disinhibition, especially early	Neurofibrillary tangles

* PD, Parkinson disease; DLB, Lewy body dementia.

typically with fluctuating cognitive impairment, visuospatial dysfunction, marked attentional deficits, psychiatric symptoms (especially complex visual hallucinations), and mild extrapyramidal features (Wilcock 2003).

Dopa-responsive dystonia (DRD; Segawa syndrome). This is a rare condition (prevalence 0.5–1.0 per million), but important to recognize as it is treatable. Onset is usually in childhood/adolescence and dystonia is the presenting feature. Parkinsonism may also occur. Reflexes may become brisk with extensor plantars. The phenotype in childhood may resemble athetoid cerebral palsy and all children with this condition should have a trial of L-dopa.

Inheritance is usually AD with reduced penetrance. The gene *GCH1* codes for an enzyme in the tetrahydrobiopterin pathway. An AR type is due to mutation in the tyrosine hydroxylase gene.

Spinocerebellar ataxia (SCA2 and SCA3). SCA patients present with gait ataxia that is slowly progressive. See 'Ataxic adult' page 50.

AR juvenile parkinsonism. Rare condition presenting at <40 years with no Lewy bodies or Lewy neuritis at autopsy and caused by loss of function mutations in *parkin*, an E3 ubiquitin ligase. Homozygous mutations in parkin are found in ~50% of patients with Parkinson disease in childhood and adolescence but only ~5% of young adults with the disease.

Benign essential tremor. A common disorder inherited as a late-onset AD condition. May be mistaken for PD.

Genetic advice

Inheritance and recurrence risk

An increasing number of genes have been recently been associated with Parkinson disease (Hardy *et al.* 2003). There are a few families with a clearly Mendelian pattern of inheritance (AR or AD) or a defined disease-causing mutation and, in those, counsel as appropriate. For the remainder, advice is based on empiric data.

A threefold increase in risk for first-degree relatives of patients with classical Parkinson disease seems appropriate (Kurtz *et al.* 2003; Payami *et al.* 2002). Given the fairly low prevalence of Parkinson disease in the population, i.e. 0.5–1% at age 65–69 years and 1–3% amongst persons of 80 years and older, the absolute risks remain fairly low.

A 7.75-fold increase in risk may be appropriate in first-degree relatives of patients with onset of Parkinson disease before the age of 50 years (Payami *et al.* 2002).

Variability and penetrance

Penetrance is age-dependent. Factors influencing penetrance are poorly understood.

Prenatal diagnosis

Theoretically possible by chorionic villus sampling (CVS) for families in which the causative mutation(s) has been identified. However, this is unlikely to be requested unless there is a family history of exceptionally early onset disease.

Predictive testing

Theoretically possible if the familial mutation is known and could be offered to at-risk adult members of the family using an approach modelled on the Huntington disease predictive testing programme.

Natural history and management

The early treatment of Parkinson disease involves education for the patient and family, access to support groups, regular exercise, and good nutrition. Dopamine agonists rather than levodopa should be the initial symptomatic therapy (Koller 2002). There is active research into disease-modifying therapies that will provide neurorescue or neuroprotection.

Support group: Parkinson's Disease Society <www.parkinsons.org.uk>, Tel. 0808 800 0303.

Expert adviser: Andrea Németh, Consultant and Lecturer in Clincal Genetics, University of Oxford, Oxford, England.

References

Burke RE. Alpha-synuclein and parkin: coming together of pieces in puzzle of Parkinson's disease [commentary]. *Lancet* 2001; **358**: 1567–8.

Hardy J, Cookson MR, Singleton A. Genes and parkinsonism. *Lancet Neurol* 2003; **2**: 221–8.

Kobayashi H, Kruger R, et al. Haploinsufficiency at the alpha-synuclein gene underlies phenotypic severity in familial Parkinson's disease. *Brain* 2003; **126** (pt. 1): 32–42.

Koller WC. Treatment of early Parkinson's disease. *Neurology* 2002; **58** (4 suppl. 1): S79–86.

Kurz M, Alves G, et al. Familial Parkinson's disease; a community-based study. *Eur J Neurol* 2003; **10**: 159–63.

Lucking CB, Durr A, et al. Association between early-onset Parkinson's disease and mutations in the *parkin* gene. *New Engl J Med* 2000; **342**: 1560–7.

Maher NE, Currie LJ. Segregation analysis of Parkinson disease revealing evidence for a major causative gene. *Am J Med Genet* 2002; **109**: 191–7.

Nussbaum RL, Ellis CE. Alzheimer's disease and Parkinson's disease. *New Engl J Med* 2003; **348**: 1356–64.

Payami H, Zareparsi S, et al. Familial aggregation of Parkinson disease; a comparative study of early-onset and late-onset disease. *Arch Neurol* 2002; **59**: 848–50.

Samii A, Nutt JG, et al. Parkinson's disease (Seminar). *Lancet* 2004; **363**: 1783–93.

Polymeropoulos MH, Lavedan C, et al. Mutation in the alpha-synuclein gene identified in families with Parkinson's disease. *Science* 1997; **276**: 2045–7.

Singleton AB, Farrer M, et al. Alpha-synuclein locus triplication causes Parkinson's disease. *Science* 2003; **302**: 841.

Wilcock GK. Dementia with Lewy bodies. *Lancet* 2003; **362** (9397): 1689–90.

Retinitis pigmentosa (RP)

RP is the most common inherited retinal dystrophy, or degeneration, affecting about 1 in 4000. It is genetically heterogeneous following autosomal dominant (AD), autosomal recessive (AR), and X-linked recessive (XLR) inheritance, and also being a frequent manifestation of mitochondrial disease. Approximately 15% of patients with RP have X-linked retinitis pigmentosa (XLRP), which is a severe form consistently symptomatic in early childhood.

In RP there is early loss of rod function followed by impaired peripheral cone function (causing field loss); foveal cones are affected late in the disease. In RP the loss of rods leads to early symptoms of night blindness and later there is loss of the peripheral visual fields, often starting in the mid-periphery. Examination of the fundus shows pigmentary changes in the mid-peripheral retina.

In individuals with RP impaired visual function is associated with the loss of rod and photoreceptors. The disorder is progressive. Central vision is lost later in the disease.

Note that the following are used interchangeably: rod–cone dystrophy = rod–cone degeneration = RP.

To date, 39 loci have been implicated in non-syndromic RP, for which 30 of the genes are known. Many of these can be grouped by function, giving insights into the disease process. These include components of the phototransduction cascade, proteins involved in retinol metabolism and cell–cell interaction, photoreceptors, structural proteins and transcription factors, intracellular transport proteins, and splicing factors (Hims *et al.* 2003).

RP may be isolated or occur as part of systemic disease or syndrome. This section deals only with isolated RP. For RP occurring as part of a systemic disease or syndrome, please see 'Retinal receptor dystrophies (cone and rod dystrophies, retinitis pigmentosa, and macular dystrophy)' page 232.

Clinical approach

The main issues are to: (1) determine that the RP is isolated, rather than part of a syndrome or systemic condition (for the latter, see 'Retinal receptor dystrophies (cone and rod dystrophies, retinitis pigmentosa, and macular dystrophy)' page 232, 'Clinical approach'); (2) confirm that the diagnosis is valid and determine the mode of inheritance; and (3) assess the risk to other family members and to offspring.

History: key points

- Three-generation family tree, or more if there is a suggestion of X-linkage.
- Age of onset and rate of progression.
- Registered as totally or partially sighted?
- Any variability in severity between males and females (suggesting X-linked inheritance).
- Other medical problems?
- Deafness?

Examination: key points

- Visual fields and fundal examination, if appropriate.
- Features of coexisting conditions (see 'Retinal receptor dystrophies (cone and rod dystrophies, retinitis pigmentosa, and macular dystrophy)' page 232).

Investigation

- Electroretinography (ERG) and full ophthalmological evaluation of affected individuals. See below for advice on carrier testing.
- DNA testing/storage (mutation analysis may be available for the main types of XLRP).

More extensive investigations are required in sporadically affected individuals and children to exclude syndromes and systemic conditions. See 'Retinal receptor dystrophies (cone and rod dystrophies, retinitis pigmentosa, and macular dystrophy)' page 232.

Other diagnoses/conditions to consider

Infantile receptor dystrophies. These are inherited disorders of the cones or rods. The most common are the following.

- **Leber congenital amaurosis** or congenital retinal blindness is one of the most common inherited cause of visual loss in childhood. The rods and cones are lost in the first year, or are dead and non-functional at birth. It is generally inherited as an AR trait but some AD families have been described. Several genes have been identified. It is important to exclude a number of syndromes such as Joubert, infantile Refsum, Senior–Loken, Lhermitte–Duclos, Bardet–Biedl, and Zellweger syndromes.
- **Rod monochromatism or achromatopsia** is caused by degeneration of the cones. The clinical features are poor acuity, nystagmus, early onset of photophobia, and total colour blindness. Mostly AR. Mutations in three genes *CNGA3*, *CNGB3* and *GNAT2* have been identified.
- **Congenital stationary night blindness.** The retina is structurally normal with a normal fundal appearance. Several mechanisms have been described with different genes involved as AD, AR, and XL families have been reported.

Macular degeneration or dystrophy. The rods and cones of the central retina, the macula, are lost to a greater degree than those of the retinal periphery.

Cone-rod dystrophy

Optic atrophy may be hereditary, congenital, or acquired.

Genetic advice

Inheritance and recurrence risk

All forms of autosomal inheritance have been found. In approximately 20% the inheritance is known to be AR, 20% AD, and 15% XL. In 50% of cases there is no family history. Many of these individuals may have AR disease, but some will represent *de novo* AD mutations, AD disease with incomplete penetrance, or X-linked disease. The AR and XL types are associated with more severe disease with an earlier age of onset.

Affected individuals with RP and known mode of inheritance. Discuss:

- offspring risks;
- possibility of predictive genetic testing in large families and/or those with a known mutation;
- prenatal diagnosis only available if known mutation.

Sporadic cases. The following are the *most likely* modes of inheritance.

- Mild disease, adult onset:
  - male: new AD mutation possible but may need to assess other family members;
  - female: could be AD or a carrier of X-linked gene.

- Severe disease of early onset:
  - male: AR or XL inheritance;
  - female: AR inheritance.

XLRP. Two major loci. RP2 (gene *RP2*) at Xp11.23 causes disease in ~15% of XLRP families and RP3 (gene *RPGR*) at Xp21.1 causes disease in ~75% of XLRP families. Some patients with mutations in *RGPR*, which localizes to the photoreceptor connecting cilia, may have more wide-spread ciliary dysfunction, e.g. deafness and recurrent sinorespiratory infection (Zito *et al.* 2003).

The great majority of *RPGR* mutations are predicted to result in premature termination of translation. An alternatively spliced exon, ORF15, is essential for retinal function. Exon ORF15 is a 'hot spot' for mutation harbouring 80% of the mutations found within a series of 47 XLRP patients (Vervoort and Wright 2002). Most *RPGR* mutations are unique to single families.

AD retinitis pigmentosa (ADRP). ADRP is genetically very heterogeneous. Three genes *RHO* (rhodopsin), *RDS* (peripherin) and *RP1* account for 25–30%, 5–10% and 5–10% of ADRP cases respectively (Berson).

Variability and penetrance

In general, the earlier onset the poorer the prognosis. There is often considerable intrafamilial variability. Some families show non-penetrance.

Prenatal diagnosis

Only possible for those with a known mutation.

Predictive testing of apparently unaffected individuals, other family members

- Carrier risk may be determined from the pedigree and female carriers of XLRP can often be detected clinically. Female carriers of XLRP display a broad spectrum of fundus appearance from normal to extensive retinal degeneration. 90% of female carriers have fundus and/or ERG abnormalities.
- Arrange for ophthalmological assessment of at-risk individuals. ERG and other investigations are required to detect the early stages of the disease. Note the age of onset in the family when making an assessment of risk.

If the presentation has been in childhood then a normal examination at age 20 is more reassuring than if the disease is of adult onset.

- May be possible by genetic testing in large families and/or those with a known mutation.
- See guidelines regarding informed consent.

Natural history and management

- **Potential long-term complication.** Progressive loss of vision.
- **Surveillance.** By an ophthalmologist.

Support group: British Retinitis Pigmentosa Society <www.brps.org.uk>, Tel. 01280 860363; Foundation Fighting Blindness (US) <www.blindness.org>.

Expert adviser: Anonymous.

References

Berson EL, Grimsly JL, *et al.* Clinical features and mutations in patients with dominant retinitis-pigmentosa-1 (RP1). *Invest Ophthalmol Vis Sci* 2001; **42**: 2217–24.

Bird AC, Jay B. Diagnosis in inherited retinal disorders. In *Molecular genetics of inherited eye disorders* (ed. A.F. Wright and B. Jay), Vol 2, pp. 53–88. Harwood Academic Publishers, Chur, Switzerland, 1994.

Cremers FPM, van den Hurk JAJM, den Hollander AI. Molecular genetics of Leber congenital amaurosis. *Hum Mol Genet* 2002; **11**: 1169–76.

Fazzi E, Signorini SG, *et al.* Leber's congenital amaurosis: an update. *Eur J Paediatr Neurol* 2003; **7** (1): 13–22.

Hims MM, Diager SP, Inglehearn CF. Retinitis pigmentosa: genes, proteins and prospects. *Dev Ophthalmol* 2003; **37**: 109–25.

Pacione LR, Szego MJ, *et al.* Progress toward understanding the genetic and biochemical mechanisms of inherited photoreceptor degenerations. *Annu Rev Neurosci* 2003; **26**: 657–700.

Rivolta C, Sharon D, De Angelis MM, Dryja TP. Retinitis pigmentosa and allied diseases, genes and inheritance patterns. *Hum Mol Genet* 2002; **11**: 1219–27.

Vervoort R, Wright AF. Mutations of *RPGR* in X-linked retinitis pigmentosa (RP3). *Hum Mutat* 2002; **19** (5): 486–500.

Zito I, Downes SM, *et al.* RPGR mutation associated with retinitis pigmentosa, impaired hearing and sinorespiratory infections. *J Med Genet* 2003; **40**: 609–15.

Rett syndrome

A severe, non-progressive neurodevelopmental disorder that almost exclusively affects females. Prevalence 1/10 000 female births. This remains a clinical diagnosis (see table), although mutations are found in the *MECP2* gene in ~80% of females with features of classic Rett syndrome. Important groups of females with atypical Rett syndrome—less commonly associated with *MECP2* mutations—include those with a congenital onset, often with early seizures, and those with a mild course and developmental stagnation rather than a marked regression.

Located on Xq28, *MECP2* encodes an abundant DNA binding protein that may act to maintain the repression of transcription of inactive genes through binding to methylated CpG groups. The range of phenotypes associated with *MECP2* mutations has broadened since the association between such mutations and Rett syndrome was first reported. The phenotypic spectrum now includes females with mild, non-progressive intellectual disability, those who previously had a clinical diagnosis of Angelman syndrome (AS) or autism, males with severe neonatal encephalopathy, and males with severe mental retardation and progressive spasticity.

MECP2 *mutations in mental retardation*

Females. Mutations in *MECP2* are involved in a broad spectrum of phenotypes from classical Rett syndrome to mild intellectual difficulties. The diagnostic yield in those without features of classic Rett syndrome is much lower. Kleefstra *et al.* (2003) reviewed a cohort of females with unexplained mental retardation and identified 2 mutations amongst 63 girls who had been tested for AS and had negative *SNRPN* (small nuclear ribonuclear protein-associated polypeptide N) methylation studies (~7%). One mutation was found in 92 girls who tested negative for *FRAXA* (~1%), and no mutations in girls who had been investigated for Prader–Willi syndrome and had negative *SNRPN* methylation studies (0%). These results support *MECP2* testing of girls with features suggestive of AS, who have negative *SNRPN* methylation studies. In girls with unexplained mental retardation, additional clinical features should determine whether analysis of *MECP2* is undertaken.

Males. Mutations in *MECP2* have been identified in males with classic Rett syndrome, when somatic mosaicism or Klinefelter syndrome is usually a feature and also in a few males with neonatal encephalopathy. Recently it was suggested that mutations in *MECP2* can cause non-specific mental retardation in males and could be responsible for up to 2% of X-linked mental retardation. Bourdon *et al.* (2003) undertook a careful review of 354 boys with mental retardation and identified only one potentially pathogenic *MECP2* sequence variation (0.28%), suggesting that the true incidence of *MECP2* mutations in males with non-syndromic mental retardation is likely to be very low. Within the group of males with PPM-X (X-linked psychosis–pyramidal signs–macroorchidism syndrome; also parkinsonian features), however, some may be found with the specific missense mutation A140V.

Clinical approach
History: key points
- Perinatal history.
- Occipital-frontal circumference (OFC) at birth.
- Developmental milestones (usually normal for first 6–18 months).
- Age at which concerns were first apparent.
- Loss of acquired skills (usually loss of any speech that has been acquired, although sometimes a few words are retained).
- Seizures.

Examination: key points
- Eye contact.
- Observe for stereotypical hand movements (hand wringing and flapping).
- Observe for periodic ventilation (episodes of hyperventilation and breath-holding).
- Gait. Usually wide-based dyspraxic/ataxic.
- OFC.
- Examine for altered tone especially in lower limbs (tone and deep tendon reflexes (DTRs)).

Investigation
- *MECP2* mutation analysis (detection rate ~85% in sporadic cases).
- If no mutation in *MECP2*, the clinical diagnosis should be reconsidered and further investigations undertaken, especially chromosome analysis and *SNPRN* methylation studies for Angelman syndrome.
- Consider mutation analysis of *STK9* if early-onset infantile spasms (Tao).

Other diagnoses/conditions to consider
Angelman syndrome (AS). Severe mental retardation, rarely with speech, ataxia, dysmorphic facial features, seizures with characteristic electroencephalogram (EEG), stereotyped hand movements, flapping. Birth OFC normal with deceleration; 30% microcephalic. See 'Angelman syndrome', page 272.

Genetic advice
More than 99% are *de novo*, with mutations usually arising on the paternal chromosome. Familial cases are very rare (only five have been demonstrated to have a familial mutation), and have so far always been connected through the female line.

Diagnostic criteria for Rett syndrome

Necessary criteria	Supportive criteria
Apparently normal prenatal and perinatal development	Seizures
Loss of acquired skills, e.g. communication and speech	Abnormal EEG
Normal OFC at birth with deceleration in head growth	Breathing dysfunction with breath-holding and hyperventilation
Marked developmental delay	
Loss of hand skills	Scoliosis/kyphoscoliosis
Stereotypic hand movements	Growth retardation
Social withdrawl during phase of regression	Cold feet
Autistic-like features	Altered muscle tone with muscle wasting
Gait/truncal apraxia/dyspraxia	Bruxism
	Disturbed sleep/wake cycle
	Spontaneous outbursts laughter/crying
	Reduced pain response

Mutation screening of *MECP2* currently identifies mutations in ~80% of girls with classic Rett syndrome. Most screening methods are polymerase chain reaction (PCR)-based and restricted to the coding part of the gene and therefore prone to miss gross rearrangements. Large deletions (at least >1 kb, and often of at least one exon) may be recognized by Southern blot or quantitative PCR techniques and can be found in females with classic or atypical Rett syndrome.

Inheritance and recurrence risk
If a mutation is identified check DNA sample from parents. If *de novo*, recurrence risk is that of germline mosaicism (i.e. very small, but has been described).

Variability and penetrance
90% of affected girls have random X-inactivation. Several apparently normal mothers have been shown to have the same *MECP2* mutation as their affected daughters, but have extremely skewed X-inactivation. In the few familial cases described, less extreme skewing may cause a milder phenotype.

Prenatal diagnosis
If a mutation is known in the proband, it is possible to offer prenatal diagnosis. Since familial cases are so rare, the risk of recurrence needs to be balanced against risks of invasive testing. However, many parents may wish testing for reassurance in a subsequent pregnancy (perhaps by amniocentesis).

Other family members
If a mutation is identified, check DNA samples from sisters, to exclude tiny risk that they are gene carriers (arising from parental germline mosaicism) who are normal due to skewed X inactivation.

Natural history and management
Potential long-term complications
Cass et al. (2003) undertook a comprehensive assessment of 87 females with Rett syndrome aged from 2 to 44 years. Levels of dependency in individuals with Rett syndrome are high. Almost all have fixed joint deformities and scoliosis in adulthood. Increasingly poor growth is another near universal feature in older children. Feeding difficulties increased into middle childhood and then reached a plateau. Improvements in mobility into adolescence were followed by a decline in those skills in adulthood. Despite the presence of repetitive hand movements, a range of hand-use skills was seen in individuals of all ages. Cognitive and communication skills were limited, but there was little evidence of deterioration of these abilities with age (Cass *et al.* 2003). There is an increased mortality rate associated with the diagnosis of Rett syndrome, perhaps related to the autonomic disturbance of ventilation and to seizures. This amount to ~1.2% per annum.

Support group: Rett Syndrome Association UK <www.rettsyndrome.org.uk>.

Expert advisers: Angus Clarke, Professor in Clinical Genetics, University of Wales College of Medicine, Cardiff, Wales, Alison Kerr, Consultant Paediatrician and Senior Lecturer, Department of Psychological Medicine, University of Glasgow, Glasgow, Scotland, and Hilary Cass, Wolfson Centre, Great Ormond Street Children's Hospital NHS Trust, London, England.

References
Bourdon V, Philippe C, *et al. MECP2* Mutations or polymorphisms in mentally retarded boys: diagnostic implications. *Mol Diagn* 2003; **7** (1): 3–7.

Cass H, Reilly S, *et al.* Findings from a multidisciplinary clinical case series of females with Rett syndrome. *Dev Med Child Neurol* 2003 May; **45** (5): 325–37.

Clarke A. Rett syndrome. *J Med Genet* 1996; **33**: 693–9.

Gill H, Cheadle JP, *et al.* Mutation analysis in the MECP2 gene and genetic counselling for Rett syndrome. *J Med Genet* 2003; **40** (5): 380–4.

Kerr A, Witt Engerstron I (eds). *Rett disorder and the developing brain.* Oxford University Press, Oxford, 2001.

Kleefstra T, Yntema HG, *et al. MECP2* analysis in mentally retarded patients: implications for routine DNA diagnostics. *Eur J Hum Genet* 2004; **12** (1): 24–8.

Schollen E, Smeets E, *et al.* Gross rearrangements in the MECP2 gene in three patients with Rett syndrome: implications for routine diagnosis of Rett syndrome. *Hum Mutat* 2003; **22** (2): 116–20.

Wan M, Lee SSJ, Zhang X, *et al.* Rett syndrome and beyond: recurrent spontaneous and familial MeCP2 mutations at CpG hotspots. *Am J Hum Genet* 1999; **65**: 1520–9.

Webb T, Latif F. Rett syndrome and the MeCP2 gene. *J Med Genet* 2001; **38**: 217–23.

Sensitivity to anaesthetic agents

There are two main types of inherited sensitivity to anaesthetic agents: suxamethonium sensitivity and malignant hyperthermia/hyperpyrexia.

Suxamethonium sensitivity
Pseudocholinesterase deficiency, butyrylcholinesterase deficiency.

Suxamethonium (succinylcholine) is a drug used in general anaesthesia to induce to neuromuscular blockade to facilitate tracheal intubation. Suxamethonium is metabolized in the plasma by the non-specific esterase pseudocholinesterase. Normally this happens quickly and the neuromuscular blockade lasts less than 5 minutes. Patients who are homozygous or compound heterozygotes for some pseudocholinesterase (BChE) variants produce pseudocholinesterase of abnormal affinity and reduced amount and metabolize the suxamethonium only slowly resulting in markedly prolonged neuromuscular blockade and paralysis. Artificial ventilation is used to support the patient until the neuromuscular blockade wears off (usually ~90 min after succinylcholine and ~5 hours after mivacurium). Apnoea after suxamethonium can last for up to 3 days in a highly sensitive individual.

Affected individuals are otherwise entirely asymptomatic (although they may be sensitive to cocaine). The condition follows autosomal recessive (AR) inheritance and therefore siblings are at 1 in 4 risk. The gene encoding pseudocholinesterase is *CHE1* on 3q26.1

Various low activity variants are defined on the basis of levels of cholinesterase and degree of inhibition by dibucaine, fluoride, and propan-1-ol, e.g. A, F, K, J (see table). 'Silent' alleles are also found, due to nonsense mutations/deletions in the *CHE1* gene. Using biochemical assays the patient's phenotype can be defined. It is often not possible to ascribe a definitive genotype without performing family studies and therefore usually only the phenotype is reported. Molecular genetic studies may be available in some centres.

The frequency of the atypical variant (A) is 0.017 in Caucasians giving a homozygous frequency of ~1/3500.

Cholinesterase levels can also be reduced in pregnancy, liver disease, and by other drugs. However, any clinical prolongation of effect is small.

Malignant hyperthermia (MH)
MH is a dangerous hypermetabolic state after anaesthesia with suxamethonium and/or volatile halogenated anaesthetic agents such as halothane and methoxyflurane. It affects ~1/20 000 anaesthetized patients and is inherited in an autosomal dominant (AD) manner. MH may also be triggered in susceptible individuals by severe exercise in hot conditions, infections, neuroleptic drugs, and overheating in infants and the overall prevalence is estimated at 1/10 000. The body temperature rises acutely to 40°C or 41°C with muscle stiffness, tachycardia, sweating, cyanosis, and tachypnoea. Hyperkalaemia, acidosis, and hypercapnia alert the anaesthetist as well as the fever. Dantrolene, which decreases the amount of calcium released from the sarcoplasmic reticulum, is an effective treatment that has reduced case fatality from 70% to 5%.

MH myopathy has a variety of clinical presentations including heatstroke, gross rhabdomyolysis after a variety of triggers, a chronically raised serum creatine kinase (CK), muscle pain, neuroleptic malignant syndrome, and sudden infant death.

The inherited abnormalities in MH-susceptible individuals lie in the regulation of myoplasmic Ca. Malignant hyperpyrexia is triggered by a rapid, sustained rise in myoplasmic Ca. Ryanodine, a plant alkaloid that effects Ca release from the sarcoplasmic reticulum (the main store for intracellular Ca), binds to a skeletal muscle calcium release channel, the ryanodine receptor (RYR). Approximately 20–40% of families with MH have mutations in *RYR1*. MH appears to be genetically heterogeneous.

Four clinical myopathies that predispose to MH have been defined:

- **Evans myopathy.** By far the most common myopathy predisposing to MH, also known as MH myopathy. It follows AD inheritance. Usually subclinical, but some muscle wasting may occur especially in the lower thigh. Serum CK may be raised, but is often normal. Muscle histology is non-specific and variable.

- **King–Denborough syndrome.** Very rare myopathy found in children, usually boys. Unusual facies, low set-ears, ptosis, short stature, thoracic kyphosis, and lumbar lordosis and pectus carinatum. Inheritance uncertain, possibly AR.

- **Central-core disease (CCD).** All members of a family in which central-core disease has been diagnosed should be regarded as susceptible to MH. Histochemistry shows striking non-staining lesions extending along type 1 fibres, and there is often type 1 atrophy.

- **Minicore myopathy.** Some patients have mutations in *RYR1*.

Classification of pseudocholinesterase variants by biochemical phenotype, genotype, and clinical sensitivity to suxamethonium*

Phenotype	Genotype	Sensitivity
U, Usual	U/U, U/S, U/J, U/K, U/A, U/F	Normal
K, Kalow (66% activity)(common)	A/K	Occasionally increased
J, J variant (33% activity)	A/J	Moderately increased
F, Fluoride-resistant (rare except in Africans)	F/F, F/S, A/F	Moderately increased
A, Atypical (dibucaine-resistant)	A/A, A/S	Markedly increased
S, Silent (no activity)	S/S	Extremely increased

* K is in strong linkage disequilibrium with A and is present in most A and J variants, reducing enzyme activity without changing its affinity. The designation AK is often used. ~90% of atypical cholinesterase gene variants are AK and only ~10% are A.

Clinical approach

History: key points

- Three-generation family tree with specific enquiry about anaesthaesia.
- Detailed history from the proband regarding experience following anaesthaesia.
- For MH enquire specifically about muscle pains after exercise or episodes of rhabdomyolysis (myoglobinuria).

Investigation

- 5 ml EDTA (ethylenedinitrilotetraacetate) sample for molecular genetic analysis if available (e.g. *CHE1* in suxamethonium sensitivity or *RYR1* in MH).
- For suxamethonium sensitivity, 1–2 ml serum or heparinized plasma (the sample should not be taken in the immediate postoperative period).
- For MH measure plasma CK.
- For MH consider *in vitro* contracture test (increased contractility of skeletal muscle in response to halothane and to caffeine). This provides a specific test to identify susceptibility to MH, but requires a muscle biopsy. Molecular genetic analysis is far more accurate, when available.

Genetic advice

Inheritance and recurrence risk

- **Suxamethonium sensitivity.** AR, with 25% risk to siblings.
- **MH.** AD, 50% risk to offspring of an affected individual.

Other family members

- **Suxamethonium sensitivity.** All siblings should be tested biochemically (and molecularly if available). Parents should also be tested, both to help define the phenotypes and also because the relatively high carrier rate in Caucasians means there is a small chance they too could be affected.
- **MH.** Parents and offspring should be offered *in vitro* muscle testing if an *RYR1* mutation that would enable predictive genetic testing is not identified within a short time.

Natural history and management

Individuals with suxamethonium sensitivity and susceptibility to MH should carry a laminated warning card and consider wearing a Medic-Alert bracelet.

Expert adviser: Gilbert Park, Director of Intensive Care Research, Addenbrooke's Hospital, Cambridge, England.

References

Cerf C, Mesguish M, *et al.* Screening patients with prolonged neuromuscular blockade after succinylcholine and mivacurium. *Anesth Analg* 2002; **94**: 461–6.

Denborough M. Malignant hyperthermia. *Lancet* 1998; **352**: 1131–6.

Girard T, Urwyler A, *et al.* Genotype–phenotype comparison of the Swiss malignant hyperthermia population. *Hum Mutat* 2001; **18**: 357–8.

Robinson R, Hopkins P, *et al.* Several interacting genes influence the malignant hyperthermia phenotype. *Hum Genet* 2003; **112**: 217–18.

Schriver CR, Beaudet AL, Sly WS and Valle D (Eds). Metabolic Basis of Inherited Diseases Chapter 4. *Pharmacogenetics* pp303–09.

Spinal muscular atrophy (SMA)

SMA is an autosomal recessive (AR) disorder characterized by symmetrical proximal muscle weakness as a consequence of degeneration of the anterior horn cells of the spinal cord. Three classical types are recognized (see below) but these are somewhat arbitrary and there is, in fact, a continuum of clinical severity. Intelligence is unaffected.

- **Type I SMA: severe (Werdnig–Hoffmann).** Onset of severe muscle weakness and hypotonia in the first few months of life; never able to sit or walk. Fatal respiratory failure usually occurs by age 2 years and often before 6 months of age. Nearly all present by 6 months and in one-third abnormal fetal movements are reported.
- **Type II SMA: intermediate.** Onset before 18 months of age (median age 8 months). Ability to sit but not to walk unaided; survival into adult life is usual.
- **Type III SMA: mild (Kugelberg–Welander).** Onset of proximal muscle weakness after 2 years, ability to walk independently initially; survival into adult life.

In addition to the three classical types there is the following.

- **Type 0 SMA.** A severe form of SMA that is usually fatal in the first months of life. These children present with arthrogryposis multiplex congenita and respiratory compromise. Approximately 50% have homozyous SMN1 deletions; the remainder are not linked to 5q of which some have mutations in the gene for infantile SMA with respiratory distress type 1 (SMARD1) which is *IGHMBP2* on chromosome 11q13 (Grohmann *et al.* 2003).

In type I SMA, the absence or dysfunction of *SMN1* is reflected in enhanced neuronal death that is already detectable by 12 weeks gestation. This is associated with a progressive loss of motor neurons towards the neonatal period. The combined birth incidence or early childhood prevalence of all types of SMA is ~1/10 000. All three types are associated with deletions and small intragenic mutations in the survival motor neuron gene *SMN1* on 5q13. Wirth (2000) found that 94% of individuals with clinically typical SMA were homozygous for an exon 7 deletion of *SMN1*, and some of the remaining 6% had one deletion allele and one intragenic mutation. The proportion of disease alleles with SMN1 deletions is highest in type I and lowest in type III. Of individuals with SMA of all three classical types who have identifiable *SMN1* mutations, 98% of disease alleles were exon 7 deletions and 2% were small intragenic mutations.

Carrier rate is estimated at 1/50. Most carriers have only one copy of *SMN1*. However, some unaffected individuals have two copies of *SMN1* on one chromosome 5 and no copies on the homologue, complicating carrier detection by dosage analysis. Approximately 7% of unaffected individuals without a family history of SMA have 3 or 4 copies of SMN1, suggesting that the 2-copy allele is not uncommon (estimated at 3.3% of *SMN1* alleles overall).

SMN2 (*SMNc*) is highly homologous to its centromeric neighbour *SMN1* (*SMNt*) and is one factor underlying the variable phenotype of SMA. Individuals with type III SMA have, on average, more copies of *SMN2* than those with type II or type I disease. However, ~5% of normal individuals lack both copies of *SMN2*. There are occasional case reports of asymptomatic individuals with homozygous *SMN1* deletions—most have an affected sibling and it is likely that the variable severity reflects variable copy number of *SMN2* amongst other factors, and that mild SMA may develop eventually.

The *SMN1/SMN2* gene cluster is prone to gene conversion (a non-reciprocal recombination process that results in an alteration of the sequence of a gene to that of its homologue).

Distal SMA encompasses a heterogeneous group of neuromuscular disorders caused by progressive anterior horn cell degeneration and characterized by progressive motor weakness and muscular atrophy, predominantly in the distal parts of the limbs. One AR variety maps to 11q13.

Clinical approach

History: key points

- Three-generation family tree with specific enquiry about consanguinity, SMA, and unexplained infant deaths.
- Pregnancy history (reduced fetal movements late in pregnancy?) and delivery.
- Development milestones.
- Subsequent progress. Age of onset of symptoms, loss of mobility, scoliosis, etc.?
- Current level of function.

Examination: key points

- **Infant.** Assess posture. Infants with type I SMA often lie in a 'frog-leg' posture due to weakness of hip girdle muscles. Assess tone (floppy); look for spontaneous movement. Typically, there is preservation of extra-ocular movement and small movements of the fingers and toes, but absence of large movements of the limbs. Poor or absent kick with weak or absent withdrawl of the limb in response to pain. Facial muscles are involved, but usually there is some preservation of facial expression. Look carefully for fasciculation. Deep tendon reflexes (DTRs) are ususally absent in types 0 and I.
- **Child/adult.** Careful neurological examination to confirm diagnosis. DTRs may be diminished rather than absent in types II and III. May present with delayed motor milestones or proximal muscle weakness (Gower's manoeuvre).

Investigation

- EDTA (ethylenedinitrilotetraacetate) sample for *SMN1* deletion assay (and mutation analysis).
- Creatine kinase (CK) to exclude a muscular dystrophy, unless proven molecular diagnosis of SMA.

Other diagnoses/conditions to consider

See 'Floppy infant' page 118.

Genetic advice

A result showing that an individual with clinically typical SMA is homozygously deleted for SMN1 confirms the diagnosis. Approximately 3.6% of patients with SMN1-related SMA will be compound heterozygotes for an SMN1 deletion and an intragenic mutation.

There is some genetic heterogeneity in SMA and Wirth *et al.* (1999) calculated that, in ~1.9% of type I, 1.6% of type II, and 13% of type III patients with typical SMA including electromyography (EMG) and muscle biopsy results, genes other than SMN1 are likely to be responsible.

Inheritance and recurrence risk
AR for all except distal SMA which may be AD, AR, or X-linked (?).

NB. A *de novo* deletion occurs in ~1.7% of individuals with SMA. Carrier testing of parents is important as this will have an important effect on recurrence risk and on the counselling and testing of other family members.

Variability and penetrance
Usually the type of SMA will be consistent within sibships, but with some variability. Within wider families, any type of SMA may occur, i.e. if counselling the uncle of a child who died from SMA type I, the risk that he will have a child with SMA *of any type* will be $(1/2 \times 1/50 \times 1/4 = 1/400)$ assuming no consanguinity and negative family history in his partner.

Prenatal diagnosis
Possible by chorionic villus sampling (CVS) at 11 weeks gestation if mutational basis of the SMA in the family is known. Need to genotype both parents prior to CVS.

Carrier testing
If an individual at population risk (negative family history) has 2 copies of SMN1 on carrier testing, the residual probability that he/she is a carrier is 1/820. If an unaffected sibling of an individual with a homozygous SMN deletion has two copies, the chance that he/she is a carrier reduces from 2/3 to 1/13 (but could be reduced to negligible if it were known that both parents were single-copy carriers).

Other family members
Cascade carrier testing can be offered and is especially important if there is consanguinity.

Natural history and management

Type I SMA. Conventionally, infants with a confirmed diagnosis of SMA type I have been offered palliative and terminal care via hospital and community paediatric teams. A recent publication from the US (Bach *et al.* 2000) challenged this approach showing that long-term ventilation with feeding and physiotherapy support has resulted in prolonged survival (although no improvement in neuromuscular function). Intercurrent chest colds may necessitate periods of hospitalization and intubation, but Bach *et al.* (2000) found in a small retrospective series of 11 children that tracheostomy can be avoided throughout early childhood in some children with SMA type I. Cognitive development in SMA is normal.

Type II SMA.
- **Impaired mobility.** Patients require specialized physiotherapy and seating input appropriate to the level of disability. Although SMA is said to be a non-progressive disease, many patients do notice a deterioration of mobility with time.

- **Feeding difficulty.** Patients with type II SMA are at risk of feeding difficulties, e.g. aspiration, which may manifest as recurrent chest infections,and some may require gastrostomy feeding.
- **Respiratory insufficiency.** Some may experience progressive respiratory failure (a severe scoliosis may exacerbate this) and ultimately may require assisted nocturnal ventilation.
- **Scoliosis.** Monitoring of scoliosis and appropriate intervention is important in preserving respiratory function in patients with type II SMA, all of whom have pronounced weakness of trunk muscles.
- **Cognitive function.** In von Gontard *et al.*'s (2002) study, environmentally mediated aspects of intelligence were higher in adolescent patients with SMA than in controls.
- **Pregnancy.** Successful pregnancy has been reported in women with SMA type II. Pulmonary function may remain stable throughout pregnancy, although it may deteriorate temporarily after delivery.

Type III SMA. The complications listed under type II SMA are much less common in type III.

Support group: The Jennifer Trust <www.jtsma.org.uk>.

Expert adviser: Kate Bushby, Action Research Professor in Neuromuscular Genetics, Institute of Human Genetics, Newcastle upon Tyne, England.

References
Bach JR, Niranjan V, *et al.* Spinal muscular atrophy type 1: a noninvasive respiratory management approach. *Chest* 2000; **117**: 1100–5.

Emery AEH. Population frequencies of inherited neuromuscular diseases—a world survey. *Neuromuscul Disord* 1991; **1**: 19–29.

Grohmann K, Varon R, *et al.* Infantile spinal muscular atrophy with respiratory distress type 1 (SMARD1). *Ann Neurol* 2003; **54**: 719–24.

Munsat TL, Davies KE. International SMA consortium meeting. *Neuromuscul Disord* 1992; **2**: 423–8.

Ogino S, Leonard DGB, *et al.* Genetic risk assessment in carrier testing for spinal muscular atrophy. *Am J Med Genet* 2002; **110**: 301–7.

Rudnik-Schoneborn S, Breuer C, Zerres K. Stable motor and lung function throughout pregnancy in a patient with infantile spinal muscular atrophy type II. *Neuromuscul Disord* 2002; **12**: 137–40.

von Gontard A, Zerres K, *et al.* Intelligence and cognitive function in children and adolescents with spinal muscular atrophy. *Neuromuscul Disord* 2002; **12**: 130–6.

Wirth B. An update on the mutation spectrum of the survival motor neuron gene (SMN1) in autosomal recessive spinal muscular atrophy (SMA). *Hum Mutat* 2000; **15**: 228–37.

Wirth B, Herz M, *et al.* Quantitative analysis of survival motor neuron copies: identification of subtle SMN1 mutations in patients with spinal muscular atrophy, genotype–phenotype correlation, and implications for genetic counselling. *Am J Hum Genet* 1999; **64**: 1340–56.

Stickler syndrome

Hereditary arthro-ophthalmopathy.

Stickler syndrome is a dominantly inherited disorder of collagen, resulting in a congenital vitreous gel anomaly, myopia, variable orofacial features, deafness, and arthropathy. It affects approximately 1/10 000 individuals, but the frequent experience of diagnosing several family members once the diagnosis is made in the proband suggests that the condition is underdiagnosed. The major risk is of retinal detachment, particularly through a giant tear, which can occur at any age. In Stickler *et al.*'s (2001) survey of 316 patients, 95% had eye problems (retinal detachment in 60%, myopia in 90%, blindness in 4%), 84% had problems with facial structure such as a flat face, small mandible, or cleft palate, 70% had hearing loss, and 90% had joint problems, primarily laxity and early joint pain from degenerative joint disease. See the table for proposed diagnostic criteria.

The condition exhibits wide inter- and intrafamilial variability. Clefts in Stickler syndrome may be submucous or wide U-shaped, or narrow V-shaped.

Type II collagen (a homotrimer of *COL2A1*) is present in both cartilage and the vitreous of the eye. Mutations in genes encoding the alpha 1 chain of type II collagen (*COL2A1*) and the A1 chain of type XI collagen (*COL11A1*) cause type I (STL1) and type 2 (STL2) Stickler syndrome respectively and the majority of patients exhibit the former. Exon 2 of the *COL2A1* gene is alternatively spliced and primarily expressed in the eye, so that exon 2 mutations result in a predominantly 'ocular only' phenotype with minimal systemic manifestations. In these cases, the diagnosis may easily be overlooked without vitreous examination. A third subgroup (non-ocular Stickler syndrome, OSMED (otospondylomegaepiphyseal dysplasia), STL3) is caused by mutations in the gene encoding the alpha 2 chain of type XI collagen, which is not expressed in the eye (*COL11A2*).

Clinical approach

History: key points

Three-generation family tree with specific reference to congenital or early-onset myopia, retinal detachment, deafness, joint laxity in youth, premature arthritis in 3rd–4th decade, hip and knee problems, and cleft palate.

Examination: key points

- Facial features. Flat midface with a depressed nasal bridge, reduced nasal protrusion, anteverted nares, and micrognathia (most evident in childhood and becoming less distinctive with age).

Proposed diagnostic criteria for Stickler syndrome (after Snead and Yates 1999)

Congenital vitreous anomaly plus any of:

1 Myopia with onset before 6 years

2 Rhegmatogenous retinal detachment or paravascular pigmented lattice degeneration

3 Joint hypermobility with abnormal Beighton score ± radiological evidence of joint degeneration

4 Audiometric confirmation of sensorineural hearing defect

5 Midline clefting

6 First-degree relative with a diagnosis of Stickler syndrome (i.e. meeting above diagnostic criteria)

* A tear or hole in the retina allows fluid from the vitreous cavity to seep beneath the retina.

- Myopia.
- Examine palate. Submucous cleft often undiagnosed; 25% have a palatal anomaly.
- Joint hypermobility including hyperextensibility of knees and elbows (abnormal Beighton score).
- Habitus. Slender extremities, long fingers, and normal height.

Investigation

- Ophthlamological assessment by vitreoretinal specialist.
- Audiometry very useful to pick up high-tone loss—patients frequently asymptomatic.
- DNA for COL2A1 mutation analysis (congenital 'membranous' anomaly of the vitreous or 'afibrillar' vitreous gel) or COL11A1 ('beaded' vitreous phenotype).

Other diagnoses/conditions to consider

Perthes disease. Perthes disease of the hip can occur in families segregating in an apparently autosomal dominant (AD) fashion with incomplete and variable penetrance. Exclude other familial causes of a dysplastic femoral head, such as multiple epiphyseal dysplasia (MED).

SEDC (spondyloepiphyseal dysplasia congenita). Patients are very small with a short trunk and marked lordosis. Myopia, cleft palate, and deafness can occur. Onset is at birth, but severe short stature may not be obvious until 2–3 years of age. In infancy the vertebral bodies are ovoid or pear-shaped but later platyspondyly with irregular endplates develops. Odontoid hypoplasia may be a problem. Bone age is markedly delayed and the epiphyses are flattened and fragmented. The capital femoral epiphysis is severely affected. Caused by mutations in *COL2A1*.

Kniest dysplasia. AD condition with myopia, macrocephaly, platyspondyly, joint enlargement and limitation, lordosis, and atlanto-axial instability.

OSMED (STL3). Otospondylomegaepiphyseal dysplasia also known as Weissenbacher–Zweymüller syndrome. Eyes are normal. Mutations in *COL11A1*.

Wagner hereditary vitreoretinopathy/erosive retinopathy appears predominantly 'ocular' with minimal systemic involvement. AD eye disorder resembling Stickler but with nyctalopia and with less common retinal detachment.

Marshall syndrome. The original pedigree is still unlinked to any known gene. Most 'Marshalls syndrome' in the literature, based on facial features, would appear to probably be type 2 Stickler syndrome.

Genetic advice

Inheritance and recurrence risk

AD. 50% risk to offspring of affected individuals.

Variability and penetrance

Wide inter- and intrafamilial variability.

Prenatal diagnosis

Technically feasible in families with a known mutation, but rarely requested.

Predictive testing
Prophylactic retinopexy is appropriate to reduce the risk of retinal detachment. Predictive testing could be used in families with a known mutation to target this more effectively.

Other family members
All first-degree relatives should be examined and offered an expert eye assessment.

Natural history and management

Potential long-term complications
- **Eye.** Moderate/severe myopia (>–5 D) is common and, in combination with the abnormal vitreous, can result in retinal detachment. Prophylactic retinopexy should be considered in types 1 and 2 Stickler syndrome. There is also an increased risk for cataract and glaucoma.
- **Ear.** Conductive loss due to glue-ear is common in young children with Stickler, particularly those with cleft palate. Szymko-Bennett *et al.* (2001) found some sensorineural hearing loss in 60% of adult patients with Stickler. It is milder in type 1 Stickler than in type 2 and generally no more progressive than age-related loss.
- **Joint.** Joint discomfort from degenerative joint disease is a problem for many Stickler patients in adult life. In one study 80% of adults had chronic hip pain. 16% had a history of abnormal development of the femoral head in childhood.

Surveillance
Periodic (at least annual) ophthalmological review from infancy.

Support group: The Stickler syndrome support group <www.sticklers.org>.

Expert adviser: Martin Snead, Consultant Ophthalmologist, Addenbrooke's Hospital, Cambridge, England.

References
Richards AJ, Scott JD, Snead MP. Molecular genetics of rhegmatogenous retinal detachment. *Eye* 2002; **16**: 388–92.

Snead MP, Yates JRW. Clinical and molecular genetics of Stickler syndrome. *J Med Genet* 1999; **5**: 353–9.

Stickler GB, Hughes W, *et al.* Clinical features of hereditary progressive arthro-ophthalmopathy (Stickler syndrome): a survey. *Genet Med* 2001; **3**: 192–6.

Szymko-Bennett YM, Mastroianni MA, *et al.* Auditory dysfunction in Stickler syndrome. *Arch Otolaryngol Head Neck Surg* 2001; **127**: 1061–8.

Wilkin DJ, Liberfarb RM, *et al.* Stickler syndrome. In *Management of genetic syndromes* (ed. S.B. Cassidy and J.E. Allanson), Chapter 24, pp. 405–16. Wiley-Liss, New York, 2001.

Thrombophilia

Individuals with thrombophilia have blood that clots more easily than normal. In the normal state there is a balance between the natural clotting and anticoagulant systems. Both of these systems may be affected by either inherited or acquired (including both intrinsic and environmental) defects. The most common manifestation of thrombophilia is venous thrombosis. The incidence of venous thrombosis is about 1 per 1000 person-years. In the US this leads to 50 000 deaths annually. Venous thromboembolism (VTE) is a multifactorial disorder, with well-characterized examples of gene–gene and gene–environment interactions underlying its pathogenesis. Genetic causes are present in approximately 25% of unselected venous thrombosis cases and up to 63% of familial cases.

Genetic causes of inherited thrombophilias (hypercoagulabilities) include the following.

- **Factor V Leiden** (R506Q mutation), causing activated protein C (APC) resistance, was discovered in 1994 and is the most common genetic risk factor for venous thrombosis. 20% of individuals with an idiopathic first venous thrombosis have this mutation, and 60% of pregnant women with a venous thrombosis have this mutation. Factor V Leiden has also been associated with an increased risk of recurrent pregnancy loss and placental infarction. 4.4% of Europeans and White Americans carry the factor V Leiden mutation.
- **Prothrombin 20210A** mutation (factor II Leiden) is carried by 1–2% of Europeans and White Americans.
- **Antithrombin III deficiency.**
- **Deficiency of protein C.** Purified human activated protein C selectively destroys factors Va and VIII:C in human plasma and thus has an important anticoagulant role.
- **Deficiency of protein S.** Protein S is a vitamin K-dependent plasma protein that inhibits blood clotting by serving as a cofactor for APC. Makris *et al.* (2000) showed that relatives of a symptomatic individual with protein S deficiency who were also carrying a *PROS1* mutation had an ~fivefold relative risk of VTE.

Overall, ~1/3000 individuals has a heritable deficiency of antithrombin III or protein C or protein S.

Acquired or environmental causes include the following.

- **Surgical, e.g. postoperative or associated with trauma.** Only major surgery is associated with a risk, e.g. abdominal surgery under general anaesthetic or an orthopaedic operation.
- **Pregnancy** (high factor VIII levels).
- **Oestrogens**, e.g. oral contraceptive use, hormone replacement therapy (HRT).
- **Malignancy.**
- **Immobility**, e.g. plaster casts, long-haul flights, stroke with limb weakness.

Patients with postoperative VTE have a very low risk of recurrence and a low incidence of thrombophilic defects (Baglin *et al.* 2003). Patients with an unprecipitated VTE have a 20% cumulative recurrence rate at 2 years; however, despite 27% of such patients having heritable thrombophilic defects, thrombophilia testing does not allow prediction of a high risk of recurrence (Baglin *et al.* 2003).

The clinical utility of testing for thrombophilia in patients with VTE is highly contentious. Middeldorp *et al.* (2001) concluded that the absolute annual incidence of spontaneous VTE in asymptomatic carriers of the factor V Leiden mutation is low and does not justify routine screening of the families of symptomatic patients. Simioni *et al.* (2002) in a prospective cohort study confirmed that the absolute risk of VTE in heterozygotes for the factor V Leiden mutation is low with an annual incidence of spontaneous VTE of 0.17% (95% confidence interval (CI), 0.02–0.6) in carriers compared with 0.1% (95% CI, 0.003–0.56) in non-carriers. However risk period-related VTE occurred with an incidence of 18% and 5% per risk period in heterozygous carriers and in non-carriers, respectively.

Testing in patients from thrombosis-prone families may be warranted in order to identify individuals who might benefit from thromboprophylaxis during risk periods. If such testing is offered, the clinician needs to have a clear idea before initiating testing in asymptomatic family members that the results will inform clinical management in each individual case. Discuss with colleagues in haematology. See the table for the American College of Medical Genetics (ACMG) guidelines on testing for factor V Leiden.

Clinical approach

History: key points

- Three-generation family tree with specific enquiry regarding:
  - venous thrombosis (note age of affected individual and site of thrombosis). Younger age of onset may indicate homozygosity, particularly for protein S or C deficiency;
  - pulmonary embolus;
  - pregnancy loss and pre-eclampsia;
  - myocardial infarction, particularly in those aged <50 years and women;
  - persistent leg ulcers;
  - childhood stroke.

Ask if there were known additional risk factors at the time of the event such as trauma, pelvic, vascular, or orthopaedic surgery, tumour, immobilization, pregnancy, oestrogen treatment, other medical conditions.

- Acquired/environmental risk factors affecting the consultant or other affected family members:
  - smoking history;
  - diabetes;
  - lupus.

Examination: key points

Assess for chronic venous hypertension and post-phlebitic syndrome as this is a risk factor for recurrent VTE.

Investigation

- Factor V Leiden or APC resistance is usually perfomed initially. Patients testing positive for factor V Leiden or APC resistance should be considered for testing for the most common other thrombophilias with overlapping phenotype, and for which testing is easy and readily available.
- Prothrombin 20210A variant. The DNA test can be multiplexed with that for factor V Leiden.
- Protein S, protein C, and antithrombin III deficiencies are too genetically heterogeneous for routine molecular genetic testing, but testing by functional coagulation

Testing for factor V Leiden (Grody *et al.* 2001)

Testing should be performed in the following circumstances
- Age <50 years, any venous thrombosis
- Venous thrombosis in unusual sites (such as hepatic, mesenteric, and cerebral veins)
- Recurrent venous thrombosis
- Venous thrombosis and a strong family history of thrombotic disease
- Venous thrombosis in pregnant women or women taking oral contraceptives
- Relatives of individuals with venous thrombosis under age 50 years
- Myocardial infarction in female smokers under age 50 years

Testing may also be considered in the following situations
- Venous thrombosis, age >50 years, except when active malignancy is present
- Relatives of individuals known to have factor V Leiden. Knowledge that they have factor V Leiden may influence management of pregnancy and may be a factor in decision-making regarding oral contraceptive use
- Women with recurrent pregnancy loss or unexplained severe pre-eclampsia, placental abruption, intrauterine fetal growth retardation, or stillbirth. Knowledge of factor V Leiden carrier status may influence management of future pregnancies

Random screening of the general population for factor V Leiden is *not* recommended

Routine testing is *not* recommended for patients with a personal or family history of arterial thrombotic disease

Physicians ordering factor V Leiden testing on a venous thrombosis patient for any of the indications recommended here should also consider the utility of functional, biochemical, and molecular screening for other heritable thrombophilic factors, especially prothrombin 20210A and plasma homocysteine levels

---

assays may be considered, especially if there is a strong family history of venous thrombosis.
- Plasma homocysteine levels. Elevation of homocysteine is another potential risk factor in those found to be positive for factor V Leiden.
- Anti-phospholipid antibodies can cause APC resistance. Also consider anticardiolipin antibodies and anti-beta 2 glycoprotein antibodies.

Other diagnoses/conditions to consider

Medical conditions that can cause activation of APC such as lupus.

Homocystinuria. Patients with classic homocystinuria (autosomal recessive (AR)) are at extremely elevated risk of thromboembolism and should probably be tested for other available thrombophilic risk factors. See 'Marfan syndrome', page 380.

Genetic advice

Inheritance and recurrence risk
The genetic thrombophilias are usually inherited as an autosomal dominant (AD) trait. If both parents are carriers for the same disorder, then there is a 1 in 4 risk of a homozygous affected child.

Variability and penetrance
Clinical expression is variable. Although, the relative risk of venous thrombosis is increased between 4- and 8-fold for factor V Leiden heterozygotes, the majority of heterozygous individuals never have a thrombotic event. The relative risk depends on gene–gene interaction and gene–environment interaction, so that individuals who carry more than one genetic cause and have additional environmental risks face increasing risks. Homozygotes have an 80-fold risk of venous thrombosis.

Prenatal diagnosis
Not offered for factor V Leiden or prothrombin 20210A.

Predictive testing and testing of other family members
Routine testing of at-risk family members is not recommended for factor V Leiden or prothrombin 20210A

as there is only a mildly increased risk for the individual and testing does not decrease morbidity or mortality (see above). As a general rule young children should not be tested. Children have special defences against forming blood clots and it is not until they reach puberty that their risk of blood clots due to thrombophilia begins to increase. Teenage daughters of patients with thrombophilia can be considered for testing if the results would influence decisions relating to contraceptive use. For some individuals there is an indication to test, such as management of a pregnancy or avoidance of hormonal medication (oral contraceptive pill, HRT), and predictive testing can be offered to adults within families with known mutations after appropriate consent is obtained.

Natural history and management
Potential long-term complications

Pregnancy. Heterozygosity for factor V Leiden has been linked to 2–3× risk of late pregnancy loss and has been associated with a higher risk of pre-eclampsia, abruption, intrauterine growth retardation (IUGR), and stillbirth, though the risk varies between studies. Individual assessment is required to assess whether the risk of thromboembolism, fetal loss, and pre-eclampsia is greater than the risks related to anticoagulation. Warfarin is a known teratogen with a recognizable embryopathy. Heparin prophylaxis is preferred for those at high risk.

Homozygotes for factor V Leiden have a higher overall risk of recurrence of VTE than heterozygotes (relative risk, 1.8; 95% confidence interval (CI), 1.0–6.17; Procare Group 2003). Balancing the risk of recurrence against the risk of major bleeding from oral anticoagulation therapy, it appears that factor V Leiden homozygotes with a first VTE are unlikely to benefit from long-term full-dose oral anticoagulant treatment. All these patients should receive short-term prophylaxis during risk situations, particularly during pregnancy (Procare Group 2003). This is also the case for venous thrombosis patients heterozygous for both factor V Leiden and the prothrombin 20210A mutation (co-inheritance occurs 1 in 1000 of the population but in

1 in 50 of patients with thromboembolism) in whom recurrence risk has been shown to be high.

Surveillance

- Patients on anticoagulants require regular surveillance.
- Advice should be given on ways to modify environmental risks and to report signs or symptoms of thrombosis.

  - **Surgical, e.g. postoperative or associated with trauma.** Only major surgery is associated with a risk, e.g. abdominal surgery under general anaesthetic or an orthopaedic operation. Heparin injections may be given to reduce thrombosis risk. Minor surgery, such as dental surgery or biopsies under local anaesthetic, are not high-risk situations.
  - **Pregnancy** (high factor VIII levels).
  - **Oestrogens.** Consider alternative forms of contraception or progesterone-only preparations if oral contraceptive use is desired. HRT generally confers a 2–3-fold increased risk for VTE. Early evidence suggests an interaction of HRT with thrombophilic states such as the factor V Leiden mutation, resulting in a synergistic increase in the risk of VTE (Peverill 2003).
  - **Immobility**, e.g. long-haul flights (ensure adequate hydration and exercise and wear venous compression stockings).

Support group: Thrombophilia: Information for patients and their relatives <www.bcshguidelines.com>; Thrombophilia support <www.fvleiden.org>.

Expert adviser: Trevor Baglin, Consultant Haematologist, Addenbrooke's Hospital, Cambridge, England.

References

BaglinT, Luddington R, et al. Incidence of recurrent venous thromboembolism in relation to clinical and thrombophilic risk factors: prospective cohort study. *Lancet* 2003; **362**: 523–6.

British Committee for Standards in Haematology. *Guideline on thrombophilia: information for patients and their relatives.* <www.bcshguidelines.com>, 2003.

Greaves M, Baglin T. Laboratory testing for heritable thrombophilia: impact on clinical management of thrombotic disease annotation. *Br J Haematol* 2000; **109** (4): 699–703.

Grody WW, Griffin JH, Taylor AK, Korf BR, Heit JA (American College of Medical Genetics (ACMG) Factor V Leiden Working Group). *American College of Medical Genetics consensus statement on factor V Leiden mutation testing.* ACMG, Bethesda, Maryland, 2001.

Kujovich JL, Goodnight SH. Factor V Leiden thrombophilia. In *GeneReviews* <www.geneclinics.org>, 1999–2001.

Makris M, Leach M, et al. Genetic analysis, phenotypic diagnosis, and risk of venous thrombosis in families with inherited deficiencies of protein S. *Blood* 2000; **95**: 1935–41.

Middeldorp S, Meinhardi JR, et al. A prospective study of asymptomatic carriers of the factor V Leiden mutatation to determine the incidence of venous thromboembolism. *Ann Intern Med* 2001; **135**: 322–37.

Peverill RE. Hormone therapy and venous thromboembolism. *Best Pract Res Clin Endocrinol Metab* 2003; **17** (1): 149–64.

Procare Group. Is recurrent venous thromboembolism more frequent in homozygous patients for the factor V Leiden mutation than in heterozygous patients? *Blood Coagul Fibrinolysis* 2003; **14** (6): 523–9.

Reich LM, Bower M, Key NS. Role of the geneticist in testing and counseling for inherited thrombophilia. *Genet Med* 2003; **5** (3): 133–43.

Seligsohn U, Lubetsky A. Medical progress: genetic susceptibility to venous thrombosis. *New Engl J Med* 2001; **344**: 1222–31.

Simioni P, Tormene D, et al. Incidence of thromboembolism in asymptomatic family members who are carriers of factor V Leiden: a prospective cohort study. *Blood* 2002; **99**: 1938–42.

Zotz RB, Gerhardt A, Scharf RE. Inherited thrombophilia and gestational venous thromboembolism. *Best Pract Res Clin Haematol* 2003; **16**: 243–59.

Tuberous sclerosis (TSC)

Tuberous sclerosis complex (TSC), epiloia, Bourneville disease, Pringle disease.

TSC is a multisystem disorder characterized by hamartomas (tumour-like lesions) in the brain, skin, and other organs and often associated with seizures and mental retardation. The prevalence is ~1/10 000. It can present at any age from fetal to late adult life and is characterized by highly variable expressivity. The most common presentation is with infantile spasms or seizures in early childhood. TSC follows autosomal dominant (AD) inheritance with a high proportion of cases (60%) caused by new mutations.

TSC is caused by mutations in *TSC1* on 9q (hamartin) or *TSC2* on 16p (tuberin). Tuberin and hamartin form a tumour suppressor heterodimer that has an important role in the phosphoinositide 3-kinase (PI3K) signalling pathway and inhibits the mammalian target of rapamycin (mTOR). This pathway is a critical regulator of cell growth and proliferation. The patchy nature of the pathology in TSC appears to be due to somatic mutation with germline inactivation of one copy of either *TSC1* or *TSC2* in all cells (first hit) and subsequent inactivation of the second copy by somatic mutation (second hit).

Dabora *et al.* (2001) undertook a molecular and genetic analysis of a cohort of 224 TSC probands. Sporadic patients with *TSC1* mutations had, on average, milder disease in comparison to patients with *TSC2* mutations, despite being of similar age. They had a lower frequency of seizures and moderate-to-severe mental retardation, fewer subependymal nodules and cortical tubers, less severe kidney involvement, and less severe facial angiofibroma.

Clinical approach

History: *key points*

- Three-generation family tree with careful enquiry for TSC, infantile spasms, epilepsy, learning disability, facial angiofibromata.
- Specific enquiry for seizures.
- Detailed developmental and behavioural history.

Examination: *key points*

- **Angiofibromata** ('adenoma sebaceum') are rarely obvious at <2 years of age and may not appear until middle age. They occur in 85% of affected individuals in 'butterfly' distribution over nose, nasolabial folds, and cheeks—also chin. Differentiate from acne by close inspection showing lack of involvement of sebaceous glands and absence of infection. Unlike acne, angiofibromata persist in the same location and do not resolve. They may coexist with acne causing diagnostic uncertainty.
- **Hypomelanotic macules** ('ash-leaf' spots) occur in 95% of affected individuals by the age of 5 years, and are usually the earliest skin feature. They may be present from birth or develop in infancy. 0.8% of normal neonates have similar macules, but rarely >3. Typically oval. May need Wood's light (360 nm wavelength ultraviolet (UV)) to visualize them.
- **Forehead fibrous plaque.** Smooth, raised flesh-coloured or yellowish-brown waxy-looking lesion (a few mm to several cm across) present on forehead (look under fringe!). Usually develop in later childhood.
- **Shagreen patches.** Discoloured, thickened leathery patches of skin (resembling orange peel) usually over

lumbar region, slightly to one side of midline. Usually multiple and varying in size from a few mm to several cm. Can appear at any age from infancy to puberty and are present in ~50% of cases by early adult life.

- **Ungual fibromata** occur in up to 88% of adults. Look carefully at all fingernails and toenails for pink or red nodules arising in the angle of the nailbed and often causing ridging or guttering of the nail. Usually multiple and more common on the toenails where they may bleed if knocked.
- **Dental pits** due to enamel hypoplasia. Can occur in normal individuals so not very specific for TSC. Fibromata similar to the ungual fibromata can occur between teeth.

Investigation

- Refer for **ophthalmology assessment**. Retinal astrocytic hamartomas are found in 40–50%. They are often multiple and bilateral and can take several forms. The most common are relatively flat, smooth oval lesions that are semitransparent and similar in colour to the fundus. Less common are the classic 'mulberry' lesions, which are raised opaque multinodular calcified hamartomas most commonly found in the vicinity of the optic disc. Retinal hamartomas are almost always asymptomatic and only interfere with vision if overlying the macula (rare).
- **Cranial imaging**
  - Computerized tomography (CT) will often show **subependymal nodules** (SENs) along the lateral walls of the lateral ventricles or in the vicinity of the caudate nucleus particularly if they are calcified. These are the most diagnostic cerebral lesions of TSC and are seen in ~80% of cases. SENs may grow in size and have the propensity to develop into **subependymal giant cell astrocytomas** (SEGAs). SEGAs typically occur in the head of the caudate nucleus and present with symptoms of hydrocephalus due to obstruction of the foramina of Munro (see below).
  - CT may demonstrate **cortical tubers** (seen in ~two/thirds of cases), but these are better visualized by magnetic resonance imaging (MRI) when they are seen in ~95% of cases. FLAIR (fluid-attenuated inversion recovery) sequences are the best MRI modality for visualizing cortical tubers. Most patients have 1–10 tubers, but some have more. Tubers may be associated with abnormalities of the underlying white matter such as migration lines. These radial migration lines are seen in ~20% of MRI scans and are thought to represent hypomyelination and white matter heterotopia.
  - Consider diagnostic specificity, radiation exposure, and availability when assessing whether MRI or CT is preferable. In infants <18 months old, in whom myelination is incomplete, MRI may be less good at visualizing tubers and CT may be the preferred investigation if a diagnosis of TS is suspected on clinical grounds.
- Consider **mutation analysis** of *TSC1* and *TSC2*. In Dabora *et al.*'s (2001) series of 224 index cases, mutations were identified in 83% of cases, comprising 138 small *TSC2* mutations, 20 large *TSC2* mutations, and 28 small *TSC1* mutations. The bias in favour of

TSC2 reflects both the larger size of the gene and an intrinsically higher mutation rate.

- **Renal ultrasound scan (USS).** Angiomyolipomata (AMLs) are the most common renal manifestation of TSC (see below). Renal cysts occur in 17–47% of patients with TSC and are often present from early childhood. They are usually multiple and bilateral. In infants a renal USS is used to identify the small minority who have a contiguous *TSC2–ADPK1* gene deletion (see below).
- In infants consider an echocardiogram as cardiac rhabdomyomas are common at this age in children with TSC and may be very helpful in making the diagnosis.
- In adult women with TSC a one-off chest CT scan may be considered to screen for lymphangiomyomatosis (LAM; Recommendation of TS Consensus Conference 1998 given in Roach *et al.* 1999).

Other diagnoses/conditions to consider

See 'Patchy hypomelanotic skin lesions' page 208.

Contiguous gene deletion involving *TSC2-ADPK1*. A small minority of patients with TSC have a contiguous gene deletion involving *TSC2* and *ADPKD1*, one of the genes encoding autosomal dominant polycystic kidney disease (ADPKD). Such patients usually present with severe early-onset renal cystic disease, renal enlargement, and radiological appearances of advanced ADPKD with a poor prognosis for renal function leading to end-stage renal failure in late childhood or early adult life.

Isolated cardiac rhabdomyoma. Cardiac rhabdomyomas identified as an unexpected finding on a routine 2nd or 3rd trimester USS (not in the context of prenatal diagnosis for TSC) is a well recognized presentation of TSC and the chance of the baby being affected by TSC in this situation is 39–86%.

Periventricular nodular heterotopia (PVNH) or bilateral periventricular nodular heterotopia (BPNH). Rare X-linked dominant (XLD) condition causing a localized neuronal migration disorder in females usually associated with seizures (88% are focal) and prenatal lethality in males. Cranial imaging shows uncalcified periventricular nodules that could be confused with those of TSC (Jardine *et al.* 1996). PVNH is caused by mutations in filamin A (*FLNA*), which encodes a widely expressed protein that regulates re-organization of the actin cytoskeleton and hence has an important role in cell migration. Additional, possibly autosomal recessive (AR) gene(s) are likely to be involved in causing PVNH non-linked to *FLN1*.

Genetic advice

Inheritance and recurrence risk

AD inheritance, but 60% of cases arise as a result of a new mutation. Germline mutations are less common in *TSC1* than in *TSC2*.

- **Affected parent.** If one parent is affected, the risk of inheriting TSC is 50% to each offspring. In view of the variation in disease severity (expressivity), the overall risk of having a child with mental retardation is likely to 25% or less (since 50% or less of individuals with TSC are mentally retarded).
- **Parents unaffected.** If neither parent is affected with TSC the risk is 2% due to germline mosaicism (this has been reported for both *TSC1* and *TSC2* and can be either maternal or paternal). Unless the causative mutation is known, parents of an apparently sporadic case should be evaluated by:
  - detailed family tree;
  - detailed skin examination including Wood's light exam;
  - expert ophthalmological assessment of the fundi;
  - consider cranial imaging (CT or MRI);
  - consider renal USS.
- **Apparently unaffected siblings** should be offered a similar evaluation before they plan a family of their own (unless the causative mutation is known in which case genetic testing should be offered). If both parents of the affected individual have been thoroughly investigated and are unaffected, the need for cranial imaging in the siblings is arguable as the prior risk, with normal clinical examination, can be estimated to be of the order <0.2% (2% risk arising from germline mosaicism, with >90% penetrance for skin features, e.g hypomelanotic macules).

The risk of a *TSC* mutation in the phenotypically normal adult offspring of an affected patient, or the phenotypically normal adult sibling of a sporadic case, is close to that of the general population; hence risk to their offspring is close to population risks. (This assumes the adult offspring/siblings have been determined to be phenotypically normal after clinical examination, including dermatological and ophthalmic assessment and cranial CT/MRI scan.)

With the increasing availability of mutation analysis, this may replace detailed clinical evaluation in the assessment of apparently unaffected relatives. Note germline mosaicism risk, so if a *de novo* mutation is identified (i.e. not present in either parent), genetic testing should still be offered to siblings.

Variability and penetrance

TSC is highly penetrant by adult life; true non-penetrance is extremely rare. TSC is highly variable; hence the need for comprehensive clinical assessment of apparently unaffected relatives (or molecular testing if the familial mutation is defined).

Prenatal diagnosis

Possible by chorionic villus sampling (CVS) where a mutation is known. The risk of a second affected child being born to the phenotypically normal parents (determined to be phenotypically normal after clinical examination, including dermatological and ophthalmic assessment and cranial CT/MRI scan) of an apparently sporadic case remains significant (2%), and prenatal diagnosis may be offered if a mutation has been identified in the affected child.

Natural history and management

Life expectancy is usually normal, even in those with severe learning difficulties, but they can die prematurely from epilepsy, cardiac arrhythmias, renal involvement, or complications of giant cell astrocytoma or pulmonary LAM.

Learning disability. 50% of individuals with TSC have normal intelligent quotient (IQ). The majority of people who are seizure-free have normal intelligence. Learning disability can be mild to severe. Severe learning disability is not thought to occur in the absence of seizures. Two-thirds of individuals with TSC who have epilepsy also have learning disability. Children who present with seizures, particularly infantile spasms, in the first 2 years of life are more likely to have learning disability than those who develop seizures later. Onset >5 years is very unlikely to be associated with

Diagnostic criteria for tuberous sclerosis (TSC; after Roach *et al.* 1999)

Requirements for a clinical diagnosis of TSC:

Definite TSC	*Either* 2 major features *or* 1 major and 2 minor features
Probable TSC	1 major and 1 minor feature
Possible diagnosis of TSC	*Either* 1 major feature *or* 2 minor features

Major features	Minor features*
Central nervous system	
Cortical tuber	Cerebral white matter radial migration lines (should not be counted as a minor feature if a cortical tuber is used as a major feature)
Subependymal nodule	
Subependymal giant cell astrocytoma	
Skin	
Facial angiofibromata or forehead plaque	'Confetti' skin lesions
Ungual fibroma (non-traumatic)	
Hypomelanotic macules (3 or more)	
Shagreen patch	
Ocular	
Multiple retinal nodular hamartomata	Retinal achromic patch
Cardiac	
Cardiac rhabdomyoma (single or multiple)	
Renal	
Angiomyolipoma (AML)[†]	Multiple renal cysts (interpret with caution in adults as may be a chance finding in older people)
Respiratory	
Pulmonary lymphangiomyomatosis (LAM)[†]	
Skeletal	
	Bone cysts
Oral/dental	
	Multiple randomly distributed pits in dental enamel (fairly common in general population)
	Gingival fibromas
Gastrointestinal	
	Hamartomatous rectal polyps
Other	
	Non-renal hamartoma

*In using these diagnostic criteria, the emphasis should be on the major features. The presence of one major feature raises a possible diagnosis of TSC and warrants further investigation. The minor features are much less specific for TSC.

[†]There is a recognized association between renal AML and pulmonary LAM so if both are present they should be counted together as one major feature.

learning difficulties unless non-convulsive status epilepticus occurs. Patients with mental retardation have significantly more cortical tubers than those with normal intelligence.

Behavioural problems are common. Learning disabilities frequently occur in conjunction with behavioural problems, but this need not always be so. Autism is seen in ~25–61% and more broadly defined pervasive developmental disorders in ~50–86%. The risk of autism is particularly high if there are tubers in the temporal lobes combined with temporal lobe epileptiform discharges and and early-onset persistent infantile spasms. Disruptive behavioural disorders characterized by marked hyperactivity and/or attention deficits are common, occurring in 43–59%. Sleep disturbance is very common, especially if a child's epilepsy is poorly controlled.

Seizures occur in 80% of individuals with TS (Joinson). The best estimate of the frequency of seizures in familial cases is ~62% (Webb)—the frequency of seizures in familial cases is likely to be lower than in sporadic cases for several reasons including a lower proportion of *TSC2* mutations. A great variety of seizure types can occur including simple and complex partial (focal) seizures, generalized tonic and tonic–clonic seizures, atonic seizures ('drop attacks'), myoclonic seizures, and infantile spasms. Seizures typically begin in infancy, often in the first few months. The pattern of seizure changes through early childhood. Seizure control can be very difficult and 85% of children who develop seizures still have them by age 5 years. Most respond at least to some extent to anticonvulsants, but a small minority have epilepsy that is refractory to anticonvulsant therapy.

Potential long-term complications

- **Giant cell astrocytomas** occur in 10–15%. Peak incidence is late childhood through adolescence. Cases present with symptoms of raised intracranial pressure (headaches, vomiting) due to obstruction of foramina of Munro.

- **AMLs** of the kidney are common and usually multiple and bilateral, increasing in size and number with age. They are readily identified on renal USS. Usually asymptomatic, but can cause renal pain, haematuria, and even intrarenal or retroperitoneal haemorrhage. They are present in 17%, 42%, 65%, and 92% of individuals with TS by <2 years, 2–5 years, 9–14 years, and 14–18 years, respectively (Jozwiak *et al.* 2000).

- **Renal cysts** occur in 17–47% and are often present from early childhood. They are usually multiple and bilateral. If cysts are numerous, consider the possibility of a contiguous *TSC2 ADPKD1* gene deletion.
- Symptomatic **LAM** is uncommon and occurs almost exclusively in adult females. Prognosis can be poor if lung involvement is extensive. It usually presents in adult life, but can present earlier. Can cause progressive respiratory impairment with emphysematous change, loss of lung volume, and risk of pneumothorax. If symptomatic, consider spirometry, chest X-ray, high-resolution CT, and refer to chest physician.
- **Cardiac rhabdomyomas** may be identified on USS in fetal life or cause outflow obstruction or arrhythmias in the neonatal period. They usually regress in number and size with age.
- **Hepatic hamartomas** are present in 25% and are usually of no clinical significance.

Support groups: UK Tuberous Sclerosis Association <www.tuberous-sclerosis.org>, Tel. 01527 871898; Tuberous Sclerosis Alliance (US) <www.tsalliance.org>, Tel. (toll-free). (800) 225 6872.

Expert adviser: John R.W. Yates, Professor of Medical Genetics, University of Cambridge, Cambridge, England.

References

Dabora SL, Jozwiak S, *et al.* Mutational analysis in a cohort of 224 tuberous sclerosis patients indicates increased severity of TSC2, compared with TSC1, disease in multiple organs. *Am J Hum Genet* 2001; **68** (1): 64–80.

Gamzu R, Achiron R, *et al.* Evaluating the risk of tuberous sclerosis in cases with prenatal diagnosis of cardiac rhabdomyoma. *Prenat Diagn* 2002; **22** (11): 1044–7.

Jardine PE, Clarke MA, *et al.* Familial bilateral periventricular nodular heterotopia mimics tuberous sclerosis. *Arch Dis Child* 1996; **74**: 244–6.

Joinson C, O'Callaghan FJ, *et al.* Learning disability and epilepsy in an epidemiological sample of individuals with tuberous sclerosis complex. *Psychol Med* 2003; **33**: 335–44.

Jozwiak S, Schwartz RA, Janniger CK, Bielicka-Cymerman J. Usefulness of diagnostic criteria of tuberous sclerosis complex in pediatric patients. *J Child Neurol* 2000; **15** (10): 652–9.

Osborne JP. *Tuberous sclerosis complex. What you should know—a practitioners guide.* Tuberous Sclerosis Association, London, 2001.

Osborne JP, Jones AC, Burley MW, *et al.* Non-penetrance in tuberous sclerosis. *Lancet* 2000; **355**: 1698.

Pipitone S, Mongiovi M, *et al.* Cardiac rhabdomyoma in intrauterine life: clinical features and natural history. A case series and review of published reports. *Ital Heart J* 2002; **3** (1): 48–52.

Roach ES, Gomez MR, *et al.* Tuberous sclerosis complex consensus conference: revised clinical diagnostic criteria. *J Child Neurol* 1999; **13**: 624–8.

Tee AR, Manning BD, *et al.* Tuberous sclerosis complex gene products, tuberin and hamartin, control mTOR signaling by acting as a GTPase-activating protein complex toward Rheb. *Curr Biol* 2003; **13** (15): 1259–68.

UK Tuberous Sclerosis Association (TSA). *Clinical guidelines.* <www.tuberous-sclerosis.org/professionals/guidelines.shtml>.

Webb DW, Fryer AE, *et al.* On the incidence of fits and mental retardation in tuberous sclerosis. *J Med Genet* 1991; **28**: 417–19.

Yates JRW. Tuberous sclerosis. In *Management of genetic syndromes*, 2nd edn (ed. SB Cassidy and JE Allanson). Wiley, New York, 2004.

Cancer

Chapter contents

BRCA1 and BRCA2 *426*
Breast cancer *430*
Cancer surveillance methods *434*
Colorectal cancer (CRC) *436*
Confirmation of diagnosis of cancer *440*
Cowden syndrome (CS) *442*
Familial adenomatous polyposis (FAP) *444*
Gastric cancer *450*
Gorlin syndrome *452*
Hereditary nonpolyposis colorectal cancer (HNPCC) *454*
Juvenile polyposis syndrome (JPS) *460*
Lifestyle factors in cancer: smoking, alcohol, obesity, diet, and exercise *462*
Li–Fraumeni syndrome (LFS) *464*
Multiple endocrine neoplasia (MEN) *466*
Neurofibromatosis type 2 (NF2) *470*
Ovarian cancer *472*
Peutz–Jeghers syndrome (PJS) *474*
Phaeochromocytoma *478*
Retinoblastoma *480*
von Hippel–Lindau (VHL) disease *484*
Wilms tumour *486*

BRCA1 and BRCA2

The majority of families with a clearly dominant predisposition to breast and/or ovarian cancer are known to harbour germline mutations in either *BRCA1* or *BRCA2*. The combined contribution of *BRCA1* and *BRCA2* to overall breast cancer is <2%.

BRCA1 is a large gene with 22 exons, with exon 11 comprising ~60% of the coding sequence. Most mutations are scattered throughout the gene. 87% of mutations identified are predicted to result in protein truncation or absence of BRCA1 protein. The BRCA1 protein is involved in many important cellular pathways including DNA repair and regulation of transcription. Several founder mutations are common in specific populations: ~1% of Ashkenazi Jewish women carry the 185delAG mutation; 5382insC is common in Ashkenazim and parts of Eastern Europe; and the missense mutation C61G is also common in Eastern Europe. 185delAG accounts for ~20% of early-onset breast cancer amongst Ashkenazim.

BRCA2 is also a large gene, with exons 10 and 11 comprising ~60% of the coding sequence. Mutations are scattered throughout the gene and most are truncating. The BRCA2 protein is involved in DNA repair and biallelic mutations in *BRCA2* cause Fanconi anaemia. The mutation 6174delT is found in 1–1.5% of Askenazi Jews and accounts for ~8% of early-onset breast cancer in that ethnic group. A single mutation, 999del5, accounts for the majority of Icelandic early-onset familial breast cancer.

Most missense mutations in *BRCA1/2* are of uncertain significance. Reference to websites such as the Breast Cancer Information Core (BIC) database may help with interpretation.

Cancer risks associated with *BRCA1*. Female carriers with a mutation in *BRCA1* have an average risk of breast cancer to age 70 of 65% (range 44–78%), and a 39% (range 18–54%) average risk to age 70 of ovarian cancer (including the fallopian tubes)(see 'Patterns of cancer' page 690). Where there are multiple affected family members, the risk estimates from the upper end of these ranges are likely to be appropriate due to co-inheritance of possible modifier genes and shared environmental exposure. The relative risk of breast cancer in *BRCA1* carriers, relative to the general population, declines with age from >30-fold below age 40 years to 14-fold above age 60 years. As a consequence of this, the incidences in *BRCA1* carriers rise to a plateau of ~3–4% per annum in the 40–49 year age group. There is a high risk of contralateral breast cancer in affected carriers. Ovarian cancer risks in *BRCA1* carriers are low (in absolute terms) below age 40 years; thereafter the incidences are ~1% per annum between 40 and 59 years and 2% after age 60. *BRCA1* mutation carriers are also at increased risk of pancreatic, prostate, endometrial, and cervical cancer.

Cancer risks associated with *BRCA2*. Female carriers of a mutation in *BRCA2* have a 45% (confidence interval (CI), 31–56%) risk of breast cancer to age 70 years and an 11% (CI, 2.4–19%) risk for ovarian cancer (including the fallopian tubes). Where there are multiple affected family members, the risk estimates from the upper end of these ranges are likely to be appropriate due to co-inheritance of possible modifier genes and shared environmental exposure. The relative risk of breast cancer in *BRCA2* carriers is ~11-fold in all age groups above 40 years, and is not significantly higher at younger ages. As a consequence of this, the incidences in

BRCA2 carriers show a pattern parallel to that in the general population, rising steeply up to age 50 years and more slowly thereafter. There is a high risk of contralateral breast cancer in affected carriers. Ovarian cancer risks in *BRCA2* carriers are in contrast very low below age 50 years but then increase sharply in the 50–59 year age group, perhaps declining somewhat thereafter. Male mutation carriers are also at increased risk of breast cancer (~6% by 70 years).

BRCA2 mutation carriers are also at increased risk of prostate and pancreatic cancer and possibly also gall bladder/bile duct cancer and malignant melanoma. The cumulative risk for prostate cancer is 0.1% by age 50 years, 1.6% by age 60 years, 7.5% by age 70 years, 19.8% by age 80 years, and the cumulative risk for all cancers in male mutation carriers is 4% by age 50 years, 13% by age 60 years, and 32% by age 70 years.

Clinical approach

History: key points
Three-generation family tree with specific enquiry for breast, ovarian, prostate, and other associated cancers.

Examination: key points
Usually not necessary for evaluation purposes.

Genetic advice
Counsel a *BRCA1/2* carrier regarding risks to his/her own health and arrange appropriate screening and/or prophylactic surgery(Lobb). Identify other 'at risk' members of the family and ensure that the offer of genetic advice, screening, and/or predictive testing is made available to all at-risk relatives from an appropriate age in early adult life.

Penetrance
Women who are contemplating prophylactic surgery may appreciate an individualized assessment of their risk.

Calculation of the lifetime risk of developing cancer in a *BRCA1/2* mutation carrier. For a BRCA1 mutation carrier age *n* years and unaffected, the chance of developing a breast cancer in remaining life (i.e. to 80 years) is:

$$1 - (100 - \text{risk of cancer by age 80 years})/(100 - \text{risk of cancer by age } n \text{ years}).$$

As an example, for a *BRCA1* mutation carrier age 50 years and unaffected, the chance of developing a breast cancer in remaining life (i.e. to 80 years) is:

$$1 - (100 - 74)/(100 - 41)$$

where 74% is penetrance to age 80 years, and 41% is penetrance to age 50 years. The result of the calculation is:

$$1 - 26/59 = 0.56 \text{ or } 56\%.$$

See table for risks calculated in this way.

Calculation of the risk of developing a second breast cancer in a *BRCA1/2* mutation carrier with breast cancer (see table). For a 50-year-old *BRCA1* mutation carrier who has already had a breast cancer and had a mastectomy, the chance of her getting another primary breast cancer over her remaining lifetime (i.e. to 80 years) is:

$$1 - (100\% - \text{risk of contralateral breast cancer by 80 year})/(100\% - \text{risk of contralateral breast cancer by 50 years}),$$

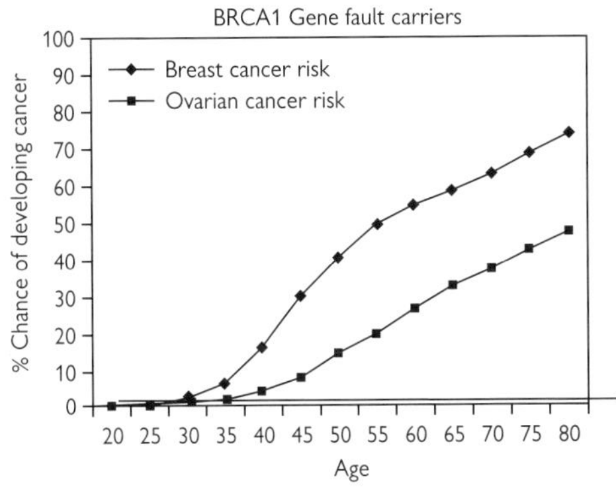

Figure 4a.1

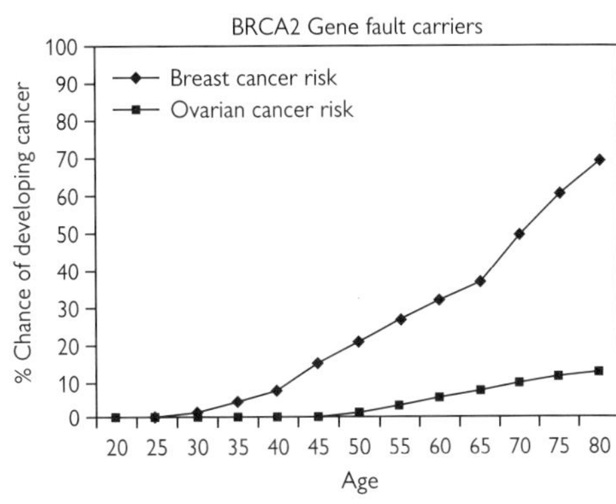

Figure 4a.2

Table showing risk of cancer by age in *BRCA1/2* carriers

	Risk (%) in **BRCA1** carrier of		Risk (%) in **BRCA2** carrier of	
Age (years)	**Breast cancer**	**Ovarian cancer**	**Breast cancer**	**Ovarian cancer**
25	0	0	0	0
30	2	1	1	0
35	7	2	4	0
40	16	4	7	0
45	30	8	14	0
50	41	15	20	1
55	50	20	26	3
60	55	27	31	5
65	59	33	36	7
70	64	38	49	9
75	69	43	60	11
80	74	48	69	12

Risk (%) of developing a second contralateral breast cancer by age in a **BRAC1/2** carrier with breast cancer

	Risk (%) of developing 2nd contralateral breast cancer in	
Age (years)	**BRCA1 carrier**	**BRCA2 carrier**
40	33	18
50	50	37
60	60	48
70	65	52
80	70	57

i.e.

$$1 - (100 - 70)/(100 - 50) = 0.4 \text{ or } 40\%.$$

For a 50-year-old *BRCA1* mutation carrier who has already had a breast cancer but had conservative surgery and has both breasts still, the chance of her getting another primary breast cancer over her remaining lifetime (i.e. to 80 years) is:

$$1 - (100\% - \text{chance of getting contralateral breast cancer})^2,$$

i.e.

$$1 - (1 - 0.4)^2 = 1 - 0.6^2 = 1 - 0.36 = 0.64 \text{ or } 64\%.$$

Predictive testing

When a familial mutation has been defined, predictive testing can be offered to members of the extended family. Since the consequences of the results are profound it would be appropriate to follow an approach similar to that developed for Huntington disease (see 'Testing for genetic status' page 28 and 'Huntington disease (HD)' page 354, especially the section on 'Predictive testing').

Management

Prophylactic salpingo-oophorectomy. In Kauff *et al.*'s (2002) prospective study of 170 carriers of *BRCA* mutations with a mean follow-up of 2 years, there was an important reduction in breast cancer risk with breast cancer developing in only 4.3% of the women who had undergone oophorectomy compared with 12.9% in the surveillance group. Ovarian cancer developed in 3.1% of women who underwent prophylactic oophorectomy compared with 6.9% of women who underwent surveillance. Rebbeck *et al.* (2002) in a retrospective analysis of *BRCA* mutation carriers obtained similar results with prophylactic oophorectomy reducing the risk of breast cancer by 53% and of ovarian cancer by 96%.

Present evidence suggests that all women who are carriers of a *BRCA1* or *BRCA2* mutation should strongly consider this intervention once their families are complete. (In Rebbeck *et al.*'s (2002) study mean age of diagnosis of ovarian cancer was 50 years). Opinion is divided on the use of hormone replacement therapy (HRT) after prophylactic oophorectomy; the decision to use oestrogens should be based on a consideration of symptoms that affect future health and the quality of life. (Rebbeck *et al.* (2002) state that some centres routinely recommend HRT after prophylactic oophorectomy until the age of 50 years.)

Prophylactic mastectomy. Meijers-Heijboer *et al.* (2001) studied 139 women with *BRCA1* or *BRCA2* mutations. 76 women chose prophylactic mastectomy, and the remainder chose surveillance (annual mammography and clinical exam). Meijers-Heijboer *et al.* (2001) followed them for ~3 years. No cases of breast cancer occurred in the mastectomy group, whereas 8 breast cancers occurred in the surveillance group. On the basis of an exponential model the yearly incidence of breast cancer in the surveillance group was 2.5%. Prophylactic mastectomy has an efficacy of at least 90% in women classified as high risk on the basis of a family history of breast cancer (Hartmann *et al.* 1999).

Prophylactic mastectomy is a highly personal decision. Up to 30% of women who undergo the procedure will have surgical complications. The protective effects must be weighed against possible surgical complications and psychological problems and the toxicity of treatment and chance of dying from a diagnosed breast cancer.

Chemoprevention. Various agents are under trial. A retrospective case-analysis showed that treatment of BRCA1 and BRCA2 mutation carriers with tamoxifen after surgery for breast cancer reduced the incidence of cancer in the contralateral breast by 50% (Narod *et al.* 2000).

Physical exercise and avoidance of obesity in adolescence. King *et al.* (2003) in a large study of Ashkenazi Jewish women with inherited mutations in *BRCA1/2* found that physical exercise and lack of obesity in adolescence were associated with significantly delayed breast cancer onset.

Oral contraceptive pill (ocp). A case-control study (Narod *et al.* 1998) showed a 60% reduction in frequency of ovarian cancer after 6 years use, but there are concerns that ocps could also increase the risk of breast cancer in women with a family history of the disease. Narod *et al.* (2002) have shown that women who are *BRCA1* mutation carriers who have ever used the ocp, or who used the ocp for $\geq$ 5 yrs, may have an increased risk for early-onset breast cancer (RR 1.2 and 1.33 respectively).

Surveillance strategies
See also 'Cancer surveillance methods', page 434.

- **Mammography** has a proven survival advantage in women in the age group 50–65 years.

- **Breast ultrasound scan (USS)** is used diagnostically to evaluate palpable breast lumps or mammographic abnormalities. Sometimes used for screening very young women (<30 years of age) with a very early onset family history, but there is no clinical evidence base for using it as a screening tool. It will not detect microcalcification.

- **Breast magnetic resonance imaging (MRI)** may be more sensitive than mammography, especially in younger women when breast density is higher. MRI may be superior to mammography in *BRCA1/2* mutation carriers, but is not generally available. (Kriege, Liberman MARIBS).

- **Clinical breast examination.** Miller *et al.* (2000) showed that clinical examination was as sensitive as mammograms alone. In situations where mammography is contraindicated and breast MRI is not available, clinical examination by a breast surgeon may be offered.

- **CA125 (cancer antigen 125) screening and ovarian USS.** Of unproven efficacy; clinical trials are in progress and in this context this is offered from age 35 years to mutation carriers who elect against prophylactic oophorectomy.

Support group: Breakthrough Breast Cancer <www.breastcancergenetics.org.uk>

Expert advisers: Douglas Easton, Director Cancer Research UK Genetic Epidemiology Unit, Cambridge, Paul Pharaoh, Cancer Research UK Senior Clinical Research Fellow, Strangeways Research Laboratory, Cambridge, and Diana Eccles, Professor of Cancer Genetics, Southampton, England.

References

Antoniou A, Pharoah PDP, *et al.* Average risks of breast and ovarian cancer associated with mutations in *BRCA1* or *BRCA2* detected in case series unselected for family history: a combined analysis of 22 studies. *Am J Hum Genet* 2003; **72**: 1117–30.

Breast Cancer Linkage Consortium. Cancer risks in BRCA2 mutation carriers. *J Natl Cancer Inst* 1999; **91**; 1310–16.

Eisen A, Weber BL. Prophylactic mastectomy for women with BRCA1 and BRCA2 mutations—facts and controversy [editorial]. *New Engl J Med* 2001; **345**: 207–8.

Hartmann LC, Schaid DJ, *et al.* Efficacy of bilateral prophylactic mastectomy in women with a family history of breast cancer. *New Engl J Med* 1999; **340**: 77–84.

Kauff ND, Satogopan JM, *et al.* Risk-reducing salpingo-oophorectomy in women with a BRCA1 or BRCA2 mutation. *New Engl J Med* 2002; **346**: 1609–15.

Kennedy RD, Quinn JE, *et al.* BRCA1: mechanisms of inactivation and implications for management of patients [review]. *Lancet* 2002; **360**: 1007–14.

King MC, Marks JH, *et al.* Breast and ovarian cancer risks due to inherited mutations in BRCA1 and BRCA2. *Science* 2003; **302**: 643–6.

Kriege M, *et al.* Efficacy of MRI and mammography for breast cancer screening in women with a familial or genetic predisposition. *NEJM* 2004; **351**: 427–37.

Lobb E, Meiser B. Genetic counseling and prophylactic surgery in women from families with hereditary breast or ovarian cancer (Commentary). *Lancet* 2004; **363**: 1841–2.

Liberman L. Breast cancer screening with MRI — What are the data for patients at high risk? *NEJM* 2004; **351**: 497–500.

MARIBS Study group. Screening with magnetic resonance imaging and mammography of a UK population at high familial risk of breast cancer: a prospective multicentre cohort study (MARIBS). *Lancet* 2005; **365**: 1769–78.

Meijers-Heijboer H, van Geel, B, *et al.* Breast cancer after prophylactic bilateral mastectomy in women with a BRCA1 or BRCA2 mutation. *New Engl J Med* 2001; **345**: 159–64.

Miller AB, To T, *et al.* Canadian National Breast Screening Study-2. 13-year results of a randomized trial in women aged 50–59 years. *J Natl Cancer Inst* 2000; **92**: 1490–9.

Narod S. What options for treatment of hereditary breast cancer? [editorial]. *Lancet* 2002; **359**: 1451.

Narod SA, Dube MP, *et al.* Oral contraceptives and the risk of breast cancer in *BRCA1* and *BRCA2* mutation carriers. *J Natl Cancer Inst* 2002; **94**: 1773–39.

Narod SA, Risch H, *et al.* Oral contraceptives and the risk of hereditary ovarian cancer. *New Engl J Med* 1998; **339**: 424–8.

Narod SA, Brunet JS, *et al.* Tamoxifen and risk of contralateral breast cancer in BRCA1 and BRCA2 mutation carriers: a case-control study. *Lancet* 2000; **356**: 1876–81.

Rebbeck TR, Lynch HT, *et al.* Prophylactic oophorectomy in carrieras of BRCA1 or BRCA2 mutations. *New Engl J Med* 2002; **346**: 1465–71.

Tabar L, Fagerberg G, *et al.* Efficacy of breast cancer screening by age. New results from the Swedish Two-County Trial. *Cancer* 1995; **75**: 2507–17.

The W, Wilson AR. The role of ultrasound in breast cancer screening. A consensus statement by the European Group for Breast Cancer Screening. *Eur J Cancer* 1998; **34**: 449–50.

The Breast Cancer Information Core (BIC) database www.nchgr.nih.gov/Intramural_research/Lab-transfer/Bic

Warner E, Plewes DB, *et al.* Comparison of breast magnetic resonance imaging, mammography, and ultrasound for surveillance of women at high risk for hereditary breast cancer. *J Clin Oncol* 2001; **19**: 3524–31.

Breast cancer

Breast cancer is the most common form of cancer affecting women. The cumulative incidence of breast cancer in developed countries is 6.3 per 100 women by age 70 years, with a lifetime risk of approximately 9–11%. The Western diet is associated both with earlier menarche and with post-menopausal obesity, which, combined with low parity, later first childbirth, and shorter breastfeeding, perhaps largely account for the much higher incidence of breast cancer in the developed world than in many developing countries.

Factors proven to affect breast cancer risk in the general population

Pregnancy and parity. Breast cancer incidence is transiently increased by pregnancy but is permanently lowered by high parity. The relative risk of breast cancer decreases by 7% for each birth. Breast cancer incidence is reduced by early first childbirth. Women having their first child at >30 years have double the risk of women having their first child at <20 years.

Breastfeeding. The longer women breastfeed, the more they are protected against breast cancer. The lack of or short duration of breastfeeding typical of women in developed countries makes a major contribution to the high incidence of breast cancer in these countries. The relative risk of breast cancer decreases by 4.3% for every 12 months of breastfeeding. This is in addition to a decrease of 7.0% for each birth. This protective effect is more marked in women having a later first pregnancy.

Menarche and menopause. Cumulative breast cancer incidence is permanently lowered by late menarche and early menopause.

Obesity. Obesity is associated with an increased risk for postmenopausal breast cancer. Regular exercise probably reduces the risk of breast cancer although the quantitative effect is uncertain and the evidence is weak.

Alcohol. Compared with non-drinkers, the relative risk of breast cancer amongst women drinking 35–44 g alcohol/day was 1.32, and for ≥45 g alcohol/day was 1.46. The relative risk increased by 7% for each additional 10 g/day (i.e. for each unit or drink of alcohol consumed on a daily basis. The data suggests that ~4% of breast cancer in developed countries may be attributed to alcohol. The effect of alcohol needs to be interpreted in the context of its beneficial effects in moderation on cardiovascular disease.

Oral contraceptive pill (ocp). A meta-analysis suggested that, both for current users and for up to 10 years post-use, there may be a 24% increase (relative risk (RR), 1.24) in risk of breast cancer Collaborative Group or Hormonal Factors in Breast Cancer 1996. Marchbanks *et al.* (2002) undertook a case-control analysis of 4575 women with breast cancer aged 35–64 years. Overall use of ocps by women with a family history of breast cancer (affected mother, sister or daughter) was *not* associated with an increased risk of breast cancer (odds ratio (OR), 0.8). In Marchbanks *et al*'s (2002) study the RR of breast cancer in women 35–44 years with a family history of breast cancer and who had ever used ocps was higher (1.4) than among older women (45–64 years) with a family history, but this difference did not reach significance. Narod *et al.* (2002) have shown that women who are *BRCA1* mutation carriers who have ever used the ocp or who used the ocp for ≥5 years may have an increased risk of early-onset breast cancer (RR, 1.2 and 1.33, respectively).

Hormone replacement therapy (HRT). For women in the general population postmenopausal combined oestrogen and progestin replacement therapy results in an increased risk of breast cancer of 5% per year of use. The risk is substantially higher than for oestrogen replacement therapy alone and does not appear to be influenced by a family history of breast cancer in a first-degree relative (mother, sister, daughter; Ursin *et al.* 2002) The added risk disappears within ~5 years of cessation of use. In the Million Women study of breast cancer and HRT (Million Women Study 2003), current users were more likely than never users to develop breast cancer (RR, 1.66) with the risk increasing with total duration of use. 10 years use of HRT is estimated to result in 19 additional breast cancers per 1000 users of oestrogen–progesterone combinations and 5 additional breast cancers per 1000 users of oestrogen-only preparations.

Factors suggesting a familial susceptibility gene

- Large number of individuals with breast/ovarian/prostate cancer in the family (on one side of the family).
- Multiple generations affected.
- Young average age at which the breast cancers were diagnosed (>25% of breast cancer diagnosed at <30 years is due to a mutation in a dominant gene; 50% of all breast cancers in the general population are diagnosed after 65 years of age).
- Pattern of different types of cancers occurring within the family.
- Multiple primary cancers in one individual with early age of onset (usually first primary at <50 years).

The combined contribution of *BRCA1* on 17q and *BRCA2* on 13q to overall breast cancer is 2–3%. Close to 10% of women diagnosed at less than 40 years are likely to carry a germline mutation in one of the known high-risk genes, but most of these will have a positive family history. The vast majority (>90%) of families with a clearly dominant predisposition to breast and ovarian cancer are known to harbour germline mutations in either BRCA1 or BRCA2 but, for breast cancer-only families with three or more affected individuals, <50% have mutations in these known genes. Other high penetrance breast cancer genes are likely to be discovered.

Other cancer-predisposing syndromes with an increased risk of breast cancer include:

- Peutz–Jeghers syndrome (PJS);
- Li–Fraumeni syndrome, which is associated with childhood soft tissue sarcomas, lung cancer, and adreno-cortical carcinoma with early age of onset (<<1% of all breast cancers);
- Cowden syndrome, which is associated with macro-cephaly, tricholemmomas, mucosal neuromas (<<1%);
- Ataxia telangiectasia (AT). Heterozygous carriers for AT are at a 3.6-fold risk of breast cancer and may account for a few per cent of dominant families.

Breast cancer in males

Breast cancer in men is rare accounting for ~0.8% of diagnoses of all breast cancers. Risk factors include testicular disease, benign breast conditions, age, Jewish ancestry, family history, and the Klinefelter syndrome (Giordano *et al.* 2002). *BRCA2* mutations predispose men to breast cancer and may account for 4–14% of all cases.

Clinical approach

History: key points

- Detailed three-generation family tree noting in affected relatives their full name and date of birth, the type of cancer, age at diagnosis of cancer, hospital where treated, and, when relevant, age at death. Extend the family tree back as far as possible on the relevant side of the family. Ask questions about the type of treatment relatives have had as such questions may give a clue as to how accurate the reported information is likely to be.
- Check ethnicity. Three mutations in *BRCA1/2* in the Ashkenazi Jewish population (*BRCA1* 185delAG, 5382insC, and *BRCA2*, 6174delT) occur with a combined frequency of 2.5% and may account for >90% of highly penetrant families in that population.

Examination: key points

Examination rarely gives diagnostic information except where a rare condition such as Cowden syndrome or PJS is suspected

Special investigations

- Confirmation of diagnosis. Reported cases of breast cancer in close relatives are rarely wrong. Reported cases of ovarian cancer, even in close relatives, are often wrong (e.g. cervical, endometrial). Aim to confirm all diagnoses of ovarian cancer and at least one diagnosis of breast cancer in a family at high/high–moderate risk or in any individual where management decisions hinge on the risk assessment.
- DNA for *BRCA1* and *BRCA2* mutation analysis in an affected member of families meeting the criteria stated below under 'Diagnostic testing'.
- Consider DNA storage from a key affected individual if she/he has advanced cancer.

Genetic advice

Averaged across all ages, the risk of breast cancer to the sister, mother, or daughter of an isolated case is increased about 2-fold (1.5–3-fold). The risk then increases with increasing numbers of affected relatives, and also with young age at diagnosis of affected relatives.

Risk assessment

Breast cancer is a common disease amongst women in late middle-age and old age in the developed world. The risk that women in the general population will be diagnosed with breast cancer is 1 in 11 (9%) to age 80 years. This provides a benchmark against which to evaluate the additional (and sometimes larger) risk attributable to the family history (see table). Generally, for women seeking advice about a family history of breast cancer, risk estimates will vary between 9% (population risk, e.g. 3rd-degree relative was only family member affected) and 40% (50% probability of inheriting an 80% penetrant gene mutation). Higher risks are only applicable when a woman is shown to have a germline mutation, or to have proliferative breast disease.

Penetrance

See discussion in 'BRCA1 and BRCA2', page 426.

Predictive testing

Possible if there is a known familial mutation. Usually only offered to adults and often deferred until a time at which surveillance may be initiated or intervention such as prophylactic oophorectomy may be considered.

Diagnostic testing

Guidelines for consideration of *BRCA1* and *BRCA2* testing in an affected family member are as follows.

- High and high/moderate risk where a DNA sample from an informed affected relative is available (use the table to determine the likelihood of identifying a mutation based on the family history, and to prioritize which gene to screen first).
- For Ashkenazi Jewish individuals, one or more relative with breast or ovarian cancer at any age can be offered testing for the Ashkenazi mutations only.

Management

Breast awareness

A large well-conducted population-based randomized controlled trial from Shanghai (Thomas *et al.* 2002) shows conclusively that regular breast self-examination does not lead to a reduction in mortality due to breast cancer compared to no screening at all. Furthermore, women who regularly self-examined had more breast biopsies and diagnoses of benign breast disease than women who did not. 'Breast awareness' should be encouraged instead, so that women understand the importance of seeking prompt advice if they notice any unusual changes in their breasts.

Surveillance strategies

Screening should take place in properly conducted studies that are fully audited. See also 'Cancer surveillance methods', this chapter.

Mammographic surveillance

A widely adopted pragmatic approach is to offer mammography where the risk due to the family history for a woman <50 years of age is at least equivalent to the risk for a woman >50 years of age in the general population. This roughly equates to a threefold increased risk of breast cancer by the age of 50 years compared with the general population. Although it is clear that cancers can be successfully detected and, in a non-randomized series, are on average diagnosed at earlier stages, conclusive evidence of a mortality reduction from screening women at increased risk of breast cancer at ages younger that 50 years does not exist (Lucassen *et al.* 2001). For *BRCA1* mutation carriers other imaging techniques (e.g. magnetic resonance imaging (MRI)) may offer better sensitivity in the younger breast in particular (Warner *et al.* 2001).

According to the triage criteria suggested above, women in the 'high', 'high/moderate' risk categories would usually be offered annual mammography from ~35 years, reducing to every 18 months from 50 years. Those in the moderate risk category may be offered mammography from 40 years. Those in the 'slightly increased risk' and 'population risk' groups will be encouraged to take up the 3 yearly mammography from 50 years offered as part of the NHS breast screening programme (NHSBSP). A typical mammographic screening strategy is shown in the table.

Further data is urgently needed to clarify the optimum type of screening (e.g. mammography or MRI), the age groups in which it is most efficacious, and to evaluate the possible benefits to women at high risk (as distinct from those at population risk).

Reassurance

Reassurance is currently the appropriate management for women where:

- there has been one family member diagnosed with breast cancer at age >40 years;

Criteria for evaluating a family history of breast cancer (adapted from Eccles *et al.* 2000)

Important guidance for using the table

- Work from the *top of the table down* in assessing risk (risk assigned is then the highest level of risk consistent with the family history)
- **Average age** is a simple arithmetic mean, i.e. a woman with relatives affected at 48 years and 39 years (mean 87/2 = 43.5 year) falls in the bracket 2 relatives diagnosed at 40–49 years
- '**Relative**' includes first-degree relative (mother, father, brother, sister, child) and their first-degree relatives. For the purposes of this analysis, female relatives linked through a male are included because the penetrance of breast cancer genes is so much lower in males than in females. A history of breast cancer in a paternal aunt age 39 years and paternal grandmother age 47 years would be equivalent to half the risk of a woman with a mother and maternal aunt or grandmother at an average age of 44 years, assuming that a dominant gene is the underlying cause of the paternal family history
- Affected relatives should be on the same side of the family. If there are relevant cancers on both maternal and paternal sides of the family, evaluate both sides separately. The estimate will then depend on whether either side looks like it might be due to a dominant gene or whether both sides look like isolated cases. Non-genetic approaches to risk estimation (such as the Gail method) may then be more helpful
- A relative with clearly **bilateral breast cancer** (ie two primaries) should be viewed as two relatives for simplicity
- A **male breast cancer** can be counted as a young female (<30 years)
- Figures in square brackets [ ] refer to the cumulative risk of developing breast cancer over the decade between age 40 and 50 years where early mammography may be appropriate
- Early-onset prostate cancer (and other BRCA1/2 associated cancers) in a male relative may be significant
- Family size is important in assessment of risk, e.g. in very large sibships the significance of 2 affected relatives diagnosed at a 50–60 years is lessened; the maximum risks in the table assume no modifying unaffected relatives

High risk (>1 in 3 lifetime risk) criteria

- Clearly dominant pattern of early onset breast and/or ovarian cancer with an affected first-degree relative
- First-degree relatives where the pattern is consistent with a diagnosis of Li–Fraumeni syndrome

High/moderate risk (>1 in 4 lifetime risk) criteria

- Clearly dominant pattern of breast and/or ovarian cancer with affected 2nd-degree relatives on the paternal side of the family
- First-degree relative with breast and ovarian cancer with age at diagnosis of first cancer <50 years
- 3 relatives diagnosed with breast cancer and/or ovarian cancer, with the breast cancer at average age of 50–60 years (1 in 4 risk) [6–7%]
- 2 relatives (one first-degree) with breast cancer diagnosed <40 years

Moderate risk (>1 in 6 lifetime risk) criteria

- 2 relatives diagnosed with breast cancer at any age (1 in 4–1 in 6 risk) [4%]
- 1 first-degree relative diagnosed with breast cancer <40 years (maximum 1 in 6 risk) [4%]
- 1 male relative diagnosed with breast cancer at any age (maximum 1 in 6 risk) [3–4%]
- 1 relative with both breast and ovarian cancer (diagnosed at any age)

Slightly increased risk (<1 in 6 lifetime risk) criteria

- 1 first-degree or a few distant relatives with no clearly dominant pattern of inheritance and age at onset > 50 years
- 1 first-degree relative diagnosed >40 years (assuming negative family history) (1 in 6–1 in 12) [2–3%]

Population risk (1 in 11 lifetime risk) criterion

- No family history of breast or ovarian cancer and an average environmental risk profile [1%]

Scoring system for the likelihood of identifying a *BRCA1* or *BRCA2* mutation based on evaluation of family history (Evans *et al.* 2004)*

		Score	
Type of cancer	Age at diagnosis (years)	BRCA1	BRCA2
Female breast cancer	< 30	6	5
Female breast cancer	30–39	4	4
Female breast cancer	40–49	3	3
Female breast cancer	50–59	2	2
Female breast cancer	> 59	1	1
Male breast cancer	< 60	5[†]	8
Male breast cancer	> 59	5[†]	5
Ovarian cancer	< 60	8	5[‡]
Ovarian cancer	> 59	5	5[‡]
Pancreatic cancer	Any	0	1
Prostate cancer	< 60	0	2
Prostate cancer	>59	0	1

* In bilateral disease, each breast cancer is counted separately. Ductal carcinoma *in situ* (DCIS) is included. Scores should be summed counting each cancer in a direct lineage (i.e. on the same side of the family). The scoring system includes a cut-off at 10 points for each gene. This equates to >10% probability of a pathogenic mutation in *BRCA1* and *BRCA2* individually.

[†] If *BRCA2* already tested.

[‡] If *BRCA1* already tested.

A typical mammographic screening strategy for women at high risk* (Cambridge 2003)

Age (years)	Strategy
< 30	No mammography
30–34	No mammography unless youngest affected relative diagnosed at < 39 years in which case start 5 years earlier than age of diagnosis
35–49	Annual mammography
50 and over	Mammography every 18 months interleaving 3 yearly mammograms within the NHSBSP and 3 yearly additional mammograms. Continue until age 69 years. Thereafter, patients can self-refer to continue 3 yearly screening as part of NHSBSP

* Moderate risk women join the NHBSP at 50 yrs. Current multicentre trials are assessing the efficacy of mammography for moderate risk women aged 40–49 years.

- there have been two family members diagnosed with breast cancer at age > 60 years; *provided that* there has been no bilateral breast cancer, no male breast cancer, and no ovarian cancer.

Standard reassurance (NICE familial breast cancer guideline 2004) should include written information giving:

- risk information about population level and family history levels of risk;
- breast awareness information;
- lifestyle advice about breast cancer risk including information about HRT, ocps, breastfeeding, lifestyle including diet and alcohol, etc.;
- advice that, if the family history changes, the genetics team should be contacted for an update of the risk assessment.

Support group: Breakthrough breast cancer <www.breastcancergenetics.org.uk>. Cancerline UK <www.cancerlineuk. net/index.asp>

Professional guidelines: <http://www.nice.org.uk/ pdf/CG014quickrefguide.pdf>

Expert advisers: Diana Eccles, Professor of Cancer Genetics, University of Southampton, Southampton and Gareth Evans, Professor of Cancer Genetics, University of Manchester, Manchester, England.

References

American College of Medical Genetics. *Genetic susceptibility to breast and ovarian cancer: assessment, counselling and testing guidelines 1999.* <www.faseb.org/genetics/acmg>.

Antoniou A, Pharoah PDP, *et al.* Average risks of breast and ovarian cancer associated with mutations in *BRCA1* or *BRCA2* detected in case series unselected for family history: a combined analysis of 22 studies. *Am J Hum Genet* 2003; **72**: 1117–30.

Collaborative Group on Hormonal Factors in Breast Cancer. Breast cancer and hormonal contraception: collaborative reanalysis of individual data on 53,297 women with breast cancer and 100,239 women without breast cancer from 54 epidemiological studies. *Lancet* 1996; **347**: 1713–27.

Collaborative Group on Hormonal Factors in Breast Cancer. Breast cancer and breastfeeding: collaborative reanalysis of individual data from 47 epidemiological studies in 30 countries, including 50 302 women with breast cancer and 96 973 women without the disease. *Lancet* 2002; **360**: 187–95.

Eccles D, Evans D, *et al.* Guidelines for managing women with a family history of breast cancer. UK Cancer Family Study Group (UKCFSG). *J Med Genet* 2000; **37**: 203–9.

Emery J, Lucassen A, *et al.* Common hereditary cancers and implications for primary care. *Lancet* 2001; **358**: 56–63.

Evans DGR, Lalloo F. Risk assessment and management of high risk familial breast cancer. *J Med Genet* 2002; **39**: 865–71.

Evans DGR, Eccles DM, *et al.* A new scoring system for the chances of identifying a *BRCA1/2* mutation outperforms existing models including BRACAPRO. *J Med Genet* 2004; **41** (6): 474–80.

Geoffroy-Perez B, Janin N, *et al.* Variation in breast cancer risk of heterozygotes for ataxia-telangiectasia according to environmental factors. *Int J Cancer* 2002; **99**: 619–23.

Giordano SH, Buzdar AU, *et al.* Breast cancer in men. *Ann Intern Med* 2002; **137** (8): 678–87.

Hamajima N, Hirose K, *et al.* Alcohol, tobacco and breast cancer—collaborative reanalysis of individual data from 532 epidemiological studies, including 58,515 women with breast cancer and 95,067 women without the disease. *Br J Cancer* 2002; **87**: 1195–6.

Lucassen A, Watson E, Eccles D. Evidence based case report: advice about mammography for a young woman with a family history of breast cancer. *Br Med J* 2001; **322** (7293): 1040–2.

Marchbanks PA, *et al.* Oral contraceptives and the risk of breast cancer. *New Engl J Med* 2002; **346**: 2025–32.

Million Women Study Collaborators. Breast cancer and hormone-replacement therapy in the Million Women study. *Lancet* 2003; **362**: 419–27.

Narod SA, Dube MP, *et al.* Oral contraceptives and the risk of breast cancer in BRCA1 and BRCA2 mutation carriers. *J Natl Cancer Inst* 2002; **94**: 1773–9.

National Institute of Clinical Excellence (NICE). *Clinical guidelines for the classification and care of women at risk of familial breast cancer in primary, secondary and tertiary care breast cancer.* NICE, 2004. Available at <www.nice.org.uk>.

NICE familial breast cancer guideline June 2004 <www.nice.org.uk/pdf/CG014quickrefguide.pdf>

Thomas DB, Gao DL, *et al.* Randomised trial of breast self-examination in Shanghai: final results. *J Natl Cancer Inst Cancer Spectrum* 2002; **94**: 1445–57.

Ursin G, Tseng CC, *et al.* Does menopausal hormone replacement therapy interact with known factors to increase risk of breast cancer? *J Clin Oncol* 2002; **20**: 699–706.

Warner E, Plewes DB, *et al.* Comparison of breast magnetic resonance imaging, mammography, and ultrasound for surveillance of women at high risk for hereditary breast cancer. *J Clin Oncol* 2001; **19**: 3524–31.

Cancer surveillance methods

Gastrointestinal (GI) surveillance

Colonoscopy

Bleeding occurs in 30/10 000 colonoscopies, the perforation rate is 10/10 000 colonoscopies, and death results from 1/10 000 colonoscopies. Complications are more likely in the elderly and those with co-morbidity or existing disease, e.g. ulcerative colitis, and also include sedative complications (NB. chest disease).

Patients scheduled for colonoscopy have bowel preparation beforehand, consisting of a low residue diet for 48 hours and then a liquid diet for 24 hours before the procedure, followed by laxatives, e.g. Picolax. Most are lightly sedated for the procedure, which, although it is usually uncomfortable to some degree, is only rarely painful. If suspicious lesions are seen they can be biopsied. Small polyps are usually excision biopsied; those with a stalk can be snared; larger polyps can often be removed piecemeal if snaring is not possible. Polypectomy is painless, but is associated with complications: perforation rate after polypectomy 22/10 000; post-polypectomy bleeding 89/10 000. Mortality after polypectomy is 3.9/10 000, with most fatalities arising in older patients.

Colonoscopy and flexible-sigmoidoscopy are both more difficult in women who have had a hysterectomy and this should be discussed. It is a factor to consider in hereditary nonpolyposis colorectal cancer (HNPCC; see 'Hereditary nonpolyposis colorectal cancer (HNPCC)', page 454) where prophylactic hysterectomy may be considered in women who warrant frequent colonoscopy, because of their endometrial cancer risk. Removing the risk of one cancer may predicate detecting another.

NB. Colonoscopy will miss approximately 6% of polyps, usually those <1 cm (Rex et al. 1997; Postic et al. 2002).

The background rate of death from colorectal cancer (CRC) at age 50–54 years is 1.8/10 000).

Flexible sigmoidoscopy

Requires less bowel preparation than a colonoscopy (e.g. sachet of Picolax on day before study or phosphate mini-enema on morning of study). Reaches, at the most, as far as the splenic flexure. Procedure takes ~10 minutes and is usually performed without sedation. Polypectomy as for colonoscopy, except that if significant lesion/s are found (CRC, polyps larger than 5 mm, three or more adenomas, adenomas 5 mm or smaller with a villous component of more than 20%, or severe dysplasia) then a colonoscopy will be required to examine the rest of the colon. Flexible sigmoidoscopy may be of considerable utility for population screening, but is not recommended as a surveillance method in familial CRC instead of colonoscopy (Atkin et al. 2001). It may be used in screening for polyps in famial adenomatous polyposis (FAP), but this will be as part of a surveillance programme also involving proctoscopy, rigid sigmoidoscopy, and colonoscopy.

Upper GI endoscopy

The complication rate of upper GI endoscopy performed for surveillance is unknown, largely because there is no evidence that it is efficacious and hence the vast majority of such examinations are performed in symptomatic individuals for diagnosis. The complication rate associated with diagnostic upper GI endoscopy is necessarily high, because of the nature of diseases necessitating such examination, e.g. oesophageal varices, bleeding peptic ulcers, late-presenting cancers. Thus, for example, the death rate in the 30 days following such an examination is about 1/200. There is some evidence to suggest that establishing a baseline in conditions associated with upper GI polyposis is worthwhile, but that continuing upper GI surveillance should be restricted to those with the most severe disease (Debinski et al. 1995; Wallace and Phillips 1999).

Expert adviser: Ian M. Frayling, Consultant in Clinical Genetics and Director of Clinical Genetics Laboratory, University Hospital of Wales, Cardiff, Wales.

Endometrial surveillance

There is currently no proven efficacious method of surveillance for endometrial cancer in HNPCC (see 'Hereditary nonpolyposis colorectal cancer (HNPCC)', page 454). Various forms of biopsy-based surveillance are possible, e.g. pipelle aspiration, but the evidence base for the use of these is lacking. Progestagen-containing intrauterine devices, e.g. Mirena coil, may prove to be efficacious but, again, studies need to be carried out. Prophylactic hysterectomy after the menopause or after a woman has completed her family is a possibility, but it should be noted (see above) that this can complicate surveillance for bowel cancer, and should not be underestimated (Adams et al. 2003).

Expert adviser: Ian M. Frayling, Consultant in Clinical Genetics and Director of Clinical Genetics Laboratory, University Hospital of Wales, Cardiff, Wales.

Breast surveillance

Mammographic screening has been shown to reduce mortality in women aged 50–64 years from the general population. (Kerlikowske et al. 1995) Current possible methods for surveillance in those at increased familial risk include mammography, ultrasound (USS), and magnetic resonance imaging (MRI). The efficacy of such techniques in younger women at increased risk is still to be established. However, the NICE guidelines for the care of women at risk of familial breast cancer (NICE 2004) include recommendations on surveillance. Briefly, surveillance is not recommended for women at increased risk under age 30. For those at increased risk aged 30–39, it should only be performed as part of approved research studies, e.g. UK MRI study. For those at increased risk aged 40–49 years annual mammography should be offered, but only after provision of written information on the positive and negative aspects of surveillance. Mammographic surveillance over the age of 50 can be performed every 3 years, e.g. as for all women as part of the UK NHS Breast Screening Programme. More frequent surveillance over age 50 should only be carried out as part of a research study. More individualized strategies will need to be established for those at risk due to *BRCA1/2* or *TP53* mutations. There is currently no evidence for routine screening by MRI and/or USS under the age of 50 years, although it may be useful diagnostically.

Breast MRI

Contrast enhanced magnetic resonance imaging (CEMRI) provides information about tissue vascularity that is not available from mammography. In many breast cancers there is neovascularity and the pattern and time course of enhancement after injection of iv contrast material (eg. gadolinium) can determine the likelihood of malignancy.

MRI can detect otherwise occult breast cancer in high-risk patients and is probably most beneficial in those at highest risk eg. carriers of *BRCA* mutations (Kriege, MARIBS). Studies that have cumulatively evaluated breast MRI in >1000 high-risk patients found that the technique identified cancer that was not seen on mammography in 4% of cases (Liberman).

Breast self-examination

A large well-conducted randomized control trial from Shanghai (Thomas *et al.* 2002) shows conclusively that regular breast self-examination does not lead to a reduction in mortality due to breast cancer compared with no screening at all. Moreover, self-examination leads to more breast biopsies and diagnoses of benign breast disease. Nonetheless, 'Breast awareness' should be encouraged so that women understand the importance of promptly reporting any unusual changes in their breasts to their doctor.

Expert adviser: Susan Thomas, Information Team, Breast Test Wales, Cardiff, Wales.

Ovarian surveillance

Routine ovarian cancer screening for the general population is not currently recommended as there is no research evidence to date to support its use.

Potential screening methods for ovarian cancer are either transvaginal ovarian USS or detection of elevated levels of the tumour marker CA125 in the blood. The small proportion of patients diagnosed with stage I ovarian cancer have a good prognosis in contrast to the majority with advanced disease.(Berek 1994) The relationship between survival rates and stage thus provides the rationale for such screening. However, the impact of screening on ovarian cancer mortality of any target population has yet to be confirmed.

Women from 'high risk' families with multiple ovarian and/or breast cancers have a 15–45% lifetime risk of ovarian cancer (Ford *et al.* 1994; Easton *et al.* 1995; Pharoah *et al.* 1998). High-risk women are often anxious and seek surveillance. In most countries there has been widespread introduction of ovarian cancer screening for women over 35 who are from the high-risk population, although the value of such surveillance remains unproven.

Ovarian surveillance can be problematic in the high-risk population as premenopausal women have a variety of both physiological (e.g. menstrual cycle variations) and benign conditions (e.g. endometriosis, ovarian cysts) that can give rise to false-positive abnormalities on USS and CA125 (Berek 1994). In addition, there is the operative morbidity associated with unnecessary surgery in women with false-positive results, the psychological consequences associated with false-positive results, the false reassurance in women with false-negative results, and the cost implications to the health service.

The UK Familial Ovarian Cancer Screening Study (UKFOCSS) is underway to assess the efficacy of annual surveillance with CA125 and transvaginal USS in the high-risk population. The primary objective is to develop an optimized surveillance strategy for ovarian cancer in terms of the most appropriate screening tests and criteria for interpretation of results, screening interval, morbidity, and cost in the high-risk population.

Surveillance for ovarian cancer is therefore only currently available in the UK in the context of this research study.

Expert adviser: Jessica Mozersky, Cancer Research UK and UCL Cancer Trials Centre, University College, London, England.

References

Adams C, Cardwell C, *et al.* Effect of hysterectomy status on polyp detection rates at screening flexible sigmoidoscopy. *Gastrointest Endosc* 2003; **57**: 848–53.

Atkin WS, Edwards R, *et al.* Design of a multicentre randomised trial to evaluate flexible sigmoidoscopy in colorectal cancer screening. *J Med Screen* 2001; **8**: 137–44.

Berek JS. Epithelial ovarian cancers. In *Practical gynecologic oncology*, 2nd edn (ed. J. Berek and N. Hacker), pp. 324–775. Lippincott Williams and Wilkins, Philadelphia, 1994.

Debinski HS, Spigelman A, *et al.* Upper intestinal surveillance in familial adenomatous polyposis. *Eur J Cancer* 1995; **31A**: 1149–53.

Dunlop MG. Guidance on gastrointestinal surveillance for hereditary non-polyposis colorectal cancer, familial adenomatous polyposis, juvenile polyposis, and Peutz–Jeghers syndrome. *Gut* 2000; **51** (Suppl. V): v21–v27.

Easton DF, Ford D, *et al.* Breast Cancer Linkage Consortium. Breast and ovarian cancer incidence in *BRCA1*-mutation carriers. *Am J Hum Genet* 1995; **56**: 265–71.

Ford D, Easton DF, *et al.* Breast Cancer Linkage Consortium.Risks of cancer in *BRCA1* mutation carriers. *Lancet* 1994; **343**: 692–5.

Kerlikowske K, Grady D, *et al.* Efficacy of screening mammography: a meta-analysis. *J Am Med Assoc* 1995; **273**: 149–54.

Kriege M, *et al.* Efficacy of MRI and mammography for breast cancer screening in women with a familial or genetic predisposition. *NEJM* 2004; **351**: 427–37.

Liberman L. Breast cancer screening with MRI — What are the data for patients at high risk? *NEJM* 2004; **351**: 497–500.

Lucassen A, Watson E, *et al.* Advice about mammography for a young woman with a family history of breast cancer. *Br Med J* 2001; **322**: 1040–2.

MARIBS Study group. Screening with magnetic resonance imaging and mammography of a UK population at high familial risk of breast cancer: a prospective multicentre cohort study (MARIBS). *Lancet* 2005; **365**: 1769–78.

National Institute of Clinical Excellence (NICE). *Clinical guidelines for the classification and care of women at risk of familial breast cancer in primary, secondary and tertiary care breast cancer.* NICE, 2004. Available at <www.nice.org.uk>.

Pharoah, PDP, Stratton, JF, *et al.* Screening for breast and ovarian cancer: the relevance of family history. *Br Med Bull* 1998; **54**: 823–38.

Postic G, Lewin D, *et al.* Colonoscopic miss rates determined by direct comparison of colonoscopy with colon resection specimens. *Am J Gastroenterol* 2002; **97**: 3182–5.

Rex DK, Cutler CS, *et al.* Colonoscopic miss-rates of adenomas determined by back-to-back colonoscopies. *Gastroenterology* 1997; **112**: 24–48.

Thomas DB, Gao DL, *et al.* Randomised trial of breast self-examination in Shanghai: final results. *J Natl Cancer Inst Cancer Spectrum* 2002; **94**: 1445–57.

Wallace MH, Phillips RK. Upper gastrointestinal disease in patients with familial adenomatous polyposis. *Br J Surg* 1998; **85**: 742–50.

Wallace MH, Phillips RK. Preventative strategies for periampullary tumours in FAP. *Ann Oncol* 1999; **10** (Suppl. 4): 201–3.

Woolf SH. The best screening test for colorectal cancer—a personal choice [editorial]. *New Engl J Med* 2000; **343**: 1641–3, and letters.

Colorectal cancer (CRC)

See also 'Familal adenomatous polyposis (FAP)' page 444 and 'Hereditary nonpolyposis colorectal cancer (HNPCC)', page 454.

CRC is a common disease. In incidence it is the third most common cancer in males (after lung and prostate cancers), and the second most common (after breast cancer) in females (Office of National Statistics 1996). Lifetime risks in 1996 in the UK were 1:18 for males and 1:20 for females. Genetic susceptibility accounts for 5–10% of CRC, but germline mutations in known single genes account for only 1–2% of cases. The shortfall is considered to be due to a combination of more common lower-penetrance genes that are mostly yet to be elucidated. A family history of the disease confers a significantly increased risk to relatives, confirmed in a recent meta-analysis (Johns and Houlston 2001). The challenge for the geneticist is to try to sort families into (1) those that are likely to be carrying a germline mutation in a defined gene, conferring a high lifetime risk, and (2) those with a reasonably strong genetic risk who are at moderate risk, and thus to target screening appropriately.

The hallmarks of genetic predisposition to bowel cancer are these.

- **Young age at diagnosis.** The mean age of diagnosis in sporadic CRC is 60–70 years (in HNPCC, the mean age of diagnosis of CRC is 44 years, and in FAP it is 39 years).
- **Multiple tumours.** Polyps and/or cancers.
- **Family history,** both of CRC and tumours at other sites.
- **Rare tumours,** e.g. small bowel cancers, skin sebaceous tumours, desmoids.

The geneticist's main role is to identify and diagnose those families with a high risk of CRC attributable to, e.g. FAP or HNPCC, and to establish an empiric risk for those at lesser risk to enable appropriate surveillance or reassurance.

The main approach is by integration of information from the family tree, from histopathology reports, cancer registry confirmations of diagnosis, and sometimes (e.g. Muir–Torre syndrome and FAP) from features on clinical examination.

CRC is a common disease, but the risk of developing it is markedly skewed towards elderly people: <1% of cases develop the disease <45 years (and <0.1% at <35 years). In addition, most (~70%) sporadic CRC occur in the rectum and sigmoid colon, with about 10% in the caecum and the rest elsewhere in the colon.

Adenomas and polyps. Colorectal adenomas are even more common. Up to one-third of those in their 70s may harbour one or two, but only 1:1000 of the population develop three or more. Large, multiple, dysplastic adenomas and villous (or tubulovillous) histology are all associated with empiric increased risk to the individual of a CRC. While most (>95%) CRC develop from adenomas; only a minority of adenomas develop into CRC.

Metaplastic (hyperplastic) polyps are similarly common. They are commonly found in association with adenomas, with or without a CRC, and they can undergo adenomatous change. So-called serrated adenomas have features of both adenomas and metaplastic polyps. Patients with a multiplicity of these other sorts of polyp are at increased empiric risk of CRC.

Small bowel carcinomas. Small bowel carcinomas are very rare in the general population (<0.003%), but occur in predisposition syndromes. Duodenal cancers occur in FAP, though jejunal and ileal cancers are uncommon. Jejunal and ileal carcinomas occur in HNPCC at ~300× the rate in the general population (duodenal cancers are rare in HNPCC—probably a reflection of the proportion of the small bowel that is duodenum). So, because of their rarity, small bowel cancers are very significant. However, exclude other causes such as coeliac disease and Crohn disease.

Ashkenazi Jews. CRC is significantly more common in this population group. This is probably due to a variety and combination of genetic factors. A missense mutation in the *APC* gene (I1307K) is found in 6% of the Ashkenazi Jewish population and is associated with the development of multiple adenomas and metaplastic polyps. A number of studies have found in general that it confers a non-statistically significant increased lifetime risk for CRC of 1.4–1.9, but the risk of CRC associated with this mutation is increased in those with a family history of CRC, implying other modifiers may be critical. Ashkenazim are also predisposed, at least in part, by a locus on 15q (CRAC1/ HMPS).

Mismatch repair. Defective mismatch repair occurs in ~15% of all colon cancers and can arise through either of two mechanisms. In ~5% of all tumours, it is caused by mutation in mismatch repair genes (e.g. *MLH1*, *MSH2*, *MSH6*), i.e. HNPCC, whereas in ~10% of tumours it is caused by epigenetic silencing of the promoter sequence of *MLH1* by biallelic methylation (i.e. there is no germline mutation). Defective mismatch repair is rare in rectal cancers and when it does occur it usually indicates HNPCC.

Clinical approach

History: key points

- Three-generation family tree with particular emphasis on history of tumours, benign and malignant, and documentation of age of diagnosis. Try to extend the family tree further on the relevant side if there are individuals with cancer in the grandparental generation.
- Enquire about the health of the consultand. Do they consider themselves in good health, have they any symptoms, e.g. a change in bowel habit, that are causing them concern? If yes, explore symptoms further and refer to a gastroenterologist/colorectal surgeon for further evaluation. Be aware that patients presenting to genetics who are especially worried about their family history may actually be symptomatic.
- Obtain histopathology records or cancer registry confirmation. Whenever available, sight of histopathology records can be critical. A CRC may be found to have occurred in the setting of multiple polyps, or polyps of a particular sort. Cases referred with a presumptive diagnosis of FAP usually turn out not to be FAP once the histopathology report is obtained.
- Decide who is affected, i.e. those with CRC, or at least three adenomatous polyps, or one adenomatous polyp, if it occurred at <60 years, or was 1 cm or greater in size, or had tubulo-villous/villous or severely dysplastic histology.
- Other relevant HNPCC-related (HRC) tumours, e.g. gastric, ovary, ureter/renal pelvis, brain, small bowel, hepatobiliary tract, and skin (sebaceous tumours).

Examination: key points

- Ask about skin lesions in the individual and family: most patients don't regard them as tumours and won't spontaneously report them. Refer to a dermatologist as

Family history criteria for triaging into 'high', 'moderate', and 'low' risk groups (UK Eastern Region Policy for Family History of Bowel Cancer 2000)*

High risk
Families with, or a good probability of, a hereditary CRC syndrome, either one of the polyposes, e.g. FAP, AFAP, PJS, or familial JPS, or HNPCC. See the separate sections in this chapter on HNPCC, FAP, PJS, and JPS.

Moderate risk
'Moderate risk' can be split into 'high–moderately increased risk' and 'low–moderately increased risk' subgroups as defined below with each subgroup warranting somewhat different surveillance. Note that the criteria for 'low–moderately increased risk' are exclusive, and any relevant family history over and above them will categorize the family as 'high–moderately increased risk'

Low–moderately increased risk
Two CRC-affected FDR with average age > 60 years
One CRC-affected FDR and one CRC/HRC-affected SDR (both on the same side of the family) both < 70 years old

High–moderately increased risk
For example, but not exclusively:
One CRC-affected FDR (45 years but > 35 years (if < 35 years, then > 50% chance of HNPCC, i.e. 'high risk')
Two CRC-affected FDR with average age < 60 years (including both parents)
Two CRC-affected FDR and one CRC/HRC-affected FDR or SDR (but AC2-negative)
One CRC-affected FDR and two CRC/HRC-affected FDR or SDR (but AC2-negative)
NB. These are only common examples of 'high–moderately increased risk' and this list is not exhaustive. Clinical judgement will be required in situations where the family history is more than 'high–moderately increased risk', but does not satisfy high risk/HNPCC criteria.

Low risk
One CRC-affected FDR aged > 45 years and no CRC/HRC-affected SDR
No affected FDR and only one or two affected SDR

* CRC, Colorectal cancer; FAP, familial adenomatous polyposis; AFAP, attenuated FAP; PJS, Peutz–Jeghers syndrome; JPS, juvenile polyposis; HNPCC, hereditary nonpolyposis CRC; FDR, first-degree relative; SDR, second-degree relative; HRC, HNPCC-related cancer; AC2.

appropriate—sebaceous adenomas often masquerade as common skin lesions.
- In suspected Peutz–Jeghers (PJS) polyposis, also check for perioral/axillary/inguinal/perianal freckling.
- Ask about and look for dental anomalies—extra/missing teeth, dentiginous cysts, osteomas of the jaw (and other sites).
- In suspected FAP it may be worth looking for congenital hypertrophy of the retinal pigment epithelium (CHRPE). Refer to an opthalmologist.
- Perhaps the key examination is pathological examination— histopathological reports (medical records, death certificates, cancer registry entries). It can well be worthwhile asking a pathologist with a specialist interest in, e.g. colorectal or skin pathology, to review histology.

Genetic advice
Risk assessment
First, sort out high-risk families.
- Ask the question 'Does or could the family have a defined polyposis?' If so proceed appropriately for FAP, attenuated (A)FAP, PJS, etc.
- Ask the question 'Does or could this family have HNPCC?' See section below. If so proceed appropriately.
- Ask the question 'Could they have some other cancer genetic syndrome, and the CRC in the family is unrelated to it?' (It is also worth considering whether the family history might be due to more than one syndrome, if it is very strong, on both sides, or very early onset.)

If the family history doesn't fit with any of the above and it largely or solely consists of CRC, then triage the family into 'high–moderate', 'low–moderate', or 'low' risk, as in the table. Use clinical commonsense. Use the patterns of cancer table and consider carefully whether there may be

Odds ratio and lifetime risk of dying from CRC

Risk group*	Odds ratio	Lifetime risk of dying from CRC (%)
General population	1.0	2
Any family history	1.8	5.9
One affected FDR (any age)	2.8	—
One affected FDR <45y	3.7	10
Two affected FDR	5.7	16.7

* FDR, First-degree relative.

an alternative genetic explanation conferring a significant genetic risk.

Penetrance
For FAP and HNPCC see 'Familal adenomatous polyposis (FAP)' page 444 and 'Hereditary nonpolyposis colorectal cancer (HNPCC)', page 454. St John et al. (1993) calculated the odds ratio for developing CRC, and Houlston estimated the lifetime risk of dying given a family history of CRC (see table).

Management
Surveillance
See also 'Cancer surveillance methods', page 434.
Note that it may not be necessary at the outset to embark on a lifetime regime of colorectal surveillance in those at risk. Consider the possible use of, at least at the outset, one-off colonoscopies to determine if, for example, polyps are present, perhaps at a young age, in other members of the family. A family at a low/low–moderate level of risk may thus be elevated into a higher risk group. Not

infrequently relatives may be having somewhat different surveillance regimes when dealt with in other regions—a pragmatic approach may be best. Also bear in mind that, given the pace of advance in imaging techniques and advanced molecular methods of stool analysis, colonoscopy may well become obsolete as the primary method of surveillance in those at increased risk, in their lifetime. An upper age when surveillance might cease of 70–75 years is suggested.

Surveillance regimes for moderately increased risk of CRC are not absolutely established. Dunlop (2002), for example, has published guidelines, but these are by no means universally accepted. The following is based on the UK Eastern Region Policy for Family History of Bowel Cancer (October 2000):

- **High-risk.** HNPCC: colonoscopy every 2 years, starting at 25–30 years, but see 'Familal adenomatous polyposis (FAP)' page 444, 'Hereditary nonpolyposis colorectal cancer (HNPCC)', etc., page 454.
- **High–moderate risk..** Colonoscopy every 5 years starting at 45 years (or 5 years before age of earliest onset CRC in family, whichever is the later).
- **Low–moderate risk.** One-off colonoscopy at 55 years. If an adenomatous polyp should be found, then adenoma surveillance guidance applies. Note that a single small adenoma found in a member of the general population does not warrant follow-up more frequently than another colonoscopy 10 years later, but if an individual found to have an adenoma has a family history the risk is sufficient to warrant colonoscopy 3 years later (Nusko et al. 2002).
- **Low risk.** Those whose empiric risk does not justify screening intervention should be reassured that their level of risk does not merit surveillance over and above that recommended for the general population. If population screening is available then individuals should be encouraged to participate.

Predictive testing

Not currently feasible, unless a condition with a known genetic basis has been diagnosed, e.g. FAP, HNPCC, in which case see relevant section.

Education

Educate your patient about the symptoms of CRC so that he/she is aware when to seek medical advice and investigation. The most significant symptoms are:

- rectal bleeding;
- a persistent change in bowel habit, usually to looser or more frequent bowel actions;
- abdominal mass;
- unexplained anaemia.

Diet and other environmental or lifestyle influences

As well as a family history, there are numerous other genetic/environmental influences on CRC risk that patients increasingly ask about, some of which are summarized in the table below. The magnitude of risk associated with, for example, a diet rich in red meat, or, probably more importantly, poor in fruit and vegetables is about the same as having a single first-degree relative with an adenoma, i.e. 2×, and not quite as great as having a single first-degree relative with CRC (2.8×). How much effect these factors have in those individuals with high penetrance genes, rather then those with 'moderate' risk, remains to be established, but undoubtedly common genetic variation plays an important part in how an individual interacts with environmental factors. There is no evidence that proprietary dietary supplements make any difference.

Update family history

Emphasize the importance of notifying the genetics dept of any new diagnoses in the family as these may significantly change the risk assessment.

Support group: Cancerline UK `www.cancerlineuk.net/index.asp`.

Expert adviser: Ian M. Frayling, Consultant in Clinical Genetics and Director of Clinical Genetics Laboratory, University Hospital of Wales, Cardiff, Wales.

References

de la Chapelle A. Microsatellite instability [perspective]. *New Engl J Med* 2003; **349**: 209–10.

Dunlop MG. Guidance of large bowel surveillance for people with two first degree relatives with colorectal cancer or one first degree relative diagnosed with colorectal cancer under 45 years. *Gut* 2002; **51** (Suppl. V): v17–v20.

Giardiello FM, Brensinger JD, Petersen GM. AGA technical review on hereditary colorectal cancer and genetic testing. *Gastroenterology* 2001; **121**: 198–213.

International Society for Gastrointestinal Hereditary Tumours (InSIGHT) `www.insight-group.com`

Jenkins MA, et al. After hMSH2 and hMLH1—what next? Analysis of three-generational, population-based, early-onset colorectal cancer families. *Int J Cancer* 2002; **102**: 166–71.

Johns LE, Houlston RS. A systematic review and meta-analysis of familial colorectal cancer risk. *Am J Gastroenterol* 2001; **96**: 2992–3003.

Lindgren G, et al. Adenoma prevalence and cancer risk in familial non-polyposis colorectal cancer. *Gut* 2002; **50**: 228–34.

Lynch HT, de la Chapelle A. Hereditary colorectal cancer. *New Engl J Med* 2003; **348**: 919–32.

Nusko G, et al. Risk related surveillance following colorectal polypectomy. *Gut* 2002; **51**: 424–8.

Ransohoff DF, Sandler RS. Screening for colorectal cancer. *New Engl J Med* 2002; **346**: 40–4.

St John DJB, et al. Cancer risk in relatives of patients with common colorectal cancer. *Ann Intern Med* 1993; **118**: 785–90.

Vasen HFA, et al. New clinical criteria for hereditary non-polyposis colorectal cancer (HNPCC, Lynch Syndrome) proposed by the ICG-HNPCC. *Gastroenterology* 1999; **116**: 1453–6.

Wijnen JT, et al. Clinical findings with implications for genetic testing in families with clustering of colorectal cancer. *New Engl J Med* 1998; **339**: 511–18.

Winawer SJ, et al. Risk of colorectal cancer in the families of patients with adenomatous polyps. National Polyp Study Workgroup. *New Engl J Med* 1996; **334**: 82–7.

Confirmation of diagnosis of cancer

In cancer genetics, risk assessment usually depends critically on the information reported in the family history. If management decisions, e.g. prophylactic surgery or invasive screening procedures, are going to be based on that information it is important to confirm its accuracy. In a perfect world every cancer diagnosis would be confirmed but, in practice, limited time and resources mean that this is usually impracticable.

Reported cases of breast cancer in close relatives are rarely wrong (inaccurate in 5% in Douglas *et al.*'s (1999) study), but reported cases of abdominal and especially gynaecological cancers often are (inaccurate in 20% in Douglas *et al.*'s (1999) study). 'Stomach' cancer can mean almost anything abdominal. 'Liver' cancer is usually secondary. 'Womb' cancer includes cervical as well as endometrial tumours. Douglas *et al.* (1999) found that management of 11% of families was changed by information obtained from cancer confirmation.

In practice it may be reasonable, at least in high-risk families, to confirm:

- all cases of colorectal and gastrointestinal tract cancer;
- all cases of ovarian cancer;
- at least one diagnosis in a family where prophylactic surgery or screening is being considered;
- at least one diagnosis in a family where mutation screening is instituted on the basis of the family tree (rather than immunohistochemical or other histopathological findings in the tumour or clinical features in the proband).

Hierarchy of reliability of confirmation

1 Pathology report. This is the 'gold standard'.
2 Cancer Registry report.
3 Hospital discharge summary.
4 Death certificate. For relatives who died a long time ago, this may be the only accessible document.

References

Douglas FS, O'Dair LC, *et al.* The accuracy of diagnoses as reported in families with cancer: a retrospective study. *J Med Genet* 1999; **36**: 309–12.

Cowden syndrome (CS)

Diagnostic criteria for Cowden syndrome (International Cowden Consortium 2000)

Pathognomonic criteria
- Mucocutaneous lesions: facial trichilemmomas, acral keratoses, papillomatous papules, mucosal lesions

Major criteria
- Breast cancer
- Thyroid cancer (non-medullary), especially follicular thyroid cancer
- Macrocephaly (> 95th centile)
- Lhermitte–Duclos disease (LDD)—dysplastic gangliocytoma of the cerebellum
- Endometrial carcinoma

Minor criteria
- Other thyroid lesions (e.g. adenomas, multinodular goitre)
- Mental retardation (IQ < 75)
- Gastrointestinal hamartomas
- Fibrocystic disease of the breast
- Lipomas
- Fibromas
- Genitourinary tumours (especially renal cell cancer, uterine fibroids) or malformation

Making a diagnosis based on the above criteria
1. Mucocutaneous lesions alone if there are: (a) 6 or more facial papules, of which 3 must be trichilemmomas, or (b) cutaneous facial papules and oral mucosal papillomatosis, or (c) oral mucosal papillomatosis and acral keratoses, or (d) 6 or more palmoplantar keratoses *or*
2. 2 major criteria but one must include macrocephaly or LDD *or*
3. 1 major and 3 minor criteria *or*
4. 4 minor criteria *or*
5. Family member meeting CS criteria above + the pathognomonic criterion *or*
6. Family member meeting CS criteria above + any one major criterion *or*
7. Family member meeting CS criteria above + two minor criteria

PTEN hamartoma tumour syndrome (PHTS), Cowden syndrome (CS).

PTEN is a tumour suppressor gene on 10q23.3 that mediates cell-cycle arrest and/or apoptosis. Germline mutations in *PTEN* cause a bewildering array of features that fall into four main clinical groupings: Cowden syndrome, Bannayan–Riley–Ruvalcaba (BRR) syndrome, Proteus syndrome, and Proteus-like syndrome. The criteria for making a diagnosis of CS are outlined in the table. CS and BRR have been observed in different members of the same family. This has led to the proposal to amalgamate these disorders into one, under the umbrella heading of PHTS.

Prevalence is difficult to determine since, due to the enormous variability of expression, age-dependent penetrance, and the subtlety of some of the features, it is likely to be underdiagnosed. Prevalence is likely to be >1/200 000.

Lhermitte–Duclos disease (LDD). LDD, or dysplastic gangliocytoma of the cerebellum, is an unusual hamartomatous overgrowth disorder. LDD can be familial or, more commonly, sporadic. It has been only recently recognized that LDD may be associated with CS. Recent work using immunohistochemistry and mutation analysis shows that loss of PTEN function is sufficient to cause LDD (Zhou *et al.* 2001). There is a high frequency of germline *PTEN* mutations in patients presenting with apparently isolated LDD. Individuals with LDD, even without apparent CS features, should be counselled as in CS.

Bannayan–Riley–Ruvalcaba syndrome (BRR). Autosomal dominant (AD) disorder consisting of macrocephaly, vascular malformations, lipomas, pigmented macules on the shaft of the penis. It is associated with malignancies (breast, thyroid, endometrial, and gut hamartomas). Birthweight usually >4000 g, occipital-frontal circumference (OFC) often >4.5 SD. Hypotonia, gross motor delay (60% have a mild proximal myopathy, a lipid myopathy with type I fibre enlargement), learning disability, and speech delay occur in 70%. 25% have seizures. Patients may have mild hypertelorism. 60% have mutations in *PTEN*.

Clinical approach
History: key points

Three-generation family tree with specific enquiry about breast and thyroid problems, large head size, and learning disability.

Examination: key points
- OFC for macrocephaly.
- Careful examination of skin and oral mucosa for characteristic 'cobblestone' mucocutaneous lesions.
- Careful examination of neck for goitre or nodularity.

Investigation

PTEN mutation analysis
- 85% mutation frequency for CS (this includes promoter analysis (Zhou 2003))
- 65% mutation frequency for BRRS (this includes large deletions)
- 20% mutation frequency for Proteus (Zhou 2001).

Genetic advice
Risk assessment

AD; 50% risk to offspring. Adults with CS are at risk of having children with BRR as well as CS.

Penetrance

Mucocutaneous lesions are found in >90% of mutation carriers and may be the only manifestation. Two-thirds have breast or thyroid disease or both.

Predictive testing

Offer cascade screening to family members once they are approaching an age to participate in screening.

Prenatal diagnosis

Technically possible by chorionic villus sampling (CVS) if a familial mutation has been identified,

Management

Surveillance strategies

All those with a germline *PTEN* mutation or clinical diagnosis of CS should be offered the following.

- From 18 years of age, annual examination of skin and thyroid (or when aged 5 years younger than youngest diagnosis of PTEN-related cancer in the family).
- For females from 25 years of age, clinical breast exam with annual mammography from 30 years (or when aged 5 years younger than youngest diagnosis of breast cancer in the family).
- From 35 years, annual dipstick urine for haematuria and for women consider screening for endometrial cancer.

Expert adviser: Charis Eng, Professor and Director, Clinical Cancer Genetics Program, Ohio State University, Columbus, Ohio, USA.

References

Celebi JT, Tsou HC, *et al*. Phenotypic findings of Cowden syndrome and Bannayan–Zonana syndrome in a family associated with a single germline mutation in *PTEN*. *J Med Genet* 1999; **36**: 360–4.

Eng, C. Will the real Cowden syndrome please stand up: revised diagnostic criteria [commentary]. *J Med Genet* 2000; **37**: 828–30.

Eng C. Invited Mutation Update. PTEN: One gene, many syndromes. *Hum Mutat* 2003; **22**: 183–98.

Pilarski R, Eng C. Commentary: Will the real Cowden syndrome please stand up (again)? Expanding mutational and clinical spectra of the PTEN hamartoma tumour syndrome. *J Med Genet* 2004; **41**: 323–6.

Smith JM, Kirk EPE, *et al*. Germline mutation of the tumour suppressor *PTEN* in Proteus syndrome. *J Med Genet* 2002; **39**: 937–40.

Waite KA, Eng C. From developmental disorder to heritable cancer: it's all in the BMP/TGF-beta family. *Nat Rev Genet* 2003; **4**: 763–73.

Zhou XP, Hampel H, *et al*. Association of a germline mutation in the *PTEN* tumour suppressor gene and Proteus and Proteus-like syndromes. *Lancet* 2001; **358**: 210–11.

Zhou XP, Marsh DJ, *et al*. Germline inactivation of PTEN and dysregulation of the phosphoinositol-3-kinase/Akt pathway cause human Lhermitte–Duclos disease in adults. *Am J Hum Genet* 2003; **73**: 1191–8.

Zhou XP, Waite KA, *et al*. Germline PTEN promoter mutations and deletions in Cowden/Bannayan–Riley–Ruvalcaba syndrome result in aberrant PTEN protein and dysregulation of the phosphoinositol-3-kinase/Akt pathway. *Am J Hum Genet* 2003; **73**: 404–11.

Familial adenomatous polyposis (FAP)

Familial polyposis, Gardner syndrome (old term for FAP with extracolonic features), familial (adenomatous) polyposis coli (FPC/FAPC), adenomatous polyposis coli (APC).

- **Classical FAP** is defined when >100 polyps are found in the colorectum at endoscopy (sigmoidoscopy or colonoscopy) or on pathological examination of the colon (after colectomy). Complete ascertainment by the Danish FAP Registry has shown the prevalence to be 1:8500, while the incidence appears to be 1.3 new cases per million population per year.
- **Colorectal adenomas.** Up to 30% of the general population will develop an adenoma or two by the age of 70 years, but only 1:1000 of the population will develop more than two adenomas. Multiplicity of adenomas is empirically associated with a significantly increased risk of colorectal cancer (CRC).
- **Attenuated FAP (AFAP).** There are a considerable number of individuals and families with generally <100 but > 2 adenomas. These are grouped under the term 'attenuated FAP'.

Dominantly inherited classical FAP is caused by mutation in the *APC* gene, and somatic mutations in this gene are also seen in the early stages of sporadic colon cancer. *APC* functions in the Wnt signalling pathway to regulate the degradation of beta-catenin. APC also binds to and stabilizes microtubules in the cell, which have an important role in chromosome segregation during mitosis. Truncating mutations in *APC* that eliminate microtubule binding may contribute to chromosomal instability in cancer cells (Kaplan *et al.* 2001).

FAP/AFAP is genetically heterogeneous: APC and MUTYH

Until very recently, FAP was considered to be solely due to autosomal dominant (AD) inheritance of germline mutations in the *APC* gene at 5q22.2. On the basis of the number of cases without antecedent family history the supposed new mutation rate was variously estimated at 10–30%. Many cases are undoubtedly due to new *APC* mutations, but there is emerging evidence that a significant proportion of such cases is due to autosomal recessive (AR) inheritance of mutations in *MUTYH* (*MYH*), a DNA repair gene involved in the repair of oxidation damage, at 1p34.1. Early estimates are that, in the UK at least, about 25% of those with >9 adenomas (i.e. AFAP) and no evidence of a dominant family history are due to *MUTYH* mutations. Up to 400 adenomas have been described in those with two *MUTYH* mutations, so the *MUTYH*-associated phenotype clearly overlaps both AFAP and FAP. There are two common mutations in Northern Europeans (see below) and, although risks to *MUTYH* carriers are undefined, they appear to be low. Some extracolonic features, such as are observed in FAP due to *APC* mutations, have been reported to occur in a few individuals with *MUTYH*-associated polyposis, specifically upper gastrointestinal tumours and congenital hypertrophy of the retinal pigment epithelium (CHRPE; see below). Therefore, the job of the geneticist is now to distinguish those families with AD FAP/AFAP due to *APC* from those due to the AR locus *MUTYH*.

In Ashkenazim, an additional locus associated with a form of adenomatous polyposis has been described on 15q13–q22, termed *CRAC1*. This is now known to be the locus responsible for HMPS (hereditary mixed polyposis syndrome). A missense mutation (*APC* I1307K) has been associated with an AFAP-like phenotype in Ashkenazi Jews, while another missense (E1317Q) has been variably associated with multiple adenomas in non-Jewish Europeans (as well as being found in 1% of Ashkenazim). However, the association with E1317Q may be because it is in linkage disequilibrium with a nonsense mutation at the 5'end of the gene.

Multisystem disease: extracolonic features

FAP due, at least, to germline *APC* mutations is associated with a number of extracolonic features (see table); indeed APC-associated FAP is a multisystem disorder. Individuals develop multiple adenomas of both the colorectum and duodenum, with concomitant risk of cancer. Fundic gland polyps develop in the stomach. Desmoid tumours are liable to develop in connective tissue and mesentery, especially in or around the trunk. Characteristic CHRPE develops in the eye. Sebaceous cysts (distinct from the sebaceous adenomas that can develop in hereditary nonpolyposis colorectal cancer (HNPCC)/Muir–Torre; see 'Hereditary nonpolyposis colorectal cancer (HNPCC)', this chapter) occur at greater frequency, as do osteomata, dental (dentiginous) cysts, and supernumerary teeth. (NB. Individuals referred as possible FAP because of multiple sebaceous cysts may have steatocystoma multiplex due to keratin 17 mutations.) An increased risk of cancer at several extracolonic sites is also observed, e.g. adrenals, primary brain, thyroid (papillary cancer), primary liver (hepatoblastoma), and hepatobiliary tree.

Extracolonic features in FAP (after Giardiello *et al.* 2001)

Cancers	Other lesions
Brain (medulloblastoma; Crails syndrome)	Congenital hypertrophy of the pigment epithelium (CHRPE)
Thyroid (e.g. papillary)	Nasopharyngeal angiofibromas
Duodenal (jejunum very rare)	Osteomas
Periampullary	Radioopaque jaw lesions
Pancreas	Supernumerary teeth
Hepatoblastoma (1/150 <5 years)	Lipomas, fibromas, epidermoid cysts
Biliary tree	Desmoid tumours
	Gastric adenomas/fundic gland polyps
	Duodenal, jejunal, ileal adenomas

Brain tumours plus polyposis: Turcot syndrome

Turcot described a syndrome in which colorectal adenomatous polyposis occurred together with a predisposition to primary brain cancers. It has subsequently been shown that Turcot is genetically heterogeneous: some cases are due to *APC* mutations; others to HNPCC (see 'Hereditary nonpolyposis colorectal cancer (HNPCC)', this chapter). Quite what proportion might be due to *MUTYH* mutations remains to be determined, but the association of colorectal polyposis and brain cancers in the first decade of life is certainly associated with inheritance of two HNPCC mutations at the same locus, i.e. a constitutional deficiency of DNA mismatch repair. (see 'Hereditary nonpolyposis colorectal cancer (HNPCC)', page 454). Primary brain cancers in FAP, although rare, are more likely to be medulloblastomas, but all types occur.

APC mutations

There are three common FAP-associated *APC* mutations: two recurrent 5 bp deletions, one at codon 1061, the other at codon 1309, and deletion of the whole gene. Together they account for about 25–30% of mutations, the rest are essentially private point mutations. Less than 1% of cases are due to cytogenetically visible chromosomal mutations involving 5q22, but these are usually associated with a contiguous gene syndrome causing dysmorphic features and learning difficulties, particularly delayed speech. The hallmark of all FAP-associated *APC* mutations is that they are null, nonsense, or frameshifting.

The spectrum of *APC* mutations associated with FAP shows a number of genotype–phenotype correlations. *APC* consists of 2843 codons. Mutations located between, approximately, codons 160 and 1600 are associated with hundreds of adenomas: classical FAP. Mutations occurring at or near to codon 1300 are associated with thousands of adenomas (and the highest colorectal cancer (CRC) risk, as well as more extracolonic signs). Mutations located 5' of codon 160 or 3' of codon 1600 are associated with AFAP. Polyp numbers are related to CRC risk: untreated, those with thousands of polyps develop CRC at a mean age of 28 years, whereas the mean age in those with hundreds of polyps is 44 years, and in those with AFAP is 55 years. Mutations 3' of codon 1400 are especially associated with desmoid tumours. Indeed, one mutation at codon 1942 (5826_5829delCAGA) has been associated with **familial infiltrative fibromatosis**, a variant of FAP in which the risk from desmoid tumours is greater than that from gastrointestinal tract cancers. Mutations located 5' of exon 9 (codons 312–438) are not associated with CHRPE (except for some mutations in exon 6), whereas those located 3' of exon 9 usually are associated with CHRPE. Mutations located in exon 9 (which is alternately spliced) are not only variably associated with CHRPE, but also with reduced polyp numbers (AFAP). The number of polyps associated with AFAP mutations is highly variable: some individuals may develop no polyps, some > 100, others between 1 and 100. Only about 10% of those with AFAP have demonstrable APC mutations; the condition is genetically heterogeneous (*APC, MUTYH, CRAC1*/HMPS, at least).

MUTYH mutations

There are two common *MUTYH* point mutations in Northern Europeans, Y165C and G382D, that together account for approximately 85% of mutant alleles. The remaining 15% are other point mutations of all classes. Although the number of individuals tested from other population groups is small, E466X appears to be the prevalent Indian mutation (all 4 unrelated individuals tested were E466X homozygotes), while a single Pakistani has been found to be homozygous for Y90X, neither mutation being found in Caucasians. The frequency of larger-scale mutations involving whole exons has yet to be determined.

Clinical approach

History: key points

- Three-generation family tree with particular emphasis on history of tumours, benign and malignant, and documentation of histological proof of diagnosis, i.e. >100 adenomas. It is critical to determine the apparent mode of inheritance, i.e. AD or not.
- Ascertain who has had screening or operations for what and when and where.

- Is the family already known to a familial cancer or polyposis registry?
- Ask about possible extracolonic features, e.g. upper gastrointestinal disease, sebaceous cysts, desmoids/ 'fibromatosis', osteomata, dental history, ophthalmic history.
- History of learning difficulties?

Examination: key points

- Check for sebaceous cysts, especially scalp and trunk: most patients don't regard them as tumours and won't spontaneously report them.
- Examine the mouth and jaws: teeth, cysts, osteomata.
- Head/neck/trunk/abdominal wall/limb swellings. Desmoids? If so, refer to surgeon.
- If patient declares or is found to have an abdominal mass refer to a gastroenterologist or colorectal surgeon.
- Gastrointestinal tract. Refer to a gastroenterologist or colorectal surgeon (see below under 'Surveillance and management').

Special investigations

- **Histopathology.** There must be over 100 adenomas in the colorectum to diagnose FAP. If there are fewer than 100 adenomas then AFAP or 'multiple adenomas' can be diagnosed. Microadenomas in the colorectal mucosa, i.e. adenomas confined to a single crypt ('monocryptal' or 'single-crypt' adenomas), are a hallmark of FAP/AFAP (but they are found in both *APC*- and *MUTYH*-associated polyposis). Multiple fundic gland polyps in the stomach are characteristic of FAP, but entirely benign.
- **Ophthalmology.** CHRPE. A single large pigmented lesion with a pale halo is diagnostic of FAP. Smaller, generally hyperpigmented, lesions are not uncommon in the general population, but are found at increased frequency in FAP, where they are typically multiple/bilateral. The number of lesions tends to be concordant within families, and correlates with site of *APC* mutation, NB. while the presence of significant CHRPE indicates FAP, their absence does not exclude it. See 'Predictive testing' below. Refer to an opthalmologist with expertise in this area.
- **APC mutation detection.** The laboratory will wish to know the phenotype, i.e. FAP or AFAP, whether CHRPE are known to be expressed, or the polyp numbers are especially dense, or the family have a particular predilection to desmoids as this will help them to direct mutation detection to the appropriate part of the gene. Similarly, it will help them in detection and interpretation to know if there is a dominant family history or not.
- **MUTYH mutation detection.** The laboratory will wish to know the pattern of inheritance, the ethnic background of the proband/family and if there is a possibility of consanguinity, and whether the phenotype is FAP or AFAP. Blood from parents and/or other relatives may be useful, together with details of their phenotype.
- **Chromosome analysis** in cases with learning disability and/or dysmorphic features.

Genetic advice

Risk assessment

- If FAP phenotype and AD inheritance, then a presumptive diagnosis of *APC*-associated FAP can be made, and appropriate counselling given regarding inheritance and possible genetic testing.

- If FAP phenotype, but AD inheritance cannot be demonstrated, i.e. isolated case or affected sibship, then disease is probably due to *APC* mutation, but may be due to *MUTYH*.
- If AFAP phenotype, and AD inheritance can be demonstrated, then may be due to *APC* mutation (approximately 10% of cases), but in most cases (90%) the cause is, as yet, elusive (though note that Ashkenazim may have the HMPS/*CRAC1* locus on 15q).
- If AFAP phenotype (with > 9 adenomas) but AD inheritance cannot be demonstrated, i.e. isolated case or affected sibship, then disease is more likely due to *MUTYH* (approximately 25% of cases) with AR inheritance, but an *APC* mutation cannot be ruled out. However, except in Ashkenazim, the cause in the rest is, as yet, elusive.

NB. The pattern of inheritance in a particular family may not be obvious until the proband's first-degree relatives have undergone colonoscopy or some other form of diagnostic examination, e.g. for CHRPE.

Mutations. There is usually little difficulty with the interpretation of FAP-related *APC* mutations, as they are almost always (possibly exclusively) null, nonsense, or splice/frameshifting. In cases of apparently new mutation, the recurrent 5 bp mutations at codons 1061 and 1309 are more likely (with the proviso that such individuals may have *MUTYH* mutations).

Linkage. In the absence of an *APC* mutation it is possible to carry out 5q22 linkage studies in families with AD FAP, preferably with flanking markers. However, given the discovery of *MUTYH* as an alternative cause, all concerned will wish to be absolutely convinced that there is a clearcut AD family history with histological proof of phenotype, as well as gathering in samples from as many relatives as possible, preferably from more than one generation.

Penetrance

There is almost complete penetrance with 50% of FAP patients developing polyps by 15 years and 95% by 35years.

Burn *et al.* (1991) determined penetrance figures for adenomas in *APC*-associated FAP, which can be combined with CHRPE data to give an age-related risk of being a gene carrier. The accompanying chart gives the FAP carrier risk for an individual at 50% prior risk of FAP and found to be free of polyps on sigmoidoscopy at a given age.

Risks can be adjusted in families that express CHRPE. Expression of CHRPE indicates gene carriers, with the proviso that the correct type and/or number of CHRPE are observed (see above). Non-expression of CHRPE occurs in 1 in 12 gene carriers, so those who do not have CHRPE have a reduced (but not zero) risk of being a carrier. By means of a Bayesian calculation a final risk can be calculated if an individual is polyp-free at a given age and CHRPE-negative (at any age), as shown in the chart.

An individual at-risk of FAP and found to have either CHRPE or a single adenoma on surveillance at a young age must be regarded as a carrier. An adenoma found in an at-risk individual at an older age may be sporadic, but continued surveillance should indicate whether or not this was the case.

Prenatal diagnosis

Technically possible if the familial *APC* mutation is known.

Surveillance and management

See also 'Cancer surveillance methods', this chapter.
Surveillance of those at risk of FAP can cease when the carrier risk drops below 1%. In the absence of CHRPE data, the residual risk of a polyp-free individual being an FAP carrier drops below 1% at age 40 years. In a family in which CHRPE are found, the residual risk of a CHRPE-negative and polyp-free individual being an FAP carrier drops below 1% at age 24 years.

Colorectal surveillance

Most individuals with *APC*-associated FAP will start to develop colorectal adenomas in their teens. Thus, surveillance is geared to the detection of these in those at risk with a view to offering prophylactic surgery at the earliest convenient time. In those with FAP who have not had a

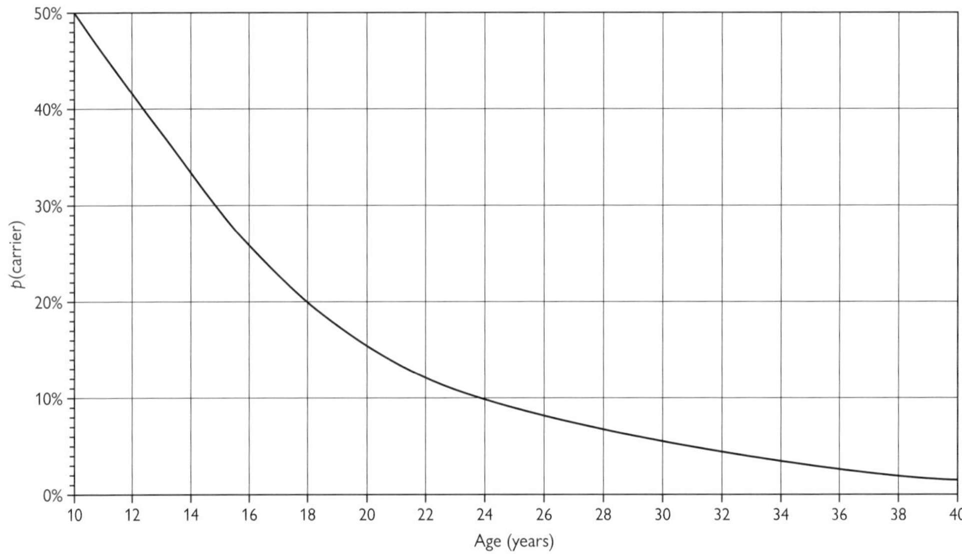

FAP carrier risk given polyp-free, at a given age. (Adapted from Burn *et al.* (1991).)

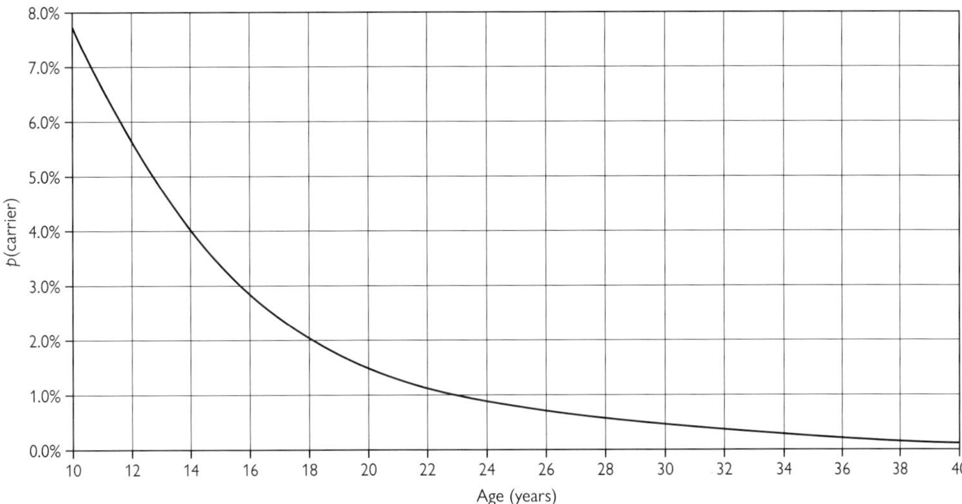

FAP carrier risk given polyp-free, at a given age, and CHRPE-negative (in families where CHRPE are expressed). (Adapted from Burn *et al.* (1991).)

prophylactic colectomy CRC can occur under 20 years of age. This is more likely in those with *APC* mutations at or around codon 1300.

There are subtle differences in the endoscopic methods of polyp surveillance. Most patients will develop polyps detectable on rigid sigmoidoscopy, i.e. in the rectum and sigmoid colon. However, rectal sparing is described, especially in AFAP. Therefore, although rigid sigmoidoscopy is quick and easy to perform, there is a place for flexible sigmoidoscopy (which can also be performed in out-patients, and can approach the splenic flexure) and colonoscopy, the latter requiring more extensive preparation and involving day-care admission.

Surveillance strategy will depend on local resources and discussion with the surgical team/endoscopist.

For **FAP** alternatives are:

- Annual or 6-monthly sigmoidoscopy from early/mid-teenage. Cover for the possibility of rectosigmoid sparing with occasional colonoscopy. Gradually extend the screening interval to 3-yearly as the patient gets older. Reassure and discharge when residual risk drops below 1% (i.e. age 40 years in the absence of CHRPE data, but see below).
- Annual flexible sigmoidoscopy from 13–15 years of age in at-risk family members until 30 years, and then at 3–5-yearly intervals until 60 years of age.

NB. This surveillance is *not* appropriate for those at risk of **AFAP**, because they often exhibit late-onset polyps, rectosigmoid sparing, and wide individual variation in expressivity/penetrance. In such cases a regime similar to that for HNPCC is more appropriate, i.e. 2-yearly colonoscopy.

Surgical management

Surgical opinion varies, but most plan for prophylactic colectomy in affected individuals between the ages of 16 and 20 years to minimize risk of malignancy. Restorative procto-colectomy with ileoanal pouch may be the operation of choice for most patients in view of the long-term risk of rectal

cancer (12–29%). However, Patients with the most severe dense polyposis, e.g. those with mutations at or around codon 1300, may be given their increased short-term risk of rectal cancer, best managed by restorative proctocolectomy with formation of an ileoanal pouch. However, for the majority of patients colectomy and ileorectal anastamosis, with rectal surveillance until mid-life when a proctectomy with ileoanal pouch formation is performed, may be preferred. Undoubtedly, best results are obtained in specialist centres and it is important for FAP patients to engage with the care of an appropriate surgical team at an early stage.

Upper gastrointestinal tract

There is no established practice as regards the surveillance and management of upper gastrointestinal polyposis in FAP. Most patients will have gastric fundic polyps, which are entirely benign, but the significant lesions are duodenal adenomas. Now that patients are avoiding colorectal cancer by prophylactic colectomy, the overall risk of duodenal cancer is 3–4%, so upper gastrointestinal disease is increasingly significant. Intensive, e.g. annual, upper gastrointestinal endoscopy is unpleasant and not without its own risks. There seems to be little point in the surveillance of those with few, less dysplastic adenomas as they are unlikely to develop duodenal cancer. However, those with more advanced duodenal polyposis (multiple, large, severely dysplastic adenomas) may benefit from some degree of upper gastrointestinal surveillance, but this remains to be proven. An upper gastrointestinal endoscopy at around 30 years may be reasonable to establish the baseline. Those with lesser disease can be left alone, while those with more advanced disease can be offered surveillance.

Desmoid tumours

FAP patients are at significantly increased risk of desmoid tumours, and about 10% will develop clinically evident disease. Desmoids are histologically benign, but may become clinically malignant as they encroach on and encase vital organs and structures, particularly in the case of intraabdominal tumours. They are indolent, difficult to surgically excise completely, and refractory to treatment with chemo- or radiotherapy. Together with upper gastrointestinal tract disease they are now one of the leading causes of premature death in FAP.

- Sporadic desmoids are more likely to occur peripherally (limbs), whereas FAP-associated desmoids more commonly arise centrally (head/neck/trunk/abdominal wall/intraabdominal).
- Families with mutations at or beyond codon 1400 have the highest risk of desmoids, perhaps up to 30–40%. There is no established form of surveillance for occult desmoids, though imaging by computerized tomography (CT) or magnetic resonance imaging (MRI) may be useful in surgical management.
- A number of FAP families have now been described in which the diagnosis only became apparent when children presented with desmoids.

Nonsurgical treatment

Although surgical management of FAP is the mainstay, a number of trials have been or are being carried out into possible chemotherapeutic options. Nonsteroidal anti-inflammatory drugs (NSAIDs) reduce CRC risk in the general population and there is evidence that they reduce the numbers of rectal polyps in those with ileorectal anastomoses, but not the risk of cancer. Nonetheless, selective cyclooxygenase 2 (COX-2) inhibition appears to have some effect on upper gastrointestinal tract disease, and Celecoxib is the first specific COX-2 inhibitor to be licensed for FAP, though not in the UK.

Support group: FAP Support group <www.fapsupportgroup.org>.

Expert adviser: Ian M. Frayling, Consultant in Clinical Genetics and Director of Clinical Genetics Laboratory, University Hospital of Wales, Cardiff, Wales.

References

Al-Tassan N, et al. Inherited variants of MYH associated with somatic G:C → T:A mutations in colorectal tumors. Nat Genet 2002; **30**: 227–32.

Burn J, et al. The UK Northern Region genetic register for FAP: use of age of onset, CHRPE and DNA markers in risk calculations. J Med Genet 1991; **28**: 289–96.

Chung DC, Mino M, et al. Case 34–2003: A 45-year-old woman with a family history of colonic polyps and cancer. New Engl J Med 2003; **349**: 1750–60.

Clark SK, Phillips RK. Desmoids in familial adenomatous polyposis [review]. Br J Surg 1996; **83**: 1494–504.

Cole TRP, Sleightholme HV. ABC of colorectal cancer: the role of clinical genetics in management. Br Med J 2000; **321**: 943–6.

Dunlop MG. Guidance on gastrointestinal surveillance for hereditary non-polyposis colorectal cancer, familial adenomatous polyposis, juvenile polyposis, and Peutz–Jeghers syndrome. Gut 2000; **51**(Suppl. V): v21–v27.

Friedl W, et al. Can APC mutation analysis contribute to therapeutic decisions in familial adenomatous polyposis? Experience from 680 FAP families. Gut 2001; **48**: 515–21.

Giardiello FM, Brensinger JD, Petersen GM. AGA technical review on hereditary colorectal cancer and genetic testing. Gastroenterology 2001; **121**: 198–213.

Healy JC, et al. MR appearances of desmoid tumors in familial adenomatous polyposis. Am J Roentgenol 1997; **169**: 465–72.

Hyer W. Polyposis syndromes: pediatric implications [review]. Gastrointest Endosc Clin N Am 2001; **11**: 659–82, vi–vii.

International Society for Gastrointestinal Hereditary Tumours (InSIGHT) www.insight-group.com

Jaeger EEM, et al. An ancestral Ashkenazi haplotype at the HMPS/CRAC1 locus on 15q13–q14 is associated with hereditary mixed polyposis syndrome. Am J Hum Genet 2003; **72**: 1261–7.

Jones S, et al. Biallelic germline mutations in MYH predispose to multiple colorectal adenoma and somatic G:C → T: A mutations. Hum Mol Genet 2002; **11**: 2961–7.

Kaplan KB, Burds AA, et al. A role for the adenomatous polyposis coli protein in chromosome segregation. Nat Cell Biol 2001; **3**: 429–32.

Sampson JR, et al. Autosomal recessive colorectal adenomatous polyposis due to inherited mutations of MYH. Lancet 2003; **362**(9377): 39–41.

Sieber OM, et al. Whole-gene APC deletions cause classical familial adenomatous polyposis, but not attenuated polyposis or 'multiple' colorectal adenomas. Proc Natl Acad Sci, USA. 2002; **99**: 2954–8.

Sieber O, Lipton L, Heinimann K, Tomlinson I. Colorectal tumourigenesis in carriers of the APC I1307K variant: lone gunman or conspiracy? J Pathol 2003a; **199**: 137–9.

Sieber OM, Lipton L, et al. The multiple colorectal adenoma phenotype, Familial adenomatous polyposis and germline mutations in MYH. New Engl J Med 2003b; **348**: 791–9.

Tomlinson I, Rahman N, Frayling I, Mangion J, et al. Inherited susceptibility to colorectal adenomas and carcinomas: evidence for a new predisposition gene on 15q14–q22. Gastroenterology 1999; **116**: 789–95.

Whitelaw SC, et al. Clinical and molecular features of the hereditary mixed polyposis syndrome. Gastroenterology 1997; **112**: 327–34.

Gastric cancer

Gastric cancer is the second largest cancer burden worldwide. In the UK, the lifetime risk in the general population is 2.3% for males, and 1.2% for females. Average age at diagnosis in men is 72 years (range 65–80 years), and in women 75 years (range 70–85 years). Survival rates are low (10% at 5 years) due to late presentation and diagnosis. In contrast to the West, Japan has introduced systematic mass screening programmes with oesophagogastroduodenoscopy (OGD), leading to the increased detection of gastric cancers confined to the mucosa or submucosa. Survival rates for patients with early gastric cancer are > 90% at 5 years.

Gastric cancer can be classified histopathologically into two distinct types: intestinal and diffuse (linitis plastica type). The major risk factor for intestinal gastric cancer identified so far is *Helicobacter pylori* infection. However, whether *H. pylori* eradication is an effective cancer prevention measure is not yet proven.

Approximately 10% of cases of gastric cancer involve familial clustering. Cancer predisposition syndromes to consider include:

- **hereditary nonpolyposis colorectal cancer (HNPCC).** ~5% lifetime risk. See 'Hereditary nonpolyposis colorectal cancer (HNPCC)', this chapter.
- **familial adenomatous polyposis (FAP).** See 'Familal adenomatous polyposis (FAP)', this chapter.
- **Peutz–Jeghers syndrome** See 'Peutz–Jeghers syndrome (PJS)', this chapter.
- **hereditary diffuse gastric cancer.** ~70–80% lifetime risk. See below.
- **BRCA2.** See 'BRCA1 and BRCA2', this chapter.

Most large familial gastric cancer kindreds show no evidence of HNPCC, and molecular genetic studies show only a low frequency (~10%) of E-cadherin mutations. Mean age at diagnosis is ~54 years, but there is wide variation. No close association with *H. pylori* has been demonstrated to date.

Hereditary diffuse gastric cancer (HDGC). HDGC accounts for just 1–3% of gastric adenocarcinomas. Histology is diffuse or 'linitis plastica' type. Hereditary diffuse cancer has a high penetrance (70–80%) and a high mortality rate. It is autosomal dominant (AD) and caused in ~35% of kindreds by inactivating mutations in *CDH1* (E-cadherin). (The overall mutation detection rate in gastric cancer families is ~10%). It has a strikingly young age of onset, with average age at diagnosis of 38 years compared with 60–70 years for sporadic gastric cancer. Screening gastroscopy and random biopsy is ineffective (as shown by the high incidence of tumour in gastrectomy specimens after prophylactic surgery in patients who have undergone surveillance). Following predictive genetic testing, prophylactic total gastrectomy is recommended in mutation carriers.

Women with *CDH1* mutations appear to have an increased risk of lobular breast cancer, with a cumulative risk of 39% by age 80 yrs.

The diagnostic criteria for HDGC are as follows.

1 Two or more documented cases of diffuse gastric cancer in first- or second-degree relatives, with at least one diagnosed at <50 years.

2 Three or more documented cases of diffuse gastric cancer in first- or second-degree relatives, independently of age of onset.

Oesophageal cancer—tylosis. Tylosis is a rare syndrome presenting with hyperkeratosis of the palms and soles of the feet. AD with variable penetrance.

- Type A tylosis presents in adolescence and is associated with a high risk for oesophageal cancer. Approximately 20% of individuals with type A develop oesophageal cancer (especially in smokers). Onset of malignancy is typically from 50 years. Annual OGD surveillance is recommended.
- Type B tylosis has a neonatal presentation and affected individuals are not at increased risk for oesophageal cancer. Two North American kindreds spanning 5 and 7 generations confirm the benign nature of type B (Maillefer *et al.* 1999). No surveillance is indicated.

The locus for focal palmoplantar keratoderma (tylosis) associated with squamous cell oesophageal cancer (TOC; type A tylosis) has been mapped to chromosome 17q25, a region frequently deleted in sporadic squamous cell oesophageal tumours.

Clinical approach
History: key points
At least three-generation family tree with specific enquiry for all forms of cancer, with age at diagnosis. Note names, dates of birth, and hospital where the diagnosis was made. This information may be helpful in confirming the family history prior to risk assessment.

Examination: key points
Not usually appropriate in an asymptomatic family member, unless there is a family history of oesophageal cancer (examine palms and soles for hyperkeratosis).

Genetic advice
Risk assessment
Relatives of gastric cancer patients have a two- to threefold increased risk of developing gastric cancer. The risk is elevated for both genders (Imsland *et al.* 2002). The lifetime risk in the general population is 2.3% for males and 1.2% for females.

- The risk with two affected relatives is 1 in 8 to 1 in 10.
- The risk with 3 affected relatives is 1 in 3.
- The risk in HDGC is AD.

Penetrance
Penetrance in HDGC is high at 70–80% for gastric cancer and ~39% for breast cancer in females.

Predictive testing
Predictive testing is possible if the familial mutation is known. In HDGC this is used where possible to determine which individuals should be offered prophylactic gastrectomy since the procedure has a high morbidity with some patients having difficulty maintaining adequate nutrition postsurgery.

Management
Surveillance strategies
See also 'Cancer surveillance methods', this chapter.
- Consider *H. pylori* screening and eradication.
- Consider regular endoscopy (ineffective for diagnosis of diffuse gastric cancer).
- Consider prophylactic total gastrectomy in HDGC.

Expert adviser: Carlos Caldas, Professor, Cancer Genomics Programme, Department of Oncology, University of Cambridge, Cambridge, England.

References

Fitzgerald RC, Caldas C. E-cadherin mutations and hereditary gastric cancer: prevention by resection. *Dig Dis* 2002; **20**: 23–31.

Huntsman DG, Carneiro F, *et al.* Early gastric cancer in young, asymptomatic carriers of germ-line E-cadherin mutations. *New Engl J Med* 2001; **344**: 1904–9.

Imsland AK, Eldon BJ, *et al.* Genetic epidemiologic aspects of gastric cancer in Iceland. *J Am Coll Surg* 2002; **195**: 181–6; discussion, 186–7.

Maillefer RH, Greydanus MP. To B or not to B: is tylosis B truly benign? Two North American genealogies. *Am J Gastroenterol* 1999; **94**: 829–34.

Risk JM, Evans KE, *et al.* Characterization of a 500 kb region on 17q25 and the exclusion of candidate genes as the familial tylosis oesophageal cancer (TOC) locus. *Oncogene* 2002; 21: 6395–402.

Weitzel LN, McCahill LE. The power of genetics to target surgical prevention. *New Engl J Med* 2001; **344**: 1942–4.

Gorlin syndrome

Basal cell naevus syndrome, naevoid basal cell carcinoma syndrome.

Gorlin syndrome is an autosomal dominant (AD) condition caused by mutations in the tumour suppressor gene *PTCH* on 9q22.3, which functions as a receptor for hedgehog. Basal cell carcinomas (BCCs) and other tumours in Gorlin syndrome show loss of heterozygosity (LOH) for *PTCH* (i.e. the tumours are the consequence of a second hit). The congenital malformations (affecting 5% of patients) are thought to be due to alterations of gene dosage in the dosage-sensitive hedgehog signalling pathway. Gorlin syndrome affects ~1/50 000 individuals.

The diagnostic criteria for Gorlin syndrome are given in the table.

Clinical approach
History: key points
- Three-generation family tree with specific enquiry about skin cancer, jaw cysts, and large head size.
- Past medical history, including any previous surgery.

Diagnostic criteria (based on Evans *et al.* 1993 and Kimonis *et al.* 1997)

Diagnosis is based on two major or one major + two minor criteria

Major criteria

More than 2 basal cell carcinomas (BCCs), or one at < 20 years, or > 10 basal cell naevi

Odontogenic keratocyst or polyostotic bone cyst

3 or more palmar/plantar pits

Bilamellar or early (20 years) calcification of falx cerebri

A first-degree relative with Gorlin syndrome

Minor criteria

Congenital skeletal anomaly: bifid, fused, splayed, or missing rib or fused vertebrae

Macrocephaly (adjusted for height) with bossing

Congenital malformation: cleft lip/palate (3–8%), pre- or postaxial polydactyly

Ovarian/cardiac fibroma

Childhood medulloblastoma

Lymphomesenteric cysts

Ocular anomalies (cataract, developmental defects)

Examination: key points
- Occipital-frontal circumference (OFC; and height to determine whether there is relative macrocephaly).
- Face for mild hypertelorism and frontal bossing.
- Skin for BCCs (may appear in early childhood, but usually proliferate from puberty onwards). There may be few to many 100s of BCCs, but many stay quiescent. More common on face and sun-exposed areas, but also occur on trunk. They are raised lesions (1–10 mm diameter) with a pearly to flesh-coloured to pale brown coloration. Skin tags on the neck that histologically have the appearance of a BCC but do not behave aggressively.
- Palms. Examine for palmar pits, small circular depressions (1–2 mm) in the hard skin of the palms (and sometimes soles), present in 65–80%. Age-dependent.
- Patients who are the first person in their families to be affected may have milder signs because of somatic mosaicism.

Investigations
- DNA (EDTA (ethylenedinitrilotetraacetate) blood sample) for *PTCH* mutations analysis—if diagnosis secure.
- Chest X-ray to look for bifid, fused, or splayed ribs and hemivertebrae (if diagnosis not secure).
- Skull X-ray (anteroposterior (AP) and lateral) to look for lamellar falx calcification (present in over 90% patients by age 20 years) and bridging of sella turcica.
- Orthopantogram (OPG) in individuals older than 7 years to look for jaw cysts (see below).

Genetic advice
Risk assessment
AD; 50% risk to offspring of an affected individual. High new mutation rate: 35–50% of affected individuals have *de novo* mutations.

Penetrance
Penetrance is complete, but there is marked intra- and interfamilial variation in expressivity.

Predictive testing
Possible if the familial mutation is known or the family is informative for linkage markers.

Prenatal diagnosis
Possible by chorionic villus sampling (CVS) if the familial mutation is known or the family is informative for linkage markers.

Management
Surveillance strategies
- **Skin.** BCCs may become locally invasive from puberty onwards. Refer to a dermatologist for annual (or more frequent) monitoring from age 12 years. BCCs are more florid in sun-exposed areas and much less common in those with black skin. Advise liberal use of sun-block, peaked caps, T-shirts, avoidance of midday sun, etc. Avoid treatment by radiation as most (but not all) families respond with multiple new lesions in the treatment field.
- **Jaw cysts.** Odontogenic keratocysts of both upper and lower jaws occur from age 7 years. Refer for annual dental screening (OPG) from age 8 years. Cysts have an age-dependent penetrance of 80% by 20 years and > 90% by 40 years. Make the patient's dentist aware of the diagnosis or possible diagnosis of Gorlin syndrome.
- **Medulloblastoma** affects ~3% and usually presents at ~2.5 years. It is more common in boys than girls (3M:1F). Investigate by magnetic resonance imaging (MRI; avoid computerized tomography (CT) if possible as ionizing radiation increases risk for BCCs). *Avoid* radiotherapy if possible in treatment as this can result in profuse BCCs in the radiation field.

Support group: Gorlin Syndrome Support Group (UK) <www.gorlingroup.co.uk>, Tel. UK 01772 517624; Basal Cell Carcinoma Nevus Syndrome/Gorlin Syndrome Homepage <www.hometown.aol.com/budcaruso/skinindex.html>, Tel. US 708–756–3410.

Expert advisers: Robert J. Gorlin, Professor (retired), Department of Oral Pathology and Genetics, University of Minnesota, Minneapolis, Minnesota, USA and Peter Farndon, Professor of Clinical Genetics, University of Birmingham, Birmingham, England.

References

Evans DG, Ladusans EJ, *et al.* Complications of the naevoid basal cell carcinoma syndrome: results of a population based study. *J Med Genet* 1993; **30**: 460–4.

Gorlin RJ. Nevoid basal cell carcinoma syndrome. *Dermatol Clin* 1995; **13**: 113–25.

Kimonis VE, Goldstein AM, *et al.* Clinical manifestations in 105 persons with nevoid basal cell carcinoma syndrome [review]. *Am J Med Genet* 1997; **69**: 299–308.

Hereditary nonpolyposis colorectal cancer (HNPCC)

Lynch syndrome type 1: site-specific colorectal cancer; Lynch syndrome type 2: family cancer syndrome

HNPCC is due to the autosomal dominant (AD) inheritance of a mutation in one of the components of the DNA mismatch repair (MMR) system. Germline mutations in *MSH2* (2p21) and *MLH1* (3p22.3) account roughly equally for > 90% HNPCC. A small number of families (<5%) have mutations in *MSH6* (2p16.3; but only 300 kb from *MSH2*), while <1% have mutations in *PMS2* (7p22.1). If *PMS1* and *MSH3* germline mutations are a cause of HNPCC then they are very rare. It is therefore distinct from the set of autosomal recessive (AR) constitutional DNA repair deficiency diseases that generally manifest with a propensity to multiple tumours and death at an early age. However, there are (often consanguineous) families that have now been described in which children develop colorectal adenomatous polyposis, primary brain cancers, leukaemia, and an neurofibromatosis type 1 (NF1)-like skin phenotype, because they are homozygous or compound heterozygous for mutations in an HNPCC gene. This phenotype is quite distinct from HNPCC and may well be the cause of at least some cases of Turcot syndrome (see below). It is noteworthy that AR inheritance of mutations in *MUTYH*, a DNA repair gene, also predisposes to colorectal adenomatous polyposis (see 'Familial adenomatous polyposis (FAP)', this chapter).

All classes of mutation are associated with HNPCC. Nonsense, frameshift, splice, and missense point mutations all occur, while an increasing number of whole exon deletions/duplications and rearrangements are being found, especially in *MSH2* where they may account for perhaps a third or more of mutations at that locus. Only one kindred has so far been described with a large chromosomal defect, a 10 Mb paracentric inversion of 2p with a breakpoint involving *MSH2*.

HNPCC accounts for about 1% of colorectal cancers, and its prevalence is of the order of 1:3000. Some populations, e.g. Finns, show a founder effect.

Muir–Torre syndrome (MTS). MTS is the co-occurrence of skin sebaceous tumours, (adenomas, epitheliomas, or carcinomas), with internal malignancy; sebaceous skin tumours are rare and consistently empirically associated with a high risk of internal cancer. A subset, probably most of MTS, is due to HNPCC, but the literature abounds with an association with breast cancer, so HNPCC may not be the sole cause of MTS. Other skin tumours, such as keratoacanthomas, are associated with MTS, but there can often be a fine histological distinction between keratoacanthomas and squamous carcinomas, which may account for the latter also being associated with MTS.

Turcot syndrome. Turcot syndrome is the co-occurrence of colorectal adenomatous polyposis and primary brain cancers. Considered by some to be an AR condition, it is now known that it can be caused by mutations in either *APC* or one of the HNPCC genes; indeed, some cases may be due to AR inheritance of two mutations in the same HNPCC gene (see above).

Pathogenesis

Microsatellite instability

Loss of MMR in a tumour manifests as microsatellite instability (MSI). MSI is defined as the presence of extra alleles at a microsatellite when compared with normal DNA from the same individual. It is due to insertion/deletion mutations at repeats, but it should be borne in mind that, in a cell that has lost MMR, point mutations are occurring all over the genome, somewhat preferentially at repeats. Microsatellites vary in their propensity to show instability, and the frequency with which the same microsatellite is affected in different tumour types also varies. Instability is observed best at di- and mononucleotide repeats, with instability at mononucleotide repeats being somewhat more significant than at dinucleotide repeats.

It is important to realize that about 15–20% of sporadic *colon* cancers show MSI, usually due to epigenetic downregulation of MLH1 by methylation. Thus unselected colon cancers with MSI have a poor positive predictive value (PPV) for HNPCC, although lack of MSI confers a reasonably good negative predictive value (NPV). MSI in *rectal* cancers, however, is rare and strongly associated with HNPCC, which can be exploited clinically as it gives an excellent PPV for HNPCC (and NPV when not present). Similarly, MSI is rare in adenomas outside of HNPCC, so giving good values for PPV/NPV. Approximately 15% of sporadic tumours of the types associated with HNPCC also show MSI, e.g. endometrial and gastric tumours. The significance of MSI testing is increased when more than one tumour can be tested from the same individual and/or family.

Immunohistochemistry

It is possible to test tumours for loss or abnormality of MMR protein expression by means of immunohistochemistry (IHC). Abnormality can include patchy expression with loss of nuclear staining as well as complete loss of expression. Approximately 30% of HNPCC tumours that have lost MMR and have MSI do not show any abnormality on IHC. However, when an IHC abnormality is found it is always associated with MSI. If it is desired to exclude HNPCC and a tumour shows normal IHC then it will be necessary to carry out MSI testing. The major advantage of IHC testing is that it has the power to indicate the gene that is involved. Its value is considerably enhanced by testing more than one tumour from the same family and/or individual, especially if these are types with a high PPV or are otherwise rare, e.g. rectal cancers, colorectal adenomas, small bowel cancers, sebaceous skin tumours, etc. (as for MSI testing). Consistent IHC abnormality of one MMR protein is excellent evidence for the pathogenicity of a mutation in that gene, which is important given the number of missense and other difficult to interpret mutations that occur in HNPCC.

If a family can be confidently diagnosed clinically as having HNPCC then the value lies in IHC indicating which gene is at fault. Whereas, in families that have a lower chance of being due to HNPCC, e.g. high–moderate bowel cancer risk, the greater value lies in excluding HNPCC by not finding MSI. Nevertheless, if an IHC abnormality should be found then MSI can be implied, and the family dealt with accordingly.

Pathology

Multiple adenomas are uncommon in HNPCC, but they do occur. However, if more than, say, half a dozen should be found and there are no other non-colorectal HNPCC-associated tumour types in the family it would be worth exploring the possibility of attenuated FAP (see FAP). It is important to note the presence of metachronous or synchronous cancers or adenomas, multiple bowel cancers in particular being a good indicator of HNPCC (see below).

Although HNPCC does not generally predispose to an obvious excess of adenomas, individuals are, nonetheless, predisposed to colorectal cancer. This may be because their adenomas are more likely to progress to carcinomas, and more quickly, than in the general population.

The endometrial cancers in HNPCC are likely to be endometrioid. Urothelial cancers in HNPCC are typically transitional cell carcinomas. Primary brain cancers are more likely to be astrocytomas/glioblastomas, but all types occur.

NB. Unusual, strange, rare tumours may occur in HNPCC (just as they can in any cancer genetic syndrome).

Tumour spectrum

The major predisposition conferred by HNPCC is to adeno-carcinomas of the colon and rectum in both sexes and to endometrial cancer in females. Unlike in the general population, where most bowel cancers occur in the rectum and sigmoid colon, in HNPCC they occur equally through-out the large bowel, thus appearing to have a propensity for 'right-sided' lesions. The young age of onset of cancers in HNPCC is commonly stressed, but it is important to realize that there may be bias introduced by selection of families for young onset, and a late-onset tumour cannot be dismissed as sporadic without supporting, e.g. molecular, evidence. As well as colorectal and endometrial cancer, HNPCC also predisposes to a wide variety of tumours at other sites (see table). Lifetime risk/penetrance figures vary, inevitably, between studies and populations, some-times widely, indicating the importance of modifiers, both environmental and genetic. The figures given in the table are working averages for use in the clinic.

The issue of breast cancer risk in HNPCC is somewhat contentious. There does not appear to be a strong general predisposition to breast cancer in HNPCC, although one study has shown that, while there is no association with *MSH2* mutations, there is a small but statistically significant increase with *MLH1* or 'neither *MSH2* nor *MLH1*' mutations, though probably not enough to warrant screening. (But see 'Muir–Torre syndrome' above.)

Genotype–phenotype

There is evidence that *MSH2* mutations confer a greater risk than *MLH1* of developing any cancer. However, when the risks are subdivided by site the differences generally lose statistical significance, except for urinary tract cancers, which are more common with *MSH2* mutations. *MSH6* mutations, however, seem to be associated with a reduced propensity to colorectal cancer, but an increased risk of endometrial as well as urothelial cancer.

Clinical approach

History: key points

- Three-generation family tree with particular emphasis on history of tumours, benign and malignant. Obtain names and dates of birth of affected relatives, age at diagnosis, and, if possible, details of the hospital where they were treated.
- Ascertain who has had screening or operations for what and when and where.

Tumour risk in HNPCC

Site	Risk in HNPCC	Approximate increase over general population	Lifetime UK general population risk*
Colorectum	Males: 45% (by 50 years), 70% (by 70 years), 80% (lifetime)	~200× 16×	5.5% (1 in 18)
	Females: 20% (by 50 years), 35% (by 70%), 40% (lifetime)	100× 8×	5.0% (1 in 20)
Endometrium	Females: 10% (by 50 years), 40% (by 70 years), 50% (lifetime)	35×	1.4% (1 in 70)
Gastric	ca. 5%	~2–3×	Males: 2.3% (1 in 45) Females: 1.2% (1 in 90)
Ovarian	ca. 4%	~2–3×	2.1% (1 in 50)
Pancreas	2%?	~2–3× (?)	1.0% (1 in 100)
Urothelial (especially ureter/renal pelvis)	2–6%	~2–3×	Males: 3.3% (1 in 30) Females: 1.3% (1 in 80)
Renal (not urothelial)	1–2%	~2–3× (?)	Males: 1.1% (1 in 90) Females: 0.6% (1 in 160)
Brain/central nervous system	3%	4×	0.7% (1 in 150)
Lymphoproliferative (not Hodgkin's)	2–3%	~2–3× (?)	1.3% (1 in 75)
Small bowel	1%	~300×	<0.003%
Hepatobiliary system (gall bladder/bile duct)	1% (?)	~2–3× (?)	

* Source: Office of Population Censuses and Surveys (1996).

- Documentation of histology or cancer registry confirmation:
  - is the family already known to a familial cancer or polyposis registry?

Examination: key points

- Ask about skin lesions in the individual and family: most patients don't regard them as tumours and won't spontaneously report them. Refer to a dermatologist as appropriate—sebaceous adenomas often masquerade as common skin lesions.
- If patient declares or is found to have a mass refer to a surgeon as appropriate.

Special investigations: key points

- **Histopathology.** When asking for reports on a known tumour, it is also worth asking if the pathology laboratory has any reports on other, perhaps undeclared, tumours on the same patient, e.g. skin tumours. Ask for histological review in unusual cases. Note the presence of synchronous cancers or adenomas in bowel cancer reports—each one counts as an independent primary tumour, especially for the purposes of molecular testing, e.g. IHC and MSI. Ask for immunohistochemistry of MMR proteins and/or MSI testing.
- **Tumour testing.** Tumour testing should be done by or in conjunction with an appropriate molecular or histopathologist. For MSI testing it is useful to have normal DNA for comparison, ideally from blood, but this is not absolutely essential. Normal DNA may be obtainable from normal tissues, but it is almost never suitable for germline mutation detection unless derived from fresh frozen, rather than formalin-fixed material.
- **Germline mutation detection.** The laboratory will wish to know about any tumour testing for MSI or IHC that has been carried out in the family. Blood should be taken for DNA testing from at least one affected family member, when possible. It is often useful to have samples from more than one individual in case segregation studies are needed to determine pathogenicity, or an individual proves to be a phenocopy. If the family is likely to have a mutation (see below) but no point mutation is found, then they may well harbour a large-scale mutation, e.g. whole exon(s) deleted. *De novo* mutations have been described, but they are difficult to spot clinically.

Diagnosis: the Amsterdam criteria

It is important to note that the Amsterdam criteria (see table) were originally only designed to select families for linkage studies and not to diagnose HNPCC clinically. As such they had to be necessarily specific, at an acceptable cost to sensitivity. A family with, e.g. only colorectal cancer, and that only just fulfils the AC, may have odds of a mutation of only 10% or so, whereas a non-AC familial cluster, say, of a woman who has had both endometrial and colorectal cancer and a close relative with a small bowel or ureteric cancer, is highly likely to be due to HNPCC.

HNPCC can be diagnosed either on clinical grounds (Amsterdam Criteria), on clinicopathological grounds (see table), e.g. after tumour testing, or by a germline mutation in a DNA mismatch repair gene.

A familial cluster of HNPCC-related tumours (HRC) is more significant than a family history of colorectal cancer alone; young-onset cancers don't always occur, though they are reasonably good indicators. Note a very young onset case, e.g. 35 years, is highly likely to be due to

Amsterdam criteria 2 ('AC2')

All criteria must be satisfied:

- At least 3 separate relatives* with colorectal cancer (CRC) or HNPCC-related cancer (HRC; see item 2 in the ICG-HNPCC's clinical definition in the following table)
- One relative must be a first-degree relative of the other two
- At least two successive generations affected
- At least one cancer (CRC or HRC) diagnosed at <50 years of age
- Familial adenomatous polyposis (FAP) excluded in CRC case(s)
- Tumours pathologically verified

* NB. Affected individuals should all be on the same side of the family, e.g. maternal or paternal relatives of the consultand.

International Collaborative Group on Hereditary Non-Polyposis Colorectal Cancer (ICG-HNPCC)'s clinical definition of HNPCC (after Vasen et al. 1999)

Any combination of points 1 to 9 may be present, but 9 alone defines HNPCC.

1. Familial clustering of colorectal and/or endometrial cancer
2. Associated HNPCC-related cancers (HRCs): gastric, ovary, ureter/renal pelvis, brain, small bowel, hepatobiliary tract, and skin (sebaceous tumours)
3. Development of cancer at an early age
4. Development of multiple cancers
5. Features of colorectal cancer (CRC): (a) predilection for proximal (right-sided) colon; (b) improved survival; (c) multiple CRC; (d) increased proportion of mucinous tumours, and tumours with marked host-lymphocytic infiltration and lymphoid aggregation at the tumour margin
6. Features of colorectal adenoma: (a) the numbers vary from one to a few; (b) increased proportion of adenomas with villous histology; and (c) high-grade dysplasia; (d) probably rapid progression from adenoma to carcinoma
7. High frequency of microsatellite instability (MSI)
8. Immunohistochemistry: loss of MLH1, MSH2, or MSH6 protein expression in tumours
9. Germline mutation in MMR gene: MSH2, MLH1, MSH6, PMS2

HNPCC, even in the absence of a family history. A rare, characteristic tumour, e.g. small bowel cancer, ureter transitional cell carcinoma (TCC), skin sebaceous adenoma, is very significant, and synchronous or metachronous bowel cancers are significant. Double primaries, especially colorectal and endometrial, are significant and remember that non-penetrance is common (hence strict adherence to the Amsterdam Criteria is insensitive).

Genetic advice

HNPCC is an AD disorder, although (often consanguineous) families have now been described in which children develop colorectal adenomatous polyposis, primary brain cancers, leukaemia, and an NF1-like skin phenotype (i.e. café-au-lait patches (CALs)), because they are homozygous or compound heterozygous for mutations in an HNPCC gene. This phenotype is quite distinct from HNPCC and may well be the cause of at least some cases of Turcot syndrome (see above).

Penetrance is incomplete and age-dependent—see table of tumour risk in HNPCC above.

Management
Surveillance
See also 'Cancer surveillance methods', this chapter.

Colorectum.
- Generally accepted practice is to carry out colonoscopy every 2 years from the age of 25 to 30 years in those at 100% (i.e. already affected by an HRC) or 50% prior risk of HNPCC.
- There is good evidence that surveillance intervals longer than 3 years result in a significant number of so-called interval cancers.
- Consider examination by barium enema if colonoscopy fails to reach the caecum.
- Don't forget those who have already developed one (bowel) cancer—they should not be discharged from follow-up.
- Liaison with colorectal surgeons is important—an individual with HNPCC who presents with a second bowel cancer may wish to consider the option of a more extensive resection as prophylaxis, e.g. panproctocolectomy rather than hemicolectomy.

Endometrium. Lifetime risk for endometrial cancer (50%) exceeds that for colorectal cancer (40%) in women with HNPCC. There is no proven method of surveillance for endometrial cancer, so women should be warned of its risk and advised to seek help in case of irregular/post-menopausal bleeding, etc. In some centres screening may be offered by means of, eg. pipelle biopsy, but this is not proven to be of benefit. Women who have completed childbearing may wish to consider a hysterectomy, though it should be borne in mind that pelvic surgery can make colonoscopy more difficult. Prophylactic hysterectomy with bilateral salpingo-oophorectomy may be an effective strategy for preventing endometrial and ovarian cancer in women with HNPCC (Schmeler), but results of current prospective cohort studies are needed in order to adequately assess the risks and benefits of prophylactic surgery against those of gynaeological screening (Offit).

Ovaries. Surveillance by means of annual ultrasound scan (USS) and serum CA125 level is possible but, like endometrial screening, it is not of proven benefit. It may be possible to offer such screening as part of a clinical trial. Ovariectomy, possibly at the time of hysterectomy, is something to be considered in conjunction with a gynaecologist (Schmeler).

Urothelial tumours. One proposed regime is:
- annual haematuria testing, 25–40 years of age;
- annual urine cytology, 40–65 years of age (perhaps with cystoscopy every 1–2 years);
- annual renal USS, 40–65 years of age.

Such surveillance is generally only offered to families in which such tumours have already occurred (as with ovarian cancer), but there is no definite genotype–phenotype or family concordance data to back this up, albeit that those with *MSH2* or *MSH6* mutations might be somewhat more prone to urothelial tumours than those with *MLH1* mutations.

Stomach. There is no regime of gastric surveillance that is of proven benefit.

Skin. Refer to a dermatologist for management of skin lesions if these are present.

Surveillance in general. HNPCC gene carriers are at increased risk of many tumour types, for most of which it is not possible to offer surveillance of proven efficacy. Counsel patients that they should have a low threshold for presentation and their doctors that they should have a low threshold for onward referral. Members of HNPCC families commonly recall stories of delays in diagnosis, especially in individuals who developed cancer at a young age.

Education
Educate your patient about the symptoms of colorectal cancer so that he/she is aware when to seek medical advice and investigation. The most significant symptoms are:
- rectal bleeding;
- a persistent change in bowel habit, usually to looser or more frequent bowel actions;
- abdominal mass;
- unexplained anaemia.

Future developments
It is important to let those at risk of HNPCC know that current recommendations and surveillance regimes are liable to change or revision as knowledge of the disorder advances. Indeed, they may welcome invitations to take part in clinical trials. There is currently an International trial (CAPP2) in progress to determine whether aspirin and/or resistant starch can reduce the risk of colorectal cancer in those with HNPCC. It is likely that advances in imaging techniques, e.g. colonography by CT or MR, will eventually replace colonoscopy, and so those at risk of HNPCC embarking on a theoretical lifetime of biennial colonoscopy are unlikely actually to have a lifetime of colonoscopy. It may be, if CAPP2 demonstrates a benefit, that chemoprophylaxis of bowel cancer will become a treatment option in HNPCC. Some form of effective endometrial surveillance may also be determined, and a trial of, e.g. a prostagen-containing intrauterine device, is being considered.

Support group: Hereditary Colon Cancer <www.mtsinai.on.ca/familialgicancer/Diseases/HNPCC/default.htm>.

Expert adviser: Ian M. Frayling, Consultant in Clinical Genetics and Director of Clinical Genetics Laboratory, University Hospital of Wales, Cardiff, Wales.

References
Berends MJ, et al. Molecular and clinical characteristics of MSH6 variants: an analysis of 25 index carriers of a germline variant. *Am J Hum Genet* 2002; **70**: 26–37.

Boland CR, et al. A NCI workshop on microsatellite instability for cancer detection and familial predisposition: development of international criteria for the determination of microsatellite instability in colorectal cancer. *Cancer Res* 1998; **58**: 5248–57.

Dunlop MG. Guidance on gastrointestinal surveillance for hereditary non-polyposis colorectal cancer, familial adenomatous polyposis, juvenile polyposis, and Peutz–Jeghers syndrome. *Gut* 2000; **51**(Suppl. V); v21–v27.

Frayling IM. Microsatellite instability. *Gut* 1999; **45**: 1–4.

Giardiello FM, Brensinger JD, Petersen GM. AGA technical review on hereditary colorectal cancer and genetic testing. *Gastroenterology* 2001; **121**: 198–213.

Halford S, et al. Low-level microsatellite instability occurs in most colorectal cancers and is a nonrandomly distributed quantitative trait. *Cancer Res* 2002; **62**: 53–7.

International Society for Gastrointestinal Hereditary Tumours (InSIGHT) www.insight-group.com

Jarvinen HJ, Aarnio M, et al. Controlled 15-year trial on screening for colorectal cancer in families with hereditary nonpolyposis colorectal cancer. *Gastroenterology* 2000; **118**: 829–34.

Lindgren G, et al. Adenoma prevalence and cancer risk in familial non-polyposis colorectal cancer. *Gut* 2002; **50**: 228–34.

Liu B, *et al.* Genetic instability occurs in the majority of young patients with colorectal cancer. *Nat Med* 1995; **1**: 348–52.

Loukola A, *et al.* MSI in adenomas as a marker for HNPCC. *Am J Pathol* 1999; **155**: 1849–53.

Lynch HT, De La Chapelle A. Genetic susceptibility to non-polyposis colorectal cancer. *J Med Genet* 1999; **36**: 801–18.

Lynch HT, *et al.* Hereditary factors in cancer: study of two large midwestern kindreds. *Arch Intern Med* 1966; **117**: 206–12.

Lynch HT, Smyrk T, Lynch JF. Molecular genetics and clinical-pathology features of HNPCC (Lynch syndrome): historical journey from pedigree anecdote to molecular genetic confirmation. *Oncology* 1998; **55**: 103–8.

Nilbert M, *et al.* MSI is rare in rectal carcinomas and signifies hereditary cancer. *Eur J Cancer* 1999; **35**: 942–5.

Park JG, *et al.* Gene–environment interaction in hereditary non-polyposis colorectal cancer with implications for diagnosis and genetic testing. *Int J Cancer* 1999; **82**: 516–19.

Offit K, Kauff ND. Reducing the risk of gynecologic cancer in the Lynch syndrome (Editorial). *NEJM* 2006; **354**: 293–5.

Schmeler KM, Lynch HT, *et al.* Prophylactic surgery to reduce the risk of gynecologic cancers in the Lynch syndrome. *N Engl J Med.* 2006; **354**: 261–9.

Scott RJ, *et al.* Hereditary nonpolyposis colorectal cancer in 95 families: differences and similarities between mutation-positive and mutation-negative kindreds. *Am J Hum Genet* 2001; **68**: 118–27.

Torre D. Multiple sebaceous tumors. *Arch Dermatol* 1968; **98**: 549–51.

Trimbath JD, *et al.* Café-au-lait spots and early onset colorectal neoplasia: a variant of HNPCC? *Fam Cancer* 2001; **1**: 103–8.

Vasen HF, *et al.* The risk of brain tumours in hereditary non-polyposis colorectal cancer (HNPCC). *Int J Cancer* 1996; **65**: 422–5.

Vasen HFA, *et al.* New clinical criteria for hereditary non-polyposis colorectal cancer (HNPCC, Lynch syndrome) proposed by the ICG-HNPCC. *Gastroenterology* 1999; **116**: 1453–6.

Vasen HF, *et al.* MSH2 mutation carriers are at higher risk of cancer than MLH1 mutation carriers: a study of hereditary nonpolyposis colorectal cancer families. *J Clin Oncol* 2001; **19**: 4074–80.

Wagner A, *et al.* Atypical HNPCC owing to MSH6 germline mutations: analysis of a large Dutch pedigree. *J Med Genet* 2001; **38**: 318–22.

Warthin AS. Heredity with reference to carcinoma, as shown by the study of the cases examined in the pathological laboratory of the University of Michigan, 1895–1913. *Arch Intern Med* 1913; **12**: 546–55.

Wijnen JT, *et al.* Clinical findings with implications for genetic testing in families with clustering of colorectal cancer. *New Engl J Med* 1998; **339**: 511–18.

Winawer SJ, Fletcher RH. Colorectal cancer screening: clinical guidelines and rationale. *Gastroenterology* 1997; **112**: 594–642.

Juvenile polyposis syndrome (JPS)

Juvenile polyps occur sporadically in childhood. They are delicate structures that are prone to haemorrhage, prolapse, and auto-amputation: they not uncommonly give rise to anaemia. Colonoscopic surveys show that they occur throughout the colorectum, albeit with a slight preponderance of lesions in the rectosigmoid colon. However, there is a group of individuals who develop multiple juvenile polyps, often with a family history of the same or bowel cancer—this is familial juvenile polyposis syndrome (JPS). JPS is an autosomal dominant (AD) condition associated with an increased risk of colorectal cancer (CRC; 10–38%) and of gastric and duodenal cancer (15–21%). The condition is genetically heterogeneous. Germline mutations in *SMAD4/MADH4/DPC4*, *BMPR1A*, and *PTEN* have all been described in JPS, and the latter is consistent with it overlapping, or being associated, with Cowden/Bannayan–Riley–Ruvalcaba syndrome (CS/BRRS). Juvenile polyps are also described in Gorlin syndrome (GS) due to *PTCH* mutations. The condition is uncommon, with a prevalence of ~1/50 000.

Diagnostic criteria. More than five juvenile polyps has been used as a definition of JPS, but more than two has also been used. JPS, however, is frequently associated with other features and/or conditions. A *SMAD4* mutation has been identified in one individual with as few as four juvenile polyps, plus a family history of JPS. Thus a pragmatic approach might be to regard as significant:

- more than 3 juvenile polyps in an isolated case without any other signs or family history; *or*
- 1 or 2 juvenile polyps in the context of related signs/conditions or a family history.

Associated clinical features. Clinically, JPS falls into two groups: (1) those individuals with only juvenile polyposis of the gastrointestinal (GI) tract; (2) those with juvenile polyposis of the GI tract plus other features. Some of the latter group are undoubtedly due to families with *PTEN*-related hamartomatous disease, i.e. CS/BRRS, or Gorlin syndrome, due to *PTCH* mutations, in which juvenile polyps have occurred. However, cases of JPS due to *SMAD4* or *BMPR1A* mutations have been described in which dysmorphic/extracolonic features have occurred, suggestive of CS/BRRS. Hereditary haemorrhagic telangectasia (HHT) has been described in several families with JPS. This appears to be a real, if rare, association, though the underlying genetic defect(s) is(are) unclear.

There is wide variation in the phenotype, both inter- and intrafamilial, perhaps not surprising given the genetic heterogeneity. Apart from juvenile polyps in the GI tract, stomach, and colorectum, other clinical features that have been associated with JPS are given in the table.

Genetics. Mutations in:

- *SMAD4* on 18q21.1 account for 30–50% of families. One recurrent 'hotspot' mutation, 1372–1375delACAG, accounts for about half of *SMAD4* cases, i.e. 15–25% of all JPS.
- *BMPR1A/ALK3* on 10q23.2 (87.4 Mb) account for about 40% of families.
- *PTEN* on 10q23.31 (88.5 Mb) account for a small number of families with features of CS/BRRS.
- *PTCH* on 9q22.32 account for a few families with Gorlin syndrome in which juvenile polyps have occurred.

Other, as yet unidentified, loci may account for other cases, perhaps those associated with HHT.

Chromosomal mutations, e.g. del 10q23.2–q23.33 and del 10q22.3–q24.1, have been found in JPS patients, a region encompassing both *PTEN* and *BMPR1A*.

Genotype–phenotype. Mutations in *SMAD4* are associated with massive gastric polyposis, whereas families with mutations in *BMPR1A* or undetectable mutations in either gene are not, although such individuals are still liable to low numbers of gastric lesions.

Features of CS/BRRS or GS in JPS may point to *PTEN* or *PTCH*, respectively, but are also described in JPS due to *SMAD4* or *BMPR1A* mutations.

Differential diagnosis. The association of JPS with CS/BRRS and Gorlin syndrome has been mentioned above. Although 90% of polyps in children up to 10 years of age are juvenile polyps, other causes of intestinal polyposis in children include:

- **Peutz–Jeghers syndrome (PJS),** but this has characteristic histology.
- **familial adenomatous polyposis (FAP).** Rare instances of polyposis before the age of 10 years are described, but the histology is of adenomas.

Clinical features associated with JPS

Feature	Mutations in				No mutation identified*
	SMAD4	BMPR1A	PTEN	PTCH	
Macrocephaly, hypertelorism	Yes	Yes	Yes	Yes	
Mental retardation	Yes		Yes	Yes	Yes
Pulmonary arteriovenous fistulae	Yes				
Ventricular septal defect (VSD)	Yes	Yes			Yes
Other cardiac defects		Yes			Yes
Thoracic skeletal anomalies	Yes			Yes	
Haemangiomata			Yes	Yes	
Lipomata			Yes	Yes	
Hypospadias					Yes
Genital freckling			Yes	Yes	
Telangiectasia	Yes				

* But not necessarily looked for, when reported.

Clinical approach

History: key points

Three-generation family tree with careful enquiry about possible features of CS/BRRS, Gorlin syndrome, and HHT (note the table above). Take a detailed history of cancer/tumours in other family members (don't forget benign tumours, e.g. haemangiomata, lipomata, etc.).

Examination: key points

- Check for skin, skeletal, neurological, cardiopulmonary, and genitourinary signs (genital freckling?).
- Mouth. Cowden syndrome signs?
- Head circumference.
- Surgical scars, e.g. skin lesions removed and since forgotten about.

Special investigations

- Upper and lower GI endoscopy.
- Radiology/imaging. Intracranial calcification, skeletal anomalies, or abnormal vertebrae?
- Cranial imaging if cerebellar signs (Lhermitte–Duclos disease is a term for dysplastic gangliocytoma of the cerebellum—see 'Cowden syndrome (CS)', page 442).
- Specialist review of histopathology. Polyps, skin lesions.
- Genetic testing. Be guided by the clinical features.
  - In cases without features suggestive of CS/BRRS or Gorlin syndrome, carry out germline mutation detection in first *SMAD4* and then *BMPR1A*. If no mutation detected in either gene, review and consider *PTEN* or *PTCH* testing.
  - In cases with features of CS/BRRS look in *PTEN*, and then *SMAD4* and *BMPR1A*.
  - In cases with features of Gorlin syndrome look in *PTCH*, and then *SMAD4, BMPR1A*, and *PTEN*.
- Have a low threshold for checking the karyotype.

Genetic advice

Risk assessment

AD, with 50% risk of transmission.

Penetrance

Uncertain, and expressivity highly variable and dependent on underlying cause/gene. Lifetime risk of CRC between 10% and 38% (relative risk (RR) 2–8) and gastric cancer 15–21% (RR > 10), though these are overall figures and not subdivided by genotype.

Predictive testing

Possible in families with an identified germline mutation. Linkage not feasible except in large kindreds, given genetic heterogeneity and loci probably yet to be identified.

Prenatal diagnosis

Possible in families with identified germline mutation.

Management

Surveillance strategies

See also 'Cancer surveillance methods', this chapter. Proven surveillance strategies in JPS are not established; however, Dunlop (2002) has recommended:

- 1–2 yearly colonoscopy from 15–18 years of age (or earlier if presenting with symptoms) until 35 years. From 35 years of age screening interval can be extended, but surveillance should continue until 70 years. Prophylactic surgery is a consideration.
- 1–2 yearly upper GI endoscopy from 25 years of age.

In cases of JPS due to CS/BRRS or Gorlin syndrome, specific anti-cancer surveillance directed at sites other than the GI tract should be considered and implemented as appropriate.

Expert adviser: Ian M. Frayling, Consultant in Clinical Genetics and Director of Clinical Genetics Laboratory, University Hospital of Wales, Cardiff, Wales.

References

Dunlop MG. Guidance on gastrointestinal surveillance for hereditary non-polyposis colorectal cancer, familial adenomatous polyposis, juvenile polyposis, and Peutz–Jeghers syndrome. *Gut* 2002; **51**(Suppl. 5): v21–7.

Friedl W, *et al.* Juvenile polyposis: massive gastric polyposis is more common in MADH4 mutation carriers than in BMPR1A mutation carriers. *Hum Genet.* 2002; **111**: 108–11.

Gallione CJ, Repette GM. A combined syndrome of juvenile polyposis and hereditary haemorrhagic telangiectasia associated with mutations in *MADH4* (SMAD4). *Lancet* 2004; **363**: 852–59.

Howe JR, Mitros FA, Summers RW. The risk of gastrointestinal carcinoma in familial juvenile polyposis [review]. *Ann Surg Oncol* 1998; **5**: 751–6.

Howe JR, *et al.* Common deletion of SMAD4 in juvenile polyposis is a mutational hotspot. *Am J Hum Genet.* 2002; **70**: 1357–62.

Hyer W. Polyposis syndromes: pediatric implications [review]. *Gastrointest Endosc Clin N Am* 2001; **11**: 659–82, vi–vii.

Merg A, Howe JR. Genetic conditions associated with intestinal juvenile polyps (Seminar). *Am J Med Genet* 2004; **129C**: 44–55.

Sayed MG, *et al.* Germline SMAD4 or BMPR1A mutations and phenotype of juvenile polyposis. *Ann Surg Oncol* 2002; **9**: 901–6.

Wirtzfeld DA, Petrelli NJ, Rodriguez-Bigas MA. Hamartomatous polyposis syndromes: molecular genetics, neoplastic risk, and surveillance recommendations [review]. *Ann Surg Oncol* 2001; **8**: 319–27.

Zhou XP, *et al.* Germline mutations in BMPR1A/ALK3 cause a subset of cases of juvenile polyposis syndrome and of Cowden and Bannayan–Riley–Ruvalcaba syndromes. *Am J Hum Genet.* 2001; **69**: 704–11.

Lifestyle factors in cancer: smoking, alcohol, obesity, diet, and exercise

Smoking

Carcinogenic effects of tobacco cause cancer of the lung, pancreas, bladder and kidney, and (synergistically with alcohol) the larynx, mouth, pharynx (except nasopharynx), and oesophagus. Recent evidence suggests that the prevalence of several other types of cancer (stomach, liver, and (probably) cervix) is also increased by smoking.

About 60% of cancers amongst smokers are due to smoking and tobacco causes one-third of all cancer deaths in developed countries. The rapid increase in the lung cancer incidence rate among continuing smokers ceases when they stop smoking—the rate remaining roughly constant for many years in ex-smokers.

Alcohol

Alcohol increases the risk of cancers of the oral cavity, pharynx, larynx, oesophagus, liver, and breast.

Obesity

There is now a consensus that cancer is more common in those who are overweight. The evidence on weight is strongest for postmenopausal breast cancer and cancers of the endometrium, gall bladder, and kidney.

A US study (Calle *et al.* 1999) estimated that ~10% of all cancer deaths among American non-smokers (7% in men and 12% in women) are caused by overweight. Bergstrom *et al.* (2001) have estimated that 5% (3% in men and 6% in women) of all incident cancers in the European Union might be prevented if no one had a body mass index (BMI) > 25.

Diet

Diet-related factors are thought to account for ~30% of cancers in developed countries (Key 2002). Adequate intakes of fruit and vegetables probably lower the risk for several types of cancer, especially cancers of the gastro-intestinal tract (Key 2002). The significance of other factors, e.g. meat, fibre, and vitamins, is currently unclear.

Exercise

Regular exercise reduces the risk of colon cancer and probably also of breast cancer, although the quantitative effect is uncertain.

General lifestyle advice

Advice to members of the general population is not to smoke and 'to maintain a healthy weight, restrict alcohol consumption and select a conventionally balanced diet ensuring an adequate intake of fruit, vegetables and cereals' (Key 2002). The extent to which such advice can modify the risk of cancer in individuals who carry or are at risk of carrying a mutation in a cancer-predisposing gene is uncertain. However, any reduction in risk, even if very small, may be of benefit.

References

Bergstrom A, Pisani P, *et al.* Overweight as an avoidable cause of cancer in europe. *Int J Cancer* 2001; **91**: 421–30.

Calle EE, Thun MJ, *et al.* Body-mass index and mortality in a prospective cohort of US adults. *New Engl J Med* 1999; **341**: 1097–105.

Key TJ. Effect of diet on risk of cancer. *Lancet* 2002; **360**: 861–8.

Peto J. Cancer epidemiology in the last century and the next decade. *Nature* 2001; **411**: 390–5.

Li–Fraumeni syndrome (LFS)

LFS is a rare autosomal dominant (AD) disorder of familial and intraindividual clustering of a wide spectrum of neoplasia occurring in children and young adults. Some affected individuals develop multiple primaries. In most families LFS is caused by germline mutations in *TP53*, a tumour suppressor gene encoding a transcription factor with a crucial role in regulation of the cell cyle and apoptosis when DNA damage occurs.

TP53 activity is commonly lost by a two-hit process during tumourigenesis in a wide variety of sporadic tumours. In LFS, with a germline *TP53* mutation, loss of heterozygosity leading to inactivation of the wild-type allele by deletion or mutation initiates tumourigenesis.

The diagnostic criteria for classical LFS are as follows.

- Proband with sarcoma diagnosed at <45 years of age *and*
- At least one first-degree relative with any cancer diagnosed at <45 years of age *and*
- Another first- or second-degree relative in the lineage with any cancer at <45 years of age or sarcoma at any age.

Although a wide variety of tumours can be seen in LFS kindreds (see table), common cancers such as lung, colon, bladder, prostate, cervix, and ovary are not found to excess. Breast cancer and sarcomas are numerically the most frequent tumour types, but the greatest increased risk relative to general population rates is for adrenocortical cancer and phyllodes tumour. (Phynodes tumours are fibroepithelial tumours which range in behaviour from benign (most) to malignant.)

Tumour types associated with LFS

Strong association	Breast cancer, soft tissue sarcomas (e.g. leiomyosarcoma), osteosarcoma, brain tumours, adrenocortical cancer, Wilms tumour, and phyllodes tumour
Moderate association	Pancreatic cancer, gastric cancer
Weak association	Leukaemias and neuroblastoma

Clinical approach

History: key points

Three-generation family tree with specific enquiry for cancers, including age at diagnosis, multiple primaries in one individual. Try to obtain full names, dates of birth, and hospital where the diagnosis was made and treatment given in order to facilitate confirmation.

Examination: key points

Usually not contributory.

Special investigations

DNA for mutation analysis of *TP53*. Mutation detection rate in families fulfilling classical criteria is ~75%. While there is a need to recognize potential new mutations in families that do not meet LFS criteria, there is a low rate of *TP53* germline mutations in breast/sarcoma families not fulfilling classical criteria for LFS. Consider mutation analysis for all children with adrenocortical cancer (some without a family history will have a 'de novo' *TP53* mutation).

Genetic advice

Risk assessment

AD with 50% risk to offspring of an affected individual.

Penetrance

Cancer risk in *TP53* mutation carriers has been estimated to be 73% in males and nearly 100% in females (the difference being due to breast cancer).

Predictive testing

Diagnostic testing may be appropriate in an affected child, but predictive testing should be restricted to adults.

Prenatal diagnosis

Possible by chorionic villus sampling (CVS) if the familial mutation is known.

Management

Surveillance for individuals who are affected by LFS or at high risk is highly problematical. Seek guidance from a unit with expertise in this area. Consider breast screening for females using MRI.

Expert adviser: Gareth Evans, Professor of Medical Genetics, University of Manchester, Manchester, England.

References

Birch JM, Alston RD, *et al.* Relative frequency and morphology of cancers in carriers of germline TP53 mutations. *Oncogene* 2001; **20**: 4621–8.

Chompret A. The Li–Fraumeni syndrome. *Biochimie* 2002; **84**: 75–82.

Evans DG, Birch JM, *et al.* Low rate of *TP53* germline mutations in breast cancer/sarcoma families not fulfilling classical criteria for Li–Fraumeni syndrome. *J Med Genet* 2002; **39**: 941–4.

Multiple endocrine neoplasia (MEN)

Multiple endocrine neoplasia type 1 (MEN1)

Wermer syndrome.

MEN is an autosomal dominant (AD) cancer syndrome affecting primarily parathyroid, enteropancreatic, endocrine, and pituitary tissues. MEN1 is caused by inactivating germline mutations in *MEN1*, a tumour suppressor gene encoding menin, a novel nuclear protein. Menin specifically interacts with FANCD2, a protein encoded by a gene involved in DNA repair and mutated in patients with an inherited cancer-prone syndrome, Fanconi anemia, playing a critical role in repair of DNA damage in concert with FANCD2 (Jin *et al.* 2003). MEN1 accounts for ~10% of patients with primary hyperparathyroidism who require surgery. In most patients hyperparathyroidism is the first manifestation of MEN1, but this is not the case in up to 10% of mutation carriers. Unlike sporadic cases of primary hyperparathyroidism, tumours are typically present in one or more parathyroid glands and present at a young age (typically 25–35 years). Disease-specific mortality in MEN1 is significant arising largely from the effects of pancreatic islet cell tumours (e.g. gastrinomas and insulinomas) and malignant thymic carcinoid.

Anterior pituitary tumours occur in 30% of MEN1 patients (most are prolactinomas (60%), somatotrophinomas (growth hormone; 20%), and corticotrophinomas and non-functioning tumours (<15%)). Associated tumours that occur in MEN1 include adrenal cortical tumours (5%), carcinoid tumours (4–10%), lipomas (1%), facial angiofibromas (88%), and collagenomas (72%).

Screening for MEN1 should be undertaken in:

- any patient with 2 or more MEN1-associated endocrine tumours;
- any patient <30 years of age with one MEN1-associated tumour;
- any first-degree relative of someone with MEN1.

Multiple endocrine neoplasia type 2 (MEN2)

Mucosal neuroma syndrome or Sipple syndrome.

MEN2 is an AD cancer predisposition syndrome characterized by the association of medullary thyroid cancer (MTC) and phaeochromocytoma. It is caused by activating germline mutations in the *RET* protooncogene. MEN2 is subdivided into three subtypes, MEN2A, MEN2B, and FMTC (familial MTC) all with a high risk for MTC arising in the C-cells (calcitonin-producing cells) of the thyroid. The usual age of onset of MTC in MEN2A is in early adult life, in MEN2B in early childhood, and in FMTC in midlife. MEN2 has a prevalence of ~1/30 000. Approximately 60–90% of MEN2 cases are MEN2A, 5% are MEN2B, and 5–35% are FMTC. In MEN2A, signs or symptoms of hyperparathyroidism or phaeochromocytoma rarely present before those of MTC. MTC can occur at an extremely young age in MEN2B and screening is usually commenced at 6 months of age. A recent study from the Netherlands (Kahraman) found that, in patients with MEN2A, MTC can be present as early as 4 years of age.

The ability of an MTC to oversecrete calcitonin, occasionally together with other hormonally active peptides, e.g. adrenocorticotrophic hormone (ACTH) or calcitonin-gene related peptide (CGRP), leads to unexplained diarrhoea, symptoms of Cushing's syndrome, or facial flushing in many patients with advanced disease. Metastatic spread occurs both locally to regional lymph nodes and to distant sites, e.g. the liver in advanced disease.

Screening for MEN2 should be undertaken in:

- any patient with MTC or two or more MEN2-associated endocrine tumours;
- any patient <30 years of age with one MEN2-associated endocrine tumour;
- any patient with mucosal neuromas or somatic features of MEN2B;
- any individual with a first-degree relative with MEN2.

The table summarizes the diagnosis of the different types of MEN.

Other conditions to consider

Familial medullary thyroid carcinoma (FMTC). A subtype of MEN2. An AD condition characterized by MTC, usually diagnosed in middle-age, without other features of MEN2. Caused by mutations in the *RET* proto-oncogene.

Diagnosis of multiple endocrine neuroplasia (MEN)*

MEN1	MEN2A	MEN2B	Carney
Gene			
MEN1 (Menin)	*RET*	*RET*	*PKAR1A*
Locus			
11q13	10q11	10q11	17q22–24
Clinical features			
Parathyroid hyperplasia (95%)	MTC (penetrance 90–95%)	MTC (penetrance 100%)	Lentigines
Pituitary adenomas (30%): (prolactin used for surveillance)	Phaeochromocytomas (50%) Parathyroid hyperplasia (20–30%)	Phaeochromocytomas (50%) Mucosal neuromas (e.g. lips and tongue)	Cardiac myxomas PPNAD Endocrine tumours
Pancreatic adenomas (40%): insulinomas gastrinoma (duodenal) VIPoma (rare) glucagonoma (rare)		Marfanoid habitus Medullated corneal nerve fibres Multiple diverticulae and megacolon	

* MTC, Medullary thyroid carcinoma; PPNAD, primary pigmented adrenocortical disease; VIP, vasoactive intestinal peptide.

Familial isolated hyperparathyroidism (FIHP). AD condition characterized by uniglandular or multiglandular parathyroid tumours that occur in the absence of other endocrine tumours. Recently, mutations in *MEN1* have been identified in some families and it seems likely that FIHP is a distinct allelic variant of MEN1.

Hyperparathyroidism–jaw tumour syndrome (HPT-JT). Caused by mutations in the parafibromin gene (*HRPT2*). An AD disease characterized by the occurrence of parathyroid tumours and fibro-osseous tumours of the jaw bones (mandible and maxilla). Some HPT-JT patients may also develop various cystic and neoplastic renal abnormalities that include Wilms tumours, hamartomas, and polycystic disease. Parathyroid tumours often occur asynchronously in patients with HPT-JT syndrome and, although most of the tumours are benign, the incidence of malignant parathyroid carcinomas is markedly increased in these patients (Shattuck *et al.* 2003).

Thyroid cancer. Thyroid cancer accounts for roughly 1% of all new malignant disease. Of these ~94% are differentiated thyroid cancer (occasionally occurring as a component of Cowden syndrome (*PTEN*) or familial adenomatous polyposis (FAP)). Another 5% are MTC, derived from the neuroendocrine C-cells (calcitonin-producing cells) of the thyroid and 1% are anaplastic. Sporadic disease accounts for ~80% of MTC with presentation usually in fifth or sixth decade. 20% of MTC occurs in the context of an inherited tumour predisposition syndrome, e.g. MEN2A, MEN2B, or FMTC.

Carney complex (CNC). Carney complex is a rare multiple neoplasia syndrome that consists of endocrine (thyroid, pituitary, adrenocortical, and gonadal), nonendocrine (myxomas, particularly atrial myxomas), and neural (schwannomas) tumours. Typically, there are cutaneous pigmented lesions (multiple blue naevi and lentigines). Primary pigmented nodular adrenocortical disease (PPNAD) is the most common endocrine manifestation of CNC. CNC is caused by mutations in *PRKAR1A*, a critical component of the cAMP (cyclic adenosine monophosphate) signalling pathway or another gene (CNC2) on 2p16.

Sporadic parathyroid cancer. Shattuck *et al.* (2003), in an analysis of 15 patients with apparently sporadic parathyroid cancer (no family history and no features of HPT-JT or MEN1, etc.), identified three patients with germline mutations in *HRPT2* (the gene mutated in HPT-JT), suggesting that certain patients with apparently sporadic parathyroid carcinoma may have the HPT-JT syndrome or a phenotypic variant.

Clinical approach

History: key points

Three-generation family tree with specific enquiry for presence of endocrine tumours, age of death, and cause of death.

Examination: key points

In MEN without a known *RET* mutation examine for physical features of MEN2B, i.e. mucosal neuromas on lips and tongue, full lips, Marfanoid habitus.

Special investigations

DNA for mutation analysis of *MEN1* in MEN1, and of exons 10 and 11 of *RET* in MEN2A, exons 10, 11, 13, and 14 of *RET* in FMTC, and exon 16 of *RET* in MEN2B.

Genetic advice

MEN1. AD with 50% risk to offspring of an affected individual or mutation carrier. More than 80% of the germline mutations in *MEN1* are inactivating and each kindred has a private mutation. No genotype–phenotype correlation is apparent.

MEN2. AD with 50% risk to offspring of an affected individual or mutation carrier. For MEN2A, MEN2B, and FMTC, mutations in the tyrosine kinase proto-oncogene *RET* are detectable in 98% of affected family members. Mutations of codon 634 Cys occur in ~85% of MEN2A families. ~95% of individuals with MEN2B have an M918T mutation in exon 16.

Approximately 6% of patients with clinically sporadic MTC carry a germline *RET* mutations and so genetic testing is offered to all new patients at diagnosis. Initial analysis of the *RET* gene targets exons 10 and 11, the most common site of mutation. If no mutation is identified proceed to analyse exons 13–16.

The probability of a *de novo* gene mutation in an index case of MEN2A is 5% and in an index case of MEN2B is 50%.

Penetrance

- In MEN1 most are penetrant by 20 years and > 90% are penetrant by 30 years; but recent data show that as many as 40% do not present with their first feature of MEN1 until after age 40 years.
- In MEN2 penetrance is 70% by 70 years.

Predictive testing

- **MEN1.** Genetic testing for MEN1 in the index cases gives useful information and confirms the clinical diagnosis but rarely alters management. However, predictive genetic testing for at-risk family members is of great value in determining which family members are at risk and should be offered annual biochemical surveillance.
- **MEN2 and familial MTC.** *RET* testing has replaced calcitonin in determining which family members are at risk and should be offered prophylactic thyroidectomy.

Prenatal diagnosis

Technically feasible by chorionic villus sampling (CVS) if the familial mutation is known.

Management

Surveillance strategies

MEN1.

- Clinical assessment looking for symptoms and signs of hypercalcaemia, nephrolithiasis, peptic ulcer disease, neuroglycopenia, hypopituitarism, galactorrhoea and amenorrhoea in women, acromegaly, Cushing disease, visual field loss, subcutaneous lipomas, facial angiofibromas, and collagenomas.
- Annual serum calcium and prolactin from 5 years of age (hypercalcaemia is the first manifestation in 90% of MEN1 patients). Measurement of gastrointestinal hormones and specific endocrine function tests should be reserved for individuals who have symptoms and signs of a MEN1-associated tumour.

MEN2 and FMTC. Where the familial mutation is known, predictive genetic testing should be offered at a young age. Prophylactic thyroidectomy is the cornerstone of management for individuals with a *RET* mutation predisposing to MEN2A, MEN2B, or FMTC, but the timing of surgery is controversial and should be guided by the genotype (see Brandi *et al.* 2001 for further details).

In families where the genotype is unknown, screening is recommended in early childhood from age 5 years or earlier in FMTC and MEN2A and from age 6 months in MEN2B. MTC and C-cell hyperplasia are suspected in the presence of elevated plasma calcitonin concentration.

- 6-monthly clinical assessment looking for symptoms and signs of MTC (lumps in the neck, diarrhoea, dysphagia), phaeochromocytoma (hypertension, headaches, palpitations, sweating), hypercalcaemia.
- 6-monthly measurement of serum calcitonin levels, basal and after stimulation with pentagastrin.
- 6-monthly urine catecholamines and/or metanephrines (phaeochromocytoma).
- 6-monthly measurement of serum calcium and parathyroid hormone levels.

HPT-JT. Surveillance protocols are being established. The following is a suggested scheme.
- Annual serum calcium and parathyroid hormone (PTH).
- Surveillance for renal neoplasia, e.g. annual renal ultrasound scan (USS).
- Awareness of risk for jaw tumours (seek specialist evaluation if symptomatic and consider a magnetic resonance imaging (MRI) scan or orthopantogram (OPG)).

Interventions
- **MEN1.** Surgery includes subtotal or total parathyroidectomy, parathyroid cryopreservation, and thymectomy. Proton pump inhibitors or somatostatin analogues are the main management for oversecretion of most enteropancreatic tumours except insulin. Surgery on gastrinomas is generally not indicated, and surgery for other enteropancreatic tumours is controversial.
- **MEN2 and FMTC.** The specific *RET* codon mutation correlates with the age of onset of MTC and the aggressiveness of the tumour and is used to guide management decisions such as whether and when to perform thyroidectomy (Brandi *et al.* 2001). Two

strategies are offered to asymptomatic mutation carriers:
- six-monthly clinical and biochemical surveillance as above, with recourse to prophylactic thryoidectomy as soon as an abnormal pentagastrin result is obtained (usually around 10–13 years) *or*
- total thyroidectomy at 5 years in MEN2A following a predictive test indicating that the child is a mutation carrier (5 years is the earliest age at which metastases have been reported). In MEN2B, metastasis has been reported as young as 2 years and the total thyroidectomy at an earlier age is advocated by some.

Support group: Association for Multiple Endocrine Neoplasia Disorders (AMEND) <www.amend.org.uk>.

Expert adviser: Rajesh Thakker, May Professor of Medicine, University of Oxford, Oxford, England.

References

Brandi ML, Gagel RF, *et al.* Guidelines for diagnosis and therapy of MEN type 1 and type 2. *J Clin Endocrinol Metab* 2001; **86**: 5658–71.

Cavaco BM, Barros L, *et al.* The hyperparathyroidism–jaw tumour syndrome in a Portuguese kindred. *Quart J Med.* 2001; **94** (4): 213–22.

Glascock MJ, Carty SE. Multiple endocrine neoplasia type 1: fresh perspective on clinical features and penetrance. *Surg Oncol* 2002; **11**: 143–50.

Jin S, Mao H, *et al.* Menin associates with FANCD2, a protein involved in repair of DNA damage. *Cancer Res* 2003; **63**: 4204–10.

Kahraman T, de Groot JW. Acceptable age for prophylactic surgery in children with multiple endocrine neoplasia type 2a. *Eur J Surg Oncol* 2003; **29**: 331–35.

Pannett AA, Kennedy AM, *et al.* Multiple endocrine neoplasia type 1 (*MEN1*) germline mutations in familial isolated primary hyperparathyroidism. *Clin Endocrinol* 2003; **58**: 639–46.

Sandrini F, Stratakis C. Clinical and molecular genetics of Carney complex. *Mol Genet Metab* 2003; **78**: 83–92.

Shattuck TM, Valimaki S, *et al.* Somatic and germ-line mutations of the *HRPT2* gene in sporadic parathyroid carcinoma. *New Engl J Med* 2003; **349**: 1722–9.

Sherman SI. Thyroid carcinoma. *Lancet* 2003; **361**: 501–11.

Thakker RV. Multiple endocrine neoplasia. *Medicine* 2001; **29** (12): 45–8.

Neurofibromatosis type 2 (NF2)

Central neurofibromatosis, bilateral acoustic neurofibromatosis.

NF2 is an autosomal dominant (AD) disorder caused by inactivating mutations in the tumour suppressor gene merlin (schwannomin) on 22q. Merlin's function as a tumour suppressor has not been elucidated. Schwannomas are benign solitary tumours of the peripheral nerve sheaths. The occurrence of multiple Schwannomas usually implies hereditary disease. Vestibular Schwannomas (acoustic neuromas), intracranial meningiomas, spinal tumours, peripheral nerve tumours, and presenile lens opacities are common in NF2. The morbidity and mortality of NF2 are largely due to bilateral vestibular Schwannomas. These present with hearing loss and tinnitus or vertigo. The diagnostic criteria for NF2 are given in the table.

Diagnostic criteria for NF2 (Evans et al. 1992b)*

A diagnosis of NF2 is made if *one* of the following criteria is met

- Bilateral vestibular Schwannomas, either proven histologically or seen by MRI with gadolinium enhancement
- A parent, sibling, or child with NF2 and either:
  - (a) a unilateral vestibular Schwannoma *or*
  - (b) 2 or more of: meningioma, glioma, Schwannoma, posterior subcapsular lenticular opacities, cerebral calcification
- Unilateral vestibular Schwannoma and 2 or more of: meningioma, glioma, Schwannoma, posterior subcapsular lenticular opacities, cerebral calcification
- Multiple meningiomas (2 or more) and one or more of: glioma, Schwannoma, posterior subcapsular lenticular opacities, cerebral opacification

* NB. None of the existing sets of criteria is adequate at initial assessment for diagnosing people with NF2 who present without bilateral vestibular Schwannomas, particularly if there is a negative family history.

In Baser *et al.*'s (2002a) study of 368 patients, the mean age of first symptoms was 22 years and the mean age of diagnosis was 27 years; 31.5% of patients were diagnosed at <20 years. Life expectancy may be shortened. The risk of mortality increases with decreasing age at diagnosis and is greater in people with intracranial meningiomas compared with those without meningiomas. The risk of mortality is lower in people with constitutional *NF2* missense mutations than in those with other types of mutations (e.g. nonsense or frameshift mutations or large deletions). The clinical features of NF2 are summarized in the table.

Some patients present young and have an aggressive course, others present in middle life and may have a very slow and indolent course. Two subtypes are recognized.

- **Mild** (Gardner, type A). Onset > 15 years and usually > 25 years. Presenting symptoms usually due to bilateral vestibular Schwannomas. Skin manifestations minimal and other central nervous system (CNS) tumours are rare.
- **Severe** (Wishardt, type 2B). Onset <30 years and usually <25 years. Meningiomas and spinal tumours occur in large numbers.

Other conditions to consider

The only genetic disorders in which Schwannomas occur are: NF2, multiple Schwannomatosis is and Carney complex.
Neurofibromatosis type 1 (NF1). Important distinguishing features are axillary freckling and Lisch nodules—both are commonly present in NF1, but are very rarely seen in NF2. Spinal neurofibromas seen in NF1 can appear identical to the spinal Schwannomas seen in NF2, both radiologically and at surgery. They are distinct histologically, but may need expert review by a neuropathologist for definitive diagnosis.

Multiple schwannomas. (Isolated familial schwannomatosis) An AD disorder defined as multiple pathologically proven schwannomas without the vestibular tumours diagnostic of NF2. Linkage to 22q, but not to the NF2 locus (MacCollin).

Carney complex (CNC). AD condition characterized by skin-pigmentary anomalies, myxomas, endocrine tumours or overactivity and schwannomas. See 'MEN syndromes' in cancer section.

Clinical approach

History: key points

Three-generation family history with specific enquiry for diagnosis of neurofibromatosis, deafness, neurosurgery.

Examination: key points

- Careful examination of the skin for NF2 plaques, café au lait spots (CALs), cutaneous neurofibromas, Schwannomas.
- Ophthalmological assessment for posterior subcapsular and cortical cataracts and congenital hypertrophy of the retinal pigment epithelium (CHRPE) or astrocytic hamartomas.

Clinical features of NF2 (after Evans et al. 1992a)*

Clinical feature	Frequency of symptomatic lesions (%)[†]
CNS tumours	
Bilateral vestibular Schwannomas	85
Unilateral vestibular Schwannoma	6
Meningiomas	45
Spinal tumours (meningiomas, Schwannomas)	26
Astrocytomas (usually in brainstem =/– upper cervical cord)	4
Ependymomas (usually in brainstem =/– upper cervical cord)	2.5
Peripheral nervous system	
Peripheral Schwannomas	68
NF2 plaques (slightly raised roughened skin lesions that may be slightly pigmented; overlying skin is often hairy)	48
Nodular Schwannomas	43
NF-like cutaneous neurofibromas	27
Peripheral neuropathy (glove and stocking or mononeuritis)	3
Café au lait (CAL) spots	
1–6 spots (only 4% had > 3spots, 0 had > 6)	43
Eyes	
Posterior subcapsular cataracts	72.4
Cortical cataracts	41.4
Retinal hamartomas (CHRPEs or astrocytic hamartomas)	8.6

* CHRPE, Congenital hypertrophy of the retinal pigment epithelium.
[†] NB. A higher frequency of all tumours in found on cranial and spinal magnetic resonance imaging (MRI); some remain aymptomatic.

Special investigations
- DNA for mutation analysis of *NF2*. In apparently sporadic cases, consider starting with mutation analysis of the tumour.
- Cranial and spinal magnetic resonance imaging (MRI) with gadolinium enhancement (if not already performed).
- Audiometry.

Genetic advice
- **Familial.** AD with 50% risk to offspring. There is strong intrafamilial correlation in the course of the disease, but marked interfamilial variability.
- ***De novo.*** About half of all patients are founders with clinically unaffected parents. Kluwe *et al.* (2003) identified mutations in *NF2* in 52% in their cohort of NF2 founders with bilateral vestibular Schwannomas and estimated the rate of mosaicism to be 24.8% (58/233). Almost all individuals with mosaicism have relatively mild disease.

Risk assessment
AD with 50% risk to offspring of an affected individual.

De novo. There has only been one report of possible germline mosaicism in NF2. If parental skin and eye examinations and head and spine MRIs are normal, the recurrence risk is very low, i.e. <1% (Ruggieri *et al.* 2001).

Penetrance
Penetrance is age-dependent and is almost complete by 60 years.

Predictive testing
Possible if the familial mutation is known. If there is no mutation, but there are several affected members and the diagnosis is typical with bilateral vestibular Schwannomas, it may be possible to do predictive testing by linkage.

Predictive testing in childhood is warranted since surveillance of 'at risk' individuals begins in early childhood.

Other family members
If there is no family history, parents <60 years of age should be screened by:
- careful examination of skin;
- ophthalmological assessment for posterior subcapsular and cortical cataracts and CHRPE or astrocytic hamartomas;
- cranial and spinal MRI with gadolinium enhancement.

Management
Patients with NF2 need care from a team with expertise in skull-base surgery, usually comprising a neurosurgeon, ear, nose, and throat (ENT) surgeon, audiologist, etc. NF2 patients who are treated in specialist centres have a significantly lower risk of mortality than those treated in non-specialist centres (Baser *et al.* 2002a). Vestibular Schwannoma growth rates in NF2 are generally higher in younger people, but are highly variable, even among multiple NF2 patients of similar ages in the same family. Early microsurgery for small tumours results in optimal preservation of hearing and facial nerve function. Complete removal of a large vestibular Schwannoma usually renders the patient completely deaf on the side of surgery. Brainstem implants may offer hope for some patients. Stereotactic Radiotherapy is best reserved for NF2 patients who have particularly aggressive tumours, those who are poor surgical risks, those who refuse surgery, or the elderly.

Surgery for lesions other than vestibular Schwannomas is usually undertaken only when indicated by symptoms.

Surveillance strategies
For mutation carriers and 'at risk' individuals, i.e. offspring of an affected parent in whom predictive genetic testing is declined or not possible:
- ophthalmological assessment in early childhood;
- annual review for symptomatic lesions until early teens;
- screening for vestibular Schwannomas from early teens;
- full cranial and spinal MRI at 15 years and again at 30 years.

If all imaging studies are normal at 30 years and no other features are present, it is likely that status is unaffected and they may be discharged from surveillance (unless the age of onset of NF2 in the family is late).

Support group: The Neurofibromatosis Association <www.nfa.zetnet.co.uk>.

Expert adviser: Gareth Evans, Professor of Medical Genetics, University of Manchester, Manchester, England.

References

Baser ME, Friedman JM, *et al.* Evaluation of clinical diagnostic criteria for neurofibromatosis 2. *Neurology* 2002a; **59**: 1759–65.

Baser ME, Friedman JM, *et al.* Predictors of the risk of mortality in neurofibromatosis 2. *Am J Hum Genet* 2002b; **71**: 715–23.

Baser ME, Evans DG, *et al.* Neurofibromatosis 2. *Curr Opin Neurol* 2003; **16**: 27–33.

Evans DGR, Huson SM, *et al.* A clinical study of type 2 neurofibromatosis. *Quart J Med* 1992a; **304**: 603–18.

Evans DGR, Huson SM, *et al.* A genetic study of type 2 neurofibromatosis; II guidelines for genetic counselling. *J Med Genet* 1992b; **29**: 847–52.

Kluwe L, Mautner V, *et al.* Molecular study of frequency of mosaicism in neurofibromatosis 2 patients with bilateral vestibular schwannomas. *J Med Genet* 2003; **40** (2): 109–14.

MaCollin M, Willatt C *et al.* Familial Schwannomatosis: exclusion of the NF2 as the germline event. *Neurology* 2003; **60**: 1968–74

Ruggieri M, Huson SM. The clinical and diagnostic implications of mosaicism in the neurofibromatoses. *Neurology* 2001; **56** (11): 1433–43.

Ovarian cancer

The lifetime risk of ovarian cancer in the general population is ~1 in 70 or 1.4%. The majority of women with a family history of ovarian cancer have a single first-degree relative affected with ovarian cancer. If there is no significant cancer history in other members of the family (e.g. breast or bowel), the estimated relative risk of developing ovarian cancer is fairly small at 3.1. In Northern Europe and North America this equates to a cumulative risk of 4% by age 70 years (Stratton et al. 1999). The relative risk of ovarian cancer in a monozygotic (MZ) twin of an affected woman is 6, i.e. twice the sibling risk, indicating that much of the excess familial risk is due to genetic factors rather than shared environmental factors.

Inherited mutations of BRCA1 in particular, also BRCA2, and to a lesser extent the mismatch-repair (MMR) genes are known to confer predisposition to ovarian cancer. Together they account for close to half of the excess familial risk of ovarian cancer. No gene that confers increased susceptibility to ovarian cancer alone has yet been identified.

Mutations in BRCA1 are thought to be responsible for the majority of families with breast/ovarian and site-specific ovarian cancer. Approximately 6–8% of all cases of ovarian cancer are attributable to BRCA mutations. Mutations in BRCA1 are associated with increased risk for ovarian cancer, especially when mutations occur in the first two-thirds of the gene. Carriers with a mutation in BRCA1 have a 65% (confidence interval (CI), 44–78%) risk of breast cancer to age 70 years and a 39% (CI, 18–54%) risk to age 70 years of ovarian cancer. Women with a mutation in BRCA2 also have a 45% (CI, 31–56%) risk of breast cancer to age 70 years, but an 11% (CI, 2.4–19%) risk to age 70 years of ovarian cancer.

Criteria for defining high-risk women

- A first-degree relative of a woman with ovarian cancer at any age who herself has a first-degree relative* with breast cancer diagnosed at <50 years
- A first-degree relative of a woman with breast cancer diagnosed at <50 years who herself has a first-degree relative* with ovarian cancer at any age
- A first-degree relative of a woman with ovarian cancer who herself has a first-or second-degree relative with ovarian cancer

* Families in which the affected individuals are connected by a second-degree relationship through an unaffected male are also eligible.

Chance of identifying a BRCA1/2 mutation according to family history (after Pharaoh and Ponder 2002)

Family history	Chance (%) of identifying mutation in BRCA1/2
At least 2 cases of ovarian cancer and at least 2 cases of breast cancer	61
At least 3 cases of ovarian cancer and no more than 1 case of breast cancer	70
2 cases of ovarian cancer and 1 case of breast cancer	47
2 cases of ovarian cancer and no cases of breast cancer	20

Ovarian cancer risks in BRCA1 carriers are low (in absolute terms) below age 40 years; thereafter the incidences are ~1% between 40 and 59 years and 2% after age 60 years. Ovarian cancer risk in BRCA2 carriers are, in contrast, very low below age 50 years but then increase sharply in the 50–59 year age group, perhaps declining somewhat thereafter.

Early age at diagnosis is not a feature of familial ovarian cancer. Stratton et al. (1999) found that, of 202 well-documented families with at least two confirmed cases of epithelial ovarian cancer, only 1.6% were diagnosed at <30 years of age. See the table for criteria used to establish high risk of ovarian cancer.

Clinical approach

Where possible try to obtain confirmation of the diagnosis of ovarian cancer. Ovarian cancer is easily misreported by families (the actual diagnosis may prove to be a benign lesion, teratoma, adenocarcinoma of the bowel, uterine cancer, etc.). Krukenberg tumour refers to secondary tumours in the ovaries usually arising from a gastric primary.

History: key points
Three-generation family tree with particular emphasis on history of cancer (especially ovarian, breast, and bowel) and documentation of age of diagnosis. Try to extend the family tree further on the relevant side if there are individuals with cancer in the grandparental generation.

Examination: key points
Not usually appropriate

Special investigations
- DNA for BRCA1/2 mutation analysis from an affected member of a family meeting the high-risk criteria, page 426.
- DNA for MMR genes if the family meets Amsterdam criteria (see table in 'Hereditary nonpolyposis colorectal cancer (HNPCC)', page 454).

Genetic advice
Risk assessment
- **Single relative affected <30 years with no other significant family history** (e.g. breast cancer or other cancers suggestive of a familial cancer syndrome). Stratton et al. (1999) found no BRCA1/2 mutations amongst 101 women with ovarian cancer diagnosed at <30 years and no tendency to greater familiality. Overall risks are likely to be similar to those of the sister of an older proband, i.e. 2–3-fold increased lifetime risk for ovarian cancer.
- **Single relative affected >30 years with no other significant family history** (e.g. breast cancer or other cancers suggestive of a familial cancer syndrome). Sister of a woman with 'sporadic' ovarian cancer has a 3-fold increased lifetime risk for ovarian cancer (Stratton et al. 1998).
- **High-risk women** (see criteria for 'high risk' in table above). High chance of a dominant genetic susceptibility to ovarian and breast cancer.

Penetrance
The risks of both breast and ovarian cancer are higher in BRCA1 carriers than BRCA2 carriers, but the difference is much more marked for ovarian cancer and for breast cancer at younger ages than for breast cancer above 50 years.

Predictive testing
Possible for those families in whom the causative mutation has been defined.

Management

Women with a single affected relative

Whilst the risk of developing ovarian cancer is higher than those of a similar age who are at population risk (relative risk (RR) 3 for first-degree relatives), this increased risk amounts to a cumulative risk of ~4% by age 70 years. In the absence of formal evidence of its efficacy, screening is not currently recommended at this level of risk.

High risk women and BRCA1/2 carriers

The risk of ovarian cancer among *BRCA1* or *BRCA2* mutation carriers decreases with parity (reduction in the odds of ovarian cancer is 12% per birth). Whether the oral contraceptive pill (ocp) confers a protective effect on ovarian cancer risk is controversial. Modan *et al.* (2001) found no protective effect of ocp in *BRCA* carriers, but Narod *et al.* (1998) did.

Prophylactic laparoscopic salpingo-oophorectomy. Although the risk of ovarian cancer in carriers of BRCA mutations is considerably lower than the risk of breast cancer in these carriers, the absence of reliable methods of early detection and the poor prognosis of advanced ovarian cancer make prophylactic salpingo-oophorectomy an option that all female carriers should consider after their families are complete. Kauff *et al.* (2002) in a prospective study of 170 carriers of BRCA mutations with a mean follow-up of 2 years found an ovarian cancer hazard ratio of 0.15 after prophylactic bilateral salpingo-oophorectomy (BSO), compared with the surveillance-only group There was also an important reduction in breast cancer risk with a breast cancer hazard ratio of 0.32 after prophylactic BSO compared with the surveillance-only group.

Salpingo-oophorectomy should be considered rather than oophorectomy given reports of tumours arising in the fallopian tubes in carriers of BRCA mutations. There is a residual risk for primary peritoneal ovarian cancer after oophorectomy.

The risk of developing ovarian cancer at <40 years is low, even in women at high genetic risk. Oophorectomy in premenopausal women precipitates an abrupt menopause. Important side-effects include hot flushes, disturbed sleep, vaginal dryness, and increased risk of osteoporosis and heart disease. Hormone replacement therapy (HRT) may be needed in the short term to counteract these side-effects.

The NIH Consensus Statement on Ovarian Cancer (1995) recommended that women at risk of inherited ovarian cancer undergo prophylactic oophorectomy after completion of child-bearing or at age 35 years.

Chemoprevention. Although the combined oral contraceptive pill (ocp) reduces the risk of ovarian cancer in the general population and in women with a family history of ovarian cancer and possibly in BRCA1/2 carriers, concerns about enhanced breast cancer risk mean that the ocp should not currently be recommended as an option for reducing the risk of ovarian cancer.

Surveillance strategies

See also 'Cancer surveillance methods', page 434.

- **Breast surveillance**. Site-specific ovarian cancer and breast/ovarian cancer are currently regarded as a continuum. Due to the high incidence of BRCA1/2 mutations in high-risk ovarian cancer families (see above), even those in whom an affected family member screens negative for BRCA1/2 mutations should be managed as if they were at high risk of breast cancer.
- **Serum CA-125 estimation and ovarian ultrasound scan (USS).** Early-stage cancers can be identified by a programme of annual serum CA-125 estimation and ovarian ultrasonography (transvaginal USS), but there is a high false-positive rate (with consequent anxiety and surgical intervention). This approach may also fail to detect ovarian cancers at a curable stage (significant false-negative rate). The outcomes of current trials are urgently needed to inform practice in this area.

Expert advisers: Bruce Ponder, Professor of Oncology, University of Cambridge, Cambridge and Paul Pharaoh, Cancer Research UK Senior Clinical Research Fellow, Strangeways Research Laboratory, Cambridge, England.

References

Antoniou A, Pharoah PDP, *et al.* Average risks of breast and ovarian cancer associated with mutations in *BRCA1* or *BRCA2* detected in case series unselected for family history: a combined analysis of 22 studies. *Am J Hum Genet* 2003; **72**: 1117–30.

Kauff ND, Satogopan JM, *et al.* Risk-reducing salpingo-oophorectomy in women with a BRCA1 or BRCA2 mutation. *New Engl J Med* 2002; **346**: 1609–15.

Modan B, Hartge P, *et al.* Parity, oral contraceptives and the risk of ovarian cancer among carriers and noncarriers of a BRCA1 or BRCA2 mutation. *New Engl J Med* 2001; **345**: 235–40.

Narod SA, Risch H, *et al.* Oral contraceptives and the risk of hereditary ovarian cancer. *New Engl J Med* 1998; **339**: 424–8.

NIH Consensus Development Panel on Ovarian Cancer. NIH consensus conference. Ovarian cancer. Screening treatment and follow-up. *J Am Med Assoc* 1995; **273**: 491–7.

Pharaoh PDP, Ponder BAJ. The genetics of ovarian cancer. *Best Pract Res Clin Obstet Gynaecol* 2002; **16** (4): 449–68.

Stratton JF, Pharaoh PDP, *et al.* A systematic review and meta-analysis of family history and risk of ovarian cancer. *Br J Obstet Gynaecol* 1998; **105**: 493–9.

Stratton JF, Thompson D, *et al.* The genetic epidemiology of early-onset epithelial ovarian cancer: a population-based study. *Am J Hum Genet* 1999; **65**: 1725–32.

Peutz–Jeghers syndrome (PJS)

Autosomal dominant (AD) syndrome consisting of characteristic gastrointestinal (GI) hamartomas, mucocutaneous pigmentation, and predisposition to GI, breast, and other cancers. Patients with PJS are at increased risk of GI intussusception and the development of a variety of malignancies, especially of the GI tract, but also including pancreas, breast, uterine, and gonadal tumours. Prevalence estimates for PJS vary between ~1/8300 and 1/29 000. About half of PJS is caused by mutations in *LKB1* (STK11) a serine/threonine kinase on 19p13.3.

Pigmentation. The characteristic freckling of the lips and perioral region develops during childhood, but usually fades from the third decade onwards (less so on buccal mucosa). It is highly variable and not universally present in PJS: in some patients the freckling is florid; in others it can be extremely subtle.

Polyps. There is a great variation in phenotype between PJS families, which is probably due, at least in part, to genetic heterogeneity. 70–90% of PJS patients have hamartomatous polyps in the small bowel, 50% have colorectal polyps, and 25% have gastric polyps. The number of polyps per patient is variable, but many fewer than in familial adenomatous polyposis (FAP). PJS polyps tend to be large and pedunculated and PJS patients may present as surgical emergencies in childhood with intussusception, small bowel obstruction, bleeding per rectum, and volvulus. Most polyps do not cause complications but may cause non-specific abdominal pain. The jejunum is the most common site for PJS polyps. Polyps and cancers occur outside of the GI tract, e.g. nose, respiratory tract, uterus, urinary tract, and gall bladder/biliary tree.

Pathology. The histology of PJS polyps is characteristic and diagnostic, consisting of a branched or frond-like pattern in the stroma, termed arborization.

PJS-associated cancers. Figures naturally vary between studies, but data (mostly) from Spigelman *et al.* (1989) and Giardiello *et al.* (2000) are given in the table. The average age of first cancer diagnosis is the mid-40s (Giardiello *et al.* 2000). Retrospective estimates of the risk of dying from any cancer in PJS range from 38.5% by age 60 to 48% by age 57. Renal cancers have been reported to be associated with PJS, as well as a number of one-off case reports of unusual, rare, or strange tumours.

Genetic heterogeneity. Boardman *et al.* (2000) found that, in both familial and apparently sporadic cases of PJS, germline LKB1 mutations could only be found in a minority (2/5 with a family history, 4/23 isolated cases), and alerted to the possibility of overlap with other hamartomatous syndromes, such as Cowden, juvenile polyposis syndrome (JPS), and Carney complex (CNC; see 'Multiple endocrine neoplasia (MEN)', page 466). Stratakis et al. (1998) have shown that two families with CNC who presented with PJS features, but which were unlinked to the CNC locus on 2p16, were also unlinked to either LKB1 or PTEN. Olschwang et al. (2001) has reported that PJS families unlinked to LKB1 are at especial risk of biliary cancer. Women with PJS-likemucocutaneous pigmentation in the absence of polyps are at increased risk of breast and

Risk of PJS-associated cancers (based on data from Spigelman *et al.* 1989 and Giardiello *et al.* 2000)

Site	Relative risk	95% confidence interval (CI)	Absolute risk (15–64 years)
All sites	15	12–19	93
Non-GI tract	9	4.2–17	
GI tract	13	2.7–38	
Oesophagus	57	2.5–557	0.5
Stomach	213	96–368	29
Small bowel—duodenum, jejunum, ileum	520	220–1306	13
Large bowel	84	47–137	39
Pancreas	132	44–261	36
Gall bladder/biliary tree*			
Breast[†]	15	7.6–27	54
Uterus/Fallopian tube	16	1.9–56	9
Cervix[‡]	1.5	0.3–4.4[‖]	10
Ovary (SCTAT)[§]	27	7.3–68	21
Testis[¶]	4.5	0.1–25[‖]	9
Lung	17	5.4–39	15

* Although Olschwang (2001) found the risk of a biliary tree cancer to be significantly raised in PJS unlinked to *LKB1*, the absolute risk is nonetheless small (0.1–0.2%, *p* < 0.0001).

[†] 3/9 cases bilateral.

[‡] Most cervical cancers in PJS are of the rare type adenoma malignum ('minimal deviation adenocarcinoma'; histologically benign but biologically malignant), which, therefore, probably does make this a significantly associated tumour type.

[§] Sex cord tumour with annular tubules (SCTAT) is a rare ovarian tumour, and when it occurs in association with PJS is usually benign. It may produce symptoms such as precocious puberty and menstrual irregularity due to hyperoestrogenism. SCTAT in women with PJS are bilateral multifocal processes that cause only modest (< 3 cm) ovarian enlargement. The lesion has been found in almost all female patients with PJS in whom the ovaries have been examined, and half of all cases of SCTAT are associated with PJS. A small number of male patients with PJS have similar oestrogen-secreting tumours (presenting with gynaecomastia, rapid growth, advanced bone age) variously described as large cell Sertoli cell tumours or resembling SCTAT.

[¶] All Sertoli cell tumours.

[‖] Not significant.

genital tract cancers and this may be a function of the genetic heterogeneity in PJS.

Diagnostic criteria for PJS. The following are based on Tomlinson and Houlston (1997).

- Either 2 or more PJS polyps in the GI tract *or* one PJS polyp in the GI tract together with either classical PJS pigmentation or a family history.
- A presumptive diagnosis can be made with classical PJS pigmentation and a family history.

Differential diagnosis

- **JPS** (see 'Juvenile polyposis syndrome (JPS)', this chapter) may be confused with PJS, but the histology of the polyps is distinct, although it may necessitate the opinion of a histopathologist specializing in GI pathology. It is well worth asking for histological review.
- **Hereditary mixed polyposis syndrome** (HMPS/*CRAC1*: see 'Familial adenomatous polyposis (FAP)', page 444) is not associated with pigmentation and includes adenomas and, so far, has only been described in Ashkenazi Jews.
- **LEOPARD syndrome** (lentigines–ECG abnormalities–ocular hypertelorism–pulmonary stenosis–abnormal genitalia–retardation of growth–deafness) shows abnormal pigmentation, but not the same pattern as in PJS, and is also not associated with polyps.

Clinical approach

History: key points

Three-generation family tree with careful enquiry about perioral freckling, recurrent abdominal pain, abdominal surgery. Take a detailed history of cancer in other family members (especially breast, GI, pancreas).

Examination: key points

- Look carefully for freckling of the lips, buccal mucosa, vulva, anus, fingers, and toes.
- Note skin lentigines.
- Be alert to endocrine signs of sex cord tumours with annular tubules (SCTATs), especially in children, e.g. precocious puberty, oestrogenization, etc.

Special investigations

- Histopathology of polyps/tumours. Consider opinion of specialist GI pathologist.
- DNA sample for *LKB1* mutation analysis from affected members of the family.

Genetic advice

PJS is genetically heterogeneous (see above). Mutations in *LKB1* are found in 40% of affected individuals; most mutations clearly predict protein truncation. There is marked inter- and intrafamilial variability of expression in PJS kindreds.

Risk assessment

AD, 50% risk of inheritance. About 10–20% have apparent new mutations; the remainder are familial. However, bear in mind that the genetic basis of most (80%) isolated/sporadic cases of PJS is not known, and might be due to an as yet unidentified autosomal recessive (AR) locus.

Penetrance

Almost complete penetrance: 0/17 clinically unaffected at-risk relatives in Ylikorkala *et al.*'s (1999) series showed the disease-associated haplotype. More than 90% have

mucocutaneous melanin pigmentation. Though again, bear in mind the genetic heterogeneity in PJS.

Predictive testing

Possible by direct mutation analysis, if mutation known in the family, or by haplotype analysis if family large enough to establish linkage to 19p13.

Individuals in whom predictive testing has not been possible and in whom screening has shown no polyps and who have no freckling can probably discontinue screening from age 30 years.

Prenatal diagnosis

Technically possible by chorionic villus sampling (CVS) if the familial mutation is known.

Management

The relative risk for cancer differs in males and females. In both sexes there is an increased risk for GI tumours, but women have a heightened risk because of a strongly increased risk of breast and gynaecological cancer. Men with PJS have an overall relative risk for cancer of 6.2 compared with 18.5 for women. Aside from anticancer surveillance the other important part of the management of PJS patients is that they should avoid repeated laparotomies for the removal of single, usually small bowel polyps: if a laparotomy is performed then the aim should be to remove all polyps, not just the one intussuscepting. Referral to and management by a surgical/gastroenterological team experienced in looking after PJS patients is recommended and should be considered.

Surveillance strategies

See also 'Cancer surveillance methods', page 434.
For *all* patients, the following is advised.

- Increased vigilance and low threshold for investigation for any clinical abnormality, whether inside or outside the GI tract, that raises the question of malignancy.
- Annually. Review with enquiry about abdominal pain, GI bleeding, jaundice, operations and/or tumours, update of family history. Check haemoglobin.
- Two-yearly. Gastroscopy, colonoscopy, and barium meal and follow-through (or abdominal computerized tomography (CT)/magnetic resonance imaging (MRI)) and increasingly capsule endoscopy. In an asymptomatic child, a one-off top and tail endoscopy and barium meal and follow-through might be done at the time of diagnosis. If they remained asymptomatic, it may be appropriate to wait until teenage years before instituting 2-yearly studies.
- Recommended polyp management. Remove all polyps > 5 mm found at gastroscopy/colonoscopy. Perform laparotomy and peroperative enteroscopy for small bowel polyps > 15 mm seen on barium follow-through, or for smaller polyps with abdominal pain.

In addition, for *females*, the following is advised.

- Check cervical smears are up to date.
- Consider annual mammography from 35 years.
- Consider ovarian/endometrial screening.

Support group: <www.epigenetic. org/~pjs/ homepage.html> (information for both clinicians and patients).

Expert advisers: Robin Phillips, Professor, St Mark's Hospital, London, England and Ian M. Frayling, Consultant in Clinical Genetics and Director of Clinical Genetics Laboratory, University Hospital of Wales, Cardiff, Wales.

References

Boardman LA, *et al*. Association of Peutz–Jeghers-like mucocutaneous pigmentation with breast and gynecologic carcinomas in women. *Medicine (Baltimore)* 2000; **79**: 293–8.

Giardiello FM, Brensinger JD, *et al*. Very high risk of cancer in familial Peutz–Jeghers syndrome. *Gastroenterology* 2000; **119** (6): 1447–53.

McGarrity TJ, Kulin HE, *et al*. Peutz–Jeghers syndrome. *Am J Gastroenterol* 2000; **95**: 596–604.

Olschwang S, Boisson C, Thomas G. Peutz–Jeghers families unlinked to STK11/LKB1 gene mutations are highly predisposed to primitive biliary adenocarcinoma. *J Med Genet* 2001; **38**: 356–60.

Spigelman AD, Murday V, Phillips RK. Cancer and the Peutz–Jeghers syndrome. *Gut* 1989; **30**: 1588–90.

Stratakis CA, *et al*. Carney complex, Peutz–Jeghers syndrome, Cowden disease, and Bannayan–Zonana syndrome share cutaneous and endocrine manifestations, but not genetic loci. *J Clin Endocrinol Metab* 1998; **83**: 2972–6.

Stratakis CA, Kirschner LS, Carney JA. Clinical and molecular features of the Carney complex: diagnostic criteria and recommendations for patient evaluation [review]. *J Clin Endocrinol Metab* 2001; **86**: 4041–6.

Tomlinson IPM, Houlston RS. Peutz–Jeghers syndrome. *J Med Genet* 1997; **34**: 1007–11.

Westerman AM, Wilson JH. Peutz–Jeghers syndrome: risks of a hereditary condition [review]. *Scand J Gastroenterol Suppl* 1999; **230**: 64–70.

Wong SS, Rajakulendran S. Peutz–Jeghers syndrome associated with primary malignant melanoma of the rectum. *Br J Dermatol* 1996; **135**: 439–42.

Ylikorkala A, Avizienyte, E, *et al*. Mutations and impaired function of LKB1 in familial and non-familial Peutz–Jeghers syndrome and a sporadic testicular cancer. *Hum Mol Genet* 1999; **8**: 45–51.

Phaeochromocytoma

The adrenal medulla and ganglia of the sympathetic nervous system are neural crest derivatives. They synthesize and secrete catecholamines (adrenaline, noradrenaline, etc.). Phaeochromocytomas usually arise in the adrenal medulla, but can arise outside the adrenal, in the sympathetic chain, where they may be called paragangliomas. Paragangliomas that originate in the sympathetic nervous system are most comonly found in the retroperitoneum, but can also occur in the thorax. Paragangliomas that originate in the parasympathetic nervous system can occur adjacent to the aortic arch, neck, skull base as local 'non-functioning' masses, also called 'glomus tumours' or chemodectomas. Germline mutations in the succinate dehydrogenase subunit genes (*SDHB* and *SDHD*) can cause susceptibility to both phaeochromocytomas (adrenal and extraadrenal) and parasympathetic-derived head and neck paraganglionomas. Classical clinical symptoms of phaeochromocytoma are paroxysmal headache, sweating, and palpitations accompanied by hypertension due to the pressor effects of catecholamine release.

Although traditionally ~10% of phaeochromocytomas have been considered to have a genetic origin, in Neumann *et al.*'s (2002) study of 271 patients with apparently sporadic phaeochromocytomas, 66 (24%) had germline mutations in *VHL*, *RET*, *SDHB*, and *SDHD* (50% were in *VHL* with the rest equally distributed). 84% of multifocal tumours and 59% of phaeochromocytomas presenting at <19 years of age were due to germline mutations.

Recent studies suggest that germline *SDHD* and *SDHB* mutations are an important cause of familial and isolated phaeochromocytoma. See the table for a summary of genetic conditions predisposing to phaeochromocytoma.

Clinical approach

History: key points

Three-generation family tree with specific reference to tumour types and features listed in the above table.

Examination: key points

- Marfanoid body habitus and mucosal neuromas (multiple endocrine dysplasia (MEN2B).
- Thyroid mass (MEN2).
- Carotid-body tumour (familial paraganglioma).
- Café au lait spots (CALs), axillary freckling, and dermal neurofibromas (neurofibramotosis type 1 (NF1)).

- Observe gait, and observe eyes for nystagmus and past-pointing/dysdiadochokinesia (cerebellar signs in Von Hippel–Lindau (VHL) secondary to cerebellar haemangioblastoma).

Special investigations

- DNA for mutation analysis if specific syndrome identified or ready access to mutation analysis of *VHL*, *RET*, *SDHB/D*.
- Ophthalmology referral for retinal angiomas (VHL) if no specific syndrome identified.
- Most patients with phaeochromocytoma will have had recent intraabdominal imaging (usually magnetic resonance imaging (MRI)) as part of their diagnosis which should identify pancreatic cysts, renal-cell cancers (VHL).

Genetic advice

Risk assessment

If specific syndrome, or germline mutation identified, offer screening to all first-degree family members.

Penetrance

See table above.

Predictive testing

If a specific germline mutation is identified (and you are certain it is disease-causing), offer predictive testing to first-degree relatives in order to target subsequent surveillance.

Management

Surveillance strategies

In genetic conditions predisposing to phaeochromocytoma, screening is usually acomplished by vanillylmandelic acid (VMA) analysis of 24 hour urine samples

Expert adviser: Eamonn Maher, Professor of Medical Genetics, University of Birmingham, Birmingham, England.

References

Dluhy RG. Phaeochromocytoma—death of an axiom [editorial]. *New Engl J Med* 2002; **346**: 1486–8.

Maher ER, Eng C. The pressure rises: update on the genetics of phaeochromocytoma. *Hum Mol Genet* 2002; **11**: 2347–54.

Neumann HPH, *et al.* Germ-line mutations in nonsyndromic phaeochromocytoma. *New Engl J Med* 2002; **346**: 1459–66.

Genetic conditions predisposing to phaeochromocytoma (after Dluhy 2002)

Syndrome*	Gene	Features[†]	Risk (%) of phaeochromocytoma
MEN2A	*RET*	MTC, hyperparathyroidism	50
MEN2B	*RET*	MTC, multiple mucosal neuromas, Marfanoid habitus, hyperparathyroidism	50
Familial paraganglioma	*SDHB* *SDHD*[‡]	Cervical paragangliomas and chemodectomas	20
VHL	*VHL*	Cerebellar and CNS haemangioblastoma, renal-cell cancer, pancreatic and renal cysts, retinal angiomas	10–20
NF1	*NF1*	CALs, axillary freckling, dermal neurofibromas	1

* MEN, Multiple endocrine dysplasia; VHL, Von Hippel–Lindau syndrome; NF1, neurofibromatosis type 1.

[†] MTC, Medullary thyroid cancer; CNS, central nervous system; CALs, café au lait spots.

[‡] Familial glomus tumours due to mutations of *SDHD* are maternally imprinted.

Retinoblastoma

Retinoblastoma (RB) is an embryonic neoplasm of retinal origin caused by mutations in the tumour suppressor gene *RB1* on 13q14. RB affects approximately 1/20 000 livebirths and arises predominantly in children <7 years of age (90% of diagnoses are made at <5 years). It can rarely occur antenatally.

The predisposition to RB is inherited as an autosomal dominant (AD) trait. Penetrance can vary. Most mutations are associated with a high (> 90%) penetrance, but some mutations have a much lower penetrance. An RB develops according to Knudson's two-hit hypothesis (see figure) when both RB1 alleles are deleted or mutated.

In genetic RB, the first hit is most commonly a mutation (~90–95%) or a deletion (5–10%). The second event is most commonly loss of heterozygosity (LOH) at syntenic loci over a large segment of 13q (~70%). Less frequently there is a separate somatic mutation (~30%) or hypomethylation (a few %) There is a high new mutation rate in RB1 and 85% of new germline mutations arise in the paternally derived allele.

The role of the geneticist is to:

1 provide information to the family, GP, and other clinicians on aetiology, recurrence risks for different family members, and second tumours;

2 arrange genetic testing if appropriate on the affected child and convey results to the family, GP, and other medical teams;

3 arrange genetic testing on the wider family if appropriate, conveying results to family and GP;

4 arrange prenatal testing if requested by the family and convey the results to appropriate clinicians.

Terminology. Many of the terms used in the literature overlap and can be confusing.

- **Unifocal:** one tumour in one eye.
- **Unilateral,** often used synonymously with unifocal: one eye affected.
- **Multifocal:** many separate tumours in one eye.
- **Bilateral:** tumours in both eyes.
- **Trilateral:** bilateral RB plus a pineoblastoma. Pineoblastomas can, very rarely, develop without obvious tumours in the eyes.
- **Genetic or hereditary RB** is defined when there is a germline *RB1* mutation affecting all cells in the body and a single somatic hit to the *RB1* gene then initiates tumourigenesis. This will include all trilateral, bilateral, and multifocal RB. It will also include ~10% of unilateral/unifocal RB.
- **Nongenetic/nonhereditary RB** occurs when the two hits to the *RB1* gene have occurred only in the tumour and are not present in other cells. This will include the majority of unilateral/unifocal RB.
- **Sporadic** is used in different contexts, meaning either that there is no family history of RB or being synonymous with nongenetic.
- **Mosaicism** can be found and can be associated with either unilateral or bilateral RB depending on the nature of the mutation and the proportion of affected cells.

Second tumours. Survivors of RB who carry a germline mutation in *RB1* are at greatly increased risk for a variety of other tumours which include:

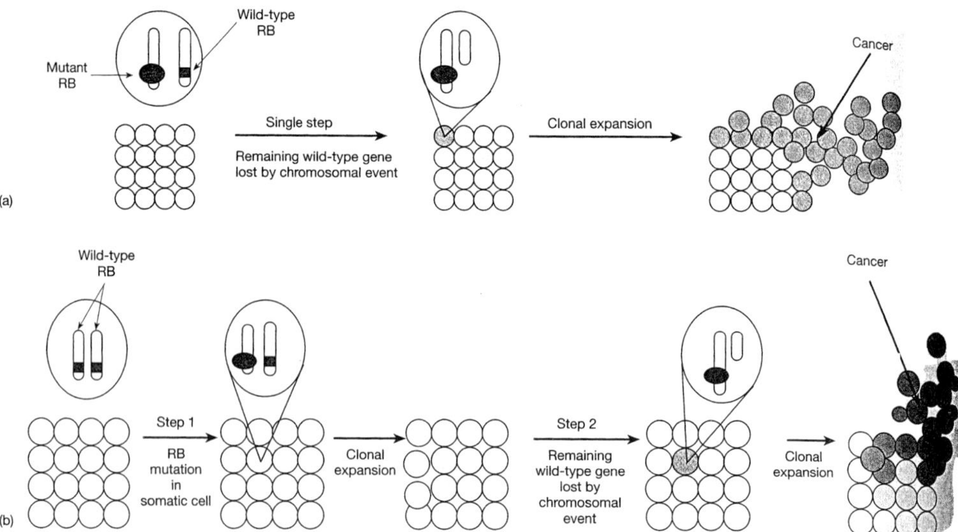

Knudson's hypothesis. (a) In individuals with an inherited predisposition to retinoblastoma every somatic cell contains one intact *Rb* allele and one mutant *Rb* allele. A single somatic mutation is therefore sufficient for loss of *Rb* activity, with subsequent clonal expansion of the double mutant cell and tumour formation. (b) In normal individuals both copies of *Rb* must be targeted by somatic mutation for *Rb* function to be disrupted. Since the somatic mutation rate is low the risk of two *Rb* mutations occurring in the same cell is low. This explains the later onset and unifocal nature of retinoblastoma cases that occur in the absence of a family history. (Taken from Warrell (2003), p. 230, by permission of Oxford University Press.)

- osteosarcoma (relative risk (RR), 200–500; 37% of second primaries), especially if treated with radiotherapy;
- other sarcomas, e.g. soft tissue sarcoma, fibrosarcomas, chrondrosarcomas (14% of second primaries);
- malignant melanoma (7%);
- brain tumours (4.5%; excludes pinealoblastoma, i.e. trilateral RB, which is not a second primary and occurs in 2.4%).

Widely varying estimates for the probablity of a second non-ocular primary in patients with germline RB1 mutations are found in the literature. Radiotherapy as part of RB treatment further increases the mortality from second tumours. Moll *et al.* (1997) estimate the cumulative incidence of second primary tumours to be 19% at the age of 35 years (RR, 15). The tumours most commonly develop in the second to fourth decades. Overall, there is an ~40% lifetime risk of any second tumour, incorporating the background risk for cancer in the general population (~30%) and the excess RB risk (6–10%).

Clinical approach

History: key points

Three-generation (or more extensive) family tree documenting RB and all other types of tumour.

Examination: key points

- Brief examination of skin of older patients with hereditary RB if appropriate.
- Parents of a child with RB should always be examined by an experienced ophthalmologist to look for spontaneously regressed tumour.

Special investigations

- DNA sample for *RB1* mutation analysis. Mutation identifiable in ~90% of families with bilateral or familial RB. For children with unilateral RB, mutation analysis will have a pick-up rate of only ~8%.
- Karyotype with fluorescent *in situ* hybridization (FISH) for *RB1*. Approximately 3% have an interstitial deletion of 13q14 (many of the children with deletions do have associated dysmorphic features and/or developmental delay, but a significant proportion do not). Such deletions are not detected by conventional molecular genetic techniques and so karyotyping with FISH should be performed on all affected children.
- Consider linkage exclusion testing (see below) alongside mutation analysis, e.g. if several siblings are being screened as a result of a new diagnosis in a child, or if particular family circumstances make sibling screening difficult.
- Tumour mutation analysis. This should be considered when mutation testing on blood is negative. If a mutation is found in tumour but not in blood, the mutation cannot have been inherited from a parent and other siblings do not need to be screened or tested. There is a possibility of low-level mosaicism in the affected child and that child's future offspring should be offered mutation analysis. (Tumour testing can only be performed if an eye has been enucleated, not from a biopsy sample.)

Genetic advice

Patients with hereditary RB (familial, bilateral, unilateral multifocal, or unilateral, or, rarely, trilateral or non-penetrant) can transmit the initial *RB1* mutation as an AD trait. Alternatively, the initial *RB1* mutation can arise in retinal cells or their embryonic precursors and not involve the germline. This is the genetic basis for nonhereditary RB (unilateral, unifocal). In ~10% of families with hereditary RB, mosaicism for the initial mutation is found either in the proband or in one of the proband's parents. The possibility of mosaicism should always be considered during the genetic counselling of newly identified families with RB.

Empiric risk assessment

- Bilateral retinoblastoma.
  - Siblings of an affected child (parent unaffected): 5%.
  - Offspring of an affected individual 50% of whom inherit mutation: 45% chance of developing RB (assuming 90% penetrance).
- Unilateral retinoblastoma.
  - Siblings of affected child (parents unaffected): 1%.
  - Offspring of affected individual: 5%. This will include both unilateral and bilateral RB in an affected offspring.

Risk assessment incorporating results of genetic testing

1 **Sporadic bilateral RB or multifocal RB.** Assumption is that these are germline RB1 mutation carriers with a RR to offspring of 45% (AD inheritance with 90% penetrance). In a few instances these patients are in fact somatic or gonosomal mosaics with a lower offspring risk. In Sippel *et al.*'s (1998) study all germline mosaics had an initial mutation that was detectable in blood, but there was insufficient data for this to be reliable.

2 **Unilateral simplex RB with *de novo RB1* mutation in blood.** Even if the mutation appears *de novo*, i.e. is not detectable in either parent, the possibility of parental germline mosaicism exists and *RB1* testing should be offered to siblings. Offspring risk is 45%.

3 **Unilateral RB with no detectable *RB1* mutation in blood.** Estimated risk for developing a tumour in the other eye is 3–5% (because of somatic mosaicism) so regular eye surveillance must be continued. Some risk of germline mosaicism exists, but offspring risk is likely to be small. Consider looking for LOH and *RB1* mutations in tumour tissue. If two intragenic mutations are identified in tumour tissue, but neither is present in blood — a postzygotic origin has to be assumed and sibs are not at risk.

4 **RB1 mutation not detectable in a sporadic individual with bilateral or multifocal disease.** Consider looking for LOH and *RB1* mutations in tumour tissue. Could be due to an undetectable mutation or mosaicism. NB. There is still an offspring risk because of the possibility of germline mosaicism, but this may be <45%.

Penetrance and expressivity

For inactivating mutations penetrance is estimated at 90%. Approximately 30% have a unilateral RB and the rest have bilateral RB. Individuals with partial loss of function mutations in RB1 have a lower penetrance and a higher incidence of unilateral disease. Mosaic individuals have reduced penetrance (60%) and expressivity.

Families suggestive of reduced penetrance. A very rough way of calculating penetrance in a particular family is to calculate the percentage of eyes affected with RB divided by the number of eyes in obligate mutation carriers, e.g. if a grandparent had unilateral RB, a parent was unaffected, and a child had bilateral RB, there are 3 affected eyes in 3 people (i.e. 6 eyes altogether) so the penetrance in that family is 50%. NB. The grandfather may have been a germline mosaic.

Predictive testing

Where a mutation is identified, cascade testing of the family is indicated, starting with parents and siblings and including the extended family as indicated. Parents who do not carry an RB mutation present in their affected child should be given a low (not negligible) risk of recurrence as germline mosaicism can occur.

Predictive testing of 'at risk' neonates is appropriate because of the burden of frequent screening by examination under anaesthesia (EUA) in the early years of life. Those defined as not at risk by mutation analysis or linkage can be excluded from screening.

Linkage analysis can be helpful in families where there is clearly familial RB but no mutation has been identified. **Linkage exclusion testing** can also be helpful for families with either bilateral or unilateral RB when no mutation has been identified. Comparing the RB genotypes in unaffected parents, affected children, and unaffected children gives a 1 in 4 chance of being able to exclude a sibling from screening.

Strategy for assessing risk to siblings and future pregnancies

1 Screen for RB1 mutations in blood of affected child. If a mutation is identified, parents can be tested to determine whether it is *de novo* or inherited and siblings can be tested.
2 Linkage exclusion testing: see above.
3 Genetic analysis of tumour: linkage exclusion testing. If there is LOH, this is presumed to be the result of the 'second hit' and linkage analysis is possible based on the RB genotype, which defines those individuals 'at risk' and enables those not sharing the haplotype to be exempt from/discontinue screening. Offspring will have a low recurrence risk because of the possibility of mosaicism in the affected individual.
4 Genetic analysis of tumour: mutation analysis. If it is possible to identify the mutations in the tumour tissue and these are not present in the affected child's blood, these define a *de novo* somatic change as the cause of the RB with no increased risk to siblings who can then be exempt from/discontinue screening.

Prenatal diagnosis

Prenatal diagnosis by chorionic villus sampling (CVS) is available in those families in which the RB1 mutation is known or when a family is informative for linkage.

Management

Treatment

At present chemotherapy is the first-line treatment, followed by local treatments such as plaques or cryotherapy for accessible tumours or lens-sparing radiotherapy. Enucleation is usually offered as a first-line treatment for a large unilateral tumour or if disease is hard to control by other treatments.

Surveillance strategies

- **Screening of children at risk of RB (i.e. sibling or child of an affected individual).** Any child with an increased risk of RB (including siblings of a child with isolated unilateral RB in whom the risk is only 1%) should be offered EUAs from the age of 2–3 weeks until the age of 5 years. The examinations are offered at decreasing frequency and most children undergo 14 EUAs.
- **Surveillance for second non-RB primaries.** Increased level of awareness by patient and GP (with accelerated referral if any concern) and regular skin check for malignant melanoma (can usually be done by patients or their partner, but if there is visual impairment it could be done by GP/dermatologist).

Support group: Retinoblastoma Society <www.rbsociety.org.uk>, Tel. 020 7600 3309.

Expert adviser: Elisabeth Rosser, Consultant Clinical Geneticist, Great Ormond Street Hospital, London, England.

References

Eng C, Li FP, *et al.* Mortality from second tumours among long-term survivors of retinoblastoma. *J Natl Cancer Inst* 1993; **85**: 1121–8.

Lohmann DR, Gerick M, *et al.* Constitutional RB1-gene mutations in patients with isolated unilateral retinoblastoma. *Am J Hum Genet* 1997; **61**: 282–94.

Mohney BG, Robertson DM, *et al.* Second nonocular tumours in survivors of heritable retinoblastoma and prior radiation therapy. *Am J Ophthalmol* 1988; **126**: 269–77.

Moll AC, Inhof SM, *et al.* Second primary tumours in patients with retinoblastoma. A review of the literature. *Ophthalmic Genet* 1997; **18**: 27–34.

Sippel KC, Fraioli RE, *et al.* Frequency of somatic and germ-line mosaicism in retinoblastoma: implications for genetic counselling. *Am J Hum Genet* 1998; **62**: 610–19.

Vogel F. Genetics of retinoblastoma. *Hum Genet* 1979; **52**: 1–54.

Warrell D. (ed.). *Oxford textbook of medicine*, 4th edn. Oxford University Press, Oxford, 2003.

von Hippel–Lindau (VHL) disease

VHL disease is an autosomal dominant (AD) disorder characterized by a predisposition to a wide variety of tumours, most frequently haemangioblastomas of the cerebellum and spinal cord, retinal angiomas, renal cell carcinoma, phaeochromocytomas, and renal, pancreatic, and epididymal cysts. The gene for VHL on 3p25 encodes a tumour-suppressor protein pVHL. pVHL is the recognition component of the E3–ubiquitin ligase complex involved in the degradation of hypoxia-inducible factor-1 (HIF) alpha-subunits, a process regulated by oxygen availabiliy and blocked by disease-causing pVHL mutations.

The most frequent initial manifestations of VHL are retinal angiomatosis, followed by cerebellar haemangioblastoma, renal cell carcinoma, and phaeochromocytoma (see table). The probabilty of a patient with VHL developing a cerebellar haemangioblasoma, retinal angioma, or renal cell carcinoma by age 60 years is 84%, 70%, and 69%, respectively. The most frequent causes of death are renal cell carcinoma and central nervous system (CNS) haemangioblastomas. Haemangioblastomas of the CNS are the most common tumour in VHL, affecting 60–80% of all patients. The average age of presentation for cerebellar haemangioblastomas is 33 years. These tumours are benign, but are a major cause of morbidity. Tumours of the endolymphatic sac are rare neuroectodermal neoplasms in the petrous bone originating from inner ear structures, which occur at increased frequency in VHL (Lonser). They may present with hearing loss, tinnitus and vertigo. Pancreatic neuroendocrine tumours and cysts, epididymal cystadenomas, and broad ligament cystadenomas are all less common features of VHL.

Most germline VHL mutations are inactivating (frameshift, nonsense, and deletions of one or more exons). Approximately 30% are missense mutations. There is a strong association between specific missense mutations and susceptibility to phaeochromocytoma.

Clinically, VHL can be subdivided into type 1 (no phaeochromocytoma) and type 2 (phaeochromocytoma present). Most families with a VHL type 2 phenotype also show renal cancer (type 2B), but rare families do not (type 2A). Rare mutations can produce a predisposition to phaeochromocytoma without other manifestations of VHL (type 2C).

Clinical approach

History: key points

- Detailed three-generation family tree with specific enquiry about renal tumours, brain tumours, and visual loss. Extend the family tree of affected individuals as far as possible.
- Detailed past medical history.
- Enquiry re current symptoms

Examination: key points

- Blood pressure (BP).
- If diagnosis is suspected, careful neurological examination, especially for cerebellar signs.
- Fundoscopy.

Special investigations

If diagnosis is suspected arrange:

- DNA sample (EDTA (ethylenedinitrilotetraacetate)) for VHL mutation screening.
- Ophthalmology opinion with direct and indirect fundoscopy for retinal angioma.
- Brain and abdominal magnetic resonance imaging (MRI) scans.
- 24 hour urine for vanillylmandelic acid (VMA).

Genetic advice

Approximately 20% are due to new dominant mutations.

Risk assessment

AD, with 50% risk that offspring will inherit the disease-causing mutation. There is considerable variation within families carrying the same mutation.

Penetrance

Penetrance is age-dependent. Mean age at first diagnosis is ~25 years. The proportion of patients who have presented by age 20 years is 65%, by 40 years 85%, by 50 years 95%, and by 60 years 98%.

Predictive testing

Possible if the familial mutation is known. Usually considered just prior to the commencement of regular surveillance at 5 years of age.

Prenatal diagnosis

Technically feasible by chorionic villus sampling (CVS) at 11 weeks gestation if the familial mutation is known, but not commonly requested.

Management

Surveillance strategies

- Annual BP from age 5 years.
- Annual direct and indirect ophthalmoscopy for detection of retinal angiomas from age 5 years. More frequent screening may be indicated if angiomas are present.
- Annual renal imaging (MRI or ultrasound scan (USS)) from age 16 years. More frequent renal USS or follow-up MRI imaging may be indicated if there are abnormalities on the renal scan.

Major complications of VHL and their frequency

Major complications of VHL	Frequency of clinical disease in cross-sectional studies
Retinal angioma	58% (may cause visual loss if not treated, e.g.with laser therapy)
Cerebellar haemangioblastoma	56% (multiple or recurrent in 1/3rd of cases)
Spinal cord haemangioblastoma	14%
Renal cell carcinoma	25% (mean age at diagnosis, 44 years)
Phaeochromocytoma	17% (NB. wide interfamilial differences in frequency)

- Annual 24 hour urine collection for VMA from 11 years.
- MRI brain scans every 3 years from age 15 years. Patients should be aware that in many centres CNS lesions are only removed if symptomatic.

Cerebellar haemangioblastoma

Approximately 30% of all cerebellar haemangioblastomas occur as part of VHl and full clinical evaluation combined with mutation screening should be undertaken in all patients presenting with apparently sporadic cerebellar haemangioblastoma. The younger the patient at diagnosis, the more likely that the patient has VHL. Most haemangioblastomas of the craniospinal axis can be safely and completely excised by surgery. Haemangioblastomas in the CNS often grow at several sites simultaneously, new lesions can arise with time, and the growth pattern of these tumours can be unpredictable. Therefore resection is deferred until the onset of symptoms to avoid unnecessary surgery (Lonser et al. 2003).

Solitary retinal angioma

Solitary retinal angiomas can occur sporadically or be associated with VHL disease. In addition to clinical evaluation, genetic testing should be considered to exclude VHL disease with a high level of certainty. Virtually all patients with multiple retinal angiomas have VHL.

Renal cysts and renal cell carcinoma

Renal cysts may be detected from the second decade; early renal cell carcinoma has been detected as early as 16 years. Renal cell carcinoma is often, but not invariably associated with cysts. Renal cell carcinoma may be multifocal and bilateral in VHL. Tumours are usually treated with partial nephrectomy; ongoing surveillance is crucial because of the risk of further renal tumours.

Support group: VHL Family Alliance <www.vhl.org>.

Expert adviser: Eamonn Maher, Professor of Medical Genetics, University of Birmingham, Birmingham, England.

References

Lonser RR, Glenn GM, et al. von Hippel–Lindau disease [seminar]. *Lancet* 2003; **361**: 2059–67.

Lonser RR, Kim HJ, et al. Tumors of the endolymphatic sac in von Hippel–Lindau disease. *NEJM* 2004; **350**: 2481–86.

Maher ER, Yates JRW, et al. Clinical features and natural history of von Hippel–Lindau disease. *Quart J Med* 1990; **283**: 1151–63.

Pugh CW, Ratcliffe PJ. The von Hippel–Lindau tumour suppressor, hypoxia-inducible factor-1 (HIF-1) degradation, and cancer pathogenesis. *Semin Cancer Biol* 2003; **13**: 83–9.

Singh AD, Ahmad NN, et al. Solitary retinal capillary hemangioma. Lack of genetic evidence for von Hippel–Lindau disease. *Ophthalmic Genet* 2002; **23**: 21–7.

Wilms tumour

Nephroblastoma.

Wilms tumour is an embryonal tumour of the kidney, occurring in 1 in 10 000 children. Most cases present between the ages of 3 and 4 years with an abdominal mass. 90% present by age 7 years. More than 90% are unilateral. Pathology is complex and typically includes blastemal, stromal, and epithelial elements. (triphasic). Stromal-predominant tumours are more common in *WT1* syndromes. Nephrogenic rests (NR), which are considered to the precursor cells for Wilms tumour, may be identifiable. A post-mortem study found that these cells are found in about 1 in 100 neonates against an incidence of Wilms tumour of 1 in 10 000 children. The position of NRs can differ in Wilms tumour syndromes, e.g. intralobar nephrogenic rests (ILNRs) are common in the *WT1* syndromes and perilobar nephrogenic rests (PLNR) are common in Wilms tumours found in overgrowth conditions, trisomy 18 and trisomy 13.

Many genes and syndromes have been reported to be associated with Wilms tumour; however, less than 5% of children with Wilms tumour have a recognizable congenital malformation syndrome. Screening for Wilms tumour in conditions with increased risk has been advocated and is widely practised, although its efficacy is unproven. As the survival of Wilms tumour is so high (90% for localized Wilms tumour and 70% for metastatic disease), an important aim of screening is early detection so that treatment reduction and consequent decreased treatment-induced morbidity is possible.

Clinical approach

History: key points

- Three-generation family tree.
- Specific enquiry regarding family history of cancer (familial Wilms tumour, Li–Fraumeni syndrome (LFS), hyperparathyroidism–jaw tumour (HPT–JT) syndrome).
- Pathology report for verification of diagnosis. NB. Stromal-predominant pathology, particularly with rhabdomyoblastic differentiation, is associated with *WT1* syndromes.
- Birth history. Birthweight increased in Beckwith–Wiedemann syndrome (BWS), Simpson–Golabi– Behmel (SGB) syndrome, and Perlman syndrome; decreased in mosaic variegated aneuploidy (MVA), Fanconi anaemia (FA), Bloom syndrome, Mulibrey (muscle–liver–brain–eye) nanism (MUL). Neonatal hypoglycaemia (BWS). Feeding difficulties due to tongue enlargement (BWS).
- Renal impairment and glomerulosclerosis (*WT1* syndromes). Mesangial sclerosis (Denys–Drash syndrome (DDS)). Focal-segmental sclerosis (Frasier syndrome).
- Genitourinary abnormalities (*WT1* syndromes), FA
- Developmental delay (WAGR (Wilms tumour–aniridia– genitourinary anomalies–mental retardation), MVA, Perlman, MUL).
- Dysmorphic features (Perlman, SGB, MVA, FA, Bloom).

Examination: key points

To exclude syndromic associations

- Height, weight, occipital-frontal circumference (OFC: increased in BWS, SGB, Perlman; decreased in MVA, FA Bloom, MUL).
- Eyes. Aniridia (WAGR), cataracts (MVA).

- Hemihypertrophy (BWS, isolated hemihypertrophy (IHH)).
- Macroglossia (BWS).
- Abdominal examination for organ enlargement, umbilical hernia (BWS).
- Genitourinary abnormalities, e.g cryptorchidism, hypospadias, genital ambiguity.
- Skeletal abnormalities (FA).
- Document any dysmorphic features.
- Blood pressure (BP) and urinalysis for proteinuria.
- Review imaging and operation notes for evidence of genitourinary malformation.

Special investigations

- Karyotype. XY phenotypic females (DDS), 11p abnormalities (11p13 *WT1*, 11p15 BWS), mosaic aneuploidies (MVA), premature centromere separation (MVA), chromosome breakage (FA, Bloom), trisomies (13, 18), del 2q37.
- Fluorescent *in situ* hybridization (FISH) 11p13 probes, if aniridia present.
- *WT1* mutation screening (DDS, Frasier; consider in bilateral Wilms tumour cases with genitourinary abnormalities).
- Mutation screening if features of BWS (UPD 11p15, *KvDMR1* methylation defect), SGB (*GPC3*) FA-D1 (*BRCA2*), MVA (*BUB1B*). LFS (*TP53*), Bloom (*BLM*), HPT-JT (*HRPT2*), MUL (*TRIM37*).
- Renal investigations may be indicated.

Syndromic diagnoses to consider

The WT1 syndromes

WAGR (Wilms tumour–aniridia–genitourinary anomalies–mental retardation). A syndrome due to a micro deletion on 11p13. There is deletion of the Wilms tumour gene, *WT1*, and the adjacent aniridia gene, *PAX6*, on chromosome 11p13. Children have a 30% risk of Wilms tumour and gonadoblastoma also reported. The mean age of diagnosis of Wilms tumour is 29 months. Usually occurs *de novo* but occasional familial cases reported.

Denys–Drash syndrome (DDS). Classic triad includes Wilms tumour, genitourinary abnormalities that can be severe in males leading to pseudohermaphroditism, and renal impairment that presents with hypertension and proteinuria leading to progressive renal failure. Kidneys show mesangial sclerosis. Caused by constitutional *WT1* mutations, particularly (but not exclusively) in the DNA-binding zinc fingers encoded by exons 7–10. The median age at diagnosis of Wilms tumour is 16 months. Usually occurs *de novo*, but non-penetrance in carrier parents has been reported.

Frasier syndrome. Typical features are renal impairment with focal-segmental glomerulosclerosis and gonadoblastoma. Wilms tumour less common but can occur. Caused by constitutional *WT1* mutations in intron 9 that alter the ratio of *WT1* splicing isoforms.

Familial Wilms tumour. Only a very small proportion of Wilms tumour families are due to *WT1* mutations, 2 out of 39 in a UK series. Genitourinary abnormalities in males are usually present.

Non-syndromic Wilms tumour. A small proportion of isolated non-syndromic Wilms tumour cases carry constitutional *WT1* mutations. Both the US and UK data suggest less than 5%. Bilateral tumours, genitourinary abnormalities, such as undescended testes, and stromal-predominant histology are all associated with increased risk of *WT1* mutation, but there are no current recommendations that any non-syndomic Wilms tumour cases should have *WT1* mutation screening.

Non-syndromic nephropathy. Some children with kidney impairment and either mesangial sclerosis or focal segmental glomerulosclerosis, but without the other features of DDS or Frasier syndrome, have been found to carry constitutional *WT1* mutations.

Other syndromes

Familial Wilms tumour. 1–3% of Wilms tumour cases cluster in families. The majority are autosomal dominant (AD) with reduced and variable penetrance. Genitourinary abnormalities suggest *WT1*. Loci on 17q21 (*FWT1*) and 19q13 (*FWT2*) have been mapped, but genes not yet identified. Some families are unlinked to all known loci indicating further heterogeneity. Age of onset, bilateral disease, metastatic disease, and/or specific pathology can cluster in some families, but there is extensive intra- and interfamilial variability.

Beckwith–Wiedemann syndrome (BWS). Macrosomia, anterior abdominal wall defects, macroglossia, anterior ear lobe creases, and posterior helical pits. Caused by dysregulation of imprinted genes on 11p15. Overall risk of Wilms tumour is ~7% with median age of diagnosis ~3 years. There is also an increased risk of other embryonal tumours such as hepatoblastoma. Risk may differ according to underlying molecular cause and appears to be higher for those with uniparental disomy (UPD) 11p15, hemihypertrophy, and lower in cases with *KvDMR1* methylation defects or *CDKN1C* mutations. However, these associations are not currently robust enough to alter management in different individuals. See 'Beckwith–Wiedemann syndrome (BWS)' page 278.

Simpson–Golabi–Behmel syndrome (SGB). X-linked recessive (XLR) disorder due to mutations and deletion in *glypican 3* (Xq26). High birthweight, heavy facies, supernumerary nipples, cryptorchidism, mild/moderate learning disability. See 'Overgrowth' page 206. Risk of Wilms tumour and other embryonal tumours.

Isolated hemihypertrophy (IHH). Poor clinical definition and true tumour risk uncertain. In Hoyme *et al.*'s (1998) study, tumours developed in 9/168 patients (5.9%). Risk is for embryonal tumours as for BWS and SGB.

Perlman syndrome. Autosomal recessive (AR) condition with macrosomia and a high incidence of Wilms tumour. Distinctive facial features and high neonatal mortality; learning disability is common.

Fanconi Anaemia (FA-D1). AR condition characterised by skeletal abnormalities, short stature, dysmorphic facies, hypersensitivity to DNA cross linking agents and haematological malignances. Eleven subtypes are known. Only subtype D1, which is due to biallelic *BRCA2* mutations, have increased risk of Wilms tumour.

Mosaic variegated aneuploidy (MVA). AR condition due to mutations in *BUB1B*. Characterised by microcephaly, developmental delay, growth retardation, and cataracts. Karyotype shows multiple mosaic monosomies and trisomies sometimes with premature chromatid separation (PCS). Some cases show only PCS. High incidence of cancer, particularly Wilms tumour.

Li–Fraumeni syndrome (LFS). AD cancer syndrome due to mutations in *TP53* (17p13) characterised by brain tumours, sarcomas, adrenocortical carcinoma, leukaemia, and young-onset breast cancer. Incidence of Wilms tumour is also increased.

Trisomy 18/trisomy 13. Trisomy 18 and trisomy 13 survivors are at increased risk of both Wilms tumour and hepatoblastoma. No increased risk of embryonal tumours in trisomy 21.

Hyperparathyroidism–jaw tumour syndrome (HPT-JT). AD condition due to mutations in *HRPT2* (1q24) characterized by hyperparathyroidism due to parathyroid tumours, ossifying fibromas of the mandible and maxilla, and renal lesions such as cysts, hamartomas, or Wilms tumour.

Bloom syndrome. AR condition due to mutations in *BLM* (15q26). Characterized by growth retardation, dysmorphic facies, sunlight-sensitive rash especially on the face, immune deficiency, and malignancies in 20% including Wilms tumour. Elevated frequency of chromosomal breaks with increased sister-chromatid exchange.

Mulibrey-nanism (MUL). AR condition, enriched in Finland, caused by mutations in *TRIM37* (17q22). Characterized by prenatal growth failure, constrictive pericarditis, dysmorphic features, and hypoplasia of various endocrine glands causing hormonal deficiency. About 4% of MUL patients develop Wilms tumour.

Genetic advice
Recurrence risk
As appropriate for specific disorder.

For a family with an isolated unilateral Wilms tumour case, the recurrence risk is very low and screening for siblings not recommended. Recurrence risk in families with non-syndromic bilateral cases without additional features or family history is also very low and no screening is recommended in relatives. Offspring risk for individuals with Wilms tumour, particularly bilateral cases, is less clear as it is only in recent generations that appreciable number of survivors are having children, but currently appears to be <5%. No current recommendations for screening of offspring.

Carrier detection
As for the specific disorder.

Prenatal diagnosis
Only possible in families with a known mutation.

Natural history and further management (preventative measures)
For *WT1* syndromes long-term monitoring of renal function with annual BP and urinalysis recommended for those without nephropathy, as they may develop renal impairment in adulthood.

Surveillance for Wilms tumour in at-risk individuals
Due to the rarity of Wilms tumour cases occurring in at-risk individuals it has not been possible to perform randomized studies to evaluate surveillance strategies. In the US, recommendations based on retrospective studies of BWS and WAGR are for ultrasound screening (USS) every 3–4 months until 7–8 years, for individuals deemed to be at increased risk. In UK, children at >5% risk of Wilms Tumour should be offered screening (*WT1* syndrome,

familial Wilms tumour, BWS, SGB, Perlman, MVA, FA-D1). Screening should be 3–4 monthly until 5 years in all conditions except BWS and some familial Wilms tumour pedigrees where it should continue until 7 years.

Support group: Many of the individual syndromes have their own support group: see <www.cafamily.org.uk>; Beckwith–Wiedemann support network <www.geocities.com/bwsn/index.html>.

Expert advisers: Nazneen Rahman, Consultant Geneticist, and Kathy Pritchard-Jones, Senior Lecturer and Honorary Consultant in Paediatric Oncology, Institute of Cancer Research and Royal Marsden Hospital, London, England.

References

Hoyme HE, Seaver LH, Jones KL, *et al.* Isolated hemihyperplasia (hemihypertrophy): report of a prospective multicenter study of the incidence of neoplasia and review. *Am J Med Genet* 1998; **79**: 274–8.

McNeil DE, Brown M, *et al.* Screening for Wilms tumour and hepatoblastoma in children with Beckwith–Wiedemann syndrome: a cost-effective model. *Med Pediatr Oncol* 2001; **37**: 349–56.

National Wilms Tumour Study Group <http://www.nwtsg.org>.

Pritchard-Jones K. Controversies and advances in the management of Wilms tumour. *Arch Dis Child* 2002; **87**: 241–4.

UK Children's Cancer Study Group (UKCCSG) <http://www.ukccsg.org>.

Chapter 5

Chromosomes

Chapter contents

22q11 deletion syndrome 490
47,XXX 494
47,XXY 496
47,XYY 498
Autosomal reciprocal translocations—background 500
Autosomal reciprocal translocations—familial 504
Autosomal reciprocal translocations—postnatal 506
Autosomal reciprocal translocations—prenatal 508
Cell division—mitosis, meiosis, and non-disjunction 510
Chromosomal mosaicism—postnatal 514
Chromosomal mosaicism—prenatal 516
Deletions and duplications 520
Down syndrome (trisomy 21) 524
Edwards' syndrome (trisomy 18) 526
Inversions 528
Mosaic trisomy 8 530
Mosaic trisomy 16 532
Patau syndrome (trisomy 13) 534
Prenatal diagnosis of sex chromosome aneuploidy 536
Ring chromosomes 538
Robertsonian translocations 540
Sex chromosome mosaicism 544
Submicroscopic chromosomal abnormalities and the chromosomal phenotype 546
Supernumerary marker chromosomes (SMCs)—postnatal 552
Supernumerary marker chromosomes (SMCs)—prenatal 554
Triploidy (69,XXX, 69,XXY, or 69,XYY) 556
Turner syndrome, 45,X and variants 558
X-autosome translocations 562

22q11 deletion syndrome

Includes DiGeorge syndrome (DGS), Shprintzen or velocardiofacial syndrome (VCFS), conotruncal anomaly face syndrome; MIM (Mendelian Inheritance in Man database) no. 188400.

Hemizygous deletion of chromosome 22q11 (del 22q11.2) may cause any combination of the following: cardiac defects; thymic hypoplasia; velopharyngeal insufficiency with cleft palate; parathyroid dysfunction with hypocalcaemia; and a distinctive facial appearance. Microdeletions of 22q11.2 usually encompass ~3 Mb of genomic DNA and are detectable by fluorescent *in situ* hybridization (FISH) analysis. There are several low-copy repeats (LCRs) on chromosome 22 (LCR22). Those flanking the 22q11 deletion region appear to facilitate homologous recombination; however misalignment between blocks of LCR22s is likely to facilitate the deletion. Most VCFS/DGS patients have a 3 Mb deletion, some have a nested distal deletion breakpoint resulting in a 1.5 Mb deletion, and a few rare patients have unique deletions, translocations, or point mutations of *TBX1* (Yagi *et al.* 2003). Overall, ~96% of patients have a defined 1.5–3 Mb deletion including 24–30 genes.

The phenotype (heart outflow tract, velopharyngeal, ear, thymic, and parathyroid abnormalities) arises from a failure to form derivatives of the third and fourth branchial arches during development. Haploinsufficiency of *TBX1* appears to be the major contributor to the phenotype seen with del 22q11 (Yagi *et al.* 2003), but *VEGF* (vascular endothelial growth factor) is likely to be an important modifier, with certain *VEGF* promoter haplotypes associated with an increased risk for cardiovascular birth defects in del 22q11 individuals. Rare patients with a *TBX1* mutation appear to have a full pharyngeal phenotype, but without the mild learning difficulties often seen in the full del 22q11. The diagnosis should be considered in any child with congenital heart disease (CHD), cleft palate, or palatal insufficiency. In approximately 94% the deletion is *de novo*, with 6% being inherited from a parent.

Occasionally, the diagnosis of del 22q11 is made antenatally during investigation of a pregnancy in which CHD or a structural renal anomaly (e.g. renal agenesis or multicystic dysplastic kidney) has been identified.

Clinical features

There is marked intrafamilial variability in expression. For example, a parent may have a cleft palate and CHD, and a child may have developmental delay, but a normal heart and palate.

Growth. Growth retardation is common. 83% have heights/weights < 50th centile and 36% are < 3rd centile for either height or weight.

Development. Reduced intelligence quotient (IQ) scores compared with other members of the family are usual. Severe mental retardation is only found in a small percentage of children with del 22q11. Individuals with 22q11 tend to have specific difficulty with abstract reasoning and have poor problem-solving skills. They often find maths and reading comprehension particularly challenging. Children with del 22q11 will often require special educational support, especially when these cognitive problems exist in combination with communication difficulties (see below).

- Normal development in 32%, although one-third of these had speech delay.
- Learning difficulties in 68%, of which 30% had mild learning problems, 18% had moderate/severe learning difficulties, and 20% were not classified.
- Hence, overall, 62% are developmentally normal or have mild learning difficulties.

Communication. In excess of 90% have some communication difficulties. These are multifactorial with hypernasality and mild cognitive and language delay all being important factors contributing to speech delay. Early speech milestones are typically delayed by several months, but use of phrases and sentences may be delayed until 3 years of age or so. Between 3 and 4 years of age there is often a rapid acceleration in language development.

Behavioural, psychological, and psychiatric problems. Patients have difficulties in establishing and maintaining friendships. Psychiatric disorders (including bipolar affective disorder and schizophrenia) are described in up to 18% of adults (overall, 6.5% of adults with 22q11 had experienced at least one episode of psychosis). 22q11 deletions account for <2% of individuals with schizophrenia in the general population.

Cardiovascular anomalies.
- 75% have significant CHD.
- Nearly 20% have tetralogy of Fallot.
- Ventricular septal defect (VSD) and interrupted aortic arch were the next most common defects.
- A wide variety of cardiac anomalies have been described including atrial septal defect (ASD), truncus arteriosus, right-sided aorta, pulmonary stenosis, aortic valve anomalies, aberrant subclavian arteries, vascular ring, anomalous origin of the the carotid artery, transposition of the great arteries (TGA), and tricuspid atresia. (As many as 10% of infants with CHD may have del 22q11 depending on the study.)
- Anomalies of the internal carotid arteries and other major neck arteries are frequent.

Otolaryngeal anomalies (Ryan *et al.* 1997).
- Cleft palate in 9% (± velopharyngeal insufficiency).
- Submucous cleft palate in 5%.
- Velopharyngeal insufficiency in 32%.
- 75% have chronic serous otitis media. Sensorineural loss, often unilateral and mild/moderate, may occur in up to 15%.

Genitourinary anomalies.
- 36% have structural renal tract anomalies including renal agenesis and multicystic dysplastic kidneys, hydronephrosis, and vesicoureteric reflux.
- Amongst male patients Wu *et al.* (2002) found a slightly increased incidence of undescended testes (6%) and hypospadias (8%).

Endocrine function.
- 60% are hypocalcaemic at some time, mostly in the neonatal period, and some have neonatal seizures secondary to hypocalcaemia that cease with calcium supplementation. A few patients have latent or late-onset hypocalcaemia. Taylor *et al.* (2003) and Greenhalgh *et al.* (2003) found hypocalcaemia in ~30% and ~42% of children, respectively, outside the neonatal period.

- Hypothyroidism is uncommon but occurs at a higher incidence than in the general population (Kawame *et al.* 2002).

Immune and haematological status.
- Patients with del 22q11 have a variable defect in cell-mediated immunity. Most patients will recover normal or near normal T-cell numbers and function by age 2 years; however, a small group experiences persistent and profound T-cell dysfunction (DGS). There is preliminary data that T-cell number and function may occasionally drop again in adolescence.
- Only 1% have a major abnormality of immune function (Ryan *et al.* 1997).
- Many had a history of recurrent minor infection in the first 2 years of life, which then resolved (Ryan *et al.* 1997).
- Mild thrombocytopenia is common. Idiopathic thrombocytopenia purpura (ITP) is also associated (Levy *et al.* 1997) and idiopathic thrombocytopenia with autoimmune haemolytic anaemia has also been reported (Kratz *et al.* 2003). Lawrence found that, even after the exclusion of patients with ITP, the mean platelet count was approximately 70% of the control population.
- Autoimmune disorders appear to be more common in children with 22q11 deletions than in the general population (Perez and Sullivan 2002). Haemolytic anaemia, type 1 diabetes mellitus (Elder *et al.* 2001), and hypothyroidism–Graves disease (Kawame *et al.* 2001) have all been reported (Perez and Sullivan 2002).

Craniofacial.
- Subtle dysmorphic features (see below).
- Approximately 1% have craniosynostosis.

Other. Pachygyria and polymicrogyria (especially bilateral perisylvian polymicrogyria) have both been reported in children with 22q11 deletions (Ehara *et al.* 2003).

Clinical approach

History: key points
- Neonatal problems. Feeding problems (e.g. mild regurgitation through nose), seizures.
- CHD. Management, e.g. previous surgery.
- Developmental progress particularly speech.
- History of infections.
- Family history of CHD, cleft palate, psychosis.

Examination: key points
- Growth parameters. Height, weight, occipital-frontal circumference (OFC).
- Face. Short palpebral fissures with telecanthus, wide and prominent nasal bridge and root, small mouth. Ears are round in shape with deficient upper helices.
- Heart. Careful clinical examination.
- Palate. Can the child speak clearly or is his/her speech nasal in quality? Is there a cleft uvula or submucous cleft palate?

Special investigations
- **Echocardiogram** (unless previously done).
- **Renal ultrasound scan (USS).**
- **Audiometry.** Children with 22q deletion have a high incidence of communication problems. These are multifactorial, but glue ear is a common and treatable cause. Those with sensorineural loss may benefit from hearing aids.
- **Plasma Ca.** Check at least once during infancy, childhood, adolescence, and pregnancy. It may be a sensible precaution to check plasma Ca on any hospital admission, particularly those for cardiac or palate surgery, or alongside other blood tests whenever these are being performed. Greenhalgh *et al.* (2003) found hypocalcaemia in 42% of school-age children with 22q11.
- **Immunology.** Full blood count (FBC) with platelets and T, B, and NK (natural killer) lymphocyte subsets (if abnormal discuss management with immunologist).
- In children older than 4 months, serum immunoglobulins and tetanus, diptheria, and Hib (*Haemophilus influenzae* type b) antibody titres (if abnormal discuss management with immunologist).
- Consider referral to speech therapy and/or to cleft team for palatal assessment.
- **Parental chromosome analysis**. FISH for 22q11.2 deletion in both parents.

Pregnancy/neonatal diagnosis
If the diagnosis is made prenatally, fetal echocardiography should be arranged (if not already performed) and plans should be made to anticipate possible problems in the neonatal period arising from:
- CHD (arrange echocardiogram in neonatal period);
- hypocalcaemia—check plasma Ca on day 1;
- feeding problems related to palatal abnormalities, e.g. nasal regurgitation, weak and slow sucking (examine for submucous cleft).

Consider prophylaxis with co-trimoxazole pending results of immune function (discuss with immunologist)

In Ryan *et al.*'s (1997) series, 8% of patients died, most within 6 months of birth; all but one death was the result of severe CHD.

Immunizations
No live vaccines should be given (i.e. oral polio, BCG (bacille Calmette–Guérin)) until immune function has been checked. Then the following should be done.
- MMR (measles, mumps, rubella) vaccine. On a pragmatic basis offer at 18 months of age to those who have 75% normal T-cell count, and who have responded normally to tetanus and Hib vaccines.
- Use inactivated polio vaccine instead of oral one (since Sep '04 the infant immunisation schedule (tetanus, diphtheria, polio, Hib and meningococcus C) in the UK includes no live vaccines) and UK babies with del 22q11 should receive their infant immunisations as usual.
- Varicella immunization (as for MMR).
- BCG vaccine should not be given until a risk assessment is carried out that establishes that potential benefit outweighs risk.

Transfusions
Any transfusion products should be cytomegalovirus (CMV)-negative and irradiated for children <6 months of age or if there is T-lymphopenia, e.g. CD4 count <500.

Genetic counselling
If either parent is found to carry the 22q-deletion, the recurrence risk is 50% for future pregnancies. The affected child will have a 50% risk of transmitting the deletion to his/her offspring in any pregnancy.

If neither parent carries the 22q-deletion, the recurrence risk is very small (~1%), but note that there are 2 reported cases of sibling recurrence presumed due to gonadal mosaicism.

Prenatal diagnosis

Possible by chorionic villus sampling (CVS) or amniocentesis. Some parents may elect for detailed fetal echocardiography in addition to or as an alternative to an invasive procedure (75% of patients with 22q11 will have a cardiac defect, some of which will be detectable by fetal echocardiography).

Support groups: Max appeal `<www.maxappeal.org.uk.; The 22q11 Group, www.vcfs.net>`; Velo-Cardio-Facial Syndrome Education Foundation `<www.vcfsef.org>`.

Expert advisers: Judith Goodship, Professor of Medical Genetics, University of Newcastle, Newcastle-upon-Tyne and Ann Harding-Bell, Speech Therapist to the Eastern Region Cleft Network, Addenbrooke's Hospital, Cambridge, England.

References

Driscoll D, Salvin J, *et al.* Prevalence of 22q11 microdeletions in DiGeorge and velocardiofacial syndromes: implications for genetic counselling and prenatal diagnosis. *J Med Genet* 1993; **30**: 813–17.

Dyce O, McDonald-McGinn D, *et al.* Otolaryngologic manifestations of the 22q11.2 deletion syndrome. *Arch Otolaryngol Head Neck Surg* 2002; **128**: 1408–12.

Ehara H, Maegaki Y, *et al.* Pachygyria and polymicrogyria in 22q11 deletion syndrome. *Am J Med Genet* 2003; **117A**: 80–2.

Elder DA, Kaiser-Rogers K, *et al.* Type I diabetes mellitus in a patient with chromosome 22q11.2 deletion syndrome. *Am J Med Genet* 2001; **101** (1): 17–19.

Garabedian M. Hypocalcaemia and chromosome 22q11 microdeletion. *Genet Couns* 1999; **10**: 389–94.

Goodman FR. Congenital abnormalities of body patterning: embryology revisited. *Lancet* 2003; **362**: 651–62.

Greenhalgh KL, Aligianis IA, *et al.* 22q11 deletion: a multisystem disorder requiring multidisciplinary input. *Arch Dis Child.* 2003; **88** (6): 523–4.

Hatchwell E, Long F, *et al.* Molecular confirmation of germ line mosaicism for a submicroscopic deletion of chromosome 22q11. *Am J Med Genet* 1998; **78**: 103–6.

Kawame H, Adachi M, *et al.* Graves' disease in patients with 22q11.2 deletion. *J Pediatr* 2001; **139** (6): 892–5.

Kratz CP, Niehues T, *et al.* Evans syndrome in a patient with chromosome 22q11.2 deletion syndrome: a case report. *Pediatr Hematol Oncol* 2003; **20** (2): 167–72.

Lawrence S, McDonald-Mcginn DM, *et al.* Thrombocytopenia in patients with chromosome 22q11.2 deletion syndrome. *J Pediat* 2003; **143**: 277–78.

Levy A, Michel G, Lemerrer M, Philip N. Idiopathic thrombocytopenic purpura in two mothers of children with DiGeorge sequence: a new component manifestation of deletion 22q11? *Am J Med Genet* 1997; **69** (4): 356–9.

McDermid HE, Morrow BE. Genomic disorders on 22q11. *Am J Hum Genet* 2002; **70**: 1077–88.

Perez E, Sullivan KE. Chromosome 22q11.2 deletion syndrome (DiGeorge and velocardiofacial syndromes). *Curr Opin Pediatr* 2002; **14** (6): 678–83.

Perez EE, Bokszczanin A, *et al.* Safety of live viral vaccines in patients with chromosome 22q11.2 deletion syndrome (DiGeorge syndrome/velocardiofacial syndrome). *Pediatrics* 2003; **112** (4): e325.

Ryan AK, Goodship JA, Wilson DI, *et al.* Spectrum of clinical features associated with interstitial chromosome 22q11 deletions: a European collaborative study. *J Med Genet* 1997; **34**: 798–804.

Sandrin-Garcia P, Macedo C, *et al.* Recurrent 22q11.2 deletion in a sibship suggestive of parental germline mosaicism in velocardiofacial syndrome. *Clin Genet* 2002; **61**: 380–3.

Stalmans I, Lambrechts D, *et al.* VEGF: a modifier of the del 22q11 (DiGeorge) syndrome? *Nat Med* 2003; **9**: 173–82.

Taylor SC, Morris G, *et al.* Hypoparathyroidism and 22q11 deletion syndrome. *Arch Dis Child.* 2003; **88** (6): 520–2.

Tobias ES, Morrison N, *et al.* Towards earlier diagnosis of 22q11 deletion. *Arch Dis Child* 1999; **8**: 513–14.

Wu HY, Rusnack SL, *et al.* Genitourinary malformations in chromosome 22q11.2 deletion. *J Urol* 2002; **168**: 2564–65.

Yagi H, Furutani Y, *et al.* Role of *TBX1* in human del 22q11.2 syndrome. *Lancet* 2003; **362**: 1366–73.

47,XXX

Triple X syndrome.

47,XXX may be diagnosed incidentally at amniocentesis/chorionic villus sampling (CVS). It occasionally comes to light later in life, but usually as an incidental finding. Mosaic karyotypes with combinations of 47,XXX/46,XX/45,X, due to postzygotic non-disjunction may be found.

The incidence is 1/1000 to 1/1200 female births. There is a significant maternal age effect, with 47,XXX being more common with advanced maternal age, increasing from 1/2500 livebirths at maternal age 33 years to 1/450 at 43 years (Hook 1992). It is substantially underascertained and the majority of 47,XXX women are unaware of their karyotype.

Clinical features

Physical. A normal female appearance is usual. Tall stature is a consistent finding (>80th percentile). The mean occipital-frontal circumference (OFC) is 10th centile. The frequency of structural urogenital anomalies may be slightly increased.

Puberty. Sexual development and puberty are normal.

Educational. Full-scale intelligence quotient (IQ) averages 10–15 points less than that of siblings. Mental retardation is not associated with 47,XXX. There is an increased risk for speech and language delay and some may require additional learning support, either part-time or full-time, but usually in a mainstream school. As for 46,XX girls there is wide variation in ability and attainment.

Behavioural. No consistent findings. An American survey of 11 XXX women showed that during adolescence and young adult life they were less well adapted and experienced more stress, work, and relationship problems than their XX siblings. However, overall they were mostly self-sufficient and functioning reasonably well. Sexual orientation is normal.

Fertility. Most 47,XXX women are fertile and have chromosomally normal babies. There may be a slightly increased risk for premature ovarian failure (POF).

Adult life. There may be a modest increase in risk for cardiovascular disease (Swerdlow *et al.* 2001).

Clinical approach

History: key points (postnatal presentation)
Developmental milestones, speech and language development, schooling.

Examination: key points (postnatal presentation)
Height.

Management

- Advise parents that if their daughter shows developmental, behavioural, or educational difficulties they should have a low threshold for asking for professional help, as early intervention can improve outcome.
- There is no indication for medical surveillance over and above that routinely offered to all children.
- In general, disclosure of the karyotype on a 'need to know' basis is advised so that the child is not treated differently or regarded differently by others. Telling a child about their 47,XXX karyotype should be a gradual process extending over many years, with parents being supported in this by health professionals. See Linden *et al.* (2002) for a full discussion of this topic.

Genetic advice

Recurrence risk
Parents of girls with 47,XXX are not routinely karyotyped. The recurrence risk is low, <1%.

Offspring risk
The risk for chromosome anomaly in women with 47,XXX is very low, <1%.

Prenatal diagnosis
Prenatal diagnosis should be offered to parents and to women with 47,XXX but there is a fine balance between the very small risk of recurrence and the risk of procedure-associated pregnancy loss.

Lay group contact: In the UK via Unique Rare Chromosome Disorders <www.rarechromo.org>.

Expert adviser: Mary Linden, Genetic Counsellor, Kimball Genetics Inc., Denver, Colorado, USA.

References

Christian SM, Koehn D, Pillay R, MacDougall A, Wilson RD. Parental decisions following prenatal diagnosis of sex chromosome anomalies, a trend over time. *Prenat Diagn* 2000; **20**: 37–40.

Harmon RJ, Bender BG, Linden MG, Robinson A. Transition from adolescence to early adulthood: adaptation and psychiatric status of women with 47,XXX. *J Am Acad Child Adolesc Psychiatry* 1998; **37**: 286–91.

Hook EB. Chromosome abnormalities: prevalence, risks and recurrence. In *Prenatal diagnosis and screening* (ed. D.L.H. Brock, C.H. Rodeck, and M.A. Ferguson-Smith), pp. 351–92. Churchill Livingstone, Edinburgh, 1992.

Linden MG, Bender BG. Fifty-one prenatally diagnosed children and adolescents with sex chromosome anomalies. *Am J Med Genet* 2002; **110**: 11–18.

Linden MG, Bender BG, Robinson A. Intrauterine diagnosis of sex chromosome aneuploidy. *Obstet Gynecol* 1996; **87**: 468–75.

Linden MG, Bender BG, Robinson A. Genetic counselling for sex chromosome abnormalities. *Am J Med Genet* 2002; **110**: 3–10.

Ratcliffe S. Long term outcome in children of sex chromosome abnormalities. *Arch Dis Child* 1999; **80**: 192–5.

Swerdlow AJ, Hermon C, *et al.* Mortality and cancer incidence in persons with numerical sex chromosome abnormalities: a cohort study. *Ann Hum Genet* 2001; **65** (Pt. 2): 177–88.

47,XXY

Klinefelter syndrome.

Klinefelter syndrome has a prevalence of 1/600–1/800 male births. There is a significant maternal age effect, with 47,XXY being more common with advanced maternal age, increasing from 1/2500 livebirths at maternal age 33 years to 1/300 at 43 years (Hook 1992).

47,XXY is usually either diagnosed prenatally as an unexpected finding at amniocentesis/chorionic villus sampling (CVS) or in adult life during investigation of male infertility. The majority are probably never diagnosed. Males with Klinefelter syndrome have a normal lifespan.

Clinical features

Physical. Babies appear normal at birth, although there may be an increased incidence of undescended testes (one-third required orchidopexy in Ratcliffe's (1999) study). Men with 47,XXY tend to be rather tall with final adult height 186 cm (compared with 177 cm for 46,XY). There is an increased risk for transient gynaecomastia. If troublesome, surgical reduction can be performed but is rarely necessary (1/19 in Ratcliffe's (1999) study).

Puberty and sexual development. Boys enter puberty normally. By midpuberty the testes begin to involute, and boys develop hypergonadotrophic hypogonadism with decreased testosterone production. Testes are small in adult life and men with Klinefelter syndrome are, with occasional exceptions, infertile. 47,XXY males are no more likely to be homosexual than 46,XY males. Men with 47,XXY have, with the exception of small testes, normal genitalia and normal sexual relations.

Educational. There is a modest decrement in intelligence quotient (IQ) of 10–15 points when compared with siblings, but IQ varies widely (as for 46,XY) and in Linden and Bender's (2002) study the range was 67–133. The majority of 47,XXY (two-thirds) will have more problems with reading and spelling than their 46,XY peers. In Linden and Bender's (2002) study, 70% received additional educational support (usually part-time support in mainstream school).

Behaviour. A tendency towards passive and unassertive behaviour has been frequently noted. Gender orientation is normal and there is no evidence for increased aberrant sexual behaviour.

Employment. Ratcliffe (1999) noted that most XXY boys have less skilled jobs than their fathers, but there was no increase in unemployment. Variation is wide and some 47,XXY men will follow professional careers.

Fertility. 47,XXY men are generally infertile. Occasionally, men with 47,XXY have a few sperm in their testes, even when none are present in the ejaculate. Testicular sperm extraction and intracytoplasmic sperm injection (ICSI) with in vitro fertilization (IVF) offer hope of biological fatherhood to some. Currently, it is not possible to predict which men will have testicular sperm. Artificial insemination by donor (AID) and adoption remain important options. Exceptionally, fertility has been reported, but is probably the result of a cryptic 47,XXY/46,XY karyotype.

Adult life. There may be a modest increase in risk for diabetes and diseases of the cardiovascular, respiratory, and digestive systems (Swerlow *et al.* 2001).

Clinical approach

History: key points (postnatal presentation)

Developmental milestones, speech and language development, schooling.

Examination: key points (postnatal presentation)

- Height.
- Pubertal development (depending on age).

Management

- Advise parents that, if their son shows developmental, behavioural, or educational difficulties, they should have a low threshold for asking for professional help, as early intervention can improve outcome.

- In general, disclosure of the karyotype on a 'need to know' basis is advised so that the child is not treated differently or regarded differently by others. Telling a child about his 47,XXY karyotype should be a gradual process extending over many years, with parents being supported in this by health professionals. See Linden *et al.* (2002) for a full discussion of this topic.

- Refer to a paediatric endocrinologist at around 10 years of age for monitoring of growth and measurement of testosterone, follicle-stimulating hormone (FSH), and luteinizing hormone (LH). If studies suggest hypergonadotrophic hypogonadism, testosterone supplementation should be offered. Testosterone supplementation (usually given as intramuscular (IM) injections every few weeks or transdermal patches applied daily) improves self-esteem, facial hair growth, and libido. It also has a protective effect in reducing the risk of osteoporosis.

- For management of infertility, refer to a reproductive medicine specialist for consideration of AID or assisted conception with IVF and ICSI. Sperm for ICSI may be obtained from ejaculate or testicular biopsy.

- Some of the literature mentions an increased risk of cancer in 47,XXY males. A Danish study of 696 men with Klinefelter found that the overall cancer incidence is not increased and concluded that no routine cancer screening seems justified (Hasle *et al.* 1995). Breast cancer is more common in XXY men than in XY men (relative risk 20); however, mean age at diagnosis was 72 years and the actual risk (approximately 3%) remains lower than in normal females. There is a very small (<1%) risk of primary mediastinal germ cell tumours that may present with precocious puberty, or respiratory symptoms at age 10–30 years.

Genetic advice

Recurrence risk

Parents of boys with XXY are not routinely karyotyped. The recurrence risk is low, <1%.

Offspring risk

There may be an increased risk of aneuploidy (both for sex chromosomes and for +21) and pre-implantation genetic diagnosis (PGD) or prenatal diagnosis should be offered.

Hennebicq *et al.* (2001) found a higher frequency of 24,XX and 24,XY sperm than in controls and also a much higher frequency of disomy 21 (6.2% versus 0.4%).

Prenatal diagnosis

Prenatal diagnosis should be offered to parents, but there is a fine balance between the very small risk of recurrence and the risk of procedure-associated pregnancy loss. Prenatal diagnosis is indicated if a patient with Klinefelter fathers a pregnancy because of the increased risk for aneuploidy (see above).

Support group: Klinefelter's syndrome association UK <www.ksa-uk.co.uk>; Klinefelter Syndrome and Associates <www.genet.org/ks>.

Expert adviser: Mary Linden, Genetic Counsellor, Kimball Genetics, Inc., Denver, Colorado, USA.

References

Hasle H, Mellemgaard A, Nielsen J, Hausen J. Cancer incidence in men with Klinefelter syndrome. *Br J Cancer* 1995; **71**: 416–20.

Hennebicq S, Pelletier R, Bergues U, *et al.* High risk for trisomy 21 for ICSI conceptus of a Klinefelter patient. *Lancet* 2001; **357**: 2104–5.

Hook EB. Chromosome abnormalities: prevalence, risks and recurrence. In *Prenatal diagnosis and screening* (ed. D.L.H. Brock, C.H. Rodeck, and M.A. Ferguson-Smith), pp. 351–92. Churchill Livingstone, Edinburgh, 1992.

Horowitz M, Wisheart JM, *et al.* Osteoporosis and Klinefelter's syndrome. *Clin Endocrinol* 1992; **36**: 113–18.

Hultborn R, Hanson C, Kopf I, *et al.* Prevalence of Klinefelter's syndrome in male breast cancer patients. *Anticancer Res* 1997; **17**: 4293.

Linden MG, Bender BG. Fifty-one prenatally diagnosed children and adolescents with sex chromosome anomalies. *Am J Med Genet* 2002; **110**: 11–18.

Linden MG, Bender BG, Robinson A. Intrauterine diagnosis of sex chromosome aneuploidy. *Obstet Gynecol* 1996; **87**: 468–75.

Linden MG, Bender BG, Robinson A. Genetic counselling for sex chromosome abnormalities. *Am J Med Genet* 2002; **110**: 3–10.

Ratcliffe S. Long term outcome in children of sex chromosome abnormalities. *Arch Dis Child* 1999; **80**: 192–5.

Robinson A, Bender BG, Linden MG. Klinefelter syndrome. In *Management of genetic syndromes* (ed. S.B. Cassidy and J.E. Allanson), pp. 195–206. Wiley-Liss, New York, 2001.

Swerdlow AJ, Hermon C, *et al.* Mortality and cancer incidence in persons with numerical sex chromosome abnormalities: a cohort study. *Ann Hum Genet* 2001; **65** (pt. 2): 177–88.

47,XYY

An extra Y chromosome is found in approximately 1 in 1000 male births. There is no advanced paternal age effect. At least 85% are undiagnosed either pre- or postnatally. Fryns and Kleczkowska (1995) found 75 males with XYY karyotype amongst nearly 100 000 karyotypes performed in the Leuven cytogenetics laboratory. This is very close to the incidence of XYY in newborn studies and indicates that the frequency of mental retardation (MR)/multiple congenital anomaly (MCA) syndromes is not increased in XYY males in general.

Referrals come from two main sources:

- prenatal identification after chorionic villus sampling (CVS)/amniocentesis for maternal age or suspected fetal abnormality, where the 47,XYY karyotype is truly an incidental finding.
- from the investigations of boys with learning and behavioural difficulties where the finding may be of clinical significance (see below).

The most common mechanism to produce the extra Y is non-disjunction at meiosis II after a normal chiasmate meiosis I. Postzygotic mitotic errors and non-disjunction at meiosis II after a nullichiasmate meiosis I are also possible.

Clinical features

Physical. At birth, height, weight, and head circumference show no difference from those of controls. From the age of 2 years the growth velocity increases until puberty. Boys enter puberty 7–8 cm taller than controls. There are no dysmorphic features.

Puberty. The growth spurt is prolonged with a final height mean of 188 cm (91st–98th centile). Secondary sexual development is normal, but the onset may be delayed by about 6 months compared to that of controls.

Educational. There is a small but significant lowering of the intelligence quotient (IQ) scores, with the mean 10–15 points lower than that of siblings, but remaining within the normal range. There is an increased incidence of mild speech/language delay. Most boys with 47,XYY will attend mainstream school. In Ratcliffe's (1999) study of 19 boys, 54% of the XYY boys had reading difficulties compared to 18% of controls. Severe mental retardation is rarely found.

Behaviour. Behavioural problems are more common in males with XYY, especially in those with learning difficulties. There is no typical behavioural phenotype for XYY and sexual orientation is normal. Problems reported in childhood include temper tantrums and defiant behaviour. 47% of the XYY boys in Ratcliffe's (1999) series of 19 boys had been referred to a psychiatrist (control, 9%). There is improvement when appropriate psychological and educational help is given.

Much attention has been paid to the association of criminal behaviour and XYY. The mean IQ scores are lower in those with criminal convictions (mainly property offences rather than crimes against persons), and lowered intelligence appears to be the major risk factor for antisocial and criminal behaviour. There is no association between 47,XYY *per se* and criminality.

Employment. Men with XYY were found to move jobs more frequently than controls. The range of jobs described is wide and most XYY males should have normal employment prospects.

Fertility. Most men with XYY are fertile and the majority of sperm in 47,XYY men are chromosomally normal. This may be because XY bivalents and Y univalents are lost during spermatogenesis, or by the loss of the additional Y in some primitive sperm cells and a proliferative advantage of XY cells.

Clinical approach (postnatal presentation)

History: key points
Developmental delay, schooling difficulties, behavioural problems.

Examination: key points (postnatal presentation)
Height.

Management
- **Prenatal detection.** Boys detected prenatally have a milder phenotype. This is due to unbiased ascertainment. Advise parent that, if their son shows developmental, behavioural, or educational difficulties, they should have a low threshold for asking for professional help, as early intervention can improve outcome.
- **Postnatal detection.** Chromosome testing has often been initiated because of developmental or behavioural difficulties and these boys require careful assessment. If a boy with XYY has dysmorphic features or malformations, they should not be attributed to the 47,XYY karyotype.
- **Disclosure of karyotype.** See Linden *et al.* (2002) for a full discussion of this topic. In general, disclosure of the karyotype on a 'need to know' basis is advised so that the child is not treated differently or regarded differently by others. Telling a child about his 47,XYY karyotype should be a gradual process extending over many years, with parents being supported in this by health professionals.

Genetic advice

Recurrence risk
Fathers of boys with XYY are not routinely karyotyped. The recurrence risk is low, <1%.

Offspring risk
The majority of sperm in 47,XYY men is chromosomally normal and XYY men are not reported to have an increased risk of sons with XYY or XXY.

Prenatal diagnosis
Prenatal diagnosis should be offered, but there is a fine balance between the very small risk of recurrence and the risk of procedure-associated pregnancy loss.

Lay group contact: In the UK via Unique Rare Chromosome Disorders <www.rarechromo.org>.

Expert adviser: Mary Linden, Genetic Counsellor, Kimball Genetics, Inc., Denver, Colorado, USA.

References
Fryns JP, Kleczkowska A. XYY syndrome and other Y chromosome polysomies. Mental status and psychosocial functioning. *Genet Couns* 1995; **6** (3): 197–206.

Gotz MJ, Johnstone EC, Ratcliffe SG. Criminality and antisocial behaviour in unselected men with sex chromosome abnormalities. *Psychol Med* 1999; **29**: 953–62.

Linden MG, Bender BG. Fifty-one prenatally diagnosed children and adolescents with sex chromosome anomalies. *Am J Med Genet* 2002; **110**: 11–18.

Linden MG, Bender BG, Robinson A. Intrauterine diagnosis of sex chromosome aneuploidy. *Obstet Gynecol* 1996; **87**: 468–75.

Linden MG, Bender BG, Robinson A. Genetic counselling for sex chromosome abnormalities. *Am J Med Genet* 2002; **110**: 3–10.

Martin RH, Shi Q, Field LL. Recombination in the pseudoautosomal region in a 47,XYY male. Hum Genet 2001; **109**: 143–5.

Ratcliffe S. Long term outcome in children of sex chromosome abnormalities. *Arch Dis Child* 1999; **80**: 192–5.

Robinson DO, Jacobs PA. The origins of the extra Y chromosome in males with a 47,XYY karyotype. *Hum Mol Genet* 1999; **8**: 2205–9.

Swerdlow AJ, Hermon C, *et al.* Mortality and cancer incidence in persons with numerical sex chromosome abnormalities: a cohort study. *Ann Hum Genet* 2001; **65** (Pt. 2): 177–88.

Autosomal reciprocal translocations—background

Chromosome rearrangements are described as balanced or unbalanced. In a balanced rearrangement the individual has a normal amount of chromosomal material (genes), but a child or adult with an unbalanced rearrangement has additional and/or missing genetic material.

Rearrangements that appear balanced using conventional cytogenetic techniques are described in reports as 'apparently balanced' because small amounts of imbalance, below the resolution of the light microscope, cannot be detected by such techniques (Ness *et al.* 2002). Typical resolution with Giemsa (G)-banding is ~5 Mb. When an apparently balanced rearrangement is detected in a phenotypically normal individual it is assumed to be truly balanced.

In general, a deficiency (monosomy) causes more problems than a similarly sized duplication (trisomy). Chromosome imbalance is usually associated with learning disability with/without congenital anomalies. Dosage-sensitive genes play a critical role in development, and any such genes that are under- or overexpressed will result in phenotypic abnormality. Most published cases (95%) of viable autosomal imbalance fall within a triangle delimited by 4% trisomy and 2% monosomy (see figure); chromosomal imbalance falling outside this triangle is likely to result in spontaneous pregnancy loss.

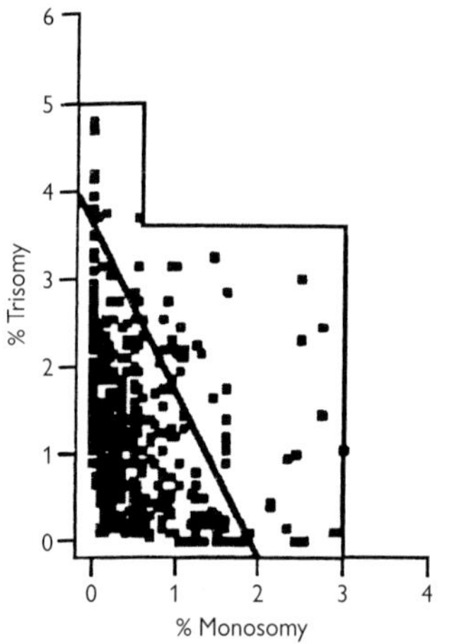

Viability of combined duplication/deletion states, according to the amount of imbalance, measured as % haploid autosomal length (HAL). Most (96%) fall within the triangular area whose hypotenuse lies between 4% duplication/0% deletion and 2% deletion/0% duplication, and a few outliers define an envelope of viable imbalances. (From Cohen *et al.* (1994), courtesy O. Cohen, and with the permission of Springer-Verlag.)

Balanced autosomal reciprocal translocations are common and carried by >0.1% of the population. In simplistic terms there are four possible outcomes to any pregnancy of a carrier of a balanced autosomal reciprocal translocation. These are a pregnancy with:

- a normal karyotype;
- a balanced autosomal reciprocal translocation (as in the parent);
- an unbalanced product of the translocation resulting in spontaneous pregnancy loss, e.g. miscarriage;
- an unbalanced product of the translocation that is viable resulting in a child with a high likelihood of learning disability with/without congenital anomalies.

One of the important roles of the geneticist is to assess the likelihood of a viable unbalanced outcome. This is likely to be a major factor governing decisions regarding invasive prenatal diagnostic tests (e.g. amniocentesis, chorionic villus sampling (CVS)).

Chromosomes are not uniform structures and this creates problems in devising methods for predicting the risk of a viable unbalanced outcome. Some regions of the chromosomes are much more gene-rich than others, and none of the computational approaches to this problem are able to account for this. Alternative approaches based on observed outcomes to pregnancies are rather cumbersome and may be subject to ascertainment bias. In practical terms, precision in calculating the likelihood of a viable unbalanced outcome is neither feasible nor necessary. Couples contemplating pregnancy and prenatal diagnosis do not make decisions based on values to two decimal places, they need 'ball-park' figures that they can evaluate alongside the risks of invasive procedures such as CVS/amniocentesis. Our practice is to define bands of risk: <0.5%; 0.5–1%; 1–5%; 5–10%; >10%.

Viable imbalance risk

In practice four different, but complementary approaches are used to assess the likelihood of a viable unbalanced outcome and determine the risk band.

- Assessment of the family history. Any family ascertained through the birth of a child with an unbalanced product (or termination of a pregnancy with multiple congenital anomalies) is likely to have a high or very high risk (5–10% or >10%). Taking all factors into consideration it would probably be unwise ever to advise a risk figure below 1% in this situation.
- Calculation of the haploid autosomal length (HAL) of the imbalance (p. 676). Risks for viability are highest with breakpoints located closest to the telomere, which yield the smallest imbalance.
- Reference to empiric data compiled by Stengel-Rutkowski.
- Literature search using PubMed and Schinzel (2001) to determine whether a viable outcome has been previously reported and, if so, the phenotype.

Different centres use different approaches and most clinicians use a combination to arrive at a risk estimate for a particular family.

Pachytene diagram

This is the key to understanding how unbalanced products can arise during meiosis (see figure). To construct a pachytene diagram (see next figure) you need to know the breakpoints and have access to a karyotype ideogram so that you can identify appoximately where along the length of the chromosomes involved the breakpoints lie (e.g. Gardner and Sutherland 2004, p. 376).

The segregation (separation of chromosomes) producing the smallest imbalance is usually found by drawing a line between the homologous segments of the two longest arms of the quadrivalent.

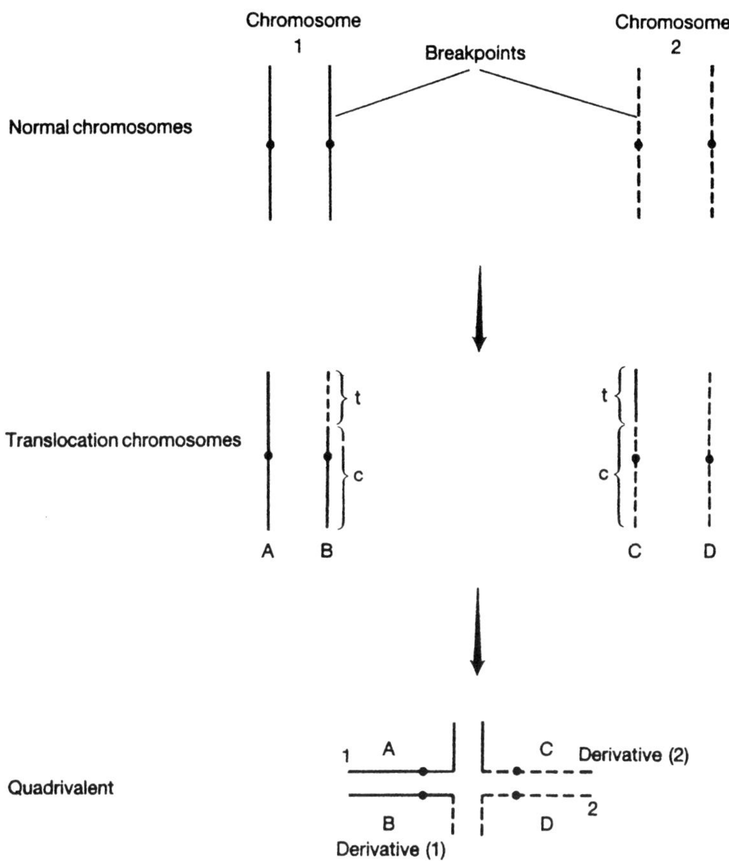

This figure shows generation of a balanced reciprocal translocation between chromosomes 1 and 2, and formation of a quadrivalent in meiosis. t, Translocated segment; c, centric segment. (From fig. 8.1, p. 136 of Young (1999) with the permission of Oxford University Press.)

The following are important general principles.

- **Alternate segregation** produces gametes with normal chromosomes (A + D) or the balanced reciprocal arrangement (B + C) present in the parent.
- **Adjacent-1 segregation** creates the smallest imbalance when the translocated segments are shorter than the centric segments (A + C and B + D). Overall, it is the most common segregation pattern producing viable imbalance (70%).
- **Adjacent-2 segregation** creates the smallest imbalance when the translocated segments are longer than the centric segments (A + B and C + D). It is a relatively uncommon segregation pattern to produce viable imbalance (5%).
- **3:1 segregation** tends to give rise to the smallest imbalance when one of the non-translocation or derivative chromosomes is very small. (A + B + C) or (B + C + D) give rise to interchange trisomy and (A + B + D) or

(A + C + D) give rise to tertiary trisomy—as a mechanism it accounts for ~25% of viable imbalance. 3:1 segregation is more common in female carriers of a balanced translocation than in male carriers.

Assessing the likelihood of viability

- Risks of viable imbalance are highest with breakpoints located closest to the telomere; the shorter the chromosome segment involved, the more likely it is to be viable.
- Monosomy is much less likely to be viable than trisomy. Monosomy for any whole autosome is not viable; trisomy for whole autosomes is only viable in the case of trisomies 13, 18, and 21.
- Most published cases (96%) of viable autosomal imbalance comprise up to 4% trisomy and up to 2% monosomy with combinations viable when they fall within a triangle delimited by 4% trisomy/0% monosomy and 2% monosomy/0% trisomy.

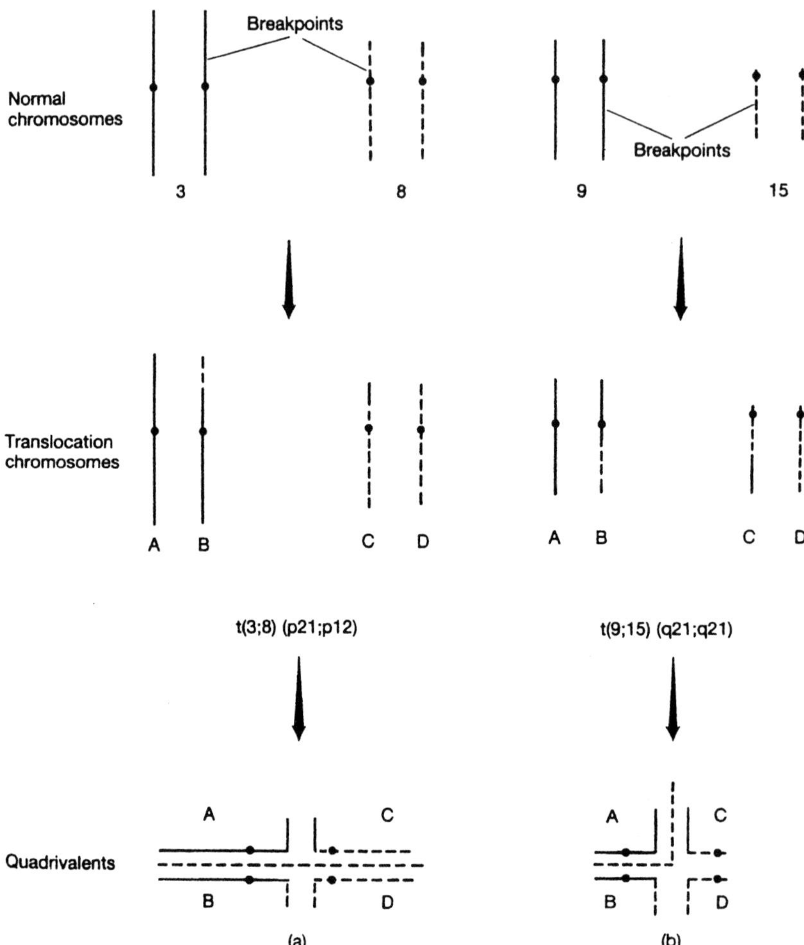

Pachytene diagrams drawn to scale for two reciprocal translocations. The bold dashed line indicates the pattern of segregation that will produce the smallest imbalance. In (a) this will be adjacent-1 segregation and in (b) 3 to 1 segregation resulting in interchange monosomy/trisomy. (From fig. 8.3, p. 139 of Young (1999) with the permission of Oxford University Press.)

Support group: Unique—The Rare Chromosome Disorder Support Group <www.rarechromo.org>, Tel. 01883 330766.

Expert adviser: Ian D. Young, Consultant Clinical Geneticist, Leicester, England.

References

Cohen O, Cans C, et al. Viability thresholds for partial trisomies and monosomies. A study of 1,159 viable unbalanced reciprocal translocations. *Hum Genet* 1994; **93**: 188–94.

Gardner RJM, Sutherland GR. *Chromosome abnormalities and genetic counselling*, Oxford Monographs on Medical Genetics no. 31, 3rd edn. Oxford University Press, New York, 2004.

Jacobs PA. Recurrence risks for chromosome abnormalities. *Birth Defects Orig Art Ser* 1979; **15** (5C): 71–80.

Lindenbaum RH, Bobrow M. Reciprocal translocations in man. 3:1 Meiotic disjunction resulting in 47- or 45-chromosome offspring. *J Med Genet* 1975; **12**: 29–43.

Ness GO, Lybaek H, Houge G. Usefulness of high-resolution comparative genomic hybridization (CGH) for detecting and characterizing constitutional chromosome abnormalities. *Am J Med Genet* 2002; **113** (2): 125–36.

Schinzel A. *Catalogue of unbalanced chromosome aberrations in man*, 2nd edn. de Gruyter, Berlin, 2001.

Stene J, Stengel-Rutowski S. Genetic risks of familial reciprocal and Robertsonian translocation carriers. In *The cytogenetics of mammalial autosomal rearrangements* (ed. A. Daniel), pp. 3–72. A.R. Liss, New York, 1990.

Young ID. *Introduction to risk calculation in genetic counselling*, 2nd edn. Oxford University Press, Oxford 1999. See especially Chapter 8.1, pp. 135–45.

Autosomal reciprocal translocations—familial

See also 'Autosomal reciprocal translocations—background', page 500.

Most rearrangements are unique to a family, but there are a few that appear recurrently, particularly a common translocation (t) between chromosomes 11 and 22. This t(11;22)(q23;q11) is the most frequently occurring non-Robertsonian translocation.

Clinical approach

For use when an individual is known to either carry, or be at risk of carrying, a balanced autosomal reciprocal translocation. Ask your colleagues in cytogenetics to produce an annotated photograph together with an ideogram of the chromosomes involved in the translocation. This is an invaluable aid to counselling.

History: key points

- Draw a three-generation family tree (or larger if indicated) and enquire about pregnancy loss, stillbirth, neonatal death, and family members with learning disability or congenital anomalies.
- Confirm that the consultand has no health problems or learning disability attributable to the translocation.

Examination: key points

Examine if there are specific indications from the history.

Special investigation

Karyotype your patient if:

- their status is unknown but they are 'at risk' from the family tree and old enough to give their consent and engage with the testing process (see 'Testing for genetic status' page 28).
- they are a known carrier of a balanced rearrangement where you do not have access to a cytogenetics report defining the breakpoints (especially important if investigation of other family members or prenatal diagnosis is planned).

Genetic advice

There is no indication that parents with a structural abnormality are at an increased risk of producing a child with a chromosomal abnormality independent of the parental rearrangement (Jacobs 1979).

Recurrence risk

The main issue is to determine the risk of viable imbalance. A suggested approach (see 'Autosomal reciprocal translocations—background', this chapter) is the following.

1 Determine breakpoints and construct a pachytene diagram using different coloured pens for the two different chromosomes involved in the translocation.

2 Make a rough risk assessment based on knowledge of family history, length of translocated segments involved.

3 Determine whether the product with the smallest imbalance could be viable.

4 Determine if a 3:1 segregation (meiotic disjunction) is a likely outcome (more likely when acrocentric chromosomes are involved in the translocation).

Carriers of t(11;22)(q23;q11) are at risk of 3:1 meiotic disjunction, which is found in 5–10% of the offspring of female carriers resulting in dup(11)(q23-qter) and dup22(pter-q11).

5 If risk of viable imbalance exists, refine the risk assessment by determining the approximate risk of viable imbalance using a combination of computerized risk assessment based on haploid autosomal length (HAL; see Appendix) or Stengel-Rutkowski tables and a literature search.

6 Classify the risk of viable imbalance into one of the risk bands for the purposes of counselling, e.g. <0.5%, 0.5–1%, 1–5%, 5–10%, >10%.

Prenatal diagnosis

The mainstay of prenatal diagnosis is by amniocentesis/chorionic villus sampling (CVS). If the unbalanced product would result in a very subtle anomaly only just detectable on a karyotype prepared from blood, discuss with the lab whether they need to work up fluorescent *in situ* hybridization (FISH) probes in order to make a confident prenatal diagnosis on preparations from CVS/amniocentesis.

For couples with adverse obstetric histories where segregation appears skewed towards unbalanced products, e.g. multiple pregnancy losses due to miscarriage or termination of pregnancy (TOP), *in vitro* fertilization (IVF) with pre-implantation genetic diagnosis (PGD) may be an option to consider. See 'Assisted reproductive technology: *in vitro* fertilization (IVF), intracytoplasmic sperm injection (ICSI), and pre-implantation genetic diagnosis (PGD)' page 568.

Support group: Unique—The Rare Chromosome Disorder Support Group <www.rarechromo.org>, Tel. 01883 330766.

Expert adviser: Ian D. Young, Consultant Clinical Geneticist, Leicester, England.

References

Cohen O, Cans C, *et al.* Viability thresholds for partial trisomies and monosomies. A study of 1,159 viable unbalanced reciprocal translocations. *Hum Genet* 1994; **93**: 188–94.

Gardner RJM, Sutherland GR. *Chromosome abnormalities and genetic counselling*, Oxford Monographs on Medical Genetics no. 31, 3rd edn. Oxford University Press, New York, 2004.

Jacobs PA. Recurrence risks for chromosome abnormalities. *Birth Defects Orig Art Ser* 1979; **15** (5C): 71–80.

Lindenbaum RH, Bobrow M. Reciprocal translocations in man. 3:1 Meiotic disjunction resulting in 47- or 45-chromosome offspring. *J Med Genet* 1975; **12**: 29–43.

Ogilvie CM, Braude P, Scriven PN. Successful pregnancy outcomes after preimplantation genetic diagnosis (PGD) for carriers of chromosome translocations. *Hum Fertil (Cambridge)* 2001; **4** (3): 168–71.

Stene J, Stengel-Rutowski S. Genetic risks of familial reciprocal and Robertsonian translocation carriers. In *The cytogenetics of mammalial autosomal rearrangements* (ed. A. Daniel), pp. 3–72. A.R. Liss, New York, 1990.

Young ID. *Introduction to risk calculation in genetic counselling*, 2nd edn. Oxford University Press, Oxford 1999. See especially Chapter 8.1, pp. 135–45.

Autosomal reciprocal translocations—postnatal

See 'Autosomal reciprocal translocations—background' page 500 and 'Autosomal reciprocal translocations—familial', page 504.

Autosomal reciprocal translocations may come to light during the investigation of babies and children with congenital malformations, developmental delay, and/or learning disability, or in the work-up of patients with recurrent miscarriage or subfertility. The terminology is as follows.

- **De novo.** If the abnormality is not found in either parent it is described as *de novo* (also consider the possibility of non-paternity).
- **Familial.** Inherited from a parent.

Normal phenotype. If the child/adult is phenotypically normal this is likely to be an incidental finding; see 'Autosomal reciprocal translocations—familial', this chapter.

Abnormal phenotype. If the child has an abnormal phenotype, continue reading this section.

Clinical approach

History: key points

- Draw a three-generation family tree (or larger if indicated) and enquire about pregnancy loss, stillbirth, neonatal death, and family members with learning disability or congenital anomalies.
- Document all known malformations in the child and anthropomorphic data.
- Presence of developmental delay.

Examination: key points

Full clinical examination and documentation of dysmorphic features.

Special investigations

- Arrange for parental chromosome analysis.
- Clinical photography.
- Consider analysis of genes at the breakpoint(s).

Genetic advice

In the following it is assumed that the autosomal reciprocal translocation is associated with phenotypic abnormalities.

Apparently balanced rearrangement

This may be an incidental finding if a normal parent carries the same rearrangement.

If it is *de novo*, the chance of the chromosome translocation being the cause is much greater and the following points also need to be considered.

- The translocation is actually unbalanced.
- Unmasking of a recessive allele on the normal homologue.
- There is abnormal gene function as a consequence of the break.
- Imprinting problems depending on the chromosomes involved. (See 'Imprinting' in Chapter 1, 'Introduction' for map of known imprinted genes.)

Consider additional chromosome analysis (e.g. fluorescent *in situ* hybridization (FISH) or painting or microarray comparative genomic hybridization (CGH)) to search for imbalance, and search the literature for relevant genes at the breakpoints. If familial with no phenotype in other family members consider the possibility of uniparental disomy (UPD).

Unbalanced rearrangement

This may be found in an infant with multiple malformations or, if the imbalance is smaller, in an older child with milder manifestations. Ascertain if the translocation has been described in the literature and evaluate if the phenotype is compatible. The features, for example, of an autosomal deletion (monosomy), may be modified by duplication of the other autosomal segment (trisomy).

Recurrence risk

- **De novo.**
  - **Sibling risk.** The chance of another affected pregnancy is very small, but offer prenatal diagnosis.
  - **Offspring risk.** See 'Autosomal reciprocal translocations—familial', this chapter.
- **Familial.** If one parent carries a translocation, see 'Autosomal reciprocal translocations—familial', this chapter.

Prenatal diagnosis

- **De novo.** Although the chance of another affected pregnancy is low some families opt for an amniocentesis for reassurance.
- **Familial.** If one parent carries a translocation, see 'Autosomal reciprocal translocations—familial', this chapter.

Management

If a baby with a *de novo* chromosome abnormality dies, ask permission for a full post-mortem examination and book a follow-up genetic appointment to counsel about the risks of recurrence and offer family follow-up.

For children with chromosome rearrangements ensure that

- the child's medical notes (e.g. GP or family practice notes) are marked with this information;
- the child's parents know that they should request an appointment in the genetics clinic when the child is in his/her mid-teens.

Support group: Unique—The Rare Chromosome Disorder Support Group <www.rarechromo.org>, Tel. 01883 330766.

Expert adviser: Ian D. Young, Consultant Clinical Geneticist, Leicester, England.

References

Gardner RJM, Sutherland GR. *Chromosome abnormalities and genetic counselling*, Oxford Monographs on Medical Genetics no. 31, 3rd edn. Oxford University Press, New York, 2004.

Ness GO, Lybaek H, Houge G. Usefulness of high-resolution comparative genomic hybridization (CGH) for detecting and characterizing constitutional chromosome abnormalities. *Am J Med Genet* 2002; **113** (2): 125–36.

Warburton D. *De novo* balanced chromosome rearrangements and extra marker chromosomes identified at prenatal diagnosis: clinical significance and distribution of breakpoints. *Am J Hum Genet* 1991; **49**: 995–1013.

Autosomal reciprocal translocations—prenatal

See also pages 500 and 504.

Autosomal reciprocal translocations are sometimes identified on karyotyping performed for maternal age indications, increased nuchal translucency, or abnormal ultrasound scan (USS) findings. Determining whether the finding is incidental or, in the case of investigation of abnormal USS findings, causative is crucial.

Clinical approach

History: key points

Draw a three-generation family tree (or larger if indicated) and enquire about pregnancy loss, stillbirth, neonatal death, and family members with learning disability or congenital anomalies.

Examination: key points

Fetal USS (fetal size and presence of any anomalies).

Special investigations

Arrange for urgent rapid parental chromosome analysis.

Genetic advice

Associated with fetal abnormality

Unbalanced rearrangement. This is likely to be the cause of the fetal abnormality whether familial or *de novo*. Define the malformations as well as possible by detailed anomaly scanning. Do a literature search for similar karyotypic abnormalities.

Apparently balanced rearrangement. It is imperative to ascertain whether it is *de novo*. If *de novo* then there may be chromosomal loss that is not detectable cytogenetically, which may be the cause of the abnormalities. Check the breakpoints for developmental genes and literature reports that may explain the fetal appearance. Counselling will discuss the fact that the chromosome abnormality is likely to be causative, in the absence of another explanation, but there is a chance that it is an incidental finding. If *familial*, consider if a mechanism such as uniparental disomy (UPD) could be the cause of the abnormalities.

Apparently normal fetus on scan

Usually the indication for pregnancy testing has been an increased risk of Down syndrome. This is a difficult counselling situation. Parental anxiety is high and there may be no absolute answers.

Unbalanced rearrangement

There is a high risk of disability in a liveborn child. Find out about the phenotype associated with the cytogenetic abnormality to aid in counselling the parents and to inform detailed fetal anomaly USS. A further normal USS at approximately 20 weeks gestation does not exclude abnormalities presenting later in pregnancy (e.g. polyhydramnios from oesophageal atresia) nor will it help refine the risks of mental handicap or sensory impairment (e.g. hearing, vision). Small size for gestation may be an indicator of chromosome imbalance and the presence of 'soft markers' is relevant in this situation.

If there is, or has been, a previous child/pregnancy in the kindred with the same unbalanced product of the translocation, this information can be used to counsel regarding the likely effects of the chromosome imbalance. If familial, arrange follow-up for 'at risk' members of the family (see 'Autosomal reciprocal translocations—familial', this chapter).

Apparently balanced translocation

De novo apparently balanced autosomal reciprocal translocation. The best study is that of Warburton (1991). She found 1 in 2000 pregnancies had a *de novo* balanced translocation. If truly balanced, then the risk of abnormality is small. The following also need to be considered as all could lead to problems.

- The translocation is actually unbalanced. Newer methodology such as microarray comparative genomic hybridization (CGH) may permit higher-resolution cytogenetic analysis (Ness *et al.* 2002).
- Unmasking a recessive allele on the normal homologue.
- There is abnormal gene function as a consequence of the break.
- The potential implications if the breakpoints involve an imprinted region of the genome.

Even though Warburton's (1991) study involved collecting data from many North American laboratories, the amount of information about follow-up is sparse because of the rarity of the occurrence and the lack of information about the effect on neurological development if the pregnancy was terminated.

When the USS was normal, 6.1% of pregnancies had abnormalities at birth or on post mortem, against the background abnormality rate of approximately 3%. The 6.1% figure does not include later onset problems caused by the chromosome imbalance, and the risk of problems, in particular developmental delay, is higher. A *two- to threefold risk over the background risk* of developmental problems is used (5–10%) when a detailed fetal scan has shown no structural abnormalities and the head size and growth are normal, but parents should understand how the risk figure has been derived.

Familial apparently balanced autosomal reciprocal translocation. If found in a parent, reassure that the translocation is unlikely to have a phenotypic affect on the fetus. Organize genetic follow-up to discuss risks of chromosome imbalance in future pregnancies and remember that at some time in the future the fetus will be an adult requiring counselling before pregnancy.

Recurrence risk

- **De novo.** The chance of another affected pregnancy is very small (parental germline mosaicism risk).
- **Familial.** If one parent carries a translocation refer to 'Autosomal reciprocal translocations—familial', this chapter.

Prenatal diagnosis

- **De novo.** Although the chance of another affected pregnancy is low some families opt for an amniocentesis for reassurance.
- **Familial.** If one parent carries a translocation refer to 'Autosomal reciprocal translocations—familial', this chapter.

Management

If the pregnancy is terminated, arrange for a full post-mortem examination including clinical photographs and book a follow-up genetic appointment to counsel about the risks of recurrence and family follow-up. If abnormalities are found, these may confirm the effect of the chromosomal abnormality.

If the pregnancy continues and the fetus is carrying a balanced translocation ensure that:

- the child is carefully examined at birth;
- the child's medical notes (e.g. GP or family practice notes) are marked with this information;
- the child's parents know that they should request an appointment in the genetics clinic when the child is in his/her mid-teens.

Support group: ARC (Antenatal Results and Choices) <www.arc-uk.org>, Tel. 020 7631 0285.

Expert adviser: Ian D. Young, Consultant Clinical Geneticist, Leicester, England.

References

Gardner RJM, Sutherland GR. *Chromosome abnormalities and genetic counselling*, Oxford Monographs on Medical Genetics no. 31, 3rd edn. Oxford University Press, New York, 2004.

Ness GO, Lybaek H, Houge G. Usefulness of high-resolution comparative genomic hybridization (CGH) for detecting and characterizing constitutional chromosome abnormalities. *Am J Med Genet* 2002; **113** (2): 125–36.

Warburton D. *De novo* balanced chromosome rearrangements and extra marker chromosomes identified at prenatal diagnosis: clinical significance and distribution of breakpoints. *Am J Hum Genet* 1991; **49**: 995–1013.

Cell division—mitosis, meiosis, and non-disjunction

Mitosis

See figure.

Somatic recombination

Pairing of homologous chromosomes, followed by recombination (crossing-over), is a central feature of meiosis. In contrast, chromosomes do not generally pair during mitotic cell division, and recombination (homologous or heterologous) is a rare event. Occasional cells do, however, undergo recombination events and this can be an important mechanism in disease. For example, mosaicism for paternal uniparental isodisomy (UPD) occurring as a result of somatic recombination may underlie some cases of Beckwith–Wiedemann syndrome (BWS; Kotzot 2001).

Somatic recombination can cause loss of heterozygosity (LOH), which is often an important step in tumour development.

Meiosis

See figure.

Female meiosis

Meiosis begins in the fifth month of fetal life in females. When the egg is fertilized it triggers successive rounds of mitotic cell division. In the fifth month of fetal life, approximately 33 rounds of mitotic division since fertilization, the fetal ovaries together contain several million oocytes. At this stage there is a switch from mitosis to meiosis. After progressing through

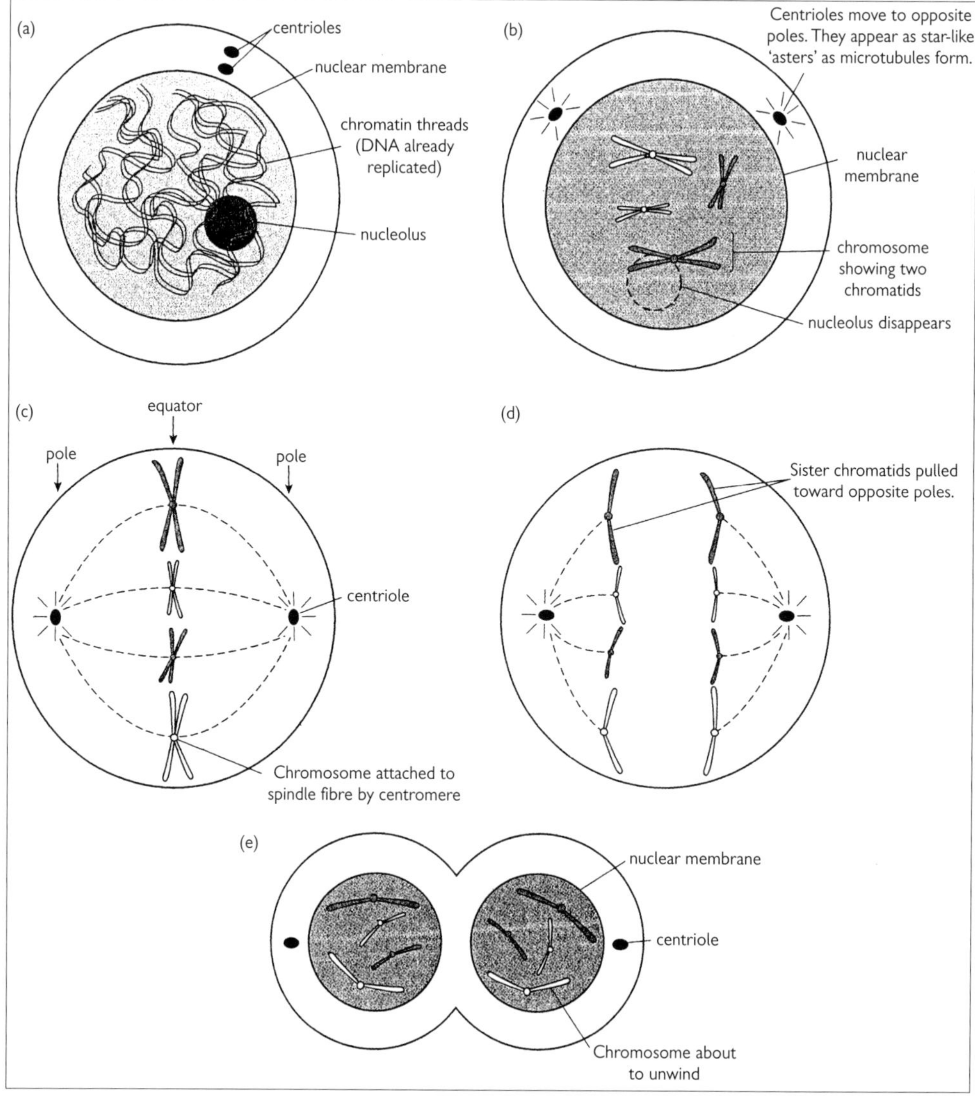

The process of mitosis: (a) Cell at the end of interphase (b) Prophase (c) Metaphase (d) Anaphase and (e) Telophase. (Adapted from Bradfield *et al.* (2001) with permission from Pearson Educational Limited © 2001.)

Table showing a comparison of Mitosis and Meiosis

Mitosis	Meiosis
Occurs in somatic cells	Occurs in the germline during oogenesis and spermatogenesis
Produces diploid (2n) cells which are genetically identical to each other and to the parent cell	Produces haploid (n) gametes (oocytes and spermatozoa) which are genetically unique because of recombination and independent assortment
Somatic recombination events are rare, but can be an important mechanism in disease	Pairing of homologous chromosomes and recombination are key features of meiosis and important in generating genetic diversity
Prophase is short (~30 minutes)	Prophase is extremely long in female meiosis and lasts from fetal life until puberty and beyond

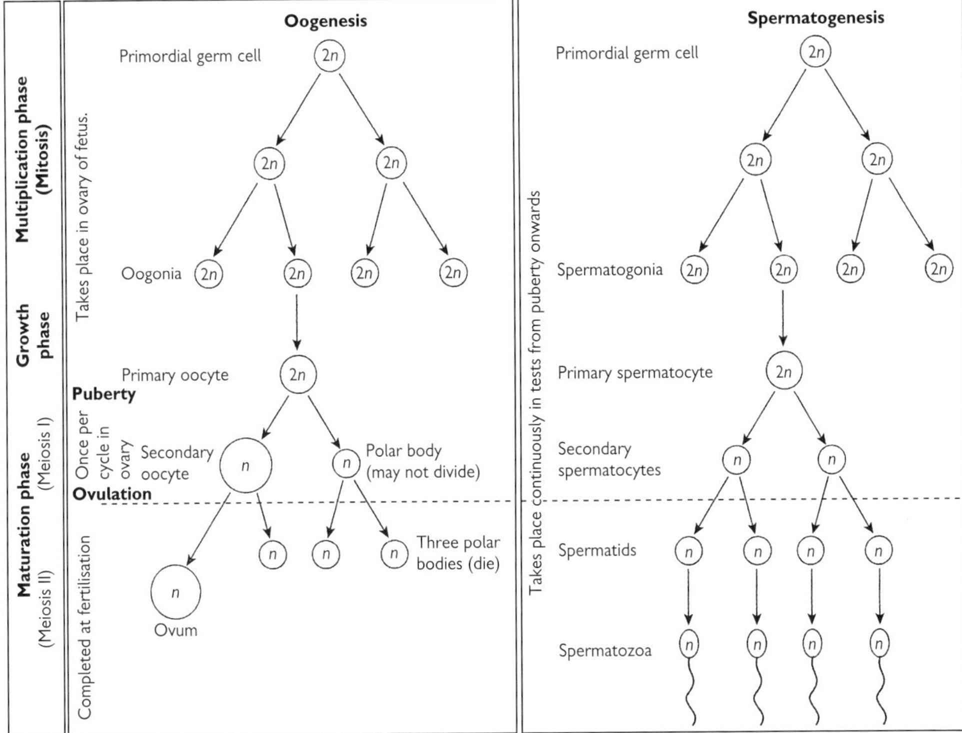

Gametogenesis—a comparison between oogenesis and spermatogenesis. (Reproduced from Bradfield *et al.* (2001) with permission from Pearson Education Limited © 2001.)

pachytene and into diplotene by the sixth month of fetal life, all of the oocytes are arrested in prophase I.

This phase lasts until puberty and beyond. During a woman's reproductive life cohorts of oocytes are released from meiotic arrest by progesterone stimulation in each menstrual cycle. The oocytes continue through the first meiotic division but arrest again in metaphase II until fertilization.

At the onset of meiosis in the fifth month of fetal life, the ovaries contain approximately 8 million oocytes; by the time of birth this has fallen to 1–2 million as a result of apoptosis. In each monthly cycle, ovulation is accompanied by a wave of apoptosis in oocytes in partially mature follicles.

See the figure for a comparison between oogenesis and spermatogenesis.

Male meiosis

In males mitotic divisions continue to occur in germline stem cell spermatogonia throughout adult life. In a 25-year-old man, about 265 rounds of spermatogonial mitotic divison have occurred since fertilization. Gene mutations usually arise as copying errors during replication, and this nearly ninefold greater number of cell divisions in the male germline before gamete formation is thought to be the basis for the mutation rate being observed to be higher in males than in females.

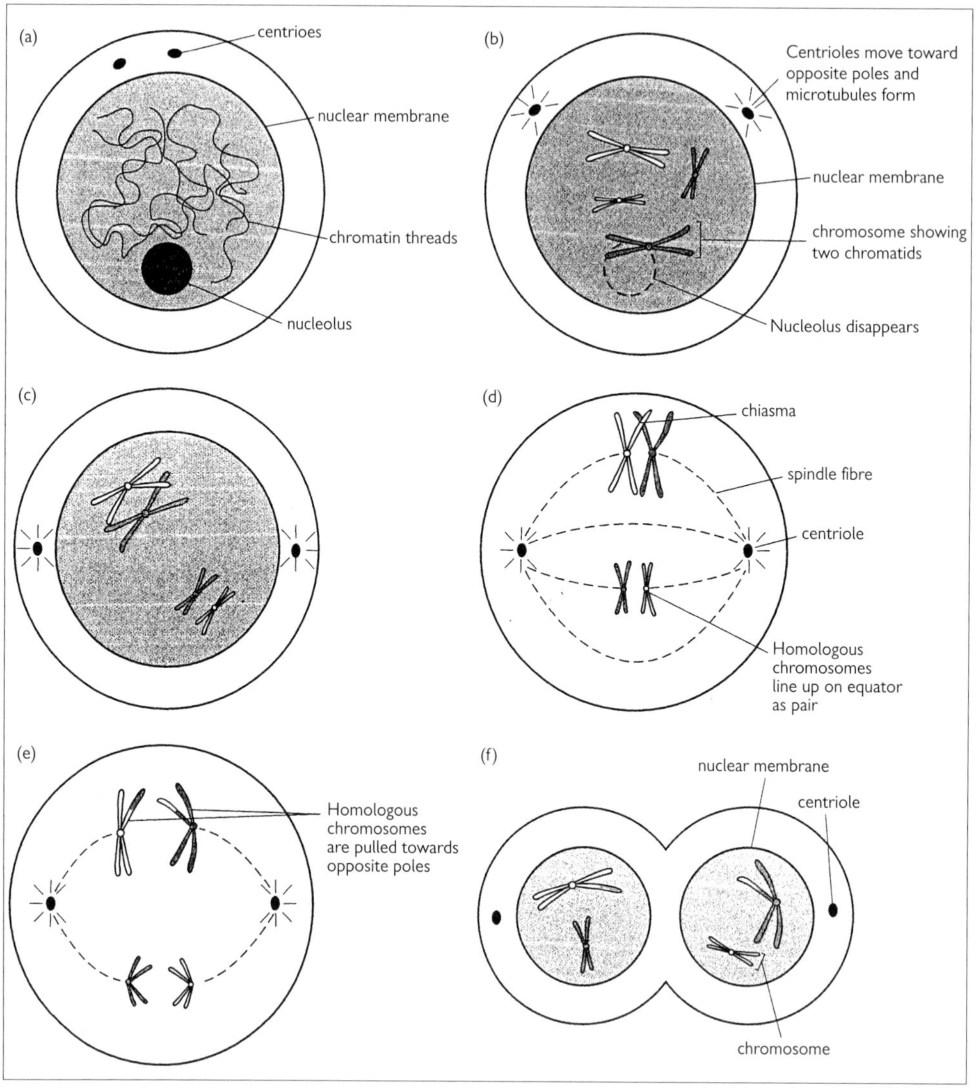

(a)

centrioes

nuclear membrane

chromatin threads

nucleolus

(b)

Centrioles move toward opposite poles and microtubules form

nuclear membrane

chromosome showing two chromatids

Nucleolus disappears

(c)

(d)

chiasma

spindle fibre

centriole

Homologous chromosomes line up on equator as pair

(e)

Homologous chromosomes are pulled towards opposite poles

(f)

nuclear membrane

centriole

chromosome

The Process of Meiosis: Meiosis 1
(a) Cell at the end of interphase (b) Early prophase 1 (c) Mid prophase 1 (d) Metaphase 1 (e) Anaphase 1 (f) Telophase 1. (Adapted from Bradfield *et al.* (2001) with permission from Pearson Educational Limited © 2001.)

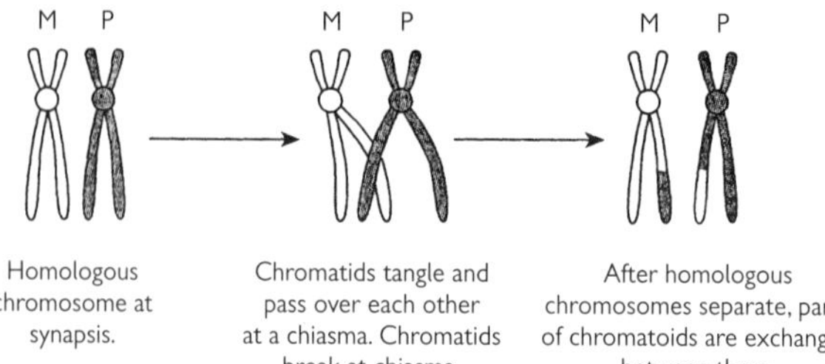

Homologous chromosome at synapsis.

Chromatids tangle and pass over each other at a chiasma. Chromatids break at chiasma.

After homologous chromosomes separate, parts of chromatoids are exchanged between them.

M = maternal chromosome
P = paternal chromosome

Diagram to illustrate 'Crossing over' (recombination) occuring in late prophase 1 i.e. between (c) and (d) above

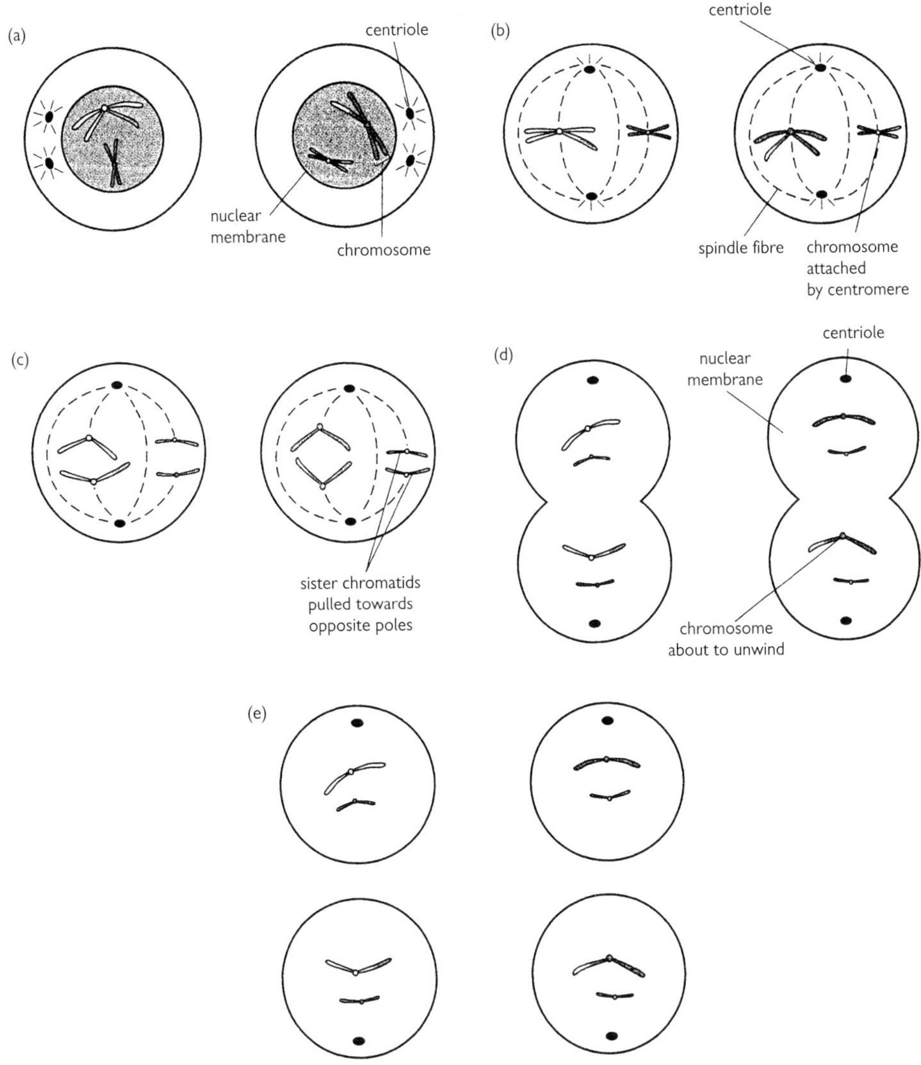

The Process of Meiosis: Meiosis 2
(a) Prophase 2 (b) Metaphase 2 (c) Anaphase 2 (d) Telophase 2 (e) Cytokinesis producing 4 haploid daughter cells. (Adapted from Bradfield *et al.* (2001) with permission from Pearson Educational Limited © 2001.)

Meiosis is initiated at puberty when, under hormonal influence, type A spermatogonia switch to type B spermatogonia (germline stem cells). The switch from mitosis to meiosis in type B spermatagonia only occurs in one of the two daughter cells (which becomes a primary spermatocyte) produced at each type B spermatogonial division (the other stays as a germline stem cell).

Throughout adult life men produce many tens of millions of spermatogonia, primary spermatocytes, and sperm each day.

Non-disjunction

See figure in 'Patau Syndrome' page 535.

Expert adviser: Martin Bobrow, Professor of Medical Genetics, University of Cambridge, Cambridge, England.

References
Bradfield P, *et al. AS level biology*. Longman, London, 2001.
Gardner RJM, Sutherland GR. *Chromosome abnormalities and genetic counselling*, 3rd edn, Oxford Monographs on Medical Genetics no. 31. Oxford University Press, New York, 2004.
Kotzot D. Complex and segmental uniparental disomy (UPD): review and lessons from rare chromosomal complements. *J Med Genet* 2001; **38**: 497–507.

Chromosomal mosaicism—postnatal

Mosaicism is defined as the presence of two or more cell populations derived from the same conceptus that have subsequently acquired a genetic difference. Mitotic non-disjunction, trisomy rescue, or occurrence of a somatic new mutation can lead to the development of two (or more) genetically distinct cell lines. When post-mitotic non-disjunction involving an autosome occurs, the monsomy cell line is invariably lost and a trisomy lineage exists together with the euploid line, e.g. 47,XY + 8/46,XY. When post-mitotic non-disjunction involving an X chromosome occurs, the monosomy line may persist, e.g. 45,X/46,XX/47,XXX.

Children may be referred after the laboratory has noted mosaicism, but note that screening for mosaicism is not routinely performed except in girls with Turner syndrome.

More commonly, the geneticist is requesting additional investigations because there are clinical signs suggestive of chromosome imbalance or mosaicism.

Clinical approach

History: key points

- Raised maternal age is a risk factor for trisomy (trisomic rescue can lead to mosaicism).
- Seizures common with some autosomal mosaic karyotypes.

Examination: key points

- Milder phenotype of known chromosomal condition (often mosaic trisomy 21 is detected in this way).
- Asymmetry, particularly noticeable in the limbs.
- Patchy or streaky skin pigmentary changes (hypomelanosis of Ito, diploid/triploid mosaicism).
- Sparse hair in the temporal region (Pallister–Killian syndrome).
- Ear malformation and pre-auricular tags (mosaic trisomy 22).
- Syndactyly and contractures of the fingers and toes.
- Deep creases on the soles of the feet and hypoplastic patellae (mosaic trisomy 8).
- Extra nipples.

Special investigations

- Ask for an increased number of cells to be analysed. If 30 cells are analysed with no evidence of mosaicism, then this excludes 10% mosaicism with 95% confidence limits.
- Karyotype another cell lineage, usually skin biopsy to give a fibroblast culture. Fluorescent *in situ* hybridization (FISH) analysis of a buccal smear may be helpful if you suspect a recognized mosaic phenotype.
- Clinical photographs.

Recognizable mosaic phenotypes

Diploid/triploid mosaicism arises from partial 'rescue' of a triploid conception with extrusion of the surplus pronucleus at the first cleavage stage and reincorporation at a subsequent cell division so the morula is mosaic (3*n*/2*n*). The affected fetus may not survive pregnancy or may survive to term. Characteristic findings are syndactyly especially of fingers 3,4 and toes 2,3, with bulbous ends of the toes and clinodactyly. There may be body asymmetry and streaky skin hyper- or hypopigmentation. Skin chromosomes may be required to make the diagnosis.

Genetic counselling is as for full triploidy. See 'Triploidy (69,XXX, 69,XXY, or 69,XYY)', this chapter.

Mosaic tetrasomy 12p (Pallister–Killian syndrome). As this mosaicism is not detected on routine lymphocyte testing, clinical recognition of the features is necessary in order that a fibroblast sample is analysed or FISH analysis of a buccal smear (Manasse *et al.* 2000) is performed. There is profound developmental delay and seizures are common. The prenatal features are listed in 'Chromosomal mosaicism—prenatal', this chapter. The facial features are characteristic. The forehead appears large, partly because there is a high hairline and sparse hair over the temples. The mouth is large and the philtrum appears full. Some children have mild coarseness of the facial features.

Mosaic trisomy 8. See 'Mosaic trisomy 8', this chapter. The clinical features that suggest the diagnosis are deep longitudinal creases on the soles of the feet, absent or hypoplastic patellae, and contractures of the fingers. There may be no developmental delay or mental retardation of varying degree. An association with haematological neoplasia and other malignancies has been reported. A fibroblast culture is needed to confirm the condition.

Mosaic trisomy 22. The phenotype is variable. Most typical are auricular, cardiac, and renal anomalies, anal atresia, and radial hypo/aplasia. A Turner-like phenotype is also reported and the degree of mental retardation is difficult to predict. The mosaicism is easier to detect on fibroblasts than in lymphocytes.

Mosaic marker 22. Most cases of cat-eye syndrome (CES) are *de novo*, but familial transmission is possible. Urioste *et al.* (1994) reported a girl, her sister, and her mother who had a supernumerary marker chromosome 22 in mosaic form. Parental karyotypes are important as some patients with mosaicism for a marker 22 have a normal phenotype (Crolla *et al.* 1997), and prenatal diagnosis should be considered.

Hypomelanosis of Ito. Large areas of the skin may be affected by hypopigmented streaks or whorls distributed along the lines of Blaschko. It may be particularly striking over the trunk. The streaks are mainly present on the limbs and the whorls on the trunk. The lesions are much easier to see under ultraviolet (UV) light. Swirly hyperpigmentation may also be seen. Seizures and developmental delay are often found. Brain imaging may reveal a migrational abnormality. A mosaic chromosomal aetiology has been found to be the cause in ~60% of reported individuals. The myriad of associated features reflects the extensive variety of aneuploid conditions seen. This pigment pattern can also be seen in otherwise apparently normal individuals. Its cause in them is unknown, but it is presumed to be due to mosaicism for single genes controlling pigment production.

Distinguish from incontinentia pigmenti (IP). See 'Unusual hair, teeth, nails, and skin' page 256.

Mosaic variegated aneuploidy (MVA). Autosomal recessive (AR) condition predisposing to mitotic non-disjunction. Affected individuals have growth failure, microcephaly, and mental retardation often with other congenital malformations, e.g. congenital heart disease (Lane *et al.* 2002) and childhood cancers (eg rhabdomyosarcoma, Wilms tumour, leukaemia). Chromosome analysis reveals a heterogeneous mix of aneuploidies, sometimes with a gain or loss of 2 or 3 different autosomes in a single cell. Premature centromere separation is a feature in some, but not all individuals. MVA is caused by biallelic mutations in *BUB1B* which encodes BUBR1, a key protein in the mitotic spindle checkpoint (Hanks).

Genetic advice

Recurrence risk

The recurrence risk is negligible for mosaicism arising from mitotic non-disjunction or somatic mutation, but a risk arises where it occurs as a result of trisomy rescue, because of the possibility of parental germline mosaicism. It is usually impossible to distinguish between mitotic non-disjunction and trisomy rescue. However, the overall risk to subsequent pregnancies is usually low except for MVA which is AR with a 25% recurrence risk.

Prenatal diagnosis

Risks of recurrence for mosaicism are usually very low (but see exception below). Prenatal diagnosis can be offered for reassurance.

Prenatal diagnosis for MVA is possible (Plaja *et al.* 2003) and should be offered because of the high recurrence risk (25%).

Lay group contact: Unique—The Rare Chromosome Disorder Support Group <www.rarechromo.org>, Tel. 01883 330766.

Expert adviser: R.J. McKinlay Gardner, Medical Geneticist, Genetic Health Services Victoria and Murdoch Children's Research Institute, Melbourne, Australia.

References

Crolla JA, Howard P, *et al.* A molecular and FISH approach to determining karyotype and phenotype correlations in six patients with supernumerary marker (22) chromosomes. *Am J Med Genet* 1997; **72** (4): 440–7.

Hanks S, Coleman K, *et al.* Constitutional aneuploidy and cancer predisposition caused by biallelic mutations in *BUB1B*. *Nat Genet* 2004; **36**: 1159–61.

Lane AH, Aijaz N, *et al.* Mosaic variegated aneuploidy with growth hormone deficiency and congenital heart defects. *Am J Med Genet* 2002; **110** (3): 273–7.

Manasse BF, Lekgate N, *et al.* The Pallister–Killian syndrome is reliably diagnosed by FISH on buccal mucosa. *Clin Dysmorphol* 2000; **9** (3): 163–5.

Plaja A, Mediano C, *et al.* Prenatal diagnosis of a rare chromosomal instability syndrome: variegated aneuploidy related to premature centromere division (PCD). *Am J Med Genet* 2003; **117A** (1): 85–6.

Schinzel A. *Catalogue of unbalanced chromosome aberrations in man*, 2nd edn. de Gruyter, Berlin, 2001.

Urioste M, Visedo G, *et al.* Dynamic mosaicism involving an unstable supernumerary der(22) chromosome in cat eye syndrome. *Am J Med Genet* 1994; **49** (1): 77–82.

Chromosomal mosaicism—prenatal

Mosaicism is defined as the presence of two or more cell populations derived from the same conceptus, but which have subsequently acquired a genetic difference. Prenatal diagnosis by chorionic villus sampling (CVS) and amniocentesis relies upon the fact that the fetus, placenta, and membranes are all derived from the fertilized egg and therefore have the same genetic constitution. Occasionally mitotic non-disjunction, trisomy rescue, or occurrence of a somatic new mutation alters this rule resulting in two (or more) genetically distinct cell lines. When post-mitotic non-disjunction involving an autosome occurs, the monosomy cell line is invariably lost and a trisomy lineage exists together with the euploid line, e.g. 47XY + 8/46XY. When post-mitotic non-disjunction involving an X chromosome occurs, the monosomy line may persist, e.g. 45X/46XX/47XXX.

See figure displaying various types of mosaicism.

Prenatal diagnosis

Mosaicism is diagnosed in 0.3% of amniocenteses and just over 2% of CVS samples (confined placental mosaicism in 1.9% and true fetal mosaicism in 0.19%). Mosaicism is often a nightmare to counsel because, although measures can be taken to reduce uncertainty, it is often not possible to provide definitive guidance on outcome. The percentage of abnormal mosaic cells identified at CVS or amniocentesis does not reliably indicate the likelihood of true fetal mosaicism or correlate with phenotypic severity if fetal mosaicism is present.

Embryonic derivations

- **CVS.** Direct (short-term culture (STC)) preparations reflect the karyotype of the chorionic cytotrophoblast; cultured CVS cells (long-term culture (LTC)) reflect the karyotype of the extra-embryonic mesoderm. Cultured chorionic villus cells come from a lineage more closely related to the fetus than direct preparations, but are less closely related than amniotic fluid cells.
- **Amniocentesis.** Cells present in amniotic fluid (amniocytes) are a mixture of cells derived from the amnion, cells shed from the fetal skin, and cells shed from the fetal urinary tract. In order to help in the evaluation of mosaicism, three independent cultures are set up when amniotic fluid cells are cultured. If an *in situ* method is used, independent colonies are assessed.

See the figure for cell lineages arising from differentiation in the very early conceptuses.

Definitions

- **Pseudomosaicism.** The mosaic cell line has arisen during laboratory culture.
- **Confined placental mosaicism (CPM).** Tissue-specific chromosomal mosaicism affecting the placenta only.
  - **Type 1 mosaicism.** Placental mosaicism confined to the cytotrophoblast.
  - **Type 2 mosaicism.** Placental mosaicism confined to the chorionic stroma (extra-embryonic mesoderm).
  - **Type 3 mosaicism.** Placental mosaicism present in both cell lineages (cytotrophoblast and extra-embryonic mesoderm).
- Classification of *in vitro* mosaicism detected at amniocentesis and CVS.

- **Level I.** A single abnormal cell in a flask or colony. Almost always a cultural artefact, and routinely not reported. (Worton and Stern (1984) found this in 7.1% of >12 000 amniocentesis samples.)
- **Level II.** Two or more cells with the same abnormality in a single flask, or a single abnormal colony in an *in situ* culture. This is nearly always **pseudomosaicism.** (Worton and Stern (1984) found this in 1.1% of >12 000 amniocentesis samples.) The decision to report this finding is based on an individual case-by-case assessment, largely based on whether the abnormality in question is ever seen in liveborns, e.g. mosaic trisomies 8, 9, 13, 18, and 21.
- **Level III.** Cells with the same abnormality present in more than one flask; two or more colonies with the same abnormality. (Worton and Stern (1984) found this in 0.3% of >12 000 amniocentesis samples.) This is likely to be a true mosaicism, although not necessarily true fetal mosaicism (see below). In Warton and Stern's (1984) study, 60% of level III mosaicism identified at amniocentesis reflected true fetal mosaicism.

Clinical approach

The finding of a mosaic karyotype on CVS or amniocentesis always requires careful evaluation of the pregnancy as a whole to determine, as far as possible, whether the aberrant cell line is present in the fetus or not and, at least in the cases of chromosome 7, 14, and especially 15, to consider the risk of syndromes associated with imprinting defects due to fetal uniparental disomy (UPD). In preparation for the consultation:

- discuss the case with your colleagues in the cytogenetics lab;
- consult a reference book, e.g. Gardner and Sutherland (2004);
- undertake a literature search, e.g. PubMed.

History: key points

- Brief family tree to include previous pregnancies.
- History of the current pregnancy.
- Raised maternal age is a risk factor for trisomy (trisomic rescue can lead to mosaicism).

Examination: key points

Detailed fetal anomaly ultrasound scan (USS) with fetal biometry and specific search for structural malformations commonly encountered in livebirths with mosaicism for the chromosome in question.

Mosaic trisomy involving an autosome

Mosaic trisomy 2. Trisomy 2 mosaicism occurs commonly in villus culture, and in most cases the +2 line is present in a small percentage of cells. True trisomy 2 mosaicism is seen in ~1/1000 CVS samples and usually represents CPM; in Sago and Chen's (1997) study, 11/11 had a normal outcome at birth. Intrauterine growth retardation (IUGR) may be a feature of some pregnancies with mosaic trisomy 2 identified at CVS (Wolstenholme *et al.* 2001). Fetal trisomy 2 mosaicism identified at amniocentesis is extremely rare; Sago and Chen (1997) report one case with mosaic trisomy 2 and multiple congenital anomalies in 58 000 amniocenteses.

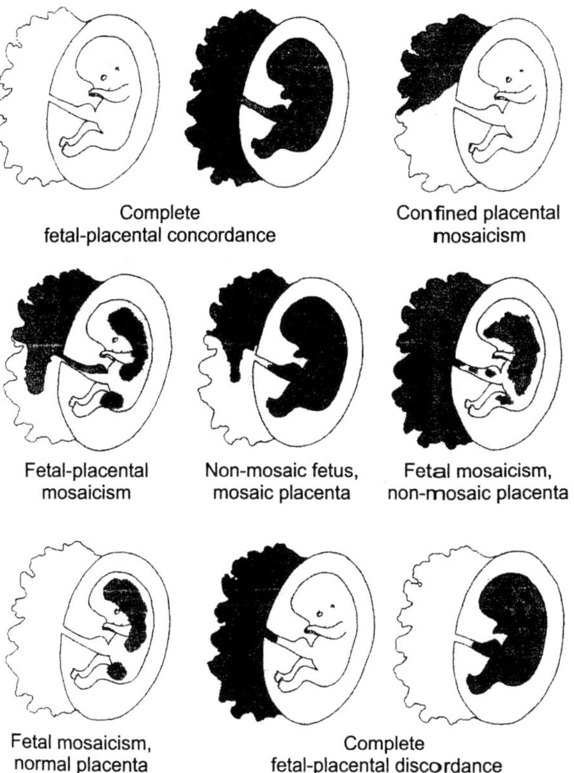

Types of mosaicism of the fetal–placental unit. Fetus is depicted enclosed in its sac at right, with the chorionic villi comprising the placenta to left. Grey areas indicate an aneuploid cell line; white areas indicate karyotypic normality. In reality, the distributions of the two cell lines are unlikely to be as clear-cut as is shown here. In the examples showing placental mosaicism, the path taken by the sampling needle will determine whether the abnormality is detected or missed at chorionic villus sampling. The cartoon of the fetus, sac, and placenta is close to the form and about two-thirds the size that actually exists at 10 weeks 0 days (gestational age as measured clinically, dated from the last menstrual period), when crown–rump length is around 30 mm. (Reproduced from fig. 25.4, p. 397 of Gardner and Sutherland (2004) with permission of Oxford University Press.)

Mosaic trisomy 7 may be identified at CVS, but is rarely confirmed at amniocentesis. Most trisomy 7 detected at CVS probably arises by mitotic non-disjunction and is present as CPM. If mosaic trisomy 7 is detected at amniocentesis, the possibility of a meiotic origin with trisomy rescue raises the possibility of UPD leading to a Silver–Russell phenotype with IUGR (Warburton 2002).

Mosaic trisomy 8. No consistent USS anomalies. No IUGR. Variable phenotype. Inconsistencies between CVS, amniocentesis, and fetal blood are reported. See 'Mosaic trisomy 8', page 530.

Mosaic trisomy 9. Cardiac, renal, and brain abnormalities, microphthalmia. Most infants with mosaic trisomy 9 have severe mental retardation.

Mosaic trisomy 13. Holoprosencephaly and midline brain defects, facial clefts, polydactyly. See Wallerstein et al. (2000) for further details; see also 'Patau syndrome (trisomy 13)', page 534.

Mosaic trisomy 15. The EUCROMIC study (Hahnemann and Vejerslev 1997) found that the trisomic cell line originates from a meiotic error in only about 50% of cases

of trisomy 15 CPM, the rest being the result of postzygotic, mitotic non-disjunction. Amniocentesis is recommended following the finding of a mosaic or non-mosaic trisomy 15 by CVS, in order to check for both UPD (risk for Angelman syndrome (paternal UPD) or Prader–Willi syndrome (maternal UPD)) and potential true fetal mosaicism.

Mosaic trisomy 16 usually arises from trisomy rescue. Placental abnormality, IUGR from 16 weeks, structural cardiac defects (particularly ventral septal defect (VSD)). See 'Mosaic trisomy 16', page 532.

Mosaic trisomy 18. IUGR, rocker bottom feet, radial defects, cardiac defects. See Wallerstein et al. (2000) for further details; see also 'Edwards syndrome (trisomy 18)', page 526.

Mosaic trisomy 20. Most cases of apparently full mosaic trisomy 20 are associated with a normal phenotype. Fetal blood sampling (FBS) is not helpful as the trisomic cells do not appear in blood. Hsu et al. (1991) reviewed 103 cases with a prenatal diagnosis of trisomy 20 mosaicism through amniocentesis. Approximately 90% were associated with a grossly normal phenotype. James et al. (2002) undertook a

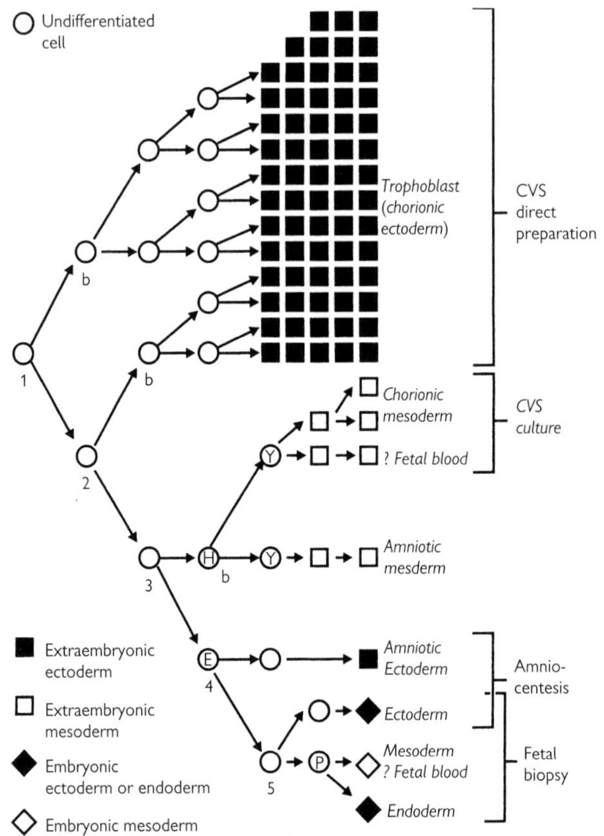

Diagram of cell lineages arising from differentiation in the very early conceptus. The fertilized egg (1) produces a trophoblast precursor (1b) and a totipotent stem cell (2) which in turn forms another trophoblast precursor (2b) and a stem cell (3) that produces the inner cell mass. The inner cell mass divides into stem cells for hypoblast (3b) and epiblast (4). The epiblast cell(s) (5) produce embryonic ectoderm and primitive streak, and the latter is the source of embryonic mesoderm and endoderm. The cell lineages sampled at various prenatal diagnostic procedures are indicated at right. E, Epiblast; H, hypoblast; P, primitive streak; Y, yolk sac. (From Bianchi *et al.* (1993) © 1993 *Am. J. Med. Genet.*, courtesy D.W. Bianchi, and with the permission of Wiley-Liss, Inc., a subsidiary of John Wiley & Sons, Inc.)

retrospective review of 14 cases (13 amniocentesis, 1 CVS) that were ascertained antenatally, all with low levels of mosaicism (8–50%). In 12 cases, the children were physically and developmentally normal, with the longest follow-up being 10 years. Minor anomalies were noted in 2 and there were no major malformations. This series confirms a much lower incidence of phenotypic abnormalities associated with mosaic trisomy 20 compared to other forms of mosaic aneuploidy. James *et al.* (2002) recommend that, if a detailed anomaly USS is normal, parents be counselled that the risk of abnormality is less than 10%. Further tests should be performed only on the basis of a clinical indication. Cytogenetic follow-up studies in liveborns should include a culture from urine sediment (Hsu *et al.* 1991).

Mosaic trisomy 21. Search for USS markers of trisomy 21. See Wallerstein *et al.* (2000) for further details; see also 'Down syndrome (trisomy 21)', page 524.

Mosaic trisomy 22. Cardiac and renal abnormalities, ear malformation, and pre-auricular tags.

Mosaic sex chromosome abnormality
See 'Sex chromosome mosaicism', page 544.

Mosaicism for a balanced or unbalanced translocation or other structural abnormality
Anomaly, cardiac, and growth scans. See 'Autosomal reciprocal translocations', page 508, for detail on *de novo* translocations.

Mosaicism for marker chromosome or ring chromosome
See 'Supernumerary marker chromosomes (SMCs)—prenatal' page 554 and 'Ring chromosomes', page 538.

Mosaic tetrasomy 12p (Pallister–Killian syndrome)
Diaphragmatic hernia, hydrops, relatively large fetal size. Detectable on amniocentesis and fibroblast culture but only rarely found in FBS or postnatal blood samples. See 'Coarse facial features' page 78 for further details.

Management
The management of each rearrangement requires specific consideration. Close discussion with the cytogeneticists is recommended to establish if further invasive tests will resolve the question of fetal involvement. In about 50%

of cases of level III mosaicism involving an autosome, the findings represent the fetal situation. Possible further investigations:

- amniocentesis if mosaicism was demonstrated in CVS. There is no indication for repeat amniocentesis if the mosaicism was detected at amniocentesis;
- FBS (cordocentesis) may be considered if the mosaicism was identified at amniocentesis or if (as in mosaic trisomy 8) there are instances of mosaicism at CVS not subsequently present in amniotic fluid, but present in fetal blood. However, in many instances a normal karyotype does not help counselling. In Hsu and Benn's (1999) series reporting mosaic trisomy 16, trisomic cells were never seen in >1% of cultured lymphocytes and so FBS is unlikely to provide helpful information in that situation;
- UPD screen when the mosaicism involves chromosomes with imprinted regions. Parental blood samples required for DNA extraction.

Important points

- If the mosaicism involves the sex chromosome there are specific issues relating to the external genitalia, fertility, and gonadal tumour risk. (See 'Sex chromosome mosaicism' page 544 and 'Turner syndrome, 45,X and variants', page 558.)
- For balanced autosomal translocations, true mosaicism is rare and the risk of an abnormal phenotype is low. (See 'Autosomal reciprocal translocations', pages 500–08 for more detail on *de novo* translocations.).
- For unbalanced rearrangements the risk is higher, and each case needs to be judged on its merits, following a thorough literature search. (See 'Autosomal reciprocal translocations', this chapter for more detail on the likely effect of unbalanced *de novo* translocations.)

Genetic advice

Recurrence risk

The recurrence risk is negligible for mosaicism arising from mitotic non-disjunction, but a risk arises where it occurs as a result of trisomy rescue, because of the possibility of parental germline mosaicism. It is usually impossible to distinguish between mitotic non-disjunction and trisomy rescue; however, the overall risk to subsequent pregnancies is usually low.

Prenatal diagnosis

Can be offered in a future pregnancy for reassurance.

Support group: ARC (Antenatal Results and Choices) <www.arc-uk.org>, Tel. 020 7631 0285.

Expert adviser: R.J. McKinlay Gardner, Medical Geneticist, Genetic Health Services Victoria and Murdoch Children's Research Institute, Melbourne, Australia.

References

Baty BJ, Olsen SB, *et al.* Trisomy 20 mosaicism in two unrelated girls with skin hypopigmentation and normal intellectual development. *Am J Med Genet* 2001; **99:** 210–16.

Bianchi DW, Wilkins-Haug L,, *et al.* Origin of extra-embryonic mesoderm in experimental animals: relevance to chorionic mosaicism in humans. *Am J Med Genet* 1993; **46:** 542–50.

Gardner RM, Sutherland GR. *Chromosome abnormalities and genetic counselling*, Oxford Monographs on Medical Genetics no. 31, 3rd edn. Oxford University Press, New York, 2004.

Hahnemann HM, Vejerslev LO. Accuracy of cytogenetic findings on chorion villus sampling (CVS)—diagnostic consequences of CVS mosaicism and non-mosaic discrepancy in centres contributing to EUCROMIC 1986–1992. *Prenat Diagn* 1997; **17:** 801–20.

Hsu LY, Kaffe S, Perlis TE. A revisit of trisomy 20 mosaicism in prenatal diagnosis—an overview of 103 cases. *Prenat Diagn* 1991; **11** (1): 7–15.

Hsu LY, Yu MT, *et al.* Rare trisomy mosaicism diagnosed in amniocytes, involving an autosome other than chromosomes 13, 18, 20 and 21: karyotype/phenotype correlations. *Prenat Diagn* 1997; **17:** 201–42.

Hsu LYF, Benn PA. Revised guidelines for the diagnosis of mosaicism in amniocytes. *Prenat Diagn* 1999; **19:** 1081–90.

James PA, Gibson K, McGaughran J. Prenatal diagnosis of mosaic trisomy 20 in New Zealand. *Aust NZ J Obstet Gynaecol* 2002; **42** (5): 486–9.

Kalousek DK, Vekemans M. Confined placental mosaicism. *J Med Genet* 1996; **33:** 529–33.

Reish O, Wolach B, *et al.* Dilemma of trisomy 20 mosaicism detected prenatally: is it an innocent finding? *Am J Med Genet* 1998; **77:** 72–5.

Robinson WP, McFadden DE, *et al.* Origin of amnion and implications for evaluation of the fetal genotype in cases of mosaicism. *Prenat Diagn* 2002; **22:** 1076–85.

Sago H, Chen E. True trisomy 2 mosaicism in amniocytes and newborn liver associated with multiple system abnormalities. *Am J Med Genet* 1997; **72** (3): 343–6.

Schinzel A. *Catalogue of unbalanced chromosome aberrations in man*, 2nd edn. de Gruyter, Berlin, 2001.

Wallerstein R, *et al.* Common trisomy mosaicism diagnosed in amniocytes involving chromosomes 13, 18, 20 and 21: karyotype–phenotype correlations. *Prenat Diagn* 2000; **20:** 103–22.

Warburton D. Trisomy 7 mosaicism: prognosis after prenatal diagnosis. *Prenat Diagn* 2002; **22** (13): 1239–40.

Wolstenholme J, White I, Sturgiss S, Carter J, Plant N, Goodship JA. Maternal uniparental heterodisomy for chromosome 2: detection through 'atypical' maternal AFP/hCG levels, with an update on a previous case. *Prenat Diagn* 2001; **21** (10): 813–17.

Worton RG, Stern R. A Canadian collaborative study of mosaicism in amniotic fluid cell cultures. *Prenat Diagn* 1984; **4** (Spec No): 131–44.

Deletions and duplications

Routine Giemsa (G)-banded karyotyping has been the 'gold-standard' in chromosome analysis for many years. The resolution of G-banding is at best ~5 Mb. New molecular cytogenetic methods, including interphase fluorescence *in situ* hybridization (FISH), primed *in situ* labelling (PRINS), multiplex ligand dependent probe amplification (MLPA), high-resolution comparative genomic hybridization (HRCGH), multicolour karyotyping, telomere FISH, genotyping, and array-CGH offer increased sensitivity and are very useful for:

1 further characterization of chromosome abnormalities as detected with routine banding analysis, including additions, duplications, deletions, translocations, markers, or complex aberrations;

2 screening for cryptic chromosome aberrations in patients with an apparently normal karyotype (Xu and Chen 2003).

Chromosome imbalance arising from segmental aneusomy may be a consequence of a deletion, duplication, or both.

Deletion. There is loss of a portion of a chromosome leading to monosomy for the deleted segment. In this deleted segment there is haploinsufficiency; those genes that are dosage-sensitive will contribute to the phenotype. Other mechanisms that may cause an abnormal phenotype are imprinting, the unmasking of a recessive mutation, and an effect on a gene not included within the deletion ('position effect'). A **contiguous gene syndrome** is a recognizable phenotype resulting from the loss of contiguous (adjacent) genes.

Microdeletion. A deletion that is sometimes detectable by high resolution banding but most commonly detected by specific FISH or PRINS testing. Array-CGH is likely to become more widely used in future. Molecular cytogenetic technology has identified a number of recurrent microdeletions as causes of clinically recognizable syndromes.

- **Interstitial deletion.** A section of the 'p' or 'q' arm is lost but the deletion does not include the telomere.
- **Terminal and subtelomeric deletions.** These may be isolated abnormalities, or may have arisen as a consequence of a reciprocal translocation, and be associated with a duplication of the reciprocal chromosome. Telomeric repeat sequences (TTAGGG) cap the termini of every human chromosome. All ends of human chromosomes must have a telomeric cap to be stable. Proximal to these repeat sequences are chromosome-specific repeat sequences, which in turn are distal to gene-rich regions. Since the density of genes in the subtelomeric regions is high, small unbalanced rearrangements, e.g. deletions, may lead to a severe phenotype. If a telomere is lost in a terminal deletion at least three mechanisms exist to maintain the chromosome end: stabilization of a terminal deletions through a process of telomere regeneration ('telomere healing'); retention of the original telomere producing an interstitial deletion; and formation of a derivative chromosomes by obtaining a different telomeric sequence through cytogenetic rearrangement ('telomere capture'; Ballif *et al.* 2000). (NB. Several subtelomeric deletions do not seem to have a phenotypic effect in all individuals, e.g. del 8pter in some and del 2qter, which can, depending on the size of the deletion, be a polymorphic variant.)

Duplication. There is duplication of a portion of a chromosome leading to trisomy for the duplicated segment. Techniques such as FISH are far less sensitive at detecting microduplications than microdeletions. With the advent of more comprehensive technology such as CGH/microarray, the number of microduplications identified is likely to increase.

- **Interstitial duplication.** Arising from an intrachromosomal duplication.
- **Direct or inverted.** In a direct duplication the duplicated segment 'ab' is in a tandem arrangement 'abab'; in an inverted duplication the duplicated segment is in an 'abba' arrangement.
- **Terminal and subtelomeric duplications.** Careful evaluation of the karyotype is required as this may be as a consequence of a reciprocal translocation and be associated with a deletion of the reciprocal chromosome.

Mechanisms of rearrangement

Recent work on genomic organization is shedding some insight into the mechanisms that underlie some recurrent rearrangements. For example, several recurrent constitutional rearrangements, including deletions, duplications, and translocations, are found at 22q11.2. These rearrangements give rise to a variety of genomic disorders, including DiGeorge/velocardiofacial syndrome (DGS/VCFS), cat eye syndrome (CES), and the supernumerary der(22)t(11;22) syndrome associated with the recurrent t(11;22). Chromosome 22-specific duplicons or low copy repeats (LCRs) have been directly implicated in these chromosomal rearrangements (Shaikh *et al.* 2001).

Three large region-specific low-copy repeat elements (LCRs), composed of different blocks (A, B, and C), flank the Williams syndrome deletion interval on 7q and are thought to predispose to misalignment and unequal crossing-over, causing the deletion (Bayes *et al.* 2003).

Prader–Willi and Angelman syndromes (PWS and AS, respectively) typically result from an approximately 4-Mb deletion of human chromosome 15q11–q13, with clustered breakpoints (BP) at either of two proximal sites (BP1 and BP2) and one distal site (BP3). Duplications in the same region are associated with autism. Pujana *et al.* (2002) have shown that clusters containing several copies of the human chromosome 15 low-copy repeat (LCR15) duplicon are located at each of these breakpoints.

Clinical approach

Ask your colleagues in cytogenetics to produce an annotated photograph together with an ideogram of the chromosome involved in the deletion/duplication. This is an invaluable aid to counselling.

History: key points

- Draw a three-generation family tree (or larger if indicated) and enquire about pregnancy loss, stillbirth, neonatal death, and family members with learning disability or congenital anomalies.
- Document all known malformations in the child and anthropomorphic data.
- Presence of developmental delay/mental retardation.

Examination: key points

Full clinical examination and documentation of dysmorphic features preferably with clinical photographs.

Special investigations

- For a terminal deletion detected on G-banding, consider FISH with subtelomeric probes. Davies *et al.* (2003) found that 3 (19%) of 16 apparently terminal deletion cases were the result of more complex rearrangements involving other chromosome subtelomeres.
- Arrange for parental chromosome analysis, with specific FISH testing if indicated. With terminal deletions, one parent could be a carrier of a balanced reciprocal translocation.
- Search the Online Mendelian Inheritance in Man (OMIM) gene map <www.ncbi.nlm.nih.gov/htbin-post/Omim/getmap> to determine whether there are any disease genes of specific relevance within the deletion, e.g. *RB1* (retinoblastoma), *APC* (familial adenomatous polyposis (FAP)), *TSC1* (tuberous sclerosis (TSC)). Tumour suppressor genes and other important dominant disease genes may need specific surveillance.

Clinical features of some interstitial microdeletion syndromes

These syndromes have a recognizable clinical phenotype and were mostly delineated before it was confirmed that the aetiology was a chromosomal microdeletion.

del (7q11.23) Williams syndrome. The microdeletion encompasses the elastin gene (*ELN*). Congenital heart disease (CHD) occurs in 80%, 75% have supravalvular aortic stenosis (SVAS), and ~25% have a discrete supravalvular pulmonary stenosis. Peripheral pulmonic stenosis is found in 50–75% of infants, but improves with time. The elastin anomaly is generalized and almost any artery can be narrowed, e.g. renal artery stenosis (40%). Aortic insufficiency (20%) and mitral valve prolapse (MVP; 15%) may occur in some adults. There are characteristic facial features. Infants and young children have periorbital fullness, bulbous nasal tip, long philtrum, wide mouth, full lips, full cheeks, and small widely spaced teeth; older children and adults have a more gaunt appearance with coarser facial features. Developmental delay with very variable mental retardation, ranging from severe to low-average with most having mild to moderate mental retardation, strengths in language but poor visuospatial skills, overfriendly personality, short attention span, and anxiety. Approximately 15% of infants have hypercalcaemia.

del (8q24) Langer–Giedion syndrome (tri-chorhinophalangeal syndrome (TRPS I), exostoses, mental retardation). TRPS is a disorder characterized by fine, sparse growing scalp hair, dystrophic brittle nails, bent fingers with cone-shaped epiphyses on X-ray, and a pear-shaped bulbous nose. When it is a part of this contiguous gene deletion syndrome it is known as TRPS II, but when isolated it is known as TRPS I, and is caused by mutation within the *TRP* gene. The *EXT1* gene is also at 8q24 and when it is deleted bony exostoses develop.

del (11p13) WAGR (Wilms tumour–aniridia–genitourinary anomalies–mental retardation). Ensure follow-up and screening up to the age of 8 years for Wilms tumour risk.

del (15q11–13) Prader–Willi syndrome (PWS). Frequency is approximately 1/10 000–1/15 000 individuals. Due to imprinting, the maternally inherited genes on 15q11 (in the PWS/AS critical region) are usually inactivated and normal development is dependent upon paternally inherited genes. 75% of patients with PWS have del 15q11–13, 24% have uniparental disomy (UPD) 15mat, only 1% have an imprinting defect (abnormal methylation but normal FISH and UPD studies). SNRPN (small nuclear ribonuclear protein-associated polypeptide N) methylation analysis detects PWS in 99%. Babies have central hypotonia and feeding difficulties with failure to thrive in infancy. There is rapid weight gain between the ages 1 and 6 years (usually 2–4 years), characterized by truncal obesity with small hands and feet, small genitalia in males, and short stature. It is the most common recognized genetic form of obesity. Typically there is insatiable appetite and food-seeking/hoarding. Most patients have intelligent quotients (IQs) in the 60s–low 70s, approximately 40% have borderline retardation or low normal intelligence, and 20% have moderate retardation. Behavioural problems can be a major issue. Most adults with PWS will require support/supervision in adult life and few will live independently. Both males and females have hypogonadotrophic hypogonadism, sexual activity is uncommon, and fertility is rare (but note, if deletion, girls are at 50% risk for child with AS—birth of an AS child to a PWS mother has been reported).

del (15q11) Angelman syndrome (AS). See 'Angelman syndrome' page 272.

del (17p11.2) Smith–Magenis syndrome (SMS). Some patients are short and obese with small hands and feet, as well as square, rather heavy facies. They may have a history of hypotonia in infancy, developmental delay, behaviour disturbance (especially affecting sleep with a disturbed day–night rhythm), and sometimes food-searching and self-injuring behaviour. Some individuals with SMS have mutations in *RAI1*, a gene encompassed by the common 17p11.2 microdeletion.

del (17p13.3) Miller–Dieker syndrome. Lissecencephaly with dysmorphic features, the microdeletion includes the *LIS1* gene. In about 12% the deletion is due to a familial chromosome rearrangement. The main features are tall prominent forehead with vertical furrowing, bitemporal narrowing, hypertelorism, upslanting palpebral fissures, short nose with anteverted nares, inverted vermilion border of upper lip with long, broad and thick upper lip. There are associated anomalies, such as CHD, omphalocele, and joint contractures.

del (22q11.2) Di George syndrome. See '22q11 deletion syndrome', page 490.

Clinical features of some interstitial microduplication syndromes

Recently reciprocal duplication syndromes have been identified for some of the well known deletions. As for the deletions, these duplications are sponsored by duplicons and occur as a result of non-homologous recombination.

dup (7q11.23) Severe expressive language delay with mild growth retardation and subtle facial dysmorphism (Somerville).

dup (22q11.2) Phenotypes range from mild to severe with considerable intrafamilial and interfamilial variability (Yobb). In some individuals mild learning disability may be the only feature, whilst at the severe end of the spectrum children can have severe congenital malformations eg. conotruncal heart disease. Velopharyngeal insufficiency appears to be common.

Terminal and subtelomeric deletions

Some have a distinctive phenotype and a specific FISH test can be requested. Subtelomeric screening in children with undiagnosed conditions has identified phenotypes with other terminal deletions. See 'Submicroscopic chromosomal rearrangements and the chromosomal phenotype', page 546.

Genetic advice

In general, duplication of chromosomal material is better tolerated than deletions. FISH and paint to fully characterize and carefully exclude deletions and parental balanced rearrangements.

- *De novo* **apparently isolated deletion or duplication.** If it is *de novo*, the chance of a chromosome deletion/duplication being the cause of the phenotype is likely, especially when the phenotype is consistent with reported cases.
- **Familial abnormality**
  - **Parent with an apparently identical deletion/duplication.** During a consultation it may become apparent that a phenotypic effect is present in a parent. If there is no phenotypic abnormality in the parent consider whether the deletion/duplication really is the cause of the phenotype, or whether it might be a polymorphism without any clinical significance. Careful study of the literature and analysis of samples from more family members may be helpful. Other less likely explanations are an imprinting effect and the unmasking of a recessive condition.
  - **Balanced rearrangement in parent.** This will usually be a balanced translocation. See 'Autosomal reciprocal translocations—familial', page 504.

Recurrence risk

- *De novo* **apparently isolated deletion or duplication.** This risk is very low, <1%, and the recurrence risk is due to mosaicism (either germline mosaicism or low-level gonosomal mosaicism) in one parent.
- **Apparently identical deletion/duplication in parent.** If an individual carrying the deletion/duplication reproduces, the risk in each pregnancy for a child carrying the deletion/duplication is ~50%.

Prenatal diagnosis

- *De novo* **apparently isolated deletion or duplication.** Possible by chorionic villus sampling (CVS)/amniocentesis. May be offered/requested for reassurance.
- **Parent with an apparently identical deletion/duplication.** Possible by CVS/amniocentesis. Offered to those families in which the deletion/duplication is the cause of abnormality. As this may involve the counselling of individuals with learning difficulties, take care to ensure that there is plenty of time for the consultation and appropriate consent for any intervention.

Support group: Unique—The Rare Chromosome Disorder Support Group <www.rarechromo.org>, Tel. 01883 330766.

Expert adviser: Bert B.A. de Vries, Clinical Geneticist, University Medical Centre, Nijmegen, The Netherlands.

References

Ballif BC, Kashork CD, Shaffer LG. FISHing for mechanisms of cytogenetically defined terminal deletions using chromosome-specific subtelomeric probes. *Eur J Hum Genet* 2000; **8** (10): 764–70.

Bayes M, Magano LF, *et al.* Mutational mechanisms of Williams–Beuren syndrome deletions. *Am J Hum Genet* 2003; **73** (1): 131–51.

Davies AF, Kirby TL, Docherty Z, Ogilvie CM. Characterization of terminal chromosome anomalies using multisubtelomere FISH. *Am J Med Genet* 2003; **120A** (4): 483–9.

De Vries BBA, Winter R, *et al.* Telomere: a diagnosis at the end of the chromosomes. *J Med Genet* 2003; **40**: 385–98.

Ensenauer RE, Adeyinka A, *et al.* Microduplication 22q11.2, an emerging syndrome: clinical, cytogenetic, and molecular analysis of thirteen patients. *Am J Hum Genet* 2003; **73** (5): 1027–40.

Gardner RM, Sutherland GR. *Chromosome abnormalities and genetic counselling*, Oxford Monographs on Medical Genetics no. 31, 3rd edn. Oxford University Press, New York, 2004.

Luciani JJ, de Mas P, *et al.* Telomeric 22q13 deletions resulting from rings, simple deletions and translocations: cytogenetic, molecular and clinical analysis of 32 new observations. *J Med Genet* 2003; **40**: 690–6.

Ness GO, Lybaek H, Houge G. Usefulness of high-resolution comparative genomic hybridization (CGH) for detecting and characterizing constitutional chromosome abnormalities. *Am J Med Genet* 2002; **113** (2): 125–36.

Pujana MA, Nadal M, *et al.* Human chromosome 15q11–q14 regions of rearrangements contain clusters of LCR15 duplicons. *Eur J Hum Genet* 2002; **10** (1): 26–35.

Shaikh TH, Kurahashi H, Emanuel BS. Evolutionarily conserved low copy repeats (LCRs) in 22q11 mediate deletions, duplications, translocations, and genomic instability: an update and literature review. *Genet Med* 2001; **3** (1): 6–13.

Sommerville MJ, Mervis CB, *et al.* Severe expressive-language delay related to duplication of the Williams-Beuren locus. *NEJM* 2005; **353**: 1694–701.

Tharapel AT, Kadandale JS, *et al.* Prader–Willi/Angelman and DiGeorge/velocardiofacial syndrome deletions: diagnosis by primed *in situ* labeling (PRINS). *Am J Med Genet* 2001; **107A**: 119–22.

Xu J, Chen Z. Advances in molecular cytogenetics for the evaluation of mental retardation. *Am J Med Genet* 2003; **117C** (1): 15–24.

Yobb TM, Somerville MJ, *et al.* Microduplication and triplication of 22q11.2: a highly variable syndrome. *Am J Hum Genet.* 2005; **76**: 865–76.

Down syndrome (trisomy 21)

The chromosomal basis for Down syndrome can be summarized as follows.

- 95% result from non-disjunction giving rise to trisomy 21.
- 2% result from Robertsonian translocation (especially 14;21) of which 50% are familial.
- 2% result from mosaicism, e.g. postzygotic non-disjunction (most common), or postzygotic loss of a chromosome 21 from a trisomic zygote (trisomy rescue).
- 1% result from a variety of chromosome rearrangements; trisomy for 21q22 confers much of the phenotype.

Rapid interphase fluorescent *in situ* hybridization (FISH) analysis is possible for confirmation of diagnosis where there is high clinical suspicion of Down syndrome. FISH is particularly liable to error in detecting mosaicism and some rearrangements causing partial trisomies. Conventional karyotyping is therefore essential to determine the genetic basis for the Down, i.e. whether there is trisomy 21, a Robertsonian translocation, mosaicism, or an unbalanced chromosome rearrangement involving 21.

The incidence of trisomy 21 conceptions increases strikingly with maternal age (see 'Maternal age' page 610). There is a high incidence of spontaneous fetal loss during pregnancy. Between ~11 weeks gestation and term, 43% of affected pregnancies are spontaneously lost, and between ~16 weeks gestation and term ~23% are lost (Hook 1992).

Clinical features

The neonate with Down syndrome typically shows marked hypotonia, small ears, upslanting palpebral fissures, flat facial profile, brachycephaly, etc. (see below under 'Examination: key points').

Development. Milestones are delayed with average age for sitting independently 6–30 months, walking 1–4 years, first words 1–3 years, toilet training 2–7 years. Mean intelligence quotient (IQ) in children and young adults with Down syndrome is 45–48, with a wide range and upper limit of ~70. There is some correlation with parental IQ. An educationally based preschool teaching service such as Portage is often of benefit.

Education. The trend is towards integration of children with Down syndrome into mainstream education with additional support, but some will benefit from education in a special school environment particularly at secondary level.

Adult life. Adults with Down syndrome generally require some form of supported accommodation and sheltered work opportunities. Most teenagers with Down syndrome will achieve a degree of independence, learning to dress themselves and speak so that their family can understand them, but even in adult life will require some level of supervision on a daily basis.

Life expectancy. Median age at death is 49 years (Yang *et al.* 2002). Survival to 60 years is 44.4% (normal population 86.4%), survival to 68 years is 13.6% (normal population 78.4%). Congenital heart disease (CHD) is a major factor in increased mortality in infancy and childhood. Survival has increased markedly over a 10–20 year view, but nonetheless there remain significant differences in life expectancy especially in those with CHD. Survival figures for patients with Down syndrome but without CHD and (with Down syndrome with CHD) are: to age 1 year 90.7% (76.3%), to 5 years 87.2% (61.8%) to 10 years 84.9% (57.1%), 30 years 79.2% (49.9%).

Cardiac defects. 40–50% have heart problems at birth, half of which are serious and require surgery. Perimembranous ventricular septal defect (VSD) is the most common defect, followed by patent ductus arteriosus (PDA) and atrial septal defect (ASD). Atrioventricular septal defect (AVSD), an endocardial cushion defect, is 1000× more common in children with Down syndrome than in the general population. Other forms of complex heart disease can occur including overriding aorta and tetralogy of Fallot.

Other congenital malformations. 45 congenital malformations occur more frequently in children with Down syndrome, including duodenal atresia or stenosis and Hirschsprung syndrome. Overall, the incidence of all congenital anomalies is increased ~twofold in children with Down syndrome.

Other medical problems, e.g. hypothyroidism, leukaemia. Hypothyroidism occurs in 20–40%. The incidence of leukaemia is about 20-fold higher than in the normal population and includes both acute lymphocytic leukaemia (ALL), which occurs in ~2%, and acute non-lymphocytic leukaemia (some of which are acute magakaryoblastic leukaemia).

Dementia. At the age of about 30–40 years some decline in cognitive ability is seen in many individuals with Down syndrome. Mean age of diagnosis of dementia is in the early 50s and dementia is an important factor in the reduced life expectancy of adults with Down syndrome. Neuropathological changes appear identical to those seen in Alzheimer disease.

Clinical approach

History: key points

- Family tree. If the karyotype is already known to be +21, only a brief family tree is required.
- Age of the mother at the time of the birth of her Down syndrome child.
- Pregnancy history.

Examination: key points

Where appropriate, use clinical photographs to supplement the examination.

- Facial features with upslanting palpebral fissures, flat facial profile, epicanthic folds, short nose with depressed nasal bridge.
- Brachycephaly and patent posterior fontanelle.
- Dermatoglyphics. Single palmar creases and sandal gap between hallux and second toe. Usually in normal individuals there are whorl patterns over the hallux and base of the first first metatarsal. In Down syndrome the hallucal whorl is often replaced by a loop and the metatarsal whorl by an open pattern with gently curved lines over the ball of the foot.
- Hypotonia, e.g. marked head lag as a newborn. Hypotonia contributes to delayed motor milestones in infancy.
- Heart. Careful clinical assessment due to high incidence of CHD (40–50%).

- Growth parameters. Height, weight, occipital-frontal circumference (OFC). Plot on Down syndrome-specific charts; see `<www.growthcharts.com>`.

Special investigations
- Karyotype of fetus/baby. Parental karyotypes not indicated if straightforward trisomy 21or mosaic trisomy 21. Parental karyotypes are essential if a translocation or other rearrangement is identified.
- If clinical diagnosis of Down syndrome seems likely, yet blood karyotype is normal, consider mosaicism screen (30 cells) and skin biopsy for fibroblast karyotype to investigate possibility of Down syndrome mosaic.
- Echocardiogram, if Down syndrome is diagnosed.

Genetic advice
Recurrence risk
Risk of recurrence of +21 is affected by maternal age and parental germline mosaicism. 10/842 (1.2%) in the Japanese series (Uehara *et al.* 1999), and 6/1211 (0.5%) in the Dutch series (Sachs *et al.* 1990) conceived another +21 pregnancy (combined risk 16/2053 is 0.8%). Data from Hook (1992) is stratified by age, but the resulting numbers are very small and hence the confidence intervals quite wide: at maternal age <30 years, 3/211 (1.4%), 30–34years, 1/145 (0.7%), 35–39 years, 0/165 (0%), >39years, 1/112 (0.9%), total 5/633 (0.8%). Overall, advising a *'slightly less than 1% recurrence risk' (0.8%) for women <39 years with an age-related risk thereafter* seems reasonable.
- Some women who have had a trisomy 21 conception may have a small increased risk for other aneuploidies (Warburton).
- If the proband has trisomy 21 there is no increased risk to second- and third-degree relatives (Berr and Borghi 1990).
- After two trisomy 21 pregnancies, a 10% + risk may be appropriate. Strongly consider the possibility of parental germline or gonosomal mosaicism. Examine parents for features of Down syndrome and do parental karyotypes with mosaicism screen. In the Dutch study (Sachs *et al.* 1990), 2/6 couples with recurrent trisomy 21 had evidence of mosaicism. If mosaicism is confined to the gonads this will not be detected—hence 10% + risk.
- *De novo* Robertsonian translocation—risk is low, but recurrence has been reported (Sachs *et al.* 1990). If parental karyotypes are normal, risk is certainly <2% (Steinberg *et al.* 1984).
- If father carries Robertsonian translocation involving 21, e.g. rob(14q21q), risk <1%.
- If mother carries Robertsonian translocation involving 21, e.g. rob(14q21q), risk 10–15%.
- If parent carries rob(21q21q) translocation, risk approaches 100% (unless trisomic rescue occurs).
- If a woman with +21 becomes pregnant, the risk of +21 in the offspring is ~50% (fertility in men with +21 is exceptionally rare).

Family history of Down syndrome
- **Single affected relative.** If a sibling, aunt, or uncle has Down syndrome, try to obtain the karyotype of the affected individual. If +21 there are no added risks to your patient arising from this. If karyotype is not obtainable and the mother was <40 years old at the time of the affected child's birth it may be reasonable to offer your patient a karyotype to exclude the very small possibility of a Robertsonian translocation involving 21.
- **More than one affected relative on same side of family** raises the possibility of a Robertsonian

translocation involving 21 (e.g. rob14;21). A karyotype of your patient is essential unless the family has already been carefully investigated.

Prenatal diagnosis
Possible by chorionic villus sampling (CVS) or amniocentesis.

Prenatal screening tests
Nuchal fold thickness at 10–13 weeks gestation, maternal serum screening (alpha-fetoprotein (AFP), beta human chorionic gonadotrophin (βhCG), unconjugated (o)estriol (uE3)) at 14–16 weeks gestation, Detailed ultrasound scan (USS; poor detection rate unless CHD is present).

Management
Referral to paediatrician at local child development centre. Involvement of paediatric cardiologist if appropriate.

The following management of Down syndrome was recommended by Roizen and Patterson (2003).
- **Evaluation.** Echocardiogram, ophthalmological assessment (refractive errors are common), hearing assessment.
- **Prevention** of obesity, periodontal disease.
- **Monitoring** of coeliac disease, thyroid function.
- **Vigilance** for arthritis, atlantoaxial subluxation, diabetes mellitus (1%), leukaemia (0.6%), obstructive sleep apnoea, seizures (8%).
- **Other.** Sexuality and reproductive health, dermatological problems, behavioural problems, development.

Support group contact: Down Syndrome Association `<www.downs-syndrome.org.uk>`; MDS UK—Mosaic Down syndrome support group `<www.mosaicdownsyndrome.org>`; US National Down Syndrome Society `<www.ndss.org>`.

Expert adviser: Martin Bobrow, Professor of Medical Genetics, University of Cambridge, Cambridge, England.

References
Berr C, Borghi E. Risk of Down syndrome in relatives of trisomy 21 children. A case-control study. *Ann Genet* 1990; **33**: 137–40.

Bray I, Wright DE, Davies C, Hook EB. Joint estimation of Down syndrome risk and ascertainment rates: a meta-analysis of nine published data sets. *Prenat Diagn* 1998; **18**: 9–20.

Hook EB. Chromosome abnormalities: prevalence, risks and recurrence. In *Prenatal diagnosis and screening* (ed. D.L.H. Brock, C.H. Rodeck, and M.A. Ferguson-Smith), pp. 351–92. Churchill Livingstone, Edinburgh, 1992.

Hunter ASGW. Down syndrome. In *Management of genetic syndromes* (ed. S.B. Cassidy and J.E. Allanson), pp. 103–29. Wiley-Liss, New York, 2001.

Pangalos CG, Talbot CC Jr, *et al.* DNA polymorphism analysis in families with recurrence of free trisomy 21. *Am J Hum Genet* 1992; **51**: 1015–27.

Roizen NJ, Patterson D. Down's syndrome [seminar]. *Lancet* 2003; **361**: 1281–9.

Sachs ES, Jahoda MG, *et al.* Trisomy 21 mosaicism in gonads with unexpectedly high recurrence risks. *Am J Med Genet Suppl* 1990; **7**: 186–8.

Steinberg C, Zackai EH, *et al.* Recurrence rate for *de novo* 21q21q translocation Down syndrome: a study of 112 families. *Am J Med Genet* 1984; **17** (2): 523–30.

Uehara S, Yaegashi N, *et al.* Risk of recurrence of fetal chromosomal aberrations: analysis of trisomy 21, trisomy 18, trisomy 13, and 45,X in 1076 Japanese mothers. *J Obstet Gynaecol Res* 1999; **25**: 373–9.

Warburton D, Dallaire L, *et al.* Trisomy recurrence: a reconsideration based on North American data. *Am J Hum Genet* 2004; **75**: 376–85.

Yang Q, Rasmussen A, *et al.* Mortality associated with Down's syndrome in the USA from 1983 to 1997: a population-based study. *Lancet* 2002; **359**: 1019–25.

Edwards' syndrome (trisomy 18)

Trisomy 18 is associated with a high rate of spontaneous loss in pregnancy and very poor outcomes in surviving infants. The spontaneous rate of pregnancy loss from the second trimester onwards is 36% (Hook *et al.* 1989). Trisomy 18 has an incidence of 1/7900 livebirths (Parker *et al.* 2003) with a strong female excess. The great majority are due to *de novo* meiotic non-disjunction. 85% are maternal in origin and there is a strong maternal age effect (as for trisomy 21).

Presentation may be:

- **Prenatal**
  - Increased nuchal translucency and/or other suspicion e.g. exomphalos at 11–13 weeks gestation.
  - Abnormal first or second trimester maternal serum screen profile (see below).
  - Unexpected result at amniocentesis for another indication at 16–18 weeks gestation.
  - Abnormal fetal ultrasound scan (USS; intrauterine growth retardation (IUGR), choroid plexus cysts, congenital heart defect (CHD; usually large ventral septal defect (VSD)), renal defects, exomphalos, overlapping fingers, rocker-bottom feet at 19–22 weeks gestation). There are usually multiple anomalies.
  - IUGR often not noted until 32 + weeks gestation, or polyhydramnios (30–60%), or intrauterine death (IUD).
- **Neonatal.** Neonate with growth retardation and dysmorphic features.

94% of infants with Edwards syndrome will have trisomy 18; the remainder have trisomy 18 mosaicism or partial 18q trisomy.

Clinical features

The most striking features in the newborn are small for dates, short sternum, and CHD.

Growth retardation. Mean birthweight 2240 g (weight, length, and occipital-frontal circumference (OFC) < 3rd centile), with postnatal failure to thrive.

Dysmorphic features. Prominent occiput, simple ears, overriding fingers, often with camptodactyly, nail hypoplasia, short hallux, irregular ribs on CXR, rocker-bottom feet (convex bottom to foot with projecting 'heel'). Very pale fundi.

Dermatoglyphics. Usually arches on all 10 digits of the hands; this is rarely found in any other condition. (The lens on an auroscope (without the ear piece) is useful for visualizing the fingerprints in a neonate.)

Congenital anomalies. At least 90% have CHD, usually VSD ± valve dysplasia. The great majority have polyvalvular dysplasia. Both spina bifida and facial clefts occur more commonly than in the general population.

Developmental disability. Developmental quotient (developmental age/chronological age) averages 0.18, i.e. severe to profound developmental delay, but falls further in older children.

Short life expectancy. Median life expectancy is 4 days (range is large from failure to establish respiration at birth through to 2+ years). Root and Carey (1994) found survival to 1 week of 45%, to 6 months of 9%, to 1 year of 5%. Longer-term survival is exceptional, but Baty *et al.* (1994a) reported a child with +18 who was 19 years old. 70% of deaths are due to cardiopulmonary arrest; central apnoea is a major factor in the neonatal period and infancy.

Clinical approach

History: key points

- Family tree. If karyotype is known to be +18, only a brief family tree is required.
- Pregnancy history.

Examination: key points

- Growth parameters.
- Dysmorphic features. See 'Clinical features' above: prominent occiput, simple ears, overriding fingers, short sternum, short hallux, rocker-bottom feet.
- Heart.

Special investigations

- Full karyotype on pregnancy/baby (parental chromosomes not indicated if straightforward +18).
- Chest X-ray usually shows irregularity of ribs.
- Consider cardiac echocardiogram.
- Clinical photographs.

Management

Nasogastric feeding is usually required initially, which may change to gastrostomy feeding in those surviving beyond 6 months. Gastro-oesophageal reflux is very common—consider prophylaxis. Older infants and children with Edwards syndrome are at increased risk for Wilms tumour and hepatoblastoma. (The kidneys usually show fetal lobulation.) Photophobia is also common in surviving children.

Genetic advice

Recurrence risk

Sibling recurrence risk is 0.55% (1/200; Baty *et al.* 1994a). (0/170 recurrences of +18 in the Japanese series (Uehara *et al.* 1999) confirm the low risk.)

Note. For mothers aged >37 years, the risk for a +21 pregnancy exceeds that for a recurrence of +18.

Prenatal diagnosis

Invasive prenatal diagnosis by chorionic villus sampling (CVS)/amniocentesis should be offered but, in view of the low recurrence risk, some couples may prefer the option of surveillance of the pregnancy by a combination of:

- First trimester screening USS at 10–14 weeks gestation (increased nuchal translucency in aneuploid pregnancies) ideally with maternal serum biochemical markers.
- Second trimester screening maternal serum screen (median levels in pregnancies affected by +18 are all reduced, alpha-fetoprotein (AFP), 0.43 MoM (multiple of the median); unconjugated oestriol (uE3), 0.43 MoM; and human chorionic gonadotrophin (hCG), 0.36 MoM). Using a prior risk of 1/200 these values can be incorporated into a serum screening algorithm to provide a revised risk estimate. (Using these parameters together with maternal age in the general population results in a 67% detection rate.);
- detailed fetal anomaly USS at 19–20 weeks gestation (high incidence of structural cardiac anomalies, choroid plexus cysts, IUGR, exomphalos, neural tube defect overlapping fingers, rocker-bottom feet).

Combining the above it should be possible to detect in excess of 80% of affected pregnancies, reducing the already low recurrence risk of 1/200 to closer to 1/1000.

Spencer and Nicolaides (2002) have devised a first trimester trisomy 13/18 risk algorithm, combining fetal nuchal translucency thickness and maternal serum free β-hCG and pregnancy-associated plasma protein A (PAPP-A), that will, for a 0.3% false-positive rate, allow 95% of these chromosomal defects to be identified at 11–14 weeks gestation.

Support group contact: SOFT UK (Support Organization for Trisomy 18, 13 and Related Disorders) <www.soft.org.uk>.

Expert adviser: John Edwards, Emeritus Professor of Genetics, University of Oxford, Oxford, England and Particia Boyd, Associate Specialist in Clinical Genetics for Prenatal Diagnosis, John Radcliffe Hospital, Oxford, England.

References

Baty BJ, Blackburn BL, Carey JC. Natural history of trisomy 18 and trisomy 13: growth, physical assessment, medical histories, survival and recurrence risk. *Am J Med Genet* 1994a; **49**: 175–88.

Baty BJ, Blackburn BL, Carey JC. Natural history of trisomy 18 and trisomy 13: psychomotor development. *Am J Med Genet* 1994b; **49**: 189–94.

Carey JC. Trisomy 18 and trisomy 13 syndromes. In *Management of genetic syndromes* (ed. S.B. Cassidy and J.E. Allanson), pp. 417–36. Wiley-Liss, New York, 2001.

Hogge WA, Fraer L, Melegari T. Maternal serum screening for fetal trisomy 18: benefits of patient-specific risk protocol. *Am J Obstet Gynecol* 2001; **185**: 289–93.

Hook EB, Topol BB, Cross PK. The natural history of cytogenetically abnormal fetuses detected at midtrimester amniocentesis which are not terminated electively: new data and estimates of the excess and relative risk of late fetal death associated with 47, +21 and some other abnormal karyotypes. *Am J Hum Genet* 1989; **45**: 855–61.

Marion RW, Chitayat D, et al. Trisomy 18 score: a rapid, reliable diagnostic test for trisomy 18. *J Pediatr* 1989; **113**: 45–8.

Palomaki GE, Haddow JE, et al. Risk based prenatal screening for trisomy 18 using alpha-fetoprotein, unconjugated oestriol and human chorionic gonadotrophin. *Prenat Diagn* 1995; **15**: 713–23.

Parker MJ, Budd JLS, Draper ES, Young ID. Trisomy 13 and trisomy 18 in a defined population: epidemiological, genetic and prenatal observations. *Prenat Diagn* 2003; **23**: 856–60.

Root S, Carey JC. Survival in trisomy 18. *Am J Med Genet* 1994; **49**: 170–4.

Spencer K, Nicolaides KH. A first trimester trisomy 13/trisomy 18 risk algorithm combining fetal nuchal translucency thickness, maternal serum free β-hCG and PAPP-A. *Prenat Diagn* 2002; **22**: 877–9.

Uehara S, Yaegashi N, et al. Risk of recurrence of fetal chromosomal aberrations: analysis of trisomy 21, trisomy 18, trisomy 13, and 45,X in 1076 Japanese mothers. *J Obstet Gynaecol Res* 1999; **25**: 373–9.

Inversions

Inversion. Arises after two breaks in a chromosome have occurred and the segment rotates 180° before reinserting. Individuals with an inversion have no phenotypic effect unless there is chromosomal loss or there is interruption to gene function

- A **pericentric inversion** contains the centromere.
- **Paracentric inversion.** The centromere is outside the inverted area; the inversion is confined to the long or short arm of the chromosome in question.

Submicroscopic inversions. Parental submicroscopic genomic inversions have recently been demonstrated to be present in several genomic disorders, e.g. Angelman syndrome (AS; Gimelli *et al.* 2003), Williams syndrome (Bayes *et al.* 2003). Some progenitor parents carry inversions of low-copy repeat (LCR) sequences and these polymorphisms facilitate misalignment and abnormal recombination between flanking segmental duplications predisposing to deletion.

De novo apparently balanced chromosome inversions associated with an abnormal phenotype. If it is *de novo*, the chance of a chromosome inversion being the cause of the phenotype is possible and the following possibilities also need to be considered.

- The inversion is actually unbalanced.
- There is abnormal gene function as a consequence of the break.
- The inversion is unmasking a recessive allele on the normal homologue.

Clinical approach

Ask your colleagues in cytogenetics to produce an annotated photograph together with an ideogram of the chromosome involved in the inversion. This is an invaluable aid to counselling.

History: key points

Three-generation family tree unless the inversion is known to be *de novo*.

Examination: key points

Ascertain that the phenotype of those carrying the inversion is normal.

Genetic advice

Familial autosomal pericentric inversions

Many pericentric inversions are not associated with a significant risk for offspring with chromosomal imbalance. Of normal offspring, half will have the inversion and half a normal karyotype. Abnormal gametes are only produced if there is a cross-over between the normal and the inverted chromosome leading to a deletion or duplication. All the recombinants have duplication of one of the non-inverted segments and deficiency of the other.

The main issue is to determine the risk of viable imbalance. The risk of a chromosomally abnormal child depends on size and type of inversion. Each individual inversion carries its own risk. This is highest when potential imbalance is small and has been documented in the literature as viable (see Ishii *et al.* 1997 or Gardner and Sutherland 2004). Recombinants of inversion involving 13, 18, and 21 may be viable so offer prenatal testing. Some general principles apply.

- **Large symmetrical pericentric inversion.** Small distal segments lead to the possibility of a viable recombinant. Larger distal segments would result in a greater degree of imbalance. This may contribute to infertility or miscarriage, but have a low risk of a liveborn child with imbalance.
- **Small inversions** are too small to allow a loop to form and the risk of a viable abnormal offspring is low.
- **'Normal variants'.** Certain pericentric inversions are considered polymorphic variants. They appear to have no effect on fertility and no excess of abnormal offspring. These inversions may not be routinely reported by the laboratory, or may be classified as a polymorphic variant on a report.

Familial autosomal paracentric inversions

Madan (1995) reviewed 184 cases and concluded that most paracentric inversions are harmless and that the risk of heterozygotes having a child with an unbalanced karyotype is low. Most paracentric inversions are found fortuitously. If recombination occurs the recombinant products would have two centromeres or no centromere at all and the risk of a viable pregnancy in most situations is low. However, in some cases, it is difficult on a G-banded karyotype to distinguish between a paracentric inversion and a paracentric insertion. The distinction is important because the risk of viable imbalance in the latter case is about 15%. Fluorescence *in situ* hybridization (FISH) or primed *in situ* labelling (PRINS) studies may be helpful.

Recurrence/offspring risk

- 10–15% in families where there has been a previous live-birth with an unbalanced recombinant karyotype.
- Discuss each case with laboratory colleagues if there is no help from the family history. The highest risk of a viable pregnancy will be in carriers of large symmetrical pericentric inversions with breakpoints close to the telomere and the recombinants of inversions involving chromosomes 13, 18, and 21.

Prenatal diagnosis

Prenatal diagnosis by chorionic villus sampling (CVS)/amniocentesis is offered when there is a significant risk of birth of a recombinant offspring.

Management

Family testing may generate unnecessary anxiety and pregnancy testing—consult with laboratory colleagues. Cascade screening of families for carriers of an inversion is not generally undertaken when the risk of viable imbalance is <0.5%.

Support group: Unique—The Rare Chromosome Disorder Support Group <www.rarechromo.org>, Tel. 01883 330766.

Expert adviser: Bert B.A. de Vries, Clinical Geneticist, University Medical Centre, Nijmegen, The Netherlands.

References

Bayes M, Magano LF, *et al.* Mutational mechanisms of Williams–Beuren syndrome deletions. *Am J Hum Genet* 2003; **73** (1): 131–51.

Gardner RJM, Sutherland GR. *Chromosome abnormalities and genetic counselling*, Oxford Monographs on Medical Genetics no. 31, 3rd edn. Oxford University Press, New York, 2004.

Gimelli G, Pujana MA, *et al.* Genomic inversions of human chromosome 15q11–q13 in mothers of Angelman syndrome patients with class II (BP2/3) deletions. *Hum Mol Genet* 2003; **12** (8): 849–58.

Ishii F, Fujita H, *et al.* Case report of rec (7)dup (7q)inv (7) (p22q22) and a review of the recombinants resulting from parental pericentric inversions on any chromosomes. *Am J Med Genet* 1997; **73** (3): 290–5.

Kaiser P. Pericentric inversions. Problems and significance for clinical genetics. *Hum Genet* 1984; **68** (1): 1–47.

Madan K. Paracentric inversions: a review. *Hum Genet* 1995; **96** (5): 503–15.

Madan K, Nieuwint AW. Reproductive risks for paracentric inversion heterozygotes: inversion or insertion? That is the question [review]. *Am J Med Genet* 2002; **107** (4): 340–3.

Mosaic trisomy 8

Mosaic trisomy 8 is a well recognized syndrome (see below) with an incidence of ~1/30 000 livebirths. The abnormal cell line tends to disappear from lymphocytes with age; a skin biopsy may be needed to make the diagnosis. There is a male:female ratio of 5:1. Life expectancy is usually normal and most infants have normal birthweight.

Clinical features

- Mental retardation. Intelligence quotient (IQ), 40–75, but occasionally near normal intelligence.
- Dysmorphic facies with a high prominent forehead and scaphocephaly.
- Contractures of fingers and toes (70%).
- Spinal deformity (65%), e.g. scoliosis, hemivertebrae.
- Cardiac anomalies (25%).
- Renal anomalies.
- Deep palmer and especially plantar creases/furrows (75%).

Identification at prenatal diagnosis (chorionic villus sampling (CVS)/amniocentesis). The identification of mosaic trisomy 8 at CVS is problematic. Empirical observations suggest that in the *majority* of cases there is confined placental mosaicism (CPM) with karyotypic discordance between the placenta and fetus and a normal fetal karyotype. However, the incidence of genuine fetal mosaicism is sufficient that further investigation, e.g. amniocentesis and/or fetal blood sampling (FBS), is indicated. Although further investigations may help to reduce uncertainty, it is not possible to completely eliminate the possibility of fetal mosaicism.

The percentage of abnormal mosaic cells identified at CVS or amniocentesis does *not* indicate the likelihood of true fetal mosaicism or correlate with phenotypic severity if fetal mosaicism is present.

Clinical approach

History: key points

- Brief family tree to include nuclear family and previous pregnancies.
- Detailed history of pregnancy and events leading to prenatal investigation. If abnormal fetal ultrasound scan (USS) was the indication, then the finding of +8 mosaicism at CVS/amniocentesis strongly indicates true fetal mosaicism. However, it is more usual that +8 mosaicism is found incidentally, during karyotyping for maternal age or increased risk based on maternal serum screening.

Examination: key points

- **Prenatal.** Detailed fetal anomaly USS with fetal biometry and specific search for spinal, cardiac, and renal malformations.
- **Postnatal.** Detailed examination with measurement of growth parameters and clinical photographs.

Special investigations

- Amniocentesis (if mosaicism was demonstrated in CVS); there is little justification for repeat amniocentesis if the initial investigation was an amniocentesis.
- FBS (cordocentesis) is strongly advocated by van Haelst *et al.* (2001) as false-negative cases of +8 mosaicism have been described following amniocentesis.

Genetic advice

Recurrence risk

Full trisomy 8 is not viable, but is sometimes seen in spontaneous pregnancy losses; it arises from errors in maternal meiosis. Mosaic trisomy 8 mainly arises from a euploid conceptus by mitotic non-disjunction, i.e. postzygotic error . Recurrence risk for mosaic trisomy 8 is therefore negligible.

Prenatal diagnosis

Following a diagnosis of mosaic trisomy 8, a discretionary amniocentesis could be offered for reassurance in a subsequent pregnancy, but recurrence risks are lower than the procedure-related risks.

Lay group contact: Unique—The Rare Chromosome Disorder Support Group <www.rarechromo.org>, Tel. 01883 330766.

Expert adviser: R.J. McKinlay Gardner, Medical Geneticist, Genetic Health Services Victoria and Murdoch Children's Research Institute, Melbourne, Australia.

References

Association of Clinical Cytogeneticists (ACC) Working Party on Chorionic Villi in Prenatal Diagnosis. Cytogenetic analysis of chorionic villi for prenatal diagnosis: an ACC collaborative study of U.K. data. *Prenat Diagn* 1994; **14** (5): 363–79.

van Haelst MM, Van Opstal D, *et al.* Management of prenatally detected trisomy 8 mosiaicism. *Prenat Diagn* 2001; **21**: 1075–8.

Webb AL, Wolstenholme J, *et al.* Prenatal diagnosis of mosaic trisomy 8 with investigations of the extent and origin of trisomic cells. *Prenat Diagn* 1998; **18**: 737–41.

Mosaic trisomy 16

Trisomy 16 is the most commonly observed trisomy in spontaneous abortions. It occurs in ~1.5% of all clinically detected pregnancies and ~7.5% of all miscarriages. In pregnancies with full trisomy 16, only minimal embryonic development occurs. In virtually all cases, a trisomy 16 conceptus arises from errors in maternal meiosis I. Mosaic trisomy 16 arises by trisomy rescue and there is therefore a risk for maternal uniparental disomy (UPD).

Trisomy 16 detected by chorionic villus sampling (CVS) most often represents confined placental mosaicism (CPM), which can be associated with intrauterine growth retardation (IUGR), but rarely other phenotypic anomalies. Even when trisomy 16 is confined to the placenta, there is a substantial risk for adverse pregnancy outcome, e.g. IUGR with intrauterine death (IUD), stillbirth, or preterm delivery (possibly due to placental malfunction).

Trisomy 16 detected at amniocentesis is often indicative of true fetal mosaicism that can lead to phenotypic anomalies. In Hsu *et al.*'s (1998) series where confirmatory chromosome analysis was conducted, 5/8 cases of mosaic trisomy 16 identified at amniocentesis represented true fetal mosaicism and 3/8 represented CPM.

Clinical features

33 cases of mosaic trisomy, of which 16 were identified at amniocentesis, were reviewed by Hsu *et al.* (1998). Of 21 continuing pregnancies, 16 (77%) had abnormal outcomes including neonatal death or liveborns with some combination of IUGR, premature delivery (high risk: 5/5 continuing pregnancies in Hsu *et al.*'s (1998) personal series were delivered at 29–36 weeks gestation), congenital heart disease (CHD), and minor anomalies. The remaining 5 pregnancies produced infants with an apparently normal phenotype at birth. 10/12 (83%) terminated fetuses had an abnormal phenotype. In 20 of the reported cases the placenta or other extraembryonic tissues were available for study and 19 (95%) had cells with trisomy 16.

Clinical approach

History: key points

- Brief family tree to include nuclear family and previous pregnancies.
- Detailed history of pregnancy and events leading to prenatal investigation. Some mosiac +16 pregnancies present with abnormal maternal serum markers (increased alpha-fetoprotein (AFP) or human chorionic gonadotrophin (hCG)).

Examination: key points

- **Prenatal.** Detailed fetal anomaly ultrasound scan (USS) with fetal biometry and specific search for structural malformations, e.g. CHD.
- **Postnatal.** Detailed examination with measurement of growth parameters and clinical photographs.

Special investigations

- Amniocentesis (if mosaicism was demonstrated in CVS). There is little justification for repeat amniocentesis if the initial investigation was an amniocentesis.
- Fetal blood sampling (FBS; cordocentesis). In Hsu *et al.*'s (1998) series, +16 cells were never seen in >1% of cultured lymphocytes and so FBS is unlikely to provide helpful information (see also table in Hsu *et al.* (1998) where +16 cells were never identified in fetal blood samples even in cases with adverse outcome, e.g. stillbirth or neonatal death).

Genetic advice

Recurrence risk

Low risk for subsequent pregnancies.

Prenatal diagnosis

Can be offered for reassurance.

Support group: ARC (Antenatal Results and Choices) <www.arc-uk.org>, Tel. 020 7631 0285.

Expert adviser: R.J. McKinlay Gardner, Medical Geneticist, Genetic Health Services Victoria and Murdoch Children's Research Institute, Melbourne, Australia.

References

Association of Clinical Cytogeneticists (ACC) Working Party on Chorionic Villi in Prenatal Diagnosis. Cytogenetic analysis of chorionic villi for prenatal diagnosis: an ACC collaborative study of U.K. data. *Prenat Diagn* 1994; **14** (5): 363–79.

Hsu W-T, Schepin Dmitriy A, *et al.* Mosaic trisomy 16 ascertained through amniocentesis: evaluation of 11 new cases. *Am J Med Genet* 1998; **80**: 473–80.

Patau syndrome (trisomy 13)

Patau syndrome is associated with a high rate of spontaneous loss in pregnancy and very poor outcomes in surviving infants. The spontaneous rate of pregnancy loss from the second trimester onwards is 64% (Hook et al. 1989). Patau syndrome, trisomy 13, has an incidence of ~1/9500 livebirths (Parker et al. 2003). 90% of cases of Patau syndrome have a trisomy 13 karyotype, whilst 5–10% are caused by a translocation, usually an unbalanced Robertsonian 13;14. A small proportion is mosaic trisomy 13. The risk of trisomy 13 increases with advanced maternal age but, even at a maternal age of 40 years, the absolute risk for a livebirth with trisomy 13 remains very low at 1/2000. Approximately 90% of trisomy 13 conceptions are due to non-disjunction (see figure) in maternal meiosis I. The majority of trisomy 13 conceptions result in spontaneous abortion.

The median survival of affected infants in a recent study (Ramussen et al. 2003) is 7–10 days, with 5–10% surviving to >12 months. Central apnoea may be an important factor in the short life expectancy. Cardiopulmonary arrest is the most common cause of death. Children surviving longer than average are more likely to be mosaic.

Clinical features

- Growth retardation.
- Holoprosencephaly (60–70%).
- Microphthalmia/anophthalmia (60–70%).
- Cutis aplasia (scalp defects).
- Cleft lip/palate (60–70%).
- Cardiac malformations (80%), e.g. atrial septal defect (ASD) or ventricular septal defect (VSD).
- Postaxial polydactyly (60–70%) and/or limb reduction defects (occasional).
- Omphalocele.
- Kidney malformations.
- Severe/profound mental retardation.

Clinical approach

History: key points

- Family tree. If karyotype is known to be trisomy 13 only a brief family tree is required.
- Maternal age.
- Pregnancy history.

Examination: key points

- Growth parameters.
- Dysmorphic features. See 'Clinical features' above: cleft lip/palate, microphthalmos, postaxial polydactyly. Supplement examination with clinical photographs where possible.

Special investigations

- Full karyotype on pregnancy/baby (parental chromosomes not indicated if straightforward trisomy 13).
- Echocardiogram.
- Cranial ultrasound scan (USS).

Management

Gastro-oesophageal reflux and feeding difficulties are almost invariable in trisomy 13. Aspiration during feeding or from reflux may cause cardiorespiratory arrest.

Genetic advice

Recurrence risk

Recurrence risk is low at ~0.5%. In one Japanese series (Uehara et al. 1999), 0/46 women with a previous trisomy 13 fetus had a recurrence. NB. For some women the maternal-age-associated risk for trisomy 21 may be higher than the recurrence risk for trisomy 13.

Robertsonian translocation (13q;14q). Carriers of a rob (13;14) translocation have a small (1% or less) risk in each pregnancy of a liveborn offspring with trisomy 13. All conceptions that are trisomy 14 will miscarry in early pregnancy. There is an additional small, <0.5% risk of uniparental disomy (UPD)14. (See 'Robertsonian translocations', page 540, for additional details and explanations.)

De novo Robertsonian translocation. It is rare for a de novo structural abnormality to recur in a future pregnancy. If parental karyotypes are normal, the risk is likely to be low, <2% (based on Steinberg et al.'s (1984) figures for de novo 21q21q Down syndrome).

Prenatal diagnosis

Possible by chorionic villus sampling (CVS) at 11 weeks gestation or amniocentesis at 15 weeks gestation. Because of the high incidence of structural malformations in trisomy 13, there is a high detection rate (~90%) on fetal anomaly USS. Given the low risks of occurrence or recurrence, some women may elect for detailed fetal anomaly USS in preference to invasive prenatal diagnosis, with recourse to invasive testing if any abnormality is suspected on scan. For a woman with a 1% risk of trisomy 13, the risk following a normal fetal anomaly USS will drop to significantly <0.5% (perhaps as low as 0.2%, based on a 1% prior risk and an 80% detection rate on USS). Spencer and Nicolaides (2002) have devised a first trimester trisomy 13/18 risk algorithm, combining fetal nuchal translucency thickness and maternal serum free beta human chorionic gonadotrophin (β-hCG) and pregnancy-associated plasma protein A (PAPP-A), that will for a 0.3% false-positive rate allow 95% of these chromosomal defects to be identified at 11–14 weeks gestation.

Support group contact: SOFT UK (Support Organization for Trisomy 18, 13 and Related Disorders) <www.soft.org.uk>.

Expert adviser: Ian D. Young, Consultant Clinical Geneticist, Leicester, England.

References

Baty BJ, Blackburn BL, Carey JC. Natural history of trisomy 18 and trisomy 13: I. Growth, physical assessment, medical histories, survival, and recurrence risk. Am J Med Genet 1994 Jan 15; **49** (2): 175–88.

Brewer CM, Holloway SH, Stone DH, Carothers AD, FitzPatrick D. Survival in trisomy 13 and trisomy 18 cases ascertained from population based registers. J Med Genet 2002; **39**: e54.

Hook EB, Topol BB, Cross PK. The natural history of cytogenetically abnormal fetuses detected at midtrimester amniocentesis which are not terminated electively: new data and estimates of the excess and relative risk of late fetal death associated with 47, +21 and some other abnormal karyotypes. Am J Hum Genet 1989; **45**: 855–61.

Parker MJ, Budd JLS, Draper ES, Young ID. Trisomy 13 and trisomy 18 in a defined population: epidemiological, genetic and prenatal observations. Prenat Diagn 2003; **23**: 856–60.

Rasmussen SA, Wong LY, Yang Q, May KM, Friedman JM. Population-based analyses of mortality in trisomy 13 and trisomy 18. *Pediatrics* 2003 ; **111**: 777–84.

Spencer K, Nicolaides KH. A first trimester trisomy 13/trisomy 18 risk algorithm combining fetal nuchal translucency thickness, maternal serum free β-hCG and PAPP-A. *Prenat Diagn* 2002; **22**: 877–9.

Steinberg C, Zackai EH, *et al.* Recurrence rate for *de novo* 21q21q translocation Down syndrome: a study of 112 families. *Am J Med Genet* 1984; **17** (2): 523–30.

Uehara S, Yaegashi N, *et al.* Risk of recurrence of fetal chromosomal aberrations: analysis of trisomy 21, trisomy 18, trisomy 13, and 45,X in 1076 Japanese mothers. *J Obstet Gynaecol Res* 1999; **25**: 373–9.

Prenatal diagnosis of sex chromosome aneuploidy

Prenatal diagnosis of sex chromosome aneuploidy is almost always incidental, occurring as an unexpected finding in a karyotype performed to investigate a risk of Down syndrome. Surveys of consecutive livebirths show that sex chromosome aneuploidy occurs in 1/400 livebirths but, outside of formal studies, sex chromosome aneuploidies are rarely ascertained at birth or in infancy. The frequency at prenatal diagnosis is even greater, estimated to be 1/250–1/300 (Ferguson-Smith and Yates 1984).

Parents are often shattered by the news of an abnormal prenatal result. Offering information about the implications of the test result for the pregnancy is entangled in the parental sense of loss for their hoped for 'normal' baby. Experienced and sensitive counselling is needed to try to help parents suffering the recoil from 'bad news' to assimilate new information about conditions most are totally unfamiliar with and to make considered and informed decisions about their pregnancy.

Clinical approach

- Take a brief history of the pregnancy, and the indications for amniocentesis/chorionic villus sampling (CVS) that led to the prenatal diagnosis. If appropriate, emphasize that the information obtained was not that for which the test was performed, e.g. increased risk of Down syndrome.
- Briefly discuss what chromosomes are and explain the unexpected findings in this pregnancy.
- Give a brief account of the particular sex chromosome aneuploidy identified (see '47,XXX' page 494, '47,XXY' page 496, '47,XYY' page 498, and 'Sex chromosome mosaicism', page 544) and what the couple might expect if they continue with the pregnancy, e.g. baby looks entirely normal (with exception of 45,X if there is a large cystic hygroma) and would expect to attend mainstream school. Outline management plans (e.g. referral of 47,XXY boy to paediatric endocrinologist at 10 years for consideration of testosterone supplementation).
- Engage the couple in discussing their hopes and fears for the pregnancy, enquire about information they have received from other sources (other health professionals, internet, libraries), and assess and comment on its validity.
- For 47,XXY and 47,XYY, and 47,XXX emphasize how infrequently these conditions are diagnosed compared to the known frequency in the general population. This

underdiagnosis reflects how infrequently individuals with sex chromosome aneuploidy come to specialist medical attention.

- Explore the choices open to the couple with regard to their pregnancy (e.g. continuing with or terminating the pregnancy) and help them to discuss their options and facilitate their decision-making. Discourage a hasty decision as the couple may need time to adjust to their new situation and assimilate the information provided.

Patients suffer a loss when they receive a prenatal diagnosis about their fetus. The loss is often not of the fetus that comes to carry the diagnosis but of the fetus the parents hoped they carried. This grief is profound yet does not preclude a woman's ability to welcome an affected fetus into the world.

(Biesecker 2001)

Genetic advice

Recurrence risks for 45,X, 47,XXX, 47,XXY, and 47,XYY are all very low and probably not discernibly increased over maternal-age-specific rates. Prenatal diagnosis in future pregnancies should be offered, but the indication for prenatal diagnosis is rather weak and there is a fine balance between the very small recurrence risks and the risk of procedure-associated pregnancy loss.

Disclosure of karyotype

See Linden *et al.* (2002) for a full discussion of this topic. In general, disclosure of the karyotype on a 'need to know' basis is advised so that the child is not treated differently or regarded differently by others.

References

Biesecker B. Prenatal diagnoses of sex chromosome conditions [editorial]. *Br Med J* 2001; **322**; 441.

Ferguson-Smith MA, Yates JRW. Maternal age specific rates for chromosome aberrations and factors influencing them: report of a collaborative European study on 52, 965 amniocenteses. *Prenat Diagn* 1984; **4** (Special issue): 5–44.

Linden MG, Bender BG. Fifty-one prenatally diagnosed children and adolescents with sex chromosome anomalies. *Am J Med Genet* 2002; **110**: 11–18.

Linden MG, Bender BG, Robinson A. Intrauterine diagnosis of sex chromosome aneuploidy. *Obstet Gynecol* 1996; **87**: 468–75.

Linden MG, Bender BG, Robinson A. Genetic counselling for sex chromosome abnormalities. *Am J Med Genet* 2002; **110**: 3–10.

Ratcliffe S. Long term outcome in children of sex chromosome abnormalities. *Arch Dis Child* 1999; **80**: 192–5.

Ring chromosomes

A ring chromosome describes the shape of the chromosome as seen by light microscopy. This section refers to individuals with a 46,r(A) karyotype, where the ring comprises a near full-length or full-length autosome. For information on supernumerary ring chromosomes (which are usually very small) please refer to 'Supernumerary marker chromosomes (SMCs)—postnatal' page 552 and 'Supernumerary marker chromosomes (SMCs)—prenatal', page 554.

Rings are created when breaks occur in the short and long arms of a chromosome with rejoining of the centric segment at the broken ends or by end-to-end fusion of the telomeres. There is monosomy for any deleted segments.

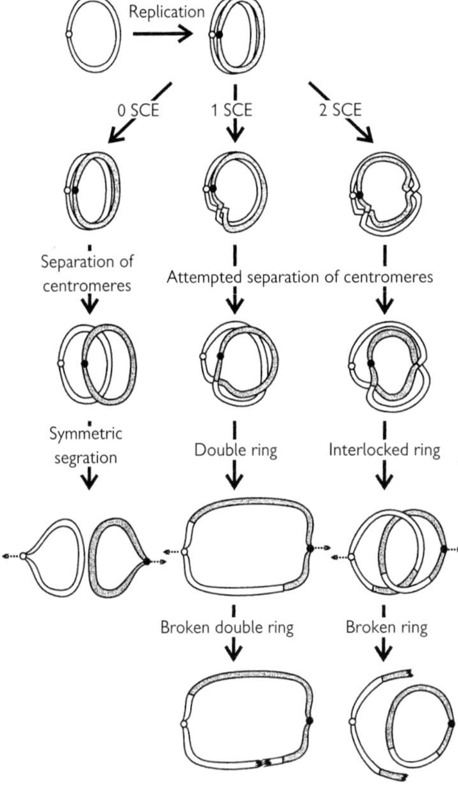

Dynamic mosaicism. The single-chromatid ring chromosome replicates during interphase. Sister chromatid exchanges (SCEs) may or may not take place. At meiosis, if there are no SCEs (left), segregation is symmetric (dotted arrows represent spindles drawing homologues to opposite poles). If there is one SCE, a double-sized ring is generated (middle). With each centromere being tugged to opposite poles at anaphase (dotted arrows), the chromosome may break. If there are two SCEs in the same direction of rotation (right), the two rings become interlocked. Breakage or other mechanical compromise is the consequence. A second SCE in the opposite direction of rotation would restore the situation. (From figure 10.2, p. 180 of Gardner and Sutherland (2004), with the permission of Oxford University Press.)

The ring may be disrupted by mitotic cell division. The larger the ring, the greater the likelihood of disruption (see below). If the ring is lost, the resulting aneuploidy is likely to be lethal to that cell lineage. Mosaicism for the ring is a frequent finding. Dynamic mosaicism (see figure) is sometimes observed, where the size of the ring chromosome varies between different cells and different tissues.

Ring chromosomes are rare and most are sporadic. The ascertainment may be:

- during the investigation of a child with developmental delay, dysmorphism and/or impaired growth—the most common presentation;
- fetal abnormality;
- an incidental finding at amniocentesis/chorionic villus sampling (CVS).

Clinical features

For all autosomal rings, including those rings that appear to have no loss of chromosomal material, there is a phenotype caused by disturbance to the growth rate. This is believed to be due to mitotic instability from abnormal segregation and sister chromatid exchange (SCE) in somatic cells. If SCE occurs, this prevents symmetrical segregation of the daughter chromosomes, predisposing to breakage of the interlocked or double ring. This is the likely mechanism underlying dynamic changes in the size of the ring chromosome, and the tendency for ring chromosome to be 'lost' during cell division. This impairment of cell division may underlie the 'ring chromosome phenotype'. The 'ring chromosome phenotype' is a general phenomenon superimposed to a greater or lesser extent on the phenotype arising from any chromosome imbalance present in the specific chromosome involved in the ring.

'Ring chromosome phenotype'.

- Growth failure/short stature.
- Microcephaly.
- Mental retardation (variable but usually moderate to severe).
- Dysmorphic facial features.

Ring X. A ring/marker X chromosome can arise from both maternal and paternal meiotic errors. Large ring X chromosomes generally produce a variant Turner syndrome phenotype and often there is mosaicism for 45,X or 46,XX. Small ring X chromosomes with absence of *XIST* gene leading to functional X disomy can produce a more severe phenotype with mental retardation, which can be severe (Kubota *et al.* 2002).

Clinical approach

Ask your colleagues in cytogenetics to produce an annotated photograph showing the ring chromosome. This is an invaluable aid to counselling.

History: key points

- Three-generation family tree (unless the ring chromosome is known to be *de novo*) with specific enquiry regarding parental health, development, and education.
- Document developmental history and medical problems of affected individuals.

Examination: key points
- **Prenatal.** Detailed fetal anomaly ultrasound scan (USS).
- **Postnatal.**
  - Anthropomorphic data: height, weight, and occipital-frontal circumference (OFC; children with ring chromosomes are usually symmetrically small except for mosaics with a normal cell line (i.e. those with rings of postzygotic origin) who may be asymmetric due to different percentages of the abnormal cell line on either side.)
  - Document and describe dysmorphic features, preferably supplementing this with clinical photographs.
  - Asymmetry or skin pigmentary abnormalities may be indicators of mosaicism.

Special investigation
- Screen 30 cells to investigate mosaicism.
- Obtain parental blood samples (Li heparin) for karyotyping. Request 30 cell screen to investigate for parental mosaicism.
- Cytogenetically characterize the ring. Use the G-banding pattern to help in identification of the origin of the ring and selection of suitable paints.
- Paint the ring or use chromosome probe arrays to try to identify the chromosome of origin.
- Consider fluorescent *in situ* hybridization (FISH; *XIST*) in girls with r(X). Structural abnormality of the X may disrupt X-inactivation causing functional X disomy.

Management

Search the Online Mendelian Inheritance in Man (OMIM) gene map at <www.ncbi.nlm.nih.gov/htbin-post/Omim/getmap> to determine whether there are any disease genes of specific relevance within the deleted regions. Tumour suppressor genes and other important dominant disease genes may need specific surveillance.

Genetic advice

99% of rings are sporadic, but there are some familial reports. In a few instances the ring chromosome has had a minimal or no phenotypic effect.

For the majority of individuals with ring chromosomes there is associated mental retardation. In 90% of the familial cases the mother has been the transmitting parent. Ring chromosomes appear to be associated with subfertility in males.

Transmission from mosaic carriers (usually the mother) to offspring may occur, and the phenotype will be difficult to predict but consider that it may be more severe than in the parent, since the child will inherit a non-mosaic 46,(r). Ring mosaicism in combination with a normal cell line has also been observed in the offspring of parents with mosaicism for a ring and is difficult to explain. This phenomenon may be due to ring opening (Speevak *et al.* 2003).

Recurrence risk
- **De novo ring.** After excluding mosaicism by karyotyping of both parents, the risk is likely to be low, <1%, but data are scant. This is presumably caused by germline association in a few instances.
- **Familial (usually maternal).** Offspring/recurrence risk is ~40%.

Prenatal diagnosis
- **De novo ring.** Prenatal diagnosis may be offered by CVS/amniocentesis for reassurance.
- **Familial (usually maternal).** As this may involve the counselling of individuals with learning difficulties, take care to ensure that there is plenty of time for the consultation and appropriate consent for any intervention.

Lay group contact: Unique—The Rare Chromosome Disorder Support Group <www.rarechromo.org>, Tel. 01883 330766.

Expert adviser: A. Schinzel, Professor, Institute of Medical Genetics, University of Zurich, Schwerzenbach, Switzerland.

References

Daniel A, Malsfiiej P. A series of supernumerary small ring marker autosomes identified by FISH with chromosome probe arrays and literature review excluding chromosome 15. *Am J Med Genet* 2003; **117A**: 212–22.

Gardner RJM, Sutherland GR. *Chromosome abnormalities and genetic counselling*, Oxford Monographs on Medical Genetics no 31, 3rd edn. Oxford University Press, New York, 2004.

Ishmael HA, Cataldi D, Begleiter ML, Pasztor LM, Dasouki MJ, Butler MG. Five new subjects with ring chromosome 22. *Clin Genet* 2003; **63**: 410–14.

Kubota T, Wakui K, *et al.* The proportion of cells with functional X disomy is associated with the severity of mental retardation in mosaic ring X Turner syndrome females. *Cytogenet Genome Res* 2002; **99** (1–4): 276–84.

Shashi V, White J, Pettenati M, Root S, Bell W. Ring chromosome 17: phenotype variation by deletion size. *Clin Genet* 2003; **64** (4): 361–5.

Speevak MD, Smart C, Unwin L, Bell M, Farrell SA. Molecular characterization of an inherited ring (19) demonstrating ring opening. *Am J Med Genet* 2003; **121A**: 141–5.

Robertsonian translocations

These are named after W.R.B. Robertson who described fusion of acrocentric chromosomes in insects. The human acrocentric chromosomes that may be involved in a Robertsonian translocation are numbers 13, 14, 15, 21, and 22. The fused chromosome contains the long arms of the two component chromosomes but lacks some or all of the short arms. The short arms contain the nucleolar organizing regions (NOR) but, as there are other copies of these genes, their loss does not have a phenotypic effect. Robertsonian translocations can be classified into two groups depending on their frequency of occurrence: common (rob(13q14q) and rob(14q21q)) and rare (all remaining possible non-homologous combinations). The common rob(13q14q) and rob(14q21q) are dicentric structures. *De novo* Robertsonian translocations most commonly arise during oogenesis (Bandyopadhyay *et al.* 2002).

The balanced carrier has 45 chromosomes. The karyotype of a Robertsomian translocation between chromosomes 14 and 21 in a female is correctly written as 45,XX,rob(14;21)(q10;q10) but often shortened to 45,XX,rob(14q21q).

Non-homologous (heterologous) translocation. Fusion of two different chromosomes, e.g. rob(13q14q).

Homologous translocation. Fusion between homologues, e.g. rob(13q13q). The two arms may derive either from fusion in the zygote of the maternal and paternal chromosomes, (in which case the recurrence risk is minimal), or from formation of an **isochromosome** (Robinson 1994). Isochromosomes, e.g. 45,i(21q), arise when maternal nondisjunction leads to the formation of a nullisomic gamete, which results in a monosomic zygote, which is 'rescued' by reduplication of the paternal homlogue and vice versa.

Frequency. Approximately 1 in 1000 individuals are carriers of a Robertsonian translocation and the most common is rob(13q14q) with a prevalence of ~1/1300.

Meoisis. Alternate segregation produces normal and balanced gametes and adjacent segregation produces disomic and nullisomic gametes. Monosomic conceptions either miscarry or do not even progress to a confirmed pregnancy. The main risk for an abnormal phenotype in the child of a balanced carrier is trisomy of 21 or 13 and uniparental disomy (UPD) of 14 or 15.

Miscarriage and subfertility. Pregnancies of balanced carriers may miscarry. Trisomies 14 and 15 will invariably fail and most trisomy 22, many trisomy 13, and some trisomy 21 pregnancies will also miscarry. When one partner has a Robertsonian translocation, some couples suffer recurrent miscarriage, although the majority do not. Males also have an increased risk of subfertility. Egozcue *et al.* (2003), using fluorescent *in situ* hybridization (FISH) to analyse decondensed sperm heads, showed that, whereas 46,XY males have a mean incidence of disomic sperm (for any chromosome) of ~6.7%, men who are carriers of a Robertsonian translocation produce from 3.4–36% abnormal spermatozoa. Munne *et al.* (2000) analysed oocytes harvested from female carriers of rob(13q14q) and rob(14q21q) who were undergoing pre-implantation genetic diagnosis (PGD) and found that rob(13q14q) generated 33% unbalanced, 51% normal, and 16% balanced oocytes (*n* = 69) and rob(14q21q) produced 42% unbalanced, 37% normal, and 21% balanced oocytes (*n* = 86). Males also have an increased risk of subfertility. This is especially true for the 13q14q translocations, which are 100 times more frequent in subfertile men than in fertile men.

Familial Down syndrome. Robertsonian translocations involving 21 are a cause of familial Down syndrome. See 'Down syndrome (trisomy 21)', this chapter.

Trisomy rescue is the 'correction' by mitotic loss of the free homologue in an unbalanced conception. After this has occurred, the fetus may have only maternal or paternal genes for that particular chromosome (uniparental disomy) but the karyotype is balanced. This is of importance in chromosomes that are imprinted (see 'Imprinting' in Chapter 1, 'Introduction') and there are recognizable syndromes associated with UPD.

Imprinting and UPD. Abnormal phenotypes in children with apparently balanced translocations may be due to genomic imprinting and UPD. Berend *et al.* (2000) identified 174 prenatally detected acrocentric rearrangements (Robertsonian translocations and isochromosomes). Only 1/168 (0.6%) non-homologous Robertsonian translocations showed UPD (in this instance UPD 13), but 4/6 (66%) of homologous acrocentric rearrangements showed UPD.

In a later study, Berend *et al.* (2002) assessed 50 individuals with a balanced isochromosome or Robertsonian translocation who had phenotypic abnormalities. 48 of these had a non-homologous Robertsonian translocation and 2 of these individuals had UPD. The two with homologous rearrangements both had UPD. Silverstein *et al.* (2002) reviewed 315 cases (including the above series) analysed for UPD after prenatal diagnosis of balanced Robertsonian translocation; of these 2 had UPD giving a risk estimate of 0.65%.

Consider UPD testing for any rearrangement involving 14 or 15, but note that the phenotype with UPD14 (maternal) is less severe than for UPD14 (paternal) and UPD15.

Clinical features

- **UPD14 (paternal).** Polyhydramnios, postnatal growth retardation, feeding difficulties, small thorax, severe developmental delay, hirsute forehead, small palpebral fissures, and joint contractures.
- **UPD14 (maternal).** Pre- and postnatal growth retardation (similar to those in Silver–Russell syndrome). Small hands and feet, hypotonia, macrocephaly, delayed closure of the anterior fontanelle, flat nasal bridge with short nose, precocious puberty in some, normal intelligence or mild delay.
- **UPD15 (maternal).** Prader–Willi syndrome. See section in Common consultations.
- **UPD15 (paternal).** Angelman syndrome. See 'Angelman syndrome' in Chapter 3, 'Common consultations'.

Clinical approach

History: key points

- Draw a three-generation family tree (or larger if indicated) and enquire about pregnancy loss, stillbirth, neonatal death, and family members with learning disability or congenital anomalies.
- Family history of infertility.
- Family history of Down syndrome (if translocation involves 21).

Examination: key points

- Document any dysmorphic features.
- Specifically consider if there are features of a UPD syndrome if the translocation involves 14 or 15.

Special investigations
- Karyotype your patient if they are 'at risk' from the family tree or the karyotype is unknown.
- Karyotype parents of children with a Robertsonian translocation.
- Consider UPD testing in children with a balanced karyotype but who have malformations and/or developmental delay consistent with a UPD phenotype. Requires an EDTA (ethylenedinitrilotetraacetate) sample from parents and child.

Genetic advice

If a *de novo* non-homologous Robertsonian translocation is identified prenatally, the risk of phenotypic abnormality is very low and arises from the small risk of UPD14 or 15, which has been estimated at 0.65% (Silverstein *et al.* 2002).

If a *de novo* homologous Robertsonian translocation has arisen in the zygote by fusion of the maternal and paternal homologues, UPD is not a concern and the recurrence risk will be minimal. However, if the translocation is an isochromosome (see above), the risk for UPD is 100%. If the translocation involves chromosomes 14 the resultant phenotype will be UPD14(maternal) or UPD14 (paternal); if it involves chromosome 15, the resultant phenotypes will be Angelman syndrome (paternal UPD) or Prader–Willi syndrome (maternal UPD). Since chromosomes 13, 21, and 22 do not appear to contain imprinted elements, a phenotypic effect would only arise in the unlikely event that the parent was a carrier for a recessive condition with a locus on the chromosomes in question that was unmasked by the UPD. All together, at least 50% of all Robertsonian translocations between homologues show UPD.

Recurrence

De novo Robertsonian translocation. The risk is low, but recurrence has been reported (Sachs *et al.* 1990). If parental karyotypes are normal, risk is certainly <2% (Steinberg *et al.* 1984). For homologous Robertsonian translocations consider using polymorphic markers to study the parental origin of the homologues since this will determine the recurrence risk (see above).

Familial Robertsonian translocation. When one parent carries a homologous Robertsonian translocation, e.g. rob(13q13q) or rob(21q21q), their reproductive future is bleak since virtually all conceptions will be either monosomic or trisomic for the chromosome in question. Conceptions trisomic for 14, 15, and most 22 will spontaneously abort, as will the majority of trisomy 13 and some trisomy 21 pregnancies. Donor gametes (artificial insemination by donor (AID), donor oocytes) or adoption may enable such a couple to become parents.

See the table for the risks of having a child with aneuploidy or UPD when one parent carries a heterologous Robertsonian translocation.

Prenatal diagnosis

rob(14q21q). As maternal transmission has a 10–15% risk of Down syndrome, invasive cytogenetic methods of prenatal diagnosis should be discussed. The risk for paternal transmission is lower but still at a level where prenatal diagnosis is offered. Nuchal and anomaly scanning and biochemical screening may be preferred by families with recurrent miscarriage or subfertility, but given the high prior risk a significant residual risk of Down syndrome will remain even if these screening tests are normal. (See 'Down syndrome (trisomy 21)', page 524.)

rob(13q14q). The main livebirth risk is for trisomy 13 but studies show this to be a risk of ~1% for rob(13q14q)mat (maternal) and <1% for rob(13q14q)pat (paternal). Unlike trisomy 21, trisomy 13 has more structural anomalies that may be detected on ultrasound scan (USS) by 20 weeks gestation when a USS has a 90% chance of detecting features of trisomy 13. In view of the low risk, and especially where there is a history of miscarriage or subfertility, amniocentesis may be preferable to chorionic villus sampling (CVS) for a definitive cytogenetic diagnosis. (See 'Patau syndrome (trisomy 13)', this chapter.)

Translocation involving 14 or 15 and UPD screening. If a balanced translocation involving chromosome 14 or 15 is identified prenatally, there is a risk (0.65%) of UPD in the fetus. It is unlikely that the fetus with UPD14 or 15 will have abnormalities that can be accurately assessed by USS, and specific testing using DNA from amniocytes and parental blood is needed to exclude UPD (Silverstein *et al.* 2002).

Management

- **Recurrent miscarriage.** If there is no other medical cause for miscarriage, reassurance that most couples will achieve a normal pregnancy eventually may be helpful to the couple. Consider confirmation of a chromosome abnormality in the products of conception.

Risks of having a child with aneuploidy or UPD when one parent carries an heterologous Robertsonian translocation (after Gardner and Sutherland 2004)

Balanced translocation	Risk (%) of trisomy 13 or 21		Risk (%) of UPD 14 or 15
	Maternal rob	Paternal rob	
rob(13q14q)	1	<1	<0.5*
rob(13q15q)	1	<1	<0.5*
rob(13q21q)	10–15	<1	—
rob(13q22q)	1	<1	—
rob(14q15q)	—	—	0.5 (mat), < 0.5* (pat)
rob(14q21q)	10–15	<1	<0.5*
rob(14q22q)	—	—	<0.5*
rob(15q21q)	10–15	<1	<0.5*
rob(15q22q)	—	—	<0.5*
rob(21q22q)	10–15	<1	—

* Silverstein *et al.* (2002) showed that the incidence of UPD was 0.65% amongst fetuses carrying a balanced Robertsonian translocation. Since some fetuses will have a normal karyotype, the overall risk for UPD is <0.5%.

- **Infertility.** When translocation couples need assisted conception for subfertility, PGD is a valuable screen for imbalance, even when the risk of viable chromosome abnormality is low.
- **PGD.** Consider referral for PGD for a couple with a non-homologous Robertsonian translocation after three or more spontaneous abortions, or if a male with a non-homologous Robertsonian translocation suffers infertility associated with oligospermia (Scriven *et al.* 2001). In practice, PGD is most likely to be considered by women with a translocation involving 21 as the livebirth risk for trisomy is low for the other translocations. It will not help carriers for (rob21q21q) and it will not detect UPD.

Family screening

- Offer chromosome analysis to adult members of the family who are 'at risk'.
- If the translocation has been identified through prenatal diagnosis or in a child, ensure that the child's medical records contain a recommendation for genetic counselling as a teenager and that parents are fully informed.

Lay group contact: Unique—The Rare Chromosome Disorder Support Group ⟨www.rarechromo.org⟩, Tel. 01883 330766; Down Syndrome Association ⟨www.downs-syndrome.org.uk⟩; Trisomy 13–SOFT (Support Organization for Trisomy 18, 13 and Related Disorders) UK ⟨www.soft.org.uk⟩.

Expert adviser: A. Schinzel, Professor, Institute of Medical Genetics, University of Zurich, Schwerzenbach, Switzerland.

References

Bandyopadhyay R, Heller A, *et al.* Parental origin and timing of *de novo* Robertsonian translocation formation. *Am J Hum Genet* 2002; **71** (6): 1456–62.

Berend SA, Bejjani BA, McCaskill C, Shaffer LG. Identification of uniparental disomy in phenotypically abnormal carriers of isochromosomes or Robertsonian translocations. *Am J Med Genet* 2002; **111**: 362–5.

Berend SA, Horowitz J, *et al.* Identification of uniparental disomy following prenatal detection of Robertsonian translocations and isochromosomes. *Am J Hum Genet* 2000; **66**: 1787–93.

Boué A, Gallano P. A collaborative study of the segregation of inherited chromosome structural rearrangements in 1356 prenatal diagnoses. *Prenat Diagn* 1984; **4**: 45–67.

Daniel A, Hook EB, Wulf G. Risks of unbalanced progeny at amniocentesis to carriers of chromosomal rearrangements: data from United States and Canadian laboratories. *Am J Med Genet* 1989: **31**: 14–53.

Egozcue J, Blanco J, *et al.* Genetic analysis of sperm and implications of severe male infertility—a review. *Placenta* 2003; **24** (suppl. 2): S62–5.

Gardner RJM, Sutherland GR. *Chromosome abnormalities and genetic counselling*, Oxford Monographs on Medical Genetics no. 31, 3rd edn. Oxford University Press, New York, 2004.

Gianaroli L, Magli MC, *et al.* Possible interchromosomal effect in embryos generated by gametes from translocation carriers. *Hum Reprod* 2002; **17** (12): 3201–7.

Kovaleva NV, Shaffer LG. Under-ascertainment of mosaic carriers of balanced homologous acrocentric translocations and isochromosomes. *Am J Med Genet* 2003; **121A** (2): 180–7.

McGowan KD, Weiser JJ, *et al.* The importance of investigating for uniparental disomy in prenatally identified balanced acrocentric rearrangements. *Prenat Diagn* 2002; **22**: 141–3.

Munne S, Escudero T, *et al.* Gamete segregation in female carriers of Robertsonian translocations. *Cytogenet Cell Genet* 2000; **90** (3–4): 303–8.

Robinson WP, Bernasconi F, *et al.* A somatic origin of homologous Robertsonian translocations and isochromosomes. *Am J Hum Genet* 1994; **54**: 290–302.

Sachs ES, Jahoda MG, *et al.* Trisomy 21 mosaicism in gonads with unexpectedly high recurrence risks. *Am J Med Genet Suppl* 1990; **7**: 186–8.

Sanlaville D, Aubry MC, *et al.* Maternal uniparental heterodisomy of chromosome 14: chromosomal mechanism and clinical follow up. *J Med Genet* 2000; **37**: 525–58.

Scriven PN, Flinter FA, Braude PR, Ogilvie CM. Robertsonian translocations—reproductive risks and indications for preimplantation genetic diagnosis. *Hum Reprod* 2001; **16** (11): 2267–73.

Silverstein S, Lerer I, *et al.* Uniparental disomy in fetuses diagnosed with balanced Robertsonian translocations: risk estimate. *Prenat Diagn* 2002; **22**: 649–51.

Steinberg C, Zackai EH, *et al.* Recurrence rate for *de novo* 21q21q translocation Down syndrome: a study of 112 families. *Am J Med Genet* 1984; **17** (2): 523–30.

Sex chromosome mosaicism

For example, 45,X/46,XY; 45,X/46,XX; 47,XXY/46,XY; 45,X/47,XXX; and 47,XXX/46,XX.

For 45,X/46,XX and 47,XXY/46,XY and 47,XYY/46,XY please see 'Turner syndrome, 45,X and variants', '47,XXY', and '47,XYY', respectively. The phenotype is generally *ameliorated* by the normal cell line. Sex chromosome mosaicism usually arises from mitotic non-disjunction arising in the postzygotic phase.

Sex chromosomes and ageing. Both sex chromosomes show an age-dependent loss. Guttenbach *et al.* (1995) found a significant correlation between X chromosome loss and ageing with the frequency of X chromosome loss ranging from 1.5% to 2.5% in prepubertal females, rising to approximately 4.5–5% in women older than 75 years. The interpretation of low-level mosaicism for a 45,X cell line during routine analysis is dependent on the age of the patient and the clinical phenotype. In males, Y hypoploidy is very low in boys < 15 years of age (0.05%) but gradually increases in frequency to 1.34% in men aged 76–80 years.

46,XX/46,XY

Apparent mosaicism of the XX/XY type is usually due to maternal cell contamination (Worton *et al.* 1984). However, it is rarely due to chimerism because of an admixture of cells from a 'vanishing twin' or because fertilization involved more than two genetically dissimilar gametes.

When detected at chorionic villus sampling (CVS)/amniocentesis arrange an anomaly ultrasound scan (USS) to confirm normal male genitalia and counsel for high probability of normal 46,XY male.

45,X/46,XY

Incidence, 1.7/10 000 amniocenteses. Individuals with a 45X/46XY karyotype can develop a wide spectrum of phenotypes, including Turner syndrome, mixed gonadal dysgenesis, male pseudohermaphroditism, and phenotypically normal men. There is considerable ascertainment bias in the literature with many cases identified following karyotyping of babies with ambiguous genitalia or severe hypospadias, but prospective studies of antenatally diagnosed cases show that a phenotypically normal male is the most likely outcome (90%).

- Chang *et al.* (1990) identified 76 cases in whom 'true mosaicism' was identified (identical chromosome anomaly in 2 or more flasks/colonies of cultured amniotic fluid cells). 75 were phenotypic males, of whom 72 (95%) had normal male genitalia and 3 had hypospadias (associated with micropenis and abnormal scrotum in 1). One of the males with normal male genitalia had a cystic hygroma. The only phenotypic female had clitoromegaly. The degree of amniotic fluid (AF) mosaicism does not predict the degree of genital/gonadal abnormality (21/23 cases with >50% 45,X were normal male phenotype, whereas the phenotypic female had only 11% 45,X). 3/11 (27%) abortuses had abnormal gonadal histology (e.g. ovotestis), of which one had a Fallopian tube on one side and epididymis on the other. If gonads are dysgenetic there is a risk for gonadoblastoma. In Chang *et al.*'s (1990) study, follow-up was available on 23 patients aged 0–4 years. Development and stature were normal except in 1 where height was <5th centile.
- Telvi *et al.* (1999) in a series of 27 prenatally diagnosed cases found no correlation between the proportion of the 45,X/46,XY cell lines in the blood or the fibroblasts and the phenotype. Mild mental retardation was present in 4 of the patients and 2 patients showed signs of autism. Three males, apparently normal at birth, developed late-onset abnormalities such as dysgenetic testes leading to infertility and Turner syndrome features.
- Hsu (1989) reviewed 54 cases with prenatal diagnosis of 45,X/46,XY mosaicism. Of 47 cases with information on phenotypic outcome, 42 cases (89.4%) were reported to be associated with a grossly normal male phenotype. Three cases (6.4%) were diagnosed as having mixed gonadal dysgenesis with internal asymmetrical gonads. Two other cases were questionably abnormal.

The approaches to 45X/47XYY and 45X/46XY/47XYY are broadly similar except that stature is difficult to predict and there may be chance of tall stature due to the XYY line as well as short stature due to 45X.

Clinical approach

See 'Turner syndrome, 45,X and variants' page 558, '47,XXY' page 496, and '47,XYY', page 498.

History: key points (postnatal presentation)

Developmental milestones, speech and language development, schooling.

Examination: key points (postnatal presentation)

- Height (short in 45,X, tall with 47,XXY and 47,XYY, but see individual sections).
- External genitalia (45,X/46,XY).
- Pubertal development (depending on age).
- Features of Turner, Klinefelter, or XYY syndromes.

Management: 45,X/46,XY

Prenatal presentation. Caution must be used in translating information derived from postnatal diagnosis to prenatal diagnosis because of ascertainment bias.

- Detailed anomaly USS to identify genitalia.
- Postnatal confirmation of karyotype.
- After birth, these children should be referred to a paediatric endocrinologist for clinical follow-up, USS, and endocrine studies to assess the growth and the risk of gonadoblastoma. In a phenotypically normal male with descended testes the risk is low but if the testes are not palpable the risk is higher.

Postnatal presentation. The main management issue is usually the risk of gonadoblastoma. Gravholt *et al.* (2000) undertook a population study in Denmark of the occurrence of gonadoblastoma in females with Turner syndrome and Y chromosome material (detected by karyotype or polymerase chain reaction (PCR)). The occurrence of gonadoblastoma amongst Y-positive patients with Turner syndrome was 7–10%. In such patients the tumour is believed to be present from birth (Gravholt *et al.* 2000).

Genetic advice

Sex chromosome mosaicism usually arises from mitotic non-disjunction arising in the postzygotic phase.

Recurrence risk

After the birth of a child (or the loss of a pregnancy) with sex chromosome mosaicism, the risk is of recurrence is very low.

Prenatal diagnosis

Recurrence risk is very low. Prenatal diagnosis is discretionary.

Support group: <www.ksa-uk.co.uk>; Klinefelter Syndrome and Associates <www.genet.org/ks>; Turner Syndrome Support Society <www.tss.org.uk>.

Expert adviser: Anonymous.

References

Chang HJ, Clark RD, Bachman H. The phenotype of 45,X/46,XY mosaicism: an analysis of 92 prenatally diagnosed cases. *Am J Hum Genet* 1990; **46** (1): 156–67.

Gravholt CH, Fedder J, *et al.* Occurrence of gonadoblatoma in females with Turner syndrome and Y chromosome material: a population study. *J Clin Endocrinol Metab* 2000; **85**: 3199–320.

Guttenbach M, Koschorz B, *et al.* Sex chromosome loss and aging: *in situ* hybridization studies on human interphase nuclei. *Am J Hum Genet* 1995; **57** (5): 1143–50.

Hsu LY. Prenatal diagnosis of 45,X/46,XY mosaicism—a review and update. *Prenat Diagn* 1989; **9** (1): 31–48.

Nance WE. Genetic tests with a sex-linked marker: glucose-6-phosphate dehydrogenase. *Cold Spring Harbor Symp Quant Biol* 1964; **29**: 415–52.

Plenge RM, Tranebjaerg L, *et al.* Evidence that mutations in the X-linked DDP gene cause incompletely penetrant and variable skewed X inactivation. *Am J Hum Genet* 1999; **64**: 759–67.

Worton RG, Stern R. A Canadian collaborative study of mosaicism in amniotic fluid cell cultures. *Prenat Diagn* 1984; **4** (Special No.): 131–44.

Telvi L, Lebbar A, Del Pino O, Barbet JP, Chaussain JL. 45,X/46,XY mosaicism: report of 27 cases. *Pediatrics* 1999; **104** (2, pt. 1): 304–8.

Submicroscopic chromosomal abnormalities and the chromosomal phenotype

Microdeletions not usually visible by routine chromosomal analysis are a major cause of human malformation and mental retardation, and preliminary data from microarray based (array-CGH) comparative genomic hybridization studies suggest that microduplications may also be important. For every microdeletion there is likely to be a microduplication. Deletion and duplication are expected to occur as reciprocal events caused by low copy repeat (LCR)-mediated non-homologous recombination. Some microduplications are already recognized, e.g. microduplication of 22q11.2 (Ensenauer *et al.* 2003), and 17p11.2 causing hereditary motor and sensory neuropathy type 1A (CMT1A). Speculatively, microduplications may turn out in general to have a milder, more benign phenotype than microdeletions, since trisomy is usually better tolerated than monosomy.

Many of the children with known microdeletion syndromes, e.g. Williams syndrome, velocardiofacial syndrome, share a similar spectrum of abnormalities, e.g. dysmorphic facial features, growth, developmental delay, and characteristic behaviour. Even though the differences between patients are enough to distinguish the conditions by clinical evaluation, a pattern emerges of features that are suggestive of a chromosomal disorder. This is called the 'chromosomal phenotype'.

'Chromosomal phenotype'. The features most commonly associated with a clinical suspicion of a chromosomal anomaly were used by de Vries *et al.* (2001) to construct a checklist of features that would help select the appropriate children for subtelomeric testing (see table).

High-resolution molecular cylogenetic analysis (UPD).

With the advent of new molecular cytogenetic technologies to investigate children for previously undetected chromosomal abnormalities, those children

Checklist* for subtelomeric studies (or chromosomal phenotype; after de Vries *et al.* 2001)

	Score[†]
Family history of mental retardation	
Compatible with Mendelian inheritance	1
Incompatible with Mendelian inheritance (including discordant phenotypes)	2
Prenatal onset growth retardation	2
Postnatal growth abnormalities	
Microcephaly (1), short stature (1)	1 or 2
Macrocephaly (1), tall stature (1)	1 or 2
Two or more facial dysmorphic features[‡]	2
Non-facial dysmorphism and congenital abnormalities[§]	2

* It is likely that certain small subtelomeric deletions with only minor (or even absent) phenotypic effects do exist, that are less suggestive of a chromosomal abnormality, and therefore could easily be missed using the checklist.

[†] Using a cut-off score of 3, no subtelomeric abnormalities were missed, using a cut-off score of 4, 11% of subtelomeric abnormalities were missed, and with a cut-off score of 6, 44% of abnormalities were missed (de Vries *et al.* 2001).

[‡] Particularly hypertelorism and nasal and ear anomalies.

[§] For each anomaly, 1 point (maximum 2). Score notably for these features: hand anomaly (1), heart anomaly (1), hypospadias ± undescended testes (1), but other anomalies can be scored up to a maximum score of 2.

Sequence organisation of human telomeres

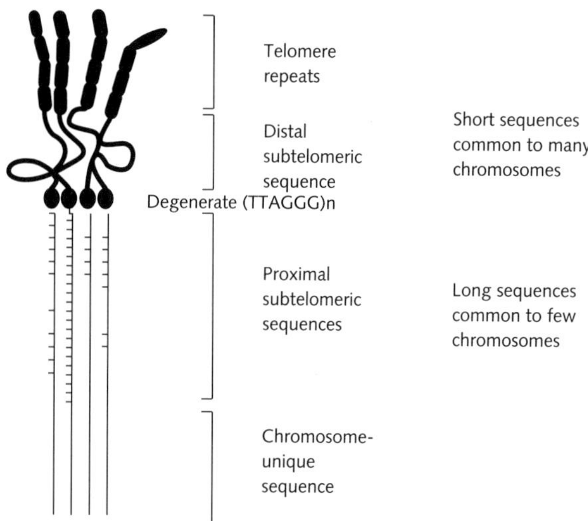

Sequence organization of human telomeres. (Courtesy of Sam Knight.)

whose features correspond to this chromosomal phenotype have been selected for research studies. The first studies concentrated on abnormalities affecting the telomeric and subtelomeric regions (Flint *et al.* 1995; Flint and Knight 2003; Knight *et al.* 1999). Over the past few years, 22 studies have reported results from 2585 patients. The prevalence of abnormalities in the entire group is 5.1%; but the figure is higher (6.8%) in individuals with moderate to severe mental retardation. About half the cases are caused by a *de novo* deletion, and about half by a balanced translocation segregating in a patient's family. More recently, Koolen has used multiplex ligation dependent amplification (MLPA) to screen for sub-telomeric deletions and duplications in 210 patients with unexplained mental retardation and identified aberrations in 6.7%.

Molecular karyotyping using arrays. Newer studies are utilising array-CGH to obtain genome-wide coverage (Lockwood). This promising new technology may further increase the diagnostic yield in patients with unexplained mental retardation. In small studies of patients with mental retardation and dysmorphic features, 'de novo' cytogenetic aberrations were identified in 14% (Vissers) and 15% (Shaw–Smith). In array-CGH, differentially labelled patient and reference DNA are hybridised to arrays consisting of thousands of genomic clones. Several different types of array have been developed and research is beginning to assess the utility of these in clinical practice:

1-Mb array. 3,000 clones are selected to provide coverage of the human genome at ~1 Mb intervals

Tiling array. >32,000 clones provide complete coverage of the human genome

Targetted array. Clones selected to target specific regions of the genome e.g. subtelomeres and known microdeletion syndromes e.g. 1p36(Yu)

SNP array. Oligonucleotides rather than clones are used to give coverage of the genome at intervals e.g. 10k SNP array which can, like genomic clone arrays, be used to identify regions of copy number change in the genome (Rauch)

Polymorphisms. Large-scale copy number variations (deletions/duplications/amplifications) varying in size from 100kb to 2Mb are widely distributed throughout the genome, and a high proportion of them, encompass known genes (Iafrate, Sebat). This unexpectedly high level of polymorphism presents challenges in interpreting the result of high-resolution genome wide techniques e.g. array-CGH (Carter). Until better data is available, parental studies are usually essential to aid interpretation of results from array-CGH.

Newer studies are currently utilizing CGH microarray technology (CGH/microarray; Yu *et al.* 2003; Vissers *et al.* 2003).

Subtelomeric rearrangements. Telomeric repeat sequences (TTAGGG) cap the termini of every human chromosome (see figure). All ends of human chromosomes must have a telomeric cap to be stable. Proximal to these repeat sequences are chromosome-specific repeat sequences, which in turn are distal to gene-rich regions. Since the density of genes in the subtelomeric regions is high, small unbalanced rearrangements, e.g. deletions, may lead to a severe phenotype. If a telomere is lost in a terminal deletion, at least three mechanisms exist to maintain the chromosome end: stabilization of a terminal deletions through a process of telomere regeneration ('telomere healing'); retention of the original telomere producing an interstitial deletion; and formation of a derivative chromosome by obtaining a different telomeric sequence through cytogenetic rearrangement ('telomere capture'; Ballif *et al.* 2004).

Terminal and subtelomeric deletions may be isolated abnormalities, or may have arisen as a consequence of a reciprocal translocation, and be associated with a duplication of the reciprocal chromosome.

Small subtelomeric deletions have been reported in a few phenotypically normal individuals, e.g. 10q and 17p (Martin *et al.* 2002). Martin *et al.* (2002) propose developing 'molecular rulers' with multiple clones spanning the

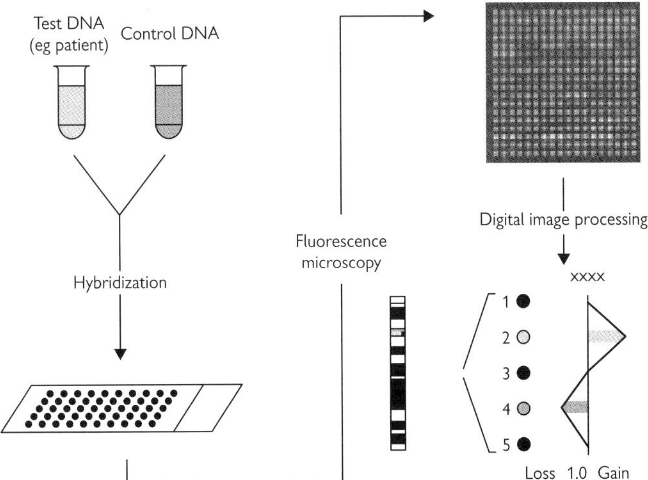

Schematic overview of the microarray-based comparative genomic hybridization technique. Test and control DNA are labeled with a green and red fluorochrome, respectively. Both DNAs are hybridized to cloned DNA fragments that have been spotted in triplicate on a glass slide (the array). Images of the fluorescent signals are captured and analyzed. Red spots indicate loss of test DNA, Green spots indicate gain of test DNA, and yellow spots indicate the presence of equal amounts of test and control DNA. For a precise evaluation, test to control fluorescence signal ratios are measured for each single clone. These results can be translated in a high-resolution overview of chromosomal changes throughout the whole genome.

subtelomeric region in order to differentiate between those telomeric rearrangements that are pathogenic and those that are benign variants. The 2q telomere also contains a polymorphic region.

Clinical features of the subtelomeric deletions

For many of these the numbers described are small (at the time of writing). In addition to features consistent with a chromosomal aetiology, those key features that may give a clinical diagnosis are listed. In many reports the phenotype due to the deletion may be modified by the presence of a duplication of a different autosome. The following descriptions are 'thumbnail sketches' of the phenotypes compiled by the authors; please refer to De Vries *et al.* (2003) for a more detailed description of each phenotype.

del (1p36). Monosomy 1p36 is the most common terminal deletion syndrome (Heilstedt *et al.* 2003). There is developmental delay and seizures are commonly present. Hypotonia is a common problem in infancy, also feeding difficulties and oropharyngeal dyscoordination. Facially, there are deep-set eyes, straight eyebrows, and some have orofacial clefts. Congenital heart disease (CHD) may be a feature and Ebstein's anomaly and other tricuspid valve defects have been particularly associated with this deletion (Slavotinek *et al.* 1999).

del(1q44). Severe cleft lip and cleft palate may be present and it is proposed that the 1q44 region may contain a gene or genes involved in normal midline development. As well as growth retardation and mental retardation, microcephaly, hypospadias, abnormal corpus callosum, and pachygyria are described.

del (2p). Sibs with mental retardation, microcephaly, and cleft lip and palate are reported.

del (2q). The key feature is brachydactyly resembling that seen in Albright hereditary dystrophy together with mental retardation. A common problem is that of 2qter deletion polymorphism, which could potentially lead to misdiagnosis. Always check the parental sample and be wary of the diagnosis of del 2q in a child with inconsistent features.

del (3p). Over 25 cases of 3p– syndrome with breakpoints at 3p25–p26 have been reported with low birthweight, microcephaly, mental retardation, growth retardation; ptosis, down-slanting palpebral fissures, and epicanthic folds are facial features. Almost all were microscopically visible deletions. CHDs occur in ~one-third of individuals with 3p– syndrome (Green *et al.* 2000), and the region includes the *CRELD1* gene, which is implicated in atrioventricular septal defects (AVSD; Robinson *et al.* 2003). Large deletions may include von Hippel–Lindau (VHL) disease gene, so consider VHL screening in these children. Knight *et al.* (1999) reported a phenotypically normal mother and child with a cryptic terminal 3p25.3 deletion.

del (3q). Single case reported with moderate mental retardation with facial dysmorphism, horseshore kidney, and hypospadias (Rossi *et al.* 2001).

del (4p) (Wolf–Hirschhorn syndrome). Characterized by low birthweight and postnatal failure to thrive, microcephaly, developmental delay, and hypotonia. There is a characteristic facial appearance with sagging everted lower eyelids, a 'Greek-helmet' profile, a short nose, and very short philtrum. Patients may have iris colobomata. Seizures are common. Some have a visible deletion with varying breakpoints on 4p; others have a cryptic deletion

requiring fluorescent *in situ* hybridization (FISH) to make the diagnosis. From Shannon *et al.*'s (2001) study, a minimum birth incidence of 1 in 95 896 was calculated. They found that the crude infant mortality rate was 17% (23/132) and, in the first 2 years of life, the mortality rate was 21% (28/132). Cases with large *de novo* deletions (proximal to and including p15.2) were more likely to have died than those with smaller deletions.

del (4q). There have been a number of reports but no consistent clinical phenotype to suggest the deletion.

del (5p) (cri du chat syndrome). This ranges from large visible deletions to smaller deletions of p15 to pter. The characteristic feature is the cat-like cry. Mainardi *et al.* (2001) investigated the genotype–phenotype correlation in 62 patients with terminal deletions. They found more severe clinical manifestation and developmental delay/mental retardation in individuals with large deletions. Their analysis of seven patients with interstitial deletions and one with a small terminal deletion confirmed the existence of two critical regions, one for the typical dysmorphic features and mental retardation in p15.2 and the other for the cat-like cry in p15.3.

del (5q). In the few reports complex cardiac defects, brachydactyly, and macrocephaly have been described, together with variable developmental delay.

del (6p). Several cases with microscopically visible, terminal 6p deletions have been described, and a distinct clinical phenotype has emerged, including developmental delay and severe language impairment, congenital heart malformations, ocular abnormalities, hearing loss, and a characteristic facial appearance (Anderlid *et al.* 2003). Macrostomia and long, down-slanting palpebral fissures may help define the phenotype. The forkhead transcription factor gene *FOXC1*, involved in a spectrum of anterior eye chamber disorders (Rieger anomaly, congenital glaucoma, and posterior embryotoxin), lies in the distal 6p25 region.

del (6q). Anderlid *et al.* (2002) reported a case with mental retardation, microcephaly, seizures, and facial dysmorphism. Lorda-Sanchez *et al.* (2000) reported a child with mental retardation and a cryptic 6q subtelomeric deletion associated with an apparently balanced paracentric inversion.

del (7p). Patients described with the deletion have the chromosomal phenotype but there are no specific diagnostic features to date.

del (7q). Sacral agenesis and anorectal malformations are associated with deletion of *HLXB9* at 7q36 (Currarino syndrome). Deletions may also take out sonic hedgehog *SHH*, and lead to holoprosencephaly. Mental retardation is also a feature.

del (8p). Behavioural and learning problems, rather than dysmorphism, appear to be found in submicroscopic deletions of 8p.

del (8q). None reported.

del (9p). This is a well-known and relatively common telomeric deletion, characterized by trigonocephaly, upward-slanting palpepral fissures, long philtrum, mental retardation, synophrys, coarse features, and epilepsy. Deletions of 9p24.3 have been associated with 46,XY gonadal dysgenesis and male–female sex reversal (Calvari *et al.* 2000).

del (9q). This is a clinically recognizable syndrome characterized by microcephaly, mental retardation, hypotonia and seizures. Facial features include a dish-shaped midfacial profile arched eyebrows, synophrys, hypertelorism, short-nose, antererted nostrils, cap mouth, protruding tonque and micrognathia. Other frequent anomalies are cardiac abnormalities, cryphorchidism and hypospadias (Iwakoshi). Considerable phenotypic overlap with Down syndrome in neonates and infants.

del (10p). There is no definable phenotype but note that microscopically visible deletions of 10p13–pter have relatively mild clinical features.

del (10q). The most consistent clinical features in Irving *et al.*'s (2003) series of microscopic terminal 10q deletions were cranial anomalies including facial asymmetry, prominent nose and nasal bridge, prominent ears, thin upper lip, along with growth retardation, developmental delay, and digital abnormalities. Martin *et al.* (2002) describes a case where a small submicroscopic telomeric deletion of 10q, size <600 kb, has been stably inherited from a normal parent.

del (11p). Only one report. Infantile spasms, epilepsy, mental retardation, and metabolic acidosis.

del (11q). Distal 11q deletions are known as Jacobsen syndrome. Thrombocytopenia/pancytopenia and cardiac defects are the cardinal features. Mild/moderate mental retardation.

del (12p). Little clinical data. Growth may be normal. Digital, dental, learning, and behavioural problems may be part of the phenotype.

del (12q). No reports.

del (13q). Mental retardation, microcephaly, low birth-weight, hypertelorism, and short fingers have been described. Several reports including that of Riegel *et al.* (2001).

del (14q). Blepharophimosis and microcephaly and variable mental retardation.

del (15q). No reports of submicroscopic deletions. Larger visible deletions may lack *IGFR1* and have features similar to those of Russell–Silver syndrome (Nagai *et al.* 2002).

del (16p) (ATR-16 syndrome). Haemoglobin H disease and mental retardation.

del (16q). No reports of pure 16q deletions from sub-telomeric investigations. Patients with ring 16 have been reported with cararacts.

del (17p) (Miller–Dieker syndrome (MDS)). The clinical features of MDS are lissencephaly, microcephaly, and severe mental retardation and the critical region is 17p13.3, which contains the *LIS1* gene. Smaller telomeric deletions of 600 kb or less have been reported in normal individuals (Martin *et al.* 2002).

del (17q). Only one report of a pure 17qter deletion-phenotype may include growth problems, as a candidate locus for Russell–Silver syndrome is at 17q25.1, and mental retardation.

del (18p). No reports of submicroscopic deletions. Microscopic deletions are associated with a 10% risk of holoprosencephaly.

del (18q) (de Grouchy syndrome). Poor growth, narrow ear canal and deafness, proximal thumbs, seizures, and mental retardation.

del (19p). No reports of submicroscopic deletions.

del (19q). No reports of submicroscopic deletions but microscopic deletions may cause a chromosomal phenotype including mental retardation and Blackfan–Diamond anaemia (red cell aplasia).

del (20p). A mother and son with moderate mental retardation, seizures, deep-set eyes, and up-slanting palpebral fissures.

del (20q). No reports of submicroscopic deletions.

del (21q). No reports of submicroscopic deletions. Visible deletions have been associated with holoprosencephaly.

del (22q13.3). All individuals reported have severe expressive language delay, behavioural disturbance (hyperactivity, aggressive outbursts), and hypotonia. The facial dysmorphic features are subtle and variable. Overgrowth has been reported. The minimal critical region is distal to the ARSA probe that is used as a 22q control for del (22q11.2). Wilson *et al.*'s (2003) comparison of clinical features to deletion size showed few correlations. Some measures of developmental assessment did correlate to deletion size; however, all patients showed some degree of mental retardation and severe delay or absence of expressive speech, regardless of deletion size.

del (Xp). The clinical phenotype of the Xpter deletion in males is well described and depends on which genes are deleted (includes *SHOX, CDPX, KAL, XLI*).

del (Xq). No reports of submicroscopic deletions.

Clinical approach

History: key points

- Draw a three-generation family tree (or larger if indicated) and enquire about pregnancy loss, stillbirth, neonatal death, and family members with learning disability or congenital anomalies.
- Document all known malformations in the child and anthropomorphic data.
- Presence of developmental delay/mental retardation.

Examination: key points

Full clinical examination and documentation of dysmorphic features (see 'Dysmorphology examination checklist' in Appendix).

Special investigations

- Note the importance of undertaking parental studies to determine whether submicroscopic chromosomal anomalies are inherited or *de novo* (remember the possibility of polymorphisms).
- Note the particular importance of parental studies for subtelomeric rearrangements, because of the possibility of a balanced cryptic translocation in one parent that may have implications for future pregnancies and for the extended family. (See 'Autosomal reciprocal translocations—familial', page 504.)

Genetic advice

Recurrence risk

- ***De novo* apparently isolated microdeletion or microduplication.** This is very low, <1%, and the recurrence risk is due to mosaicism (either germline mosaicism or low-level gonosomal mosaicism) in one parent.
- **Apparently identical microdeletion/microduplication in parent.** If an individual carrying the deletion/duplication reproduces, the risk in each pregnancy for a child carrying the deletion/duplication is ~50%. If the parent does not have any phenotypic abnormalities, consider the possibility of a polymorphism. If there is a discrepant phenotype between the parent and child,

detailed molecular studies are needed to determine whether the rearrangement is really identical or whether there has been a mutation between parent and child, e.g. a duplication in a parent becoming a triplication in the child and the clinician should consider other possibilities e.g. a microdeletion unmasking a recessive phenotype, or an imprinted gene, or complex inheritance.

Prenatal diagnosis

- *De novo* **apparently isolated microdeletion or microduplication.** Prenatal diagnosis is possible by chorionic villus sampling (CVS)/amniocentesis. May be offered/requested for reassurance. Ensure that the phenotype matches with other case reports or with the phenotype of genes known to be deleted/duplicated in the rearrangement, i.e. that the rearrangement is truly pathogenic.

- **Parent with an apparently identical microdeletion/ microduplication.** Prenatal diagnosis is possible by CVS/amniocentesis. It is offered to those families in which the deletion/duplication is the cause of abnormality. As this may involve the counselling of individuals with learning difficulties, take care to ensure that there is plenty of time for the consultation and appropriate consent for any intervention. If there is no apparent phenotype, the microdeletion/duplication may be a polymorphism for which prenatal diagnosis would not be indicated.

Support group: Unique—The Rare Chromosome Disorder Support Group <www.rarechromo.org>, Tel. 01883 330766.

Expert adviser: Bert B.A. de Vries, Clinical Geneticist, University Medical Centre, Nijmegen, The Netherlands.

References

Anderlid BM, Schoumans J, et al. Subtelomeric rearrangements detected in patients with idiopathic mental retardation. *Am J Med Genet* 2002; **107**: 275–84.

Anderlid BM, Schoumans J, et al. Cryptic subtelomeric 6p deletion in a girl with congenital malformations and severe language impairment. *Eur J Hum Genet* 2003; **11**: 89–92.

Baker E, Hinton L, et al. Study of 250 children with idiopathic mental retardation reveals nine cryptic and diverse subtelomeric anomalies. *Am J Med Genet* 2002; **107**: 285–93.

Ballif BC, Wakui K, Gajecka M, Shaffer LG. Translocation breakpoint mapping and sequence analysis in three monosomy 1p36 subjects with der(1)t(1;1)(p36;q44) suggest mechanisms for telomere capture in stabilizing de novo terminal rearrangements. *Hum Genet* 2004; **114** (2): 198–206. Epub 2003, Oct 25.

Calvari V, Bertini V, et al. A new submicroscopic deletion that refines the 9p region for sex reversal. *Genomics* 2000; **65**: 203–12.

Carter NP. As normal as normal can be? (comment) *Nat Genet* 2004; **36**: 931–32.

de Vries BBA, White SM, et al. Clinical studies on submicroscopic subtelomeric rearrangements: a checklist. *J Med Genet* 2001; **38**: 145–50.

de Vries BBA, Winter R, et al. Telomere: a diagnosis at the end of the chromosomes. *J Med Genet* 2003; **40**: 385–98.

Ensenauer RE, Adeyinka A, et al. Microduplication 22q11.2, an emerging syndrome: clinical, cytogenetic, and molecular analysis of thirteen patients. *Am J Hum Genet* 2003; **73**: 1027–40.

Flint J, Knight S. The use of telomere probes to investigate submicroscopic rearrangements associated with mental retardation. *Curr Opin Genet Dev* 2003; **13**: 310–16.

Flint J, Willkie AO, et al. The detection of subtelomeric chromosomal rearrangements in idiopathic mental retardation. *Nat Genet* 1995; **9**: 132–40.

Green EK, Priestley MD, et al. Detailed mapping of a congenital heart disease gene in chromosome 3p25. *J Med Genet* 2000; **37**: 581–7.

Heilstedt HA, Ballif BC, et al. Physical map of 1p36, placement of breakpoints in monosomy 1p36, and clinical characterization of the syndrome. *Am J Hum Genet* 2003; **72**: 1200–12.

Iafrate AJ, Fenk L, et al. Detection of large-scale variation in the human genome. *Nat Genet* 2004; **36**: 949–51.

Irving M, Hanson H, et al. Deletion of the distal long arm of chromosome 10; is there a characteristic phenotype? A report of 15 de novo and familial cases. *Am J Med Genet* 2003; **123A**: 153–63.

Iwakoshi M, Okamoto N, et al. 9q34.3 deletion syndrome in three children. *Am J Med Genet* 2004; **126A**: 278–83.

Knight SJL, Regan R, et al. Subtle chromosomal rearrangements in children with unexplained mental retardation. *Lancet* 1999; **354**: 1666–81.

Koolen DA, Nillesen WM, et al. Screening for subtelomeric rearrangements in 210 patients with unexplained mental retardation using multiple ligation dependent probe amplification (MLPA). *J Med Genet* 2004; **41**: 892–99.

Lockwood WW, Chari R, et al. Recent advances in array comparative genomic hybridization technologies and their applications in human genetics. *Eur J Hum Genet.* 2006; **14**: 139–48.

Lorda-Sanchez I, Lopez-Pajares I, et al. Cryptic 6q subtelomeric deletion associated with a paracentric inversion in a mildly retarded child. *Am J Med Genet* 2000; **95**: 336–8.

Mainardi PC, Perfumo C, Cali A, Coucourde G, Pastore G, Cavani S, Zara F, Overhauser J, Pierluigi M, Bricarelli FD. Clinical and molecular characterisation of 80 patients with 5p deletion: genotype–phenotype correlation. *J Med Genet* 2001; **38**: 151–8.

Martin CL, Waggoner DJ, et al. 'Molecular rulers' for calibrating phenotypic effects of telomere imbalance. *J Med Genet* 2002; **39**: 734–40.

Nagai T, Shimokawa O, et al. Postnatal overgrowth by 15q-trisomy and intrauterine growth retardation by 15q-monosomy due to familial translocation t (13; 15): dosage effect of IGF1R? *Am J Med Genet* 2002; **113**: 173–7.

Oostlander AE, Meijer GA. Microarray-based comparative genome hybridisation and its applications in human genetics (Review). *Clinical Genetics* 2004; **66**: 488–95.

Rauch A, Ruschendorf F, et al. Molecular karyotyping using an SNP array for genome wide genotyping. *J Med Genet* 2004; **41**: 916–22.

Riegel M, Baumer A, et al. Submicroscopic terminal deletions and duplications in retarded patients with unclassified malformation syndromes. *Hum Genet* 2001; **109**: 286–94.

Robinson SW, Morris CD, et al. Missense mutations in *CRELD1* are associated with cardiac atrioventricular septal defects. *Am J Hum Genet* 2003; **72**: 1047–52.

Rossi E, Piccini F, et al. Cryptic telomeric rearrangements in subjects with mental retardation associated with dysmorphism and congenital malformations. *J Med Genet* 2001; **38**: 417–20.

Sebat J, Lakshmi S, et al. Large-scale copy number polymorphisms in the human genome. *Science* 2004; **305**: 525–28.

Shannon NL, Maltby EL, Rigby AS, Quarrell OW. An epidemiological study of Wolf–Hirschhorn syndrome: life expectancy and cause of mortality. *J Med Genet* 2001; **38**: 674–9.

Shaw–Smith C, Redon R, et al. Microarray based comparative genomic hybridization (array-CGH) detects submicroscopic chromosomal deletions and duplications in patients with learning disability/mental retardation and dysmorphic features. *J Med Genet* 2004; **41**: 241–48.

Slavotinek A, Shaffer LG, Shapira SK. Monosomy 1p36. *J Med Genet* 1999; **36**: 657–63.

Trask BJ. Human cytogenetics: 46 chromosomes, 46 years and counting. *Nat Rev Genet* 2002; **3**: 769–78.

Vissers LEM, de Vries BBA, et al. Array-based comparative genomic hybridization for the genomewide detection of submicroscopic chromosomal abnormalities. *Am J Hum Genet* 2003; **73**: 1261–70.

Supernumerary marker chromosomes (SMCs)—postnatal

Background information for this section is in 'Supernumerary marker chromosomes (SMCs)—prenatal' on page 554. SMCs are usually found postnatally in a few children investigated for developmental delay. The incidence of SMCs in this group is about 3/1000 against the livebirth rate of 0.5/1000 (0.05%), demonstrating that *many markers have no phenotypic effect*. In approximately 30% of carriers of a small marker chromosome (excluding the ~70% SMCs derived from one of the acrocentric chromosomes), an abnormal phenotype is observed (Starke *et al.* 2003). Some SMCs have a well described phenotype that can assist counselling. The two most common are idic(15) and idic(22), where 'idic' stands for isodicentric.

idic(15) also written as idic(15)(pter-q13) or psudic(15)(pter-q12::q13-pter). A bisatellited isodicentric (idic; symmetrical) or pseudodicentric marker (psudic; asymmetrical). The facial features are not diagnostic but severe developmental delay and seizures are the usual presenting features (see below). Maternal age is increased and most markers are of maternal origin. Rapid confirmation of the origin is by fluorescent *in situ* hybridization (FISH) using the SNRPN (small nuclear ribonuclear protein-associated polypeptide N) or other probes for the Prader–Willi (PWS)/Angelman syndrome (AS) critical region. Individuals with a 15 marker that does not contain the PW/AS critical region almost invariably have a normal phenotype. Recent molecular studies have revealed a hitherto unrecognized degree of structural heterogeneity in SMCs derived from chromosome 15, and clinical evaluations show that the degree of developmental impairment is proportional to the number of additional copies and extent of the duplication, triplication, or quadruplication conferred by the presence of the chromosome 15 SMC (Roberts *et al.* 2003).

idic(22). Chromosome 22 SMCs without euchromatin have a low risk of causing abnormalities. Larger markers with euchromatin lead to a variable phenotype from apparently no phenotypic effect to cat-eye syndrome.

Cat-eye syndrome (CES): idic 22, alternatively written as idic(22)(pter-q11.2). The phenotype of CES includes the following.
- Coloboma of the iris/choroid.
- Other structural eye abnormalities.
- Pre-auricular tags and pits.
- Anal anomalies (anterior displacement of the anus, anal atresia, anal fistulae).
- Cardiac defects (total anomalous pulmonary venous drainage (TAPVD), Fallot tetralogy).
- Structural renal anomalies including atresia and ectopia.
- Variable developmental delay and mental retardation.

The prognosis for survival is good except in infants with severe cardiac and renal abnormalities. Parental age is increased and most *de novo* markers are of maternal origin.

Clinical approach

History: key points
Three-generation family tree (unless marker is known to be *de novo*) with specific enquiry regarding parental health, development, and education.

Examination: key points
Careful clinical assessment (see 'Dysmorphic child' page 102).

Special investigation
- Obtain parental blood samples (Li heparin) for karyotyping. Request 30 cell screen to investigate for parental mosaicism.
- Cytogenetically characterize the marker. Use the G-banding pattern to determine whether or not a centromere is present and whether or not it is satellited to help in identification of the origin of the marker and selection of suitable FISH probes and paints.
- Paint the marker and use chromosome-specific FISH probes to try to identify the chromosome of origin.
- If the marker contains euchromatin and is derived from an imprinted region of the genome, initiate uniparental disomy (UPD) studies (requires DNA from the proband and parents).
- Cardiac and renal ultrasound scans (USS) in children with idic(22).

Genetic advice
When the SMC has been identified, search the literature prior to counselling for details of the possible phenotypic effect of the marker. For many of the common markers there are considerable data. If the marker is mosaic, the phenotype may be modified and milder. If a parent of a child with an abnormal phenotype has an SMC, but no phenotypic features, consider whether the marker or another aetiology is causing the phenotype in the child.

Recurrence risk
- For *de novo* SMCs the recurrence risk is very low.
- For familial SMCs the risk of transmission is high but is rarely associated with phenotypic abnormality, idic(22) being an exception to this. Because of the wide phenotypic variability in idic(22), it is possible for a parent carrying the marker to have a normal phenotype and yet have a child who is severely affected (Crolla *et al.* 1997). Where the parent carries an SMC in a mosaic form, the child may inherit this in a mosaic or non-mosaic form. Where both parent and child are mosaic, there may be considerable phenotypic variability (see notes on this point in 'Supernumerary marker chromosomes— prenatal', page 554).

Prenatal diagnosis
Possible by chorionic villus sampling (CVS) or amniocentesis.

Support group: Unique—The Rare Chromosome Disorder Support Group <www.rarechromo.org>, Tel. 01883 330766.

Expert adviser: John Crolla, Clinical Molecular Cytogeneticist, Wessex Regional Genetics Laboratories, Salisbury, England.

References

Buckton K. Spowart G, Newton MS, Evans HJ. Forty four probands with additional 'marker' chromosomes. *Hum Genet* 1985; **69**: 353–70.

Crolla JA, Harvey JF, Sitch FL, Dennis NR. Supernumerary marker 15 chromosomes: a clinical, molecular and FISH approach to diagnosis and prognosis. *Hum Genet* 1995; **95**: 161–70.

Crolla JA, Howard P, *et al.* A molecular and FISH approach to determining karyotype and phenotype correlations in six patients with supernumerary marker (22) chromosomes. *Am J Med Genet* 1997; **72** (4): 440–7.

Crolla JA, Long FL, Rivers H, Dennis NR. FISH and molecular study of autosomal supernumerary marker chromosomes excluding those derived from 15. I: results of 26 new cases. *Am J Med Genet* 1998; **75**: 355–66.

Gardner RJM, Sutherland GR. *Chromosome abnormalities and genetic counselling*, Oxford Monographs on Medical Genetics no. 31, 3rd edn. Oxford University Press, New York, 2004.

Roberts SE, Maggouta F, *et al.* Molecular and fluorescence *in situ* hybridization characterization of the breakpoints in 46 large supernumerary marker 15 chromosomes reveals an unexpected level of complexity. *Am J Hum Genet* 2003; **73**: 1061–72.

Starke H, Nietzel A, *et al.* Small supernumerary marker chromosomes (SMCs): genotype–phenotype correlation and classification. *Hum Genet* 2003; **114** (1): 51–67. Epub 2003, Sept. 16.

Supernumerary marker chromosomes (SMCs)—prenatal

Supernumerary marker chromosomes occur in ~0.05% of livebirths (Buckton *et al.* 1985) and in 0.04% (Warburton 1991) to 0.08% (Hook and Cross 1987; Blennow *et al.* 1994) of prenatal diagnosis populations. In general, if it can be demonstrated that the SMC contains only heterochromatin, it will almost certainly have no phenotypic effect. A number of SMCs may comprise both heterochromatic (predominantly α-satellite DNA) and euchromatic components resulting in segmental trisomy or tetrasomy and, consequently, these may have effects resulting in developmental aberration(s).

Structurally, SMCs fall into five principal groups: (1) satellited or bisatellited; (2) small metacentrics; (3) small supernumerary ring-shaped chromosomes; (4) so-called 'minutes'; and (5) neocentromeric chromosomes. All the SMCs in group 1 are derived from the acrocentric autosomes (13, 14, 15, 21, or 22), but acrocentric SMCs from phenotypic groups 3 and 4 have also been reported.

Some marker chromosomes, e.g. the 22q derived marker found in cat-eye syndrome (CES), contain a duplicated euchromatic segment resulting in segmental tetrasomy (McDermid and Morrow 2001; Crolla *et al.* 1997). Overall, 60–80% of SMCs are derived from acrocentric chromosomes, principally 13, 14, 15, and 22, particularly 15 and 22.

About 30% of markers are familial. If the parent carrying the marker has a normal phenotype, there is a low risk of abnormality in most circumstances. Transmission from mosaic parents of SMCs derived from 22 and 15 to non-mosaic children has been reported but is extremely rare, though it may increase the risk of abnormality or uniparental disomy (UPD; for 15). Another possible scenario is a parent carrying a mosaic 'minute' (all heterochromatic) that is transmitted to the child who is a non-mosaic where the risk is still likely to be low but each case needs to considered individually.

Marker chromosomes may be ascertained in the evaluation of a pregnancy with abnormal ultrasound scan (USS) or serum screening findings, or incidentally during antenatal karyotyping. A *de novo* SMC is found in ~1/2500 amniocenteses.

The clinical outcome of some SMCs is difficult to predict as they can have different phenotypic consequences because of: (1) differences in euchromatic DNA-content; (2) different degrees of mosaicism; and/or (3) UPD of the chromosomes homologous to the SMC. Starke *et al.* (2003) attempted a genotype–phenotype classification for small marker chromosomes based on subcentromere-specific multicolour fluorescent *in situ* hybridization (FISH) and UPD analysis.

Clinical approach

History: key points
Three-generation family tree (unless marker is known to be *de novo*) with specific enquiry regarding parental health, development, and education.

Examination: key points
Detailed fetal anomaly USS.

Special investigation
- Obtain parental blood samples (Li heparin) for karyotyping. Request 30 cell screen to investigate for parental mosaicism.

- Cytogenetically characterize the marker. Use the G-banding pattern to determine whether or not it is satellited as this may help in identification of the origin of the marker and selection of suitable FISH probes.
- Use appropriate chromosome-specific FISH probes and/or paint the marker to try to identify the chromosome of origin.
- 70% of all SMCs are from the acrocentric autosomes and 60% of these will be *de novo*. Prenatal FISH studies must therefore focus on identification of the chromosomal and euchromatic content, particularly of bisatellited *de novo* SMCs.
  - Approximately 50% will be derived from chromosome 15 and, if FISH shows these to be (a) dicentric for the chromosome 15 specific alpha repeat and (b) to contain two copies of the Prader–Willi/Angelman syndrome critical region (PWACR), then this will invariably be associated with a very poor outcome characterized by severe developmental delay, autistic-like features, behavioural problems, and fitting.
  - If the SMC is a dicentric 15 but does not contain PWACR euchromatin, this will be associated with a normal outcome providing that UPD(15) is excluded for *de novo* SMC(15)s of this type. Further discrimination of empirical risk factors associated with dicentric acrocentric SMCs can be carried out using FISH in combination with chromosome 22-specific probes notably p190.22 (D22Z3, Rocchi *et al.* 1994) and cosmids cloned from the CES critical region (McDermid).
  - SMCs derived from chromosomes 14 and 13/21 (these two centromeres cannot be differentiated between using alphoid probes) are largely associated with a benign postnatal outcome (Crolla 1998).
- Risk assessment associated with non-acrocentric SMCs is more problematical and determination of the chromosomal origin (i.e. after excluding an acrocentric autosomal origin) is probably less useful. However, use of centromere-specific libraries of probes will give a chromosomal origin in most cases, and further use of the relevant chromosomal paint will help to determine (if crudely) the presence of significant additional euchromatin. In this context, Crolla (1998) refined the risk of an abnormal phenotype originally quoted by Warburton (1991) from 15% up to 30% in those cases of *de novo* autosomal (non-acrocentric) SMCs that contain demonstrable additional euchromatin.

Management
- Where a *de novo* SMC is found at chorionic villus sampling (CVS) the possibility of confined placental mosaicism (CPM) must be seriously considered, but is rarely found.
- If the SMC was identified at *follow-up* amniocentesis or fetal blood sampling (FBS) in more than one culture or colony, no further invasive prenatal tests are required.

If the SMC contains euchromatin further investigation of the pregnancy is indicated, using:
- fetal USS for structural anomalies;
- amniocentesis and/or FBS if SMC detected at CVS.

Genetic advice

When the SMC has been identified, search the literature prior to counselling for details of the possible phenotypic effect.

- Warburton (1991) reported that 13% of pregnancies with SMCs were associated with congenital abnormalities and that some abnormalities were more likely to cause developmental problems.
- Crolla (1998) gives a 30% risk in those cases of *de novo* autosomal (non-acrocentric) SMCs that contain demonstrable euchromatin.
- Daniel and Malsfiiej (2003) reviewed 77 cases with supernumerary small ring marker autosomes and reported that 30% of the prenatally ascertained cases had an abnormal phenotype attributable to the ring.

If the chromosomal origin is unknown, the likelihood of abnormality in the fetus will be increased if the SMC:

- is *de novo*;
- is large;
- contains euchromatin;
- is a ring.
- Fetal anomalies are identified on USS.

SMC associated with fetal abnormality. Define the malformations as well as possible by detailed anomaly scanning. Do a literature search for similar phenotypic abnormalities in similar markers.

Apparently normal fetus on scan. Usually the indication for pregnancy testing has been an increased risk of Down syndrome. This is a difficult counselling situation. Parental anxiety is high and there may be no absolute answers. Most of the series of prenatally identified SMCs have limited long-term developmental information. It is particularly important to have comprehensive FISH analyses performed on satellited and bi-satellited SMCs as the SMC(15) containing additional copies of the PWACR will not show abnormalities on USS.

- If the pregnancy is terminated, arrange for a full post-mortem examination and book a follow-up genetic appointment to counsel about the risks of recurrence and family follow-up.
- If the pregnancy continues and the fetus is carrying an SMC ensure:
  - that the baby is examined at birth by a paediatrician and appropriate genetic and paediatric follow-up is arranged to screen for developmental problems;
  - that the child's medical notes (e.g. .GP or family practice notes) are marked with this information;
  - that the child's parents know that they should request an appointment for genetic counselling when the child is in his/her mid-teens.

Recurrence risk

- For *de novo* SMCs the recurrence risk is very low.
- For familial SMCs the risk of transmission is high (~50% (?)) but is rarely associated with phenotypic abnormality. Where the parent carries an SMC in a mosaic form, the child may inherit this in a mosaic or non-mosaic form Where both parent and child are mosaic, there may be considerable phenotypic variability.

Prenatal diagnosis

Possible by CVS or amniocentesis.

Support group: Unique—The Rare Chromosome Disorder Support Group <www.rarechromo.org>, Tel. 01883 330766; ARC (Antenatal Results and Choices) <www.arc-uk.org>, Tel. 020 7631 0285.

Expert adviser: John Crolla, Clinical Molecular Cytogeneticist, Wessex Regional Genetics Laboratories, Salisbury, England.

References

Blennow E, Bui TH, Kristoffersson U, Vujic M, Anneren G, Holmberg E, Nordenskjold M. Swedish survey on extra structurally abnormal chromosomes in 39 105 consecutive prenatal diagnoses: prevalence and characterization by fluorescence *in situ* hybridization. *Prenat Diagn* 1994; **14** (11): 1019–28.

Buckton K., Spowart G, Newton MS, Evans HJ. Forty four probands with additional 'marker' chromosomes. *Hum Genet* 1985; **69**: 353–70.

Crolla JA (1998). FISH and molecular studies of autosomal supernumerary marker chromosomes excluding those derived from chromosome 15. II. A review of the literature. *Am J Med Genet*, 75: 367–381.

Crolla JA, Harvey JF, Sitch FL, Dennis NR. Supernumerary marker 15 chromosomes: a clinical, molecular and FISH approach to diagnosis and prognosis. *Hum Genet* 1995; **95**: 161–70.

Crolla JA, Howard P, *et al.* A molecular and FISH approach to determining karyotype and phenotype correlations in six patients with supernumerary marker (22) chromosomes. *Am J Med Genet* 1997; **72** (4): 440–7.

Crolla JA, Long FL, Rivers H, Dennis NR. FISH and molecular study of autosomal supernumerary marker chromosomes excluding those derived from 15. I: results of 26 new cases. *Am J Med Genet* 1998; **75**: 355–66.

Crolla JA, Youings SA, *et al.* Supernumerary marker chromosome in man: parental origin, mosaicism and maternal age revisited. *Eur J Hum Genet* 2005; **13**: 154–60.

Daniel A, Malsfiiej P. A series of supernumerary small ring marker autosomes identified by FISH with chromosome probe arrays and literature review excluding chromosome 15. *Am J Med Genet* 2003; **117A**: 212–22.

Gardner RJM, Sutherland GR. *Chromosome abnormalities and genetic counselling*, Oxford Monographs on Medical Genetics no. 31, 3rd edn. Oxford University Press, New York, 2004.

Hastings RJ, Nisbet DL, *et al.* Prental detection of extra structurally abnormal chromosomes (ESACs): new cases and a review of the literature. *Prenat Diagn* 1999; **19**: 436–45.

Hook EB, Cross PK. Extra structurally abnormal chromosomes (ESAC) detected at amniocentesis: frequency in approximately 75,000 prenatal cytogenetic diagnoses and associations with maternal and paternal age. *Am J Hum Genet* 1987; **40** (2): 83–101.

Li MM, Howard-Peebles PN, Killos LD, Fallon L, Listgarten E, Stanley WS. Characterization and clinical implications of marker chromosomes identified at prenatal diagnosis. *Prenat Diagn* 2000; **20**: 138–43.

McDermid HE, Morrow BE. Genomic disorders on 22q11 [review]. *Am J Hum Genet* 2002; **70**: 1077–88.

Rocchi M, Archidiacono N, Antonacci R, Finelli P, D'Aiuto L, Carbone R, Lindsay E, Baldini A. Cloning and comparative mapping of recently evolved human chromosome 22-specific alpha satellite DNA. *Somat Cell Mol Genet* 1994; **20** (5): 443–8.

Starke H, Nietzel A, *et al.* Small supernumerary marker chromosomes (SMCs): genotype–phenotype correlation and classification. *Hum Genet* 2003; **114** (1): 51–67. Epub 2003, Sept. 16.

Warburton D. *De novo* balanced chromosome rearrangements and extra marker chromosomes identified at prenatal diagnosis: clinical significance and distribution of breakpoints. *Am J Hum Genet* 1991; **49**: 995–1013.

Triploidy (69,XXX, 69,XXY, or 69,XYY)

Triploidy is usually identified after pregnancy loss. Triploidy is one of the most frequent chromosome aberrations in first trimester spontaneous abortions (see table in 'Miscarriage and recurrent miscarriage', page 616). Approximately 7.5% of all spontaneous abortions have a triploid karyotype. In contrast to aneuploidies due to non-disjunction, increased maternal age is not a risk factor and the mechanism of triploidy remains poorly understood (Brancati *et al.* 2003). The great majority of triploid conceptions are lost in the first trimester, but a few survive into the second trimester; survival into the 3rd trimester is rare and invariably leads to intrauterine or neonatal death. Fetuses with diploid/triploid mosaicism may be more likely to survive longer in pregnancy.

- **Digynic** (either 69XXX or 69XXY). The double contribution comes from the mother, and arises due to incorporation of the second polar body into the fertilized oocyte.
- **Diandric** (either 69XXX, 69XXY, or 69XYY). The double contribution comes from the father and arises due to fertilization of an oocyte by two sperm simultaneously.

Gestational trophoblastic tumour (GTT) disease

The cause of GTT remains unknown. If there is a common genetic origin for all GTT, then it is likely that a combination of an abnormality in the paternal genes associated with deletion of a maternal suppressor gene could explain the patterns seen clinically.

Partial hydatidiform mole (PM). A triploid gestation in which the extra chromosomal haploid set is of paternal origin (diandric).

Complete hydatidiform mole (CM). An androgenetic diploid pregnancy in which all the nuclear DNA is paternally derived.

Persistent gestational trophoblastic disease and choriocarcinoma. The time interval between the antecedent pregnancy and clinical presentation of choriocarcinoma ranges from a few weeks to years. After termination of a molar pregnancy, the risk of developing malignant disease, simply detected by a plateau or rising serum or urine human chorionic gonadorophin (hCG), is 8% for a CM and 0.5% for a PM. The incidence is 1/40 000–1/50 000 in patients following a full-term pregnancy. Whereas the tumour resulting from CM or PM is usually an invasive mole (which grows more slowly and metastasizes less rapidly then the highly malignant choriocarcinoma), choriocarcinoma can arise in up to 3% of CMs and ~0.1% of PMs. *All women with a CM or PM should be placed on hCG follow-up* (see `<www.hmole-chorio.org.uk>` for further details). Persistent GTT disease can follow either a normal pregnancy or, much more commonly, a molar pregnancy.

Diploid/triploid mosaisicm

Daniel studied 3*n*/2*n* mosaics and two different mechanisms of origin were identified: (1) delayed digyny, by incorporation of a pronucleus from a second polar body into one embryonic blastomere; and (2) delayed dispermy, similarly, by incorporation of a second sperm pronucleus into one embryonic blastomere. (In 3*n*/2*n* mosaicism, an origin from a diploid gamete is excluded, since all such conceptuses would be simple triploids.) In Daniel's study one fetus with apparent 3*n*/2*n* mosaicism was a chimera (formed by the fusion of two zygotes), and in another instance the 3*n* line was confined to the placenta (confined placental mosaicism (CPM)). The affected fetus with 3*n*/2*n* mosaicism may not survive pregnancy or may survive to term. Characteristic findings are syndactyly especially of fingers 3,4 and toes 2,3, with bulbous ends of the toes and clinodactyly. There may be body asymmetry and streaky skin hyper- or hypopigmentation. Skin chromosomes may be required to make the diagnosis. Genetic counselling is as for full triploidy.

Clinical features

Digynic
- More likely than diandric to survive to the 2nd trimester.
- Severe intrauterine growth retardation (IUGR).
- Disproportionately large head. May have holoprosencephaly.
- Abnormally small placenta, oligohydramnios, and abnormal placental Doppler indices.

Diandric
- Accounts for >90% of cases of partial hydatidiform moles (focal trophoblastic hyperplasia with villous hydrops together with identifiable fetal tissue).
- Symmetrical IUGR with structural anomalies (82%), e.g. neural tube defect.
- High maternal serum hCG (80%).
- Big placenta, oligohydramnios and abnormal placental Doppler indices, increased risk of pre-eclampsia.

Clinical approach

History: key points
Pregnancy history. Events leading to diagnosis of triploidy, e.g.abnormal ultrasound scan (USS), abnormal maternal serum screening analytes.

Examination: key points
Not usually relevant.

Genetic advice
Chromosome analysis of the parents is *not* indicated.

Recurrence risk
The recurrence risk for diandric triploidy with partial mole is ~1% (Berkowitz *et al.* 2000). Recurrence of triploidy of maternal origin (digynic triploidy) has been described only in a few families (Brancati *et al.* 2003). Overall, recurrence risks are generally very low and probably not much increased over background rates, given that triploidy is found in ~7.5% of all spontaneous abortions and a significant number of cleavage-stage embryos (Munne *et al.* 2002).

Prenatal diagnosis
Prenatal diagnosis in future pregnancies is discretionary and not specifically indicated given that most triploid conceptions will spontaneously fail.

Management
All women with a partial mole should be registered for ongoing hCG monitoring following the pregnancy because of the small risk (0.5%) of malignant transformation. (See `<www.hmole-chorio.org.uk>` for further details.)

Lay group contact: Unique—The Rare Chromosome Disorder Support Group <www.rarechromo.org>, Tel. 01883 330766.

Expert adviser: Anonymous.

References

Berkowitz RS, Tuncer ZS, Bernstein MR, Goldstein DP. Management of gestational trophoblastic diseases: subsequent pregnancy experience. *Semin Oncol* 2000; **27** (6): 678–85.

Brancati F, Mingarelli R, Dallapiccola B. Recurrent triploidy of maternal origin. *Eur J Hum Genet* 2003; **11** (12): 972–4.

Daniel A, Wu Z, Darmanian A, Collins F, Jackson J. Three different origins for apparent triploid/diploid mosaics. *Prenat Diagn* 2003; **23** (7): 529–34.

Daniel A, Wu Z, et al. Three different origins for apparent triploid/diploid mosaics. *Prenat Diagn* 2003; **23**: 529–34.

Fox H. Gestational trophoblastic disease. Neoplasia or pregnancy failure? [editorial]. *Br Med J* 1997; **314**: 1363.

Genest DR. Partial hydatidiform mole: clinicopathological features, differential diagnosis, ploidy and molecular studies, and gold standards for diagnosis. *Int J Gynecol Pathol* 2001; **20**: 315–22.

Jacobs PA, Wilson CM, et al. Mechanisms of origin of complete hydatidiform mole. *Nature* 1980; **286**: 714–16.

Jacobs PA, Szulman AE, et al. Human triploidy: relationship between paternal origin of the additional haploid complement and development of partial hydatidiform mole. *Ann Hum Genet* 1982; **46**: 223–31.

Jauniaux E. Partial moles: from postnatal to prenatal diagnosis. *Placenta* 1999; **20**: 379–88.

Munne S, Sandalinas M, et al. Chromosome mosaicism in cleavage-stage human embryos: evidence of a maternal age effect. *Reprod Biomed Online* 2002; **4** (3): 223–32.

Seckl MJ, Fisher RA, et al. Choriocarcinoma and partial hydatidiform moles. *Lancet* 2000; **356**: 36–9.

Turner syndrome, 45,X and variants

Turner described the features of this syndrome in 1938, and in 1959 it was found that girls with Turner syndrome (TS) had an absent X chromosome (45,X karyotype). It affects 1 in 2500 live female births. The majority (up to 99%) of TS conceptions are lost as spontaneous abortions. The rate of intrauterine lethality between 12 and 40 weeks gestation is ~65%.

In some females with TS there may be a normal X chromosome and a structurally rearranged X chromosome. In addition, mosaicism is frequently present, particularly when multiple tissues are tested.

The karyotypes in Birkebaek et al.'s (2002) study of 410 adult females with TS were as follows: 49% had 45,X; 23% had mosaicism with a structural abnormality of the second X; 19% had 45,X/46,XX mosaicism; and 9% had 46,XX and a structural abnormality of the second X (see 'Sex chromosome mosaicism', page 544).

Mosaicism 45,X/46,XY presents the additional problem of the risk of gonadoblastoma and, when detected prenatally, of the phenotypic sex of the child.

80% of the X chromosomes in 45,X are of maternal origin. The majority of TS karyotypes are thought to be the result of paternal meiotic errors that generate abnormal sex chromosomes and the 45,X line is the result of mitotic loss of the abnormal chromosome. Isochromosome Xq and ring/marker X arise from both maternal and paternal meiotic errors. A significant inverse relationship with maternal age is found for 45,X, perhaps reflecting the higher miscarriage rate with advancing maternal age for aneuploid as well as euploid conceptions

Structural abnormalities of the X chromosome found in TS include deletions, duplications, inversions, isodicentric chromosomes, translocations, and rings. Preferential inactivation of the abnormal X is the mechanism that ensures the relatively mild phenotype of Turner syndrome.

Ring X can produce a more severe phenotype, associated with mental retardation, when there is absence of the *XIST* gene leading to functional X disomy. In mosaic ring X TS females, with a 45,X/46,X,r(X) karyotype, the proportion of cells with functional X disomy may be associated with the severity of mental retardation (Kubota et al. 2002).

Sex chromosomes and ageing. Guttenbach et al. (1995) found a significant correlation between X chromosome loss and ageing with the frequency of X chromosome loss ranging from 1.5% to 2.5% in prepubertal females, rising to approximately 4.5–5% in women older than 75 years. The interpretation of low-level mosaicism for a 45,X cell line during routine analysis is dependent on the age of the patient and the clinical phenotype.

Clinical features

There is considerable phenotypic variation in TS. In some girls there may be few features other than short stature to suggest the diagnosis. The phenotype can be sufficiently subtle that a karyotype is routinely included in the evaluation of girls with short stature because otherwise this diagnosis may be missed. The presence of mosaicism affects the phenotype as does the risk of such features as coarctation of the aorta that are higher in full 45,X. Please note that many of the structural chromosomal abnormalities do have specific features; consult with the laboratory and perform a literature search for further information.

Physical features.

- **Short stature** and **gonadal dysgenesis** are the two features found in the majority of females with TS. The untreated mean adult height is 147 cm, but this is increased following growth hormone (GH) therapy in childhood. Physical features such as the short, broad webbed neck, ptosis, and low hairline are secondary to fetal oedema/hydrops. Motor milestones may be slightly delayed.
- **Cardiovascular malformations** are found in 15–50%, particularly coarctation of the aorta and ventricular septal defects (VSDs).
- **Oedema of the hands and feet** is a common finding in the newborn with TS.
- **Renal anomalies** including horseshoe kidney, other structural abnormalities, and agenesis are found in about one-third.

Puberty and sexual development. Poor growth, with no pubertal growth spurt, and absent or minimal breast development is usual. Some women have a few periods and this is more likely in the presence of a 46,XX cell line.

Education. Intelligence is usually normal but mean intelligence quotient (IQ) is generally 10–15 points lower than that of siblings. Mild speech and language delay is common. Individuals with TS have relative difficulty on measures of spatial/perceptual skills, visual–motor integration, visual memory, and attention (Ross et al. 2000). Most girls with TS attend mainstream schools.

Behaviour. Social adjustment problems are common and some girls/women with TS may have physical features that make them different from their peers. Girls with TS may also have subtle perceptual difficulties, e.g. difficulties with facial affect recognition. In comparison with a control group, McCauley et al. (2001) found that TS girls had significantly more problems in terms of social relationships and school progress. They had fewer friends and spent less time with their friends than the control group. Social difficulties appear to be an area of vulnerability for TS girls. Skuse et al. (1997) found that TS women with a paternally derived X were significantly better adjusted, with superior verbal and higher-order executive function skills that mediate social interactions than those with a maternally derived X. This observations suggests that there is a genetic locus for social cognition that is imprinted and is not expressed from the maternally derived X chromosome (Skuse et al. 1997).

Employment. Most women with TS lead independent adult lives.

Fertility. The majority of women with TS are infertile. 31 women of the 410 in the Danish survey by Birkebaek and colleagues (2002) achieved at least one spontaneous pregnancy. However, only women with 45,X/46,XX mosaicism or 46,XX and structural abnormality of the second X gave birth to live children after spontaneous pregnancies. In vitro fertilization (IVF) with donor oocytes has resulted in successful pregnancy for some women with TS. In a recent US survey, Karnis et al. (2003) ascertained 146 TS patients treated, resulting in 101 pregnancies, and drew attention to the ~2% risk for death from rupture or dissection of the aorta in pregnancy. It is imperative that patients are screened by echocardiography, assessed by a cardiologist, and advised of the potential risks before attempting to become pregnant.

Pregnancy may occur in patients with structural anomalies of the X chromosomes in which the Xq13–q26 region, containing the genes that are thought to control ovarian function, is spared; or in patients with a mosaic karyotype containing a 46,XX cell line that preserves ovarian function.

Cancer. Breast cancer is very uncommon in women with TS (women in the general population have a lifetime risk of ~10%).

Clinical approach

History: key points

- Developmental milestones. The rare presence of significant delay or mental retardation alerts to the possibility of a ring X, X-autosome translocation, or other structural abnormality of the X that alters X-inactivation or causes functional disomy.
- Deafness.

Examination: key points

- Height/length. Plot on TS-specific centile charts.
- Neck short, broad, webbed; low posterior hairline.
- Hands and feet. Puffiness/oedema. Short metacarpals metatarsals, especially 4th. Small nails.
- Chest. Widely spaced nipples; chest described as shield-shaped. Breast development.
- Cardiovascular system. Delayed femoral pulses, heart murmurs, raised blood pressure.
- Skin. Pigmented naevi.
- Secondary sexual development and external genitalia (if appropriate).

Special investigations

- Karyotype with 30 cell count to investigate possible mosaicism.
- Consider fluorescent *in situ* hybridization (FISH; *XIST*) in girls with r(X).
- Echocardiogram.
- Renal ultrasound scan (USS).
- Audiogram.
- Clinical photographs.

Management

Hall *et al.* noted in 1982 that one-third of TS was diagnosed in the neonatal period, one-third in childhood, and one-third in adolescence. Now many fetuses are found to have TS after oedema or hydrops is seen on scans performed at 12 weeks of pregnancy to measure the nuchal fold (a USS used to estimate the risk for trisomy 21). The postnatal management strategy described below is for the typical TS individual and may require modification to reflect karyotypes other than 45,X.

Antenatal. When TS has been detected due to the presence of fetal oedema/hydrops there is a high chance that the pregnancy will be lost naturally. For those women in whom the pregnancy is ongoing, scan for cardiac and renal anomalies. When detected incidentally, with no associated hydrops, the survival may be longer and the phenotype milder. For mosaic karyotypes the prognosis depends on the proportion of abnormal cells and on the cell-line involved. Discuss with the cytogenetic laboratory and use reference literature information.

Neonate. Document physical features. Renal scans and cardiovascular assessment are indicated. Give the parents information about future surveillance.

Childhood. All girls known to have TS should be under the care of a paediatric endocrinologist. Short stature, due to a combination of the loss of growth genes on the X (SHOX) and an absent pubertal growth spurt, can be partially corrected by GH in childhood, but the overall gain in height is comparatively small (<5 cm). Recurrent otitis media is common, affecting ~two-thirds of girls (Gungor *et al.* 2000), and a sensorineural dip in hearing that progresses over time has been observed as early as 6 years of age (Hultcrantz 2003). Careful surveillance for deafness is important to facilitate language acquisition and schooling.

Adolescence. Begin oestrogen replacement therapy, starting at the usual age of puberty. Continue to monitor blood pressure. Deafness and autoimmune disease may present in this age group. Schooling and emotional difficulties may require management.

Adult. In addition to primary ovarian failure, adults with TS are also susceptible to a range of disorders, including osteoporosis, hypothyroidism, and renal and gastrointestinal disease. The problems of adult life are these.

- **Primary ovarian failure.** Continue sex hormone replacement. Ovum donation provides an option for some women with TS to become pregnant (see above). The prevalence of osteoporosis and bone fractures is not increased significantly in women with TS who are treated with standard oestrogen therapy. Women less than 150 cm in height are likely to be misdiagnosed with osteoporosis when a real bone density is measured, unless adjustments for body size are made (Bakalov *et al.* 2003).
- **Autoimmune diseases.** Hypothyroidism is a common problem; also diabetes mellitus (15%) and inflammatory bowel disease.
- **Obesity.** Ensure that hypothyroidism has been excluded.
- **Deafness.** High-frequency sensorineural hearing loss is very common and may be a premature variant of presbycusis. In Gungor *et al.*'s (2000) study, only one-third had normal audiometry.
- **Reduced life expectancy.** The life expectancy in TS is reduced due to obesity and cardiovascular disease, mainly ischaemic heart disease but also aortic dissection, which is more common in individuals with pre-existing coarctation.
- **Bowel.** Bleeding and protein loss due to telangiectasiae.

Surveillance

It is recommended that women stay under the care of an endocrinologist, or specialist with experience of TS or preferably a multidisciplinary team (Elsheikh *et al.* 2002) to coordinate surveillance with the aim of improving life expectancy and reducing morbidity. Suggested screening to include:

- annual assessment of weight and blood pressure. Consider tests of glucose and bone metabolism, liver function tests, renal function if symptomatic;
- thyroid function tests—baseline and then as required;
- cardiovascular risk profile;
- bone density scan—baseline as a young adult then as required;
- hearing test (audiometry).

Genetic advice

The karyotype should include counting 30 cells to establish if there is mosaicism. Parental karyotypes are not requested in the presence of non-mosaic 45,X. Maternal karyotypes are indicated when a girl has 46,XX and a structurally abnormal second X. Mosaicism involving 46,XY in the presence of a female phenotype requires consideration of the risk of gonadoblastoma in the residual gonadal tissue (Gravholt *et al.* 2000).

Recurrence risk

After the birth of a child (or the loss of a pregnancy) with 45,X the risk is of recurrence is very low.

Women who carry a structural rearrangement of an X chromosome have a high risk of recurrence and the phenotype may be severe or, more commonly, lethal in pregnancy if the fetus is male.

Offspring risk

Natural fertility is rare. Prenatal diagnosis should be offered (Tarani *et al.* 1998) because of the increased risk for trisomy 21 and 45,X.

Women carrying structural rearrangements are at risk for a similarly affected female or a more severe problem in a male fetus, which may not be viable. Prenatal diagnosis is possible by either chorionic villus sampling (CVS) or amniocentesis.

Prenatal diagnosis

Recurrence risk is very low. Prenatal diagnosis based on this indication should be offered. USS for nuchal translucency at 10–14 weeks and later to examine for any evidence of hydrops may be considered as an alternative (Baena).

Lay group contact: Turner Syndrome Support Society <www.tss.org.uk>.

Expert adviser: Mary Linden, Genetic Counsellor, Kimball Genetics Inc., Denver, Colorado, USA.

References

Bakalov VK, Chen ML, *et al.* Bone mineral density and fractures in Turner syndrome. *Am J Med* 2003; **115** (4): 259–64.

Baena N, De Vigan C, *et al.* Turner syndrome; evaluation of prenatal diagnosis in 19 European registries. *Am J Med Genet* 2004; **129**: 16–20.

Birkebaek NH, Cruger D, Hansen J, Nielsen J, Brunn-Petersen G. Fertility and pregnancy outcome in Danish women with Turner syndrome. *Clin Genet* 2002; **61**: 35–9.

Conway GS. The impact and management of Turner's syndrome in adult life. *Best Pract Res Clin Endocrinol Metab.* 2002; **16** (2): 243–61.

Elsheikh M, Dungar DB, Conway GS, Wass JA. Turner syndrome in adulthood. *Endocr Rev* 2002; **23**: 120–40.

Gravholt CH, Fedder J, *et al.* Occurrence of gonadoblatoma in females with Turner syndrome and Y chromosome material: a population study. *J Clin Endocrinol Metab* 2000; **85**: 3199–202.

Gungor N, Boke B, *et al.* High frequency hearing loss in Ullrich–Turner syndrome. *Eur J Pediatr* 2000; **159** (10): 740–4.

Guttenbach M, Koschorz B, *et al.* Sex chromosome loss and aging: *in situ* hybridization studies on human interphase nuclei. *Am J Hum Genet* 1995; **57** (5): 1143–50.

Hall JG, Sybert VP, Williamson RA, Fisher NL, Reed SD. Turner's syndrome. *West J Med* 1982; **137**: 32–44.

Hultcrantz M. Ear and hearing problems in Turner's syndrome. *Acta Otolaryngol* 2003; **123** (2): 253–7.

Karnis MF, Zimon AE, *et al.* Risk of death in pregnancy achieved through oocyte donation in patients with Turner syndrome: a national survey. *Fertil Steril* 2003; **80** (3): 498–501.

Kubota T, Wakui K, *et al.* The proportion of cells with functional X disomy is associated with the severity of mental retardation in mosaic ring X Turner syndrome females. *Cytogenet Genome Res* 2002; **99** (1–4): 276–84.

Linden MG, Bender BG. Fifty-one prenatally diagnosed children and adolescents with sex chromosome anomalies. *Am J Med Genet* 2002; **110**: 11–18.

Linden MG, Bender BG, Robinson A. Genetic counselling for sex chromosome abnormalities. *Am J Med Genet* 2002; **110**: 3–10.

McCauley E, Feuillan P, *et al.* Psychosocial development in adolescents with Turner syndrome. *J Dev Behav Pediatr* 2001; **22** (6): 360–5.

Ranke MB, Saenger P. Turner's syndrome. *Lancet* 2001; **358**: 309–14.

Ross JL, D. Roeltgen D, Feuillan P, Kushner H, Cutler GB Jr. Use of estrogen in young girls with Turner syndrome: effects on memory. *Neurology* 2000; **54**: 164.

Ross JL, Stefanotos GA, *et al.* Persistent cognitive deficits in adult women with Turner syndrome. *Neurology* 2002; **58**: 218–25.

Saenger P. Wikland KA, *et al.* Recommendations for the diagnosis and management of Turner syndrome [review]. *J Clin Endocrinol Metab* 2001; **86**: 3061–9.

Sebire NJ, Snijders RJ, *et al.* Detection of sex chromosome abnormalities by nuchal translucency screening at 10–14/40. *Prenat Diagn* 1998; **18**: 581–4.

Skuse DH, James RS, *et al.* Evidence from Turner's syndrome of an imprinted X-linked locus affecting cognitive function. *Nature* 1997; **387** (6634): 705–8.

Swerdlow AJ, Hermon C, *et al.* Mortality and cancer incidence in persons with numerical sex chromosome abnormalities: a cohort study. *Ann Hum Genet* 2001; **65** (pt. 2): 177–88.

Sybert VP, McCauley E. Turner's syndrome. *NESM* 2004; **351**: 1227–28.

Tarani L, Lampariello S, *et al.* Pregnancy in patients with Turner's syndrome: six new cases and review of literature. *Gynecol Endocrinol* 1998; **12** (2): 83–7.

Therman E, Susman B. The similarity of phenotypic effects caused by Xp and Xq deletions in the human female: a hypothesis. *Hum Genet* 1990; **90**: 185–6.

Uematsu A, Yorifuji T, Muroi J, Mamada M, Kaji M, Yamanaka C, Momoi T, Nakahat T. Parental origin of normal X chromosome in Turner syndrome with various karyotypes: implications for the mechanism leading to generation of a 45,X karyotype. *Am J Med Genet* 2002; **111**: 134–9.

X-autosome translocations

Translocations between an X chromosome and an autosome are different to autosomal translocations, and genetic counselling is more complex, for the following reasons.

X inactivation. In women a single X chromosome is functional per diploid adult cell. The other X is described as inactive and this inactivation occurs by the second week following conception. X-inactivation in the embryo is usually a random process. Usually the ratio approximates to 50%. This process is genetically controlled from the X inactivation centre. The *XIST* gene, in the X inactivation centre at Xq13, is a *cis*-acting gene and only transcribed in the inactive X. Methylation maintains inactivation. X-inactivation patterns may be assessed by comparing the ratio of the two alleles at a highly polymorphic site, e.g. the CA repeat in the androgen receptor gene, in a non-methylation sensitive assay with the ratio of the same alleles in a methylation-sensitive assay. The genes at the tip of the short arm of the X in Xp22.3 escape inactivation; this area is known as the pseudoautosomal region (PAR).

Functional disomy. The genes on each X are active— one copy has escaped inactivation. An abnormal phenotype results from overexpression of the affected genes. An important mechanism both in females with apparently balanced X;autosome translocations and in association with X duplications.

X inactivation pattern observed in balanced female carriers

Those cells in which the intact X remained active would have functional disomy (see above) for the part of the X that is unable to inactivate because of the translocation. There is selection against this and, in the majority of balanced carriers:

- the 'normal' X that is not involved in the translocation is inactive;
- the two parts of the translocated X are active.

However, in these balanced carriers phenotypic abnormalities may arise:

- if the chromosomal breakpoint is through a gene;
- if the active X carries an X-linked mutation;
- if the 'skewing' of X-inactivation varies between different tissues (Hatchwell *et al.* 1996).

In those carriers where the intact X remains active, the genes that are functionally disomic can lead to phenotypic features and developmental delay (e.g. in hypomelanosis of Ito). Also contributing to the phenotype is the possibility of spreading inactivation of genes from the derivative chromosome carrying the X-chromosome inactivation centre (Xic) into the contiguous region of the autosome.

X inactivation pattern observed in unbalanced females

The situation is reversed and selective inactivation of the *abnormal* X (as long as it contains the Xic) gives a milder than expected phenotype. Additionally, spreading of inactivation on to the autosome results in a reduction of trisomy of that section to functional disomy. If there is no Xic in the translocated X, there will be functional partial disomy of the X and autosomal monosomy.

Clinical features

X-linked disease in a female proband. X-autosome translocations that disrupt a disease-gene on the X can result in manifestation of the disease in a female, e.g. X-autosome translocations with a breakpoint in Xp21.2 can account for clinical signs of Duchenne muscular dystrophy (DMD) and Becker muscular dystrophy (BMD). Translocations lead to skewed X-inactivation of the normal dystrophin gene at an early stage of development as there is selection for cells where the normal X is inactive.

Hypomelanosis of Ito is characterized by swirly disturbances of skin pigmentation over the trunk and linear or streaky pigmentary disturbance over the limbs. It is known to be associated in many cases with chromosomal mosaicism. While no particular pattern is generally evident for the specific chromosomes involved in such patients, a subgroup of female patients exists in whom the common factor is the presence of a balanced, constitutional X; autosome translocation, with a cytogenetic breakpoint in the pericentromeric region of the X. The phenotype in these cases may result not from the interruption of X linked genes but from the presence of mosaic functional disomy of X sequences above the breakpoint (Hatchwell 1996).

Infertility.

- **Female infertility.** Some female carriers of X-autosome translocations may be infertile. There are critical regions of the X chromosome (Xq13–q22 and Xq22–27) which, if involved with the translocation, may be associated with gonadal dysgenesis (Therman *et al.* 1990). These women are at risk from primary amenorrhoea or premature ovarian failure.
- **Male infertility.** Males with X-autosome translocations are infertile.

Clinical approach

Ask your colleagues in cytogenetics to produce an annotated photograph together with an ideogram of the chromosomes involved in the translocation. This is an invaluable aid to counselling.

History: key points

- Draw a three-generation family tree (or larger if indicated with particular attention to the maternal line) and enquire about pregnancy loss, stillbirth, neonatal death, and family members with learning disability or congenital anomalies.
- Males with infertility (carriers (?)).
- Ovarian failure.
- Presence of developmental delay.
- Conditions that may be X-linked.

Examination: key points

- Full clinical examination and documentation of dysmorphic features.
- Neurocutaneous features, especially pigmentary disturbance (hypomelanosis of Ito).

Special investigations

Arrange for parental chromosome analysis.

Genetic advice

- **De novo.** X-autosome translocations are usually of paternal origin.
- **Mother also has an X-autosome translocation.** Discuss with the laboratory the theoretical outcomes of segregation at meiosis. The differences between this

type of translocation and an autosomal translocation include the following.

- A rearrangement with functional disomy of part of the X is likely to have a phenotypic effect and this includes a risk of severe mental retardation.
- There may be partial Turner, Klinefelter, or XXX syndromes.
- The viability of an autosomal imbalance may be improved because of spreading inactivation such that the abnormality is viable but has a risk of severe phenotypic abnormality.
- Apparently balanced male hemizygotes have been reported with both normal and abnormal phenotypes making phenotypic prediction on the basis of the karyotype difficult.

Recurrence risk

- **De novo.** Very low
- **Maternal.** Although there is a high risk of imbalance, the difficulty lies in predicting the likely phenotypic effect. Even in mothers and babies with the same chromosome change the phenotype may be variable.

Prenatal diagnosis

Because of the difficulty in predicting X inactivation, only 46,XX and 46,XY are accurate predictors of a normal phenotype. Ultrasound for evidence of structural abnormality.

Support group contact: Unique—The Rare Chromosome Disorder Support Group <www.rarechromo.org>, Tel. 01883 330766.

Expert adviser: Anonymous.

References

Gardner RJM, Sutherland GR. *Chromosome abnormalities and genetic counselling*, Oxford Monographs on Medical Genetics no. 31, 3rd edn. Oxford University Press, New York, 2004.

Hatchwell E. Hypomelanosis of Ito and X; autosome translocations: a unifying hypothesis. *J Med Genet* 1996; **33:** 177–83.

Hatchwell E, Robinson D, *et al.* X inactivation analysis in a female with hypomelanosis of Ito associated with a balanced X;17 translocation: evidence for functional disomy of Xp. *J Med Genet* 1996; **33** (3): 216–20.

Powell CM, Taggart RT, *et al.* Molecular and cytogenetic studies of an X;autosome translocation in a patient with premature ovarian failure and review of the literature. *Am J Med Genet* 1994; **52** (1): 19–26.

Sharp AJ, Spotswood HT, *et al.* Molecular and cytogenetic analysis of the spreading of X inactivation in X; autosome translocations. *Hum Mol Genet* 2002; **11:** 3145–56.

Therman E, Laxova R, *et al.* The critical region on the human Xq. *Hum Genet* 1990; **85:** 455–61.

Chapter 6

Pregnancy and fertility

Chapter contents

Anterior abdominal wall defects 566

Assisted reproductive technology: *in vitro* fertilization (IVF), intracytoplasmic sperm injection (ICSI), and pre-implantation genetic diagnosis (PGD) 568

Bowed limbs 572

Club-foot (talipes) 574

Congenital cystic lung lesions, Currarino syndrome, and sacrococcygeal teratoma 576

Congenital diaphragmatic hernia 578

Cytomegalovirus (CMV) 580

Dandy–Walker malformation 582

Drugs in pregnancy 584

Female infertility and amenorrhoea: genetic aspects 586

Fetal alcohol syndrome (FAS) 588

Fetal anticonvulsant syndrome (FACS) 590

Fetomaternal alloimmunization (rhesus D and thrombocytopenia) 592

Hyperechogenic bowel 594

Hypoplastic left heart 596

Imaging in prenatal diagnosis 598

Invasive techniques and genetic tests in prenatal diagnosis 600

Low maternal serum oestriol 604

Male infertility: genetic aspects 606

Maternal age 610

Maternal diabetes mellitus and diabetic embryopathy 612

Maternal phenylketonuria (PKU) 614

Miscarriage and recurrent miscarriage 616

Oedema—increased nuchal translucency, cystic hygroma, and hydrops 618

Premature ovarian failure (POF) 620

Radiation exposure, chemotherapy and landfill sites 622

Renal tract anomalies 624

Rubella 628

Short limbs 630

Toxoplasmosis 634

Twins and twinning 636

Varicella 640

Ventriculomegaly 642

Anterior abdominal wall defects

The overall prevalence is 4.3/10 000 births. The frequent use of antenatal ultrasound scan (USS) and maternal serum alpha-fetoprotein (AFP) has increasingly led to the detection of abdominal wall defects before birth. The sensitivity of USS detection is ~95% for both gastroschisis and exomphalos (RCOG). There should be close liason with neonatal intensive care and paediatric surgery regarding perinatal management. Currently, there is no convincing evidence to support routine lower segment Caesarean section (LSCS) for most abdominal wall defects.

Gastroschisis

Gastroschisis involves herniation of gut and occasionally genitourinary tract through an abdominal wall defect to one side (usually the right) of the umbilicus. The defect arises through incomplete closure of the lateral folds of the embryo during the sixth week of gestation. No membrane covers the loops, which float free in the amniotic fluid. Intestinal atresia may occur as a complication of gastroschisis.

Gastroschisis is usually an isolated defect; only 5% of cases have other anomalies. There is no appreciable increase in the incidence of aneuploidy in isolated gastroschisis. Amniocentesis is not indicated if gastroschisis is an isolated finding.

Gastroschisis is strongly associated with young maternal age, mothers under 20 being 12 times more likely to have infants with gastroschisis. The total prevalence of gastroschisis has changed from 0.29/10 000 births in 1974 to 1.66/10 000 in 1998 (Di Tanna *et al.* 2002). The speed at which the increase has occurred suggests environmental rather than genetic risk factors. Of livebirths with isolated gastroschisis in the Northern Region study (Rankin *et al.* 1999), 92.3% were alive at 1 year. The pregnancy should be monitored closely and delivery planned for ~37 weeks gestation. Perinatal management involves normal delivery in a high-risk unit, with cling film applied over the externalized bowel loops immediately after delivery. Note the association with amyoplasia and intestinal atresia (Reid *et al.* 1986).

Exomphalos

Exomphalos (omphalocele) is a midline defect with herniation of abdominal contents into the base of the umbilical cord, confined by an amnioperitoneal membrane. In a large exomphalos, liver as well as intestine may be present in the sac. There is a high incidence of aneuploidy (30%), especially +18 and +13, and the finding of an exomphalos is an indication for karyotyping, e.g. by amniocentesis. Overall, in two-thirds of cases (including those with aneuploidy), there are other structural anomalies, often multiple, especially congenital heart disease (CHD); in one-third the exomphalos is an isolated anomaly. Of livebirths with isolated exomphalos and a normal karyotype, 95.5% were alive at 1 year.

Exomphalos is a feature of Beckwith–Wiedemann syndrome (BWS; also characterized by macrosomia, macroglossia, and nephromegaly). If any of these features or large placenta/polyhdramnios are present, carefully consider this diagnosis (see 'Beckwith–Wiedemann syndrome (BWS)' page 278).

Perinatal management involves aiming for a vaginal delivery in a hospital with a neonatal unit, unless the exomphalos is large in which case delivery should be planned at a high-risk perinatal centre. There is an increased incidence of respiratory distress syndrome, and blood sugar should be monitored in view of the association with BWS. The baby should be transferred after delivery for treatment in a paediatric surgical centre.

Bladder exstrophy

Bladder exstrophy has an incidence of 1/10 000–1/40 000 births and is more common in males (2.3M:1F). It is caused by incomplete closure of the inferior part of the anterior abdominal wall. The defect starts at 4 weeks gestation and is caused by failure of migration of mesenchymal cells between the ectoderm of the abdomen and cloaca. Separation of the pubic bones, a low-set umbilicus, and abnormal genitalia are associated anomalies. Surgical intervention is required to reconstruct the bladder, abdominal wall, and genitalia, with initial surgery usually performed within the first 48 hours after birth.

OEIS (omphalocele and epispadias–exstrophy of the bladder–imperforate anus–spinal anomalies) complex

OEIS is a spectrum of developmental anomalies of increasing severity. OEIS is rare, affecting ~1/200 000. It is probably sporadic with a low recurrence risk, but affected individuals have not reproduced. The majority of males with OEIS have extremely abnormal genitalia.

Body wall complex (Body stalk anomaly)

Presence of body wall defects with evisceration of thoracic and/or abdominal organs, often in association with neural tube defect and/or limb deficiency. Scoliosis, abnormalities of the lower extremities and a short/absent umbilical cord are common features. Maternal serum AFP is usually markedly elevated.

Clinical assessment

Examination: key points

Detailed fetal anomaly USS to search for other anomalies and assess fetal growth.

Special investigations.

Offer amniocentesis for karyotype in selected cases e.g. exomphalos.

Genetic advice and management

- **Gastroschisis.** Isolated gastroschisis has a low sibling recurrence risk of ~1%. For a parent with gastroschisis, the offspring risk is low, with only 2 reported cases of parent-child occurrence (Schmidt).
- **Exomphalos.** Isolated exomphalos has a low sibling recurrence risk of ~1%.
- **Bladder exstrophy** is usually a sporadic defect, although occasional familial cases have been reported. Recurrence risk is ~1%. For a parent with bladder exstrophy, the risk to offspring is ~1/70.
- **OEIS** is probably sporadic with a low recurrence risk, but affected individuals have not reproduced.
- **Body wall complex** is probably sporadic with a low recurrence risk.

Support group: GEEPS (Gastroschisis, Exomphalos, Extrophies Parents' Support Group) <www.geeps.org>

Expert adviser: Lyn Chitty, Consultant in Genetics and Fetal Medicine, University College Hospital, London, England.

References

Anteby EY, Yagel S. Route of delivery of fetuses with structural anomalies. *Eur J Obstet Gynecol Reprod Biol* 2003; **106**: 5–9.

Curry J, *et al.* The aetiology of gastroschisis. *Br J Obstet Gynaecol* 2000; **107**: 1339–46.

Di Tanna GL, Rosano A, Mastroiacovo P. Prevalence of gastroschisis at birth: retrospective study. *Br Med J* 2002; **325**: 1389–90.

Heider AL, Strauss RA, *et al.* Omphalocele 'Clinical outcomes in cases with normal kearyotypes. *Am J Obstet Gynecol* 2004; **190**: 135–41.

Rankin J, Dillon E, *et al.* Congenital anterior abdominal wall defects in the North of England, 1986–1996; occurrence and outcome. *Prenat Diagn* 1999; **19**: 662–8.

Reid CO, Hall JG, *et al.* Association of amyoplasia with gastroschisis, bowel atresia and defects of the muscular layer of the trunk. *Am J Med Genet* 1986; **24**: 701–10.

Salihu HM, Boos R, Schmidt W, *et al.* Omphalocele and gastroschisis. *J Obstet Gynecol* 2002; **22**: 489–92.

Schmidt AI, Gluer S, *et al.* Family cases of gastroschisis. *J Pediatr Surg* 2005; **40**: 740–1.

Stone DH, Rimaz S, Gilmour WH. Prevalence of congenital anterior abdominal wall defects in the United Kingdom: comparison of regional registers. *Br Med J* 1998; **317**: 1118–19.

Wilcox DT, Chitty LS. Non-visualisation of the fetal bladder: aetiology and management. *Prenat Diagn* 2001; **21**: 977–83.

Assisted reproductive technology: *in vitro* fertilization (IVF), intracytoplasmic sperm injection (ICSI), and pre-implantation genetic diagnosis (PGD)

Assisted reproductive technology (ART) has revolutionized the treatment of infertility. Treatment with ART now accounts for 1–3% of all births in many Western countries. In conjunction with single cell genetic analysis based on polymerase chain reaction (PCR) or fluorescent *in situ* hybridization (FISH) it has also made pre-implantation genetic diagnosis (PGD) possible for some genetic disorders. PGD has been available as a clinical service since 1990 and can be offered to some patients as an alternative to prenatal diagnosis.

In vitro fertilization (IVF)

Controlled stimulation of the ovaries with exogenous gonadotrophins leads to the recruitment of many follicles (monitored by ultrasound scan (USS)). When the number and size of the developing follicles is deemed appropriate, oocyte maturation is triggered hormonally. 34–38 hours later, the oocytes are collected by transvaginal USS-guided aspiration of the follicular fluid. The oocytes are then fertilized *in vitro* with the partner's sperm and any resulting morphologically sound embryos are transferred into the woman's uterus 2 days later.

Hansen *et al.* (2002) found that 75/837 (9.0%) of infants conceived with IVF had a major birth defect diagnosed by 1 year of age compared with 168/4000 (4.2%) of the normal population. Excess defects were observed in multiple, singleton, and term singleton births. Risk of low birth weight (not due to prematurity) was 2.6 times that of the general population for singletons.

In Schieve *et al.*'s (2002) study, infants conceived after reproductive technology (IVF, donor oocyte, ICSI) accounted for 0.6% of all infants born to mothers 20 years or older, but 3.5% of low birthweight infants, and 4.3% of very low birthweight infants. Use of ART roughly doubles the risk of having a term singleton with low birthweight or a child with a major birth defect and greatly increases the risk of multiple pregnancy with increased risk of prematurity and consequent low birthweight. A possible link has recently been made between *in vitro* conception and certain congenital abnormalities, notably Beckwith–Wiedemann syndrome (BWS; Maher *et al.* 2003; Gosden *et al.* 2003). Halliday estimates the risk of BWS after IVF to be 1 in 4,000, but no excess was seen in a large Danish Registry study (Lindegard).

Intracytoplasmic sperm injection (ICSI)

ICSI involves the injection of a single sperm directly into a mature oocyte. ICSI is favoured for fertility patients where there is male factor infertility including azoospermia, oligozoospermia, and poor morphology or motility. Additionally, ICSI is used for PCR-based PGD techniques, to avoid the risk of extracting extra sperm, buried in the zona pellucida, at embryo biopsy, which would contaminate the assay. Hansen *et al.* (2002) found that 26/301 (8.6%) of infants conceived with ICSI had a major birth defect diagnosed by 1 year of age compared with 168/4000 (4.2%) of the normal population.

Pre-implantation genetic diagnosis (PGD)

PGD is a relatively new technology, but one that is becoming more widely recognized as a valid clinical service available in many countries. It is also often a misunderstood concept and raises wide controversy amongst professionals and the public alike.

Most couples requesting PGD do so because they wish to avoid the possibility of terminating a pregnancy following prenatal diagnosis. Others may require ART anyway to circumvent a fertility problem that may be caused by a genetic disorder, e.g. congenital bilateral absence of the vas deferens (CBAVD), as well as the presence of a genetic risk to the offspring.

PGD was first introduced for sexing embryos in the case of X-linked genetic disorders in 1990 (Handyside *et al.* 1990). In 1992 the first case of a liveborn girl after successful PGD for the single gene disorder, cystic fibrosis, was reported. PGD for single gene disorders moved on a stage further in 1995 with the successful outcome of a pregnancy following PGD for Duchenne muscular dystrophy to detect the dystrophin gene deletion. This resulted in a successful non-carrier female pregnancy. Since then the worldwide development of this service has expanded and The European Society of Human Reproduction and Embryology (ESHRE) published its third report in 2002 presenting data from 25 centres across Europe, the USA, and Australia. This publication reports outcomes of 1561 cycles of PGD. The data reflect the reasons for referral, reproductive histories, and the outcome of treatment. It is clear that most of the couples requesting PGD have had at least one pregnancy previously that has resulted in a fetus or child with a genetic disorder and that most of these couples do not have any living unaffected children. Data has been collected on 451 pregnancies resulting in 251 deliveries (156 singletons, 54 twins, and 5 triplets) giving a total of 279 babies born. Four cycles resulted in an incorrect diagnosis in the fetus and in one cycle a fetus was found to have a chromosomal problem unrelated to the referral genetic diagnosis.

Outcome of liveborn babies. Evidence suggests that human embryo development *in vitro* is not affected by biopsy at the 8-cell stage (Hardy *et al.* 1990), but the authors acknowledge that on-going pregnancies should be closely monitored by USS. The need for international collaboration for long-term follow-up of children born as the result of PGD was recognized, although in the latest report from the ESHRE (2002) Consortium it is noted that there is a lack of data on outcome of the pregnancies reported and that this anomaly will be addressed in future data collection; nevertheless, data were available on 180 of the 279 babies born. The perinatal mortality rate was 3/180, prematurity was the most commonly reported neonatal complication (67/180), which in turn was related to the number of multiple pregnancies. Overall, the congenital malformation rate was 6.6% (3.9% major; 2.7% minor) (ESHRE 2002).

Worldwide, PGD is now available for a wide range of genetic disorders but, as a technically demanding procedure, its application is still limited to fewer conditions than conventional prenatal diagnosis. Setting up a pre-implantation genetic screening (see below) assay for a specific genetic mutation is time-consuming and labour-intensive. *Many centres are therefore not able to offer PGD to couples with rare mutations that may be family-specific.* The table is not designed to give an exhaustive list of conditions for which PGD is available, but it does indicate the conditions for which PGD is most widely available.

Some genetic disorders for which PGD is currently available

Autosomal dominant
Myotonic dystrophy[*]
Huntington disease[*]

Autosomal recessive
Cystic fibrosis[*]
Spinal muscular atrophy[*]
Beta thalassaemia
Sickle cell disease[*]

X-linked, direct mutation testing
Fragile X syndrome[*]
Alport syndrome
Duchenne muscular dystrophy

X-linked, embryo sexing only[†]
Duchenne/Becker muscular dystrophy[*]
Haemophilia
Hunter syndrome[*]
Ornithine transcarbamylase (OTC) deficiency[*]
Incontinentia pigmenti[*]

Chromosomal disorders[‡]
Robertsonian translocations[*]
Reciprocal translocations[*]
Other chromosomal disorders (inversions, deletions)[*]

[*] Available in the UK.
[†] The majority of serious X linked conditions will be considered for PGD by embryo sexing in UK centres.
[‡] Dependent upon the availability of FISH probes.

Regulation of PGD. The regulation of PGD worldwide varies from country to country (Geraedts *et al.* 2001). In many countries where regulations do apply, the bodies responsible for ART will also regulate PGD. The UK Human Fertilisation and Embryology Act (HFE Act 1990) came into being and, in accordance with the Act, the Human Fertilisation and Embryology Authority (HFEA) was convened in 1990. This regulates all ART including PGD in the UK.

Success rate. The pregnancy and livebirth success rates of PGD are comparable to those for infertile couples undergoing ART. The cumulative ESHRE data suggested a pregnancy success rate of 22% per embryo transferred (ESHRE 2002). Given that the majority of couples referred for PGD are fertile, the chance of success must be discussed with couples in detail prior to the start of treatment.

Side-effects of treatment. The occurrence of ovarian hyperstimulation syndrome (OHSS) is relatively common, but can vary in its clinical severity from mild to severe and life-threatening. In its mildest form it is likely to occur in 8–23% of cases and, in its severe form, in 0.1–2% of cases. In severe cases OHSS can incur a hospital admission for a woman undergoing treatment and this is of specific concern for those undertaking PGD who may have a disabled child at home requiring care.

Misdiagnosis. There have been reports of misdiagnoses in PGD cycles. The technology of single cell analysis is complex and demanding and all couples are made aware of the chance of this happening. There are several possible reasons for misdiagnosis including mosaicism, which may occur if the cell analysed is not representative of the embryo biopsied (Harper *et al.* 1995), and allele drop-out (ADO), which results in elective amplification of only one of the two parental alleles being studied. ADO could lead to misdiagnosis in a dominant disorder due to loss of the affected allele. Finally, the need to apply large numbers of PCR cycles to obtain an adequate DNA sample from the biopsied single cell creates scope for contamination.

Cost. In the UK funding for PGD is not centrally organized within the NHS. Most local health authorities will apply their policy for funding IVF treatment to PGD and this may vary from area to area. Couples who are unsuccessful in their application for health authority funding will face a costly bill of several thousand pounds per cycle, making treatment inaccessible for many.

Special issues.

- **HLA tissue typing for bone marrow transplantation (BMT).** One of the most controversial uses of PGD, for which the HFEA (UK) has just granted one ART centre a licence to practise, is that of HLA typing to provide a compatible bone-marrow-matched child for a sibling with a genetic disorder. The aim of this technology is to analyse the embryos for the genetic disorder concerned and detect an embryo that is both unaffected and an HLA type match for the affected sibling (Verlinsky *et al.* 2001). This is a highly technically demanding procedure and one that is unlikely to be available widely at the present time, but demand may grow and this in turn will generate requests for licences from other centres.

- **Pre-implantation genetic screening (PGS).** In July 2001 the HFEA approved in principle the technique of PGS or aneuploidy screening (Ferriman 2001). This technique differs from PGD as it is applied to couples who have had repeated IVF/ICSI failures. It is hoped that by screening the embryos for chromosomal abnormalities PGS will increase the pregnancy rate amongst infertile couples of 35 years and over, who are undergoing ART. A large randomized controlled study is yet to be undertaken; therefore conclusive evidence that PGS is beneficial is awaited.

Expert advisers: Alison Lashwood, Consultant Nurse in Preimplantation Genetic Diagnosis, Guy's Hospital, London and Frances Flinter, Consultant Clinical Geneticist, Guy's Hospital, London, England.

References

ESHRE Preimplantation Genetic Diagnosis Consortium. Data collection III (May 2001). *Hum Reprod* 2002; **17**: 233–46.

Ferriman A. UK approves preimplantation genetic screening technique. *Br Med J* 2001; **323**: 125.

Geraedts JPM, *et al.* Preimplantation genetic diagnosis (PGD), a collaborative activity of clinical genetic departments and IVF centres. *Prenat Diagn* 2001; **21**: 1086–92.

Gosden R, Trasler J, *et al.* Rare congenital disorders, imprinted genes, and assisted reproductive technology. *Lancet* 2003; **361**: 1975–7.

Halliday J, Oke K *et al.* Beckwith-Wiedemann syndrome and IVF: a case-control study. *Am J Hum Genet* 2004; **75**: 526–8.

Handyside A, Delhanty J. Preimplantation genetic diagnosis: strategies and surprises. *Trends Genet* 1997; **13**: 270–5.

Handyside AH, Kontogianni, EH, *et al.* Pregnancies from biopsied human preimplantation embryos sexed by Y specific DNA amplification.*Nature* 1990; **244**: 768–70.

Hansen M, Kurinczuk JJ, *et al.* The risk of major birth defects after intracytoplasmic sperm injection and *in vitro* fertilisation. *New Engl J Med* 2002; **346**: 725–30.

Hardy K, Martin K, *et al.* Human preimplantation development *in vitro* is not adversely affected by biopsy at the 8 cell stage. *Hum Reprod* 1990; **5**: 708–14.

Harper JC, Coonen E, *et al.* Mosaicism of autosomes in morphologically normal, monospermic preimplantation human embryos. *Prenat Diagn* 1995; **15**: 41–9.

Lindegaard O, Pinborg A, *et al.* Imprinting diseases and IVF: Danish National IIVF cohort study. *Hum Reprod* 2005: Jan 21.

Maher ER, Brueton LA, *et al.* Beckwith–Wiedemann syndrome and assisted reproduction technology (ART). *J Med Genet* 2003; **40**: 62–4.

Schieve LA, *et al.* Low and very low birth weight in infants conceived with use of assisted reproductive technology. *New Engl J Med* 2002; **346**: 731–7.

Sermon K, van Steirteghem A, *et al.* Preimplantation diagnosis (Review). *Lancet* 2004; **363**: 1633–41.

Verlinsky Y, *et al.* Preimplantation diagnosis for Fanconi anemia combined with HLA matching. *J Am Med Assoc* 2001; **285**: 3130–3.

Bowed limbs

The femur length is measured routinely during the anomaly ultrasound scan (USS) at 18–20 weeks gestation to compare with other fetal measurements such as head circumference and abdominal circumference to assess proportionate growth. Bowing of all the long bones, or an isolated long bone, may be seen at this scan. Alternative terms for bowing include bent or angulated. Bowing is often seen in association with limb shortening.

Clinical assessment

History: key points

- Maternal factors; e.g. insulin-dependent diabetes mellitus (an association with femoral hypoplasia unusual facies).
- Three-generation family history. Note a history of skeletal abnormality, brittle bones/osteogenesis imperfecta (OI), previously affected sibling(s), stillbirth, or neonatal death.
- Consanguinity (autosomal recessive (AR) dysplasias and syndromes).
- Establish an accurate gestational age for the pregnancy (use earliest available USS).

Examination: key points

- Measurements of all long bones and head and abdominal circumference.
- Is there any evidence of asymmetry?
- Are all the bones bowed, or is only one limb or one bone affected?
- If the femora are bowed check the spine and kidneys.
- *If the features are consistent with a skeletal dysplasia* follow the protocol in 'Short limbs', page 630 to ensure accurate assessment of the fetus.

The particular features to assess in association with bowing are:
- Undermineralization of skull (OI, hypophosphatasia);
- symmetrical bowed femora are most commonly due to campomelic dysplasia or OI types III and IIb
- short 'crumpled' limbs (OI types IIa and IIc);
- very short limbs and ribs; bowing most obvious in the femora (thanatophoric dysplasia (TD));
- beaded ribs (caused by fractures; OI types IIa and IIc);
- tibia most affected by bowing (campomelic dysplasia (talipes, sex reversal, cardiac defects), OI type IIb, Beemer–Langer syndrome).

A suspected chromosomal disorder or malformation syndrome requires thorough examination of the fetus (see 'Short limbs', this chapter).

Special investigations

Referral to a specialist centre for scanning may be indicated.

- In fetuses with features of a malformation syndrome offer Chromosome analysis by chorionic villus sampling (CVS)/amniocentesis/fetal blood (depending on the gestation and the need for rapid results).
- Comparison of the phenotypic sex with the chromosomal sex to exclude sex reversal (campomelic dysplasia). Specifically request a careful analysis of the 17q24–25 region as abnormalities have been reported in association with campomelic dysplasia.
- Request that DNA is stored for future DNA testing,

- **Molecular analysis.** Rapid molecular testing in pregnancy to confirm a skeletal dysplasia is only available for a limited number of conditions. However, genetic-based diagnosis may be possible in future pregnancies if DNA is stored from the affected fetus.

Diagnoses to consider

There is considerable overlap with the discussion in 'Short limbs', page 630.

Campomelic dysplasia. The tibia shows the most marked bowing. Sex reversal is commonly found as this dysplasia is caused by haploinsufficiency of the SRY-related gene *SOX9* or by rearrangements and deletions of the 17q24–5 region. Cytogenetic analysis is indicated. The abnormality may not disrupt or delete the *SOX9* gene but may exert a position effect. Parental chromosomes should be performed if the fetus has an chromosome abnormality. Recurrences are due to germline mosaicism for a *SOX9* mutation, or chromosome imbalance.

Osteogenesis imperfecta (OI). Severe forms, e.g. type II, present with short deformed limbs often with bowing, angulation, and/or fractures. The fetus may have a narrow chest and some have undermineralization of the skull. Mostly due to dominant mutations in genes encoding type I collagen. Recurrence risk is due to parental germline mosaicism and is estimated at ~7% (Cole). In Pepin *et al.*'s (1997) series of prenatal diagnoses for type II OI, of the 50 couples who had had one previous affected pregnancy, one had a second affected pregnancy, a rate of 2%. Two of the 7 unaffected couples (28%) who had had two previous affected pregnancies with OI type II had a third affected pregnancy. See 'Fractures' in Chapter 2, 'Clinical approach'.

Infantile hypophosphatasia. AR condition characterized by severe deficiency of chondro-osseous mineralization and caused by mutations in the tissue non-specific alkaline phosphatase gene *TNSALP* on 1p34–36. There is deformity and fracture of the long bones and the skull is undermineralized assuming a globular shape. Most cases are lethal in the neonatal period. However, there are reports of a good prognosis following the observation of severe long bone bowing in prenatal scans with evidence for autosomal dominant (AD) transmission. Consult the literature prior to counselling. The blood alkaline phosphatase level is extremely low or undetectable.

Thanatophoric dysplasia (TD). Curved ('telephone receiver') femora found in TD type 1. TD is a sporadic neonatal lethal skeletal dysplasia caused by *de novo* dominant mutations in *FGFR3* (1/20 000). See 'Short limbs', page 630.

Undiagnosed skeletal dysplasias. Rare dysplasias have additional skeletal features but the precise diagnosis may not be made until after birth. An estimation of whether the condition is likely to be lethal in the neonatal period is needed for counselling purposes and to advise neonatal colleagues. See 'Short limbs', page 630 for USS predictors of a lethal dysplasia.

Genetic advice and management

Advise as appropriate for the specific condition diagnosed.

- **Investigation of the fetus and baby with a skeletal dysplasia.** A diagnosis is vitally important in order to be able to advise about appropriate management and also recurrence risks. If the pregnancy is terminated or the baby is stillborn, it is possible to get most of the information required even if a post-mortem examination is refused. See 'Short limbs', page 678 for a list of important investigations.

- **Asymmetrical and/or single bone involvement.** This is more likely to be due to a sporadic, vascular, or environmental factor than a genetic syndrome.

Support group: Many of the syndromes have their own support groups. See <www.cafamily.org.uk>; ARC (Antenatal Results and Choices) <www.arc-uk.org>, Tel. 020 7631 0285.

Expert adviser: Lyn Chitty, Consultant in Genetics and Fetal Medicine, University College Hospital, London, England.

References

Cole WG, Dalguish R, *et al.* Perinatal lethal osteogenesis imperfecta. *J Med Genet* 1995; **22**: 284–89.

Moore CA, *et al.* Mild autosomal dominant hypophosphatasia: *in-utero* presentation in 2 families. *Am J Genet* 1999; **86**: 410–15.

Parilla BV, Leeth EA, *et al.* Antenatal detection of skeletal dysplasias. *J Ultrasound Med* 2003; **22**: 255–8.

Pepin M, Atkinson M, Starman BJ, Byers PH. Strategies and outcomes of prenatal diagnosis for osteogenesis imperfecta: a review of biochemical and molecular studies completed in 129 pregnancies. *Prenat Diagn* 1997; **17** (6): 559–70.

Wynne-Davies R, Hall CM, Hurst JA Radiological diagnosis of the skeletal dysplasias presenting at birth. Occasional Publication (2000).

Club-foot (talipes)

Club-foot usually occurs as an isolated anomaly (77%), but it may reflect an underlying neurological or neuromuscular disorder. It may also be a feature of a chromosomal disorder (e.g. trisomy 18), syndrome, or neural tube defect (NTD). Club-foot may be a consequence of oligohydramnios. Careful assessment is therefore indicated when club-foot is identified antenatally on ultrasound scan (USS).

Bakalis undertook a retrospective study of >100,000 pregnancies undergoing routine ultrasound scanning at 18–23 weeks gestation. The incidence of fetal talipes was 0.1%. Talipes was bilateral in ~60% and unilateral in ~40%. In nearly half of cases, talipes was of complex aetiology, occurring in association with other defects, while in the other half it was idiopathic (isolated). In 19% of cases, an initial diagnosis of idiopathic talipes was changed to complex, because of the subsequent identification of associated features. Adverse outcomes were more frequently associated with bilateral talipes than with unilateral talipes (odds ratio 3.4).

Talipes equinovarus (TEV). Both the forefoot and the hindfoot are in equinus (plantar-flexed) and varus (rotated towards the midline). Prevalence is 1.6/1000 livebirths, with male preponderance (male:female ratio 2:1). The spectrum of disorder ranges from mild positional deformity that corrects easily in the first week or two of life to completely rigid deformity. Approximately 50% respond to conservative treatment (stretching exercises and strapping/splinting) and 50% require surgery which often has to be repeated.

Talipes calcaneovalgus. The forefoot is dorsiflexed and everted. Often responds to gentle stretching exercises. Male:female ratio 0.6:1.

Clinical assessment

History: key points

- Three-generation family tree with specific enquiry about relatives with club-foot, contractures (distal arthrogryposis), etc.
- History of oligohydramnios (early amniocentesis <14 weeks (Philip), liquor leak, renal abnormality).

Examination: key points

- Detailed fetal anomaly USS.
  - Careful assessment of whole fetus with special attention to brain and spinal (exclude NTD) and fetal movement, range of movement of joints (exclude arthrogryposis).
  - If additional features are identified the possibility of a syndrome or chromosomal anomaly is increased.
  - Check amniotic fluid volume.
  - Assess if there are features of a skeletal dysplasia.
- Check maternal serum screening results and combine with maternal age in algorithm to determine risk for Trisomy 18 (see Edwards' syndrome page 526).
- Assess mother for myotonic dystrophy.

Special investigations

- Consider karyotype (especially if there are other risk factors for aneuploidy, e.g. soft markers on USS, advanced maternal age, abnormal serum screen).

- Consider DNA testing for myotonic dystrophy in the mother if any suggestive features on history/examination.

Genetic advice and management

Prenatally detected club-foot. In the Oxford series (Boyd, personal communication), of 149 cases (1991–2003) identified prenatally, there were 6 false positive diagnoses with either no abnormality at birth or positional clubfoot only and 110/149 (74%) were isolated anomalies. In the Harvard series (Shipp and Benacerraf 1998) of 68 fetuses, 8 (11.8%) were false-positive diagnoses and 4 (5.9%) had abnormal karyotypes (+21, +18,47,XXY, 47,XXX). In Malone et al.'s (2000) series of 51 cases of club-foot identified from 27 000 targeted USS, all were confirmed postnatally and no additional malformations were detected. Mean gestation at diagnosis was 21 weeks gestation. In Carroll et al.'s (2001) series, follow-up was available on only 31/40 livebirths. Two were false-positive diagnoses, but, of the remainder, 26/29 had a structural defect, for which 21 required surgery, and 3/29 a positional defect. The largest study is that of Bakalis (see above). Note the significant proportion of cases thought to be idiopathic at presentation which had additional features when reassessed on subsequent scan or postnatally.

Isolated talipes equinovarus. The recurrence risk for sibs in isolated TEV is 3% (risk for sibs of a male patient is 2%; risk for sibs of a female patient is 5%).

Isolated talipes calcaneovalgus. Recurrence risk for sibs is 4.5%.

Support group: STEPS <www.steps-charity.org.uk>, Tel. 0871 717 0044.

Expert advisers: Lyn Chitty, Consultant in Genetics and Fetal Medicine, University College Hospital, London and Patricia Boyd, Associate Specialist in Clinical Genetics for Prenatal Diagnosis, John Radcliffe Hospital, Oxford, England.

References

Bakalis S, Sairam S, et al. Outcome of antenatally diagnosed talipes equinovarus in an unselected obstetric population. *Ultrasound Obstet Gynecol* 2002; **20**: 226–9.

Boyd PA, Chamberlain P, et al. 6-year experience of prenatal diagnosis in an unselected population in Oxford, UK. *Lancet* 1998; **352**: 1577–81.

Carroll SGM, Lockyer H, et al. Outcome of fetal talipes following *in utero* sonographic diagnosis. *Ultrasound Obstet Gynecol* 2001; **18**: 437.

Malone FD, Marino T, et al. Isolated clubfoot diagnosed prenatally: is karyotyping indicated? *Obstet Gynecol* 2000; **95**: 437.

Philip J, Silver RK, et al. Late first-trimester invasive prenatal diagnosis: results of an international randomized trial. *Obstet Gynecol* 2004; **103**: 1164–73.

Shipp TD, Benacerraf BR. The significance of prenatally identified isolated clubfoot: is amniocentesis indicated? *Am J Obstet Gynecol* 1998; **178**: 600.

Wynne-Davies R. Family studies and the cause of congenital club foot, talipes equinovarus, calcaneovalgus and metatarsus varus. *J Bone Joint Surg* 1964; **46B**: 445–63.

Congenital cystic lung lesions, Currarino syndrome, and sacrococcygeal teratoma

Congenital cystic lung lesions

These are rare and present on ultrasound scan (USS) as a cystic or solid mass in the chest, which needs to be differentiated from a congenital diaphragmatic hernia. Causes of congenital cystic lung lesions include: congenital cystic adenomatoid malformation (CCAM); pulmonary sequestration; congenital lobar emphysema (CLE); and bronchogenic cysts. Most cases fare well, but if hydrops is present the prognosis is worse. CCAM is diagnosed in ~1/25 000– 1/35 000 pregnancies (Laberge et al. 2001). Many cases of CCAM improve spontaneously or resolve apparently completely *in utero*. Postnatal management is difficult as the majority are clinically asymptomatic and natural history studies are lacking. Sauvat et al. (2003) reviewed 29 cases of CCAM identified antenatally. The first chest X-ray was normal in 12 (~40%), but computerized tomography (CT) showed abnormality in 25. Only 10% of patients were symptomatic postnatally. CCAM vanished postnatally in 6. The treatment of asymptomatic CCAM is controversial. Surgery may be advocated because of the low morbidity and the prevention of late complications. The surgical indications for asymptomatic lesions should be discussed on a case-by-case basis with the parents (Sauvat et al. 2003). Parents should be counselled by a respiratory paediatrician.

Fetuses with a significant lesion, particularly if associated with mediastinal shift in the third trimester, should be delivered in a unit with facilities for neonatal intensive care and respiratory support as early surgical treatment may be required. Karyotyping is not indicated. 'Bilateral' lesions may represent laryngeal/tracheal atresia (consider autosomal recessive (AR) Fraser-cryptophthalmos syndrome).

Currarino syndrome

Autosomal dominant (AD) sacral agenesis is characterized by a partial agenesis of the sacrum typically involving sacral vertebrae S2–S5 only. Associated features include anorectal malformation, a presacral mass, and urogenital malformation. Together, these features have been defined as the Currarino syndrome which is caused by dorsal-ventral patterning defects during embryonic development. Some have an anterior sacral meningocele or a skin dimple. Severe constipation is a common symptom in cases diagnosed postnatally. The syndrome occurs in the majority of patients as an AD trait associated with mutations in the homeobox gene *HLXB9* that encodes the nuclear protein HB9. In Kochling et al.'s (2001) study, highly variable phenotypes and a low penetrance with half of all carriers being clinically asymptomatic were found in three families, whereas affected members of one family showed almost identical phenotypes. See Lynch et al. (2000) for further details.

Sacrococcygeal teratoma

A sacrococcygeal teratoma is a germ cell tumour composed of tissues that orginate from each of the three layers of the embryonic disc. The incidence is 1/35 000–1/40 000 livebirths. It is more common in females (1M:4F). Sacrococcygeal teratomas are highly vascular tumours that can grow very rapidly. There may be associated malformations of the sacrum, vertebrae, and gastrointestinal or genitourinary tracts. Only a minority of tumours are malignant.

Sacrococcygeal teratomas are classified as follows.

- Type I. Predominantly external with only a minimal presacral component (40%).
- Type II. Significant intrapelvic extension (36%).
- Type III. Largest portion of the tumour within the pelvis.
- Type IV. Whole of the tumour within the pelvis and abdominal cavity.

The pregnancy should be monitored closely for signs of mirror syndrome. The prognosis will depend on the type of lesion, gestational age and size of the lesion at delivery.

The great majority of cases are sporadic. However, familial teratoma with an AD mode of inheritance has been reported.

Expert adviser: Lyn Chitty, Consultant in Genetics and Fetal Medicine, University College Hospital, London, England.

References

Kochling J, Karbasiyan M, Reis A. Spectrum of mutations and genotype–phenotype analysis in Currarino syndrome. *Eur J Hum Genet* 2001; **9** (8): 599–605.

Laberge JM, Flageole H, et al. Outcome of prenatally diagnosed congenital cystic adenomatoid lung malformation: a Canadian experience. *Fetal Diagn Ther* 2001; **16**: 178–86.

Lynch SA, Wang Y, Strachan T, Burn J, Lindsay S. Autosomal dominant sacral agenesis: Currarino syndrome. *J Med Genet* 2000; **37** (8): 561–6.

Sauvat F, Michel JL, et al. Management of asymptomatic neonatal cystic adenomatoid malformations. *J Pediatr Surg* 2003; **38** (4): 548–52.

Congenital diaphragmatic hernia

The diaphragm develops in early embryonic life and is usually fully formed by 9 weeks gestation. Congenital diaphragmatic hernia occurs when any of the four components making up the diaphragm (the septum transversum, pleuroperitoneal membranes, dorsal mesentry of the oesophagus, and body wall) fail to grow toward each other or to fuse by the 8th week after conception (Wenstrom *et al.* 1991). The most common site for diaphragmatic hernia is the left side, through which stomach, bowel, spleen, and liver can pass. Poor prognostic features include early diagnosis, and liver in chest. The main cause of death is pulmonary hypoplasia, due to constrained development of the fetal lungs *in utero*.

Congenital diaphragmatic hernia occurs in ~1/3700 livebirths (Wenstrom *et al.* 1991). The overall prenatal detection rate by ultrasound scan (USS) is ~60%. They are most commonly detected at the 20 weeks gestation fetal anomaly scan, but some may present late. In a series of 31 prenatally diagnosed cases from France (Betremieux *et al.* 2002), 10 fetuses (32%) had associated anomalies of which four had chromosomal anomalies (trisomy 18, 22q11 deletion) and 4 had Fryns syndrome. Enns *et al.* (1998) reviewed 60 prenatal diagnoses of congenital diaphragmatic defect and also found that 33% had additional anomalies on prenatal USS.

Congenital diaphragmatic hernia with an abnormal karyotype or other major structural abnormalities e.g. heart, brain, has a poor outcome. Isolated congenital diaphragmatic hernia, when delivered in a tertiary unit with access to expert neonatal intensive care and paediatric surgical facilities has a survival rate in excess of 50%. Long term complications including feeding difficulties, respiratory problems and intellectual delay may occur and parents should be referred to a paediatric surgeon for consultation and discussion of prognosis as soon as possible after prenatal diagnosis.

Other causes of a mass in the fetal chest. In the West Midlands Perinatal Institute's (2003) review, 14/121 (12%) prenatal diagnoses of congenital diaphragmatic hernia made in a fetal medicine centre were false-positive diagnoses. It is important to consider this possibility when counselling parents prenatally. Final diagnoses in the false-positive cases included: congenital cystic adenomatoid malformation (CCAM), bronchogenic cyst, hydrothorax, pleural effusions, lung sequestration, duodenal atresia, and gut malrotation. Fetal magnetic resonance imaging (MRI) may be helpful in making the correct diagnosis in difficult cases.

Clinical assessment

History: key points

Three-generation family tree with enquiry about consanguinity.

Examination: key points

- Detailed fetal biometry.
- Detailed anomaly USS to detect other structural anomalies.

Special investigations

- Amniocentesis or placental biopsy for karyotype. Karyotyping is indicated as +18 and +13 are associated with diaphragmatic hernia and, overall, 14% of pregnancies with diaphragmatic hernia had a chromosomal abnormality in the West Midlands Perinatal Institute's (2003) study.
- Fetal echocardiography. 16% have cardiac malformations.

Some diagnoses to consider

Trisomy 18. See 'Edwards syndrome (trisomy 18)' page 526.

Trisomy 13. See 'Patau syndrome (trisomy 13)' page 534.

Pallister–Killian syndrome (tetrasomy 12p) is due to mosaicism for an isochromosome of 12p that is present in skin fibroblasts but not in blood lymphocytes. Other USS anomalies such as increased nuchal translucency, congenital diaphragmatic hernia, polyhydramnios, rhizomelic limb shortening, and abnormal facial profile with prominent philtrum in association with fetal overgrowth are very suggestive of the syndrome, but they are inconstant and may even be absent. Doray *et al.* (2002) propose that, in cases where USS indicators are present, the first investigation should be chorionic villus sampling (CVS) or placental biopsy and then amniocentesis if the first cytogenetic result is normal. FBS is the least indicated method because of the low frequency of the isochromosomes in lymphocytes. In this cytogenetic strategy, fluorescent *in situ* hybridization (FISH) and especially interphase FISH on non-cultured cells increase the probability of identifying the isochromosome. See also 'Coarse facial features' in Chapter 2, 'Clinical approach'.

Fryns syndrome. Fryns syndrome is a rare autosomal recessive (AR) disorder of multiple congenital abnormalities. Major diagnostic criteria include congenital diaphragmatic hernia, distal limb and nail hypoplasia, and abnormal facies. More than 70 cases have been reported since the first report in 1979, 86% of which have been associated with an early lethal outcome.

Simpson–Golabi–Behmel (SGB) syndrome. X-linked recessive (XLR) disorder due to mutations in *glypican 3* (Xq26). Overgrowth is of prenatal onset and continues postnatally. Birthweight and birth occipital-frontal circumference (OFC) of affected males are usually both > 97th centile. May have cardiac/gastrointestinal malformations. See 'Overgrowth' page 206.

Cornelia de Lange syndrome. Birth incidence ~1 in 50,000. Intrauterine growth retardation (IUGR; often developing in the third trimester) with limb anomalies ranging from short forearms with small hands and tapering fingers to severe limb reduction defects. Upper limb defects are very much more common than lower limb defects. Distinctive craniofacial features (microbrachycephaly, depressed nasal bridge with anteverted nares, long smooth philtrum, and micrognathia). A gene for de Lange syndrome was recently identified as *NIPBL* on 5p13.1. See 'Limb reduction defects' page 152.

Donnai–Barrow syndrome. Rare AR condition characterized by diaphragmatic hernia, exomphalos, absent corpus callosum, hypertelorism, myopia, and sensorineural deafness (Chassaing *et al.* 2003).

Meacham syndrome. Rare disorder characterised by congenital diaphragmatic hernia, cardiac and pulmonary malformations with sex reversal (normal female external genitalia with abnormal male gonads) (Killeen).

Lethal multiple pterygium syndrome (LMPS) is an uncommon fetal-onset disorder of unknown aetiology. LMPS results from fetal akinesia commencing in the first or early second trimester. In the majority of cases, the precise underlying cause will not be identified; however, occasionally a metabolic or neurodevelopmental disorder or a specific primary myopathy may be demonstrated, providing adequate autopsy investigations are undertaken (Cox *et al.* 2003).

Genetic advice and management

For isolated congenital diaphragmatic hernia the sibling recurrence risk is very low at ~1%.

Repair

The repair is usually through the abdomen with reduction of herniated contents and excision of any sac preceding repair. The defect may be closed primarily, or a muscle patch or inert graft may be needed. Sometimes there is intestinal malrotation requiring a Ladd's procedure to place the intestine in the non-rotated position.

Information for families: <www.cafamily.org.uk/Direct/d28.html>.

Expert adviser: Lyn Chitty, Consultant in Genetics and Fetal Medicine, University College Hospital, London, England.

References

Betremieux P, Lionnais S, *et al.* Perinatal management and outcome of prenatally diagnosed congenital diaphragmatic hernia: a 1995–2000 series in Rennes University Hospital. *Prenat Diagn* 2002; **22**: 988–94.

Chassaing N, Lacombe D, Carles D, Calvas P, Saura R, Bieth E. Donnai–Barrow syndrome: four additional patients. *Am J Med Genet* 2003; **121A** (3): 258–62.

Cox PM, Brueton LA, *et al.* Diversity of neuromuscular pathology in lethal multiple pterygium syndrome. *Pediatr Dev Pathol* 2003; **6** (1): 59–68.

Doray B, Girard-Lemaire F, *et al.* Pallister–Killian syndrome: difficulties of prenatal diagnosis. *Prenat Diagn* 2002; **22** (6): 470–7.

Enns GM, Cox VA, *et al.* Congenital diaphragmatic defects and associated syndromes, malformations, and chromosome anomalies: a retrospective study of 60 patients and literature review. *Am J Med Genet* 1998; **79** (3): 215–25.

Garne E, Haeusler M, *et al.* Congenital diaphragmatic hernia: evaluation of prenatal diagnosis in 20 Euopean regions. *Ultrasound Obstet Gynecol* 2002; **19**: 329–33.

Harrison MR, Keller RL, *et al.* A randomised trial of fetal endoxcopic tracheal occlusion for severe fetal congenital diaphragmatic hernia. *New Engl J Med* 2003; **349**: 1916–24.

Huddy CL, Boyd PA, Wilkinson AR, Chamberlain P. Congenital diaphragmatic hernia: prenatal diagnosis, outcome and continuing morbidity in survivors. *Br J Obstet Gynaecol* 1999; **106** (11): 1192–6.

Killeen OG, Kelehan P, *et al.* Double vagina with sex reversal, congenital diaphragmatic hernia, pulmonary and cardiac malformations—another case of Meacham syndrome. *Clin Dysmorphol* 2002; **11**: 25–28.

Lally KP. Congenital diaphragmatic hernia. *Curr Opin Paediatr* 2002; **14**: 486–90.

Marino T, Wheeler PG, *et al.* Fetal diaphragmatic hernia and upper limb anomalies suggest Brachmann–de Lange syndrome. *Prenat Diagn* 2002; **22** (2): 144–7.

Paladini D, Borghese A, *et al.* Prospective ultrasound diagnosis of Pallister–Killian syndrome in the second trimester of pregnancy: the importance of the fetal facial profile. *Prenat Diagn* 2000; **20** (12): 996–8.

Stege G, Fenton A, Jaffray B. Nihilism in the 1990s: the true mortality of congenital diaphragmatic hernia. *Pediatrics* 2003; **112** (3, pt. 1): 532–5.

Wenstrom KD. Fetal surgery for congenital diaphragmatic hernia [perspective]. *New Engl J Med* 2003; **349**: 1887–8.

Wenstrom KD, Weiner CP, Hanson JW. A five-year statewide experience with congenital diaphragmatic hernia. *Am J Obstet Gynecol* 1991; **165** (4, pt. 1): 838–42.

West Midlands Perinatal Institute. *West Midlands Congenital Anomaly Register. Congenital Diaphragmatic Hernia 1995–2000.* West Midlands Perinatal Institute 2003.

Williams HJ, Johnson KJ. Imaging of congenital cystic lung lesions. *Paediatr Respir Rev* 2002; **3**: 120–7.

Cytomegalovirus (CMV)

Congenital CMV is diagnosed, investigated, and managed by fetal medicine specialists, paediatricians, and specialists in infectious diseases with laboratory diagnostic support. The geneticist may be involved prior to a definitive diagnosis because the phenotype may overlap with genetic disorders. Therefore, a brief summary of the condition is included in this section. CMV is by far the most common serious intrauterine infection with an incidence of symptomatic disease at birth of 0.1% (Spagno 2001). The severity of infection appears related to gestation at the time of infection: those fetuses acquiring infection in the first trimester have relatively severe consequences, whereas those infected during the third trimester may be asymptomatic.

CMV is a member of the herpesvirus family. There can be both primary and recurrent disease but primary disease is more likely to lead to congenital infection than recurrent infection. In children and adults most infections are subclinical. The virus is transmitted by close personal contact (saliva, genital tract, breast milk).

CMV is commonly acquired at birth and through the first few months of life and it is often difficult to distinguish serologically between congenital and perinatally acquired infection.

The *in utero* risk of congenital transmission is not gestation-dependent. The majority of congenitally infected babies do not have any clinical signs and have a good prognosis, though deafness may be late-presenting. Of the 10% with signs, there is a significant mortality and about 20% with typical features die in the perinatal period. Typical features are low birthweight, lethargy, poor feeding, thrombocytopenia, hepatosplenomegaly, intracranial calcification, and chorioretinitis (see table).

Clinical and laboratory findings in neonates with symptomatic CMV infection (after Azam *et al.* 2001)

Finding	Percentage of cases
Prematurity (<38 weeks gestation)	34
Intrauterine growth retardation (IUGR)	50
Microcephaly	53
Jaundice	67
Petechiae	76
Purpura	13
Hepatosplenomegaly	60
Thrombocytopenia (platelet count < 100 000/mm^3)	77
Haemolytic anaemia	51
Raised alanine aminotransferase (>55 U/l)–mild hepatitis	83

Approximately 60% of survivors with symptomatic neonatal infection have sensorineural hearing deficit and ~70% have microcephaly, seizures, motor abnormalities, developmental delay, or other cognitive impairment such that, overall, 90% of survivors with symptomatic neonatal infection will have a sensory deficit or cognitive impairment.

As CMV is usually subclinical, it is more likely that the condition is considered when scan abnormalities are seen or in babies with features of congenital CMV.

Clinical assessment

History: key points, postnatal
- Birthweight, occipital-frontal circumference (OFC).
- Lethargy, poor feeding.

Examination: key points, postnatal
- Microcephaly and neurological abnormalities.
- Petechiae.
- Hepatosplenomegaly and jaundice.

Special investigations
- Prenatal
  - Ultrasound scan (USS): fetal ascites, poor fetal growth, intracranial calcification, brain cysts, ventriculomegaly, oligohydramnios.
  - Polymerase chain reaction (PCR) for CMV in amniotic fluid.
  - Maternal CMV serology.
- Postnatal
  - Isolate virus from urine or perform CMV PCR in the first 2 weeks of life.
  - Serological testing e.g., for toxoplasmosis, syphilis, varicella zoster virus, parvovirus, rubella virus and cytomegalovirus.
  - Liver function tests, full blood count (FBC), and platelets (thrombocytopenia).
  - Brain imaging of all symptomatic babies (typical features of congenital CMV infection are intracranial calcifications that are predominantly periventricular, periventricular pseudocysts, polymicrogyria, and cerebellar hypoplasia).
  - Audiological assessment and follow-up.
  - Ophthalmology referral (chorioretinitis).

Genetic advice and management

Children with proven congenital CMV are not managed by geneticists but the following points may be useful.
- If there are no clinical signs at birth the prognosis for normal development is good; ~90% have no problems. Hearing loss may develop so screen throughout infancy and early childhood.
- There is a high risk of neurological deficits in babies with typical clinical features of congenital CMV. Microcephaly is the most specific predictor of mental retardation (see table).
- Recurrences have been reported due to reactivation of maternal disease but, in general, the risk for developmental problems is very low in recurrent disease.

Neurodevelopmental outcome in symptomatic CMV infection (after Noyola *et al.* 2001)[*]

Symptoms	Outcome
Microcephaly + abnormal CT scan	Mean IQ < 50; major motor deficit in 75%
Normal OFC + abnormal CT scan	Mean IQ 70–80; major motor deficit in 37%
Normal OFC + normal CT scan	Mean IQ >90; no major motor deficit

[*] CT, Computerized tomography; IQ, intelligence quotient; OFC, occipital-frontal circumference.

- Consider the autosomal recessive (AR) condition of pseudo-TORCH/microcephaly–intracranial calcification in babies with signs of congenital infection, but in whom there are no serological features or no virus identified.
- Please refer to the appropriate eye or brain section of Chapter 2, 'Clinical Approach', for discussion of other syndromes with some of the features of congenital infections.

Expert advisers: Donald Peebles, Consultant in Fetal Medicine, University College Hospital, London and Tim Wreghitt, Consultant Virologist, Addenbrooke's Hospital, Cambridge, England.

References

Azam A, Vial Y, et al. Prenatal diagnosis of congenital cytomegalovirus infection. *Obstet Gynecol* 2001; **97**: 443–8.

Jones CA, Isaacs D. Predicting the outcome of symptomatic congenital cytomegalovirus infection. *J Paeditr Child Health* 1995; **31**: 70–71.

Modlin JF, Grant PE, et al. Case 25–2003: A newborn boy with petechiae and thrombocytopenia. *New Engl J Med* 2003; **349**: 691–700.

Noyola DE, Demmler GJ, et al. Early predictors of neurodevelopmental outcome in symptomatic congenital cytomegalovirus infection. *J Pediatr* 2001; **138**: 325–31.

Spagno S. Cytomegaloviruses. In *Infectious diseases of the fetus and newborn infant*, 5th edn (ed. J.S. Remington and J.O. Klein), pp. 389–424. W.B. Saunders, Philadelphia, 2001.

Dandy–Walker malformation

Includes Dandy–Walker syndrome, Dandy–Walker variant, Dandy–Walker complex. See 'Cerebellar anomalies' in Chapter 2, 'Clinical approach'.

Dandy–Walker malformation (DWM) is a developmental anomaly of the posterior fossa. It is characterized by:
- cystic dilatation of the fourth ventricle;
- complete or partial agenesis of the cerebellar vermis;
- enlargement of the posterior fossa with upward displacement of the tentorium.

DWM is heterogeneous in aetiology. Nearly half of fetuses with DWM have a chromosome anomaly, and DWM is listed as a feature of 80 syndromes in the London Dysmorphology Database (e.g. 3C (craniocerebellocardiac) dysplasia, Joubert syndrome, hydrolethalus, Walker–Warburg syndrome (WWS), Smith–Lemli–Opitz (SLO), Meckel– Gruber). DWM should not be diagnosed prior to 18 weeks gestation (although it may be suspected earlier). The cerebellar vermis does not finish its development until 17–18 weeks gestation and at 15–16 weeks it is not uncommon to find the cerebellar vermis incompletely formed.

Clinical outcome varies from normal development, to severe handicap and perinatal death. Poor fetal or perinatal outcome may be related to extra-central nervous system (CNS) malformations, e.g. cardiac defects. One series (Aletebi and Fung 1999) found neurodevelopmental delay in 80% of survivors with follow-up to 4 years of age.

Clinical assessment

History: key points
Take a detailed three-generation family history and enquire carefully about consanguinity.

Examination: key points
If identified at 19 weeks gestation, fetal anomaly ultrasound scan (USS):
- look carefully for other CNS malformations, e.g. ventriculomegaly (32%), agenesis of corpus callosum, holoprosencephaly, lissencephaly, occipital meningocele, or encephalocele;
- look carefully for extra-CNS malformations, e.g. cardiac defects (40%; chromosomal anomaly or 3C), polydactyly (+13, Joubert), renal anomaly.

Special investigations
- Offer karyotype (46% had abnormal karyotype in Ecker *et al.*'s (2000) series).
- TORCH (toxoplasmosis–other (including syphilis, varicella zoster, parvovirus)–rubella–cytomegalovirus–herpes simplex virus) screen.

Genetic advice and management
- If a chromosome anomaly is identified, counsel as appropriate.
- If additional findings on USS, this strongly increases the possibility of a syndromic association (e.g. 3C, hydrolethalus, WWS, SLO, Meckel–Gruber). Since many of these conditions follow autosomal recessive (AR) inheritance there is often a high recurrence risk.
- When the evidence suggests that DWM has not occurred as part of a Mendelian or chromosomal disorder then the recurrence risk is relatively low, on the order of 1–5% (Murray *et al.* 1985).

Expert adviser: Lyn Chitty, Consultant in Fetal Medicine, University College Hospital, London, England.

References

Aletebi FA, Fung KF. Neurodevelopmental outcome after antenatal diagnosis of posterior fossa abnormalities. *J Ultrasound Med* 1999; **18**: 683–9.

Ecker JL, Shipp TD, Bromley B, Benacerraf B. The sonographic diagnosis of Dandy–Walker and Dandy–Walker variant: associated findings and outcomes. *Prenat Diagn* 2000; **20**: 328–32.

Kolble N, Wisser J, *et al.* Dandy–Walker malformation: prenatal diagnosis and outcome. *Prenat Diagn* 2000; **20**: 318–27.

Murray JC, Johnson JA, Bird TD. Dandy–Walker malformation: etiologic heterogeneity and empiric recurrence risks. *Clin Genet* 1985; **28** (4): 272–83.

Parisi MA, Dobyns WB. Human malformations of the midbrain and hindbrain: review and proposed classification scheme. *Mol Genet Metab* 2003; **80**: 36–53.

Drugs in pregnancy

Sometimes enquiries relate to a drug exposure in an ongoing pregnancy. In this instance, seek advice from the UK National Teratology Information Service (NTIS), which provides information and advice about all aspects of toxicity of drugs and chemicals in pregnancy throughout the UK, or its equivalents in Europe, the USA, and Canada. More typically, the geneticist is asked to assess a child with a congenital malformation, dysmorphic features, or developmental delay and to assess whether a known drug exposure during pregnancy is relevant to the child's problems.

Angiotensin-converting enzyme inhibitors (ACE inhibitors)
Prolonged renal failure and hypotension in the newborn, decreased skull ossification, hypocalvaria, and renal tubular dysgenesis. The features of ACE inhibitor fetopathy suggest that the underlying pathogenetic mechanism is fetal hypotension, which may also result from other exposures (Barr 1994), although oligohydramnios with fetal compression may be a contributory factor.

Anticonvulsants
See 'Fetal anticonvulsant syndrome (FACS)', this chapter.

Carbimazole
Choanal atresia, hypoplastic nipples and developmental delay may occur after first trimester exposure to carbimazole (or its active metabolite methimazole), used in the treatment of maternal hyperthyroidism (e.g. Graves' disease) (Wilson). This is likely to be a rare but significant effect.

Cocaine
An increased incidence of spontaneous abortion, placental abruption, prematurity, intrauterine growth retardation (IUGR), and neurological deficits has been documented. Hoyme et al. (1991) report congenital limb deficiency and intestinal atresia in offspring of mothers who abused cocaine and suggests that these are a consequence of drug-induced fetal vascular disruption. Exposure to cocaine and its derivatives, e.g. 'crack', is connected with clear drug-induced effects; an increased incidence of abruptio placentae, maternal and neonatal intracranial haemorrhage, and possibly urogenital defects.

Fluconazole
Risk of Antley–Bixler craniosynostosis after high dose in first trimester (see 'Cramiosynosphosis' page 288).

Lithium
Initial reports from the Danish Register of Lithium Babies indicated significantly increased rates of cardiovascular malformations (Schou et al. 1973). A recent review of pooled data suggests a more modest risk of Ebstein anomaly of the tricuspid valve (10–20 times that in the general population where it occurs in 1/20 000 cases). A prospective controlled study of 148 women, found a relative risk of 1.2 for all congenital anomalies and of 3.5 for cardiac anomalies in the babies exposed to lithium (Jacobsen et al. 1992). Lithium has also been reported to affect neonatal thyroid function. A 5-year follow-up of 60 children exposed to lithium in the second and third trimesters found no significant differences in developmental anomalies compared with non-exposed siblings (Schou 1976). The animal and human data following lithium exposure have been extensively reviewed by Moore (1995)—see Shepard et al. (2002).

Oral contraceptive pill (ocp)
No association between first trimester exposure to oral contraceptives and malformation in general (Bracken 1990) or external genital malformations (Raman-Wilms et al. 1995) was noted in two meta-analyses.

Retinoids
The introduction in 1984 of isotretinoin (Roaccutane) for oral treatment of severe acne and etretinate for psoriasis led to a spate of birth defects. Etretinate is fat-soluble with an elimination half-life of 120 days or more (and has been taken off the market in the UK because of its teratogenic effects). Acitretin was introduced to replace etretinate since it is excreted from the body rapidly with a half-life of 50–60 hours.

Retinoid embryopathy results in some or all of the following abnormalities: CNS defects (hydrocephalus, optic-nerve blindness, retinal defects, microphthalmia, posterior fossa defects, and cortical and cerebellar defects); craniofacial defects (microtia or anotia, low-set ears, hypertelorism, depressed nasal bridge, microcephaly, micrognathia, and agenesis or stenosis of external ear canals); cardiovascular defects (transposition of the great arteries (TGA), tetralogy of Fallot, ventricular septal defect (VSD), atrial septal defect (ASD)); thymic defects (ectopia and hypoplasia or aplasia; and miscellaneous defects (limb reduction, decreased muscle tone, spontaneous abortion, and behavioural anomalies).

Warfarin
Warfarin and other coumarin derivatives cross the placenta and can cause bleeding in the fetus and, after exposure at 6–12 weeks gestation, an embryopathy (chondrodysplasia punctata with nasal hypoplasia and/or stippled epiphyses). In addition, CNS malformations can occur after exposure during any trimester. The risk of a poor outcome is 80% when the mean daily dose of warfarin is >5 mg, but <10% when the mean daily dose is <5 mg. Warfarin does not induce an anticoagulant effect in an infant who is breastfed and therefore can safely be used post-partum. (Nevertheless, to be on the safe side, the infant should receive 1 mg vitamin K orally 2–3 times a week in the first 4 weeks of life. To avoid any possible complication, the coagulation status should be checked at about 10–14 days, at least in premature infants (Schaefer 2001).)

Unfractionated and low molecular weight heparins do not cross the placenta and are not secreted into breast milk.

Patients with prosthetic heart valves. Pre-pregnancy counselling from a cardiologist and obstetrician with expertise in fetomaternal medicine is advised. The precise safety of warfarin during pregnancy continues to be debated, but it is probably appropriate to withhold warfarin between 6 and 12 weeks gestation because of the risk of embryopathy and from 34 weeks gestation because of the risk of post-partum haemorrhage (PPH). Recommended options include:

- once daily low molecular weight heparin to maintain the activated partial thromboplastin time (APTT) within therapeutic range throughout the pregnancy;

- warfarin throughout the pregnancy except for the first trimester (either for the entire trimester or between 6 and 12 weeks gestation) and from 34 weeks gestation when warfarin should be replaced by unfractionated or low molecular weight heparin.

When coumarins have been used after 6 weeks post-conception or throughout pregnancy, fetal risks should be assessed by detailed ultrasound scan (USS), but termination of pregnancy is not necessarily to be recommended (Reuvers 2001).

Clinical assessment

History: key points

- What drugs/exposures occurred?
- At what gestation was the pregnancy exposed?
- Family tree to determine whether any malfomations noted may have a genetic rather than a teratogenic basis.

Examination: key points

Detailed fetal anomaly USS with careful search for structural malformation.

Special investigations

Contact NTIS for an individual risk assessment.

Genetic advice and management

For women who have an affected infant, the recurrence risk is likely to be *high* if they stay on the same medication at the same dose. *Serious consideration must be given to revising her medication in advance of another pregnancy, in conjunction with her physician.*

Nevertheless, while the overall risk is high, the exact risk may be somewhat unpredictable since it is influenced by the pharmacometabolism of the feto-placental complex which is in part genetically determined and may vary between siblings. For example, a woman may stay on the same dose of sodium valproate in three pregnancies, but only have one child who is adversely affected.

Information sources: UK: National Teratology Information Service (NTIS) <www.ncl.ac.uk/pharmsc/entis.htm> Tel. 0191 232 1525; Europe: European Teratology Information Services (ENTIS) <www.entisorg.com>; Canada: Motherisk Program <www.motherisk.org>, Tel. (416) 813 6780; USA: OTIS Organisation of Teratology Information Services <www.otispregnancy.org> Tel. (866) 626 6847.

Expert adviser: Patricia McElhatton, Consultant Teratologist and Head of National Teratology Information Service, Newcastle-upon-Tyne, England.

References

Austin M-PV, Mitchell PB. Pschotropic medications in pregnant women: treatment dilemmas. *Med J Australia* 1998; **169**: 428–31.

Barr M Jr. Teratogen update: angiotensin-converting enzyme inhibitors. *Teratology* 1994; **50**: 399–409.

Bracken MB. Oral contraception and congenital malformations in offspring: a review and meta-analysis of the prospective studies. *Obstet Gynecol* 1990; **76**: 552–7.

Cotrufo M, de Feo M, *et al.* Risk of warfarin during pregnancy with mechanical valve prostheses. *Obstet Gynecol* 2002; **99**: 35–40.

Holmes LB. Teratogen-induced limb defects. *Am J Med Genet* 2003; **112**: 297–303.

Hoyme HE, Jones KL, *et al.* Prenatal cocaine exposure and fetal vascular disruption. *Pediatrics* 1991; **87**: 416–18.

Jacobson SJ, Jones K, *et al.* Prospective multicentre study of pregnancy outcome after lithium exposure during first trimester. *Lancet* 1992; **339**: 530–3.

Jilma B, Kamath S, *et al.* ABC of antithrombotic therapy. Antithrombotic therapy in special circumstances. I Pregnancy and cancer. *Br Med J* 2003; **326**: 37–40.

Koren G, Pastuszak A, Ito S. Drugs in pregnancy [review]. *New Engl J Med* 1998; **338**: 1128–37.

Moore JA. An assessment of lithium using the IEHR evaluative process for assessing human developmental and reproductive toxicity of agents. IEHR Expert Scientific Committee. *Reprod Toxicol* 1995; **9** (2): 175–210.

Raman-Wilms L, Tseng AL, *et al.* Fetal genital effects of first trimester sex hormone exposure: a meta-analysis. *Obstet Gynecol* 1995; **85**: 141–9.

Reuvers M. Anticoagulants and antifibrinolytics. In *Drugs during pregnancy and lactation* (ed. C. Schaefer), pp. 85–92. Elsevier, Amsterdam, 2001.

Schaefer C. Anticoagulants and antifibrinolytics. In *Drugs during pregnancy and lactation* (ed. C. Schaefer), pp. 312–13. Elsevier, Amsterdam, 2001.

Schou M. What happened to the lithium babies? A follow-up study of children born without malformations. *Acta Psychiatr Scand* 1976; **54**: 193–7.

Schou M, Goldfield MD, *et al.* Lithium and pregnancy. I. Report from the Register of Lithium Babies. *Br Med J* 1973; **2**: 135–6.

Shepard TH, Brent RL, *et al.* Update on new developments in the study of human teratogens. *Teratology* 2002; **65**: 153–61.

Wilson LC, Kerr BA, *et al.* Choanal atresia and hypothelia following methimagole exposure in utero: a second report. *Am J Med Genet* 1998; **75**: 220–22.

Female infertility and amenorrhoea: genetic aspects

Infertility is defined by the failure to conceive after 12 months of unprotected intercourse and affects an estimated 14% of the population of reproductive age in the UK (Templeton *et al.* 1990). Despite advances in the diagnosis of causes of subfertility, inability to conceive remains unexplained in 25–30% of fully investigated couples. The conditions listed here are those that tend to be referred to the genetics clinic for advice; they affect only a small minority of women presenting with infertility.

Primary amenorrhoea. The four most common causes of primary amenorrhea are gonadal dysgenesis (48.5%), congenital absence of the uterus and vagina (CAUV; 16.2%), gonadotrophin-releasing hormone (GnRH) deficiency (8.3%), and constitutional delay of puberty (6.0%) (Timmreck and Reindollar 2003). For further information on ovarian failure, see 'Premature ovarian failure', page 620, and 'Turner syndrome, 45, X and variants' page 558.

Clinical assessment

History: key points
- Three-generation family history.
- Birth history and early development.
- Enquire about breast development, menarche, and menstruation.

Examination: key points
- Detailed assessment is usually undertaken by a gynaecologist/fertility specialist. This includes a general physical exam, assessment of secondary sex characteristics, and pelvic exam.
- Assess whether the neck is short or whether there is any limitation of movement (MURCS (Müllerian duct anomalies–renal aplasia–cervicothoracic somite dysplasia)).

Special investigations
- Usually baseline investigations (e.g. day-3 serum follicle-stimulating hormone (FSH), luteinizing hormone (LH), prolactin, and thyroid function tests; day-21 serum progesterone (as well) and a pelvic ultrasound scan (USS) or magnetic resonance imaging (MRI)) will have been undertaken by the reproductive medicine team. Ovarian and adrenal androgens may also have been measured. In primary amenorrhoea spot measurements of hormone levels are taken as, without an established menstrual cycle, it is not possible to date the measurements.
- Karyotype.

Diagnoses to consider

Turner syndrome. 45,X karyotype giving rise to female phenotype with short stature and streak gonads. See 'Turner syndrome, 45,X and variants' page 558.

Congenital adrenal hyperplasia (CAH). Non-classical CAH may present with subfertility in adult life. See 'Congenital adrenal hyperplasia (CAH)' page 282.

Congenital absence of uterus and vagina (CAUV). Also known as Mayer–Rokitansky–Kuster–Hauser syndrome or Müllerian aplasia. Prevalence is 1/4000–1/5000 females. Patients with CAUV are genetically and phenotypically female, with 46, XX karyotype, normal ovaries, breast development, and female patterns of body hair. In most CAUV patients, the uterus, cervix, and upper two-thirds of the vagina are absent; normal Fallopian tubes may be present and caudally attached to two small muscular buds. Most cases are isolated with only occasional reports of familial occurrence. Elias *et al.* (1984) found only 1/37 female sibs to have a symptomatic uterine anomaly (2.7%), and 0/24 mothers, 0/45 maternal aunts, and 0/50 paternal aunts. Petrozza *et al.*'s (1997) survey of 17 female infants born through surrogacy to CAUV women did not reveal any CAUV offspring, suggesting it rarely follows autosomal dominant (AD) inheritance.

There is a high incidence of associated anomalies.
- Renal malformations in 30%, e.g. unilateral renal agenesis or ectopia of one or both kidneys. Arrange renal USS.
- Skeletal anomalies including spinal and limb defects in 11–12%. Arrange cervical spine films.
- Cardiac and hearing defects have also been described but are uncommon.

MURCS (Müllerian duct anomalies–renal aplasia–cervicothoracic somite dysplasia (Klippel–Feil anomaly)) is thought to be a sporadic disorder.

Complete androgen insensitivity syndrome (CAIS). Female phenotype with 46,XY karyotype characterized by primary amenorrhoea due to absent uterus and absent/sparse pubic and axillary hair. CAIS is due to mutations in the androgen receptor gene. See 'Androgen insensitivity syndrome (AIS)' page 270.

Gonadal agenesis/dysgenesis (including 46,XY).
- *SRY* mutations or deletions of SRY (explains only 15–20% of XY females).
- Approximately 80% of XY females with gonadal dysgenesis are of unknown aetiology. They often have uterus and streak gonads.

Hypogonadotrophic hypogonadism. The genetic basis for idiopathic hypogonadotropic hypogonadism is largely unknown. Genes currently recognized to be involved were reviewed by Silveira *et al.* (2002) and include *KAL-1* (associated with X-linked Kallmann syndrome), GnRH receptor, gonadotrophins, pituitary transcription factors (*HESX1*, *LHX3*, and *PROP-1*), orphan nuclear receptors (*DAX-1*, associated with X-linked congenital adrenal hypoplasia, and *SF-1*), and three genes also associated with obesity (leptin, leptin receptor, and prohormone convertase 1 (*PC1*)). Treatment comprises induction of puberty and maintenance replacement therapy. Fertility induction treatment is sometimes possible with gametogenesis induced by either exogenous gonadotrophin or pulsatile GnRH therapy. Since pregnancy is dependent on assisted reproductive technology (ART) and has only recently become available to affected women, there are very few data on offspring risks.

Kallmann syndrome (KS) is a genetic condition characterized by the association of hypogonadotrophic hypogonadism and anosmia with or without other anomalies. It is much less common in females than in males and affects ~1/40 000 females. See 'Male infertility: genetic aspects', page 606.

Genetic advice and management
- The geneticist's role is to explain the genetic basis of the disorder causing infertility/amenorrhoea. Depending on the specific diagnosis, if ART using the patient's own ova

could be used to achieve a pregnancy, then advice about reproductive implications is also appropriate.

- Management of the amenorrhoea and infertility is the remit of a specialist in reproductive medicine.
- ART enables pregnancy in some patients. Women with ovarian failure may use donated ovum to achieve a pregnancy. Women with CAUV may undergo oocyte retrieval and *in vitro* fertilization (IVF) and have their fetus carried by a surrogate mother.

Support groups: Müllerian aplasia <rosagroup@yahoo.co.uk>; CHILD:The National Infertility Support Network <www.child.org.uk>, Tel. 01424 732361.

Expert advisers: Melanie Davies, Consultant Obstetrician and Gynaecologist (Reproductive Medicine) and Ozkan Ozturk, Senior Lecturer in Obstetrics and Gynaecology (Reproductive Medicine), both at University College Hospital, London, England.

References

Elias S, Simpson JL, *et al*. Genetics studies in incomplete müllerian fusion. *Obstet Gynecol* 1984; **63**: 276–9.

Evers JLH. Female subfertility [seminar]. *Lancet* 2002; **360**: 151–9.

Kobayashi A, Behringer RR. Developmental genetics of the female reproductive tract in mammals. *Nat Rev Genet* 2003; **4**: 969–80.

Petrozza JC, Fray MR, *et al*. Congenital absence of the uterus and vagina is not commonly transmitted as a dominant genetic trait: outcomes of surrogate pregnancies. *Fertil Steril* 1997; **67**: 387–9.

Resendes BL, Sohn SH, *et al*. Role for anti-Müllerian hormone in congenital absence of the uterus and vagina. *Am J Med Genet* 2001; **98**: 129–36.

Silveira LF, MacColl GS, Bouloux PM. Hypogonadotropic hypogonadism. *Semin Reprod Med* 2002; **20** (4): 327–38.

Templeton A, Fraser C, Thompson B. The epidemiology of infertility in Aberdeen. *Br Med J.* 1990; **301** (6744): 148–52.

Timmreck LS, Reindollar RH. Contemporary issues in primary amenorrhea. *Obstet Gynecol Clin North Am* 2003; **30** (2): 287–302.

Fetal alcohol syndrome (FAS)

Sometimes the geneticist is asked to evaluate a child to determine whether his/her learning difficulties or short stature are related to prenatal alcohol exposure. This opinion may be used in court proceedings or care orders and it is important that it is as accurate as possible. It is also crucial to establish this diagnosis because of the potential for preventing recurrence in future pregnancies if the maternal alcohol problems can be treated.

On other occasions, the history of maternal alcohol exposure is not forthcoming and has to be carefully sought during the evaluation of a child presenting with developmental delay. The incidence of FAS varies depending on geographical location but, according to Sampson *et al.* (1997), the incidence per thousand livebirths in Seattle (US) was 2.8 and in Cleveland (US) was 4.6. The combined rate of FAS and alcohol-related neurodevelopmental disorder (ARND) in Seattle was estimated at nearly 1% of all livebirths. The reduced brain mass and neurobehavioural disturbances associated with human FAS may be related to the recent observation in rats that ethanol can trigger widespread apoptotic neurodegeneration (Ikonomidou *et al.* 2000).

Quantitative structural MRs in children with FAS has shown structural abnormalities in several regions of the brain, including the cerebellum, corpus callosum and the basal ganglia. The changes are more frequent and severe in children with dysmorphic facial features (Riley).

- Both high regular intake of alcohol and binge drinking can cause FAS and ARND.
- The critical time period extends throughout pregnancy.
- FAS is associated with high-dose exposure (estimated blood alcohol concentrations to ≥ 150 mg/dl) delivered at least weekly for at least several weeks in the first trimester, or chronic ingestion of at least 2 g/kg/day of alcohol. (1 unit (10 g alcohol) = 1 glass of table wine = 0.5 pint of beer, lager, or cider = 1 measure of sherry or vermouth. Standard bottle of spirits = 32 units; standard bottle of wine = 8 units; can of extra strong lager = 4 units.)
- There is a continuum of risk with population-based studies showing that chronic low-dose exposures to 15 cc absolute alcohol per day can be associated with reduction in intelligence quotient (IQ) and increased rates of attention and learning problems. These changes are too subtle to detect in an individual, but at higher levels of exposure probably merge with ARND.

The table gives the clinical features of FAS.

Diagnostic categories (Stratton et al. *1996*)

1 FAS with confirmed maternal alcohol exposure.
- Face, central nervous system (CNS) neurodevelopmental and growth anomalies.
- Clear history of alcohol exposure (substantial regular intake or heavy episodic drinking; there may be a history of drunken episodes, withdrawal symptoms, social problems related to drinking, assault, liver problems).

2 FAS without confirmed maternal alcohol exposure.
- Face, brain, and growth anomalies.
- Fostered or adopted child without pregnancy history available.

3 Partial FAS with confirmed maternal alcohol exposure.

Clinical features of FAS

Facial features*
Short palpebral fissures
Flat midface
Long and flattened philtrum
Thin vermilion of upper lip

Growth retardation
Low birthweight for gestational age (less than 2.5 centile)
Decelerating weight over time not due to nutrition
Disproportionately low weight to height relationship

CNS neurodevelopmental anomalies
Microcephaly or decreased cranial size at birth
Structural brain anomalies, e.g. partial or complete agenesis of corpus callosum, cerebellar hypoplasia
Impaired fine motor skills, sensorineural deafness, poor hand–eye coordination, poor tandem gait

Behavioural/cognitive/learning deficits
Complex pattern of behaviour or cognitive abnormalities that are inconsistent with developmental level and cannot be explained by family background or environment alone, such as learning difficulties, deficits in school performance, poor impulse control, problems in social perception, deficits in higher-level receptive and expressive language, poor capacity for abstraction, specific deficits in mathematical skills, or problems in memory, attention, and judgement

* Moore *et al.* (2001) have identified 6 craniofacial measurements that could differentiate individuals with and without prenatal alcohol exposure with 96% accuracy, 98% sensitivity, and 90% specificity.

- Some facial features.
- Growth retardation or CNS neurodevelopmental abnormalities or behavioural/ cognitive/learning deficits.

4 Alcohol related birth-defects, e.g. congenital heart disease (CHD), developmental anomalies of the renal tract, etc. This may coexist with category 5.

5 ARND. CNS neurodevelopmental anomalies or behavioural/cognitive/learning deficits; may coexist with category 4.

Clinical assessment

History: key points
- Draw a brief family tree and document parental heights (useful for calculating target parental centile range in assessment of short stature).
- Obtain a detailed account of maternal alcohol intake throughout pregnancy. If you strongly suspect FAS clinically, you may need to seek information on maternal alcohol intake from several sources, e.g. relatives, obstetric record, or GP.
- Take a careful history of exposures in pregnancy including medical and recreational drugs.
- Document the birthweight. Are other birth measurements recorded, e.g. occipital-frontal circumference (OFC)?
- Developmental history.

Examination: key points
- Growth parameters. Height, weight, OFC (measure head size and height of parents for comparison).

- Facial features (see table above).
- Neurological examination including developmental assessment.

Special investigations

Whether or not to do further investigations is a matter for individual clinical judgement, and will be in part dictated by how compelling the evidence for FAS is. It is our usual practice to do the following investigations.

- Karyotype.
- FRAX (fragile X syndrome) unless microcephalic.
- Consider magnetic resonance imaging (MRI) scan.

Genetic advice and management

Unless the maternal alcohol problem is successfully treated the recurrence risks in a subsequent pregnancy are high.

Support group: Fetal alcohol syndrome trust <www.medicouncilalcol.demon.co.uk/FAST/fast.htm>.

Expert adviser: Lewis B. Holmes, Professor of Pediatrics, Harvard Medical School and Chief, Genetics and Teratology Unit, Massachusetts General Hospital for Children, Boston, Massachusetts, USA.

References

Astley SJ, Clarren SK. A case definition and photographic screening tool for the facial phenotype of fetal alcohol syndrome. *J Pediatr* 1996; **129**: 33–41.

Ikonomidou C, Bittigau P, *et al.* Ethanol-induced apoptotic neuro-degeneration and fetal alcohol syndrome. *Science* 2000; **287**: 1056–60.

Mattson SN, Riley EP, *et al.* Heavy prenatal alcohol exposure with or without physical features of fetal alchol syndrome leads to IQ deficits. *J Pediatr* 1997; **131**: 718–21.

Moore ES, Ward RE, *et al.* The subtle facial signs of prenatal exposure to alcohol: an anthropometric approach. *J Pediatr* 2001; **139** (2): 215–19.

Riley EP, McGee CL, *et al.* Teratogenic effects of alcohol: a decade of brain imaging. *Am J Med Genet* 2004; **127c**: 35–41.

Sampson PD, Streissguth AP, *et al.* Incidence of fetal alcohol syndrome and prevalence of alcohol-related neurodevelopmental disorder. *Teratology* 1997; **56**: 317–26.

Stratton K, Howe C, Battaglia F (Eds.). *Fetal alcohol syndrome: diagnosis, epidemiology, prevention and treatment,* Institute of Medicine Committee to study fetal alcohol syndrome. National Academy Press, Washington DC, 1996.

Fetal anticonvulsant syndrome (FACS)

Seizure disorders are one of the most common neurological problems affecting women of child-bearing age. Approximately 0.4% of pregnant women take anticonvulsant medication during pregnancy. Sodium valproate (Epilim), phenytoin (Epanutin), carbamazepine (Tegretol), and phenobarbitone all have teratogenic potential. A range of newer anticonvulsant agents such as lamogitrine, vigabactrin, topiramate, etc. have been introduced over the past 10–15 years, but experience in pregnancy is slight and their teratogenic potential is unclear.

For any woman with epilepsy who is contemplating pregnancy, the risks of anticonvulsant therapy must be weighed against the risks of seizure-induced morbidity and mortality, both to the mother and the unborn fetus. Maternal morbidity includes the physical risks of accidents and the social consequences of active epilepsy (e.g. loss of driving licence) and the risk of sudden unexplained death in epilepsy (SUDEP), a documented cause of death in maternal mortality statistics in recent years. Fetal morbidity in epilepsy is largely related to the risks of the mother falling, the risks of status epilepticus during pregnancy and seizures during delivery (1–2% of women with epilepsy will have a convulsion during delivery), and the risks due to teratogenic effects of anti-epileptic drugs.

Main features of anticonvulsant embryopathy

Major malformations. The major malformations seen most often in anticonvulsant-exposed children are those that also occur commonly in unexposed children: heart defects, hypospadias, club-foot, and cleft lip or palate (the risk for cleft lip is increased 3-fold after exposure to phenobarbital as monotherapy, but is increased only slightly after exposure to phenytoin). The risk for neural tube defects appears to be ~5% with valproate exposure, ~1% with carbamazepine exposure, and not increased for other drugs

Microcephaly (?noted only after polytherapy)

Growth retardation

Midface hypoplasia, e.g. depressed bridge of the nose, short nose with anteverted nostrils, and long upper lip; less commonly, a broad bridge of the nose, thin vermilion, small mouth, and a wide philtrum

Hypoplasia of the fingers, e.g. arch patterns on >5 fingers and/or stiff interphalangeal joints; nail hypoplasia

Overall, there is a fairly solid consensus that treastment with anticonvulsants in pregnancy for whatever reason, i.e. epilepsy or mood disorder, is associated with an *overall two- to threefold increased risk of congenital malformation* (see table) compared to the risk in the general population (Dolk and McElhatton 2002). The actual risks in a given pregnancy are somewhat idiosyncratic, being dependent on the specific drug, individual maternal and fetal metabolism, and genetic susceptibility—factors not yet clarified. Hence there are no hard and fast rules about teratogenic thresholds. The risks are greater for combination therapy and for higher doses. The lowest risks are with exposure to monotherapy at the lowest dose compatible with adequate seizure control.

Recently, concern is emerging about important adverse effects on *cognitive development and behaviour*. In a retrospective study of 57 children with FACS who were ascertained through the FACS support group (introducing ascertainment bias to the study, which would tend to increase the frequency of reporting of developmental abnormalities), Moore et al. (2000) found 46/57 (81%) reported behavioural problems, e.g. hyperactivity and poor concentration, 46/57 had speech delay, 44/57 (77%) had learning problems, and 6/57 (11%) had a diagnosis of autism or Asperger syndrome. Reinisch et al. (1995) provides convincing evidence of significantly lower verbal intelligence scores (−0.5 SD) after *in utero* exposure to phenobarbital, with the effect most marked for exposure in the third trimester. The anticonvulsant-exposed child with midface hypoplasia has an increased risk of having deficits in cognitive function in comparison to the exposed child with a normal face (Holmes).

The pathogenesis of congenital heart disease (CHD) in FACS is not understood and a variety of defects are seen including ventricular septal defect (VSD), aortic stenosis, pulmonary stenosis, and patent ductus arteriosus (PDA).

In one recent study (Holmes et al. 2001), the combined frequency of anticonvulsant embryopathy was 20.6% (odds ratio (OR), 2.8) in children exposed to monotherapy, and 28% (OR, 4.2) in children exposed to 2 or more drugs versus 8.5% in unexposed controls (children whose mothers did not have epilepsy). This study showed that there is a pattern of effects, not just major malformations. This pattern with cognitive deficits should be considered to be 'fetal anticonvulsant syndrome'.

Clinical assessment

History: key points

- Three-generation family tree.
- Detailed enquiry about the precise dose and type of anticonvulsant taken during pregnancy (may need to request mother's obstetric notes for this information).
- Enquiry about other potential teratogenic exposures during pregnancy, e.g. alcohol, maternal illness.
- Detailed history of delivery and perinatal period including birthweight. Were there symptoms of neonatal withdrawal, e.g. jitteriness, seizures, poor feeding?
- Detailed developmental and behavioural history of the child.

Examination: key points

- Height, weight, occipital-frontal circumference (OFC).
- Eyes. Assess for prominence of metopic ridge, hypertelorism/telecanthus, epicanthic folds, infraorbital groove.
- Mouth and nose. Assess shortness of nose, length of philtrum, smoothness of philtrum, thinness of upper lip, left lip/palate.
- Hands and feet for joint laxity, nail hypoplasia, stiffness of interphalangeal joints, long overlapping fingers.
- Heart for murmur.
- Hypospadias.

Special investigations

If there is developmental delay with dysmorphic features:

- chromosomes;
- FRAXA (fragile X syndrome);
- urine amino and organic acids.

Genetic advice and management

Sibling recurrence risk is estimated at 39–55% (Dean et al. 2002).

If there is a possibility of a subsequent pregnancy refer to a neurologist for assessment as to whether it is appropriate to consider: withdrawal of anticonvulsants (if the mother has not had a seizure for several years); simplification of therapy (monotherapy rather than polytherapy); or, if the seizures are well controlled, a reduction in dose. The total dose of valproate (and possibly other drugs) should be divided and given 3 to 4 times a day to minimize high peak concentrations of the parent drug or its metabolites. Slow-release preparations are available. Emphasize to the mother that she should not stop or change her medication without prior discussion with her neurologist.

Child with FACS

- Consider referral for vision screening (high incidence of refractive error in FACS, e.g. myopia in 50% of those exposed to valproate).
- Consider referral for audiometry (glue ear in 33%)
- Consider referral to child development centre if developmental delay.

Future pregnancy

- Screening for neural tube defects (NTDs: alpha fetoprotein (AFP) and ultrasound scan (USS)) and cardiac defects (fetal echocardiography) can be offered.
- With the exception of a major structural malformation, it is not currently possible to offer prenatal diagnosis for FACS.
- Consider periconceptual high-dose folic acid supplementation (4 mg/day) because valproate (VPA), carbamazepine, phenytoin, phenobarbitone, and primidone are all folate antagonists (although Hernandez-Diaz et al. (2000) did not find a protective effect of multivitamin supplementation).
- Take anticonvulsant therapy as monotherapy and keep the dose as low as possible (divide doses through the day; see above).
- Vitamin K should be given to the baby at birth by intramuscular (IM) injection.

Features associated with specific anticonvulsant drugs

- **Valproate.** Tenfold increase in incidence of NTDs. In Kozma's (2001) survey the most commonly observed musculoskeletal abnormalities include contractures of small joints and presence of long overlapping fingers (36%), foot deformity (30%), thumb abnormalities (17%), and radial defects (16%). Trigonocephaly or a prominent metopic suture is common. There appears to be a significant risk for cleft palate without cleft lip. The teratogenic effects of VPA are related to dose in the first trimester and large daily doses of VPA (>1000 mg) have a higher risk of causing malformations and NTDs than smaller doses. In the Australian study (Vajda et al. 2003) the dose of VPA taken was higher in pregnancies with birth defects compared to those without (mean 2081 mg versus 1149 mg; $p < 0.0001$). High daily doses at the end of pregnancy increase the likelihood of fetal withdrawal symptoms such as irritability, jitteriness, and neonatal seizures.

  In 2005, Wyszynski reported a 10.7% prevalence of major malformations in babies exposed to VPA monotherapy in the first trimestere of pregnancy, compared with 2.9% in offspring of women exposed to all other antiepileptic drugs and 1.6% in the normal new born population.

- **Carbamazepine.** Some increased risk for NTDs, but less than for VPA. Hypoplastic nails have been specifically noted after carbemazepine therapy. Facial features are less obvious than with VPA.
- **Lamotrigine.** In 2002, Tennis reported the rate of major malformations was 1.8% among 168 monotheraphy-exposed infants. The UK Epilepsy and Pregnancy Registry reported 2.1% among 390 monotherapy-exposed infant. (Morrow). There is currently no long-term follow-up data available regarding neurodevelopmental outcome.

Support group: National Fetal Anti-convulsant Syndrome Association <www.facsline.org>.

Expert advisers: Jill Clayton-Smith, Consultant Clinical Geneticist, St Mary's Hospital, Manchester, England and Lewis B. Holmes, Professor of Pediatrics, Harvard Medical School and Chief, Genetics and Teratology Unit, Massachusetts General Hospital for Children, Boston, Massachusetts, USA.

References

Dean JCS, Hailey H, et al. Long term health and neurodevelopment in children exposed to antiepileptic drugs before birth. *J Med Genet* 2002; **39**: 251–9.

Dolk H, McElhatton P. Assessing epidemiological evidence for the teratogenic effects of anticonvulsant medications. *J Med Genet* 2002; **39**: 243–4.

Glover SJ, Quinn AG, et al. Ophthalmic findings in fetal anticonvulsant syndrome(s). *Ophthalmology* 2002; **109**: 942–7.

Hernandez-Diaz S, Werler MM, et al. Folic acid antagonists during prenancy and the risk of birth defects. *New Engl J Med* 2000; **34**: 1608–14.

Holmes LB. The teratogenicity of anticonvulsant drugs; a progress report [commentary]. *J Med Genet* 2002; **39**: 245–7.

Holmes LB, Coull BA, et al. The correlation of deficits in IQ with midface and digit hypoplasia in children exposed in utero to anticonvulsant drugs. *J Pediatr* 2005; **146**: 118–22.

Holmes LB, Harvey EA, et al. The teratogenicity of anticonvulsant drugs. *New Engl J Med* 2001; **344**: 1132–8.

Kozma C. Valproic acid embryopathy: report of two siblings with further expansion of the phenotypic abnormalities and a review of the literature. *Am J Med Genet* 2001; **98**: 168–75.

Moore SJ, Turnpenny P, et al. A clinical study of 57 children with fetal anticonvulsant syndromes. *J Med Genet* 2000; **37** (7): 489–97.

Morrow JI, et al. *Epilepsia* 2003; **44** (suppl 8); (Abstract PO96).

Reinisch JM, Sanders SA, et al. In utero exposure to phenobarbital and intelligence deficits in adult men. *J Am Med Assoc* 1995; **274** (19): 1518–25.

Shorvon S. Antiepileptic drug therapy during pregnancy: the neurologist's perspective [commentary]. *J Med Genet* 2002; **39**: 248–50.

Tennis P, Eldridge RR, et al. Preliminary results on pregnancy outcome in women using lamiotrigine, *Epilepsia* 2002; **43**: 1161–67.

Vajda FJ, O'Brien TJ, et al. The Australian registry of anti-epileptic drugs in pregnancy: experience after 30 months. *J Clin Neurosci* 2003; **10**: 543–9.

Williams G, King J, et al. Fetal valproate syndrome and autism: additional evidence of an association. *Dev Med Child Neurol* 2001: **43**: 202–6.

Wyszynski DF, Nambisan M, et al. Increased rate of major malformations in offspring exposed to valproate during pregnancy. *Neurology* 2005; **64**: 961–65.

Fetomaternal alloimmunization (rhesus D and thrombocytopenia)

Alloimmunization against blood cell alloantigens

Blood cell alloantigen incompatibility between fetus and mother may occur where the fetus possesses a blood cell alloantigen derived from the father that is not present on the maternal blood cells. Blood cell alloantibodies of the IgG class will cross the placenta and bind their cognate alloantigen. If the expression of the alloantigen is restricted to one type of blood cell, then IgG-mediated blood cell destruction may ensue, resulting in anaemia, thrombocytopenia, or neutropenia, respectively.

Red cell blood groups

- **Rhesus D (RhD).** About 15 % of Caucasian women are RhD negative. Immunization against RhD is rare because of the introduction of RhD prophylaxis. Severe RhD haemolytic disease of the newborn (HDN) occurs in less than 100 cases per annum in the UK (620 000 live births).
  - Alloimmunization against red cell alloantigens occurs as a consequence of fetomaternal haemorrhage, which is generally below 4 ml of fetal erythrocytes. The amount of fetomaternal haemorrhage needs to be measured in RhD negative women within 48 hours after delivery of a RhD positive baby so that the amount of RhD prophylaxis can be adjusted in case of bleeds exceeding 4 ml. Abdominal trauma, complications of pregnancy such as vaginal bleeding and abruption, and any invasive procedures carry an increased risk of significant fetomaternal haemorrhage. Such events in RhD negative women need to be covered with RhD prophylaxis.
  - Prevention of RhD immunization is by injection of anti-D immunoglobulin G (RhD prophylaxis) to all RhD negative pregnant women at specified times during pregnancy and after delivery in case of a RhD positive baby. Once sensitization occurs, RhD prophylaxis is no longer effective.
- **Red cell alloantigens other than RhD.** HDN because of immunization against red cell blood groups other then RhD is rare but may be severe, i.e. in the case of K(ell) immunization. ABO incompatibility cannot cause severe anaemia in the fetus, but frank haemolysis may occur in the group A or B neonate born to a group O mother.

A routine screening programme to identify women with immunization against red cell alloantigens other than A and B and to identify all RhD negative women is in place. The aim of this screening programme is to prevent morbidity and mortality due to severe HDN and to provide compatible transfusion support for alloimmunized women. Good antenatal care should prevent the occurrence of hydrops fetalis and cases of severe HDN should be managed in partnership with a fetal medicine team with an interest in HDN and the National Blood Service. Monitoring of the severity of RhD immunization is by measuring the concentration of anti-D in the maternal serum. In case of a RhD heterozygous partner, RhD genotyping can be performed on maternal plasma from late in the first trimester.

Clinical features in the fetus

- The fetus becomes anaemic due to haemolysis caused by the maternal IgG anti-D.
- The severity of the anaemia can be determined by periumbilical blood sampling (PUBS).
- Before correction of fetal anaemia became feasible by the transfusion of RhD negative donor blood, cardiac failure developed as the fetus becomes more anaemic and, in severe cases, progressed to hydrops fetalis.

The management of the at-risk fetus. Since the technical advance of PUBS, survival rates of severe cases have been excellent. Precise data on mortality are lacking but are in the UK thought to be as low as 10 per annum. The following investigations are routine.

- Prior history of HDN.
- Maternal anti-D quantitation in IU/ml.
- RhD phenotyping of the partner.
- In case of a heterozygous partner, RhD genotyping of the fetus on maternal plasma.
- Ultrasound (USS) fetal assessment.
- Fetal haemoglobin (Hb) estimation by PUBS and, if required, correction of anaemia by intrauterine, intravascular transfusion.
- Amniocentesis has become less popular as the method of spectrophotometry for bilirubin (Liley index) has its limitations.

The management of the neonate
- RhD antigen and direct antiglobulin test.
- Full blood count and bilirubin levels.
- Severe HDN may become apparent by the baby rapidly becoming jaundiced, as the immature liver is unable to adequately conjugate the bilirubin and levels of unconjugated bilirubin rise. This is toxic to the brain and unless treated may lead to kernicterus. Exchange transfusion is used both to treat the anaemia and lower the level of bilirubin.

The management of the at-risk neonate. When it is expected that an infant may be severely affected, the paediatricians, haematologist, and the National Blood Service (NBS) should be aware of the likely delivery date so that preparations for an immediate exchange transfusion at birth (if necessary) have been made. Group O RhD negative blood from specially selected donors is available from the NBS and must be crossmatched against the serum of the mother. Exchange transfusion because of RhD disease is nowadays rare as the majority of severe cases will have been transfused *in utero*.

Neonatal alloimmune thrombocytopenia (NAIT)

NAIT is defined as an isolated thrombocytopenia with a count $<150 \times 10^9/l$ and caused by maternal IgG alloantibodies against platelet-specific alloantigens. So-called human platelet antigen (HPA) antibodies cause severe thrombocytopenia in approximately 1 per 1200 live births in Caucasians and this is the most frequent cause of severe thrombocytopenia in the otherwise healthy term infant.

In sharp contrast to HDN, NAIT is *frequently observed in a first pregnancy*. No screening for HPA immunization is place. The presentation is usually through an infant with thrombocytopenic purpura, petechiae, and/or other signs of bleeding. The main clinical concern is the risk of an intracranial haemorrhage during pregnancy, delivery, or in the neonatal period. In Caucasoids the most commonly encountered HPA antibody is against HPA-1a (formerly P1^{A1}, Zw^a).

The management of the pregnant woman who is known to be alloimmunized against HPA-1a is complex and there are several options. A choice must be based on the history of previous pregnancies (in > 90% of cases the severity of thrombocytopenia will be as or more severe). For high-risk cases the following approaches are possible.

- HPA genotype the partner and, if heterozygous, determine the HPA genotype of the fetus from a sample of amniotic fluid.

If the amniotic fluid is positive for the cognate HPA antigen the following is suggested.

- Weekly infusion of high-dose intravenous immunoglobulin G (IV IgG) with or without corticosteroids given to the mother (the preferred approach in North American centres), *or*
- repeated *in utero* transfusions of HPA-compatible platelets from highly selected donors (the preferred treatment approach in some European centres).
- The least traumatic route of delivery. Generally, a planned Caesarean section is chosen but there is no good evidence that this reduces the risk of an intracranial bleed in the 'at risk' neonate.
- The paediatrician, haematologist, and transfusion service should be informed prior to delivery so that compatible HPA-matched platelets are available to treat the baby.

The management of a new index case is on basis of the clinical signs of bleeding and the platelet count. In case of overt bleeding or a platelet count < 20 x 10^9/l, correction of the count with HPA-1a and -5b negative donor platelets is recommended. The results of the serological investigation must not be awaited as the risk of severe bleeding is assumed to be highest in the first 48 hours after delivery.

Clinical assessment

History: key points
- Previous affected child.
- Fetal loss/miscarriage prior to any blood group testing.

- Pregnancy complications that could cause fetomaternal haemorrhage.

Examination: key points
Not part of the genetic assessment.

Special investigations
These are performed by the fetal medicine team and a blood cell genetics/immunology reference centre (see above).

Genetic advice and management

- **HDN.** A routine preventative screening programme for red blood cell alloimmunization and the risk of HDN is in place. RhD negative women require antenal RhD prophylaxis with a follow-up dose after delivery of a RhD positive infant. RhD negative is generally based on a deletion of the RhD gene and is denoted with the Rh*dd* genotype. The RhD positive father may be homozygous for D (*DD*), in which case all future children are at risk of RhD immunization, or heterozygous (*Dd*) with a 50% risk.
- **NAIT.** No screening programme in place. It is important to investigate the HPA antigen status of sisters of child-bearing age when the condition has been confirmed in an index case. Families with a severe case history need to be managed in close partnership with a fetal medicine unit and the haematologist and the NBS.

Support group: Platelet Disorder Support Association `<www.pdsa.org>`.

Expert adviser: Willem H. Ouwehand, Lecturer in Haematology, University of Cambridge, Cambridge, England.

References
Blanchette VS, Johnson J, Rand M. The management of alloimmune neonatal thrombocytopenia. *Bailliere's Best Pract Res Clin Haematol* 2000; **13** (3): 365–90.

Bowman J. The management of hemolytic disease in the fetus and newborn *Semin Perinatol* 1997; **21** (1): 39–44.

Kaplan C. Immune thrombocytopenia in the foetus and the newborn: diagnosis and therapy. *Transfus Clin Biol* 2001; **8** (3): 311–14.

Moise KJ Jr. Management of rhesus alloimmunization in pregnancy. *Obstet Gynecol* 2002; **100** (3): 600–11.

Hyperechogenic bowel

Echogenic bowel, hyperechoic bowel.
Hyperechogenic bowel is a 'soft marker', usually identified as an incidental finding at a routine antenatal ultrasound (USS) examination. Assessment of the echogenicity of the fetal bowel is subjective: to be classed as hyperechogenic the bowel should be of equivalent brightness to the iliac crests. Hyperechogenic fetal bowel is detected in 0.1–1.8% of pregnancies during the second or third trimester. In some fetuses this is a normal variant However, there is a recognized association with fetal abnormality, including:

- chromosomal anomalies;
- cystic fibrosis (CF);
- congenital infection (cytomegalovirus (CMV) and toxoplasmosis);
- adverse pregnancy outcome e.g. IUGR, fetal death.

Intra-amniotic haemorrhage with fetal ingestion of blood pigments can cause hyperechogenic bowel.

Simon-Bouy et al. (2003) published a French multicentre study of 682 fetuses with hyperechogenic bowel. Karyotyping, screening for viral infection, and screening for CF mutations were performed in all cases. Pregnancy outcome and postnatal follow-up were known in 91%. Of the 682 cases, 65.5% had a normal outcome, 6.9% had multiple malformations, 3.5% had a significant chromosome anomaly, 3% had CF, and 2.8% had a viral infection. In Al-Kouatly et al.'s (2001a) series of 175 fetuses with hyperechogenic bowel, 5 had CF (3%), 5 had an autosomal trisomy (3%), 0 had toxoplasmosis, and 1 had CMV(0.5%). In one study (Al-Kouatly et al. 2001b), there was a 5.8% incidence of intrauterine fetal demise amongst fetuses with hyperechogenic bowel after CF, aneuploidy, and CMV infection had been excluded. Elevated maternal serum alpha-fetoprotein (AFP) and SHCG were the strongest predictor of this outcome, with oligohydramnios and intrauterine growth retardation (IUGR) also being important risk factors. With aneuploidy these are usually other abnormalities or risk factors present.

Clinical approach

History: key points

- Three-generation family tree with specific enquiry for CF.
- Detailed pregnancy history noting any pregnancy bleeding, maternal illness/rash, invasive procedures, e.g. chorionic villus sampling (CVS).
- Obtain results of aneuploidy screeming e.g. maternal serum screening (if available).

Examination: key points

- Fetal biometry.
- Detailed fetal anomaly USS to confirm hyperechogenic bowel and search carefully for other signs of fetal abnormality, placental haemorrhage, etc.
- Doppler measurements—placental and fetal.

Special investigations

- Consider amniocentesis. Risk for fetal chromosome anomaly (most commonly +21). The risk increases if other anomalies or markers on USS.

- Offer parental CF carrier testing (and arrange to store amniotic fluid and cultures pending these results). 2–3% risk for CF.
- Maternal serum for investigation of congenital infection.

Genetic advice and management

- Abnormal karyotype. Counsel as appropriate.
- Single CF mutation detected in fetus. The residual risk for CF in fetus with hyperechogenic bowel can be estimated as follows. 3% of fetuses with hyperechogenic bowel have CF and of these 22% will have a single CF mutation on a 29-mutation screen (see 'Cystic fibrosis (CF)', page 292). The remaining 97% of fetuses with hyperechogenic bowel are assumed to have the same carrier frequency for CF as the general population, i.e. 4%. Thus, for fetuses with hyperechogenic bowel and a single CF mutation, the ratio of CF affected:CF non-affected is $(3 \times 22):(97 \times 4) = 66:388$, i.e. ~1:6. Hence, of all fetuses with hyperechogenic bowel and a single CF mutation, ~15% will have CF. NB. The figures given are for a northern European population and need validating in practice and depend on the accuracy of definition of echogenic bowel.
- CF mutation detected in both parents. The risk for CF in fetus with hyperechogenic bowel is very high. Amniocentesis or placental biopsy could be used for diagnostic confirmation if termination of pregnancy is being considered. Alternatively, if the pregnancy is continuing, confirmation of the neonatal genotype could be made on cord blood at term. In Al-Kouatly et al.'s (2001a) series, 5/5 fetuses where both parents carried a mutation had CF.
- If negative CF screen and normal karyotype, the risk for early-onset IUGR and adverse pregnancy outcome remains. Instigate follow-up growth scans especially if maternal serum AFP and HCG elevated or Doppler studies abnormal.

Expert adviser: Lyn Chitty, Consultant in Fetal Medicine, University College Hospital, London, England.

References

Al-Kouatly HB, Chasen ST, et al. The clinical significance of fetal echogenic bowel. Am J Obstet Gynecol 2001a; **185**: 1035–8.

Al-Kouatley HB, Chasen ST, et al. Factors associated with fetal demise in fetal echogenic bowel. Am J Obstet Gynecol 2001b; **185**: 1039–43.

Bosco AF, Norton ME, et al. Predicting the risk of cystic fibrosis with echogenic bowel and one cystic fibrosis mutation. Obstet Gynecol 1999; **94**: 1020–23.

Penna L, Bower S. Hyperechogenic bowel in the second trimester fetus: a review. Prenat Diagn 2000; **20**: 909–13.

Simon-Bouy B, Satre V, et al. Hyperechogenic fetal bowel: a large French collaborative study of 682 cases. Am J Med Genet 2003; **121A** (3): 209–13.

Strocker AM, Snijders RJ, et al. Fetal echogenic bowel: parameters to be considered in differential diagnosis. Ultrasound Obstet Gynecol 2000; **16**: 519–23.

Hypoplastic left heart

Hypoplastic left heart syndrome (HLHS).
HLHS accounts for 1% of all congenital heart disease (CHD), but is responsible for 25% of deaths from CHD in the first week of life. In addition to the hypoplastic left ventricle, there may be aortic stenosis/atresia, mitral stenosis/atresia, and/or hypoplasia of the aortic arch. At least 21% of fetuses have extracardiac anomalies, including hydrops, hydrocephalus, Dandy–Walker malformation (DWM), etc. (Tennstedt et al.1999; Brackley et al. 2000). In postnatal series, only 10–15% have extracardiac anomalies (Natowicz et al. 1988; Perez-Delboy and Simpson 2003). In Brackley et al.'s (2000) series, overall survival rate for fetuses diagnosed with HLHS antenatally was 25% (excluding termination of pregnancy (TOP) cases). The left ventricular outflow tract malformations, aortic valve stenosis coarctation of the aorta and hypoplastic left heart constitute a mechanistically defined subgroup of congenital heart defects that have substantial evidence for a genetic component (with a complex but most likely oligogenic pattern of inheritance (McBride).

Clinical assessment

History: key points

- Obtain a three-generation family tree with specific enquiry regarding CHD.
- History of maternal diabetes.

Examination: key points

- Approximately 5% will have multiple congenital malformations that suggest a specific syndrome diagnosis (Natowicz et al. 1988).
- Detailed fetal ultrasound scan (USS). 21% have extracardiac anomalies (hydrops, hydrocephalus, DWM, etc.).

Special investigations

Karyotype including 22q. Overall, 12% have a chromosomal anomaly (+13, 45,X, +21, +18, del 5, del 11, etc), but only 6% if the hypoplastic left heart is an isolated finding.

Genetic advice and management

Genetic advice

Recurrence risk for future pregnancies. No figures are available from large prospective series. Brenner et al. (1989) found CHD in 13% of first-degree relatives of hypoplastic left heart patients. Recurrence of hypoplastic left heart occurs in 2–4% in some series (Perez-Delboy and Simpson 2003; Cox and Wilson, personal communication). Bicuspid aortic valve (BAV) may occur in asymptomatic parents and first-degree relatives of probands with aortic stenosis, coarctation of the aorta, and HLHS. 0.8% of the general population have BAV, but 7.7% of HLHS relatives had left ventricular outflow tract malformations or significant congenital heart disease in McBride's study.

Management

Options open to parents include:

- TOP;
- supportive comfort care for the infant. In the Birmingham series (Brackley et al. 2000), 7/11 died in the first week of life, and a further 3 within the first 28 days;
- Norwood staged palliation procedure. Of 36 babies who had surgery postnatally, 12 survived (33%). Post-delivery the baby is duct-dependent (requires prostaglandin E2 infusion if active management is planned) and rapid transfer to paediatric cardiothoracic centre (in utero transfer may be preferred by some units).

Support group: Little Hearts Matter, 11 Greenfield Crescent, Edgbaston, Birmingham, B15 3AU, Tel. 0121 455 8982, e-mail <info@lhm.org>, website <www.lhm.org.uk>.

Expert advisers: Helen Cox, Consultant in Clinical Genetics, Birmingham Womens' Hospital, Birmingham, UK and David I. Wilson, Professor of Human Developmental Genetics, University of Southampton, Southampton, England.

References

Brackley KJ, Kilby MD, et al. Outcome after prenatal diagnosis of hypoplastic left-heart syndrome: a case series. Lancet 2000; **356**: 1143–7.

Brenner JA, Berg KA, Schneider DS, Clark EB, Boughman JA. Cardiac malformations in relatives of infants with hypoplastic left heart syndrome. Am J Dis Child 1989; **143**: 1492–5.

McBride KL, Pignatellir R, et al. inheritance analysis of congenital left ventricular outflow tract obstruction malformations: segregation, multiplex relative risk, and heritability. Am J Med Genet A 2005; Feb 2nd.

Natowicz M, Chatten J, Clancy R, Conard K, Glauser T, Huff D, Lin A, Norwood W, Rorke LB, Uri A, Weinberg P, Zackai E, Kelley RI. Genetic disorders and major extracardiac anomalies associated with the hypoplastic left heart syndrome. Pediatrics 1988; **82**: 698–706.

Perez-Delboy A, Simpson GG. Ultrasound Med Biol 2003; **29**: S134.

Tennstedt C, Chaoui R, Korner H, Dietel M. Spectrum of congenital heart defects and extracardiac malformations associated with chromosomal abnormalities: results of a seven year necropsy study. Heart 1999; **82**: 34–39.

Towbin JA, Belmont J. Molecular determinants of left and right outflow tract obstruction. Am J Med Genet 2000; **97**: 297–303.

Imaging in prenatal diagnosis

Ultrasound scanning (USS)

Targeted USS can be very useful in prenatal diagnosis or surveillance of conditions characterized by structural anomalies. The role of the geneticist is to assess the genetic risk to the pregnancy and advise the patient and obstetrician on investigations available to manage that risk.

- Detailed fetal anomaly scanning is best interpreted if there is secure dating of the pregnancy. Arrange a dating USS at 8–12 weeks gestation. At this stage in pregnancy there is a tight correlation between crown–rump length (CRL) and gestation.
- Discuss the limitations of USS. It can detect many major structural anomalies, but not all, e.g. cleft palate can often be difficult to diagnose, the sonographic signs of some anomalies may present late (hydrocephalus, microcephaly, some renal anomalies), or the condition may have a variable presentation. USS does not give information regarding cognition, vision, or hearing (except when there are obvious gross structural defects present).

Dating USS is best undertaken at 8–12 weeks gestation. At this stage in pregnancy there is a tight correlation between CRL and gestation. It is an important investigation if invasive tests are planned, e.g. chorionic villus sampling (CVS) or amniocentesis, or if scanning will subsequently be used to monitor fetal growth or limb length.

Nuchal scanning is best undertaken at 11–13 weeks gestation. Increased nuchal translucency can be an indication of a chromosomal anomaly or congenital heart disease (CHD) or a wide variety of other syndromes, but many fetuses with a mildly enlarged nuchal translucency measurement are normal at birth. See 'Oedema—increased nuchal translucency, cystic hygroma, and hydrops', page 618.

Fetal anomaly scanning. Routine anomaly USS is usually undertaken around 20 weeks. If there is a past history of specific structural anomalies, or USS is being undertaken for prenatal diagnosis rather than routine obstetric screening, scanning should be arranged in conjunction with a fetal medicine specialist as the appropriate gestational age at which to scan will vary with the particular condition (see table).

Three-dimensional USS. New developments in USS technology enable the image to be presented in three dimensions. This may be particularly valuable when assessing facial features and anomalies of the hands and feet, although advances in two-dimensional technology have improved imaging considerably.

Fetal echocardiography. Routine obstetric anomaly USS includes a minimum of the four-chamber view of the heart but, increasingly, views of the outflow tracts are included. If there is suspicion of a CHD, or scanning is being undertaken because of an increased risk of CHD (e.g. family history or increased nuchal translucency), a more comprehensive study of the fetal heart should be undertaken. Specialist fetal echocardiography includes ventricular outlet views and Doppler assessment of flow.

Fetal sexing. Up to 11–12 weeks gestation, the external genitalia appear the same in both sexes (although the orientation of the phallus differs, pointing cranially in males and caudally in females). Even up to 20 weeks gestation it

Guidelines for timing of fetal ultrasound scanning (USS) for specific congenital malformations

Feature	Time to start USS (weeks gestation)
Anencephaly	11–12
Anterior abdominal wall defects (e.g. gastroschisis/exomphalos)	12
Cleft lip (cleft palate often difficult to visualize)	from 16
Congenital heart disease	11–12 (nuchal scan) 14 (scan) 20–22 (review)
Corpus callosum	19+*
Ear anomalies (only detectable if severe)	20
Eyes and orbital spacing	12–14
Facial profile (e.g. severe micrognathia)	14
Fingers and toes (number of digits)	From 12–14
Gender assignment	From 11+[†]
Hydrocephalus	19 (serial scanning thereafter)
Kidneys	From 12–14; readily visualized from 16 weeks
Lissencephaly	From 20+[‡]
Microcephaly	19[§]
Spina bifida	From 13

* Serial scanning. Absence is usually detectable; hypoplasia is more difficult to determine reliably.
[†] Sometimes gender cannot be assigned with confidence until 20–22 weeks gestation.
[‡] See 'Lissencephaly and neuronal migration disorders' page 156. Rarely detected prenatally.
[§] With serial scanning thereafter. See 'Microcephaly' page 172.

can sometimes be difficult to reliably determine the fetal sex from the appearances of the external genitalia. In the future, a combination of USS of the genital tubercle and analysis of maternal blood for free fetal DNA may enable reliable non-invasive fetal sexing from 8 weeks gestation (Chitty, personal communication, 2004).

Indications for karyotyping. There are a few abnormalities that, when seen in isolation, do not warrant consideration of karyotyping. These include: gastroschisis or unilateral multicystic dysplastic kidney (MCDK). The majority of other anomalies will confer an increased risk for a chromosome anomaly, but the need for karyotyping should be assessed on an individual basis taking into consideration:

1 the presence or absence of other USS anomalies;
2 the detail of the USS performed;
3 other risk factors (maternal age, nuchal translucency measurement, maternal serum screen result).

Fetal magnetic resonance imaging (MRI)

Fetal MRI requires ultrafast technology to capture images to minimize movement artefact. Currently, fetal MRI is considered for the further delineation of intracranial anomalies, especially neuronal migration defects, and some other complex disorders (Garel). Interpretation of images is challenging because this is a relatively new area and there are limited data on the range of normality at specific gestations. Refer for expert advice.

Support group: ARC (Antenatal Results and Choices) <www.arc-uk.org>, Tel. 020 7631 0285.

Expert adviser: Lyn Chitty, Consultant in Fetal Medicine, University College Hospital, London, England.

References

Garne E, Loane M, *et al*. Prenatal diagnosis of severe structural congenital malformations in Europe. *Ultrasound Obstet Gynecol* 2005; **25**: 6–11.

Garel C, The role of MRS in the evaluation of the fetal brain with an emphasis on biometry, gyration and parenchyma. *Pediatr Radiol* 2004; **34**: 694–99.

Invasive techniques and genetic tests in prenatal diagnosis

Chorion villus sampling (CVS) and placental biopsy

CVS was introduced into clinical practice in the UK during the 1980s. The technique enables sampling of the chorion (developing placenta) during the first trimester of pregnancy. In the second and third trimester of pregnancy, the same technique is termed **placental biopsy**. In the first trimester both transabdominal (TA) and transcervical (TC) approaches may be used to obtain a sample. The trophoblast and embryo are both derived from the fertilized egg, and therefore share the same genetic make-up. This genetic identity is the basis for using CVS as an indirect way of determining the genetic make-up of the fetus. Trophoblast is a highly cellular tissue and ideal for DNA extraction, making this the procedure of choice for many molecular genetic investigations. The mean weight of CVS specimens varies between different centres, but in one study was 15.2 ± 6.0 mg (Brun et al. 2003). (Larger samples are sometimes needed for biochemical prenatal diagnosis requiring enzyme analysis of uncultured CVS material.)

The procedure-associated loss rate is estimated at 1.5–2% (Brambati et al. 2001; Brun et al. 2003). See table for further information and a comparison with amniocentesis. In the early 1990s two clusters of babies with limb defects following CVS were reported (Firth 1997; Burton et al. 1992), raising the possibility of a causal association between early CVS and transverse limb deficiency. The risk of limb deficiency extends through the period of limb morphogenesis and slightly beyond, falling from levels 10–20-fold above background at ≤ 9 weeks, to levels approaching (or only a few-fold above) background at 11 weeks and beyond (Firth 1997). Stoler et al. (1999) in a review of the literature found that the frequency of vascular disruption defects, e.g. gastroschisis, intestinal atresias, and club-foot, was significantly increased among CVS-exposed infants compared with a baseline unexposed population.

Comparison of chorionic villus sampling (CVS) and amniocentesis

Feature	CVS	Amniocentesis
Gestation	From 11 weeks gestation; usually 11–13 weeks gestation	From 15 weeks gestation; usually 15–17 weeks gestation
Post-procedural loss rate (miscarriage risk)	1.5–2% (Brambati et al. 2001; Brun et al.2003)	1% (Tabor et al. 1986)
Complications	Vaginal spotting/bleeding (1–4%) especially after transcervical	Amniotic fluid leak causing oligohydramnios
	(TC) procedures. Intrauterine infection (<0.1%). Amniotic fluid leak after unintentional puncture of amniotic sac (rare)	Increased risk for respiratory problems, eg. transient tachypnoea of the newborn
Culture failure	0.21% (Brun et al. 2003)*	Chorioamnionitis (rare) 0.1%*[†]
Maternal contamination	<1% after microscopic selection of the villi (Brun et al. 2003)	Very low
Mosaicism risk	Confined placental mosaicism in 1.9% and true fetal mosaicism in 0.19% (Wang et al. 1993)	0.3% (with ~50% of cases representing true fetal mosaicism)
Timescale for results[‡]	Interphase trisomy FISH or PCR-based common aneuploidy screen 2–3 days	Interphase trisomy FISH or PCR-based common aneuploidy screen 2–3 days
	Routine karyotype around 14 days (cultured cells)	Routine karyotype around 14 days (cultured cells)
	Molecular genetic analysis. CVS is the procedure of choice as DNA can be extracted directly from the trophoblast sample, e.g. fetal sexing by amelogenin probe[§] 2–3 days, routine mutation analysis 7–14 days, mutation analysis requiring Southern blotting 10–21 days	Molecular genetic analysis. Amniocentesis is usually substantially slower than CVS since any investigation requiring substantial amounts of DNA requires amniocyte culture (for 10–14 days) prior to DNA extraction. Molecular genetic analysis then takes a further period of time (see CVS column for estimates). It is usually possible to obtain sufficient DNA for a single PCR-based analysis (e.g. cystic fibrosis prenatal diagnosis) from the amniotic liquor
	Biochemical diagnosis, e.g. enzyme assay usually within 14–21days	Biochemical diagnosis, e.g. enzyme assay, usually within 14 days
Availability	Specialist centers	Most obstetric units

* Placental biopsy at late gestations, e.g. third trimester, has a higher incidence of culture failure than CVS at 11–13/40. Amniocentesis at late gestations, e.g. third trimester, also has a higher incidence of culture failure than amniocentesis at 15–17/40.

[†] Reid et al. (1996) in a small study found the frequency of an abnormal karyotype was greater in those pregnancies in which amniotic fluid culture failure occurred in comparison with those in which a cytogenetic result was obtained (six of 32 (19%) versus 149 of 4092 (4%); p < 0.001). In this series, all chromosomally abnormal fetuses had anomalies detected at ultrasonography (e.g. oligohydramnios, hydrops, and fetal growth restriction).

[‡] These are intended only as a rough guide. Check with your local laboratory before providing information to patients.

[§] Fetal sexing. The amelogenin locus is polymorphic with both an X-chromosome-specific variant and a Y-chromosome-specific variant. PCR analysis of the amelogenin locus is sometimes used for fetal sexing in the prenatal diagnosis of X-linked recessive disorders. In the future, a combination of USS of the genital tubercle and analysis of maternal blood for free fetal DNA may enable reliable non-invasive fetal sexing from 8/40 (Chitty, personal communication, 2004).

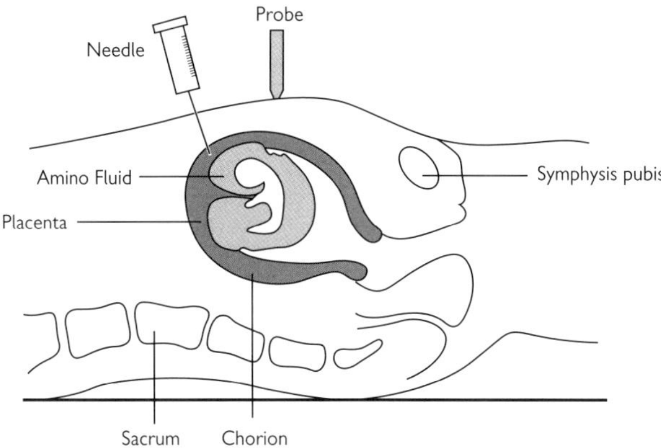

Chorion villus sampling. Adapted from Flinter, F. *et al.* (2004). *The Genetics of Renal Disease*, with permission from Oxford University Press.

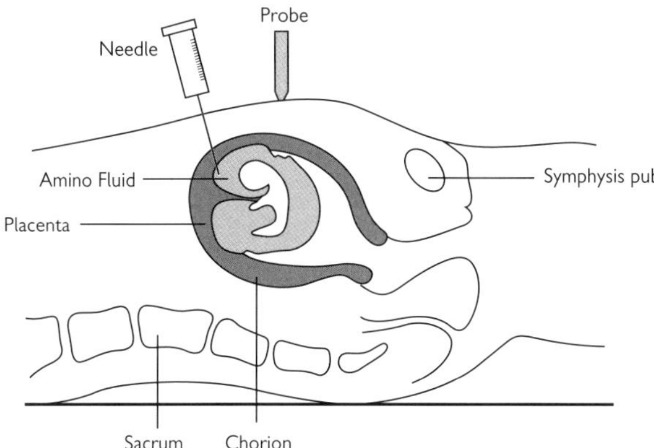

Amniocentesis. Adapted from Flinter, F. *et al.* (2004). *The Genetics of Renal Disease*, with permission from Oxford University Press.

Amniocentesis

Mid-trimester amniocentesis became established during the 1970s as the standard technique for the prenatal diagnosis of chromosome abnormalities. With amniocentesis, a 22-gauge spinal needle is directed transabdominally under ultrasound guidance through the wall of the uterus and into a pool of amniotic fluid. Usually ~15 ml of amniotic fluid is withdrawn. Horger and Finch's (2001) study of 4600 amniocenteses by a single operator (1972–2000) showed a constant procedure-related pregnancy loss rate of 0.95%. All large trials including Tabor *et al.*'s (1986) randomized study of low-risk women have shown a fairly constant risk of around 1% (fetal loss rate in women after amniocentesis was 1.7% compared with controls, 0.7%). This figure is the procedure-related risk, not the absolute risk, as there is a small risk of spontaneous loss throughout the second trimester of pregnancy. The use of ultrasound continuously throughout the procedure, operator experience, and time after gestation are the most important factors determining the risk of postprocedure loss.

A retrospective case-control study of 1296 children born following amniocentesis showed no increase in registrable disability (hearing impairment, learning disability, visual problems, and limb anomalies) over a follow-up period of 7–18 years (Baird *et al.* 1994). See table above for further information and a comparison with CVS.

Early amniocentesis. The Canadian Early and Mid-trimester Amniocentesis Trial (CEMAT) Group (1998) study showed that early amniocentesis (before 13 weeks gestation) is associated with an increased risk of fetal loss and talipes equinovarus (1.3% versus 0.1%) compared with mid-trimester amniocentesis and should be abandoned.

The Cochrane review of CVS versus amniocentesis (Alfirevec *et al.* 2000) concluded that the increase in miscarriages after CVS compared to amniocentesis appeared to be procedure-related and that second trimester amniocentesis appeared to be *safer than CVS*. Uncertain results (e.g. mosaicism) are *more frequent with CVS* than mid-trimester amniocentesis and there are fewer false-positive and false-negative diagnoses. The benefits of earlier diagnosis with CVS must be set against the greater risk of pregnancy loss and uncertain results. Jauniaux *et al.* (2000) conclude that mid-trimester amniocentesis remains the safest invasive procedure and that CVS is associated with a higher risk of subsequent pregnancy loss.

Clinical assessment

For all invasive procedures, the maternal blood group should be known prior to the procedure, and anti-D prophylaxis offered to all rhesus-negative women.

- Assess the genetic risk to the pregnancy and offer information about the procedure-related risks to help the patient to assess the risk/benefit for their individual situation.
- Mention the limitations of the technique (normal karyotype does not guarantee normal baby).
- Mention the possibility of unexpected results or results that are difficult to interpret if karyotyping is undertaken (e.g. sex chromosome aneuploidy, mosaicism). Risks are greater with CVS than amniocentesis.
- Make arrangements for communicating the results.

Special investigations
Important notes.
- **Polymerase chain reaction (PCR)-based analyses.** For all molecular genetic diagnoses involving PCR, a maternal DNA sample should be available to enable testing for maternal cell contamination.
- **Molecular diagnosis of recessive disorders.** For all molecular genetic diagnoses for autosomal recessive (AR) disorders, the molecular carrier status of each parent should be defined in advance of prenatal diagnosis.
- **For X-linked recessive (XLR) disorders.** The molecular carrier status of the mother should be defined in advance of prenatal diagnosis (but note risks arising from germline mosaicism).
- **Molecular diagnosis of deletions.** For all molecular genetic prenatal diagnoses involving PCR for detection of a large-scale deletion, e.g. spinal muscular atrophy (SMA), congenital adrenal hyperplasia (CAH), linkage analysis should be used in conjunction with mutation detection.
- **Subtle cytogenetic findings.** For all cytogenetic diagnoses involving detection of subtle rearrangements, e.g. 1p–, small interstitial deletion of 20p, or reciprocal translocations with little effect on chromosome length in the derivative chromosome, check with the laboratory in advance. Because the quality of chromosome preparations from CVS and amniocentesis is less good than that of those from blood, the laboratory may need to work up fluorescent *in situ* hybridization (FISH) probes to enable them to give a confident result.

Multiple pregnancies

First trimester ultrasound scan (USS) is necessary to delineate chorionicity; from this an assessment of the likely zygosity is possible (see 'Twins and twinning', this chapter). Brambati *et al.* (2001) found that determination of the presence or absence of the lambda sign led to a correct assignment of chorionicity in all cases in a series of >200 multiple pregnancies. With this information it is possible to estimate the likely genetic risks.

- For a monozygotic (MZ) pregnancy, the risk that both twins are affected approximates to the risk for a singleton pregnancy.
- For a dizygotic (DZ) pregnancy, each twin is assessed independently and the risk that one or both twins might be affected is *twice* that in a singleton pregnancy. Careful consideration needs to be given to the management of the pregnancy if one twin is shown to be affected, whereas the other is normal.

When an invasive procedure is indicated in twins, CVS has, over amniocentesis, the advantage of allowing selective termination to be performed in the first trimester, when the procedure-related risk of pregnancy loss is less than when performed later in pregnancy. It has the disadvantage of leading to ambiguous results in up to 2% of cases (Dommergues 2002). Selective termination in mid-trimester carries a 5–10% risk of pregnancy loss or very preterm delivery.

There is debate about choice of diagnostic procedure. Dommergues (2002) argues that CVS is the choice technique in twin pregnancies at very high risk, whilst amniocentesis is still indicated in cases at more moderate risk, whereas Brambati *et al.* (2001) state that that first-trimester TA CVS is a highly efficient, reliable, and relatively safe approach for genetic diagnosis in twin pregnancies. The overall procedure-related risk of miscarriage following sampling of a twin pregnancy is estimated to be ~5% with either CVS or amniocentesis. A precise evaluation of the relative risks of CVS and mid-trimester amniocentesis in twins must await randomized control studies.

Support group: ARC (Antenatal Results and Choices) <www.arc-uk.org>, Tel. 020 7631 0285.

Expert adviser: Lyn Chitty, Consultant in Fetal Medicine, University College Hospital, London, England.

References

Alfirevic Z. Early amniocentesis versus transabdominal chorion villus sampling for prenatal diagnosis. *Cochrane Database Syst Rev* 2000; (2): CD00077.

Alfirevic Z, Gosden CM, *et al.* Chorion villus sampling versus amniocentesis for prenatal diagnosis. *Cochrane Database Syst Rev* 2000; (2): CD00055.

Baird PA, Yee IM, Sadovnick AD. Population-based study of long-term outcomes after amniocentesis. *Lancet* 1994; **344**: 1134–6.

Brambati B, Tului L, Guercilena S, Alberti E. Outcome of first-trimester chorionic villus sampling for genetic investigation in multiple pregnancy. *Ultrasound Obstet Gynecol* 2001; **17** (3): 209–16.

Brun JL, Mangione R, *et al.* Feasibility, accuracy and safety of chorionic villus sampling: a report of 10 741 cases. *Prenat Diagn* 2003; **23** (4): 295–301.

Burton BK, Schulz CJ, Burd LI. Limb anomalies associated with chorionic villus sampling. *Obstet Gynecol* 1992; **79** (5, Pt. 1): 726–30.

Dommergues M. Prenatal diagnosis for multiple pregnancies. *Curr Opin Obstet Gynecol* 2002; **14** (2): 169–75.

Firth H. Chorion villus sampling and limb deficiency: cause or coincidence? *Prenat Diagn* 1997; **17**: 1313–30.

Horger EO, Finch H. A single physician's experience with four thousand six hundred genetic amniocenteses. *Am J Obstet Gynecol* 2001; **185**: 279–88.

Jauniaux E, Pahal GS, Rodeck CH. What invasive procedure to use in early pregnancy? *Bailliere's Best Pract Res Clin Obstet Gynaecol* 2000; **14**: 651–62.

Philip J, Silver RK, *et al.* Late first-trimester invasive prenatal diagnosis: results of an international randomized trial. *Obstet Gynecol* 2004; **103**: 1164–73.

Reid R, Sepulveda W, Kyle PM, Davies G. Amniotic fluid culture failure: clinical significance and association with aneuploidy. *Obstet Gynecol* 1996; **87** (4): 588–92.

Royal College of Obstetricians and Gynaecologists (RCOG). *Clinical guidelines: amniocentesis.* Feb, 2003 <www.rcog.uk/guidelines>.

Stoler JM, McGuirk CK, Lieberman E, Ryan L, Holmes LB. Malformations reported in chorionic villus sampling exposed children: a review and analytic synthesis of the literature. *Genet Med* 1999; **1** (7): 315–22.

Tabor A, Philip J, *et al.* Randomised controlled trial of genetic amniocentesis in 4606 low-risk women. *Lancet* 1986; **i**: 1287–93.

The Canadian Early and Mid-trimester Amniocentesis Trial (CEMAT) Group. Randomised trial to assess safety and fetal outcome of early and midtrimester amniocentesis. *Lancet* 1998; **351** (9098): 242–7.

Wang BB, Rubin CH, Williams J 3rd. Mosaicism in chorionic villus sampling: an analysis of incidence and chromosomes involved in 2612 consecutive cases. *Prenat Diagn* 1993; **13** (3): 179–90.

Wapner RJ, Evans MI, *et al.* Procedural risks versus theology: chorion villus sampling for Orthodox Jews at less than 8 weeks' gestation. *Am J Obstet Gynecol* 2002; **186**: 1133–6.

Wilson RD. Amniocentesis and chorionic villus sampling. *Curr Opin Obstet Gynecol* 2000; **12** (2): 81–6.

Low maternal serum oestriol

Maternal serum unconjugated oestriol (uE_3) is a component of many antenatal maternal serum screening programmes for Down syndrome. Occasionally, serum screening reveals very low levels of uE_3. In a large Californian programme that studied >100,000 pregnancies, 0.27% had low uE_3 levels of ≤0.2 ng/mL, or 0.15 MoM (multiples of the median). Intrauterine fetal death (IUD) occurred in 57% of the 68 women with low uE_3 and positive screening results and in 6% of women with low uE_3 levels and negative screening results. In viable pregnancies, the most common cause of a low uE_3 is X-linked ichthyosis.

X-linked ichthyosis (steroid sulphatase (STS) deficiency)

STS-deficiency or X-linked ichthyosis (XLI) is located at Xp22.3 and affects 1/1300–1/1500 males. Affected males have generalized scaling that usually begins soon after birth. There may be associated corneal opacities that do not affect vision, and there is an increased incidence of cryptorchidism.

In 85–90% of cases it is caused by a deletion that encompasses the *STS* gene. In perhaps 5% of cases the deletion is extensive enough to involve adjacent loci and may sometimes be cytogenetically visible. This can include an adjacent MRX gene giving rise to learning disability, with autistic spectrum problems and epilepsy in some (Gohlke *et al.* 2000). Around 10% of patients have point mutations or other intragenic mutations. Valdes-Flores *et al.* (2001) demonstrated by fluorescent *in situ* hybridization (FISH) analysis that most apparently 'sporadic' affected males are due to inherited deletions; 10/12 mothers of apparently sporadic males were carriers in their series. Perinatal risks in pregnancies affected by XLI include:

- failure to initiate labour with prolonged gestation (postmaturity) and small increased risk of IUD;
- failure to progress in labour.

Clinical approach

1 Exclude other causes of low uE3.
- Ultrasound scan (USS) to confirm viable pregnancy (and sex of baby).
- Check that the mother is not on dexamethasone or a similar medication.
- If viable female pregnancy, see 5 below.
- If viable male pregnancy with normal USS, the most likely diagnosis is STS-deficiency (XLI). Recalculate the Down syndrome risk using age, alpha-fetoprotein (AFP), and human chorionic gonadotrophin (hCG) and excluding uE_3. Offer amniocentesis if high risk. Continue through steps outlined below until a specific diagnosis is reached.
- Three-generation family tree with specific enquiry for a family history of XLI. Enquire about the educational attainment of affected males.
- Obtain maternal blood sample for karyotype, FISH for STS, DNA.

2 Confirmed family history of XLI with no associated learning or behavioural problems.
- Reassurance; advice about XLI.

- Advise obstetrician about perinatal risks (see above).
- Consider implications for other family members.

3 No family history of XLI; mother has FISH deletion, but no cytogenetically visible deletion.
- As above.

4 No family history of XLI and no FISH deletion in mother (uncommon). Probably the mother and baby carry a point mutation or, less likely, the baby has a new mutation that could be a deletion (maybe a large deletion).
- Offer amniocentesis for karyotype and STS FISH.
- As above, if diagnosis confirmed.
- Consider points under 5 (below).

5 Female pregnancy (rare).
- Consider autosomal recessive (AR) congenital adrenal hypoplasia (CAH; very rare and uE_3 levels not usually as low as in STS deficiency).
- Consider AR multiple sulphatase deficiency (very rare).
- Consider Smith–Lemli–Opitz (SLO) syndrome. uE_3 levels not usually as low as in STS deficiency. Detailed fetal anomaly USS and amniocentesis for 7-dehydrocholesterol.

6 Sex reversal (rare)
- Note that undetectable levels of maternal oestriol may be found in Antley-Bixler syndrome due to mutations in PDR (Cragun)—see 'Craniosynostosis' page 288. If 46,XY but female genitalia on USS, consider 17-hydroxylase deficiency, lipoid adrenal hypoplasia, and SLO.

Support group: Ichthyosis Support Group <www.ichthyosis.co.uk>, Tel. 020 7461 9034.

Expert adviser: John R.W. Yates, Professor of Medical Genetics, University of Cambridge, Cambridge, England.

References

Cragun DL, Trumpy SK, *et al.* undetectable maternal serum E_3 and postnatal abnormal sterol and steroid metabolism in Antley–Bixler syndrome. *Am J Med Genet* 2004; **129A**: 1–7.

DiGiovanna JJ, Robinson-Bostom L. Ichthyosis: etiology, diagnosis, and management. *Am J Clin Dermatol* 2003; **4** (2): 81–95.

Glass IA, Lam, RC, Chang T, *et al.* Steroid sulphatase deficiency is the major cause of extremely low oestriol production at mid-pregnancy: a urinary steroid assay for the discrimination of steroid sulphatase deficiency from other causes. *Prenat Diag* 1998; **18**: 789–800.

Gohlke BC, Haug K, *et al.* Interstitial deletion in Xp22.3 is associated with X linked ichthyosis, mental retardation, and epilepsy. *J Med Genet* 2000; **37** (8): 600–2.

Schoen E, Norem C, *et al.* Maternal serum unconjugated estriol as a predictor for Smith–Lemli–Opitz syndrome and other fetal conditions. *Obstet Gynecol* 2003; **102** (1): 167–72.

Valdes-Flores M, Kofman-Alfaro SH, Jimenez Vaca AL, Cuevas-Covarrubias SA. Deletion of exons 1–5 of the STS gene causing X-linked ichthyosis. *J Invest Dermatol* 2001; **116**: 456–8.

Male infertility: genetic aspects

For a man to be judged normally fertile, World Health Organization (WHO) criteria state that he should have a sperm count of 20×10^6/ml, and that spermatazoa should show 50% progressive motility and 30% healthy morphology. Natural pregnancy is still possible below these cut-off figures, but conception is less likely to occur. A male factor is judged to be the dominant cause of subfertility in 20–26% of couples. Despite advances in the diagnosis of causes of subfertility, inability to conceive remains unexplained in 25–30% of fully investigated couples. Referrals are usually only made to the genetics clinic when a specific diagnosis with genetic implications has been made.

The following terminology is used in sperm analysis.

- **Azoospermia.** No sperm seen in the ejaculate.
- **Severe oligozoospermia.** Sperm count $<10 \times 10^6$/ml.
- **Oligozoospermia.** Sperm concentration $<20 \times 10^6$/ml.
- **Asthenozoospermia.** <50% of sperm have normal motility or <25% have any motility.
- **Teratozoospermia.** <30% of sperm have a normal morphology.

One or more of abnormalities of sperm count, motility, or morphology is found in almost 90% of infertile males. General reviews indicate that 13.7% of non-obstructive azoospermic and 4.6% of oligospermic men have an abnormal karyotype. These mainly consist of an XXY constitution or a Robertsonian or reciprocal translocation (de Braekeleer and Dao 1991). Egozcue *et al.* (2003) have used fluorescent *in situ* hybridization (FISH) on decondensed sperm heads to analyse the chromosome constitution of spermatozoa in different populations. In normal males with 46,XY, the mean incidence of disomy in sperm (including all chromosomes) is ~6.7%. Carriers of Robertsonian translocations produce from 3.4% to 36.0% abnormal sperm, and carriers of reciprocal translocations produce from 47.5% to 81.0% abnormal spermatozoa.

Clinical assessment

History: key points

- Three-generation family tree.
- If congenital bilateral absence of the vas deferens (CBAVD), detailed enquiry about respiratory symptoms, nasal polyps, chronic sinusitis, pancreatic insufficiency, etc.

Examination: key points

Usually undertaken by an andrologist/fertility specialist, this includes a general physical examination and an assessment of secondary sex characteristics, testicular size, consistency, and presence/absence of vas deferens.

Special investigations

- Baseline investigations such as sperm count (semen analysis) will usually have been completed by the reproductive medicine team. These may include hormone tests such as testosterone, follicle-stimulating hormone (FSH), luteinizing hormone (LH), and prolactin and thyroid function tests.
- Chromosome analysis.
- Consider testing for AZF microdeletions
- DNA for mutation analysis of the cystic fibrosis (CF) gene (CFTR; 70% of males with CBAVD have mutations in both CFTR alleles). Consider partner screening if positive (see below).
- If azoospermia with normal karyotype, ultrasound scan (USS) to look for renal agenesis.

Diagnoses to consider

Congenital bilateral absence of the vas deferens (CBAVD)

Obstructive azoospermia due to absence of the vas deferens can occur as an autosomal recessive (AR) disorder due to mutations in the CF gene, CFTR. CBAVD is an almost invariable finding in males with CF. CBAVD can also occur in association with unilateral (or bilateral) renal agenesis; this condition is not associated with mutations in CFTR. Advances in reproductive medicine make it possible for some men with CBAVD to father children using percutaneous epididymal sperm aspiration (PESA), intracytoplasmic sperm injection (ICSI), and *in vitro* fertilization (IVF) techniques.

CBAVD due to CFTR. After careful exclusion of a diagnosis of non-classical CF, AR CBAVD is a more appropriate diagnostic term than 'a variant of CF' in otherwise healthy men. CBAVD males have a much higher incidence of partially functional alleles (e.g. R117H) than men with CF. The other allele may be delta F508. Hence there is a risk of classical (or non-classical) CF in offspring. In addition the inefficient 5T splice variant is commonly found in CBAVD males.

- Offer CF mutation analysis to partners of CBAVD males.

CBAVD with unilateral renal agenesis. Abnormal development of the entire mesonephric duct at a very early stage in embryonic development (< 9 weeks gestation) may lead to CBAVD and renal agenesis. This is a less common condition than CBAVD due to CFTR (Augarten) of males with CBAVD ~20%. In one series of 11 pregnancies achieved, 10 had normal renal anatomy, but one was a male pregnancy with bilateral renal agenesis and CBAVD.

- Offer detailed fetal USS of renal tract.

Chromosome anomalies

Klinefelter syndrome (47,XXY)
The most common chromosomal anomaly causing infertility and hypogonadism. See '47,XXY' page 496.

Y chromosome anomalies

Microdeletions. Approximately 10–15% of men with idiopathic azoospermia or severe oligospermia have AZF (azoospermia factor) deletions. The most frequent microdeletion is AZFc (azoospermia factor c), which removes ~4 Mb from Yq. Homologous recombination between large repeats has been shown to be a mechanism of deletion for AZFa and AZFc, but not for AZFb. However, identical sequences in AZFb and AZFc exist, and this finding could explain deletions found in these regions (Ferlin *et al.* 2003).

- Natural transmission of AZFc microdeletions from fathers to sons has been reported, but is rare as most men with AZFc deletions require ICSI with IVF to overcome their spermatogenic failure.

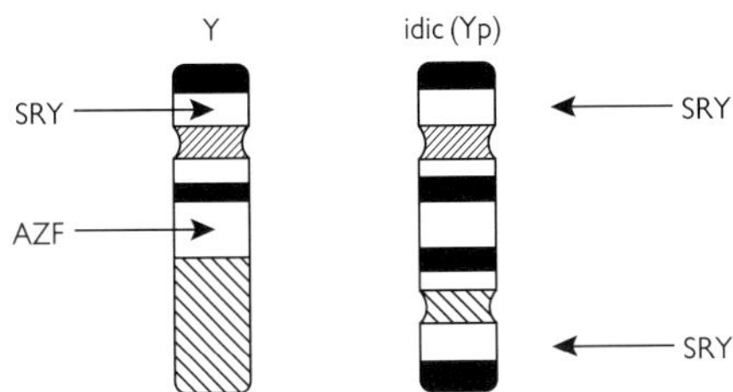

(Left) Normal Y chromosome and (right) isodicentric Y chromosome (idic (Yp)). SRY, Male-determining gene; AZF, azoospermia factor gene.

• Patsalis *et al.* (2002) report that there may be a risk of 45X/46XY or 45X karyotype in offspring of males with AZFc microdeletions. Consider offering pre-implantation genetic diagnosis (PGD) or prenatal diagnosis.

Isodicentric Y chromosome—idic(Yp). Males with an isodicentric Y chromosome have a male phenotype because of the presence of the SRY gene, but have azoospermia because they have no copies of the AZF genes that are required for spermatogenesis (see figure).

46,XX males. Prevalence is 1/20 000. This condition is usually due to:

• cryptic translocations involving SRY-bearing Y material and the X chromsomes (FISH for *SRY*);
• mosaicism for XX and cell lines involving Y chromosome material;
• true XX hermaphroditism where both testicular and ovarian tissues persist (findings are variable but may have ovary on one side and testis on the other) may be due to mosaicism or chimerism or to mutations in genes in the pathway downstream of SRY.

Monogenic conditions causing meiotic arrest

Meiosis produces haploid gametes from diploid parental cells. This process is unique to the germ cells of the gonads. The synaptonemal complex has a key role in meiosis and consists of several proteins (SYP1, 2, and 3). Miyamoto *et al.* (2003) have identified heterozygous mutations in *SYCP3* in 2/19 men with non-obstructive azoospermia showing maturation arrest.

Hypogonadotrophic hypogonadism

The clinical presentation is often with delayed puberty or lack of masculinisation (voice/sexual hair, etc.) rather than infertility. Adolescent and adult males with hypogonadotrophic hypogonadism require testosterone replacement; infertility may be treatable with gonadotrophins or GnRH.

Kallmann syndrome (KS) is a genetic condition characterized by the association of hypogonadotrophic hypogonadism and anosmia with or without other anomalies. KS affects about 1 in 8000 males and 1 in 40,000 females, with most presentations being of the 'sporadic' type. It can follow autosomal dominant (AD), AR, or X-linked inheritance. The gene underlying the X-linked form of the disease, *KAL-1*, encodes a glycoprotein, anosmin-1, that is involved in the embryonic migration of gonadotrophin-releasing hormone (GnRH)-synthesizing neurons and the differentiation of the olfactory bulbs. There is considerable phenotypic variation even within families. Massin *et al.* (2003) describe three brothers carrying an intragenic deletion of *KAL-1*; all three had a history of hypogonadotropic hypogonadism with delayed puberty. They had variable degrees of anosmia/hyposmia, but brain magnetic resonance imaging (MRI) showed hypoplastic olfactory bulbs in all three. Other problems present in only one or two of the brothers included unilateral renal aplasia, high-arched palate, brachymetacarpia, mirror movements, and abnormal eye movements. Dode *et al.* (2003) found that that loss-of-function mutations in *FGFR1* (the same gene where gain-of-function mutations cause craniosynostosis) underlie AD KS. There is good evidence for at least one more autosomal locus. Dode *et al.* (2003) propose that the *KAL-1* gene product, the extracellular matrix protein anosmin-1, is involved in fibroblast growth factor (FGF) signalling and that the gender difference in anosmin-1 dosage (because KALI partially escapes X inactivation) may explain the higher prevalance of KS in males.

Genetic advice and management

The geneticist's role is to explain the genetic basis of the disorder causing infertility. Depending on the specific diagnosis, if assisted reproductive techniques (ART) could be used to achieve a pregnancy with the patient's own sperm, then advice about reproductive implications is also appropriate. Management of the infertility is the remit of a specialist in reproductive medicine.

Support group association: CHILD: The National Infertility Support Network <www.child.org.uk>, Tel. 01424 732361.

Expert advisers: Melanie Davies, Consultant Obstetrician and Gynaecologist (Reproductive Medicine) and Ozkan Ozturk, Senior Lecturer in Obstetrics and Gynaecology (Reproductive Medicine), both at University College Hospital, London, England.

References

Augarten A, Yahav Y, et al. Congenital bilateral absence of vas deferens in the absence of cystic fibrosis. *Lancet* 1994; **344**: 1473–4.

Claustres M, Guittard C, et al. Spectrum of CFTR mutations in cystic fibrosis and in congenital absence of the vas deferens in France. *Hum Mutat* 2000; **16**: 143–56.

De Braekeleer M, Dao TN. Cytogenetic studies in male infertility: a review. *Hum Reprod* 1991; **6** (2): 245–50.

Dode C, Levilliers J, et al. Loss-of-function mutations in FGFR1 cause autosomal dominant Kallmann syndrome. *Nat Genet* 2003; **33** (4): 463–5.

Egozcue J, Blanco J, et al. Genetic analysis of sperm and implications of severe male infertility—a review. *Placenta* 2003; **24** (suppl. 2): S62–5.

Evers JLH. Female subfertility [seminar]. *Lancet* 2002; **360**: 151–9.

Ferlin A, Moro E, et al. The human Y chromosome's azoospermia factor b (AZFb) region: sequence, structure, and deletion analysis in infertile men. *J Med Genet* 2003; **40** (1): 18–24.

Hu Y, Tanriverdi F, et al. Kallmann's syndrome: molecular pathogenesis. *Int J Biochem Cell Biol* 2003; **35** (8): 1157–62.

Massin N, Pecheux C, et al. X chromosome-linked Kallmann syndrome: clinical heterogeneity in three siblings carrying an intragenic deletion of the KAL-1 gene. *J Clin Endocrinol Metab* 2003; **88** (5): 2003–8.

McCallum T, Milunsky J, et al. Unilateral renal agenesis associated with congenital bilateral absence of the vas deferens: phenotypic findings and genetic considerations. *Hum Reprod* 2001; **16**: 282–8.

Miyamoto T, Hasuike S, *et al.* Azoospermia in patients heterozygous for a mutation in *SYCP3*. *Lancet* 2003; **362**: 1714–19.

Oliveira LM, Seminara SB, *et al.* The importance of autosomal genes in Kallmann syndrome: genotype–phenotype correlations and neuroendocrine characteristics. *J Clin Endocrinol Metab* 2001; **86** (4): 1532–8.

Patsalis PC, Sismani C, Quintana-Murci L, Taleb-Bekkouche F, Krausz C, McElreavey K. Effects of transmission of Y chromosome AZFc deletions. *Lancet* 2002; **360**: 1222–4.

Maternal age

With advanced maternal age there is an increased risk for the following.

- **Subfertility.** An increasing incidence of chromosomally abnormal conceptuses with advancing age is a major factor in decline in fertility. Chromosomally abnormal embryos have a lower implantation rate than euploid embryos (Munne 2003).
- **Miscarriage.** Increased risk due to increased incidence of chromosomally abnormal conceptuses with advanced maternal age and higher miscarriage rate with advancing age for aneuploid as well as euploid conceptions. Risk of early pregnancy loss in a 40-year-old woman is 30–40%.
- **Aneuploidy** (except 45,X, 47,XYY, triploidy, and *de novo* rearrangements). Non-disjunction at meiosis I is the main age-dependent factor. Risks increase exponentially with advancing maternal age for +21, +18, +13, and also for 47,XXX and 47,XXY. For the autosomal trisomies, this rise apppears to be followed by a levelling off at the extreme upper end of the age range. Marquez *et al.* (2000) in a study of more than 1000 cleavage-stage human embryos from patients undergoing *in vitro* fertilization IVF found that aneuploidy increased with maternal age, from 3.1% in embryos from 20–34 years old patients to 17% in patients 40 years or older.
  - 80% of 45,X pregnancies show loss of paternal contribution (may occur postzygotically). A significant inverse relationship with maternal age is found for liveborn 45,X cases, perhaps reflecting the higher miscarriage rate with advancing maternal age for aneuploid as well as euploid conceptions.
- **Dizygotic twinning.**

Genetic advice and management

- Figures in the table are for livebirths. The risk for Down syndrome at chorionic villus sampling (CVS) or amniocentesis is higher, since a proportion of affected pregnancies result in spontaneous fetal loss (miscarriage or intrauterine death (IUD)). Approximately 43% of affected pregnancies would be lost spontaneously between the time of CVS and term, and approximately 23% between the time of amniocentesis and term.
- Overall, the risk for **any chromosome aneuploidy** (e.g. +21, +18, +13, 47,XXX, 47,XXY, which are age-dependent, and 45,X, 47,XYY, triploidy and *de novo* arrangements, which are not influenced by maternal age) is *approximately double the risk for Down syndrome*.

Expert adviser: Martin Bobrow, Professor of Medical Genetics, University of Cambridge, Cambridge, England.

Observed and predicted odds of Down syndrome livebirth by maternal age (after Morris et al. 2002) with suggested counselling odds for use in clinic

Maternal age at child'sbirth (years)	Counselling odds*	Observed odds	Predicted odds[†]
17	1:1550	1:1599	1:1504
18	1:1500	1:1789	1:1497
19	1:1450	1:1440	1:1488
20	1:1450	1:1441	1:1476
21	1:1450	1:1409	1:1461
22	1:1450	1:1465	1:1441
23	1:1400	1:1346	1:1415
24	1:1400	1:1396	1:1381
25	1:1350	1:1383	1:1339
26	1:1250	1:1187	1:1285
27	1:1200	1:1235	1:1219
28	1:1150	1:1147	1:1139
29	1:1000	1:1002	1:1045
30	1:950	1:959	1:937
31	1:820	1:837	1:819
32	1:700	1:702	1:695
33	1:570	1:589	1:571
34	1:440	1:430	1:455
35	1:350	1:338	1:352
36	1:260	1:259	1:266
37	1:200	1:201	1:199
38	1:150	1:162	1:148
39	1:110	1:113	1:111
40	1:85	1:84	1:85
41	1:70	1:69	1:67
42	1:55	1:52	1:54
43	1:45	1:37	1:45
44	1:40	1:38	1:39
45	1:35	1:32	1:35
46	1:30	1:31	1:31
47	1:30	1:25	1:29

* Counselling odds are 'rounded' figures for use in the clinic setting.
† Predicted odds are based on the statistical model described by Morris *et al.* (2002).

References

Ferguson-Smith MA, Yates JRW. Maternal age specific rates for chromosome aberrations and factors influencing them: report of a collaborative European study on 52,965 amniocenteses. *Prenat Diagn* 1984; **4**: 5–44.

Marquez C, Sandalinas M, *et al.* Chromosome abnormalities in 1255 cleavage-stage human embryos. *Reprod Biomed Online* 2000; **1** (1): 17–26.

Morris JK, Mutton DE, Alberman E. Revised estimates of the maternal age specific live birth prevalence of Down's syndrome. *J Med Screen* 2002; **9**: 2–6.

Munne S. Preimplantation genetic diagnosis and human implantation—a review. *Placenta* 2003; **24** (suppl. B): S70–6.

Maternal diabetes mellitus and diabetic embryopathy

The incidence of major congenital malformations amongst infants of diabetic mothers (IDMs) is 6–9%, i.e. 2–3 times background rates. Meta-analysis of 14 series totalling 4605 IDMs found a major malformation in 279 (6%). The risk is limited to patients who are diabetic at the time of conception and is not found amongst gestational diabetics. Diabetic women also have an increased risk of first trimester spontaneous abortion (approximately twofold). Risks for both complications can be reduced by improved metabolic control. With good to excellent control, risk for malformation remains elevated, whereas risk for miscarriage reduces to background levels.

The Diabetes in Early Pregnancy study showed that good maternal control is associated with normal neurodevelopmental outcomes.

Mills *et al.* (1979) showed that the malformations in infants of diabetic mothers were present by 3 to 8 weeks postfertilization. Mills *et al.* (1988) also showed that diabetic women with good metabolic control are no more likely than non-diabetic women to lose a pregnancy, but diabetic women with elevated blood glucose and glycosylated haemoglobin levels in the first trimester have a significantly increased risk of having a spontaneous abortion. The table lists some features of diabetic embryopathy.

Relative risk (compared to offspring of non-diabetic women) of having a feature of diabetic embryopathy

Feature	Relative risk
Caudal regression	211
Situs inversus	42
Arthrogryposis	28
Spinal anomalies (including vertebral anomalies)	23
Duplex ureter	23
Pseudohermaphroditism (?ambiguous genitalia)	11
Gross skeletal anomalies	10
Hydronephrosis	7
Gross skeletal and associated anomalies	6
Anencephaly	6

More recently, Greene (1999) reviewed 860 consecutive fetuses and infants of diabetic women and found three types of anomaly were all much more common in IDMs:

- anomalies of the heart and great vessels ($\times 4.5$);
- neural tube defects (NTDs; $\times 11.5$);
- bilateral renal agenesis ($\times 5$).

The mechanism of diabetic embryopathy is not well understood. The diabetic environment appears to simultaneously induce alterations in several interrelated teratological pathways (e.g. disturbances in metabolism of inositol, prostaglandins, and reactive oxygen species). Several clinical studies have not established an association between maternal hypoglycaemia and diabetic embryopathy in humans; but animal studies clearly indicate that hypoglycaemia is potentially teratogenic during embryogenesis.

Pre-existing maternal diabetes is associated with a five-fold increase in risk of cardiovascular malformations, which occur in 3.6% of babies with diabetic mothers compared with 0.74% of babies with non-diabetic mothers (odds ratio (OR), 5.0). Transposition of the great arteries (TGA), truncus arteriosus, and tricuspid atresia are overrepresented to produce a substantial excess of these malformations (Wren *et al.* 2003).

There is a high incidence of skeletal and vertebral defects in diabetic embryopathy. This group includes a variety of findings, e.g.radial aplasia/hypoplasia, ulnar aplasia/hypoplasia, preaxial polydactyly. Preaxial polydactyly of the foot with unusual proximal insertion of the preaxial digit has been suggested as a marker for diabetic embryopathy (Slee and Goldblatt 1997).

Caudal regression. Most cases of caudal regression are sporadic or associated with maternal diabetes. The condition is thought to be part of a spectrum including imperforate anus, sacral agenesis, and sirenomelia.

Clinical assessment
History: key points
- Three-generation family tree (to assess whether there is an obvious genetic explanation for any observed malformation).
- Detailed account of quality of diabetic control periconceptually. What was the HbA1c? Did she experience any hypoglycaemic episodes?
- Brief inquiry about other possible teratogenic exposures, e.g. drugs, infection, alcohol.
- If child liveborn, detailed perinatal history, birthweight, and growth parameters.

Examination: key points
If anomaly identified examine parents, e.g. if limb defect in fetus/child examine hands/feet of parents; if cardiac defect, likewise.

Special investigations
- Maternal serum screening for NTD (lab must be informed of maternal diabetes because norms for alpha-fetoprotein (AFP) need to be adjusted).
- Detailed fetal anomaly ultrasound scan (USS; Wong *et al.* (2002) found the detection rate for fetal anomalies was lower for diabetic women (30%) than for non-diabetic women (73%) with subobtimal image quality (maternal obesity) a major factor).
- HbA1c (measure of glycaemic control over previous 6–8 weeks). In one series (Wong *et al.* 2002), periconceptual HbA1c >9% was associated with a high incidence of major anomalies (14.3%).

Genetic advice and management
Insulin-dependent diabetes mellitus (TID/IDDM) follows polygenic inheritance with an important role for the immune response genes associated with the HLA complex on chromosome 6.
- 2% offspring risk if mother has TID.
- 4% offspring risk if father has TID.

Diabetic control should be optimized *before* a pregnancy and tightly monitored. All diabetic women need specialist management by an obstetrician with special expertise in fetomaternal medicine.

Expert adviser: Lewis B. Holmes, Professor of Pediatrics, Harvard Medical School and Chief, Genetics and Teratology Unit, Massachusetts General Hospital for Children, Boston, Massachusetts, USA.

References

Eriksson UJ, Borg LA, *et al.* Pathogenesis of diabetes-induced congenital malformations. *Ups J Med Sci* 2000; 105: 53–84.

Greene MF. Spontaneous abortions and major malformations in women with diabetes mellitus. *Semin Reprod Endocrinol* 1999; **17**: 127–36.

Kucera J. Rate and type of congenital anomaly among offspring of diabetic women. *J Reprod Med* 1971; **7**: 61–70.

Mills JL, Baker L, Goldman AS. Malformations in infants of diabetic mothers occur before the seventh gestational week. Implications for treatment. *Diabetes* 1979; **28** (4): 292–3.

Mills JL, Simpson JL, *et al.* Incidence of spontaneous abortion among normal women and insulin-dependent diabetic women whose pregnancies were identified within 21 days of conception. *New Engl J Med* 1988; **319** (25): 1617–23.

Schwartz R, Teramo KA. Effects of diabetic pregnancy on the fetus and newborn. *Semin Perinatol* 2000; **24**: 120–35.

Slee J, Goldblatt J. Further evidence for preaxial hallucal polydactyly as a marker of diabetic embryopathy. *J Med Genet* 1997; **34**: 261–3.

Wong SF, Chan FY, *et al.* Routine ultrasound screening in diabetic pregnancies. *Ultrasound Obstet Gynecol* 2002; **19**: 171–6.

Wren C, Birrell G, *et al.* Cardiovascular malformations in infants of diabetic mothers. *Heart* 2003; **89**: 1217–20.

Maternal phenylketonuria (PKU)

PKU is a treatable autosomal recessive (AR) inborn error of metabolism resulting from a deficiency of phenylalanine hydroxylase and characterized by mental retardation. It is caused by mutations in the *PAH* gene on 12q24.1. The newborn screening programme for PKU introduced in the 1960s means that it is now possible to prevent mental retardation in individuals with PKU by strict adherence to a phenylalanine-restricted diet; with optimal dietary control, intelligence can be normal. In a recent survey, Walter *et al.* (2002) showed that adolescents and young adults generally do not comply with recommendations for the monitoring and control of phenylalanine concentrations. *Maternal PKU can be teratogenic unless very strict dietary control is resumed prior to conception and maintained during pregnancy.* In the postnatal period, children with untreated PKU develop white matter changes identifiable by cranial MRI. Offspring of untreated mothers with PKU also have a brain effect but this occurs prenatally and is expressed as microcephaly, hypoplasia of the corpus callosum and mental retardation (but no white matter changes) (Levy).

Teratogenic effects on the offspring are very similar to those of the fetal alcohol syndrome (FAS).

- Microcephaly: present from birth.
- Mental retardation. Reduced cognitive function is a virtually constant feature in offspring of untreated maternal PKU. Also striking hyperactivity and emotional problems.
- Congenital heart disease (CHD), especially tetralogy of Fallot, and aortic coarctation.
- Intrauterine growth retardation (IUGR).
- Facial dysmorphism:
  - epicanthic folds;
  - maxillary hypoplasia;
  - flattened nasal bridge and upturned nose;
  - long philtrum and thin upper lip;
  - micrognathia.

Clinical assessment
History: key points
- Brief family tree. Enquire specifically for consanguinity.
- Enquire about pre-pregnancy diet and obtain details of the most recent pre-pregnancy maternal blood phenylalanine levels.
- Obtain accurate information about the dating of the pregnancy and dietary control and blood phenylalanine levels during the pregnancy.

Special investigations
- Maternal phenylalanine levels should be monitored weekly in pregnancy.
- Detailed ultrasound scan (USS) surveillance is usually offered but CHD is the only feature likely to be detectable on mid-trimester scan (see below).
- Refer for expert dietary advice if the pregnancy is continuing.

Genetic advice and management
- This is an example of a genetic disease (PKU) in the mother that is very harmful (teratogenic) to her unborn infant. The genetic risks are less crucial; the mother is usually a compound heterozygote for mutations in the phenylalanine hydroxylase gene.
- Risk to offspring for PKU if mother's partner is unrelated and has no family history of PKU is 1/100 (1/50 × 1/2).

- Neonatal screening by Guthrie spot on day 15 is a robust and sensitive method of diagnosis of the newborn with PKU. Levels >350 µmol/l are diagnostic (levels are usually >1000 µmol/l in newborns with PKU). In a high risk situation, some labs offer a preliminary check on a blood spot d3 (even if this is normal the routine blood spot on d5 remains essential http://newbornscreening-bloodspot.org.uk
- Close follow-up and counselling for a girl with PKU is essential to make her aware of the risk for fetal damage when pregnant and the methods for prevention.

Presentation in first trimester
In practice many women with PKU present already pregnant. Some maternal PKU pregnancies not begun on treatment until the tenth week of gestation have had good outcomes, whereas others have had very poor outcomes with full maternal PKU syndrome. Maternal phenylalanine level at presentation may help to determine the likelihood of problems (see table). Of the features of maternal PKU syndrome, only CHD is likely to be detectable on USS by 19 weeks gestation; the other features are unlikely to become apparent until the third trimester.

Teratogenic effects and the frequencies (%) relative to the degree of maternal hyperphenylalanaemia in offspring from untreated maternal phenylketonuria and hyperphenylalanaemia (Levy and Ghavami 1996)

Abnormality in offspring	Frequency (%) relative to maternal blood phenylalanine level*			
	>1200 µM	>1000 µM	>600 µM	>200 µM
Mental retardation	92	73	22	21
Microcephaly	73	68	35	24
Congenital heart disease	12	15	6	0
Low birthweight	40	52	56	13

* To convert from mg/dl to µM multiply by 0.0165.

Maximum accepted blood phenylalanine concentrations and frequency of capillary-blood sampling (adapted from Medical Advisory Panel of the National Society for Phenylketonuria 1999)

Age (years)	Blood phenylalanine concentration (µmol/l)	Frequency of capillary blood sampling
<0.5	360	Weekly
<5	360	Fortnightly
5–10	480	Monthly
>10	700	Monthly
Pregnancy	360	Weekly

Pre-pregnancy counselling
Ideally, women with PKU should receive information about the need for strict dietary control and careful supervision during pregnancy as teenagers. NB. Women with

mild hyperphenylalanaemia (blood phenylalanine level <400 µM on a normal diet are probably not at increased risk, but those with moderate hyperphenylalanaemia (blood level 400–600 µM) will need strict dietary control in pregnancy, even though they do not have PKU. The following information and management programme should be followed.

- Information about teratogenic effects of untreated maternal PKU.
- Stress the need for careful planning of pregnancies with initiation of strict dietary control at least 1 month before conception.
- Stress the need to maintain maternal blood phenylalanine level <360 µM (6 mg/dl),
- Stress the need for joint supervision by obstetrician/physician with an interest in metabolic disease during pregnancy.
- During pregnancy aim for phenylalanine level of 100–250 µM.

Support groups: National Society for PKU (NSKPU) <http://web.ukonline.co.uk/nspku>; CLIMB (Children Living with Inherited Metabolic Diseases) <www.climb.org.uk>.

Expert adviser: Lewis B. Holmes, Professor of Pediatrics, Harvard Medical School and Chief, Genetics and Teratology Unit, Massachusetts General Hospital for Children, Boston, Massachusetts, USA.

References

Levy H, Ghavami M. Maternal phenylketonuria: a metabolic teratogen. *Teratology* 1996; **53**: 176–84.

Levy HL, Lobbregt D, *et al.* Maternal phenylketonuria: magnetic resonance imaging of the brain in offspring. *V Pediatr* 1996; **128**: 770–75.

Medical Advisory Panel of the National Society for Phenylketonuria. *Management of PKU. A consensus document for the diagnosis and management of children, adolescents and adults with phenylketonuria.* The National Society for Phenylketonuria (United Kingdom) Ltd., London, 1999.

Medical Research Council Working Party on Phenylketonuria. Recommendations on the dietary management of phenylketonuria: report of Medical Research Council Working Party on Phenylketonuria. *Arch Dis Child* 1993; **68**: 426–7.

Phenylalanine hydroxylase locus knowledgebase <www.pahdb.mcgill.ca>.

Scriver CR, Hurtubise M, *et al.* PAHdb2003: what a locus-specific knowledgebase can do. *Hum Mutat* 2003; **21**: 333–44.

Walter JH, White FJ, *et al.* How practical are recommendations for dietary control in phenylketonuria? *Lancet* 2002; **360**: 55–7.

Miscarriage and recurrent miscarriage

Miscarriage is a lay term for spontaneous early pregnancy loss.

- **Early pregnancy loss (EPL).** Miscarriage or spontaneous abortion at <12 weeks gestation.
- **Spontaneous abortion.** Spontaneous pregnancy loss at <24 weeks gestation.
- **Blighted ovum.** Empty gestational sac seen on ultrasound scan (USS) with no fetal parts.
- **Missed abortion.** Fetal parts identified in gestational sac, but no cardiac activity in pregnancy <24 weeks gestation.
- **Intrauterine fetal death (IUD).** Fetal death >24 weeks gestation but before onset of labour.
- **Recurrent abortion.** Three or more consecutive spontaneous abortions.

25–30% of all pregnancies end in early pregnancy loss. The rate of EPL decreases with gestation. Gestation, maternal age, and previous history are the most important determinants of EPL (see table). Risk of miscarriage increases with maternal age: women aged 40 are twice as likely to miscarry as women aged 20, attributable in part to increased risk of chromosomally abnormal conceptus with increased maternal age.

Incidence of early pregnancy loss (EPL; after Jauniaux et *al.* 2001)

	Incidence of EPL (%)
Total loss of conceptions (includes biochemical pregnancies)	50–70
Total clinical miscarriages	25–31
Clinical miscarriages <6 weeks gestation	18
Clinical miscarriages at 6–9 weeks gestation	4
Clinical miscarriages at >9 weeks gestation	3
In primigravidas	6–10
Risk after 3 miscarriages	25–30
Risk in a 40-year-old woman	30–40

At least 50% of miscarriages have a chromosome abnormality. Higher rates to 60–70% are found with studies using chorionic villus sampling (CVS) at time of diagnosis of EPL or comparative genomic hybridization (CGH) to analyse culture failure samples) (Fritz), or array-CGH (Schaeffer). The most common findings are shown in the second table.

In Philipp et *al.*'s (2003) embryoscopic study of 233 missed abortions, 75% of cases had an abnormal karyotype and 55% had a morphological defect (including holoprosencephaly, anencephaly, encephalocele, spina bifida, microcephaly, facial dysplasia, limb reduction defect, cleft hand, syndactyly, pseudosyndactly, polydactyly, various forms of cleft lip, and an amniotic adhesion). Overall, 18% had a morphological defect with a normal karyotype, while no embryonic or chromosomal abnormality could be diagnosed in only 7% of the cases.

Recurrent miscarriage
In Stephenson et *al.*'s (2002) study of 225 products of conception (POCs) from couples with recurrent miscarriage, 225 (54%) of samples were euploid and 195 (46%) were cytogenetically abnormal (of which 66.5% were trisomic, 19% were polyploid, 9% were 45,X, 4% were unbalanced translocations, and one was 46,X+21). The distribution of

The most common chromosomal abnormalities leading to miscarriage

Chromosome abnormality	Percentage of	
	Chromosome abnormalities	Spontaneous abortions
Autosomal trisomy*	50	25
Triploidy (69,XXX, 69,XXY, 69,XYY)	15	7.5
45,X	10	5
Tetraploidy (92,XXXX or 92,XXYY)	5	2.5
Unbalanced structural chromosome abnormalities [†]	4	2

* +16 is the most common accounting for 30% of trisomies.

[†] 50% *de novo*; 50% inherited.

cytogenetic abnormalities in the recurrent miscarriage group was not significantly different from that in controls when stratified for maternal age, although slightly more unbalanced translocations were identified.

Approximately 5.5% of couples with three or more miscarriages will carry a balanced translocation (~10 x background), usually a reciprocal autosomal or a Robertsonian translocation. De Braekeleer and Dao (1990) in a large study from Quebec of ~22 000 couples with two or more spontaneous abortions found that, in 4.7%, one partner carried a chromosome rearrangement (e.g. reciprocal autosomal or Robertsonian translocation).

Robinson et *al.* (2001) undertook a study of 54 couples who were ascertained as having two or more documented aneuploid or polyploid spontaneous abortions. He found that the aetiology of trisomy is predominantly a result of meiotic errors related to increased maternal age, regardless of whether the couple has experienced one or multiple aneuploid spontaneous abortions. Furthermore, this is true even when a second spontaneous abortion involves the same abnormality. The overwhelming majority were simply a consequence of the dramatic increase of trisomic conceptions with increased maternal age, and other theoretical possiblities, such as germline mosaicism, factors affecting chromosome structure and segregation, increased sperm aneuploidy in the male partner, or accelerated 'ageing' of the ovaries, did not appear to play a significant role. (However, these data do not exclude some population variability in risk for aneuploidy.)

Clinical assessment

Recurrent miscarriage with normal parental chromosomes is not in itself an indication for referral to the genetics clinic. However, if a couple has a significant history of recurrent fetal loss and especially if cytogenetic abnormalities have been identified in POCs, the couple may be referred to the genetics clinic.

History: key points
Three-generation family tree noting history of miscarriage, stillbirth, or neonatal death or unexplained handicap/congenital anomaly.

Examination: key points
Not usually appropriate.

Special investigations

- Karyotype both partners if three or more miscarriages or if a balanced or unbalanced translocation has been identified in the POC.
- Other investigations such as antiphospholipid antibodies, lupus anticoagulant and investigations for systemic lupus erythematosus (SLE), protein C, and factor V Leiden are best undertaken in a gynaecological setting.

Genetic advice and management

- If a parental chromosome rearrangement is identified, counsel appropriately (see 'Autosomal reciprocal translocations—familial' page 504).
- If there is no parental chromosome rearrangement, the couple are best managed in a reproductive medicine clinic rather than a genetics clinic.
- If the karyotype of abortus is aneuploid, the chance of a successful next pregnancy is higher than if the abortus is euploid (68% subsequent livebirth rate versus 41% in Carp *et al.*'s (2001) series).
- Recurrent pregnancy loss of affected males can occur in some rare X-linked dominant disorders such as incontinentia pigmenti (IP), Golz syndrome (focal dermal hypoplasia), and orofaciodigital (OFD) syndrome, but it is rarely a presenting feature and together they account for only a miniscule fraction of recurrent miscarriages.

Support group: The Miscarriage Association <www.miscarriageassociation.org.uk>.

Expert adviser: Lyn Chitty, Consultant in Fetal Medicine, University College Hospital, London, England.

References

Carp H, Toder V, *et al.* Karyotype of the abortus in recurrent miscarriage. *Fertil Steril* 2001; **75**: 678–82.

De Braekeleer M, Dao TN. Cytogenetic studies in couples experiencing repeated pregnancy losses. *Hum Reprod* 1990; **5** (5): 519–28.

Fritz B, Hallermann C, *et al.* Cytogenetic analyses of culture failures by comparative genome hybridisation (CGH)—re-evaluation of chromosome aberration rates in early spontaneous abortions. *Eur J Hum Genet* 2001; **9**: 539–47.

Jauniaux E, *et al.* Early pregnancy loss. In *Emery and Rimoin's principles and practice of medical genetics*, 3rd edn (ed. D.L. Rimoin), Chapter 63. Churchill Livingstone, Edinburgh, 2001.

Ogasawara M. Aoki K, *et al.* Embryonic karyotype of abortuses in relation to the number of previous miscarriages. *Fertil Steril* 2000; **73**: 300–4.

Philipp T, Philipp K, *et al.* Embryoscopic and cytogenetic analysis of 233 missed abortions: factors involved in the pathogenesis of developmental defects of early failed pregnancies. *Hum Reprod* 2003; **18** (8): 1724–32.

Risch HA, Weiss NS, *et al.* Risk factors for spontaneous abortion and its recurrence. *Am J Epidemiol* 1988, **128**: 420–30.

Robinson WP, McFadden DE, Stephenson MD. The origin of abnormalities in recurrent aneuploidy/polyploidy. *Am J Hum Genet* 2001; **69** (6): 1245–54.

Schaeffer AJ, Chung J, *et al.* Comparative genomic hybridization-array analysis enhances the detection of aneuploidies and submicroscopic imbalances in spontaneous miscarriages. *Am J Hum Genet* 2004; **74**: 1168–74.

Stephenson MD, Awartani, *et al.* Cytogenetic analysis of miscarriages from couples with recurrent miscarriage: a case-control study. *Hum Reprod* 2002; **17**: 446–51.

Oedema—increased nuchal translucency, cystic hygroma, and hydrops

The reason that chromosomally abnormal fetuses have increased nuchal oedema, cystic hygromas, or hydrops is not well understood. Cystic hygroma *per se* seems to arise as a result of lymphatic dysplasia and is particularly associated with 45,X (Turner syndrome). Increased nuchal fold thickness/nuchal translucency may resolve spontaneously (even in a karyotypically abnormal pregnancy). Even when fetal lymphoedema resolves, dysmorphism may result from the tissue distension/displacement that occurred during fetal life, e.g. neck webbing, nuchal skin folds, hypertelorism and epicanthic folds, low set ears, wide-spaced nipples.

There is an increased risk of congenital heart disease (CHD) in karyotypically normal pregnancies with increased nuchal fold thickness/cystic hygroma/hydrops. Some structural cardiac anomalies such as coarctation of the aorta and hypoplastic left heart may be sequelae of fetal lymphoedema.

Nuchal translucency

Subcutaneous accumulation of fluid at the back of the fetal neck is visualized by ultrasound scan (USS) examination at 10–14 weeks gestation as increased nuchal translucency (NT) thickness. It is associated with chromosomal abnormalities, a wide range of cardiac defects, and genetic syndromes. Zoppi *et al.* (2001) analysed 10 001 pregnancies with known outcome and found the fetal nuchal translucency thickness was >1.5 MoM (multiples of the median) in 510 (5%) of the normal fetuses, in 52 (81%) of the trisomy 21 fetuses, and in 33 (72%) of those with other chromosomal defects. The respective values for nuchal translucency thickness >2.0 MoM were 195 (2%), 41 (64%), and 32 (70%).

Many pregnancies are now screened for chromosome anomalies (e.g. Down syndrome) using an algorithm combining nuchal fold thickness measured by USS at 10–14 weeks gestation with maternal age and maternal serum markers. Spencer *et al.* (2003) report their experience with first trimester screening of >12 000 women. The uptake of first trimester screening was 97.5% and the uptake of invasive testing in the increased risk group (risk >1/300) was 77%. Using a combination of maternal serum free beta-human chorionic gonadotrophin (hCG) and pregnancy-associated plasma protein-A (PAPP-A) and fetal nuchal translucency thickness, the rate of detection of trisomy 21 was 92% (23 of 25), of trisomy 13 or 18 was 100% (all 15), and of all aneuploidies was 96% (49 of 51). The false-positive rate was 5.2%.

Increased nuchal translucency may also be a presenting feature of CHD and a variety of disparate and rare genetic disorders including Noonan syndrome, and skeletal dysplasias, etc. Galindo *et al.* (2003) found that cardiac defects were present in 9.1% of chromosomally normal fetuses with increased nuchal translucency (>3.9 mm). The risk ranged from 5.3% in those with nuchal translucency thickness of 3.9 mm (= 95th centile) to 24% with nuchal translucency thickness of 6 mm.

Cystic hygroma

Cystic hygroma can be nonseptate or septate (divided into cystic compartments). In Tanriverdi *et al.*'s (2001) series, 56.5% had a chromosomal anomaly (e.g. 45,X, trisomy 18, and trisomy 21). There is a high fetal loss rate: in one Japanese series of 27 cases, 22 (82%) resulted in spontaneous fetal demise and 5 (18%) in livebirth (Fujita *et al.* 2001). Large size of the hygroma and presence of hydrops were adverse prognostic features. Of the livebirths, the 3 cases with chromosomal or structural abnormalities were handicapped. In Bronshtein *et al.*'s (2003) series of > 40 000 consecutive transvaginal USS assessments at 14–16 weeks gestation, all 13 fetuses with Turner syndrome (45,X) had septated cystic hygroma, severe subcutaneous oedema, and hydrops at that gestation and 12/13 had short femurs.

Hydrops

USS definition requires skin oedema >5 mm (over the skull), associated with other serous effusions (ascites, pericardial effusion, hydrothorax) and/or polyhydramnios and/or increased placental thickness (>6 cm in depth). Fetal hydrops is classified as 'immune (fetomaternal alloimmunization)' or 'non-immune'. There is a high pregnancy loss rate in pregnancies with non-immune hydrops and perinatal mortality is also very high (~87% in McCoy *et al.*'s (1995) series).

The causes of fetal hydrops are summarized in the table. Some metabolic disorders with hydrops as a feature include the following.

- Congenital disorders of glycosylation.
- Farber disease (ceraminidase deficiency).
- Galactosialidosis (Neuraminidase deficiency with β-galactosidase deficiency).
- Gaucher disease (β-glucosidase deficiency).
- Glycogen storage disease IV.
- GM_1 gangliosidosis (β-galactosidase-1 deficiency)
- I cell disease.

Causes of fetal hydrops (from Machin 1997)

Cause	Number*	%
Cardiovascular (structural defects, tachy- and bradyarrhythmias, high output cardiac failure)	370	23.3
Chromosomal (45,X and +21, triploidy, and a variety of rare chromosome rearrangements)	209	13.2
Thoracic (diaphragmatic hernia, cystic adenomatoid malformation of the lung, etc.)	152	9.6
Anaemia (e.g. homozygous alpha thalassaemia, congenital dyserythropoietic anaemia)	114	7.2
Cystic hygroma	97	6.1
Twinning	93	5.9
Fetal infections (e.g. parvovirus B19)	67	4.2
Miscellaneous	131	8.3
Unknown	318	20.1

* Total number of cases studied is 1551.

- Mucopolysaccharide (MPS) 1 (Hurler), MPS IV, MPS VII (β-glucuronidase deficiency). Can assay glycosaminoglycans (GAGs) in amniotic fluid.
- Multiple sulphatase deficiency (arylsulphatase A and other sulphatases).
- Niemann–Pick A (sphingomelinase deficiency).
- Niemann–Pick type C disease (cholesterol esterification defect).
- Salla disease and sialic acid storage disease.
- Sialidosis (neuraminidase deficiency)
- Wolman disease (acid esterase).
- (Pearson syndrome (anaemia)—a mitochondrial disorder).

Clinical assessment

History: key points
- Three-generation family tree with specific reference to previous fetal loss, family history of anaemia (e.g. thalassaemia, pyruvate kinase deficiency).
- Ethnic origin of parents (eg. α-thalassaemia, G6PD (glucose-6-phosphate dehydrogenase)).

Examination: key points
- Detailed fetal anomaly USS at 19–20 weeks gestation for the presence of structural anomalies and skeletal dysplasias.
- Detailed fetal echocardiography.

Special investigations
- Fetal karyotype (amniocentesis, chorionic villus sampling (CVS), or fetal blood sampling (FBS)). It may also be possible to arrange biochemical analysis of amniotic fluid and cultured amniocytes, e.g. for lysosomal disorders (some specialist centres offer a 'hydrops screen' for lysosomal storage disorders).
- The obstetrician should consider investigations to exclude fetomaternal alloimmunization (antibody levels), fetal infection (e.g. congenital parvovirus B19), and fetal anaemia.
- If the baby dies, arrange for clinical photography, skeletal radiograph (some skeletal dysplasias may present as

hydrops and accurate assessment of fetal limb length is made difficult in the presence of severe oedema), tissue storage (e.g. fibroblast culture), and DNA storage, and offer post-mortem examination.

Genetic advice and management
Make every effort to achieve a diagnosis and counsel as for the specific diagnosis.

Expert adviser: Lyn Chitty, Consultant in Genetics and Fetal Medicine, University College Hospital, London, England.

References

Bronshtein M, Zimmer EZ, et al. A characteristic cluster of fetal sonographic markers that are predictive of fetal Turner syndrome in early pregnancy. *Am J Obstet Gynecol* 2003; **188**: 1016–20.

Fujita Y, Satoh S, et al. *In utero* evaluation and the long-term prognosis of living infants with cystic hygroms. *Fetal Diagn Ther* 2001; **16**: 402–6.

Galindo A, Comas C, et al. Cardiac defects in chromosomally normal fetuses with increased nuchal translucency at 10–14 weeks gestation. *J Matern Fetal Neonatal Med* 2003; **13**: 163–70.

Machin GA. Hydrops, cystic hygroma, hydrothorax, pericardial effusions and fetal ascites. In *Potter's pathology of the fetus and infant* (ed. E. Gilbert-Barness), pp. 163–81. Mosby-Year Book, St Louis, 1997.

Makrydimas G, Souka A, et al. Osteogenesis imperfecta and other skeletal dysplasias presenting with increased nuchal translucency in the first trimester. *Am J Med Genet* 2001; **98**: 117–20.

McCoy MC, Katz VL, et al. Non-immune hydrops after 20 weeks' gestation: review of 10 years' experience with suggestions for management. *Obstet Gynecol* 1995; **85** (4): 578–82.

Nicolini U. Fetal hydrops and tumours. In *Fetal medicine* (ed. C.H. Rodeck and M.J. Whittle), Chapter 56, pp. 737–54. Churchill Livingstone, London, 1999.

Nyhan WL, Ozand PT. *Atlas of metabolic diseases.* Chapman and Hall Medical, London, 1998.

Spencer K, Spencer CE, et al. Screening for chromosomal abnormalities in the first trimester using ultrasound and maternal serum biochemistry in a one-stop clinic: a review of three years prospective experience. *Br J Obstet Gynaecol* 2003; **110** (3): 281–6.

Tanriverdi HA, Hendrik HJ, et al. Hygroma colli cysticum: prenatal diagnosis and prognosis. *Am J Perinatol* 2001: **18**: 415–20.

Zoppi MA, Ibba RM, et al. Fetal nuchal translucency screening in 12,495 pregnancies in Sardinia. *Ultrasound Obstet Gynecol* 2001; **18**: 649–51.

Premature ovarian failure (POF)

The median age at menopause in Western populations of women is approximately 51 years. By convention, menopause that occurs at ages 40–45 years is considered 'early' and occurs in about 5% of women. POF is defined as cessation of menses due to hypergonadotrophic amenorrhoea below the age of 40 years. It occurs in ~1% of women in the general population. Depending upon the age at diagnosis, the probability of a genetic, autoimmune, or idiopathic cause will be more or less likely. At least one-third to one-half of cases remain idiopathic.

Women with POF are usually investigated and managed by a gynaecologist, and are only referred to a geneticist if there is a strong family history or if a genetic aetiology seems likely. Normal follicle-stimulating hormone (FSH) with elevated oestrogen indicates diminished ovarian reserve. High concentrations of FSH (>20 IU/l)) associated with low concentrations of oestradiol are seen in patients with POF.

Amongst women with idiopathic sporadic POF, ~2% carry a FRAXA (fragile X syndrome) premutation. Amongst women with familial POF, ~14% carry a FRAXA premutation.

Xq26.2–Xq28 appears to contain a critical region for normal ovarian function.

Development of the ovary. After migration of the primordial germ cells into the developing ovary, the population of germ cells increases by mitosis to reach a maximum of ~8 million at around 20 weeks gestation. The population of germ cells declines steadily thereafter, by the process of atresia to reach a level of around 1–2 million at birth (Baker 1963).

Clinical assessment

History: key points

- Three-generation family tree noting age of menopause in relatives and enquiring about family history of learning disability.
- Personal history noting age of menarche and menopause.
- Past medical history. Treatment with cytotoxic agents or radiotherapy for treatment of childhood cancer?

Examination: key points

- Height.
- Examine briefly for physical features of Turner syndrome (TS), e.g. short, broad, webbed neck and low posterior hair-line. Wide carrying angle. Shield-shaped chest. Heart murmur.

Special investigations

The reproductive medicine team will usually have arranged a hormone analysis and autoimmune screen.

- Karyotype with mosaicism screen (30 cells) if early POF (Turner mosaic).
- FRAXA analysis.

Diagnoses to consider

Turner syndrome (TS). Typically, in TS menopause precedes menarche, and there is no evidence of ovarian function, but occasional individuals with TS may menstruate briefly. See 'Turner syndrome, 45,X and variants' in Chapter 5, 'Chromosomes'.

Mosaic Turner syndrome. Guttenbach *et al.* (1995) found a significant correlation between X chromosome loss and ageing with the frequency of X chromosome loss ranging from 1.5–2.5% in prepubertal females, rising to approximately 4.5–5% in women older than 75 years. Thus interpretation of the significance of low-level 45,X/46,XX mosaicism in a woman with POF can be difficult. Devi *et al.* (1998) found that, in patients with POF, the percentage of cells with a single X chromosome (mean, 5.50) was significantly greater than in the controls of similar age (mean, 2.42), implying that some cases of POF may be attributable to low-level 45,X/46,XX mosaicism.

X-chromosome rearrangements. Some X deletions and translocations are known to be responsible for POF. Xq26.2–Xq28 appears to contain a critical region for normal ovarian function.

Fragile X pre-mutation carrier. Approximately 24% of female fragile X pre-mutation carriers will undergo premature menopause (cessation of menses at <40 years). This information may be helpful to carrier women for reproductive planning. See 'Fragile X syndrome' page 324.

Survivor of radiation- and chemotherapy-treated childhood cancer. Larsen *et al.* (2003) evaluated ovarian function in 100 survivors of childhood cancer and found that one in every six female survivors had developed POF. Results from survivors with spontaneous menstrual cycles indicated a diminished ovarian reserve, with the expectation that cessation of fertility may occur at an earlier age than normal.

Galactosaemia. The development of POF in females with galactosaemia is more likely if the patient's *GALT* genotype is Q188R/Q188R and if the mean erythrocyte Gal-1-P is >3.5 mg/dl during therapy.

FSH receptor mutations. Inactivating mutations of the FSH receptor have been described in rare cases of POF. This is a rare autosomal recessive (AR) cause of POF, characterized by high plasma FSH levels associated with very low oestrogen and inhibin B levels. No biological response to high doses of recombinant FSH is detected (Meduri *et al.* 2003).

Blepharophimosis–ptosis–epicanthus inversus syndrome (BPES). In this condition there is a reduced horizontal diameter of the palpebral fissures, droopy eyelids, and a fold of skin that runs from the lower lids inwards and upwards (epicanthus inversus). Mutations in *FOXL2*, a forkhead transcription factor on 3q, are found in ~67% of patients. Intelligence is mostly normal except where there is a microdeletion encompassing the gene. In type I BPES eyelid abnormalities are associated with POF and type II has eyelid defects only. See 'Ptosis, blepharophimosis, and other eyelid anomalies' page 224.

Autoimmune polyendocrinopathy–candidiasis–ectodermal dystrophy (APECED) is a rare AR disorder caused by mutations in the autoimmune regulator (*AIRE*) gene on chromosome 21q22.3. Patients most often suffer from loss of endocrine function in the parathyroid and adrenal glands but may also develop type 1 diabetes, thyroid disease, or hypogonadism. Hypoparathyroidism is much more common in affected females than in affected males.

Genetic advice and management

Woman with POF should be given hormone replacement therapy (HRT) at least until the age of 50. HRT is preferable to the contraceptive pill, which will also provide an artificial menstrual cycle but will not allow ovulation to occur. If pregnancy is desired it can occur whilst taking HRT, even though the chances of ovulation are extremely unlikely. It is possible to have '*in vitro* fertilization' (IVF) using donated eggs that have been fertilized by the sperm of the recipient's partner and created embryos can be transferred to the recipient uterus after a special HRT regimen.

Support group: Premature Ovarian Failure Support Group <www.pofsupport.org>.

Expert advisers: Melanie Davies, Consultant Obstetrician and Gynaecologist (Reproductive Medicine) and Ozkan Ozturk, Senior Lecturer in Obstetrics and Gynaecology (Reproductive Medicine), both at University College Hospital, London, England.

References

Baker T. A quantitative and cytological study of germ cells in human ovaries. *Proc R Soc London* (B) 1963; **158**: 417–33.

Browne C, Strike P, Jacobs PA. X chromosome loss and ageing. *J Med Genet* 2002; Proceedings of BSHG SP61.

Devi AS, Metzger DA, *et al.* 45,X/46,XX mosaicism in patients with idiopathic premature ovarian failure. *Fertil Steril* 1998; **70** (1): 89–93.

Guerrero NV, Singh RH, *et al.* Risk factors for premature ovarian failure in females with galactosemia. *Pediatrics* 2000; **137**: 833–41.

Guttenbach M, Koschorz B, *et al.* Sex chromosome loss and aging: *in situ* hybridization studies on human interphase nuclei. *Am J Hum Genet* 1995; **57** (5): 1143–50.

Laml T, Preyer O, *et al.* Genetic disorders in premature ovarian failure. *Hum Reprod Update* 2002; **8**: 483–91.

Larsen EC, Muller J, *et al.* Reduced ovarian function in long-term survivors of radiation- and chemotherapy-treated childhood cancer. *J Clin Endocrinol Metab* 2003; **88**: 5307–14.

Marozzi A, Manfredini E, *et al.* Molecular definition of Xq common-deleted region in patients affected by premature ovarian failure. *Hum Genet* 2000; **107**: 304–11.

Meduri G, Touraine P, *et al.* Delayed puberty and primary amenor-rhea associated with a novel mutation of the human follicle-stimulating hormone receptor: clinical, histological, and molecular studies. *J Clin Endocrinol Metab* 2003; **88**: 3491–8.

Meyer G, Badenhoop K. Autoimmune regulator (AIRE) gene on chromosome 21: implications for autoimmune polyendocrinopa-thy–candidiasis–ectodermal dystrophy (APECED) any more common manifestations of endocrine autoimmunity. *J Endocrinol Invest* 2002; **25**: 804–11.

Santoro N. Mechanisms of premature ovarian failure. *Ann Endocrinol (Paris)* 2003; **64** (2): 87–92.

Sherman SL. Premature ovarian failure in the fragile X syndrome. *Am J Med Genet* 2000; **97**: 189–94.

Radiation exposure, chemotherapy and landfill sites

Radiation-induced heritable diseases have not been demonstrated in humans and estimates of genetic risks for protection purposes are based on mouse experiments. The most comprehensive epidemiological study is of the Japanese atomic bomb survivors and their children, which found little evidence for inherited defects attributable to parental radiation. Studies of workers exposed to occupational radiation or of populations exposed to environmental radiation appear too small and exposures too low to convincingly detect inherited genetic damage (Boice et al. 2003).

Diagnostic radiation. Radiation exposure after diagnostic imaging in pregnancy is too small to cause developmental problems. The main risk is an incremental added risk for childhood cancer.

- The background risk for childhood cancer is 1/650 (all (fatal and non-fatal) cancers in the first 15 years of life).
- Added risk of childhood cancer per millisievert (mSv) exposure is 1/17 000.
- Fetal exposure from a chest X-ray or mammogram is < 0.01 mSv.
- Background radiation in Cambridge, UK is about 2.5 mSv per annum.

Therapeutic radiation. An international study is nearing completion of over 25 000 survivors of childhood cancer in the USA and Denmark who gave birth to or fathered over 6000 children (Boise et al. 2003). Doses to gonads are being reconstructed from radiotherapy records with 46% over 100 mSv and 16% over 1000 mSv. Adverse pregnancy outcomes being evaluated include major congenital malformations, cytogenetic abnormalities, stillbirths, miscarriages, neonatal deaths, total deaths, leukaemia and childhood cancers, altered sex ratio, and birthweight. In the USA series to date, 4214 children were born to cancer survivors among whom 157 (3.7%) genetic diseases were reported in contrast to 95 (4.1%) reported conditions among 2339 children born to sibling controls. In the Denmark series the comparable figures were 82 (6.1%) birth defects among 1345 children of cancer survivors and 211 (5.0%) among 4225 children of sibling controls. Coupled with prior studies, these preliminary findings, if sustained by ongoing dose–response analyses, provide reassurance that cancer treatments including radiotherapy do not carry much if any risk for inherited genetic disease in offspring conceived after exposure.

Offspring risks to survivors of childhood cancer

Female survivors. Green et al. (2002) reviewed pregnancy outcome among female participants in the Childhood Cancer Survivor Study who returned a questionnaire. 1915 women reported 4029 pregnancies (63% live births, 1% stillbirths, 15% miscarriages, 17% abortions, 3% unknown or in gestation). There were no significant differences in pregnancy outcome by treatment. A higher, but not statistically significant, risk of miscarriage was present among women whose ovaries were in the radiation therapy field (relative risk (RR), 1.86; $p = 0.14$), were near the radiation therapy field (RR, 1.64; $p = 0.06$), or were shielded (RR, 0.90; $p = 0.88$). The rate of live birth was not lower for the patients treated with any particular chemotherapeutic agent and the study did not identify adverse pregnancy outcomes for female survivors treated with most chemotherapeutic agents. The offspring of the patients who received pelvic irradiation were more likely to weigh < 2500 g at birth (RR, 1.84; $p = 0.03$).

Male survivors. Green et al. (2003) reviewed pregnancy outcome among male participants in the Childhood Cancer Survivor Study who returned a questionnaire. 1227 men reported they sired 2323 pregnancies (69% live births, 1% stillbirths, 13% miscarriages, 13% abortions, 5% unknown or in gestation). This large study did not identify adverse pregnancy outcomes for the partners of male survivors treated with most chemotherapeutic agents. (The male:female ratio was slightly altered compared with offspring of siblings of survivors and concerns about procarbazine warrant further investigation.)

Landfill sites

80% of the population of the UK live within 2 km of a landfill site.

In Elliott et al.'s (2001) survey of >1 million livebirths in the UK, the relative risk for women resident within <2 km of a landfill site for all congenital anomalies was 1.01 (adjusted for confounders), i.e. there is a very small excess risk of congenital anomalies. Adjusted risks were 1.05 for neural tube defects (NTDs), 1.07 for hypospadias and epispadias, 1.19 for gastroschisis and exomphalos, 1.05 for low birthweight (<2.5 kg), and 1.04 for very low birthweight (<1.5 kg). There was no excess risk for stillbirth. In reality what this means is: 'this 1% higher rate of birth defects would represent about 100 cases of birth defects each year across England and Wales. This is out of a total of ~12 000 cases of birth defects expected each year in England and Wales.' (Troop 2001).

The EUROHAZCON study found a 33% increase in the risk of non-chromosomal anomalies for residents living within 3km of 21 European *hazardous waste* landfill sites. A similar effect was found for chromosomal anomalies with an odds ratio of 1.41 for chormosomal anomalies in people who lived close the sites (0–3 km) compared with those who lived further away (3–7 km) after adjustment for confounding by maternal age and socioeconomic status (Dolk et al. 1998).

Expert advisers: Karen Goldstone, Radiation Protection Advisor, Addenbrooke's Hospital, Cambridge and Patricia McElhatton, Consultant Teratologist and Head of National Teratology Information Service, Newcastle-upon-Tyne, England.

References

<www.doh.gov.uk/landfillrep.pdf> Final Landfill Report Dec 2001.

Boice JD Jr, Tawn EJ, et al. Genetic effects of radiotherapy for childhood cancer. *Health Phys* 2003; **85** (1): 65–80.

Diagnostic medical exposures: advice on exposure to ionising radiation during pregnancy. Joint Guidance from National Radiation Protection Board, College of Radiographers, Royal College of Radiographers. 1998.

Dolk H, Vrijheid M, et al. Risk of congenital anomalies near hazardous-waste landfill sites in Europe: the EUROHAZCON study. *Lancet* 1998; **352**: 423–7.

Elliott P, Briggs D, et al. Risk of adverse birth outcomes in populations living near landfill sites. *Br Med J* 2001; **323**: 363–8.

Green DM, Whitton JA, et al. Pregnancy outcome of female survivors of childhood cancer: a report from the Childhood Cancer Survivor Study. *Am J Obstet Gynecol* 2002; **187** (4): 1070–80.

Green DM, Whitton JA, et al. Pregnancy outcome of partners of male survivors of childhood cancer: a report from the Childhood Cancer Survivor Study. *J Clin Oncol* 2003; **21** (4): 716–21.

Troop P. Department of Health briefing CEM/CMO/2001/10.

Vrijheid M, Dolk H, et al. Chromosomal congenital anomalies and residence near hazardous waste landfill sites. *Lancet* 2002; **359**: 320–2.

Renal tract anomalies

Renal tract anomalies are common, comprising ~15% of all prenatally detected congenital anomalies. More than 70% are associated with other anomalies. Renal tract anomalies are found in ~250–300 syndromes and ~35% of all chromosome anomalies.

The main presentation of renal tract anomalies on fetal ultrasound scan (USS) is:

1 renal tract dilatation;

2 cystic or 'bright' kidneys;

3 oligohydramnios: fetal urine production accounts for the majority of amniotic fluid production from 14 weeks gestation. Any impairment in fetal urine output will manifest as oligohydramnios;

4 renal agenesis.

Dysplastic kidneys can be any size, ranging from massive kidneys distended with multiple large cysts up to 9 cm in diameter that are termed multicystic dysplastic kidneys (MCDK) to normal-sized or small kidneys with or without cysts that are echogenic.

In embryological terms either multicystic dysplasia or renal agenesis or both may occur if the complex morphogenesis of the kidney is disturbed. Dysplastic kidneys identified on antenatal USS may even disappear completely, both before and after birth, suggesting that many patients diagnosed with renal agenesis may orginally have had dysplasia.

Numerous kindreds have been described with autosomal dominant (AD) inheritance of aplasia, dysplasia, and other urinary tract abnormalities including vesicoureteral reflux (VUR), duplications, and horseshoe kidneys. The exact familial incidence of renal/urinary tract disease is unknown. However, Roodhooft et al. (1984) looked at index cases with bilateral agenesis/severe dysplasia and reported that 9% of relatives had renal malformations (the most common anomaly being unilateral renal agenesis).

Renal agenesis

Unilateral renal agenesis occurs in 0.15/1000 newborns, and bilateral renal agenesis affects 0.12/1000 newborns. Renal agenesis is more common in males (2.45m:1f). Bilateral renal agenesis presents with severe oligohydramnios beyond 14 weeks gestation and **Potter sequence** (pulmonary hypoplasia, micrognathia, talipes), and there is a high incidence of associated anomalies. Unilateral renal agenesis may be an incidental finding or discovered during the investigation of a renal tract disorder. There may be hypertrophy of the contralateral kidney. The ipsilateral ureter and Fallopian tube may be absent. 60% of cases of unilateral renal agenesis have an anomaly in a contiguous field.

Conditions to consider in cases of renal agenesis are the following.

- **VATER (vertebral defects–anal atresia–tracheo-oesophageal fistula–(o)esophageal atresia–renal anomalies)/VACTERL (vertebral defects–anal atresia–cardiac anomalies–tracheo-oesophageal fistula–(o)esophageal atresia–renal anomalies–limb defects).** See 'Radial ray defects and thumb hypoplasia' page 228.

- **MURCS** (Müllerian duct anomalies–renal aplasia–cervicothoracic somite dysplasia). See 'Female infertility and amenorrhoea: genetic aspects', page 586.

- **BOR syndrome (branchio-oto-renal).** See 'Ear anomalies' page 108.

- **Fraser syndrome.** Autosomal recessive (AR) disorder with cryptophthalmos and syndactyly. See 'Ptosis, blepharophimosis, and other eyelid anomalies' page 224.

Multicystic dysplastic kidney (MCDK)

MCDK most commonly presents as an incidental finding on prenatal USS. Sonographically, an MCDK is large, often very large, and irregularly bright with large cystic areas all but replacing the renal substance. Unilateral MCDK occurs in 1/3000–1/5000 births and liquor volume is usually normal. Bilateral MCDK occurs in 1/10 000 births and there is oligohydramnios.

Lazebnik et al. (1999) reviewed 102 prenatally diagnosed cases. In unilateral cases, abnormality of the contralateral kidney is common (33%). Associated nonrenal anomalies occur frequently with both unilateral (26%) and bilateral (67%) MCDK and increase the risk of a chromosome anomaly when present. Males are more likely than females to be affected (2.4M:1F), but females are twice as likely to have bilateral disease. There is a strong association between dysplasia and obstruction and the lower urinary tract should always be carefully assessed. 20–50% have a genitourinary anomaly on the contralateral side, e.g. VUR, or pelvi-ureteral junction (PUJ) obstruction. 10% have contralateral renal agenesis. Most MCDKs involute, both pre- and postnatally.

- **Unilateral MCDK.** In Lazebnik et al.'s (1999) study, unilateral MCDK without associated renal or nonrenal anomlies was not associated with an abnormal chromosome study and resulted in favourable outcomes. In Aubertin et al.'s (2002) study of 73 cases of apparently isolated MCDK, +21 was found in one fetus and genitourinary defects were subsequently identified in 33% and nonrenal abnormalities in 16%. Karyotyping is not generally undertaken in unilateral MCDK.

- **Bilateral MDK.** Karyotyping is indicated if there is bilateral renal involvement or an addditional USS finding. A wide range of chromosome anomalies are associated with MCDK including a variety of deletions/duplications that may often not be detectable on a routine antenatal karyotype. If there is an associated cardiac anomaly, offer 22q.11 fluorescent in situ hybridization (FISH).

Unilateral MCDK can be familial but is most commonly a sporadic anomaly. Belk et al.'s (2002) study did not find significant renal anomalies in any of the 94 first-degree relative of unilateral MCDK index cases, so formal screening of relatives is not recommended.

Large 'bright' or hyperechogenic kidneys

The term 'hyperechogenic' or 'bright' kidneys is used to describe renal tissue that is brighter than liver or spleen. Sonographically, polycystic kidneys are large and uniformly 'bright'. Initial kidney development is unremarkable, but subsequently cysts develop; adjacent functioning renal tissue is compromised and may eventually leading to renal insufficiency. In autosomal recessive polycystic kidney disease (ARPKD; infantile polycystic kidney disease) the cysts only arise from the collecting ducts. In autosomal dominant polycystic kidney disease (ADPKD; adult polycystic kidney disease) cysts arise from all areas of the nephron or collecting duct. There are usually numerous small cysts in ARPKD; fewer, larger cysts are more characteristic of ADPKD.

ARPKD. Incidence is ~1/20 000–livebirths. It usually presents in the 2nd or 3rd trimester with large 'bright' kidneys and progressive oligohydramnios. Prognosis is usually poor. All have hepatic and renal involvement, but the clinical spectrum is very diverse. Both kidneys are symmetrically involved and markedly enlarged. Individual cysts are not detectable on antenatal USS. It is caused by mutations in *PKHD1* ('polyductin') on 6p12, which is among the largest human genes. It has a minimum of 86 exons assembled into a variety of alternatively spliced transcripts (Onuchic). Both truncating and non-conservative missense mutations are described. All patients with two truncating mutations display a severe phenotype with perinatal or neonatal demise while patients surviving the neonatal period bear at least one missense mutation (certain misense mutations produce a severe phenotype) (Bergmann). There is a subgroup in which the disease phenotype is milder and who may survive into teenage years and early adulthood (Zerres *et al.* 1993).

ADPKD. Rarely, ADPKD may present in fetal or neonatal life with large hyperechogenic kidneys; individual cysts may also be detectable. Prognosis is good for fetal life and early childhood, unless there is oligohydramnios, which is extremely uncommon. If ADPKD does develop prenatally in a family, there is an increased likelihood that further affected children will also present early (Zerres *et al.* 1993). Individuals with ADPKD who develop cysts in fetal life may be at risk for earlier onset of complications, e.g. hypertension and renal impairment. See 'Autosomal dominant polycystic kidney disease (ADPKD)' page 262.

Other conditions causing enlarged 'bright' kidneys on antenatal USS.
- **Beckwith–Wiedemann syndrome (BWS).** Increasd renal echogenicity, hydronephrosis, and cysts may be seen in addition to large kidneys and generalized overgrowth. Other features detectable antenatally include exomphalos and large tongue and increased liquor. See 'Beckwith–Wiedemann syndrome (BWS)' page 278.
- **Bardet–Biedl syndrome (BBS).** AR syndrome characterized by polydactyly, obesity, developmental delay, hypogonadism, and a rod–cone dystrophy. Prenatally large echogenic kidneys and polydactyly are the only detectable features.
- **Oral–facial–digital (OFD) syndrome type 1 (X-linked).**
- **Meckel–Gruber.** AR disorder with occipital encephalocele, microcephaly, cleft lip and palate, large multicystic kidneys, and postaxial polydactyly. Considerable phenotypic variation is possible even between sibs. See 'Neural tube defects' page 392.
- **Trisomy 13.** Other congenital malformations are usually present, e.g. holoprosencephaly, postaxial polydactyly, orofacial clefting, and cardiac defects.
- **Zellweger.** AR peroxisome disorder with severe hypotonia, seizures, and nystagmus. Antenatally, multiple renal cysts may be seen bilaterally as may cerebral ventriculomegaly. Prenatal diagnosis is possible by quantification of very long chain fatty acids (VLCFAs) at chorionic villus sampling (CVS).

Renal tract dilatation

Mild pyelectasis. Mild pyelectasis (dilatation of the fetal renal pelvis) is a common finding, seen in 0.5–1% of pregnancies, and is often incidental, with no significant long-term sequelae. However, there is a small association with postnatal renal pathology, e.g. VUR and aneuploidy. Karyotyping may be considered if there are other risk factors present. Scott and Renwick (2001) reviewed antenatal measurements and concluded that a fetal renal pelvic diameter of >7 mm at 18 weeks gestation is likely to denote a clinically significant degree of dilatation and they recommended follow-up and postnatal investigation in such cases. Providing the renal pelvic diameter is not >15 mm at any stage in gestation, there is a low risk of clinically significant obstruction.

Congenital urethral obstruction. In males this is usually due to maldevelopment of the urethra ranging from complete urethral atresia to posterior urethral valves (PUVs) that form around the membranous/prostatic urethra. In the female bladder, outflow obstruction is rare and may be the result of 'cloacal plate abnormalities' with associated anomalies of the genital tract (e.g. vagina and uterus) and bowel. Cloacal plate anomalies can also occur in males.

According to Thomas (2001), the following are predictors of early-onset renal failure in congenital urethral obstruction.
- Dilatation detectable at <24 weeks gestation.
- Moderate/severe upper tract dilatation (renal pelvis anteroposterior diameter ≥10 mm in second trimester).
- Thick-walled bladder.
- Oligohydramnios.
- USS evidence of renal dysplasia, i.e. echogenic cortex, microcystic renal change.

Prune-belly syndrome. Abdominal muscle deficiency, megaureter, megacystis, and undescended testis affecting 1/30 000. Almost all cases are male. Sibling recurrence risk is low (<1%). Discordant monozygotic (MZ) twins have been reported.

Occasionally the bladder is enlarged due to non-obstructive causes, e.g. neuropathic bladder (consider spinal USS in early infancy) or MMIH syndrome (see next entry).

MMIH (megacystis–microcolon–intestinal hypoperistalsis) syndrome. AR. Microcolon. microileum, short bowel, intestinal malrotation, intestinal hypoperistalsis. Prognosis is poor. This should be considered when the bladder is dilated, but the kidneys and upper renal tract appear normal with normal liquor volume, especially in female fetuses.

Vesico-ureteric reflux (VUR)

VUR is common (~1% of all livebirths) and is usually an asymptomatic and self-limiting disease. Poor prognostic features are high-grade reflux and scarring at birth. Chronic pyelonephritis and reflux nephropathy remain important causes of end-stage renal failure in adult life. Medical management (prophylactic antibiotics) and surgical management are equally effective. In some families VUR appears to follow an AD pattern of inheritance with highly variable penetrance and expression; in others there may be a polygenic basis.

Risk factors for VUR are:
- dilatation of renal pelvis on antenatal USS;
- affected sibling;
- affected parent.

Management of a neonate at risk for VUR. Management is complex and optimal management varies with the sex of the baby and the severity of the antenatal findings. Prophylactic antibiotics from birth are indicated in some infants and various imaging modalities, e.g. USS, micturating cysturethrogram (MCUG), and functional scans (e.g. dimercaptosuccinic acid (DMSA) scans) are possible. This is a controversial area and neonates should be managed in conjunction with a paediatrician with expertise in this field.

Clinical assessment of pregnancy with renal tract anomalies

History: key points

- Three-generation family tree with detailed enquiry about renal tract problems, stillbirths, or neonatal deaths.
- Careful history regarding possible teratogens (alcohol, diabetes, rubella, angiotensin-converting enzyme (ACE) inhibitors).

Examination: key points

Detailed fetal anomaly USS with careful attention to the genitourinary tract and scrutiny for other malformations.

Special investigations

- Offer amniocentesis as indicated in the text.
- Consider parental USS (not indicated for unilateral MCKD or mild pyelectasis).
- If the USS suggests renal parenchymal involvement (e.g. bright kidneys) and the pregnancy fails or is terminated, strong consideration should be given to archiving DNA and obtaining a renal biopsy or full post-mortem assessment.

Genetic advice and management

Attempt to exclude monogenic, syndromic, and chromosomal causes insofar as this is possible.

Recurrence risks

- **Renal agenesis.** Recurrence risk for sibs is 3–8% for bilateral renal agenesis. There may be some additional risk for unilateral renal agenesis.
- **Perinatal lethal MCDK.** Empiric recurrence risk for sibs in 3.6%, but only 0.2% for cousins.
- **Non-lethal MCDK.** Empiric recurrence risk for normal parents of a child with isolated MCDK is small, of the order 2–3%. If one parent is affected, the recurrence risk is 15–20%.
- Conditions with **renal parenchymal cysts.** Counsel for specific diagnosis (see text).
- **Congenital urethral obstruction.** Sibling risks are small.
- **VUR.** There is a high sibling recurrence risk (20–45%) when siblings are carefully evaluated (e.g. MCUG). There is a high offspring risk for children of affected parents (~15–20%).

Expert advisers: Richard Sandford, Wellcome Trust Senior Fellow in Clinical Research and Honorary Consultant in Medical Genetics, University of Cambridge, Cambridge and Lyn Chitty, Consultant in Fetal Medicine, University College Hospital, London, England.

References

Aubertin G, Cripps S, *et al.* Prenatal diagnosis of apparently isolated unilateral multicystic kidney; implications for counselling and management. *Prenat Diagn* 2002; **22**: 388–94.

Belk RA, Thomas DF, *et al.* A family study and the natural history of prenatally detected unilateral multicystic dysplastic kidney. *J Urol* 2002; **167** (2 Pt. 1): 666–9.

Bergmann C, Senderek J, *et al.* Spectrum of mutations in the gene for autosomal recessive polycystic kidney disease (ARPKD/PKHD1). *Am Soc Nephrol* 2003; **14**: 76–89.

Bergmann C, Senderek J, *et al.* PKHDI mutations in autosomal recessive polycystic kidney disease (ARPKD). *Hum Mutat* 2004; **23**: 451–63.

Chudleigh PM, Chitty LS, Pembrey M, Campbell S. The association of aneuploidy and mild fetal pyelectasis in an unselected population; the results of a multicenter study. *Ultrasound Obstet Gynecol* 2001; **17**: 197–202.

Chudleigh T. Mild pyelectasis. *Prenat Diagn* 2001; **21**: 936–41.

De Bruyn R, Gordon I. Postnatal investigation of fetal renal disease. *Prenat Diagn* 2001; **21**: 984–91.

Lazebnik N, Bellinger MF, Ferguson JE 2nd, Hogge JS, Hogge WA. Insights into the pathogenesis and natural history of fetuses with multicystic dysplastic kidney disease. *Prenat Diagn* 1999; **19** (5): 418–23.

Onuchic LF, Furu L, *et al.* PKHD1, the polycyotic kidney and hepatic disease 1 gene, encodes a novel large protein containing multiple immunoglobulin-like plexin-transcription-factor domains and parallel beta-helix 1 repeats. *Am J Hum Genet* 2002; **70**: 1305–17.

Pilu G, Nicolaides KH. Features of chromosomal defects. *The 18–23 week scan. Diagnosis of fetal abnormalities*, pp. 99–104. Parthenon Publishing, Carnforth, Lancashire, 1999.

Roodhooft AM, Birnholz JC, *et al.* Familial nature of congenital absence and severe dysgenesis of both kidneys. *New Engl J Med* 1984; **310**: 1341–5.

Scott JE, Renwick M. Antenatal renal pelvic measurements: what do they mean? *BJU Int* 2001; **87** (4): 376–80.

Thomas DFM. Does prenatal diagnosis alter outcome? *Prenat Diagn* 2001; **21**: 1004–11.

Wellesley D, Howe DT. Fetal renal anomalies and genetic syndromes. *Prenat Diagn* 2001; **21**: 992–1003.

Winyard P, Chitty L. Dysplastic and polycystic kidneys: diagnosis, associations and management. *Prenat Diagn* 2001; **21**: 924–35.

Zerres K, Rudnik-Schoneborn S, *et al.* Childhood onset autosomal dominant polycystic kidney disease in sibs: clinical picture and recurrence risk. German Working Group on Paediatric Nephrology. *J Med Genet* 1993; **30**: 583–8.

Zerres K, Rudnik-Schoneborn S, *et al.* Autosomal recessive polycystic kidney disease in 115 children: clinical presentation, course and influence of gender (Review). Arbeitsgemeinschaft fur Padiatrische, Nephrologie. *Acta Paediatr* 1996; **85**: 437–45.

Rubella

Rubella is a mild viral illness that causes a transient fine erythematous macular rash, lymphadenopathy involving postauricular and suboccipital glands, and, occasionally in adults, arthritis and arthralgia. In unimmunized populations it is most common among children aged 4–9 years. Clinical diagnosis is unreliable as other viruses can cause a similar picture. The period of infectivity extends from 1 week before until 4 days after the onset of the rash. The incubation period is 14–21 days.

Congenital rubella syndrome (CRS)

In contrast to the mild nature of rubella in children, it can cause a devastating embryopathy (see table). Maternal rubella infection at 8–10 weeks gestation results in fetal damage in up to 90% of infants and multiple defects are common; by 16 weeks gestation the risk of damage declines to ~10–20%, and fetal damage is rare after this stage in pregnancy.

Features of congenital rubella syndrome

Growth retardation

Mental retardation

Eyes: cataract, pigmentary retinopathy*

Ears: sensorineural deafness*

Heart: patent ductus arteriosus (PDA), peripheral pulmonary
artery stenosis, septal defects (35%)

Inflammatory lesions of brain, liver, lungs, and bone-marrow

* The only defects that commonly occur in isolation are sensorineural deafness and pigmentary retinopathy.

Some affected infants appear normal at birth, but sensorineural deafness is detected later. Before immunization programmes were introduced, CRS was an important cause of congenital deafness.

Rubella re-infection can occur in individuals with either natural or vaccine-induced antibody. Occasional cases of CRS after re-infection in pregnancy have been reported. Although the risk to the fetus cannot be quantified precisely, it is considered to be low.

Rubella vaccine

- The vaccine virus is *not* transmitted from vaccinees to susceptible contacts. Thus there is no risk to pregnant women from contact with recently immunized subjects.
- Active surveillance in the USA, UK, and Germany has found no case of CRS following inadvertent immunization shortly before or during pregnancy. There is no evidence that the attenuated vaccine virus is teratogenic. Termination of pregnancy (TOP) following inadvertent immunization should *not* be recommended (UK Department of Health 1996). Nevertheless, rubella vaccine should not be given to a woman known to be pregnant and pregnancy should be avoided for 1 month after immunization (UK Department of Health 1996).

Epidemiology

Following the introduction of population vaccination programmes, rubella infection and especially CRS have become rare in the UK and most parts of the developed world. Sporadic cases occur, often associated with travel abroad. Tookey *et al.*'s (2002) population-based survey showed that, whereas <2% of British-born women were susceptible, overall susceptibility for other women was ~5%. African and Asian women had particularly high susceptibility

rates. If rubella were to re-establish itself in the UK, women who had come to Britain in later childhood or adult life would be at higher risk of acquiring infection in pregnancy than indigenous women.

CRS remains a problem in the developing world.

Clinical assessment

History: key points, postnatal

Detailed history regarding timing of exposure to rubella, or onset of rash.

Examination: key points, postnatal

- Growth parameters, including occipital-frontal circumference (OFC).
- Heart.
- Eyes for cataracts, pigmentary retinopathy.

Special investigations: prenatal

- Maternal *rubella virus* serology. (If the pregnancy may be at risk because of possible contact with a child/adult with rubella, establish the maternal status prior to invasive testing in the fetus.)
- Ultrasound (USS): growth retardation, cardiac defects.
- Fetal blood sample (FBS) for (1) polymerase chain reaction (PCR) for *rubella virus* RNA in fetal blood and (2) *rubella virus*-specific IgM. NB. No rubella *virus* RNA was detectable in amniotic fluid after a maternal rash at 15 weeks gestation, despite being present in fetal blood (Tang *et al.* 2003).

Special investigations: postnatal

- Confirmation of congenital infection. Look for rubella virus RNA in serum and urine.
- Serum for *rubella virus*-specific IgM and IgG.
- Ophthalmology referral (cataract and pigmentary retinopathy).
- Audiometry (sensorineural deafness).
- Echocardiogram.
- Consider cranial imaging. Intracranial calcification can occur (Numuzaki and Fujikawa 2003).

Genetic advice and management

- All pregnant women with suspected rubella or exposed to rubella must be investigated serologically (looking for rubella virus-specific IgM and IgG), irrespective of a history of immunization, clinical rubella, or a previous positive rubella virus antibody result (Department of Health 1996).
- In the UK, all children should be immunized with rubella virus containing vaccine (e.g. MMR (measles–mumps–rubella virus)) at 12–15 months and again at ~4 years (Department of Health 1996). This policy is intended to provide high herd immunity and thus prevent outbreaks of rubella during which susceptible pregnant women could become infected. Currently, take-up rates for immunization in the UK are below the level required for community protection.
- Women found to be rubella virus antibody negative on antenatal screening should be immunized after delivery and before discharge from the maternity unit in order to provide protection in a subsequent pregnancy (Department of Health 1996).

Expert adviser. Tim Wreghitt, Consultant Virologist, Addenbrooke's Hospital, Cambridge, England.

References

Department of Health. *Immunisation against infectious disease—Edward Jenner Bicentenary edition.* HMSO, London, 1996.

Lanzieri TM, Segatto TC, *et al.* Burden of congenital rubella syndrome after a community-wide rubella outbreak, Rio Branco, Acre, Brazil, 2000 to 2001. *Pediatr Infect Dis J* 2003; **22** (4): 323–9.

Numazaki K, Fujikawa T. Intracranial calcification with congenital rubella syndrome in a mother with serologic immunity. *J Child Neurol* 2003; **18** (4): 296–7.

Tang JW, Aarons E, *et al.* Prenatal diagnosis of congenital rubella infection in the second trimester of pregnancy. Prenat Diagn 2003; **23** (6): 509–12.

Tookey PA, Cortina-Borja M, Peckham CS. Rubella susceptibility among pregnant women in North London, 1996–1999. *J Public Health Med* 2002; **24** (3): 211–16.

Short limbs

The femur length is measured routinely during the anomaly ultrasound scan (USS) at 18–20 weeks gestation in order to compare it with other fetal measurements such as head circumference (HC) and abdominal circumference (AC) to assess proportionate growth.

A short femur may indicate/be a feature of:

- incorrect dates;
- a small normal baby;
- intrauterine growth retardation (IUGR), which would be very severe to be detected at 20 weeks;
- a chromosomal disorder;
- a skeletal dysplasia;
- a malformation syndrome with IUGR or limb reduction as one of the major features.

The clinical geneticist is asked for an opinion when the fetal medicine specialist suspects a chromosomal disorder, skeletal dysplasia, or malformation syndrome. It is more common for referrals to be made later than 20 weeks after it becomes apparent that the femur length growth is falling away from the centile chart.

See also 'Limb reduction defects' page 152 and 'Radial ray defects and thumb hypoplasia' page 228.

Clinical assessment

History: key points

- Maternal factors; age (trisomy), previous IUGR, diseases such as systemic lupus erythematosus (SLE).
- Family history of short stature (don't forget to look at the father!).
- Consanguinity (autosomal recessive (AR) dysplasias and syndromes).
- Insulin-dependent diabetes mellitus (IDDM; sacral agenesis, and an association with femoral hypoplasia, unusual facies).
- Drug exposure. Warfarin may produce a chondrodysplasia punctata (CDP) phenotype. Alcohol, phenytoin, and carbazepine may give limb reduction defects.
- Establish an accurate gestational age for the pregnancy (use earliest available USS).

Examination: key points

- Measurements of all long bones, HC, thorax, and AC.
- Is there any evidence of asymmetry?
- Are all the bones short, or is only one limb or one bone affected?

If the features are consistent with a skeletal dysplasia ensure that all the following are scanned and, where possible, measured.

- Long bones:
  - length and degree of shortening;
  - pattern of shortening (proximal, distal, or both);
  - epiphyses for stippling;
  - bowing (camptomelic dysplasia, osteogenesis imperfecta (OI) with fractures, hypophosphatasia);
  - bone density/mineralization (OI, achondrogenesis, and hypophophatasia);
  - fractures (OI, hypophosphatasia).
- Skull:
  - cranial shape (clover-leaf skull in thanatophoric dysplasia (TD));

- mineralization (reduced in hypophosphatasia, OI IIa/c, and achondrogenesis).
- Vertebral structure:
  - scoliosis;
  - hemivertebrae;
  - (platyspondyly);
  - mineralization.
- Chest:
  - cardiothoracic ratio;
  - rib length and fractures;
  - thoracic:AC ratio.
- Hands and feet:
  - trident hand (TD and achondroplasia);
  - talipes (diastrophic dysplasia, spondyloepiphyseal dysplasia congenita (SEDC));
  - polydactyly (asphyxiating thoracic dystrophy and short rib polydactyly syndromes, oral–facial–digital (OFD) syndrome);
  - absent digits;
  - hitchhiker thumb (diastrophic dysplasia).
- **Facial.** Clefts, profile, frontal bossing (achondroplasia), depressed nasal bridge (CDP), micrognathia (camptomelic dysplasia).
- **External genitalia.** Camptomelic dysplasia, Smith–Lemli–Opitz (SLO) syndrome and some short rib polydactyly syndromes may have sex reversal (Smith–Lemli–Opitz (SLO) disorder).
- **Hydrops.**
- **Polyhydramnios.**

A suspected **chromosomal disorder** or **malformation syndrome** requires thorough examination of the following.

- **Limbs** for deficiencies such as radial aplasia.
- **Intracranial anatomy** and **neural tube defects** (NTDs).
- **Cardiac** anatomy.
- **Renal** structure.
- Careful examination of the **face**.
- **Fetal size.** Many chromosomal disorders and syndromes presenting with short limbs involve low birthweight.
- **Placenta**, e.g. triploidy.

Special investigations

- Referral to a specialist centre for scanning may be indicated.
- **Chromosome analysis** by chorionic villus sampling (CVS)/amniocentesis/fetal blood sampling (FBS) depending on the gestation and the need for rapid results. If mosaicism is detected, particularly on CVS, then consult with the cytogeneticist about the possibility of uniparental disomy testing.
- **Molecular analysis.** Available for some skeletal dysplasias. In practice *FGFR3* testing for achondroplasia is often performed on fetuses with short femurs but most fetuses with achondroplasia do not have significant shortening at 20 weeks.

Genetic advice and management

Chromosomal disorders

- A short femur is one of the USS markers of **trisomy 21**.

- Fetuses with **trisomy 13** or **18** are small but have other have distinctive USS features.
- **Triploidy.** Triploid fetuses are very growth retarded; the dygynic type are more likely to survive to the 2nd trimester and have relative macrocephaly (see 'Triploidy' page 556).
- Bilateral radial ray defects are found in **Fanconi syndrome**. Routine cytogenetic analysis will not detect chromosomal breaks (see 'Radial ray defects and thumb hypoplasia' page 228 and 'DNA repair defects' page 304).

Syndromes with limb shortening

Most malformation syndromes without a family history, will not be diagnosed prenatally. It is impossible to distinguish between a malformation syndrome and chromosomal disorder by scan and cytogenetic analysis is indicated. A history of IDDM or drug exposure may be significant. If the karyotype is normal, consider the following.

Cornelia de Lange syndrome. This may present with IUGR and radial defects. Birth incidence ~1/50 000. See 'Limb reduction defects' page 152.

Seckel syndrome and microcephalic primordial dwarfism. These have extreme IUGR and microcephaly (these are very rare syndromes but included because of their extreme growth retardation). See 'Microcephaly' page 172.

Russell–Silver syndrome. This has IUGR but with a near-normal OFC. The head is proportionately large, but usually between the 3rd and 25th centiles. The face is triangular and the mouth downturned. Asymmetry is a key diagnostic feature. About 10% of children have been shown to have maternal uniparental disomy (UPD) of chromosome 7.

Smith–Lemli–Opitz (SLO) syndrome has been suspected after the detection of short limbs. Diagnostic biochemical analysis of sterols is indicated if there are other features of the syndrome. See 'Hypospadias' page 142.

Hydrolethalus syndrome. This is a rare AR condition, more common in Finland, characterized by hydrocephalus, Dandy–Walker malformation (DWM), bossed forehead, wide nasal root with short nose, micrognathia, short broad neck, small thorax with short ribs, congenital heart disease (CHD), marked limb shortening, postaxial polydactyly (80%), and polyhydramnios. The prognosis is very poor; nearly all are stillborn or succumb on the first day of life.

Skeletal dysplasias

There are some dysplasias that can be confidently diagnosed prenatally, either by the USS appearance alone, or USS plus genetic testing, e.g. TD. In some the diagnosis remains unknown though attempts should be made to place into a diagnostic group. See Appendix pages 696–99. In Parilla *et al.*'s (2003) series of 31 cases of skeletal dysplasia detected antenatally, a final diagnosis was possible in 80% with 8 cases of TD, 6 of OI, 3 of achondroplasia, 2 of Roberts syndrome, and one each of a variety of conditions including Ellis–van Creveld, spondyloepiphyseal dysplasia (SED), metaphyseal dysplasia, etc.

Thanatophoric dysplasia (TD). Sporadic neonatal lethal skeletal dysplasia caused by *de novo* dominant mutations in *FGFR3* (1/20 000). The limbs are extremely short with rolls of redundant skin, and the chest is very narrow causing death from respiratory failure in the immediate neonatal period. The head is relatively large with a prominent forehead and depressed nasal bridge. In an on-going pregnancy, confirmation of the diagnosis pre-delivery is indicated in order to plan neonatal management.

- **TD type 1.** Curved ('telephone receiver') femora and variable (mild) craniosynostosis. Several mutations: Arg248Cys (55%), Tyr373Cys (24%), Ser249Cys (6%), or mutations in the stop codon (10%).
- **TD type II.** Straight femora and clover-leaf skull (severe craniosynostosis). All have mutation Lys650Glu.

The recurrence risk is low; the possibility of gonadal mosaicism needs to be considered.

Achondroplasia. (See 'Achondroplasia' page 260, 'Common consultations'.) This is the most common survivable dysplasia and is caused by mutations in *FGFR3* gene on 4p. 80% represent new mutations. There are 2 common mutations, G1138A and G1138C, and these mutations lead to increased activity of *FGFR3*. There is a paternal age effect with mutations on the paternally derived chromosome.

The limb lengths are usually on or above the 5th centile until 24 weeks; thus many do not present until the 3rd trimester. The HC is usually around 95th centile. Observations of trident hands and frontal bossing are useful.

Osteogenesis imperfecta (OI). Severe forms, e.g. type II, present with short deformed limbs often with bowing, angulation, and/or fractures. There may be a narrow chest and some have undermineralization of the skull. See 'Fractures' page 122 and 'Bowed limbs', page 572.

Infantile hypophosphatasia. AR condition characterized by severe deficiency of chondro-osseous mineralization caused by mutations in the tissue non-specific alkaline phosphatase gene *TNSALP* on 1p34–36. There is deformity and fracture of the long bones and the skull is undermineralized assuming a globular shape. The blood alkaline phosphatase level is extremely low or undetectable.

Diastrophic dysplasia (dwarfism). The thumbs are angulated and well described as hitch-hiker thumbs. Additional skeletal features are severe bilateral talipes (club-foot), scoliosis, calcification of the costal cartilages, and short stature. The ear pinnae have cysts. Cleft palate may be present. It is an AR skeletal dysplasia caused by mutation in a sulphate transporter gene now known as *SLC26A2* but more commonly referred to as *DTDST*. Children with diastrophic dysplasia should be under orthopaedic supervision. Achondrogenesis type IB and atelosteogenesis type II are allelic.

Short rib-polydactyly syndromes. A group of lethal skeletal dysplasias with AR inheritance characterized by markedly short ribs, short limbs, usually polydactyly, and multiple anomalies of major organs. At least four types have been recognized. Diagnostic overlap between the different subtypes of the short rib-polydactyly syndrome group suggests that these may not be single entities, but rather part of a continuous spectrum with variable expressivity (Elcioglu and Hall 2002).

- Type 1 (Saldino–Noonan). Narrow thorax with protuberant abdomen and ascites. Urogenital defects and CHD are common.
- Type 2 (Majewski). Midline cleft of the upper lip and relatively normal pelvic and long bones, except for the tibiae, which are oval in shape. Affected infants may also have ambiguous genitalia.
- Type 3 (Verma–Naumoff). Very short ribs and limbs. Some overlap with type 1.

- Beemer–Langer type. Lethal short-rib dwarfism. Large head with brain anomalies, e.g. hydrocephalus, etc. Flat face. Short bowed bones. Polydactyly is an inconstant feature.

Achondrogenesis. Achondrogenesis results in stillbirth (or neonatal death) and is characterized by severe limb shortening, a relatively large head, a short neck, a short trunk, and a protuberant abdomen. Facial features include a flat nasal bridge and the whole nose is short with anteverted nostrils. Radiologically, ossification of the skull, spine, and pelvis is more deficient in type 1 than in type 2. The long bones are more severely micromelic in type 1 and there are spiky metaphyseal spurs in both, but more so in type 1. It is genetically heterogeneous. Some are due to mutations in *COL2A1* and some have mutations in *SLC26A2*.

Undiagnosed skeletal dysplasias. An estimation of whether the condition is likely to be lethal in the neonatal period is needed for counselling purposes and to advise neonatal colleagues. USS measurements of the fetus such as the cardiothoracic ratio and the presence of other malformations are used, but none are particularly accurate. Where possible, plans should be made for a senior paediatrician to be present at the delivery.

Predictors of lethal skeletal dysplasia (after Parilla *et al.* 2003) include:

- early and severe shortening of the long bones;
- femur length: AC ratio <0.16;
- small chest with short ribs and high cardiothoracic ratio;
- marked bowing or fractures.

Investigation of the fetus and baby with a skeletal dysplasia

A diagnosis is vitally important in order to be able to advise about appropriate management and also recurrence risks.

- DNA storage. Cord blood, FBS, placental tissue, and skin biopsy can all be used. An increasing number of dysplasias have known mutations.
- Chromosome analysis.
- Skin biopsy (collagen studies in OI).
- Radiology: full skeletal survey.
- Clinical photography.
- Clinical measurements.

If the baby dies it is possible to get most of the information required even if a post-mortem examination is refused. If a post mortem is performed it should include bone histology.

Support group: Many of the syndromes have their own support groups. See <www.cafamily.org.uk>.

Expert adviser: Lyn Chitty, Consultant in Fetal Medicine, University College Hospital, London, England.

References

Elcioglu NH, Hall CM. Diagnostic dilemmas in the short rib–polydactyly syndrome group. *Am J Med Genet* 2002; **111** (4): 392–400.

Parilla BV, Leeth EA, *et al.* Antenatal detection of skeletal dysplasias. *J Ultrasound Med* 2003; **22**: 255–8.

Pepin M, Atkinson M, Starman BJ, Byers PH. Strategies and outcomes of prenatal diagnosis for osteogenesis imperfecta: a review of biochemical and molecular studies completed in 129 pregnancies. *Prenat Diagn* 1997; **17** (6): 559–70.

Toxoplasmosis

Congenital toxoplasmosis is diagnosed, investigated, and managed by fetal medicine specialists, paediatricians, and specialists in infectious diseases with laboratory diagnostic support. The geneticist may be involved prior to a definitive diagnosis because the phenotype may overlap with genetic disorders; therefore a brief summary of the condition is included in this section.

Congenital toxoplasmosis is caused by a parasite, *Toxoplasma gondii*. The maternal signs and symptoms of toxoplasmosis include fever, tiredness, and lymphadenopathy, although the infection is often asymptomatic. In the pregnant mother, the infection is caught by eating anything infected or contaminated with the parasite such as:

- raw or undercooked meat;
- food contaminated with cat faeces or with contaminated soil;
- unpasteurized goats milk.

The fetus is infected across the placenta from an infected mother. The brain and retina are particularly affected and the signs of the disease in neonates and infants include chorioretinitis, hydrocephalus, intracranial calcification, and seizures.

The rate of transmission depends on the point in gestation at which the mother acquires the infection. In a recent European review (Mombro *et al.* 2003), none of the mothers infected in the first trimester had affected babies ($n = 45$); there was transmission in 17% of mothers with seroconversion *or* probable infection in the second trimester and a transmission rate of 35% with infection in the third trimester. Other studies (Martin 2001) calculate an overall 40% chance of fetal infection from affected mothers. 80–90% of infants with congenital toxoplasmosis are asymptomatic at birth and thus careful clinical assessment, particularly of the eye and central nervous system (CNS), is required. Antibiotic treatment during pregnancy can reduce the rate of complications. Spiramycin is used to decrease placental transmission, whilst a combination of pyrimethamine and sulphonamides are used to treat known fetal infection.

The majority of people with congenital toxoplasmosis have impaired sight in one or both eyes due to retinochoroiditis, which does not usually present until childhood or teens or even later. Severe damage to the brain is unusual and usually presents soon after birth. Typical features include hydrocephalus and calcification of brain tissue with developmental delay and epilepsy.

Clinical assessment

In pregnancy, the assessment should be under the supervision of the fetal medicine specialist who will decide whether invasive testing (amniocentesis, cordocentesis) and antibiotic treatment (usually spiramycin) in pregnancy is indicated. This will be influenced by the gestation, ultrasound (USS) features, and maternal serology (IgM, IgA, and IgG). Making a firm antenatal diagnosis can be problematical due to problems timing the onset of the infection, because IgM titres stay positive for years in some cases. Use of different IgM assays can help and antibody avidity testing may also be useful. Diagnosis of toxoplasmosis should be made in conjunction with colleagues in microbiology and a National Reference Laboratory.

History: key points, postnatal

- Birthweight, occipital-frontal circumference (OFC).
- Lethargy, poor feeding (signs of possible neurological involvement).

Examination: key points, postnatal

- Microcephaly and neurological abnormalities.
- Chorioretinitis.

Special investigations: prenatal

- USS: poor fetal growth, intracranial calcification, ventriculomegaly.
- Polymerase chain reaction (PCR) for *Toxoplasma gondii* DNA in amniotic fluid.
- Maternal *Toxoplasma gondii* serology.

Special investigations: postnatal

- Confirmation of congenital infection. Check if placental tissue would be of use.
- Brain imaging of all symptomatic babies (toxoplasma is typically associated with enlarged ventricles without cortical malformations).
- Ophthalmology referral (chorioretinitis).

Genetic advice and management

Proven congenital toxoplasmosis is not a genetic condition. Babies with signs of congenital infection, but in whom there are no serological features, may be referred to a geneticist for an opinion.

- Consider the autosomal recessive (AR) condition of pseudo-TORCH/microcephaly–intracranial calcification in babies with signs of congenital infection, but in whom there are no serological features to support the diagnosis.
- Please refer to the appropriate eye section or brain section of Chapter 2, 'Clinical approach', for discussion of other syndromes with some of the features of congenital infections.

Expert advisers: Donald Peebles, Consultant in Fetal Medicine, University College Hospital, London and Tim Wreghitt, Consultant Virologist, Addenbrooke's Hospital, Cambridge, England.

References

Martin S. Congenital toxoplasmosis. *Neonatal Netw* 2001; **20**: 23–30.

Mombro M, Perathoner C, Leone A, Buttafuoco, Zotti C, Lievre MA, Fabris C. Congenital toxoplasmosis: assessment of risk to newborns in confirmed and uncertain maternal infection. *Eur J Pediatr* 2003; **162** (10): 703–6.

Monatora SG, Liesenfeld O. Toxoplasmosis (Seminar). *Lancet* 2004; **363**: 1965–76.

Twins and twinning

Twins occur in 1 in 80 livebirths. They have a special place in Greek mythology and ancient legends. Classical twin studies have played a key role in defining the 'heritability' of a trait by studying the concordance in monozygotic (MZ) versus dizygotic (DZ) twins. Many aspects of twin pregnancies, including prematurity and maternal physiology, make them different from singleton pregnancies.

'Vanishing' twin
Only 29% of women with a twin pregnancy on ultrasound scan (USS) at <10 weeks gestation will give birth to twins. Hence there is an ~70% loss rate in twin pregnancies

Congenital anomalies
Congenital anomalies occur in at least 10% of all twin pregnancies. The congenital anomaly rate is probably higher in MZ than in DZ twins, partly due to the increased burden of anomalies arising from vascular disruption and possibly because, in the earliest phase of embryonic development, the cytoplasm of a single egg cell supports the nutritional requirements of two embryos prior to implantation. Both MZ and DZ twins have an increased risk for deformational congenital anomalies, associated with constraint and intrauterine crowding, such as greater moulding of the head, craniosynostosis, dislocated hips, bowing of legs, and club-feet.

Disruptions in MZ twins, including hemifacial microsomia, limb reduction defects, and amyoplasia and bowel atresia, are probably related to the shared placental circulation unique to MZ twins with differences in vascular flow leading to vascular compromise.

Dizygotic (DZ) twins ('non-identical twins')
DZ twins share the same genetic similarity as siblings, i.e. they have 50% of their nuclear DNA in common and they have a 25% risk to be concordant for autosomal recessive (AR) disorders. DZ twins have separate placentas and membranes (dichorionic diamniotic; see figure, part (a)), although they might be fused and even have vascular connections. At least 8% of DZ twins show some level of chimerism in blood lymphocytes. This is also occasionally seen in singletons (possibly arising from a 'vanished' twin). The introduction of artificial reproductive technologies (ART) has led to an 'epidemic' of DZ twins.

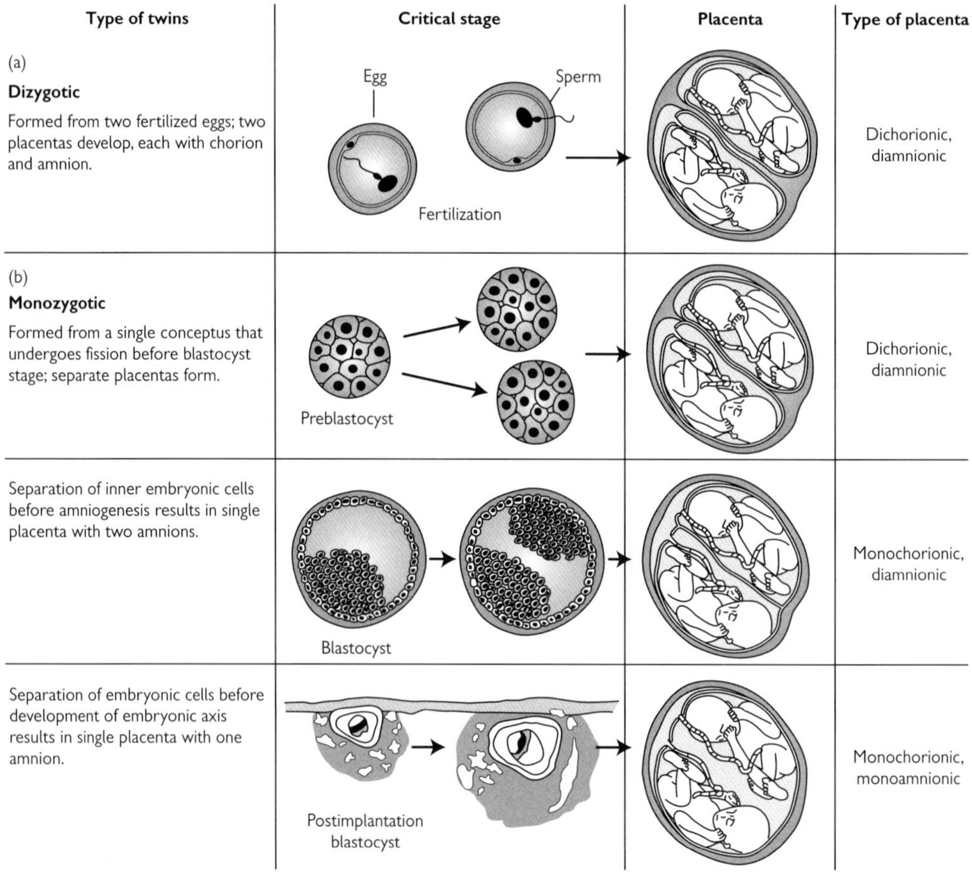

Type of twins	Critical stage	Placenta	Type of placenta
(a) **Dizygotic** Formed from two fertilized eggs; two placentas develop, each with chorion and amnion.	Egg / Sperm → Fertilization		Dichorionic, diamnionic
(b) **Monozygotic** Formed from a single conceptus that undergoes fission before blastocyst stage; separate placentas form.	Preblastocyst		Dichorionic, diamnionic
Separation of inner embryonic cells before amniogenesis results in single placenta with two amnions.	Blastocyst		Monochorionic, diamnionic
Separation of embryonic cells before development of embryonic axis results in single placenta with one amnion.	Postimplantation blastocyst		Monochorionic, monoamnionic

(a) Dizygotic twins, (b) Monozygotic twins.

There are now 6 published cases of DZ twins with a monochromic placenta. This exceptionally rare phenomenon has been documented using fibroblast DNA, and seems to be more common after ART, The bone marrow of one twin may take over both bone marrows.

Factors increasing DZ twinning rate.
- **Raised gonadotrophin levels.** Older, taller, heavier mothers and nulliparas. The peak incidence is at 37 years.
- **Fertility drugs**, e.g. clomiphene. These promote superovulation with a markedly increased risk for DZ twinning.
- **Familial factors.** Women with a family history of DZ twinning are more likely to have DZ twins.
- **Ethnicity.** The rate of DZ twinning varies widely between different populations. It is low in Asian populations with an incidence of 4/1000, intermediate in Europeans and Northern Americans at 10–14/1000, and high in Africans at 26–40/1000.

Types of DZ twinning.
- **Superfecundation.** More than one egg fertilized in same menstrual cycle.
- **Superfetation** (rare). Implantation of a second fertilized egg in a uterus containing a pregnancy.
- **Polar body twins** (rare). Fertilization of the nucleus of the egg and the polar body by two different sperm.

Monozygotic (MZ) twins ('identical twins')
MZ twins are genetically identical. MZ twinning occurs at the same rate worldwide. In MZ twinning a single egg is fertilized by a single sperm. MZ twins account for 3–4/1000 births in the UK. Manipulation of the environment around the time of conceptions can induce MZ twinning in animals; the MZ twinning rate is increased threefold in *in vitro* fertilization (IVF) pregnancies. Milki *et al.* (2003) report an MZ twinning rate of 5.6% with blastocyst transfer, compared with 2% following day 3 transfer (cleavage-stage). The placentation of MZ twinning is thought to be determined by the time at which twinning occurs following fertilization (see table and second figure). 25–30% of MZ twins have completely separate placentas and membranes, 70–75% share one placenta with monochorionic diamniotic membranes, and 1–2% have one set of membranes and one placenta (monochorionic, monoamniotic; see part (b) of first figure). Monochorionic placentas of all types are prone

Placentation of MZ twins in relationship to timing of twinning after fertilization

Placentation of MZ twins	Time of twinning after fertilization	% of all MZ pregnancies surviving to term	Comment
Dichorionic diamniotic	Separation by day 3	25	Early separation leads to completely separate placentation
Monochorionic diamniotic	4–8 days	70–75	Single placenta with separate amniotic sacs
Monochorionic monamniotic	9–12 days	1–2	Risk of tangled cords
Conjoined twins	13–14 days	Rare	75% are female

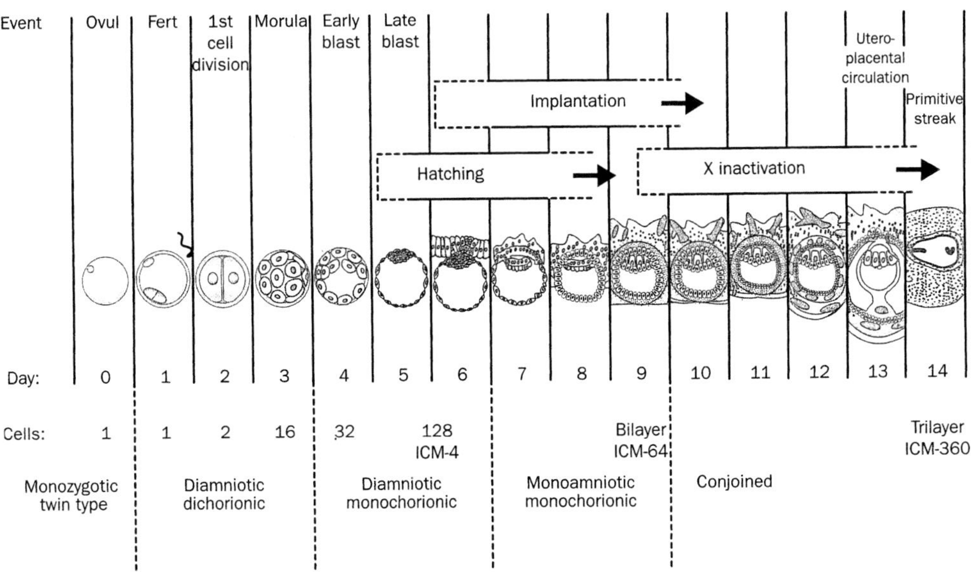

Schematic drawing of normal human embryonic development with timing of monozygotic twinning superimposed. (Reprinted from Hall (2003) with permission from Elsevier.)

to have vascular connections that can lead to twin–twin transfusion syndrome, twin reverse arterial perfusion sequence (TRAP), and to disruptive congenital anomalies (see above).

Types of MZ twin.

- **Acardiac.** ~1/35 000 births. Normal twin supports acardiac twin with risk of cardiac failure and hydrops in normal twin.
- **Fetus papyraceus.** Frequent if looked for. Co-twin dies in 2nd or 3rd trimester and is delivered at term, often attached to the placenta.
- **Concordant MZ twins.** The great majority of MZ twins.
- **Discordant MZ twins.** Due to a new dominant mutation, chromosomal aneuploidy, differential X-inactivation (Valleix *et al.* 2002), imprinting loss/gain (Weksburg *et al.* 2002), mitotic recombination.
- **Mirror image twins.** 10–15% of MZ twins. Twinning occurs late in development during the establishment of the body axis (just prior to the formation of conjoined twins).

Discordance. Discordance between MZ twins has been noted for chromosomal anomalies, single gene disorders, skewed X inactivation, genomic imprinting defects, mitochondrial disturbances, and minisatellites. These factors need to be born in mind during prenatal diagnosis, since MZ twins could be discordant for chromosomal anomalies and chromosomal mosaicism.

Vascular shunts. MZ twins are at risk of placental vascular anastomoses that may be arterioarterial, venovenous, or arteriovenous. They predispose to a variety of congenital anomalies due to vascular disruption: microcephaly; porencephaly; hydranencephaly; gastroschisis; intestinal atresia; and transverse limb reduction defects. If the co-twin dies in the 2nd or 3rd trimester, MZ twins are at greatly increased risk of cerebral palsy (perhaps due to embolization or disturbance of the coagulation balance arising from the dying/dead twin).

Clinical assessment

History: key points

- Family tree with history of twinning and determine ethnicity.
- Pregnancy and delivery. Were there separate placentas? Were there separate amniotic sacs?

- Subsequent growth and development. How similar are the twins? Can strangers tell them apart?

Examination: key points

- Careful examination of MZ (monochorionic) twins for congenital anomalies.
- Growth parameters.
- Examine as for the issue in question. Are the twins concordant or discordant for the problem?

Special investigations

DNA for zygosity testing; may need to use buccal swab or skin fibroblasts if single placenta. Documentation of zygosity at birth (using cord blood) may be considered for all same-sex dichorionic twins.

Genetic advice and management

Zygosity testing sufficient for routine clinical practice can usually be accomplished using a relatively small number (e.g. 7 or more) of highly polymorphic microsatellite markers. Microsatellite polymorphisms are based on short tandem repeats usually di-, tri-, or tetranucleotides that can be typed by polymerase chain reaction (PCR) and give a discrete allele with a precise repeat number.

Support group: Multiple Births Foundation <www.multiplebirths.org.uk>, Tel. 020 8383 3519; TAMBA (Twins and Multiple Births Association) <www.tamba.org.uk>, Tel. 0870 770 3305.

Expert adviser: Judith G. Hall, Professor of Paediatrics and Medical Genetics, University of British Columbia, Vancouver, British Columbia, Canada.

References

Glingianaia SV, Rankin J, et al. A multiple pregnancy register in the north of England. *Twin Res* 2002; **5**: 436–9.

Hall JG. Twinning [review]. *Lancet* 2003; **362**: 735–43.

Milki AA, Jun SH, et al. Incidence of monozygotic twinning with blastocyst transfer compared to cleavage-stage transfer. *Fertil Steril* 2003; **79**: 503–6.

Valleix S, Vinciguerra C. Skewed X-chromosome inactivation in monochorionic diamniotic twin sisters results in severe and mild haemophilia A. *Blood* 2002; **100**: 3034–6.

Weksberg R, Shuman C, et al. Discordant *KCNQ1OT1* imprinting in sets of monozygotic twins discordant for Beckwith–Wiedemann syndrome. *Hum Mol Genet* 2002; **11**: 1317–25.

Varicella

Varicella (chickenpox) is an acute highly infectious disease that is transmitted by personal contact or droplet spread. Secondary infection rate amongst household contacts is high at ~90%. Since chickenpox is so common in childhood, 90% of adults are immune. The incubation period is 2–3 weeks. Chickenpox is usually a mild illness in childhood, but can be more serious in adults, especially pregnant women who are at risk of fulminating varicella pneumonia.

Congenital varicella syndrome

Women who develop chickenpox during the first 20/40 of pregnancy have a 1–2% risk of having a baby with congenital varicella infection. The syndrome comprises congenital limb hypoplasia, skin scarring usually involving one or a few dermatomes, and damage to the eyes and central nervous system (CNS).

- Most cases of congenital varicella syndrome follow maternal varicella at 8–20 weeks gestation.
- The risk of congenital varicella syndrome after maternal infection at <13 weeks gestation is 0.4% (Enders *et al.* 1994).
- The risk of congenital varicella syndrome after maternal infection at 13–20 weeks gestation is 2.0% (Enders *et al.* 1994).
- The risk of congenital varicella syndrome after maternal herpes zoster is very low (0 in a series of 366 women; Enders *et al.* 1994).

Management of the pregnancy

- Detailed fetal anomaly ultrasound scanning (USS) with particular attention to the CNS and eyes.
- Repeat fetal anomaly USS at least 5 weeks after maternal infection.

- It is feasible to measure IgM in paired sera from the mother, but only important if there is doubt about the diagnosis of chickenpox and there is no history of contact or the rash or course of the illness in the mother is atypical.

Management of the mother

- Maternal varicella can be a serious and even fatal condition (risk of pneumonitis and encephalitis).
- Seek advice from an infectious diseases expert or virologist and give consideration to the use of acyclovir.
- Consider amniocentesis with varicella zoster virus (VZV) polymerase chain reaction (PCR) of amniotic fluid for rapid fetal diagnosis
- If a pregnant woman has no history of chickenpox or zoster and has recently been in contact with a case of chickenpox or zoster, take a 10 ml clotted blood sample for VZV IgG immunity check. Pregnant woman with no immunity to VZV should be offered zoster immune globulin (ZIG) in these circumstances.

Expert advisers: Donald Peebles, Consultant in Fetal Medicine, University College Hospital, London and Tim Wreghitt, Consultant Virologist, Addenbrooke's Hospital, Cambridge, England.

References

Enders G, Miller E, Craddock-Watson J, *et al.* Consequences of varicella and herpes zoster in pregnancy: prospective study of 1739 cases. *Lancet* 1994; **343**: 1547–50.

Royal College of Obstetricians and Gynaecologists (RCOG). *Clinical guidelines: Chickenpox in pregnancy.* RCOG, London, June 2001. `<www.rcog.uk/guidelines>`.

Ventriculomegaly

Ventriculomegaly in a fetus is an increase in the size of the cerebral ventricles, as measured by ultrasound scan (USS). This finding is associated with an increased risk of fetal chromosomal abnormalities, congenital anomalies and infections, syndromes, perinatal death, and childhood developmental delays (Wax *et al.* 2003). A wide range in the incidence of mild ventriculomegaly is reported in the literature (1.5–20/1000 fetuses).

- **Normal.** Axial sonograms of the brain through the atrium of the lateral ventricle demonstrate that the normal atrial diameter remains relatively constant from 14 weeks gestation. The atrium has a mean diameter of 7.6 ± 0.6 mm (standard deviation (SD)). Atrial diameters exceeding 10 mm (above 4 SDs) suggest ventriculomegaly, with a low false-positive rate (Cardoza *et al.* 1988).
- **Mild ventriculomegaly.** The lateral ventricle diameter is ≥10 mm but ≤15 mm.
- **Moderate/severe ventriculomegaly**. The lateral ventricle diameter is >15 mm.

True hydrocephalus has a birth incidence of 4–8/10 000 livebirths and stillbirths. Congenital malformations of the central nervous system (CNS; e.g spina bifida), infections (congenital infection or meningitis), and haemorrhage can all give rise to hydrocephalus.

It is important to distinguish between ventriculomegaly caused by conditions where the ventricles appear large due to poor brain growth, and ventriculomegaly caused by hydrocephalus due to cerebrospinal fluid (CSF) obstruction. In general, mild ventriculomegaly is more associated with chromosomal anomalies and syndromes and moderate/severe ventriculomegaly with hydrocephalus and structural intracranial anomalies (although there are many exceptions to this).

The prognosis for ventriculomegaly depends on the underlying diagnosis. It is important to determine if the ventriculomegaly is isolated or associated with other malformations. Sonographically isolated mild ventriculomegaly is associated with a significantly better prognosis than non-isolated mild ventriculomegaly (Goldstein *et al.* 1990). Studies have shown that the majority of fetuses with additional abnormalities can be detected with a combination of detailed scans and chromosomal analysis.

Mild ventriculomegaly may resolve with no neurological deficit. Alternatively, mild ventriculomegaly may be associated with serious neurological disability in many chromosomal and genetic disorders. Overall, isolated mild ventriculomegaly resolves in ~two-thirds before birth, with no apparent neurodevelopmental sequelae (see below). Management and counselling for mild ventriculomegaly is a challenging and difficult task.

Clinical assessment

History: key points

- Detailed three-generation family tree. Extend further on maternal side if possible. Enquire specifically for other relatives with hydrocephalus, unexplained stillbirths, spasticity, or mental handicap.
- Consanguinity. Autosomal recessive (AR) genetic syndromes.
- Enquire about infections, trauma, bleeding disorders in mother.

Examination: key points

Over 80% of fetuses with dilated cerebral ventricles have another abnormality on scan. About one-third of these are intracranial and two-thirds extracranial.

- Other intracranial anomalies. Document which ventricles are dilated.
- Detailed fetal anomaly USS looking for extracranial anomalies. Particularly examine the spine (neural tube defects (NTDs)).

Special investigations

- Karyotype. The incidence of aneuploidy if lateral ventricle diameter >15 mm is ~15% (Graham *et al.* 2001), and is also high in mild ventriculomegaly.
- Cytomegalovirus (CMV) and toxoplasmosis screen,
- Screen for neonatal alloimmune thrombocytopenia (NAIT).
- Consider fetal magnetic resonance imaging (MRI) in moderate/severe ventriculomegaly.
- Store DNA from fetus if pregnancy terminated, in case features of a single gene disorder are found at post mortem.
- Detailed post mortem, including neuropathology, in terminated fetuses. As neuropathology takes extra time (brain requires fixing), ensure that the parents give the correct consent for this procedure. Despite clear appearances of ventriculomegaly on prenatal USS, these appearances may not be confirmed at post mortem.

Diagnoses to consider

The following are conditions to consider in fetuses with ventriculomegaly.

Hydrocephalus

'True' isolated hydrocephalus. This is secondary to a relative or complete block to CSF flow. This is divided into communicating and non-communicating hydrocephalus. X-linked hydrocephalus with aqueduct stenosis may present in this way. For more details refer to 'Hydrocephalus' page 134.

After careful consideration of the differential diagnosis and a post mortem that does not reveal any features suggestive of a genetic or chromosomal disorder:

- the empiric risk for sibs of an isolated case is up to 5%, with all studies showing a higher risk for male sibs of an affected male.
- the risk for male sibs of an isolated male case with aqueduct stenosis is higher (5–10%) unless *L1CAM* has been excluded.
- children of consanguineous parents may have hydrocephalus as part of an AR condition.

If there is incomplete information the recurrence risk cannot be accurately assessed.

Hydrocephalus with an NTD. See 'Neural tube defects' in Chapter 3, 'Common consultations'.

Structural brain anomalies that may be associated with, or confused with, ventriculomegaly

Holoprosencephaly (HPE). During embryonic life the forebrain vesicle divides along the dorsal midline to form the cerebral hemispheres. Failure, or partial failure, of this cleavage results in **alobar holoprosencephaly** where the two lateral ventricles are replaced by a single midline ventricle that is often greatly enlarged, to part fusion of the frontal lobes (**lobar holoprosencephaly**). Other midline forebrain structures including the olfactory bulbs and tracts, optic bulbs and tracts, corpus callosus, thalamus, hypothalamus, and pituitary are frequently also affected.

About 50% of HPE has a chromosomal aetiology. Trisomy 13 is the most common abnormality but many other anomalies have been described. Particularly exclude loci known to have been associated with HPE. Triploidy may be found in fetuses with HPE. Consider telomere analysis in babies with HPE and other malformations/low birthweight.

The most common single gene associated with HPE is sonic hedgehog, *SHH*. See 'Holoprosencephaly' page 130.

Hydranencephaly. Scans show a small rim of cerebral cortex but the cerebellum and brainstem may be normal. Disruption to the carotid artery supply is one cause. Enquire about early pregnancy. May be confused with holoprosencephaly.

Arachnoid and porencephalic cysts. An arachnoid cyst is a cystic cavity within the arachnoid membrane. Hydrocephalus can occur by obstruction and reduced CSF resorption. The majority of arachnoid cysts are sporadic. See 'Structural intracranial anomalies (agenesis of the corpus callosum, septo-optic dysplasia, and arachnoid cysts)' page 248.

Single gene disorders

X-linked hydrocephalus. The neural cell adhesion molecule L1CAM plays a key role during neurodevelopment. The gene encoding *L1CAM* maps to Xq28, and males with mutation in this gene have a phenotype characterized by a combination of corpus callosum hypoplasia, mental retardation, adducted thumbs, spastic paraplegia, and hydrocephalus. There is a high degree of intra- and interfamilial variability. See 'Hydrocephalus' page 134.

Walker–Warburg syndrome (WWS) and muscle–eye–brain (MEB) disease. These are AR disorders that share the combination of cerebral neuronal migration defects (type II lissencephaly), ocular abnormalities, and a congenital muscular dystrophy. The features of WWS are hydrocephalus, agyria, retinal dystrophy, and sometimes an encephalocele—thus its alternative name of HARD ± E. Both syndromes are due to genes in the O-mannosylation pathway (*POMT1* gene in WWS and *POMGNT1* in MEB).

Pseudo-TORCH. An AR condition with intracranial calcification therefore mimicking congenital infection.

Chromosomal disorders

Exclude chromosomal disorders in fetuses with additional malformations. Counsel as appropriate.

Genetic advice and management

There have been a number of prospective studies to try and establish the natural history of fetal ventriculomegaly. Nevertheless, management of mild fetal ventriculomegaly and counselling of parents remain difficult as the cause of the ventriculomegaly and the absolute risk and degree of possible resulting handicap often cannot be determined with confidence (Wyldes and Watkinson 2004).

Mild ventriculomegaly

Robson *et al.* (1998) reviewed 155 fetuses with mild ventriculomegaly reported to the Northern Region of the UK fetal anomaly register. The diagnosis was confirmed by scan in 123 (80%).

Of the 123 fetuses with mild ventriculomegaly:

- 73 (60%) had another anomaly, of which 15 (12% overall) were chromosomal abnormalities and 28 (23% overall) had NTDs;
- 50 (40%) had isolated ventriculomegaly. 13 were terminated and there were 2 intrauterine deaths;
- of the 35 livebirths in the isolated ventriculomegaly group, the ventriculomegaly had resolved before delivery in 22 (63% of livebirths). These children were all normal apart from one fetus with trisomy 13 (mother had declined amniocentesis). In the remaining 13, 3 had severe disability at 2 years (i.e. 23% of those with persisting ventriculomegaly at birth): 1 child had congenital CMV, 1 had agenesis of the corpus callosum, and 1 had severe mental retardation with no additional structural brain lesions.

Fetal hydrocephalus

The study by Futagi *et al.* (2002) of 38 children with fetal hydrocephalus treated surgically in the neonatal period represents a group with more severe and persistent ventriculomegaly.

- These authors concluded that aetiology was a major determinant of the outcome.
- Neurodevelopmental outcome in the patients was normal in three patients and there was borderline intelligence in one patient, mental retardation in seven patients, and motor disturbance in 27 patients (five of whom were intellectually normal).
- An early onset and a high lateral ventricular width/ hemispheral width ratio at diagnosis of hydrocephalus were significantly correlated with a poor intellectual outcome.

Support groups: Association for Spina Bifida and Hydrocephalus (ASBAH) <www.asbah.org>, Tel. 01733 555988; ARC (Antenatal Results and Choices) <www.arc-uk.org>, Tel. 020 7631 0285.

Expert advisers: Lyn Chitty, Consultant in Fetal Medicine, University College Hospital, London, Patricia Boyd, Associate Specialist in Prenatal Diagnosis, John Radcliffe Hospital, Oxford, and Kenny McCormick, Consultant Neonatologist, John Radcliffe Hospital, Oxford, England.

References

Cardoza JD, Goldstein RB, Filly RA. Exclusion of fetal ventriculomegaly with a single measurement: the width of the lateral ventricular atrium. *Radiology* 1988; **169**: 711–14.

Futagi Y, Suzuki Y, Toribe Y, Morimoto K. Neurodevelopmental outcome in children with fetal hydrocephalus. *Pediatr Neurol* 2002; **27** (2): 111–16.

Goldstein RB, La Pidus AS, Filly RA, Cardoza J. Mild lateral cerebral ventricular dilatation *in utero*: clinical significance and prognosis. *Radiology* 1990; **176** (1): 237–42.

Graham E, Duhl A, *et al.* The degree of antenatal ventriculomegaly is related to paediatric neurological morbidity. *J Matern Fetal Med* 2001; **10**: 258–63.

Kelly EN, Allen VM, *et al.* Mild ventriculomegaly in the fetus, natural history, associated findings and outcome of isolated mild ventriculomegaly: a literature review. *Prenat Diagn* 2001; **21** (8): 697–700.

Robson S, McCormick K, Rankin J. Prenatally detected mild/moderate cerebral ventriculomegaly: associated anomalies and outcome. *Eur J Pediatr Surg* 1998; **8** (supp1): 70–1.

Robson S, Webster S, Smith M, McCormick K, Embleton N. Outcome of mild/moderate fetal cerebral ventriculomegaly. *J Obstet Gynaecol* 2003; **23** (suppl. 1): S22–S23.

Wax JR, Bookman L, *et al.* Mild fetal cerebral ventriculomegaly: diagnosis, clinical associations and outcomes. *Obstet Gynaecol Surv* 2003; **58**: 407–14.

Wyldes M, Watkinson M. Isolated mild fetal ventriculomegaly [review]. *Arch Dis Child Fet Neonat Ed* 2004; **89**: F9–13.

Appendix

Appendix contents

Bayes' theorem *646*
Behavioural pattern profile (Shalev and Hall 2004) *648*
Carrier frequency and carrier testing for autosomal recessive disorders *650*
Centile charts for boys height and weight *652*
Centile charts for girls height and weight *656*
Centile charts for occipital-frontal circumference (OFC) *660*
CK (Creatine kinase) levels in carriers of Duchenne muscular dystrophy (DMD) *662*
Conversion charts from English to metric units for height and weight *664*
Denver Developmental Screening Test *666*
Distribution of muscle weakness in different types of muscular dystrophy *668*
Dysmorphology examination checklist *670*
Embryonic fetal development (overview) *672*
Family tree sheet and symbols *674*
Haploid autosomal lengths of human chromosomes *676*
Investigation of lethal metabolic disorder or skeletal dysplasia *678*
ISCN Nomenclature *680*
Karyotypes *682*
Normal range of aortic root dimensions *684*
Paternity testing *688*
Patterns of cancer *690*
Radiological investigations including magnetic resonance imaging (MRI) *694*
Skeletal dysplasia charts *696*
Staging of puberty *700*

Bayes' theorem

Bayes' theorem as applied to X-linked recessive disorders where males do not reproduce (e.g. Duchenne muscular dystrophy (DMD)).

This provides a method of modifying the prior risk by the introduction of conditional factors (such as number of unaffected sons).

Important notes

- ν = mutation rate in male gametes and m = mutation rate in female gametes.
- For DMD, $\nu = m$.
- Prior probability that any female is a carrier of a sex-linked recessive disorder with a genetic fitness of zero = $4m$ (see Young (1999) for formal proof).
- Probability that the daughter of a non-carrier will become a carrier as a result of a new mutation is $2m$ (she has 2 X chromosomes), whereas probability that the son of a non-carrier will be affected as a result of a new mutation is m (he has one X chromosome).
- Terms of m^2 or m^3 are ignored for the purposes of these calculations as they are so small. Similarly $1-4m$ is approximated to 1 because the $4m$ term is so tiny in comparison.
- Mothers with 2 or more affected children or carrier daughters are assumed to be carriers. (The possibility of gonadal mosaicism is generally not considered in making these calculations.)
- Identify the closest female relative from whom both the consultand and all the affected male relatives are descended—the 'dummy consultand' or I1 in the worked examples.
- Information must never be used twice.

Worked examples

The five worked examples refer to parts (a)–(e), respectively, of the figure. In the figure the person for whom the genetic risk is being calculated is marked by an arrow. The roman numerals denote the row/generation (going top to bottom) and the arabic numerals the position (left to right) in that row so that III2 is the second person in the third generation (bottom row). Circles denote females and squares males. Black squares indicate affected males. The required result for the arrowed proband is given in bold face type.

1. See part (a) of the figure. II2 is a carrier as she has an affected brother and son. I1 is a carrier as she has an affected son and carrier daughter (ignoring germline mosaicism). If I1 is a carrier, her daughter has a 1/2 risk of being a carrier, and her grand-daughter has a carrier risk of **1/4**.

2. See part (b) of the figure and table (b). In this family tree, there is uncertainty as to where the dystrophin mutation has arisen. Is it present in the maternal grand-mother, or has it arisen de novo in the affected boy (III1) or in his mother (II1)? Bayes' theorem can help to establish the relative probabilities.

3. See part (c) of the figure and table (c). This family tree is similar to that shown in part (b), except for the addition of 4 unaffected boys. This substantially reduces the chance that I1 is a carrier. This 'conditional' information is put into the Bayes' calculation to derive the carrier risk.

4. See part (d) of the figure and table (d¹). This family tree is similar to that shown in part (c), but there are fewer

Table (b)

		I1 is a carrier (C)			I1 is not a carrier (NC)	
Prior probability		$4m$			$1-4m = 1$	
II1	C		NC	C		NC
Prior	1/2		1/2	$2m$		1
Conditional (1 affected son)	1/2		m	1/2		m
Joint probability	m		$(2m^2)$	m		m
Relative probability		m		:	$2m$	
Absolute probability		$m/m + 2m$			$2m/m + 2m$	
		1/3			2/3	

The probability that I1 is a carrier is 1/3; therefore theprobability that her daughter is a carrier is **1/6**.*

Table (c)

		I1 is a carrier (C)			I1 is not a carrier (NC)	
Prior probability		$4m$			$1-4m = 1$	
Conditional (4 normal sons)		$1/2 \times 1/2 \times 1/2 \times 1/2$			1	
II1	C		NC	C		NC
Prior	1/2		1/2	$2m$		1
Conditional (1 affected son)	1/2		m	1/2		m
Joint probability	$m/16$		$(m^2/8)$	m		m
Relative probability		$m/16$		:	$2m$	
Absolute probability		$m/33m$			$32m/33m$	
		1/33			32/33	

The probability that I1 is a carrier is 1/33; therefore the probability that her daughter is a carrier is **1/66**.*

Table (d[1])

		I1 is a carrier (C)			I1 is not a carrier (NC)	
Prior probability		$4m$			$1-4m = 1$	
Conditional (3 normal sons)		$1/2 \times 1/2 \times 1/2$			1	
II1	C		NC	C		NC
Prior	1/2		1/2	$2m$		1
Conditional (1 affected son)	1/2		m	1/2		m
Joint probability	$m/8$		$(m^2/4)$	m		m
Relative probability		$m/8$		:	$2m$	
Absolute probability		$m/17m$			$16m/17m$	
		1/17			16/17	

The probability that I1 is a carrier is 1/17; therefore the probability that her daughter is a carrier is **1/34**.[*]

Table (d[2])

	II5 is a carrier (C)	II5 is not a carrier (NC)
Prior probability	1/34	33/34
Conditional (1 normal son)	1/2	1
Joint probability	1/68	33/34
Relative probability	1 :	66
Absolute probability	1/67	66/67

The probability that II5 is a carrier is **1/67**.[*]

unaffected males in generation II and there is additional conditional information since the consultand has a normal son (table (d[2])).

5. See part (e) of the figure and table (e). In this family tree, there is uncertainty as to where the dystrophin mutation has arisen. Has it arisen *de novo* in the affected boy (III5) or in his mother (II1) or in the maternal grandmother (I1)? The affected boy has 4 normal brothers. This conditional information substantially reduces the chance that his mother (II1) or his maternal grandmother (I1) are carriers for a dystrophin mutations. Bayes's theorem can help to establish the relative probabilities.

Table (e)

		I1 is a carrier (C)			I1 is not a carrier (NC)	
Prior probability		$4m$			$1-4m = 1$	
II1	C		NC	C		NC
Prior	1/2		1/2	$2m$		1
Conditional (4 normal sons)	$(1/2)^4$		1	$(1/2)^4$		1
Conditional (1 affected son)	1/2		m	1/2		m
Joint probability	$m/16$		$(2m^2)$	$m/16$		m
Relative probability		m		:	$17m$	
Absolute probability		1/18			17/18	

The probability that I1 is a carrier is 1/18; therefore the probability that her daughter is a carrier is **1/36**.[*]
Note: m is a small number so $1 - m \approx 1$, $m^2 \approx 0$.

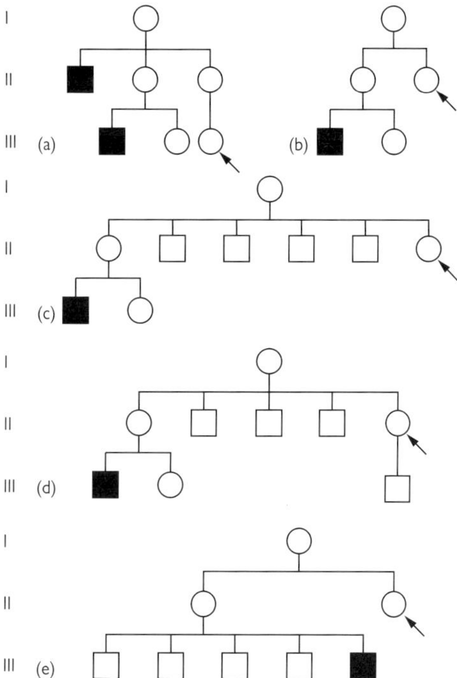

Figure: Pedigrees of Duchenne muscular dystrophy requesting the genetic risks run by the female relatives marked by arrow.[*]

[*] All figures and tables are adapted from Bundey S. Calculation of genetic risks in Duchenne muscular dystrophy by geneticists in the United Kingdom. *J Med Genet* (1978) **15**: 249–53. © BMJ Publishing Group (1978). Reproduced with permission from BMJ Publishing Group.

References

Bundey S. Calculation of genetic risks in Duchenne muscular dystrophy by geneticists in the United Kingdom. *J Med Genet* 1978; **15**: 249–53.

Young ID. *Introduction to risk calculation in genetic counselling*, 2nd edn. Oxford University Press, Oxford, 1999.

Behavioural pattern profile (Shalev and Hall 2004)

Behaviour is often an important clue to diagnosis. A structured approach to assessment may help the clinical geneticist to analyse and document an individual's behaviour. The 'Behavioural pattern profile' may be used in full (see Shalev for a form to record your assessment). Alternatively, in a time-pressured clinic setting, the main categories may serve as a prompt to documenting key features of an individual's behaviour.

Scoring
The scoring range is 0–4 to denote:

0 no deviation from normal;

1 very mild deviation from normal;

2 mild deviation from normal;

3 moderate deviation from normal;

4 severe deviation from normal.

Description of categories

1 Facial expression: description of the general appearance of the patient's face. Specific features:
   - *Decreased.* Decreased facial movements, reduced variability of facial expression as a consequence of decreased movement of facial musculature.
   - *Unusual.* Peculiar or abnormal facial movements that may be noticed while the patient is talking or eating, or during rest, including unusual appearance of emotional facial expression.
   - *Characteristics.* Free description of the typical facial expression, the predominant facial appearance of the patient, that might be observed most of the time during rest.

2 Motor milestones and daily living: the pattern of achievement, the motor skills, and daily living skills. Can be aided by developmental screening tests such as Denver Developmental Screening Test (see Appendix). Specific features:
   - *Gross motor skills.* The timing of sitting, standing, walking.
   - *Fine motor skills.* The timing of gaining skills such as grasping a rattle, passing a cube, finger–thumb grasping, scribbling.
   - *Locomotion.* The degree of patient's locomotion range when compared to normal individuals, including consideration of the level of independent moving around beyond infancy.
   - *Feeding, dressing, toilette.* The level of independent management with daily living needs.

3 Language and speech: application of human's main communicative tool by the patient. Specific features:
   - *Amount of speech.* Quantitative assessment of the amount of expressivity of language (or language-related sounds when considering babies).
   - *Expressive versus receptive language discrepancy.* The presence of an abnormal gap between the ability to produce language and the ability to understand it.
   - *Which is better?* Circle expressive or receptive.
   - *Voice quality.* The deviation of the voice character from normal, the magnitude of its peculiarity.
   - *Voice character.* Description of the voice's nature, such as hoarse, cat cry, low or high pitched, nasal speech.

- *Fluency, repetition.* The level of disruption of the articulatory flow, self-corrections, reformulations, false starts, repetition of sound, word, or phrase.
- *Overly focused on specific topic or object.* Being excessively interested and focused on a specific issue, leading to excessive expressions concentrating at the same point such as repeated questions.
- *Pattern of speech.* Assess the magnitude of the deviation of the general pattern of speech from normal.
- *Pattern characters.* Verbal description of the unusual pattern of language. Examples: fast speech, possessing rich vocabularies, inappropriate use of words and phrases, low grammatical abilities.

4 School: the specific aspects of the patient's involvement in the educational system. Specific features:
   - *School readiness.* Consider if the patient could attend the regular system at all and, if he or she does, what would be the need for special educational programmes and help.
   - *Reading.* The level of gaining reading skills compared to normal.
   - *Reading versus comprehension discrepancy.* The presence of a significant gap between the ability to narrate text and to understand its content.
   - *Which is better?* Reading or comprehension.
   - *Numbers and arithmetic.* Disabilities in quantitative assessment of objects, calculation, and other fields of arithmetic.

5 Emotions: the emotional general state and the typical pattern of emotional reaction. Specific features:
   - *Aggressive.* The tendency for wild or combative expression, including violent outbursts. Often is accompanied by irritability and frequent outbreaks of anger.
   - *Pleasant.* A kind and affectionate character.
   - *Depressive.* Lethargy, low mood and lack of happiness, reduced ability to enjoy or be satisfied.
   - *Emotional lability.* Inconsistency of emotions, a frequent shift from one specific mood to another.
   - *Anxious.* Being extremely worried, with no apparent reasonable correlation between the level of worry and its cause.
   - *Temper tantrum.* A wild episode, which is usually a reaction of anger or frustration, often characterized by excessive and aggressive motor activity (occasionally with no apparent target) It might be manifested as rolling on the ground, kicking, and boxing, accompanied by loud screaming and cry, or breath-holding.
   - *Other.* Describe any unusual emotional pattern.

6 Sociability: the pattern of interaction with the surroundings as well as the forms of relations with other people. Specific features:
   - *Disinterested in the surroundings.* Apathy, lack of interest in the close environment, including people.
   - *Response to environmental change.* The ability to adapt to changes in daily routines, to other caretakers, to new surroundings.
   - *Easily communicates.* Sociable, bonds with people quickly and willingly.

- *Social avoidance.* Profound shyness, deliberate avoidance of social bonding involving gaze, touch, or conversation.
- *Eye contact.* Unusual eye contact during communication with others.
- *Recognition of other's expression.* The ability to figure out and 'read' the mood of another person according to facial expression.
- *Other unusual social interaction.* Description of other specific pattern of impairment of social relationship, such as gaze aversion.

7 Unusual motor patterns: outline of unusual movements seen at rest and during typical reaction to stimulation. Specific features:
- *Increased activity.* Restlessness, hypermotor and hyperactive appearance.
- *Repetitive.* Specific patterned movements that are repeatedly performed by the patient, such as hand flapping, lip licking, rocking.
- *Self-injury.* Actions that are associated with self-hurt and damage, such as biting, scratching, forcing object into body orifices.
- *Tics.* Brief, involuntary spasmodic movements that repeatedly appear, such as blinking, grimacing, or sniffing.
- *Body posture.* The presence of a typical unusual position of the body during rest or activity.
- *Sitting position.* The presence of a characteristic unusual position of the body of the patient while sitting.
- *Unusual gait.* The presence of a characteristic unusual walk pattern, such as 'puppet gait'.
- *Unsteadiness.* Being unstable during activities such as sitting, standing, or walking.
- *Bruxism.* Teeth grinding, during sleep or when awake.
- *Pattern description.* Verbal illustration of any of the above-mentioned specific patterns, or others.

8 Unusual reactions to stimulation: unusual typical response to physical, emotional, or intellectual stimulation. Specific features:
- *Attention span.* The presence of shorter than normal attentive period, manifested as inability to concentrate for a reasonable duration of time on a specific activity. The patient quickly loses interest in the activity and moves on to another one.
- *Easily startled.* Immediate distraction and generation of worry and fear following mild stimulation that normally leads to minimal or no effect. The patient responds usually by startling to any stimulation.
- *Easily excited.* The generation of enthusiasm and thrill by mild stimulus that is lower or shorter than that that normally will lead to similar response. The patient responds usually with excitement to any stimulation.
- *Pain or heat threshold.* Unusually low (L) or high (H) sensitivity to pain or heat. In addition to ranking the deviation of the threshold from normal, circle low (L) or high (H).

- *Hypersensitivity to sound, touch, light.* Unusual need and enjoyment from touch, or feeling specific surface or texture, or specific sound and light. Unusual defiance to touch or natural tactile stimulation, sound, or light.
- *Specific reaction to sensory stimuli.* Verbal description of characteristic attraction or repulsion to specific visual, auditory, tactile, or olfactory stimulation. Visual stimulation includes specific colours, letters and digits, faces, squares, etc.
- *Other.* Verbal description of any other specific characteristic response to stimuli.

9 Feeding and eating: specific aspects of feeding the patient or unusual eating habits. Specific features:
- *General pattern.* Description of daily unusual characteristics of food consumption, such as feeding difficulties including prolonged feeding and need for special aid during feeding (which is usually associated with low weight), 'playing' with food, fast eating, the use of large bolus, 'passion' for food or disgust by food, 'self-imposed' diet.
- *Overeating.* Higher than usual consumption of food, usually associated with overweight.
- *Reaction to specific food product.* Verbal description of unusual attraction or repulsion to specific food products, focused on specific tastes, specific textures, food associated with pronounced odours, etc.
- *Other.* Any unusual pattern of feeding or eating.

10 Sleeping: unusual sleeping habits of the patient. Specific features:
- *Falling asleep.* Difficulties in calming and being ready for sleep, unusual pattern of falling asleep.
- *Duration.* Abnormal sleeping duration associated with abnormal waking timing, unusually shorter or longer duration of sleep.
- *Sleep/wake cycles.* Abnormal cycles of sleep and wake such as too many cycles of sleep/wake during the night, fewer cycles than usual during infancy, abnormal cycles during the day, abnormal distribution of sleep/wake cycles during day or night.
- *Nighttime waking.* Unusual pattern of nighttime waking.
- *Other.* Any unusual pattern of sleep.

11 Autonomic system abnormalities: specify unusual problems associated with probable dysfunction of the autonomic system of the patient. Examples of issues for consideration: abnormal amount or odour of sweat, gastrointestinal motility problems, bladder incontinence, unusual breathing pattern, recurrent unexplained fever, and cardiovascular manifestations such as abnormal heart rate and blood pressure instability.

12 Describe any additional unusual feature. Describe any special, unusual, or quirky behavioural feature that distinguishes the examined individual from sibs or peers.

Reference

Shalev SA, Hall JG. Behavioural pattern profile: a tool for the description of behaviour to be used in the genetics clinic. *Am J Med Genet* 2004; **128A** (4): 389–95.

Carrier frequency and carrier testing for autosomal recessive disorders

The Hardy–Weinberg equation

In a large randomly mating population with a disease caused by mutations at a single locus, it is possible to calculate the carrier frequency from a knowledge of the incidence of affected individuals in the population.

If N is the normal allele and n is the disease allele, then NN is the homozygous normal state, nn is the homozygous affected state, and Nn is the carrier state.

The frequency of the 3 genotypes can be determined from the binomial expression $(p + q)^2$, where p and q are the frequencies of the normal and disease alleles, respectively, and $p + q = 1$:

Frequency of NN = p^2 Normal

Frequency of Nn = $2pq$ Carrier

Frequency of nn = q^2 Affected

The carrier rate can be calculated as:

Carrier rate = $2pq = 2(1 - q)q = 2q - 2q^2$.

If the disease is rare, e.g. 1/1000 or less, the $2q^2$ term becomes very small and, for the purposes of clinical risk estimation, can be ignored and so the carrier rate can be approximated to $\sim2q$,

Carrier rate $\sim2(q^2)^{1/2}$, i.e. $2q$
or $2 \times$ (disease frequency for rare diseases)$^{1/2}$,

e.g. for a rare disease with a frequency of 1/90 000, the carrier rate is $2(1/90\ 000)^{1/2} = 2 \times 1/300 = 1/150$. The first table gives a guide to gene and carrier frequencies for different disease frequencies.

The following sources may be helpful in finding disease frequencies from which carrier frequencies can be derived:

The Frequency of Inherited Disorders Database (FIDD)
<http://archive.uwcm.ac.uk/uwcm/mg/fidd>
Online Mendelian Inheritance in Man (OMIM)
<www.ncbi.nlm.nih.gov>

Table to show data about carrier frequency and carrier testing for a sample of autosomal recessive disorders

See second table.

Carrier and gene frequencies for representative values of disease frequency

Disease frequency (q^2)	Gene frequency (q)	Carrier frequency ($2pq$)
1/100	1/10	2/11
1/400	1/20	~1/10
1/900	1/30	~1/15
1/1000	1/32	~1/16
1/1600	1/40	~1/20
1/2000	1/45	~1/23
1/5000	1/71	~1/35
1/10 000	1/100	~1/50
1/15 000	1/122	~1/60
1/20 000	1/141	~1/70
1/25 000	1/158	~1/80
1/30 000	1/173	~1/85
1/40 000	1/200	~1/100
1/50 000	1/224	~1/110
1/60 000	1/245	~1/125
1/70 000	1/265	~1/135
1/80 000	1/283	~1/140
1/90 000	1/300	~1/150
1/100 000	1/316	~1/160
1/150 000	1/387	~1/200
1/200 000	1/448	~1/225

Scriver CR, Beaudet AL, Sly WS, Valle D (eds). The Metabolic and molecular bases of inherited disease 8th edn McGraw-Hill, New York, 2001

Disease*	Carrier frequency in general population	Gene	Carrier testing for	
			Relatives at increased risk	Individuals at population risk
α1-antitrypsin deficiency	1/25 for Z and 1/17 for S alleles in northern European population	SERPINA1	α1-antitrypsin phenotyping on sample of clotted blood	α1-antitrypsin phenotyping on sample of clotted blood
Batten disease or juvenile neuronal lipofuscinosis (JNCL)	LB rate 0.46/10 000, i.e ~1/20000. Note genetic heterogeneity: LB rate for CLCN3 ~1/30 000 giving a carrier rate for CLCN3 of ~1/85	CLCN1 (21%), CLCN2 (7%), CLCN3 (72%)	Common 1 kb deletion of exon 7 and 8 in CLCN3	Common 1 kb deletion of exon 7 and 8 in CLCN3
Congenital adrenal hyperplasia (CAH)	1/50 for CYP21	CYP21	In classic CAH ~20–25% have a gene deletion and ~30% have an intron 2 splice-site mutation. The missense mutation V281L is the most common mutation in non-classic CAH	Possible for the common mutations
Congenital deafness: connexin 26 type	1/50 in European, North American, and Mediterranean populations	GJB2	Possible if mutations have been defined in the proband	Possible for common 35delG mutation
Cystic fibrosis (CF)	1/23 in Caucasians (see CF section in 'Common consultations' for other ethnic groups)	CFTR	Available by direct mutation analysis if mutation in proband is known	Possible using commercial multiplex mutation assay
Friedreich's ataxia	1/85	Frataxin	Analysis for triplet repeat (GAA)$_n$ expansion	Analysis for triplet repeat (GAA)$_n$ expansion
Galactosaemia	1/105	GALT1	Mutation analysis of GALT1	Screen for common Q188R mutation
Gaucher	1/25 in Ashkenazi population	GBA	Analysis of acid beta-glucosidase enzyme. Mutation analysis of GBA	4 common mutations of GBA in the Askenazi population
Haemochromatosis	1/10 in N. European populations (see 'Haemochromatosis' in 'Common consultations' for more details)	HFE	Mutation analysis for C282Y and H63D	Mutation analysis for C282Y and H63D
Hurler	1/60	IDUA	Mutation analysis of IDUA (2 common nonsense mutations, W402X and Q70X) Enzyme analysis of alpha-L-iduronidase	2 common nonsense mutations, W402X and Q70X
Krabbe	Very rare, more common in Druze and Sicilian populations	GALC	Mutation analysis of GALC Enzyme analysis of glycosylceramidase	
Metachromatic leukodystrophy	1 in 40 000 LB, 1/100	ARSA	Mutation analysis of ARSA Enzyme analysis of arylsulfatase A gene	
Phenylketonuria (PKU) 1/50		PAH	Mutation analysis of PAH Linkage analysis Enzyme analysis	Mutation analysis of PAH for common mutations
Sanfilippo [MPS III]	1/65,000 LB (all types)	SGSH (type A)	Mutation analysis of SGSH Enzyme analysis of heparan N-sulphatase	
		NAGLU (type B)	Mutation analysis of NAGLU Enzyme analysis of alpha-N-acetylglucosaminidase	
Spinal muscular atrophy (SMA)	1/50	SMN1	Mutation analysis for exon 7 deletion in SMN1	Mutation analysis for exon 7 deletion in SMN1
Tay–Sachs disease	1/30 in Ashkenazi Jewish populations	HEXA	Mutation analysis of HEXA Enzyme analysis of hexosaminidase A gene	Mutation analysis in Jewish population Enzyme analysis in non-Jewish population

* Please refer to the relevant sections of this book for a fuller account.

Centile charts for boys height, weight, and occipital-frontal circumference (OFC)

In the centile charts that follow, there is a normal distribution—approximately 68%, 95%, and 99.6% fall within the mean ±1, 2, and 3 standard deviations (SD), respectively.

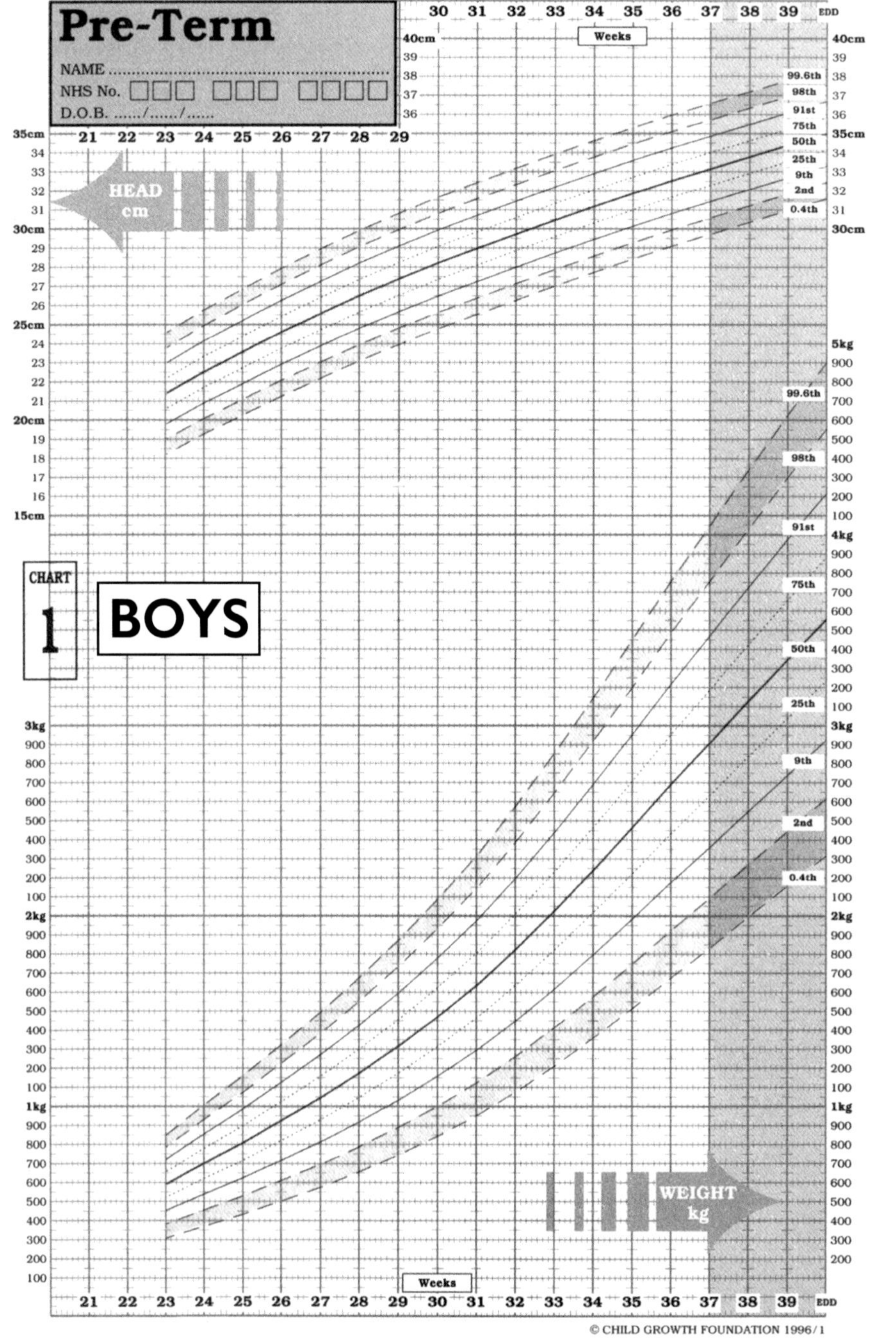

Boys: four-in-one growth charts. (1) Preterm; (2) 0–1 year; (3) 1–5 years; (4) 0–20 years. (© Child Growth Foundation 1996/2001.)

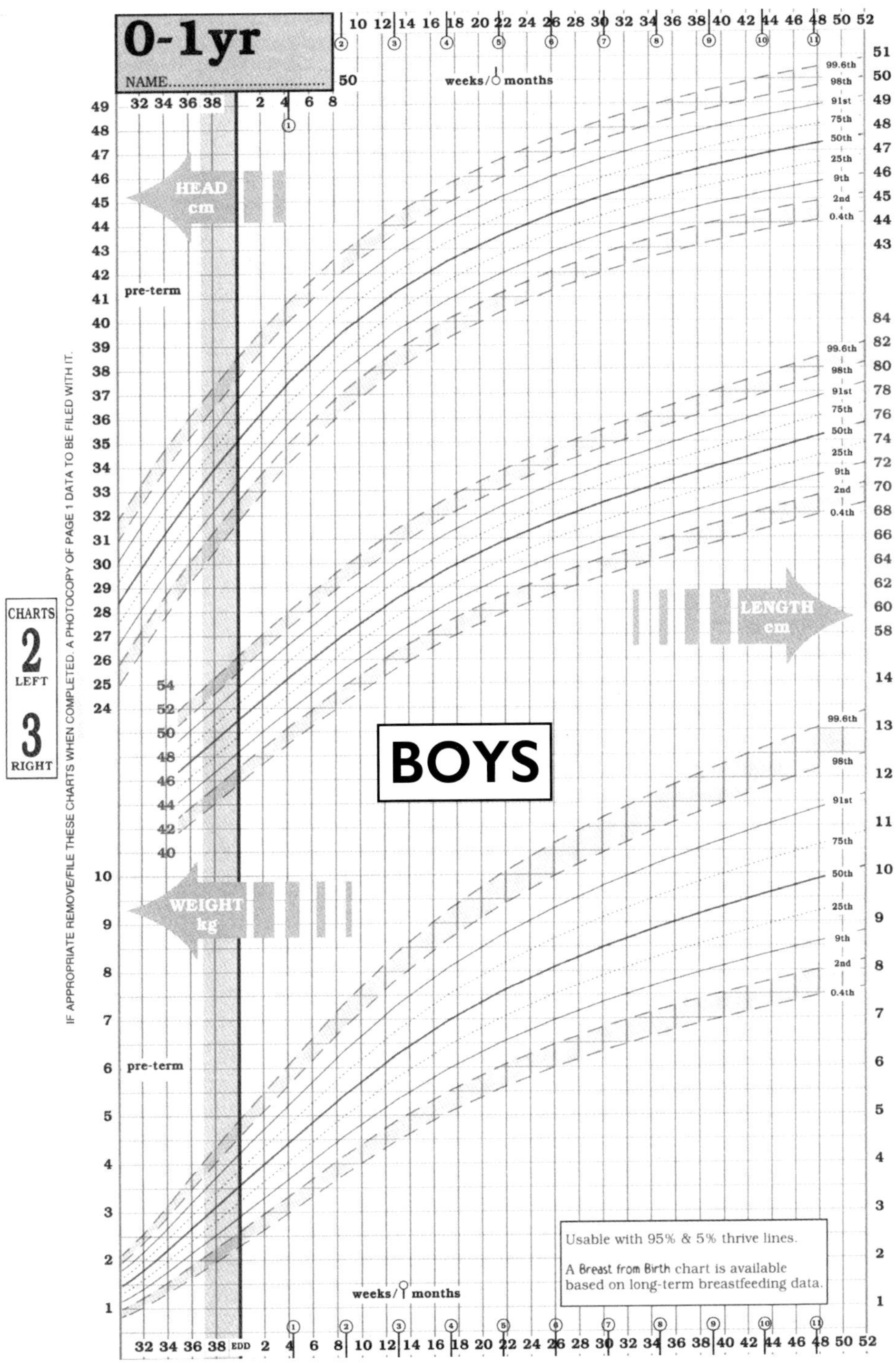

Boys: four-in-one growth charts (2) 0–1 year.

Figure *Continued.*

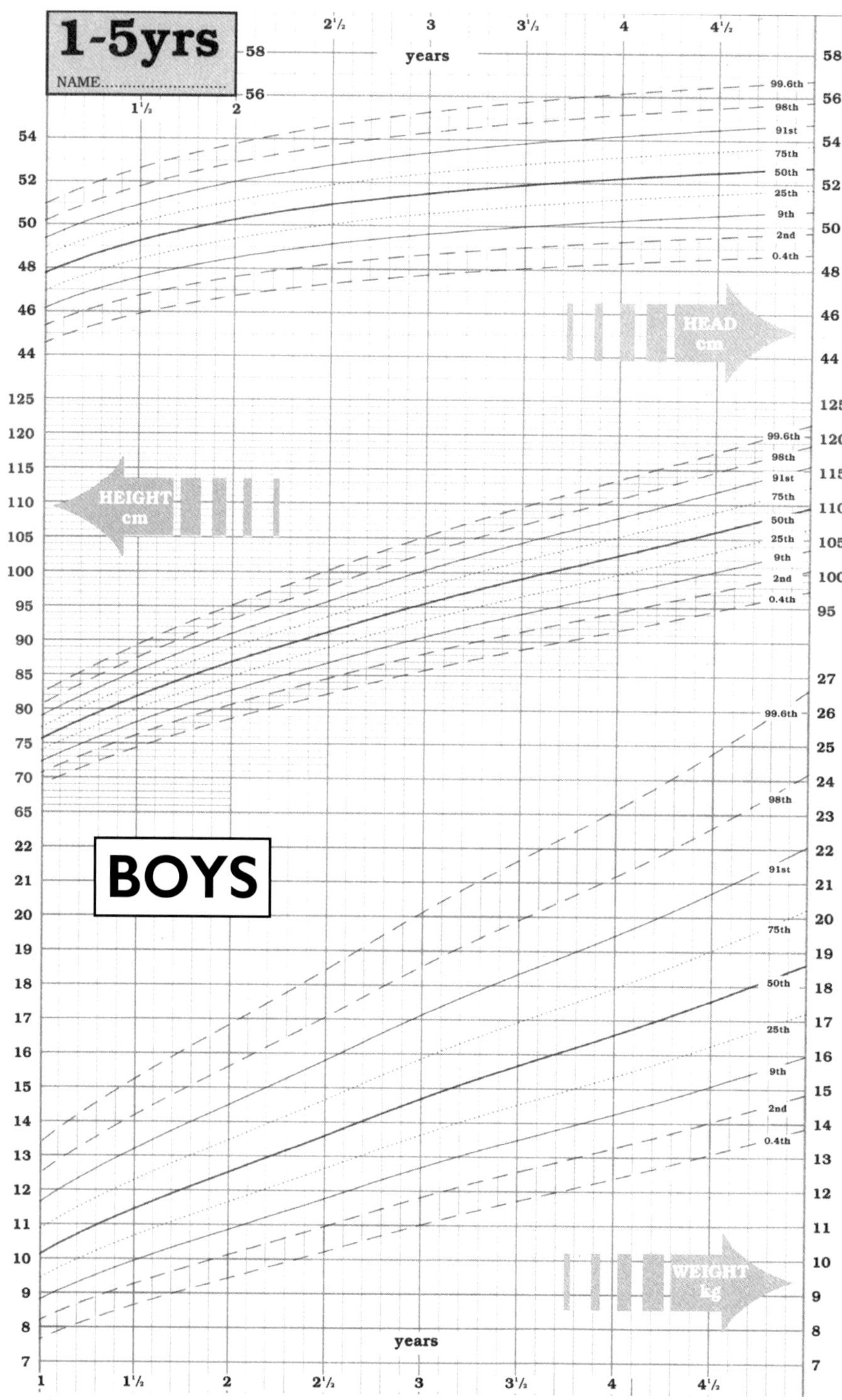

Boys: four-in-one growth charts (3) 1–5 year.

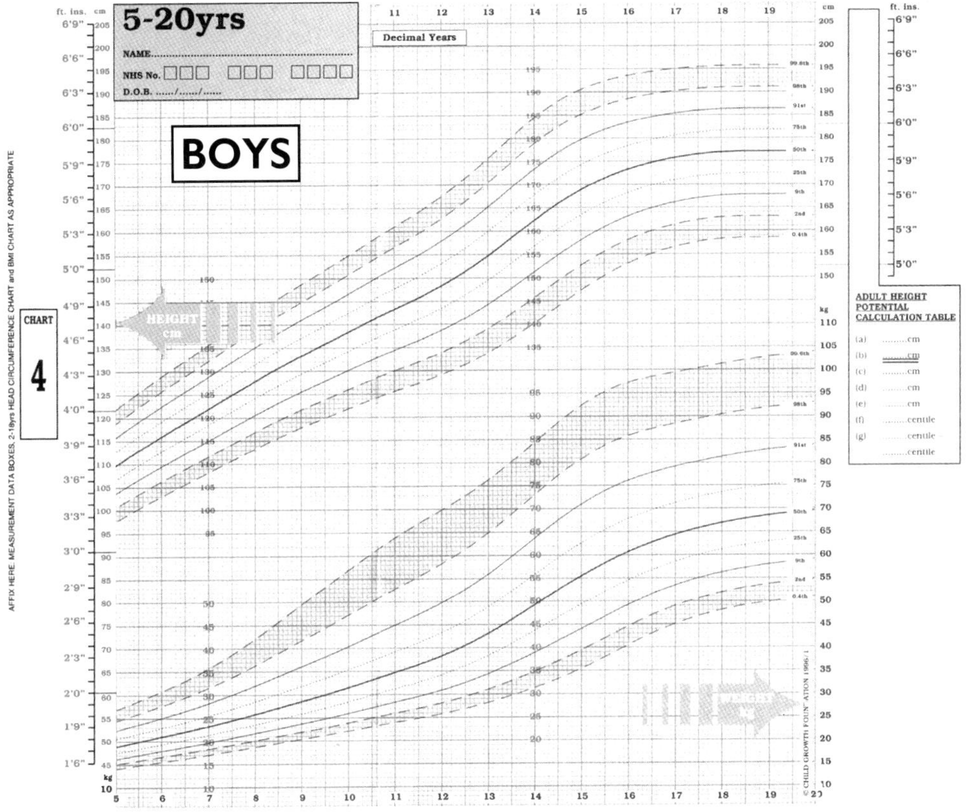

Figure *Continued.*

Centile charts for girls height, weight, and occipital-frontal circumference (OFC)

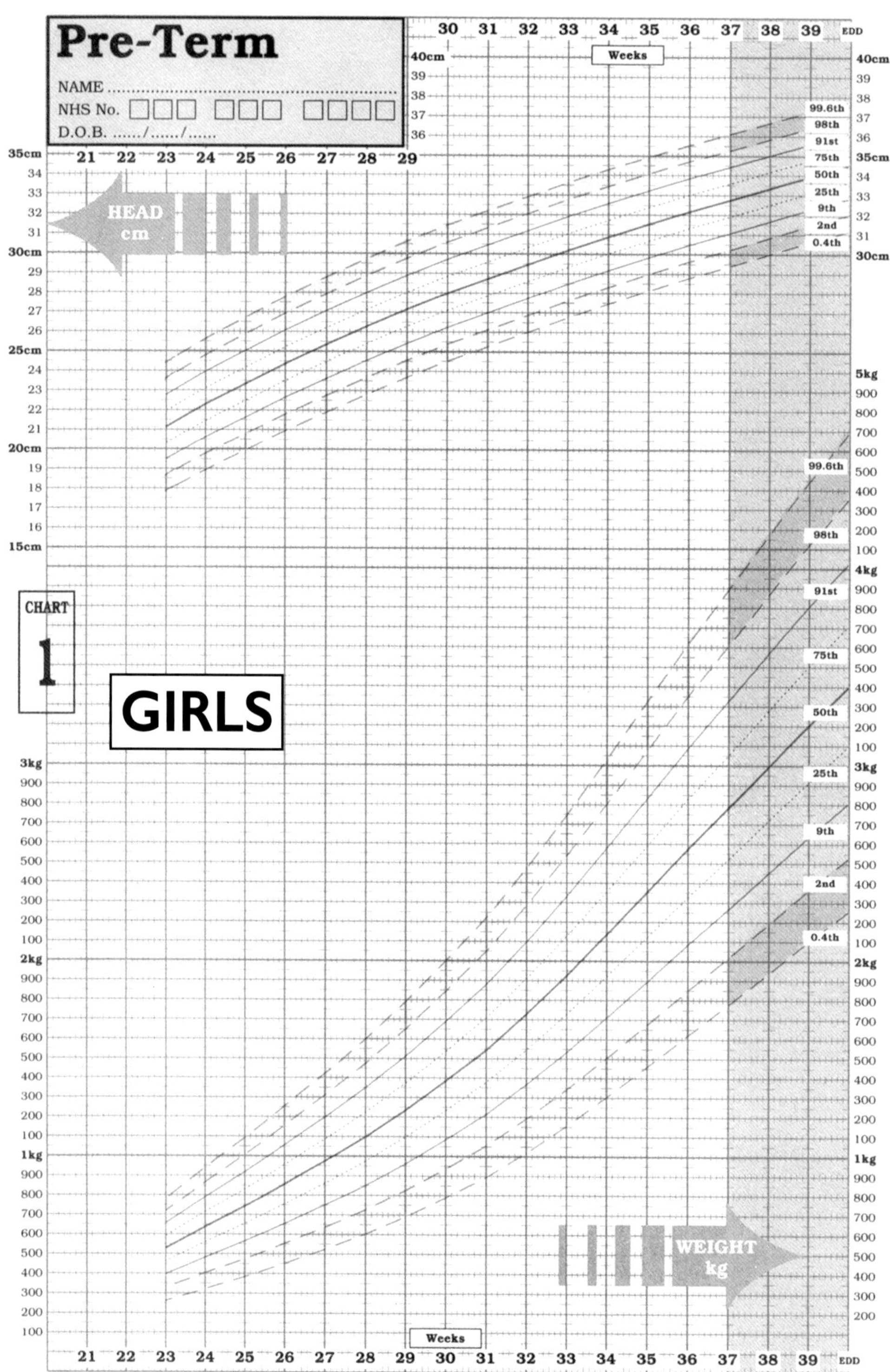

Girls: four-in-one growth charts. (1) Preterm; (2) 0–1 year; (3) 1–5 years; (4) 0–20 years. (© Child Growth Foundation 1996/2001.)

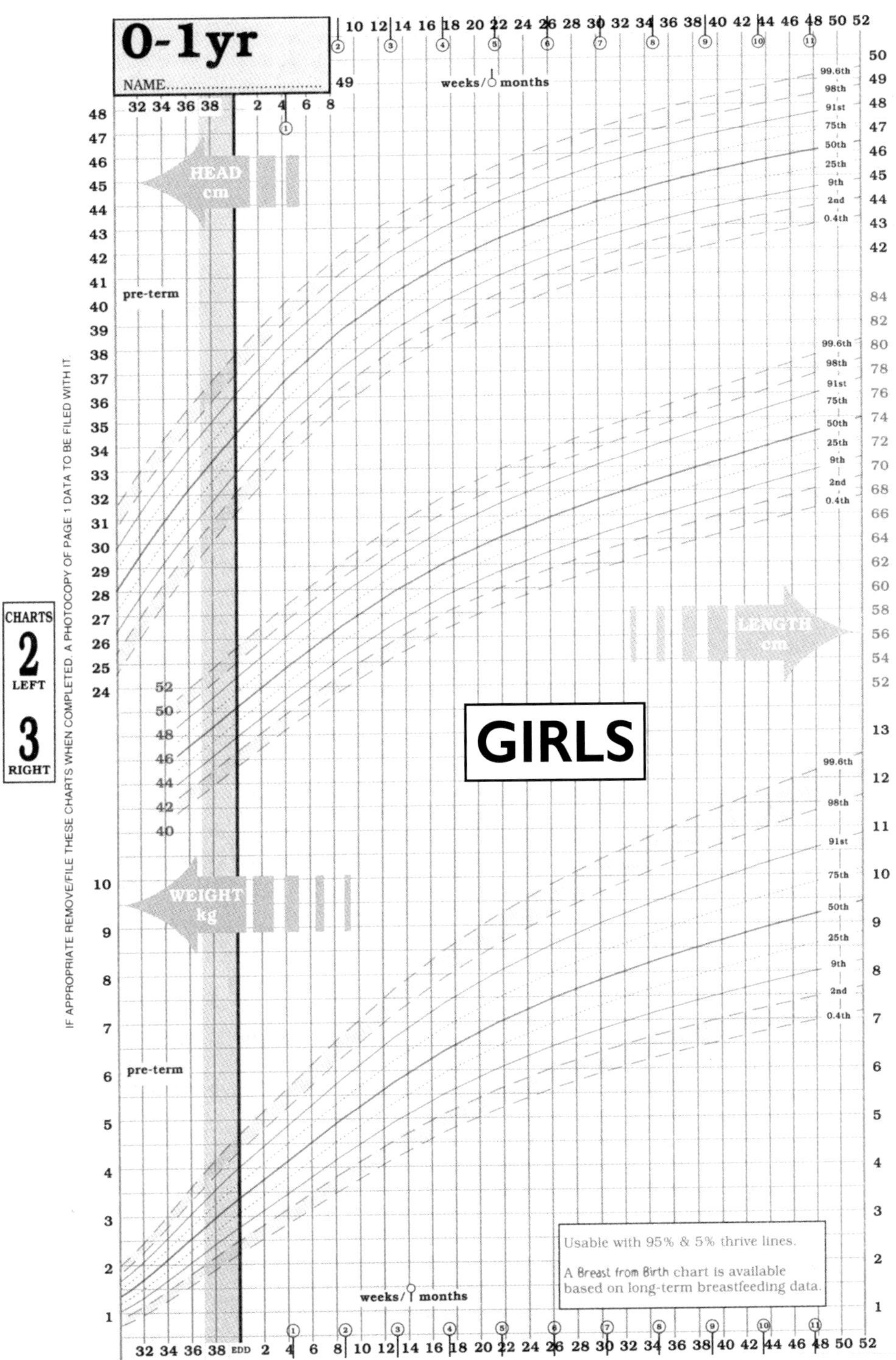

Girls: four-in-one growth charts (2) 0–1 year.

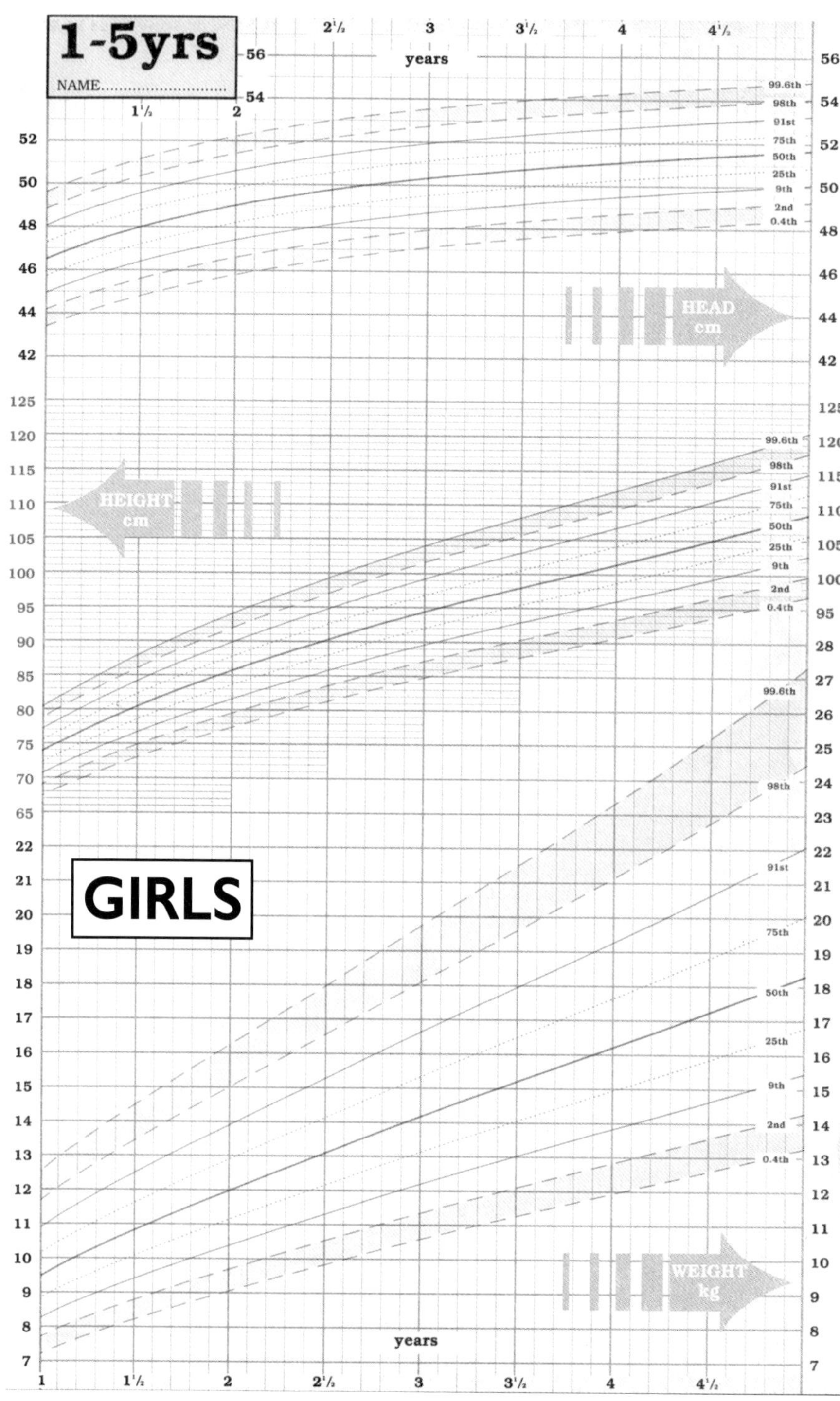

Girls: four-in-one growth charts (3) 1–5 year.

Figure *Continued*.

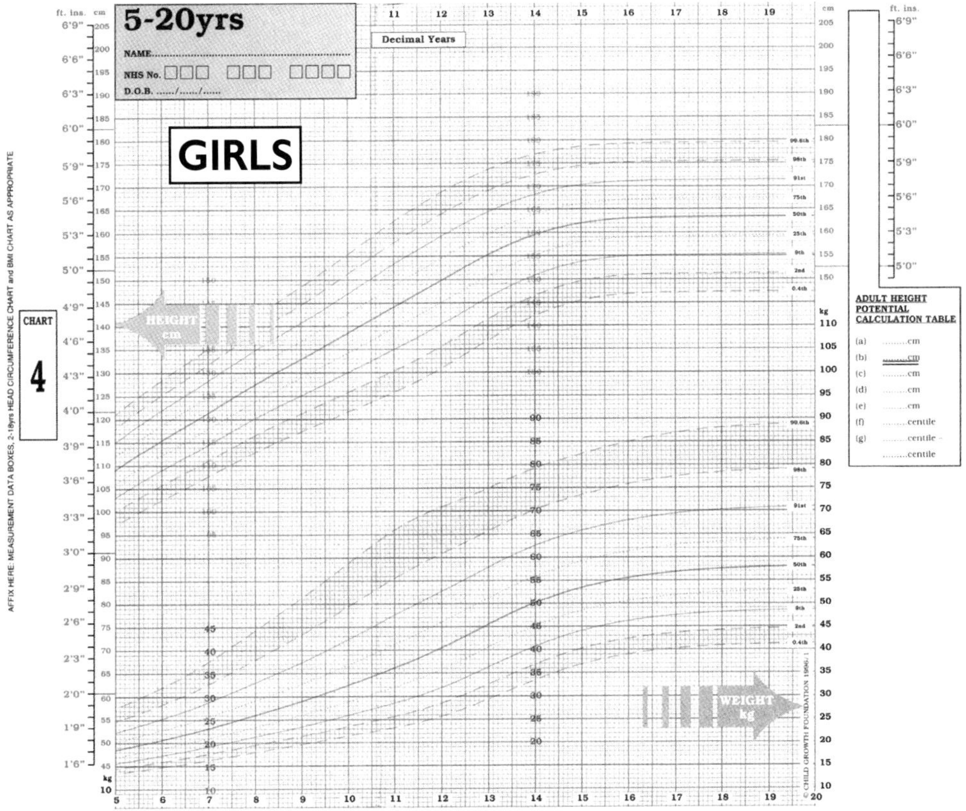

Figure *Continued.*

Centile charts for occipital-frontal circumference (OFC)

Boys: head circumference chart. Birth–18 years. (© Child Growth Foundation 1996/2001.)

• Please place a sticker (if available) otherwise write in space provided.

Surname

First names

NHS no: Local no:

G.P. Code

H.V. Code

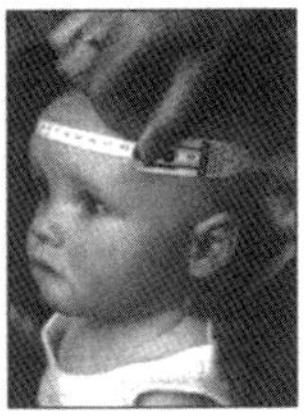

GIRLS

HEAD CIRCUMFERENCE

(BIRTH - 17 YEARS)

United Kingdom cross-sectional reference data : 1996/1

The principal chart [birth-1yr] for a girl's head circumference [OFC] is held in her Personal Child Health Record [PCHR]. The chart below is for the girl whose OFC needs to be monitored for a further year or beyond. Reconstruct her PCHR OFC curve in the extreme left section with her PCHR data. Plot from 1yr onwards in the normal way. NB The grid up to 2yrs is calibrated in months: from 2yrs onwards it is calibrated in years. Some girl's heads may still be growing after age 17 but reliable adult OFC data for the UK are not currently available. If required, record the mother's OFC and approximate centile [%] in the box below. Turn overleaf to find the father's approximate OFC %.

Technique

Measure the greatest circumference as illustrated with the tape touching the occipital prominence at the rear of the head and passing around the forehead as the midpoint between the eyebrows and the hairline. Measure to the nearest completed millimetre. The recommended **Lasso-o** tape is designed to measure both children and adults.

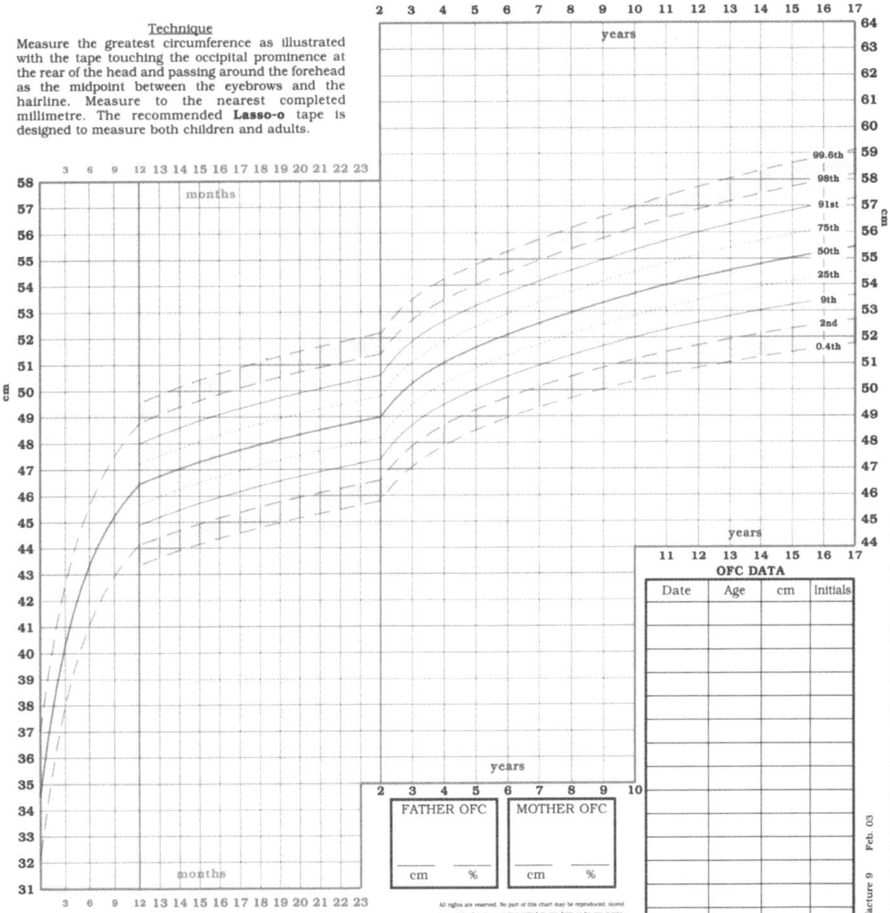

Cross-sectional stature and weight reference curves for the UK. 1990
(JV Freeman, TJ Cole, S Chinn, PRM Jones, EM White, MA Preece) *ARCH DIS CHILD* 1995: 73: 17-24

© CHILD GROWTH FOUNDATION 1996/1
(Charity Reg. No 274325)
2 Mayfield Avenue,
London W4 1PW

Printed and Supplied by
HARLOW PRINTING LIMITED
Maxwell Street ◊ South Shields
Tyne & Wear ◊ NE33 4PU

Girls: head circumference chart. Birth–17 years. (© Child Growth Foundation 1996/2001.)

CK (Creatine kinase) levels in carriers of Duchenne muscular dystrophy (DMD)

Currently, molecular genetic analysis enables detection of deletions and duplications of the dystrophin gene in ~65–70% of boys with DMD. If a dystrophin mutation is detected, this allows robust carrier detection in the families of boys (although the possibility of germline mosaicism in the mother of a sporadic case should always be remembered). In future, the ability to undertake sequencing of the dystrophin gene should enable the great majority of families to have robust carrier detection. Carrier detection by assessment of CK levels is *fallible and should only be used as a last resort* when molecular methodology has failed to identify a mutation in a boy with biopsy proven DMD.

Table of likelihood of carrier status for DMD based on serum creatine kinase (CK) level*

CK level (IU/l)*	Relative risk of being	
	Carrier	Not carrier
0–40	0.12	1
40–49	0.12	1
50–59	0.16	1
60–69	0.27	1
70–79	0.46	1
80–89	0.86	1
90–99	1.67	1
100–109	3.28	1
110–119	6.49	1
120–129	12.79	1
130–139	25.12	1
140–149	49.02	1
150–159	94.34	1
160–169	180.9	1
= 170	Carrier	

*** Important note. These data should be** *used in conjunction with analysis of the family tree* **to provide conditional information in a Bayesian calculation; they are not intended for 'stand alone' assessment of carrier status. Laboratory measurements of CK vary and these data were derived in a laboratory where an upper limit of normal (95%) for adult females was 100 IU/l. Consult with your laboratory and do not use these data if the upper limit of normal in your laboratory differs appreciably from this value. (It may be possible to adjust the value by proportion, e.g. if the upper limit of normal in your laboratory is 200 IU/l, then by dividing the CK level by 2, the table could then be used to obtain an approximation of the probability.)**

NB. Carriers of autosomal recessive (AR) limb girdle dystrophies may sometimes have a mildly elevated CK so, unless the diagnosis of DMD has been proven by molecular genetic analysis, it is important to ensure that the diagnosis in the proband is well founded and based on muscle biopsy.

Important points

- Women should refrain from intense exercise, e.g. running, aerobics for 48 hours before the sample is taken.
- CK levels should be expressed in IU/l.
- Take the average of 3 separate values—each sample taken on a different occasion and the sample should preferably be processed by the laboratory on the day of sampling. The repeat samples need to be taken some time apart, preferably at monthly intervals.
- CK levels are reduced during pregnancy. *Consistently elevated levels would be very suggestive of carrier status in an 'at risk' female*, but results within the normal range in pregnancy are probably uninterpretable.
- The proportion of carriers of BMD who show elevated levels of CK is lower than for DMD and so the same tables/graphs *cannot* be used for the two conditions.

References

Sibert JR, Harper PS, *et al.* Carrier detection in Duchenne muscular dystrophy. Evidence from a study of obligatory carriers and mothers of isolated cases. *Arch Dis Child* 1979; **54**: 534–7.

Conversion charts from English to metric units for height and weight

BSI CONVERSION CHART FOR HEIGHT AND WEIGHT

HEIGHT

ft in	m	ft in	m	ft in	m	ft in	m	ft in	m	ft in	m	ft in	m
0 0¼	0·006	1 0¼	0·311	2 0¼	0·616	3 0¼	0·921	4 0¼	1·226	5 0¼	1·530	6 0¼	1·835
0 0½	0·013	1 0½	0·318	2 0½	0·622	3 0½	0·927	4 0½	1·232	5 0½	1·537	6 0½	1·842
0 0¾	0·019	1 0¾	0·324	2 0¾	0·629	3 0¾	0·933	4 0¾	1·238	5 0¾	1·543	6 0¾	1·848
0 1	0·025	1 1	0·330	2 1	0·635	3 1	0·940	4 1	1·245	5 1	1·549	6 1	1·854
0 1¼	0·032	1 1¼	0·337	2 1¼	0·641	3 1¼	0·946	4 1¼	1·251	5 1¼	1·556	6 1¼	1·861
0 1½	0·038	1 1½	0·343	2 1½	0·648	3 1½	0·952	4 1½	1·257	5 1½	1·562	6 1½	1·867
0 1¾	0·044	1 1¾	0·349	2 1¾	0·654	3 1¾	0·959	4 1¾	1·264	5 1¾	1·568	6 1¾	1·873
0 2	0·051	1 2	0·356	2 2	0·660	3 2	0·965	4 2	1·270	5 2	1·575	6 2	1·880
0 2¼	0·057	1 2¼	0·362	2 2¼	0·667	3 2¼	0·972	4 2¼	1·276	5 2¼	1·581	6 2¼	1·886
0 2½	0·064	1 2½	0·368	2 2½	0·673	3 2½	0·978	4 2½	1·283	5 2½	1·588	6 2½	1·892
0 2¾	0·070	1 2¾	0·375	2 2¾	0·679	3 2¾	0·984	4 2¾	1·289	5 2¾	1·594	6 2¾	1·899
0 3	0·076	1 3	0·381	2 3	0·686	3 3	0·991	4 3	1·295	5 3	1·600	6 3	1·905
0 3¼	0·083	1 3¼	0·387	2 3¼	0·692	3 3¼	0·997	4 3¼	1·302	5 3¼	1·607	6 3¼	1·911
0 3½	0·089	1 3½	0·394	2 3½	0·698	3 3½	1·003	4 3½	1·308	5 3½	1·613	6 3½	1·918
0 3¾	0·095	1 3¾	0·400	2 3¾	0·705	3 3¾	1·010	4 3¾	1·314	5 3¾	1·619	6 3¾	1·924
0 4	0·102	1 4	0·406	2 4	0·711	3 4	1·016	4 4	1·321	5 4	1·626	6 4	1·930
0 4¼	0·108	1 4¼	0·413	2 4¼	0·718	3 4¼	1·022	4 4¼	1·327	5 4¼	1·632	6 4¼	1·937
0 4½	0·114	1 4½	0·419	2 4½	0·724	3 4½	1·029	4 4½	1·334	5 4½	1·638	6 4½	1·943
0 4¾	0·121	1 4¾	0·425	2 4¾	0·730	3 4¾	1·035	4 4¾	1·340	5 4¾	1·645	6 4¾	1·949
0 5	0·127	1 5	0·432	2 5	0·737	3 5	1·041	4 5	1·346	5 5	1·651	6 5	1·956
0 5¼	0·133	1 5¼	0·438	2 5¼	0·743	3 5¼	1·048	4 5¼	1·353	5 5¼	1·657	6 5¼	1·962
0 5½	0·140	1 5½	0·444	2 5½	0·749	3 5½	1·054	4 5½	1·359	5 5½	1·664	6 5½	1·968
0 5¾	0·146	1 5¾	0·451	2 5¾	0·756	3 5¾	1·060	4 5¾	1·365	5 5¾	1·670	6 5¾	1·975
0 6	0·152	1 6	0·457	2 6	0·762	3 6	1·067	4 6	1·372	5 6	1·676	6 6	1·981
0 6¼	0·159	1 6¼	0·464	2 6¼	0·768	3 6¼	1·073	4 6¼	1·378	5 6¼	1·683	6 6¼	1·988
0 6½	0·165	1 6½	0·470	2 6½	0·775	3 6½	1·080	4 6½	1·384	5 6½	1·689	6 6½	1·994
0 6¾	0·171	1 6¾	0·476	2 6¾	0·781	3 6¾	1·086	4 6¾	1·391	5 6¾	1·695	6 6¾	2·000
0 7	0·178	1 7	0·483	2 7	0·787	3 7	1·092	4 7	1·397	5 7	1·702	6 7	2·007
0 7¼	0·184	1 7¼	0·489	2 7¼	0·794	3 7¼	1·099	4 7¼	1·403	5 7¼	1·708	6 7¼	2·013
0 7½	0·190	1 7½	0·495	2 7½	0·800	3 7½	1·105	4 7½	1·410	5 7½	1·714	6 7½	2·019
0 7¾	0·197	1 7¾	0·502	2 7¾	0·806	3 7¾	1·111	4 7¾	1·416	5 7¾	1·721	6 7¾	2·026
0 8	0·203	1 8	0·508	2 8	0·813	3 8	1·118	4 8	1·422	5 8	1·727	6 8	2·032
0 8¼	0·210	1 8¼	0·514	2 8¼	0·819	3 8¼	1·124	4 8¼	1·429	5 8¼	1·734	6 8¼	2·038
0 8½	0·216	1 8½	0·521	2 8½	0·826	3 8½	1·130	4 8½	1·435	5 8½	1·740	6 8½	2·045
0 8¾	0·222	1 8¾	0·527	2 8¾	0·832	3 8¾	1·137	4 8¾	1·441	5 8¾	1·746	6 8¾	2·051
0 9	0·229	1 9	0·533	2 9	0·838	3 9	1·143	4 9	1·448	5 9	1·753	6 9	2·057
0 9¼	0·235	1 9¼	0·540	2 9¼	0·845	3 9¼	1·149	4 9¼	1·454	5 9¼	1·759	6 9¼	2·064
0 9½	0·241	1 9½	0·546	2 9½	0·851	3 9½	1·156	4 9½	1·460	5 9½	1·765	6 9½	2·070
0 9¾	0·248	1 9¾	0·552	2 9¾	0·857	3 9¾	1·162	4 9¾	1·467	5 9¾	1·772	6 9¾	2·076
0 10	0·254	1 10	0·559	2 10	0·864	3 10	1·168	4 10	1·473	5 10	1·778	6 10	2·083
0 10¼	0·260	1 10¼	0·565	2 10¼	0·870	3 10¼	1·175	4 10¼	1·480	5 10¼	1·784	6 10¼	2·089
0 10½	0·267	1 10½	0·572	2 10½	0·876	3 10½	1·181	4 10½	1·486	5 10½	1·791	6 10½	2·096
0 10¾	0·273	1 10¾	0·578	2 10¾	0·883	3 10¾	1·187	4 10¾	1·492	5 10¾	1·797	6 10¾	2·102
0 11	0·279	1 11	0·584	2 11	0·889	3 11	1·194	4 11	1·499	5 11	1·803	6 11	2·108
0 11¼	0·286	1 11¼	0·591	2 11¼	0·895	3 11¼	1·200	4 11¼	1·505	5 11¼	1·810	6 11¼	2·115
0 11½	0·292	1 11½	0·597	2 11½	0·902	3 11½	1·206	4 11½	1·511	5 11½	1·816	6 11½	2·121
0 11¾	0·298	1 11¾	0·603	2 11¾	0·908	3 11¾	1·213	4 11¾	1·518	5 11¾	1·822	6 11¾	2·127
1 0	0·305	2 0	0·610	3 0	0·914	4 0	1·219	5 0	1·524	6 0	1·829	7 0	2·134

Conversions are correct to the nearest millimetre

WEIGHT

st lb oz	kg	st lb oz	kg	st lb oz	kg	st lb oz	kg	st lb oz	kg
0 0 1	0·028	0 3 11	1·673	0 7 5	3·317	0 10 15	4·961	1 0 9	6·605
0 0 2	0·057	0 3 12	1·701	0 7 6	3·345	0 11 0	4·990	1 0 10	6·634
0 0 3	0·085	0 3 13	1·729	0 7 7	3·374	0 11 1	5·018	1 0 11	6·662
0 0 4	0·113	0 3 14	1·758	0 7 8	3·402	0 11 2	5·046	1 0 12	6·690
0 0 5	0·142	0 3 15	1·786	0 7 9	3·430	0 11 3	5·075	1 0 13	6·719
0 0 6	0·170	0 4 0	1·814	0 7 10	3·459	0 11 4	5·103	1 0 14	6·747
0 0 7	0·198	0 4 1	1·843	0 7 11	3·487	0 11 5	5·131	1 0 15	6·776
0 0 8	0·227	0 4 2	1·871	0 7 12	3·515	0 11 6	5·160	1 1 0	6·804
0 0 9	0·255	0 4 3	1·899	0 7 13	3·544	0 11 7	5·188	1 1 1	6·832
0 0 10	0·283	0 4 4	1·928	0 7 14	3·572	0 11 8	5·216	1 1 2	6·861
0 0 11	0·312	0 4 5	1·956	0 7 15	3·600	0 11 9	5·245	1 1 3	6·889
0 0 12	0·340	0 4 6	1·984	0 8 0	3·629	0 11 10	5·273	1 1 4	6·917
0 0 13	0·369	0 4 7	2·013	0 8 1	3·657	0 11 11	5·301	1 1 5	6·946
0 0 14	0·397	0 4 8	2·041	0 8 2	3·685	0 11 12	5·330	1 1 6	6·974
0 0 15	0·425	0 4 9	2·070	0 8 3	3·714	0 11 13	5·358	1 1 7	7·002
0 1 0	0·454	0 4 10	2·098	0 8 4	3·742	0 11 14	5·386	1 1 8	7·031
0 1 1	0·482	0 4 11	2·126	0 8 5	3·770	0 11 15	5·415	1 1 9	7·059
0 1 2	0·510	0 4 12	2·155	0 8 6	3·799	0 12 0	5·443	1 1 10	7·087
0 1 3	0·539	0 4 13	2·183	0 8 7	3·827	0 12 1	5·471	1 1 11	7·116
0 1 4	0·567	0 4 14	2·211	0 8 8	3·856	0 12 2	5·500	1 1 12	7·144
0 1 5	0·595	0 4 15	2·240	0 8 9	3·884	0 12 3	5·528	1 1 13	7·172
0 1 6	0·624	0 5 0	2·268	0 8 10	3·912	0 12 4	5·557	1 1 14	7·201
0 1 7	0·652	0 5 1	2·296	0 8 11	3·941	0 12 5	5·585	1 1 15	7·229
0 1 8	0·680	0 5 2	2·325	0 8 12	3·969	0 12 6	5·613	1 2 0	7·257
0 1 9	0·709	0 5 3	2·353	0 8 13	3·997	0 12 7	5·642	1 2 1	7·286
0 1 10	0·737	0 5 4	2·381	0 8 14	4·026	0 12 8	5·670	1 2 2	7·314
0 1 11	0·765	0 5 5	2·410	0 8 15	4·054	0 12 9	5·698	1 2 3	7·343
0 1 12	0·794	0 5 6	2·438	0 9 0	4·082	0 12 10	5·727	1 2 4	7·371
0 1 13	0·822	0 5 7	2·466	0 9 1	4·111	0 12 11	5·755	1 2 5	7·399
0 1 14	0·850	0 5 8	2·495	0 9 2	4·139	0 12 12	5·783	1 2 6	7·428
0 1 15	0·879	0 5 9	2·523	0 9 3	4·167	0 12 13	5·812	1 2 7	7·456
0 2 0	0·907	0 5 10	2·551	0 9 4	4·196	0 12 14	5·840	1 2 8	7·484
0 2 1	0·936	0 5 11	2·580	0 9 5	4·224	0 12 15	5·868	1 2 9	7·513
0 2 2	0·964	0 5 12	2·608	0 9 6	4·252	0 13 0	5·897	1 2 10	7·541
0 2 3	0·992	0 5 13	2·637	0 9 7	4·281	0 13 1	5·925	1 2 11	7·569
0 2 4	1·021	0 5 14	2·665	0 9 8	4·309	0 13 2	5·953	1 2 12	7·598
0 2 5	1·049	0 5 15	2·693	0 9 9	4·337	0 13 3	5·982	1 2 13	7·626
0 2 6	1·077	0 6 0	2·722	0 9 10	4·366	0 13 4	6·010	1 2 14	7·654
0 2 7	1·106	0 6 1	2·750	0 9 11	4·394	0 13 5	6·038	1 2 15	7·683
0 2 8	1·134	0 6 2	2·778	0 9 12	4·423	0 13 6	6·067	1 3 0	7·711
0 2 9	1·162	0 6 3	2·807	0 9 13	4·451	0 13 7	6·095	1 3 1	7·739
0 2 10	1·191	0 6 4	2·835	0 9 14	4·479	0 13 8	6·123	1 3 2	7·768
0 2 11	1·219	0 6 5	2·863	0 9 15	4·508	0 13 9	6·152	1 3 3	7·796
0 2 12	1·247	0 6 6	2·892	0 10 0	4·536	0 13 10	6·180	1 3 4	7·824
0 2 13	1·276	0 6 7	2·920	0 10 1	4·564	0 13 11	6·209	1 3 5	7·853
0 2 14	1·304	0 6 8	2·948	0 10 2	4·592	0 13 12	6·237	1 3 6	7·881
0 2 15	1·332	0 6 9	2·977	0 10 3	4·621	0 13 13	6·265	1 3 7	7·910
0 3 0	1·361	0 6 10	3·005	0 10 4	4·649	0 13 14	6·294	1 3 8	7·938
0 3 1	1·389	0 6 11	3·033	0 10 5	4·678	0 13 15	6·322	1 3 9	7·966
0 3 2	1·417	0 6 12	3·062	0 10 6	4·706	1 stone	6·350	1 3 10	7·995
0 3 3	1·446	0 6 13	3·090	0 10 7	4·734	1 0 1	6·379	1 3 11	8·023
0 3 4	1·474	0 6 14	3·118	0 10 8	4·763	1 0 2	6·407	1 3 12	8·051
0 3 5	1·503	0 6 15	3·147	0 10 9	4·791	1 0 3	6·435	1 3 13	8·080
0 3 6	1·531	0 7 0	3·175	0 10 10	4·819	1 0 4	6·464	1 3 14	8·108
0 3 7	1·559	0 7 1	3·203	0 10 11	4·848	1 0 5	6·492	1 3 15	8·136
0 3 8	1·588	0 7 2	3·232	0 10 12	4·876	1 0 6	6·520	1 4 0	8·165
0 3 9	1·616	0 7 3	3·260	0 10 13	4·904	1 0 7	6·549	1 4 1	8·193
0 3 10	1·644	0 7 4	3·289	0 10 14	4·932	1 0 8	6·577	1 4 2	8·221

st lb oz	kg	st lb oz	kg	st lb oz	kg	st lb oz	kg	st lb oz	kg
1 4 3	8·250	1 7 13	9·894	1 11 7	11·538	2 1 1	13·183	2 4 11	14·827
1 4 4	8·278	1 7 14	9·922	1 11 8	11·567	2 1 2	13·211	2 4 12	14·855
1 4 5	8·306	1 7 15	9·951	1 11 9	11·595	2 1 3	13·239	2 4 13	14·883
1 4 6	8·335	1 8 0	9·979	1 11 10	11·623	2 1 4	13·268	2 4 14	14·912
1 4 7	8·363	1 8 1	10·007	1 11 11	11·652	2 1 5	13·296	2 4 15	14·940
1 4 8	8·391	1 8 2	10·036	1 11 12	11·680	2 1 6	13·324	2 5 0	14·968
1 4 9	8·420	1 8 3	10·064	1 11 13	11·708	2 1 7	13·353	2 5 1	14·997
1 4 10	8·448	1 8 4	10·092	1 11 14	11·737	2 1 8	13·381	2 5 2	15·025
1 4 11	8·477	1 8 5	10·121	1 11 15	11·765	2 1 9	13·409	2 5 3	15·054
1 4 12	8·505	1 8 6	10·149	1 12 0	11·793	2 1 10	13·438	2 5 4	15·082
1 4 13	8·533	1 8 7	10·177	1 12 1	11·822	2 1 11	13·466	2 5 5	15·110
1 4 14	8·562	1 8 8	10·206	1 12 2	11·850	2 1 12	13·494	2 5 6	15·139
1 4 15	8·590	1 8 9	10·234	1 12 3	11·878	2 1 13	13·523	2 5 7	15·167
1 5 0	8·618	1 8 10	10·263	1 12 4	11·907	2 1 14	13·551	2 5 8	15·195
1 5 1	8·647	1 8 11	10·291	1 12 5	11·935	2 1 15	13·579	2 5 9	15·224
1 5 2	8·675	1 8 12	10·319	1 12 6	11·963	2 2 0	13·608	2 5 10	15·252
1 5 3	8·703	1 8 13	10·348	1 12 7	11·992	2 2 1	13·636	2 5 11	15·280
1 5 4	8·732	1 8 14	10·376	1 12 8	12·020	2 2 2	13·664	2 5 12	15·309
1 5 5	8·760	1 8 15	10·404	1 12 9	12·049	2 2 3	13·693	2 5 13	15·337
1 5 6	8·788	1 9 0	10·433	1 12 10	12·077	2 2 4	13·721	2 5 14	15·365
1 5 7	8·817	1 9 1	10·461	1 12 11	12·105	2 2 5	13·750	2 5 15	15·394
1 5 8	8·845	1 9 2	10·489	1 12 12	12·134	2 2 6	13·778	2 6 0	15·422
1 5 9	8·873	1 9 3	10·518	1 12 13	12·162	2 2 7	13·806	2 6 1	15·450
1 5 10	8·902	1 9 4	10·546	1 12 14	12·190	2 2 8	13·835	2 6 2	15·479
1 5 11	8·930	1 9 5	10·574	1 12 15	12·219	2 2 9	13·863	2 6 3	15·507
1 5 12	8·958	1 9 6	10·603	1 13 0	12·247	2 2 10	13·891	2 6 4	15·536
1 5 13	8·987	1 9 7	10·631	1 13 1	12·275	2 2 11	13·920	2 6 5	15·564
1 5 14	9·015	1 9 8	10·659	1 13 2	12·304	2 2 12	13·948	2 6 6	15·592
1 5 15	9·043	1 9 9	10·688	1 13 3	12·332	2 2 13	13·976	2 6 7	15·621
1 6 0	9·072	1 9 10	10·716	1 13 4	12·360	2 2 14	14·005	2 6 8	15·649
1 6 1	9·100	1 9 11	10·744	1 13 5	12·389	2 2 15	14·033	2 6 9	15·677
1 6 2	9·129	1 9 12	10·773	1 13 6	12·417	2 3 0	14·061	2 6 10	15·706
1 6 3	9·157	1 9 13	10·801	1 13 7	12·445	2 3 1	14·090	2 6 11	15·734
1 6 4	9·185	1 9 14	10·830	1 13 8	12·474	2 3 2	14·118	2 6 12	15·762
1 6 5	9·214	1 9 15	10·858	1 13 9	12·502	2 3 3	14·146	2 6 13	15·791
1 6 6	9·242	1 10 0	10·886	1 13 10	12·530	2 3 4	14·175	2 6 14	15·819
1 6 7	9·270	1 10 1	10·915	1 13 11	12·559	2 3 5	14·203	2 6 15	15·847
1 6 8	9·299	1 10 2	10·943	1 13 12	12·587	2 3 6	14·231	2 7 0	15·876
1 6 9	9·327	1 10 3	10·971	1 13 13	12·616	2 3 7	14·260	2 7 1	15·904
1 6 10	9·355	1 10 4	11·000	1 13 14	12·644	2 3 8	14·288	2 7 2	15·932
1 6 11	9·384	1 10 5	11·028	1 13 15	12·672	2 3 9	14·316	2 7 3	15·961
1 6 12	9·412	1 10 6	11·056	2 stone	12·701	2 3 10	14·345	2 7 4	15·989
1 6 13	9·440	1 10 7	11·085	2 0 1	12·729	2 3 11	14·373	2 7 5	16·017
1 6 14	9·469	1 10 8	11·113	2 0 2	12·757	2 3 12	14·402	2 7 6	16·046
1 6 15	9·497	1 10 9	11·141	2 0 3	12·786	2 3 13	14·430	2 7 7	16·074
1 7 0	9·525	1 10 10	11·170	2 0 4	12·814	2 3 14	14·458	2 7 8	16·103
1 7 1	9·554	1 10 11	11·198	2 0 5	12·842	2 3 15	14·487	2 7 9	16·131
1 7 2	9·582	1 10 12	11·226	2 0 6	12·871	2 4 0	14·515	2 7 10	16·159
1 7 3	9·610	1 10 13	11·255	2 0 7	12·899	2 4 1	14·543	2 7 11	16·188
1 7 4	9·639	1 10 14	11·283	2 0 8	12·927	2 4 2	14·572	2 7 12	16·216
1 7 5	9·667	1 10 15	11·311	2 0 9	12·956	2 4 3	14·600	2 7 13	16·244
1 7 6	9·696	1 11 0	11·340	2 0 10	12·984	2 4 4	14·628	2 7 14	16·273
1 7 7	9·724	1 11 1	11·368	2 0 11	13·012	2 4 5	14·657	2 7 15	16·301
1 7 8	9·752	1 11 2	11·396	2 0 12	13·041	2 4 6	14·685	2 8 0	16·329
1 7 9	9·781	1 11 3	11·425	2 0 13	13·069	2 4 7	14·713	2 8 1	16·358
1 7 10	9·809	1 11 4	11·453	2 0 14	13·097	2 4 8	14·742	2 8 2	16·386
1 7 11	9·837	1 11 5	11·482	2 0 15	13·126	2 4 9	14·770	2 8 3	16·414
1 7 12	9·866	1 11 6	11·510	2 1 0	13·154	2 4 10	14·798	2 8 4	16·443

WEIGHT

st lb oz	kg
2 8 5	16·471
2 8 6	16·499
2 8 7	16·528
2 8 8	16·556
2 8 9	16·584
2 8 10	16·613
2 8 11	16·641
2 8 12	16·670
2 8 13	16·698
2 8 14	16·726
2 8 15	16·755
2 9 0	16·783
2 9 1	16·811
2 9 2	16·840
2 9 3	16·868
2 9 4	16·896
2 9 5	16·925
2 9 6	16·953
2 9 7	16·981
2 9 8	17·010
2 9 9	17·038
2 9 10	17·066
2 9 11	17·095
2 9 12	17·123
2 9 13	17·151
2 9 14	17·180
2 9 15	17·208
2 10 0	17·236
2 10 1	17·265
2 10 2	17·293
2 10 3	17·322
2 10 4	17·350
2 10 5	17·378
2 10 6	17·407
2 10 7	17·435
2 10 8	17·463
2 10 9	17·492
2 10 10	17·520
2 10 11	17·548
2 10 12	17·577
2 10 13	17·605
2 10 14	17·633
2 10 15	17·662
2 11 0	17·690
2 11 1	17·718
2 11 2	17·747
2 11 3	17·775
2 11 4	17·803
2 11 5	17·832
2 11 6	17·860
2 11 7	17·889
2 11 8	17·917
2 11 9	17·945
2 11 10	17·974
2 11 11	18·002
2 11 12	18·030
2 11 13	18·059
2 11 14	18·087
2 11 15	18·115
2 12 0	18·144
2 12 1	18·172
2 12 2	18·200
2 12 3	18·229
2 12 4	18·257
2 12 5	18·285
2 12 6	18·314
2 12 7	18·342
2 12 8	18·370
2 12 9	18·399
2 12 10	18·427
2 12 11	18·456
2 12 12	18·484
2 12 13	18·512
2 12 14	18·541
2 12 15	18·569
2 13 0	18·597
2 13 1	18·626
2 13 2	18·654
2 13 3	18·682
2 13 4	18·711
2 13 5	18·739
2 13 6	18·768
2 13 7	18·796
2 13 8	18·824
2 13 9	18·853
2 13 10	18·881
2 13 11	18·910
2 13 12	18·937
2 13 13	18·966
2 13 14	18·994
2 13 15	19·023
3 stone	19·051
3 0 1	19·079
3 0 2	19·108
3 0 3	19·136
3 0 4	19·164
3 0 5	19·193
3 0 6	19·221
3 0 7	19·249
3 0 8	19·278
3 0 9	19·306
3 0 10	19·334
3 0 11	19·363
3 0 12	19·391
3 0 13	19·419
3 0 14	19·448
3 0 15	19·476
3 1 0	19·504
3 1 1	19·533
3 1 2	19·561
3 1 3	19·590
3 1 4	19·618
3 1 5	19·646
3 1 6	19·675
3 1 7	19·703
3 1 8	19·731
3 1 9	19·760

st lb oz	kg
3 1 10	19·788
3 1 11	19·816
3 1 12	19·845
3 1 13	19·873
3 1 14	19·901
3 1 15	19·930
3 2 0	19·958
3 2 1	19·986
3 2 2	20·015
3 2 3	20·043
3 2 4	20·071
3 2 5	20·100
3 2 6	20·128
3 2 7	20·156
3 2 8	20·185
3 2 9	20·213
3 2 10	20·242
3 2 11	20·270
3 2 12	20·298
3 2 13	20·327
3 2 14	20·355
3 2 15	20·383
3 3 0	20·412
3 3 1	20·440
3 3 2	20·468
3 3 3	20·497
3 3 4	20·525
3 3 5	20·553
3 3 6	20·582
3 3 7	20·610
3 3 8	20·638
3 3 9	20·667
3 3 10	20·695
3 3 11	20·723
3 3 12	20·752
3 3 13	20·780
3 3 14	20·809
3 3 15	20·837
3 4 0	20·865
3 4 1	20·894
3 4 2	20·922
3 4 3	20·950
3 4 4	20·979
3 4 5	21·007
3 4 6	21·035
3 4 7	21·064
3 4 8	21·092
3 4 9	21·120
3 4 10	21·149
3 4 11	21·177
3 4 12	21·205
3 4 13	21·234
3 4 14	21·262
3 4 15	21·290
3 5 0	21·319
3 5 1	21·347
3 5 2	21·376
3 5 3	21·404
3 5 4	21·432
3 5 5	21·461
3 5 6	21·489
3 5 7	21·517
3 5 8	21·546
3 5 9	21·574
3 5 10	21·602
3 5 11	21·631
3 5 12	21·659
3 5 13	21·687
3 5 14	21·716
3 5 15	21·744
3 6 0	21·772
3 6 1	21·801
3 6 2	21·829
3 6 3	21·857
3 6 4	21·886
3 6 5	21·914
3 6 6	21·943
3 6 7	21·971
3 6 8	21·999
3 6 9	22·028
3 6 10	22·056
3 6 11	22·084
3 6 12	22·113
3 6 13	22·141
3 6 14	22·169
3 6 15	22·198
3 7 0	22·226
3 7 1	22·254
3 7 2	22·283
3 7 3	22·311
3 7 4	22·339
3 7 5	22·368
3 7 6	22·396
3 7 7	22·424
3 7 8	22·453
3 7 9	22·481
3 7 10	22·510
3 7 11	22·538
3 7 12	22·566
3 7 13	22·595
3 7 14	22·623
3 7 15	22·651
3 8 0	22·680
3 8 1	22·708
3 8 2	22·736
3 8 3	22·765
3 8 4	22·793
3 8 5	22·821
3 8 6	22·850
3 8 7	22·878
3 8 8	22·906
3 8 9	22·935
3 8 10	22·963
3 8 11	22·991
3 8 12	23·020
3 8 13	23·048
3 8 14	23·076

st lb oz	kg
3 8 15	23·105
3 9 0	23·133
3 9 1	23·162
3 9 2	23·190
3 9 3	23·218
3 9 4	23·247
3 9 5	23·275
3 9 6	23·303
3 9 7	23·332
3 9 8	23·360
3 9 9	23·388
3 9 10	23·417
3 9 11	23·445
3 9 12	23·473
3 9 13	23·502
3 9 14	23·530
3 9 15	23·558
3 10 0	23·587
3 10 1	23·615
3 10 2	23·643
3 10 3	23·672
3 10 4	23·700
3 10 5	23·729
3 10 6	23·757
3 10 7	23·785
3 10 8	23·814
3 10 9	23·842
3 10 10	23·870
3 10 11	23·899
3 10 12	23·927
3 10 13	23·955
3 10 14	23·984
3 10 15	24·012
3 11 0	24·040
3 11 1	24·069
3 11 2	24·097
3 11 3	24·125
3 11 4	24·154
3 11 5	24·182
3 11 6	24·210
3 11 7	24·239
3 11 8	24·267
3 11 9	24·296
3 11 10	24·324
3 11 11	24·352
3 11 12	24·381
3 11 13	24·409
3 11 14	24·437
3 11 15	24·466
3 12 0	24·494
3 12 1	24·522
3 12 2	24·551
3 12 3	24·579
3 12 4	24·607
3 12 5	24·636
3 12 6	24·664
3 12 7	24·692
3 12 8	24·721
3 12 9	24·749
3 12 10	24·777
3 12 11	24·806
3 12 12	24·834
3 12 13	24·863
3 12 14	24·891
3 12 15	24·919
3 13 0	24·948
3 13 1	24·976
3 13 2	25·004
3 13 3	25·033
3 13 4	25·061
3 13 5	25·089
3 13 6	25·118
3 13 7	25·146
3 13 8	25·174
3 13 9	25·203
3 13 10	25·231
3 13 11	25·259
3 13 12	25·288
3 13 13	25·316
3 13 14	25·344
3 13 15	25·373
4 stone	25·401
4 0 1	25·430
4 0 2	25·458
4 0 3	25·486
4 0 4	25·515
4 0 5	25·543
4 0 6	25·571
4 0 7	25·600
4 0 8	25·628
4 0 9	25·656
4 0 10	25·685
4 0 11	25·713
4 0 12	25·741
4 0 13	25·770
4 0 14	25·798
4 0 15	25·826
4 1 0	25·855
4 1 1	25·883
4 1 2	25·911
4 1 3	25·940
4 1 4	25·968
4 1 5	25·996
4 1 6	26·025
4 1 7	26·053
4 1 8	26·082
4 1 9	26·110
4 1 10	26·138
4 1 11	26·167
4 1 12	26·195
4 1 13	26·223
4 1 14	26·252
4 1 15	26·280
4 2 0	26·308
4 2 1	26·337
4 2 2	26·365
4 2 3	26·393

st lb oz	kg
4 2 4	26·422
4 2 5	26·450
4 2 6	26·478
4 2 7	26·507
4 2 8	26·535
4 2 9	26·563
4 2 10	26·592
4 2 11	26·620
4 2 12	26·649
4 2 13	26·677
4 2 14	26·705
4 2 15	26·734
4 3 0	26·762
4 3 1	26·790
4 3 2	26·819
4 3 3	26·847
4 3 4	26·875
4 3 5	26·904
4 3 6	26·932
4 3 7	26·960
4 3 8	26·989
4 3 9	27·017
4 3 10	27·045
4 3 11	27·074
4 3 12	27·102
4 3 13	27·130
4 3 14	27·159
4 3 15	27·187
4 4 0	27·216
4 4 1	27·244
4 4 2	27·272
4 4 3	27·301
4 4 4	27·329
4 4 5	27·357
4 4 6	27·386
4 4 7	27·414
4 4 8	27·442
4 4 9	27·471
4 4 10	27·499
4 4 11	27·527
4 4 12	27·556
4 4 13	27·584
4 4 14	27·612
4 4 15	27·641
4 5 0	27·669
4 5 1	27·697
4 5 2	27·726
4 5 3	27·754
4 5 4	27·782
4 5 5	27·811
4 5 6	27·839
4 5 7	27·868
4 5 8	27·896
4 5 9	27·924
4 5 10	27·953
4 5 11	27·981
4 5 12	28·009
4 5 13	28·038
4 5 14	28·066
4 5 15	28·094
4 6 0	28·123
4 6 1	28·151
4 6 2	28·179
4 6 3	28·208
4 6 4	28·236
4 6 5	28·264
4 6 6	28·293
4 6 7	28·321
4 6 8	28·350
4 6 9	28·378
4 6 10	28·406
4 6 11	28·435
4 6 12	28·463
4 6 13	28·491
4 6 14	28·520
4 6 15	28·548
4 7 0	28·576
4 7 1	28·605
4 7 2	28·633
4 7 3	28·661
4 7 4	28·690
4 7 5	28·718
4 7 6	28·746
4 7 7	28·775
4 7 8	28·803
4 7 9	28·831
4 7 10	28·860
4 7 11	28·888
4 7 12	28·916
4 7 13	28·945
4 7 14	28·973
4 7 15	29·002
4 8 0	29·030
4 8 1	29·058
4 8 2	29·087
4 8 3	29·115
4 8 4	29·143
4 8 5	29·172
4 8 6	29·200
4 8 7	29·228
4 8 8	29·257
4 8 9	29·285
4 8 10	29·313
4 8 11	29·342
4 8 12	29·370
4 8 13	29·398
4 8 14	29·427
4 8 15	29·455
4 9 0	29·484
4 9 1	29·512
4 9 2	29·540
4 9 3	29·569
4 9 4	29·597
4 9 5	29·625
4 9 6	29·654
4 9 7	29·682
4 9 8	29·710

st lb oz	kg
4 9 9	29·739
4 9 10	29·767
4 9 11	29·795
4 9 12	29·824
4 9 13	29·852
4 9 14	29·880
4 9 15	29·909
4 10 0	29·937
4 10 1	29·965
4 10 2	29·994
4 10 3	30·022
4 10 4	30·050
4 10 5	30·079
4 10 6	30·107
4 10 7	30·136
4 10 8	30·164
4 10 9	30·192
4 10 10	30·221
4 10 11	30·249
4 10 12	30·277
4 10 13	30·306
4 10 14	30·334
4 10 15	30·362
4 11 0	30·391
4 11 1	30·419
4 11 2	30·447
4 11 3	30·476
4 11 4	30·504
4 11 5	30·532
4 11 6	30·561
4 11 7	30·589
4 11 8	30·617
4 11 9	30·646
4 11 10	30·674
4 11 11	30·703
4 11 12	30·731
4 11 13	30·759
4 11 14	30·788
4 11 15	30·816
4 12 0	30·844
4 12 1	30·873
4 12 2	30·901
4 12 3	30·929
4 12 4	30·958
4 12 5	30·986
4 12 6	31·014
4 12 7	31·043
4 12 8	31·071
4 12 9	31·099
4 12 10	31·128
4 12 11	31·156
4 12 12	31·184
4 12 13	31·213
4 12 14	31·241
4 12 15	31·269
4 13 0	31·298
4 13 1	31·326
4 13 2	31·355
4 13 3	31·383
4 13 4	31·411
4 13 5	31·440
4 13 6	31·468
4 13 7	31·496
4 13 8	31·525
4 13 9	31·553
4 13 10	31·581
4 13 11	31·610
4 13 12	31·638
4 13 13	31·666
4 13 14	31·695
4 13 15	31·723
5 stone	31·752
5 0 1	31·780
5 0 2	31·808
5 0 3	31·836
5 0 4	31·865
5 0 5	31·893
5 0 6	31·922
5 0 7	31·950
5 0 8	31·978
5 0 9	32·007
5 0 10	32·035
5 0 11	32·063
5 0 12	32·092
5 0 13	32·120
5 0 14	32·148
5 0 15	32·177
5 1 0	32·205
5 1 1	32·233
5 1 2	32·262
5 1 3	32·290
5 1 4	32·318
5 1 5	32·347
5 1 6	32·375
5 1 7	32·403
5 1 8	32·432
5 1 9	32·460
5 1 10	32·489
5 1 11	32·517
5 1 12	32·545
5 1 13	32·574
5 1 14	32·602
5 1 15	32·630
5 2 0	32·659
5 2 1	32·687
5 2 2	32·716
5 2 3	32·744
5 2 4	32·772
5 2 5	32·800
5 2 6	32·829
5 2 7	32·857
5 2 8	32·886
5 2 9	32·914
5 2 10	32·942
5 2 11	32·971
5 2 12	32·999
5 2 13	33·027

st lb oz	kg
5 2 14	33·056
5 2 15	33·084
5 3 0	33·112
5 3 1	33·141
5 3 2	33·169
5 3 3	33·197
5 3 4	33·226
5 3 5	33·254
5 3 6	33·282
5 3 7	33·311
5 3 8	33·339
5 3 9	33·367
5 3 10	33·396
5 3 11	33·424
5 3 12	33·452
5 3 13	33·481
5 3 14	33·509
5 3 15	33·537
5 4 0	33·566
5 4 1	33·594
5 4 2	33·623
5 4 3	33·651
5 4 4	33·679
5 4 5	33·708
5 4 6	33·736
5 4 7	33·764
5 4 8	33·793
5 4 9	33·821
5 4 10	33·849
5 4 11	33·878
5 4 12	33·906
5 4 13	33·934
5 4 14	33·963
5 4 15	33·991
5 5 0	34·019
5 5 1	34·048
5 5 2	34·076
5 5 3	34·104
5 5 4	34·133
5 5 5	34·161
5 5 6	34·189
5 5 7	34·218
5 5 8	34·246
5 5 9	34·275
5 5 10	34·303
5 5 11	34·331
5 5 12	34·360
5 5 13	34·388
5 5 14	34·416
5 5 15	34·445
5 6 0	34·473
5 6 1	34·501
5 6 2	34·530
5 6 3	34·558
5 6 4	34·586
5 6 5	34·615
5 6 6	34·643
5 6 7	34·671
5 6 8	34·700
5 6 9	34·728
5 6 10	34·756
5 6 11	34·785
5 6 12	34·813
5 6 13	34·842
5 6 14	34·870
5 6 15	34·898
5 7 0	34·927
5 7 1	34·955
5 7 2	34·983
5 7 3	35·012
5 7 4	35·040
5 7 5	35·069
5 7 6	35·097
5 7 7	35·125
5 7 8	35·153
5 7 9	35·182
5 7 10	35·210
5 7 11	35·238
5 7 12	35·267
5 7 13	35·295
5 7 14	35·323
5 7 15	35·352
5 8 0	35·380
5 8 1	35·409
5 8 2	35·437
5 8 3	35·465
5 8 4	35·494
5 8 5	35·522
5 8 6	35·550
5 8 7	35·579
5 8 8	35·607
5 8 9	35·635
5 8 10	35·664
5 8 11	35·692
5 8 12	35·720
5 8 13	35·749
5 8 14	35·777
5 8 15	35·805
5 9 0	35·834
5 9 1	35·862
5 9 2	35·890
5 9 3	35·919
5 9 4	35·947
5 9 5	35·976
5 9 6	36·004
5 9 7	36·032
5 9 8	36·061
5 9 9	36·089
5 9 10	36·117
5 9 11	36·146
5 9 12	36·174
5 9 13	36·202
5 9 14	36·231
5 9 15	36·259
5 10 0	36·287
5 10 1	36·316
5 10 2	36·344

st lb oz	kg
5 10 3	36·372
5 10 4	36·401
5 10 5	36·429
5 10 6	36·457
5 10 7	36·486
5 10 8	36·514
5 10 9	36·543
5 10 10	36·571
5 10 11	36·599
5 10 12	36·628
5 10 13	36·656
5 10 14	36·684
5 10 15	36·713
5 11 0	36·741
5 11 1	36·769
5 11 2	36·798
5 11 3	36·826
5 11 4	36·854
5 11 5	36·883
5 11 6	36·911
5 11 7	36·939
5 11 8	36·968
5 11 9	36·996
5 11 10	37·024
5 11 11	37·053
5 11 12	37·081
5 11 13	37·110
5 11 14	37·138
5 11 15	37·166
5 12 0	37·195
5 12 1	37·223
5 12 2	37·251
5 12 3	37·280
5 12 4	37·308
5 12 5	37·336
5 12 6	37·365
5 12 7	37·393
5 12 8	37·421
5 12 9	37·450
5 12 10	37·478
5 12 11	37·506
5 12 12	37·535
5 12 13	37·563
5 12 14	37·591
5 12 15	37·620
5 13 0	37·648
5 13 1	37·677
5 13 2	37·705
5 13 3	37·733
5 13 4	37·762
5 13 5	37·790
5 13 6	37·818
5 13 7	37·847
5 13 8	37·875
5 13 9	37·903
5 13 10	37·932
5 13 11	37·960
5 13 12	37·988
5 13 13	38·017
5 13 14	38·045
5 13 15	38·073
6 stone	38·102
6 0 1	38·130
6 0 2	38·158
6 0 3	38·187
6 0 4	38·215
6 0 5	38·244
6 0 6	38·272
6 0 7	38·300
6 0 8	38·329
6 0 9	38·357
6 0 10	38·385
6 0 11	38·414
6 0 12	38·442
6 0 13	38·470
6 0 14	38·499
6 0 15	38·527
6 1 0	38·555
6 1 1	38·584
6 1 2	38·612
6 1 3	38·640
6 1 4	38·669
6 1 5	38·697
6 1 6	38·725
6 1 7	38·754
6 1 8	38·782
6 1 9	38·810
6 1 10	38·839
6 1 11	38·867
6 1 12	38·896
6 1 13	38·924
6 1 14	38·952
6 1 15	38·981
6 2 0	39·009
6 2 1	39·037
6 2 2	39·066
6 2 3	39·094
6 2 4	39·122
6 2 5	39·151
6 2 6	39·179
6 2 7	39·207
6 2 8	39·236
6 2 9	39·264
6 2 10	39·292
6 2 11	39·321
6 2 12	39·349
6 2 13	39·377
6 2 14	39·406
6 2 15	39·434
6 3 0	39·462
6 3 1	39·491
6 3 2	39·519
6 3 3	39·548
6 3 4	39·576
6 3 5	39·604
6 3 6	39·633
6 3 7	39·661

st lb oz	kg
6 3 8	39·689
6 3 9	39·718
6 3 10	39·746
6 3 11	39·774
6 3 12	39·803
6 3 13	39·831
6 3 14	39·859
6 3 15	39·888
6 4 0	39·916
6 4 1	39·944
6 4 2	39·973
6 4 3	40·001
6 4 4	40·029
6 4 5	40·058
6 4 6	40·086
6 4 7	40·115
6 4 8	40·143
6 4 9	40·171
6 4 10	40·200
6 4 11	40·228
6 4 12	40·256
6 4 13	40·285
6 4 14	40·313
6 4 15	40·341
6 5 0	40·370
6 5 1	40·398
6 5 2	40·426
6 5 3	40·455
6 5 4	40·483
6 5 5	40·511
6 5 6	40·540
6 5 7	40·568
6 5 8	40·596
6 5 9	40·625
6 5 10	40·653
6 5 11	40·682
6 5 12	40·710
6 5 13	40·738
6 5 14	40·767
6 5 15	40·795
6 6 0	40·823
6 6 1	40·852
6 6 2	40·880
6 6 3	40·908
6 6 4	40·937
6 6 5	40·965
6 6 6	40·993
6 6 7	41·022
6 6 8	41·050
6 6 9	41·078
6 6 10	41·107
6 6 11	41·135
6 6 12	41·163
6 6 13	41·192
6 6 14	41·220
6 6 15	41·250
6 7 0	41·277
6 7 1	41·305
6 7 2	41·334
6 7 3	41·362
6 7 4	41·390
6 7 5	41·419
6 7 6	41·447
6 7 7	41·475
6 7 8	41·504
6 7 9	41·532
6 7 10	41·560
6 7 11	41·589
6 7 12	41·617
6 7 13	41·645
6 7 14	41·674
6 7 15	41·702
6 8 0	41·730
6 8 1	41·759
6 8 2	41·787
6 8 3	41·816
6 8 4	41·844
6 8 5	41·872
6 8 6	41·901
6 8 7	41·929
6 8 8	41·957
6 8 9	41·986
6 8 10	42·014
6 8 11	42·042
6 8 12	42·071
6 8 13	42·099
6 8 14	42·127
6 8 15	42·156
6 9 0	42·184
6 9 1	42·212
6 9 2	42·241
6 9 3	42·269
6 9 4	42·297
6 9 5	42·326
6 9 6	42·354
6 9 7	42·383
6 9 8	42·411
6 9 9	42·439
6 9 10	42·468
6 9 11	42·496
6 9 12	42·524
6 9 13	42·553
6 9 14	42·581
6 9 15	42·609
6 10 0	42·638
6 10 1	42·666
6 10 2	42·694
6 10 3	42·723
6 10 4	42·751
6 10 5	42·779
6 10 6	42·808
6 10 7	42·836
6 10 8	42·864
6 10 9	42·893
6 10 10	42·921
6 10 11	42·949
6 10 12	42·978

The last of the ounce columns (two short columns side by side):

st lb oz	kg	st lb oz	kg
6 10 13	43·006	6 12 7	43·743
6 10 14	43·035	6 12 8	43·772
6 10 15	43·063	6 12 9	43·800
6 11 0	43·091	6 12 10	43·828
6 11 1	43·120	6 12 11	43·857
6 11 2	43·148	6 12 12	43·885
6 11 3	43·176	6 12 13	43·913
6 11 4	43·205	6 12 14	43·942
6 11 5	43·233	6 12 15	43·970
6 11 6	43·261	6 13 0	43·998
6 11 7	43·290	6 13 1	44·027
6 11 8	43·318	6 13 2	44·055
6 11 9	43·346	6 13 3	44·083
6 11 10	43·375	6 13 4	44·112
6 11 11	43·403	6 13 5	44·140
6 11 12	43·431	6 13 6	44·169
6 11 13	43·460	6 13 7	44·197
6 11 14	43·488	6 13 8	44·225
6 11 15	43·516	6 13 9	44·254
6 12 0	43·545	6 13 10	44·282
6 12 1	43·573	6 13 11	44·310
6 12 2	43·602	6 13 12	44·339
6 12 3	43·630	6 13 13	44·367
6 12 4	43·658	6 13 14	44·395
6 12 5	43·687	6 13 15	44·424
6 12 6	43·715		

7 stone and above (st lb → kg):

st lb	kg	st lb	kg
7 1	44·906	13 8	86·183
7 2	45·359	13 9	86·636
7 3	45·813	13 10	87·090
7 4	46·266	13 11	87·543
7 5	46·720	13 12	87·997
7 6	47·174	13 13	88·450
7 7	47·627	14 st	88·904
7 8	48·081	14 1	89·358
7 9	48·534	14 2	89·811
7 10	48·988	14 3	90·265
7 11	49·442	14 4	90·718
7 12	49·895	14 5	91·172
7 13	50·349	14 6	91·626
8 st	50·802	14 7	92·079
8 1	51·256	14 8	92·533
8 2	51·710	14 9	92·986
8 3	52·163	14 10	93·440
8 4	52·617	14 11	93·894
8 5	53·070	14 12	94·347
8 6	53·524	14 13	94·801
8 7	53·978	15 st	95·254
8 8	54·431	15 1	95·708
8 9	54·885	15 2	96·162
8 10	55·338	15 3	96·615
8 11	55·792	15 4	97·069
8 12	56·246	15 5	97·522
8 13	56·699	15 6	97·976
9 st	57·153	15 7	98·430
9 1	57·606	15 8	98·883
9 2	58·060	15 9	99·337
9 3	58·513	15 10	99·790
9 4	58·967	15 11	100·244
9 5	59·421	15 12	100·698
9 6	59·874	15 13	101·151
9 7	60·328	16 st	101·605
9 8	60·781	16 1	102·058
9 9	61·235	16 2	102·512
9 10	61·689	16 3	102·965
9 11	62·142	16 4	103·419
9 12	62·596	16 5	103·873
9 13	63·049	16 6	104·326
10 st	63·503	16 7	104·780
10 1	63·956	16 8	105·233
10 2	64·410	16 9	105·687
10 3	64·864	16 10	106·141
10 4	65·317	16 11	106·594
10 5	65·771	16 12	107·048
10 6	66·224	16 13	107·501
10 7	66·678	17 st	107·955
10 8	67·132	17 1	108·409
10 9	67·585	17 2	108·862
10 10	68·039	17 3	109·316
10 11	68·492	17 4	109·769
10 12	68·946	17 5	110·223
10 13	69·400	17 6	110·677
11 st	69·853	17 7	111·130
11 1	70·307	17 8	111·584
11 2	70·760	17 9	112·037
11 3	71·214	17 10	112·491
11 4	71·668	17 11	112·945
11 5	72·121	17 12	113·398
11 6	72·575	17 13	113·852
11 7	73·028	18 st	114·305
11 8	73·482	18 1	114·759
11 9	73·936	18 2	115·212
11 10	74·389	18 3	115·666
11 11	74·843	18 4	116·120
11 12	75·296	18 5	116·573
11 13	75·750	18 6	117·027
12 st	76·204	18 7	117·480
12 1	76·657	18 8	117·934
12 2	77·111	18 9	118·388
12 3	77·564	18 10	118·841
12 4	78·018	18 11	119·295
12 5	78·472	18 12	119·748
12 6	78·925	18 13	120·202
12 7	79·379	19 st	120·656
12 8	79·832	19 1	121·109
12 9	80·286	19 2	121·563
12 10	80·739	19 3	122·016
12 11	81·193	19 4	122·470
12 12	81·647	19 5	122·924
12 13	82·100	19 6	123·377
13 st	82·554	19 7	123·831
13 1	83·007	19 8	124·284
13 2	83·461	19 9	124·738
13 3	83·915	19 10	125·191
13 4	84·368	19 11	125·645
13 5	84·822	19 12	126·099
13 6	85·275	19 13	126·552
13 7	85·729	20 st	127·006

Conversions are correct to the nearest gramme

Denver Developmental Screening Test

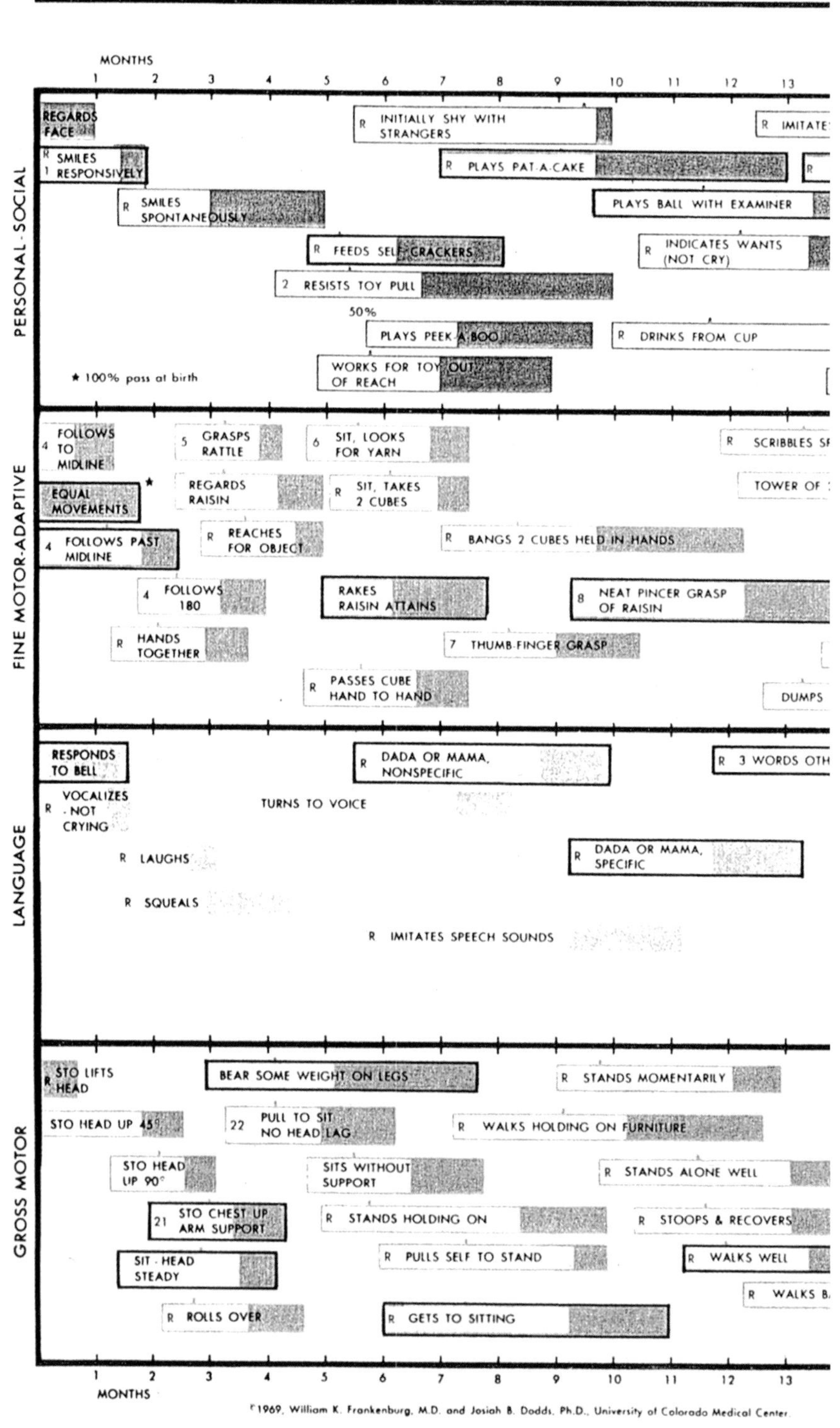

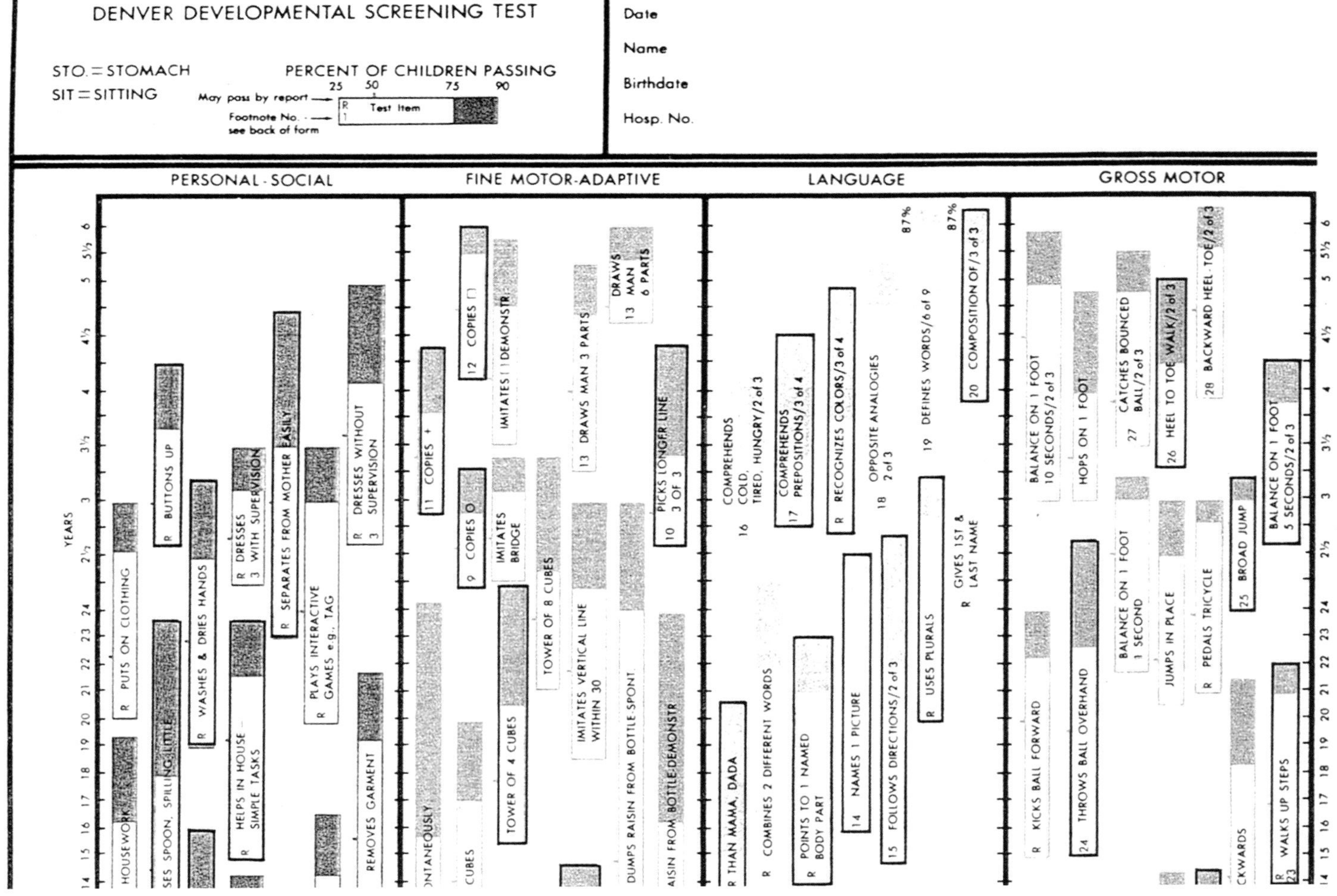
DENVER DEVELOPMENTAL SCREENING TEST
STO. = STOMACH
SIT = SITTING
PERCENT OF CHILDREN PASSING
25 50 75 90
May pass by report
R Test Item
Footnote No.
see back of form
Date
Name
Birthdate
Hosp. No.
The Denver Developmental Screening Test. (©The Test Agency Ltd.)
PERSONAL - SOCIAL
FINE MOTOR - ADAPTIVE
LANGUAGE
GROSS MOTOR
YEARS
14 15 16 17 18 19 20 21 22 23 24 2½ 3 3½ 4 4½ 5 5½ 6
HOUSEWORK
R PUTS ON CLOTHING
SES SPOON, SPILLING LITTLE
R BUTTONS UP
R WASHES & DRIES HANDS
R HELPS IN HOUSE — SIMPLE TASKS
R DRESSES 3 WITH SUPERVISION
R SEPARATES FROM MOTHER EASILY
R PLAYS INTERACTIVE GAMES e.g. TAG
REMOVES GARMENT
R DRESSES WITHOUT 3 SUPERVISION
ONTANEOUSLY
CUBES
11 COPIES +
9 COPIES O
12 COPIES ☐
IMITATES [ ] DEMONSTR
TOWER OF 4 CUBES
IMITATES BRIDGE
TOWER OF 8 CUBES
IMITATES VERTICAL LINE WITHIN 30
13 DRAWS MAN 3 PARTS
DRAWS 13 MAN 6 PARTS
DUMPS RAISIN FROM BOTTLE - SPONT.
AISIN FROM BOTTLE - DEMONSTR
10 PICKS LONGER LINE 3 OF 3
R THAN MAMA, DADA
R COMBINES 2 DIFFERENT WORDS
R POINTS TO 1 NAMED BODY PART
14 NAMES 1 PICTURE
15 FOLLOWS DIRECTIONS/2 of 3
R USES PLURALS
COMPREHENDS 16 COLD, TIRED, HUNGRY/2 of 3
COMPREHENDS 17 PREPOSITIONS/3 of 4
R RECOGNIZES COLORS/3 of 4
OPPOSITE ANALOGIES 18 2 of 3
19 DEFINES WORDS/6 of 9
87%
R GIVES 1ST & LAST NAME
20 COMPOSITION OF/3 of 3
87%
R KICKS BALL FORWARD
24 THROWS BALL OVERHAND
BALANCE ON 1 FOOT 1 SECOND
JUMPS IN PLACE
R PEDALS TRICYCLE
CKWARDS
25 BROAD JUMP
R 23 WALKS UP STEPS
BALANCE ON 1 FOOT 10 SECONDS/2 of 3
HOPS ON 1 FOOT
27 CATCHES BOUNCED BALL/2 of 3
26 HEEL TO TOE WALK/2 of 3
28 BACKWARD HEEL - TOE/2 of 3
BALANCE ON 1 FOOT 5 SECONDS/2 of 3
YEARS
14 15 16 17 18 19 20 21 22 23 24 2½ 3 3½ 4 4½ 5 5½ 6

Distribution of muscle weakness in different types of muscular dystrophy

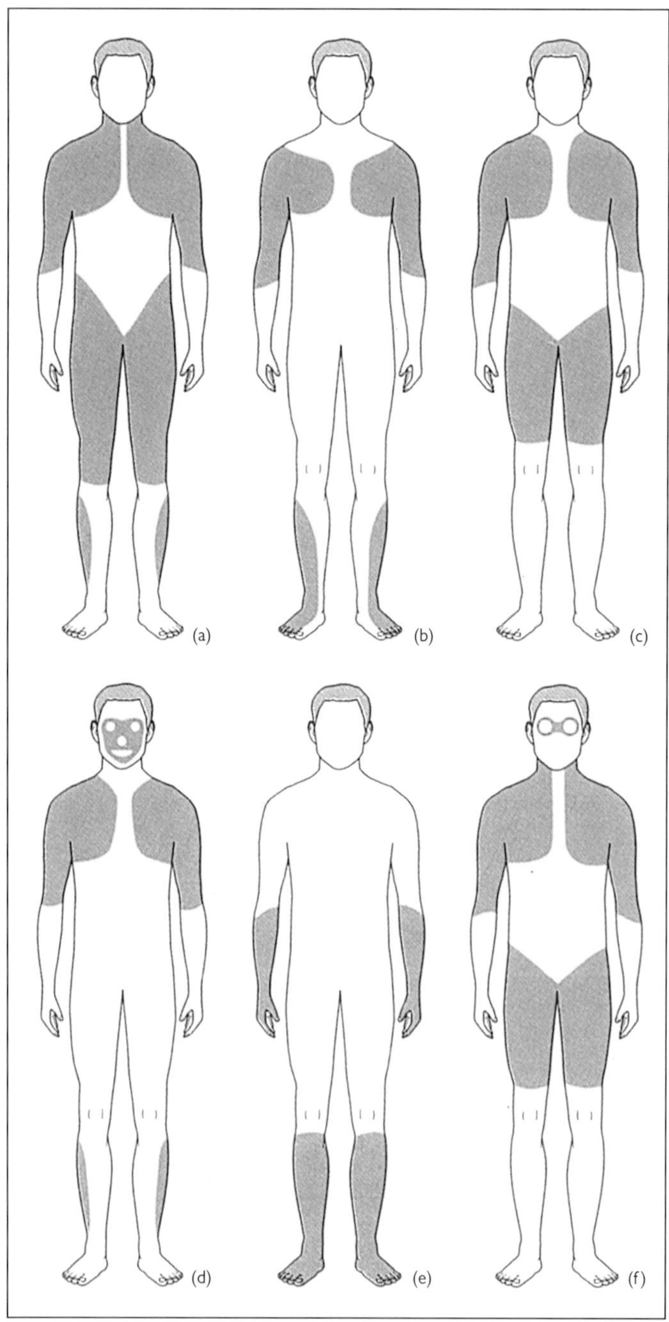

Distribution of predominant muscle weakness in different types of dystrophy: (a) Duchenne-type and Becker-type; (b) Emery–Dreifuss; (c) limb-girdle; (d) facioscapulohumeral; (e) distal; and (f) oculopharyngeal. (Reproduced from Emery (1998), fig. 1, p. 992, by permission of the BMJ Publishing Group.)

References

Emery AE. The muscular dystrophies. *Br Med J* 1998; **317**: 991–5.

Dysmorphology examination checklist

Dysmorphology examination checklist*

Growth parameters[†]	Length/height ...... cm Weight ...... kg OFC ...... cm Length/height ...... centile[†] Weight ...... centile OFC ...... centile
Stature	Proportionate ☐ Disproportionate ☐ If disproportionate, further measurements: Span ...... cm Lower segment ...... cm Upper segment ...... cm Sitting height ...... cm
Build	Normal ☐ Describe, e.g. truncal obesity
Face	Overall impression Normal ☐ Dysmorphic features, familial ☐ Dysmorphic features, non-familial ☐
Skin	Normal ☐ Describe birth marks, neurocutaneous stigmata, e.g. café au lait spots, Pigmentary anomalies, Cutis laxa, tight skin. or unusual texture
Cranium	Normal ☐ Describe skull shape, e.g. brachycephaly Fontanelle: describe if large/small/additional
Ears	Normal ☐ Describe size and position Structure, e.g. creases Pits or tags
Eyes	Normal ☐ Describe whether eyes are deepset or prominent Spacing, e.g. hypertelorism, Epicanthic folds Palpebral fissures, e.g. length/angle/everted Eyebrows, e.g. interrupted, arched, straight
Nose	Normal ☐ Describe, e.g. long/short Nasal bridge, e.g. hypoplastic/prominent Nasal tip, e.g. bulbous Nares, e.g. anteverted
Philtrum	Normal ☐ Describe, e.g. long/short/smooth
Mouth	Normal ☐ Describe, e.g. small/large Lips, e.g. thin/full/cleft Tongue, e.g. large/furrowed Palate, e.g. cleft palate Frenulum, e.g. single/missing/multiple Gums, e.g. thickened gums Teeth, e.g. size/shape/eruption
Chin	Normal ☐ Describe e.g. small chin (micrognathia), prominent chin (prognathism)
Hands/feet and limbs	Normal ☐ Describe fingers, e.g. polydactyly, syndactyly, brachydactyly Palmar and plantar creases Nails, e.g. hypoplastic, dysplastic
Chest	Normal ☐ Describe chest shape, e.g. pectus excavatum/carinatum Nipples, e.g. inverted/supranumerary
Heart	Normal ☐ Describe, e.g. murmurs
Abdomen (including genitalia)	Normal ☐ Describe, e.g. organomegaly, hypospadias
Back	Normal ☐ Describe, e.g. scoliosis
Nervous system	Normal ☐ Describe gait, e.g. ataxic, high stepping Posture, e.g. frog-legged Tone, e.g. spastic, hypotonic Reflexes, e.g. increased, diminished
Communication	Normal ☐ Record best level of communication, e.g. single words, signs, gesture
Behaviour[‡]	Normal ☐ Describe, eg. hand flapping—consider video of unusual behaviour

* Use free text/line-drawings supplemented by clinical photographs to describe any unusual features.

[†] OFC, Occipital-frontal circumference. Centiles are for chronological age, but you can also look at them for height age, for instance for a child 4 years old, but with a height age of 2 years, you can determine whether the head is normal for age or proportionate for height age.

[‡] See 'Behavioural pattern profile (Shalev and Hall 2004)' in this Appendix for more detailed assessment of behaviour.

Embryonic fetal development (overview)

Age (days)	Length (mm)	Stage * (Streeter)	Gross appearance	CNS	Eye	Ear	Face	Limbs	Heart	Gut, abdomen	Lung	Urogenital	Other
4		III	Blastocyst										Early blastocyst with inner cell mass and cavitation (58 cells) lying free within the uterine cavity
8	1	IV	Embryo, Trophoblast, Endometrium										Implantation Trophoblast invasion Embryonic disc with endoblast and ectoblast
12	2	V	Ectoderm, Amniotic sac, Endoderm, Yolk sac							Yolk sac			Early amnion sac. Extraembryonic mesoblast, angioblast Chorionic gonadotropin
19	1	IX	Ant. head fold, Body stalk, Heart	Enlargement of anterior neural plate					Merging mesoblast anterior to prechordal plate	Stomatodeum Cloaca		Allantois	Primitive streak Hensen's node Notochord Prechordal plate Blood cells in yolk sac
23	2	X Early somites	Foregut, Allantois	Partial fusion neural folds	Optic evagination	Otic placode	Mandible Hyoid arches		Single heart tube Propulsion	Foregut		Mesonephric ridge	Yolk sac larger than amnion sac
28	4	XII 21–29 somites		Closure neural tube Rhombencephalon, mesen, prosen, Ganglia V VII VIII X	Optic cup	Otic invagination	Fusion, mand. arches	Arm bud	Ventric outpouching Gelatinous reticulum	Rupture stomatodeum Evagination of thyroid, liver and dorsal pancreas	Lung bud	Mesonephric duct enters cloaca	Rathke's pouch Migration of myotomes from somites
34	7	XIV		Cerebellar plate Cervical and mesencephalic flexures	Lens invagination	Otic vesicle	Olfactory placodes	Leg bud	Auric. outpouching Septum primum	Pharyngeal pouches yield parathyroids, lat. thyroid, thymus Stomach broadens	Bronchi	Ureteral evag. Urorect sept. Germ cells Gonadal ridge Coelom, Epithelium	
38	11	XVI		Dorsal pontine flexure Basal lamina Cerebral evagination Neural hypophysis	Lens detached Pig-mented retina	Endolymphatic sac Ext. auditory meatus Tubotympanic recess	Nasal swellings	Hand plate, Mesench. condens. Innervation	Fusion mid A-V canal Muscular vent. sept.	Intestinal loop into yolk stalk Caecum Gallbladder Hepatic ducts Spleen	Main lobes	Paramesonephric duct Gonad ingrowth of coelomic epithelium	Adrenal cortex (from coelomic epithelium) invaded by sympathetic cells=medulla Jugular lymph sacs
45	17	XVIII		Olfactory evagination Cerebral hemisphere	Lens fibres Migration of retinal cells, Hyaloid vessels		Choana, 1° palate	Finger rays, Elbow	Aorta Pulmonary artery Valves Membrane ventricular septum	Duodenal lumen obliterated Caecum rotates right Appendix	Tracheal cartil.	Fusion urorect. septum Open urogenital memb., anus Epith. cords in testicle	Early muscle
51	22	XX		Optic nerve to brain	Corneal body Mesoderm No lumen in optic stalk			Clearing, central cartil.	Septum secundum			S-shaped vesicles in nephron blastema connect with collecting tubules from calyces	Superficial vascular plexus low on cranium
56	26	XXII			Eyelids	Spiral cochlear duct Tragus		Tubular bones				A few large glomeruli Short secretory tubules Tunica albuginea Testicle, interstitial cells	Superficial vascular plexus at vertex

* The embryonic ages for Streeter's stages XII–XXII have been altered in accordance with the human data from Iffy, L. *et al.* (1967). *Acta anat.* **66**, 178.

(Adapted from Smith 1982, by permission)

Age (weeks)	Length C–R	Length Tot	Weight (gm)	Gross appearance	CNS	Eye, ear	Face, mouth	Cardiovascular	Lung	Gut	Urogenital	Skeletal muscle	Skeleton	Skin	Blood, thymus lymph	Endocrine
7	2.8				Cerebral hemisphere Infundibulum, Rathke's Olfactory lobes Dura and pia mater	Lens nearing final shape	Palatal swellings Dental lamina, Epithel	Pulmonary vein into left atrium		Pancreas, dorsal and ventral fusion	Renal vesicles	Differentiation toward final shape	Cartilagnous models of bones Chondrocranium Tail regression	Mammary gland		Parathyroid associated with thyroid Sympathetic neuroblasts invade adrenal
8	3.7				Primitive cereb. cortex Spinal cord histology Cerebellum	Eyelid Ear canals	Nares plugged Rathke's pouch detach Sublingual gland	A–V bundle Sinus venosus absorbed into auricle	Pleuroperitoneal canals close Bronchioles	Liver relatively large Intestinal villi	Müllerian ducts fusing	Muscles well represented Movement	Ossification centre Sternum	Basal layer	Bone marrow Thymus halves unite Lymphoblasts around the lymph sacs	Thyroid follicles
10	6.0					Iris Ciliary body Eyelids fuse Lacrimal glands Spiral gland different	Lips, Nasal cartilage Palate		Laryngeal cavity reopened		Ovary distinguishable		Joints	Hair follicles Melanocytes	Enucleated RBCs Thymus yields reticulum and corpuscles Thoracic duct Lymph nodes; axillary iliac	Adrenalin Noradrenalin
12	8.8				Cord–cervical & lumbar enlarged, Cauda equina	Retina layered Eye axis forward	Tonsillar crypts Cheeks Dental papilla	Accessory coats, blood vessels	Elastic fibres	Gut withdrawal from cord Pancreatic alveoli Anal canal	Testosterone Renal excretion Bladder sac Müllerian tube into urogenital sinus Vaginal sacs, prostate	Perineal muscles	Tail degenerated	Corium, 3 layers Scalp, body hair Sebaceous glands Nails beginning Palm creases	Blood principally from bone marrow Thymus—medullary and lymphoid	Testicle—Leydig cells Thyroid—colloid in follicle Anterior pituitary acidophilic granules Ovary—prim. follicles
16	14				Corpora quadrigemina Cerebellum prominent Myelination begins	Scala vestibuli Cochlear duct Scala tympani	Palate complete Enamel and dentine	Cardiac muscle condensed	Segmentation of bronchi complete	Gut muscle layers Pancreatic islets Bile	Seminal vesicle Regression, genital ducts		Notochord degenerated	Dermal ridge pattern Hand creases Sweat glands Keratinization Scalp hair pattern		Anterior pituitary—basophilic granules
20						Inner ear ossified	Ossification of nose		Decrease in mesenchyme Capillaries penetrate linings of tubules	Omentum fusing with transverse colon Mesoduodenum. Sacs, desc. colon attach to body wall. Meconium. Gastric, intest. glands	Typical kidney Mesonephros involuting Uterus and vagina Primary follicles	In-utero movement can be detected	Distinct bones	Hair at eyebrow Venix caseosa Nail plates Mammary budding	Blood formation decreasing liver	
24		32	800		Typical layers in cerebral cortex Cauda equina at first sacral level	Eyelids reopen Retinal layers complete Perceive light	Nares reopen Calcification of tooth primordia		Change from cuboidal to flattened epithelium Alveoli		No further collecting tubules					Testes—decrease in Leydig cells
28		38.5	1100		Cerebral fissures and convolutions	Auricular cartilage	Taste sense		Vascular components adequate for respiration							Testes descend
32		43.5	1600	Accumulation of fat					Number of alveoli still incomplete					Nails to fingertips		
36		47.5	2600		Cauda equina, at L–3 Myelination within brain	Lacrimal duct canalized	Rudimentary frontal maxillary sinuses	Closure of foramen ovale, ductus arteriosus, umbilical vessels, ductus venosus Relative hypertrophy left ventricle			Urine osmolarity continues to be relatively low		Only a few secondary epiphyseal centre's ossified in knee	Eccrine sweat Lanugo hair prominent Nails to toe lips	Haemoglobin 17–18g Leukocytosis	
38		50	3200											New hair, gradual loss of lanugo hair		
First postnatal year +					Continuing organization of axonal networks Cerebrocortical function, motor co-ordination Myelination continues until 2–3 years	Iris pigmented, 5 months Mastoid air cells Co-ordinate vision 3–5 months Maximal vision by 5 years	Salivary gland ducts became canalized Teeth begin to erupt 5–7 months Relatively rapid growth of mandible and nose		Continue adding new alveoli				Ossification of 2nd epiph. centres hamate, capitate, proximal humerus, femur New ossif. 2nd epiph. centres till 10–12 years Ossif. of epiphyses till, 16–18 yrs		Transient (6 wk) erythroid hypoplasia Haemoglobin 11–12 g 75 gamma globulin produced by 6 weeks Lymph nodes develop cortex, medulla	Transient estrinization Adrenal—regression of fetal zone Gonadotropin with feminization of ♀ 9–12 yr (on set); masc. of ♂ 10–14 yr (on set)

(Adapted from Smith 1982, by permission)

Family tree sheet and symbols

Usage of standardized pedigree nomenclature reduces the chances for incorrect interpretation of patient and family medical and genetic information. It may also improve the quality of patient care provided by genetic professionals and facilitate communication between researchers involved with genetic family studies (Bennett *et al.* 1995).

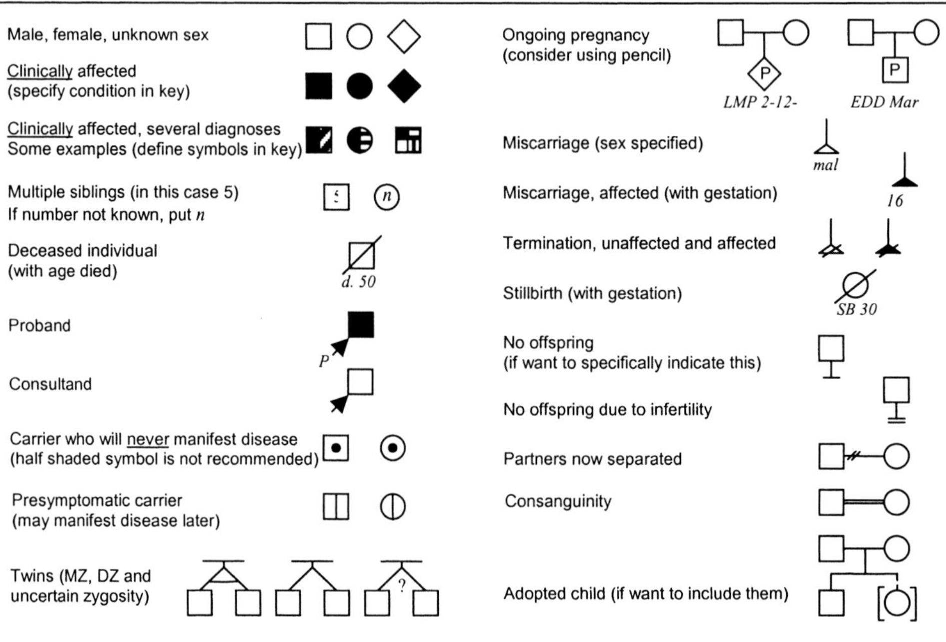

Recommended symbols for pedigree drawing.

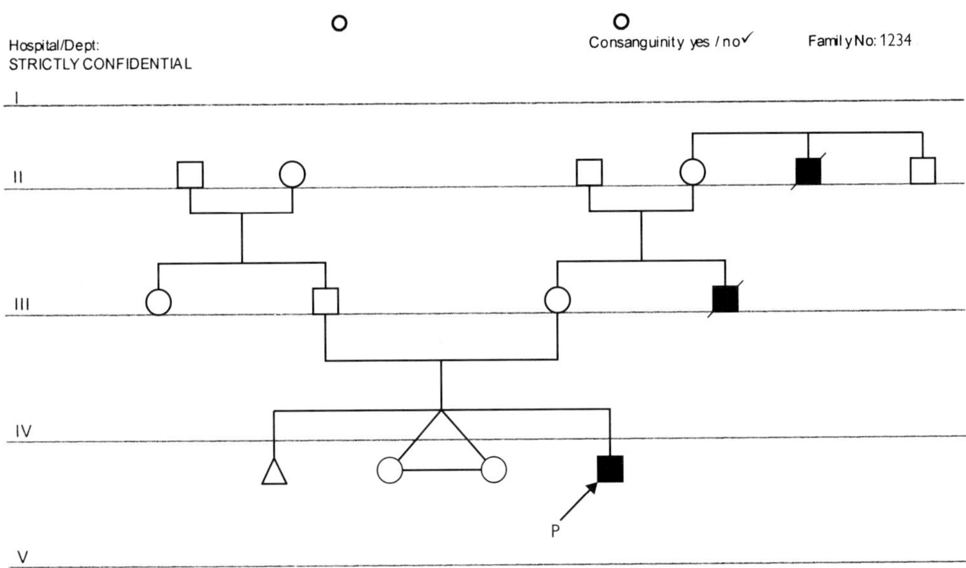

Sample sheet for drawing a pedigree.

References

Bennett RL, Steinhaus KA, et al. Recommendations for standardized human pedigree nomenclature. Pedigree Standardization Task Force of the National Society of Genetic Counselors. *Am J Hum Genet* 1995; **56**: 745–52.

Haploid autosomal lengths of human chromosomes

Daniel (1979) studied interchange segment sizes and the sizes of chromosome imbalance arising from the different modes of meiotic segregation in a selected sample of reciprocal translocations (Rcp). The study population included spontaneous abortions and children born with chromosomal imbalance. He concluded that:

1 the interchange segments were larger in the spontaneous abortion Rcp;

2 all of the imbalances observed in full-term neonates plotted close to the origin and to the left of the line joining 4% trisomy to 2% monosomy;

3 the imbalances observed in the neonates in each individual Rcp were of the smallest size possible arising by any segregation mode.

Haploid autosomal length (HAL)

To determine the amount of particular segmental imbalance as a fraction of the haploid autosomal length (HAL):

1 measure the length of the entire chromosome using a millimetre ruler;

2 measure the length of the chromosome segment involved in the imbalance using a millimetre ruler;

3 determine the percentage of the length of that specific chromosome that would be involved in the imbalance, e.g. for the segment 4q13.3–qter this represents 18% of the length of chromosome 4;

4 From the table below determine the percentage of the total HAL ie. chromosome 4 represents 6.3% of HAL, 18% x 6.3% = 1.14%, hence the imbalance represents 1.14% of HAL which falls within the envelope of potentially viable imbalance (see figure on p 500 in 'Autosomal reciprocal translocations—background').

Percentage of haploid autosomal length (HAL) that each autosome constitutes (after Daniel 1979)

Chromosome	% of HAL	Chromosome	% of HAL
1	8.44	12	4.66
2	8.02	13	3.74
3	6.83	14	3.56
4	6.30	15	3.46
5	6.08	16	3.36
6	5.90	17	3.25
7	5.36	18	2.93
8	4.93	19	2.67
9	4.80	20	2.56
10	4.59	21	1.90
11	4.61	22	2.04

Example

For the unbalanced karyotype 46,XX, der(20)t(14;20)(q24;q13.3) the segment 14q24-qter represents 33% of the length of chromosome 14, hence the imbalance represents 33% x 3.56% = 1.18% of HAL as a trisomy. In this rearrangement there is no monosomy and so it falls within the triangle of potentially viable imbalance (see figure on p 500 'Autosomal reciprocal translocations—background').

References

Daniel A. Structural differences in reciprocal translocations. Potential for a model of risk in Rcp. *Hum Genet* 1979; **51**: 171–82.

Gardner RJM, Sutherland GR. *Chromosome abnormalities and genetic counselling*, Oxford Monographs on Medical Genetics no. 31, 3rd edn. Oxford University Press, New York, 2004.

Investigation of lethal metabolic disorder or skeletal dysplasia

Metabolic autopsy

A diagnosis is vitally important in order to be able to advise about recurrence risks and possibly to offer prenatal diagnosis in a subsequent pregnancy. If it has not been possible to make a diagnosis during life and there is a suspicion of an underlying metabolic disorder, the following samples taken immediately after death can substantially increase the chance of making a diagnosis and enable the diagnostic process to continue after death.

- Plasma: heparinized, separated, and deep frozen.
- Blood spots on Guthrie card for acylcarnitine.
- Urine in plain universal container: deep frozen.
- Blood in EDTA(ethylenedinitrilotetraacetate) for DNA extraction and storage.
- Skin for fibroblast culture taken into tissue culture medium and stored in a fridge at 4–8°C.
- Liver biopsy snap frozen for histochemistry/enzymology.
- Muscle snap frozen for histochemistry/enzymology/ immunohistochemistry.
- Consider clinical photographs.
- Consider skeletal X-rays in a baby.

Investigation of the fetus and baby with a skeletal dysplasia

A diagnosis is vitally important in order to be able to advise about appropriate management and also recurrence risks.

- DNA storage. Cord blood, fetal blood sample, placental tissue and skin biopsy can all be used. An increasing number of dysplasias have known mutations.
- Chromosome analysis.
- Skin biopsy (collagen studies in OI).
- Radiology: full skeletal survey.
- Clinical photography.
- Clinical measurements.

If the baby dies it is possible to get most of the information required even if a post-mortem examination is refused. If a post mortem is performed, it should include bone histology.

References

Leonard JV, Morris AAM. Inborn errors of metabolism around the time of birth [review article]. *Lancet* 2000; **356**: 583–7.

ISCN Nomenclature

Symbols and abbreviated terms used in the description of chromosomes and chromosomal abnormalities (Mitelman 1995)

add
additional material of unknown origin
46,XX,add(1)(p36)

arrow (→)
from–to, in detailed system
46,XX,add(1)(?::p36 → qter)

brackets, square ([ ])
surround the absolute number of cells in each clone
45,X[20]/46,XX[10]

colon, single (:)
break, in detailed system
46,XX,del(6)(qter → p21:)

colon, double (::)
break and reunion, in detailed system
46,XX,del(6)(qter → p11::p21→pter)

comma (,)
separates chromosome numbers, sex chromosomes, and chromosome abnormalities
45,XX,add(1)(p36),–21

decimal point (.)
denotes subbands
46,XX,add(1)(p36.1)

del
deletion
46,XX,del(6)(qter → p21:)

de novo
designates a chromosome abnormality that has not been inherited
46,XX,del(22)(q11.2q11.2)de novo

der
derivative chromosome
46,XX,der(5)t(1;5)(p36;q24)pat

dic
dicentric
46,X,dic(X)(p11)

dup
duplication
46,XX,dup(5)(p13p23)

fra
fragile site
46,Y,fra(X)(q27.3)

h
heterochromatin, constitutive
46,XY,16qh+

hsr
homogeneously staining region
46,XX,hsr(14)(q21)

i
isochromosome
46,X,i(X)(p10)

ins
insertion
46,XX,ins(5)(q12q22q34)

inv
inversion
46,XX,inv(9)(p11q13)

mar
marker chromosome
47,XX,+mar

mat
maternal origin
46,XX,der(5)t(1;5)(p36;q24)mat

minus sign (−)
loss
45,XX, −21

p
short arm of chromosome
46,XX,add(1)(p36)

parentheses
surround structurally altered chromosome and breakpoints
46,XX,der(5)t(1;5)(p36;q24)mat

pat
paternal origin
46,XX,der(5)t(1;5)(p36;q24)pat

plus sign (+)
gain
47,XX,+21

q
long arm of chromosome
46,XX,der(5)t(1;5)(p36;q24)pat

question mark (?)
questionable identification of a chromosome or chromosome structure
47,XX,+?21

r
ring chromosome
46,X,r(X)

rec
recombinant chromosome
46,XX,rec(4)dup(4q)inv(4)(p14q34)

s
satellite
46,XX,12ps

sce
sister chromatid exchange
Sce(9)(p11p23)

semicolon (;)
separates altered chromosomes and breakpoints in structural rearrangements involving more than one chromosome
46,XX,t(1;5)(p36;q24)

slant line (/)
separates clones
45,X/46,XX

t
translocation
46,XX,t(1;5)(p36;q24)

ter
terminal (end of chromosome)
46,XX,add(1)(?::p36 → qter)

upd
uniparental disomy
46,XX,upd(15)(mat)

In situ hybridization: symbols and abbreviations (Mitelman 1995)

minus sign (−)
  absent from a specific chromosome
  46,XX.ish del(22)(q11.2q11.2)(D22S735−)
plus sign (+)
  present on a specific chromosome
  46,XX.ish del(22)(q11.2q11.2)(D22S735-,D22S422+)
multiplication sign (×)
  precedes the number of signals seen
  46,XX.ish 22q11.2(D22S735 × 2)
period (.)
  separates cytogenetic observations from results of *in situ* hybridization
  46,XX.ish del(22)(q11.2q11.2)(D22S735−)
semicolon (;)
  separates probes on different derivative chromosomes
  46,XX, t(1;5)(p36;q24).ish t(1;5)(D1S432+,D5S563−; D1S432−,D5S563)
FISH
  fluorescence *in situ* hybridization
ish
  in situ hybridization; when used without a prefix applies to chromosomes (usually metaphase or prometaphase) of
    dividing cells
  46,XX.ish del(22)(q11.2q11.2)(D22S735−)
nuc ish
  Nuclear or interphase *in situ* hybridization
  nuc ish 18cen(D18Z1 × 3)
wcp
  whole chromosome paint
  46,XX,r(9).ish r(9)(wcp9+)

Reference

Mitelman F. (ed.). ISCN (1995): an international system for human
  cytogenetic nomenclature. Karger, Basel, 1995.

Karyotypes

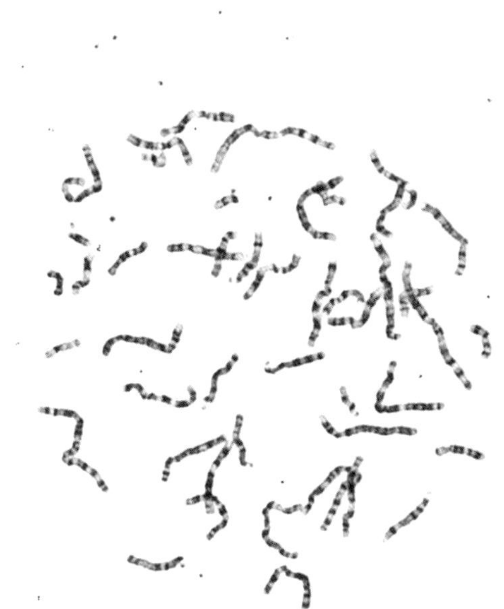

Normal metaphase spread.

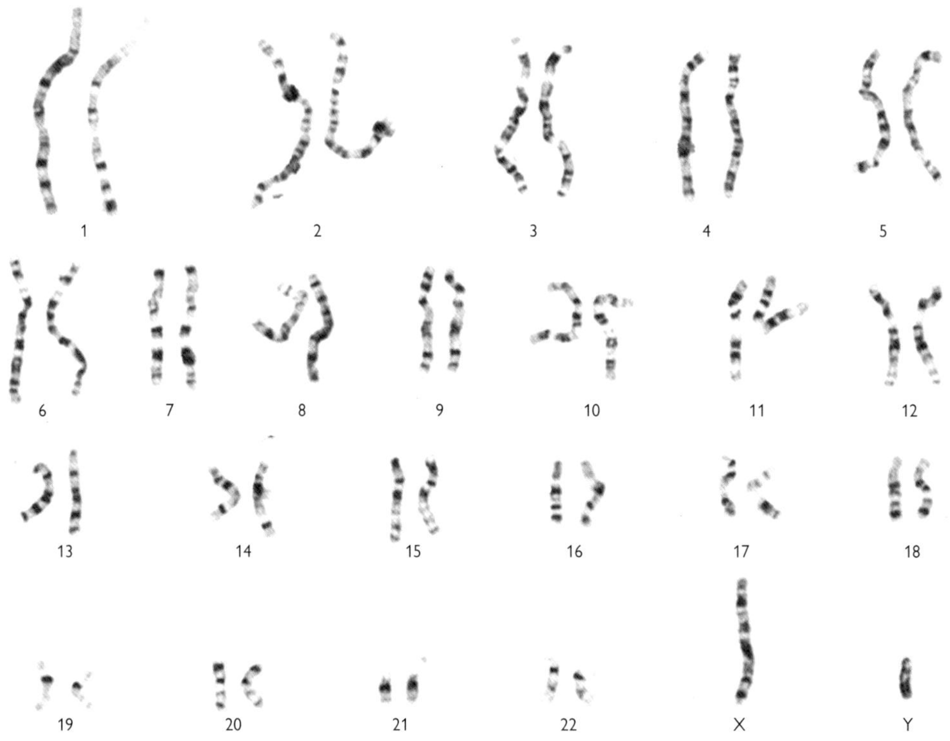

Normal male G-banded karyotype.

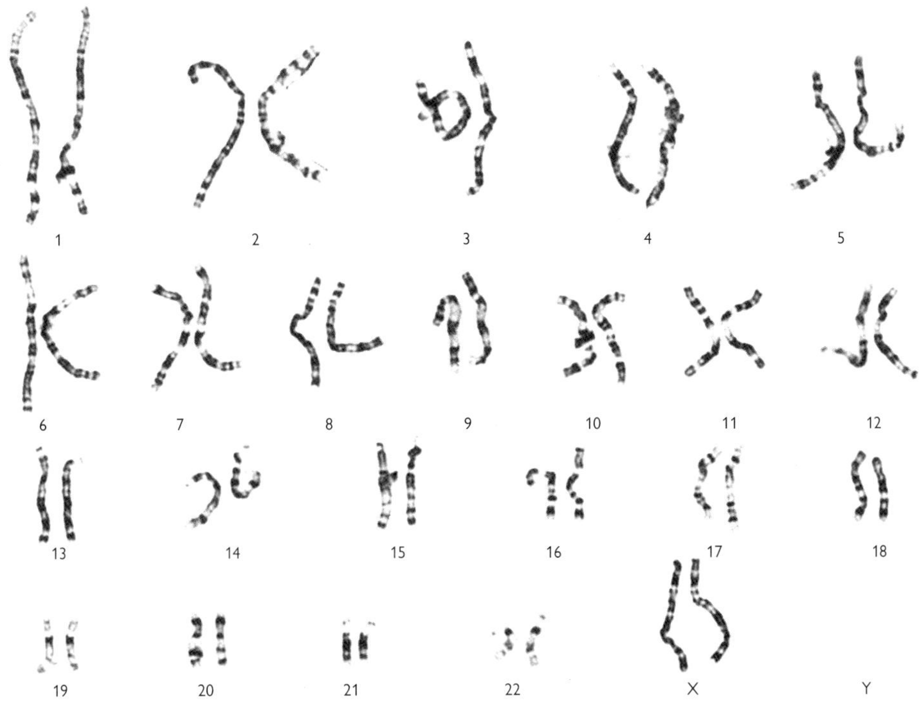

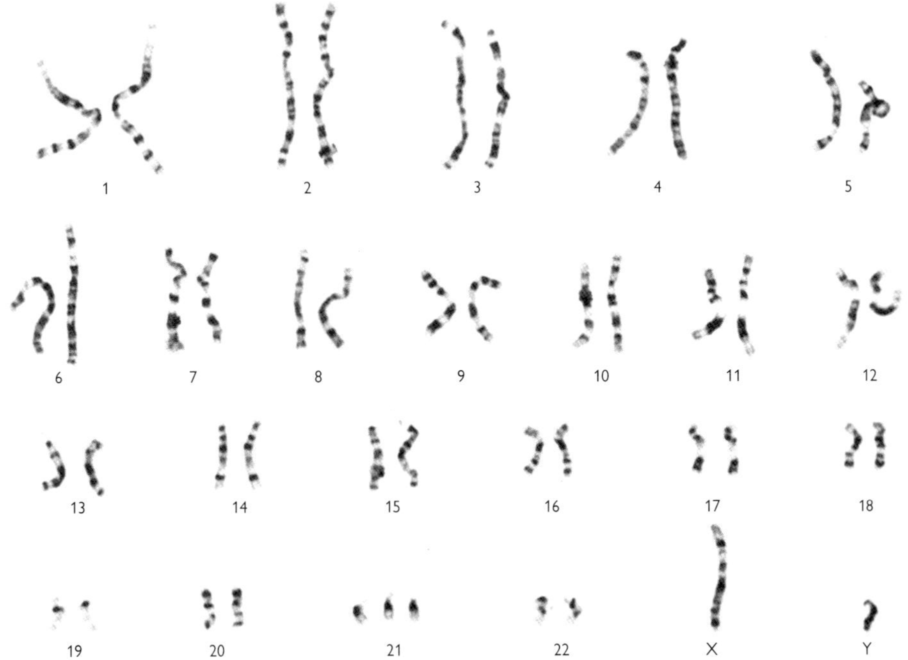

Normal female G-banded karyotype.

Trisomy 21 G-banded karyotype.

Normal range of aortic root dimensions

Nomograms standardly used to detect aortic dilatation by echocardiography in children and adults are based on M-mode data. Aortic root dilatation is overdiagnosed when two-dimensional echocardiographic data are compared with M-mode nomograms. This appendix provides nomograms devised for two-dimensional echocardiography. The first two figures give nomograms for calculation of body surface area (BSA) in children and adults, respectively. The following two figures then give 95% normal confidence limits for aortic root diameter at sinuses of Valsalva in relation to BSA in children and adults, respectively. The final figure gives normal echo values for aortic diameter as a function of BSA.

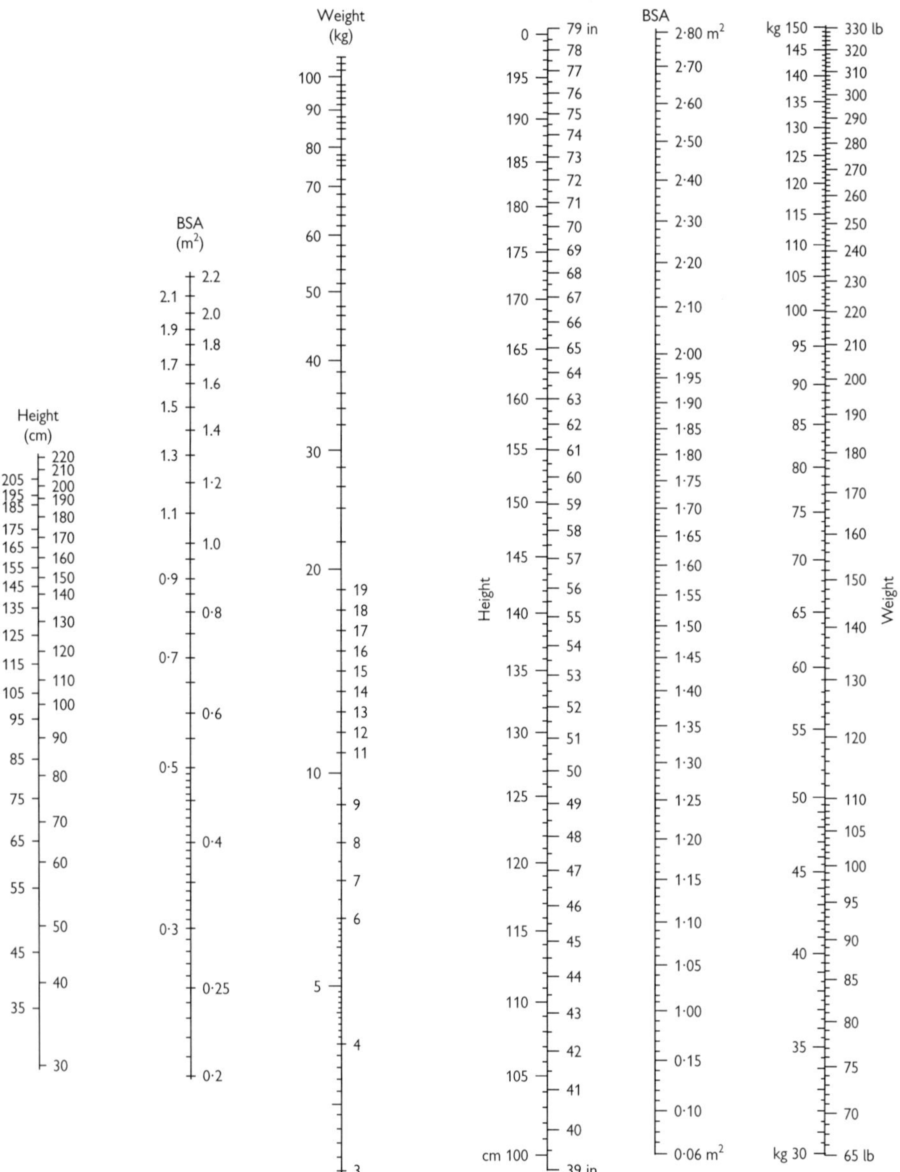

Nomogram for calculation of body surface area (BSA) in children. To use the nomogram a ruler is aligned with the height and weight on the two lateral axes. The point at which the centre line is intersected gives the corresponding value for BSA.

Nomogram for calculation of body surface area (BSA) in adults. The point at which the centre line is intersected gives the corresponding value for BSA.

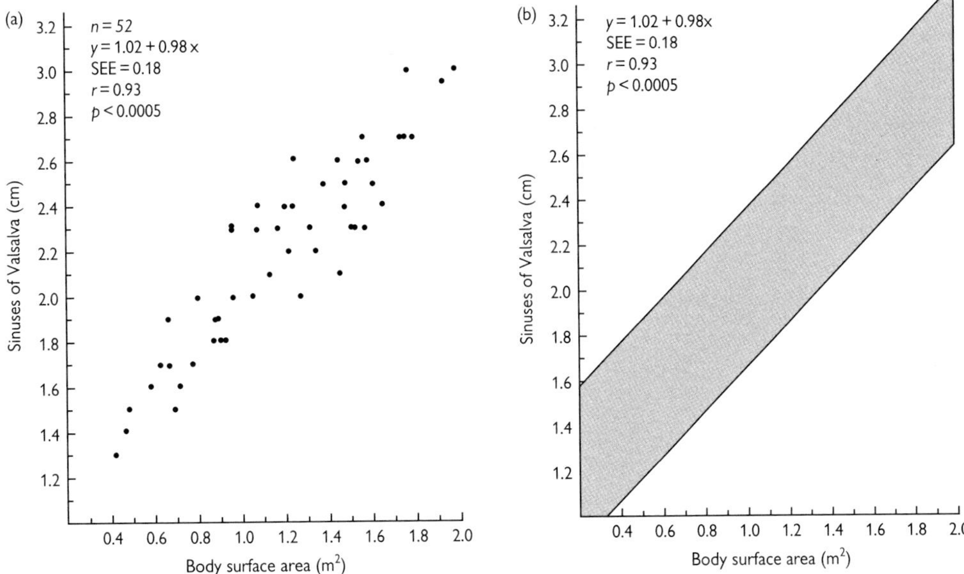

(a) Relation of body surface area (BSA) to aortic root diameter in normal infants and children. (b) The grey area represents the 95% confidence interval (CI) for aortic root diameter at sinuses of Valsalva in infants and children. (From Roman *et al.* (1989).)

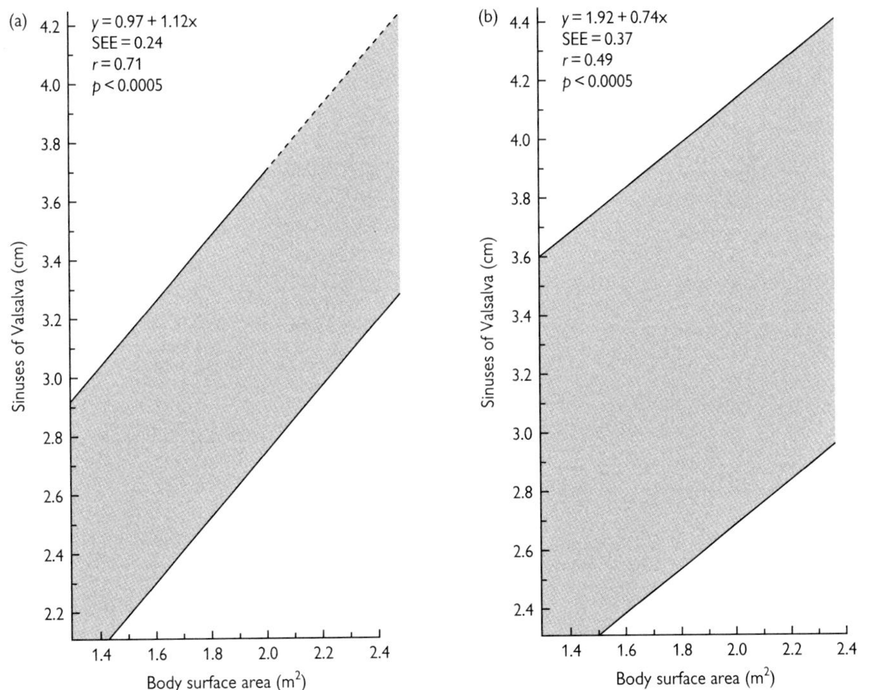

The grey area represents the 95% normal confidence limits for aortic root diameter at sinuses of Valsalva in relation to body surface area (BSA) in: (a) adults under 40 years of age; (b) adults 40 years of age and older. (From Roman *et al.* (1989).)

References

Henry WL, Ware J, Gardin JM, Hepner SI, McKay J, Weiner M. Echocardiographic measurements in normal subjects. Growth-related changes that occur between infancy and early adulthood. *Circulation* 1978; **57** (2): 278–85.

Roman MJ, *et al.* Two dimensional aortic root dimensions in normal children and adults. *Am J Cardiol* 1989; **64**: 507–12.

Paternity testing

In the UK paternity testing for social or legal indications is not undertaken as part of health care, but is available privately through several agencies (see list at end of article).

Typical testing methodology

A child inherits half of his/her DNA from each parent. DNA samples are analysed using polymerase chain reaction (PCR) and short tandem repeat (STR) profiling. Every STR marker in the child's pattern should be present in either the mother's or father's DNA. If, for example, 16 highly polymorphic STRs are used when a mother, alleged father, and child are tested, proof of paternity can be established with a minimum certainty of 99.99% or, alternatively, DNA analysis can prove non-paternity with 100% certainty.

DNA from children is often collected as a mouth swab; samples from the mother and alleged father are collected as mouth swabs or blood samples.

There are commercial operations in most developed countries. Contact your molecular genetics lab for details of reputable centres.

Patterns of cancer

	Skin		GI tract						Male genital tract	Female genital tract			
	Skin	Breast	Colorectal	Gastric	Pancreas	Liver	Hepato-biliary tract	Small bowel	Prostate	Endometrium	Myometrium	Cervix	Ovary
BRCA1		F 65% (range* 44–78%) to age 70 yr											F 39% (range* 18–54%) to age 70yr
BRCA2	Melanoma	F 45% (CI* 31–56%) to age 70 yr; M ~6% to age 70 yr							7.5% by age 70 yr				F 11% (CI* 2.4–19%) to age 70 yr
HNPCC	Sebaceous tumours, keratoacanthomas		M 80%, F 40%	~5%	~2%		~1%	1% (jejunal & ileal)		50%			~4%
FAP (APC)	Sebaceous cysts		nearly 100%	Fundic gland polyps	++	+(hepatoblastoma in children)	++	++ (duodenal 3–4%)					
PJS			29%					10%	9%	39%			SCTAT (usually benign) in 21%
Hereditary gastric (ECAD)				+++ 70–80%									
LFS		+++	++		++								
VHL													
Cowden		+++	Cowden's hamartomata							++	Fibroids		
Gorlin	+++ BCCa												
RB	++ melanoma (7% of 2nd tumours)												
MEN1					++ adenomas								
MEN2													
NF2	Neurofibromata												
Fumarase carrier												Fibroids	
Mean age of diagnosis for this type of cancer in the UK with 25th and 75th quartiles	Melanoma M 60yr (49–74yr); F 58yr (44–74yr)	F 63yr (52–75 yr)	M 71yr (64–79 yr); F 73 yr (66–83yr)	M 72 yr (65–80yr); F 75yr (70–85yr)	M 70yr (63–79yr); F 74yr (67–83yr)				M 73yr (67–80yr)	F 67yr (59–76yr)		F 52yr (37–68yr)	F 65yr (55–76yr)
Lifetime UK Population Risk (OPCS 1996) expressed as %	0.9% (Melanoma)	F 9–11%	M5.5%, F5.0%	M 2.3%, F 1.2%	1%	0.4%	0.08%	0.12%	7.3%	1.4%		F 0.9%	F 2.1%
Lifetime UK Population Risk (OPCS 1996) expressed as chance of diagnosis	1 in 117 (Melanoma)	1 in 9	M 1 in 18, F 1 in 20	M 1 in 45, F 1 in 90	1 in 100	1 in 250	1 in 1250	1 in 830	1 in 14	1 in 70		1 in 116	1 in 50

* – where there are multiple affected family members, the risk estimates from the upper end of these ranges are likely to be appropriate

Greatly increased risk +++
Moderately increased risk ++
Some increased risk

A chart giving the pattern of cancer in the UK. HNPCC, Hereditary nonpolyposis colorectal cancer; FAP, familal adenomatous polyposis; PJS, Peutz–Jeghers syndrome; LFS, Li–Fraumeni syndrome; VHL, von Hippel–Lindau; RB, retinoblastoma; MEN, multiple endocrine neoplasia; NF2, neurofibromatosis type 2; TCC, transitional cell carcinoma.

Endocrine			Nervous system		Musculoskeletal		Urinary tract		Haematological		
Parathyroid	Thyroid	Adrenal	Eye	Brain	Sarcoma	Benign	Kidney	Urothelial	Lympho–proliferative	Leukaemia	
											BRCA1
											BRCA2
				3% (astrocytomas > medulloblastoma)			1–2% RCCa	2–6% TCCa (renal pelvis and ureter)	2–3%		HNPCC
	++ papillary	+ (adren corticalca)		++ (medulloblastoma > astrocytoma)		Desmoid tumours, osteomata, odontomata					FAP (APC)
	36%						13%				PJS
											Hereditary gastric (ECAD)
		+++ (cortex)		+++	+++		+++ (Wilm's)			+	LFS
		++ (phaeochromo cytoma) 17%		+++ (cerebellar haemangioblastoma) 56%			+++ (RCCa) 25%				VHL
	+++ (non~medullary)			Lhermitte–Duclos SOL in cerebellum		Lipomata, haemangiomata	++				Cowden
				++ medulloblastoma in children							Gorlin
			+++ 90% (retinoblastoma)	+ (4.5% of 2nd tumours)	+++ (51% of 2nd tumours)						RB
+++				++ pituitary adenomas							MEN1
++ (2A not 2B)	+++ FMTC	++ (phaeochromo cytoma)									MEN2
				+++ schwannomas and meningiomas							NF2
											Fumarase carrier
				M 57yr (46–71yr); 59yr (48–74yr)			M 66yr (59– 76yr); F 68yr (60–79yr)		NHL M 64yr (54– 76yr); F 67yr (58–79yr)	M 63yr (55– 78yr); F 66yr (57–82yr)	Mean age of diagnosis for this type of cancer in the UK with 25th and 75th quartiles
				0.7%			M 1.1%, F 0.6%	M 3.3%, F 0.6%	1.3%	0.9%	Lifetime UK Population Risk (OPCS 1996) expressed as %
				1 in 150			M 1 in 90, F 1 in 160	M 1 in 90, F 1 in 160	1 in 75	1 in 110	Lifetime UK Population Risk (OPCS 1996) expressed as chance of diagnosis

Expert advisers: Ian M. Frayling, Consultant in Clinical Genetics and Director of Clinical Genetics Laboratory, University Hospital of Wales, Cardiff, Wales and Paul Pharaoh, Cancer Research UK Senior Clinical Research Fellow, Strangeways Research Laboratory, Cambridge, England.

References

<www.cancerresearchuk.org/aboutcancer/statistics/statsmisc/pdfs/cancerstats incidence.pdf>. OPCS (Office of Population Censors and Surveys) 1996.

Radiological investigations including magnetic resonance imaging (MRI)

MRI

T1-weighted sequences typically demonstrate the cerebral anatomy well and are frequently used pre- and post-intravenous contrast medium (gadolinium DTPA (diethyltriaminepentaacetic acid)) to aid identification of pathology through typical patterns of vascular enhancement, in a similar fashion to computerized tomography (CT).

T2-weighted sequences are particularly useful for demonstrating oedema and for focal tumour detection, which both have increased signal and appear 'bright' on the images. T2-weighted sequences are limited in some situations by the fact that cerebrospinal fluid (CSF) also appears with increased signal and this may mask some subtle lesion (for example cortical tubers) close to fluid-filled regions such as the ventricles. In this situation **FLAIR (fluid-attenuated inversion recovery) sequences** are helpful as they provide effective T2-weighting for oedema, tumours, and tuberous sclerosis (TS) tubers while suppressing the signal from fluid making it appear dark.

Computerized tomography (CT)
See table.

Conventional radiographs (X-rays)
See table.

Radiation dose from commonly requested computerized tomography (CT) investigations (from National Radiation Protection Board 2002)

CT examination	Effective dose (mSv)	Equivalent number of chest X-rays
Head	2	100
Abdomen	10	500

Expert advisers: David Lomas, Professor, Department of Radiology, University of Cambridge and Karen Goldstone, Radiation Protection Adviser, Addenbrooke's Hospital, Cambridge, England.

Radiation dose from commonly requested X-ray investigations (from National Radiation Protection Board 2002)

Examination*	Effective dose (mSv)	Equivalent number of chest X-rays
Skull X ray (PA and LAT)	0.06	3
Teeth panoramic views	0.01	0.5
Cervical spine (AP and LAT)	0.07	3.5
Thoracic spine (AP and LAT)	0.7	35
Lumbar spine (AP and LAT)	1.0	5
Whole spine/scoliosis (AP/PA and LAT)	0.07	3.5
Upper arm	0.0008	0.4
Hand	0.0005	0.25
Radius and ulna/forearm	0.001	0.05
Wrist	0.0005	0.025
Pelvis	0.7	35
Femur	0.0025	1.25
Tibia and fibula	0.002	1
Foot	0.0006	0.03
Skeletal survey	1.80	90
Chest X ray (PA only)	0.02	1
Abdomen (plain film)	0.7	35
Ba follow-through/small bowel meal	3	150
Ba enema	7.2	360
IVU	2.4	120
MCUG	1.1	55
Bone mineral densitometry	0.002	0.1

* PA, Posteroanterior; AP, anteroposterior; LAT, lateral; IVU, intravenous urography; MCUG, micturating cysturethrogram.

Reference
National Radiation Protection Board (NRPB). <www.nrpb.org/publications/w_series_reports/2002/nrpb_w4>.

Skeletal dysplasia charts

SKELETAL DYSPLASIAS PRESENTING AT BIRTH

DIAGNOSIS †	ALWAYS LETHAL *	LIMBS SHORT	LIMBS BENT/ANGULATED	LIMBS DISLOCATION	LIMBS FEMUR/TIBIA/FIBULA	LIMBS POLY-DACTYLY	SKULL OSSIFICATION	RIBS SHORT	RIBS BEADED/FRACTURED	SPINE PLATY-SPONDYLY	SPINE SOME ABSENT OSSIFICATION	PELVIS "TRIDENT"/"SPIKEY"	BONE DENSITY ▲▼ / + FRACTURE
ACHONDROPLASIA - HETERO:		rhizo.						+				+	
- HOMO:	+	rhizo.						+				+	
THANATOPHORIC I	+	++	+					++		++		+	
II	+	+	+				Clover leaf	+		+		+	
(Thanatophoric Variants)													
ACHONDROGENESIS I	+	++					▼	+	+		+		
II	+	++						+			+		
HYPOCHONDROGENESIS	+	+						+		+	+		
SPONDYLO-EPIPHYSEAL DYSPLASIA CONGENITA		(rhizo.)						+		+			
OSTEOGENESIS IMPERFECTA IIA	+	+	+				▼		+	+			▼ +
IIB	+	+	+						+				▼ +
IIC	+	+	+				▼		+				▼ +
III		(+)	(+)						+				▼ +
HYPOPHOSPHATASIA Lethal	+	+			Fib. ▼		▼		+	+	+		▼ +
Surviving		+											
CAMPOMELIC	+		+	+	Fib. ▼								
KYPHOMELIC		rhizo.	+										
DIASTROPHIC		+ (1st M.C. ++)		+						(+) (Scoliosis)			
METATROPIC		+			Dumb-bell			+		++			
KNIEST		+			Dumb-bell					(+)			
FIBROCHONDROGENESIS	+	+			Dumb-bell			++		++			
CHONDRODYSPLASIA PUNCTATA		rhizo. (+)											stippled ectopic calcification
OSTEOPETROSIS							▲						▲ +
PYCNODYSOSTOSIS							▲						▲ +
SHORT RIB SYNDROMES I Saldino-Noonan	+	+				+		++				+	
II Majewski	+	meso.			Oval Tibia	+		++					
III Verma-Naumoff	+	+				+		++				+	
Beemer	+	meso.				(+)		++					
Asphyxiating Thoracic (Jeune)		(+)				(+)		++				+	
Ellis van Creveld		meso.				+		++				+	
Atelosteogenesis I	+	rhizo.	+	+	Fib. ▼			+		+		+	
II	+	rhizo.		+	Fib. ▼								
III		rhizo.		+	(Fib. ▼)								
Boomerang / De La Chappelle	+	+	+		Fib. ▼			+		+	(+)	(+)	
Opsismodysplasia		+						+		+	+	+	
Schneckenbecken	+	+			Dumb-bell			+			+	+	
Dyssegmental Dysplasia I		+	+					+					
II	+	+	+					+					

All these findings should be easily observed by the non-specialist

†   Grouped according to main radiographic features and (approximately) in descending order of frequency.

⋆   Short limbs can be identified on ultrasound by 20 weeks gestation in the lethal conditions and a few non-lethal.

( )   In parenthesis – the finding may be present but mild, or absent.

▼ – indicates: 'reduced, short, hypoplastic or absent'.

▲ – indicates: 'increased, dense'.

Tissues should be stored from all these severe skeletal dysplasias to enable confirmatory genetic testing and/or prenatal diagnosis. Cryopreserved fibroblasts are suggested.

An approach to the radiological diagnosis of lethal and other skeletal dysplasias presenting at birth. (A chart prepared by R. Wynne-Davies C.M. Hall and J. Hurst for the Skeletal Dysplasia Group for Teaching and Research, Occasional publication no. 8c (2004).)

THE NON-LETHAL

DIAGNOSTIC GROUPS †	X-ray <2yrs ▼	X-ray 2yr over ▲	Stature: Increased	Trunk	Limbs	Rhizo.	Mesomelic	Size	Density	Suture Fusion (Early ▲ / Late ▼ / Wormian W)	Facial Bones	Mandible	Scoliosis/Kyphosis	Persistent Ovoid	Platyspondyly	Odontoid Dysplasia
I MULTIPLE EPIPHYS: DYS:		▲			(+)										(T.11, 12)	
HERED: ARTHRO: OPHTH:	▼	▲									▼	(▼)	(+)		+	
CHONDRO: PUNCTATA (Severe & mild forms)	▼	▲			+	(+)	(+)				(▼)		+			
(Conradi)					(Aysym:)											
II SPONDYLO-EPIPHYS: Congenita	▼			+	+	(+)					(▼)		(+)	+	+	+
Tarda – X Linked		▲		+									(+)		+	
– Dom: Rec.		▲		+									(+)		+	
– Progressive arth:		▲		(+)									(+)		+	
III METAPHYS: DYS: – SCHMID		▲			Lower									(+)		
– McKUSICK	(▼)	▲			+				(▲)					(+)		(+)
– JANSEN	▼			+	+			▼	▲	(▲)	+					
– with MALABSORP:, NEUTROPEN:		▲														
SPONDYLO-METAPHYSEAL DYS:		▲		+										(+)	+	
IV ACHONDROPLASIA	▼				+	+		▲			▼		T-L Kyphos		·	
HYPOCHONDROPLASIA		▲			+	+		(▲)			(▼)					
DYSCHONDROSTEOSIS		▲			+		+									
ACROMESOMELIA	▼				+		+				(▼)		(+)		(+)	
ACRODYSOSTOSIS		▲			(+)		(+)		(▲)		(▼)					
V PSEUDOACHONDROPLASIA		▲		+	+									+	(+) (Triangular)	(+)
DIASTROPHIC DYSPLASIA	▼			+	+								+	(+)	+	
METATROPIC DYSPLASIA	▼			+	+							(	+		++	(+)
KNIEST DISEASE	▼			+	+						▼		+		(+)	(+)
DYGGVE-MELCHIOR CLAUSEN		▲		+	+			(▼)							+	(+)
CHONDRO: ECTO: (Ellis van Creveld)	▼			(+)	+		+					Teeth ▼				
ASPHYX: THOR: DYS (Jeune)	▼	▲		(+)	+											
VIII STORAGE DISEASES																
MPS – Hurler	▼			+	+			▲	▲	Sag: ▲		Condyles ▼	(T-L Kyphos)	+	Hooked	(+)
– Hunter		▲		+	+			(▲)	(▲)				T-L Kyphos	+	Hooked	(+)
– Scheie		▲														
– Sanfilippo		▲							(▲)					+		
– Mannosidosis		▲						▲					(T-L Kyphos)			
– Maroteaux-Lamy		▲		+	+			(▲)	(▲)	Sag: ▲		Condyles ▼	T-L Kyphos	+	Hooked	(+)
– Morquio		▲		+	+								T-L Kyphos	+	Early Hooked / Later Tongued	++
MLS – GM, Gangliosidosis Type 1	▼	▲		+	+			▲	▲	▲		Condyles ▼	T-L Kyphos	+	Hooked	
IX METABOLIC BONE DISEASE																
HYPOPHOSPHATASIA	▼	▲		(+)	(+)				▲							
HYPERPHOSPHATASIA		▲		(+)	(+)			▲	▲							
HYPOPHOSPHATAEMIC RICKETS		▲			+			(▲)	(▲)	(▲)			(+)			
PSEUDO-HYPOPARATHYROID:		▲		(+)	(+)			Ectopic Cal:								
X DECREASED BONE DENSITY																
OSTEOGEN: IMPERFECTA	▼	▲		(+)	(+)			▲	(Platybasia) ▼	W ▼	▼	(Teeth)	(+)		Biconcave (+)	
IDIOPATH: JUV: OSTEOPOROSIS		▲		(+)											(+)	
OSTEOLYSIS (Hajdu Cheney)		▲							(Platybasia) ▼	W ▼						
(CLEIDOCRANIAL DYS:)		▲		(+)	(+)			▲	(▼)	W ▼			(+)			
XI SCLEROSING BONE DYSPLASIAS																
OSTEOPETROSIS – Severe	▼			+	+				▲ *			Infection				
– Mild		(▲)							(▲)							
PYCNODYSOSTOSIS	▼	▲		+	+				▲	W ▼	▼	▼ Infection				
CRANIO-METAPHYSEAL	▼							▲	▲ *		▲	▲ Teeth				
PYLE'S METAPHYSEAL DYS:		▲	(+)						▲							
FRONTO-METAPHYSEAL		▲		(+)	(+)			Frontal ▲	▲			(▼)	Segmental anomalies			
MELNICK NEEDLES		▲	(+)						▲			(▼)	(+)			
ENGELMANN		(▲)	(+)					▲	▲							
CRANIO-DIAPHYSEAL	▼			(+)	(+)			▲	▲ *		▲	▲				
OSTEOPATHIA STRIATA		(▲)							▲ *							

XII TUMOUR-LIKE DISORDERS
Diaphyseal aclasis, Ollier, Maffucci, dysplasia epiphysealis hemimelica, fibro dysplasia (myositis) ossificans progressiva, polyostotic fibious dysplasia, melorheostosis: nearly always

†   – "Lethal dwarfs" – see separate sheet; "increased limb length" – omitted
▲▼ – increase / decrease over normal
★   – wherever skull base is involved there may be cranial nerve compression

SKELETAL DYSPLASIAS

PRINCIPAL RADIOLOGICAL FEATURES

Other	Cage	Ribs	Clavicle	Wings (Ilium)	Base (Ilium)	Acetab: Under-developed ▼ / Protrusio: ▲	Epiphysis	Metaphysis	Diaphysis	Coxa vara	Malalignment	Wrist / Hands	Ossification: Advanced ▲ / Delayed ▼	Principal Associated Anomalies or Complications	Further Invest: (Radiology / Haematology / Biochemistry / Genetic)
						(▼) (▲)	+	(+)		(+)	+	(+)	▼		(G)
							+	Infancy: dumb-bell						Cleft palate. Myopia. Hearing ▼	(G)
Coronal															
Clefts							(+)	(Cupped)				(+)	Punctate Calcif:	Cataract; heart; skin lesions	B.
	Carinatum			▼			+ (less distally)	+		++			▼ (Hip)	Cleft palate; Myopia	R. (Cl.2)
Post. Vert. lump							+								(G)
							+					(MC ▼)			
							+				Contracture	+ ('Rheumatoid')	▲		
								+		+					B. (? rickets)
		▲ ant						+				▼		Blood ▼, Hair ▼	B.H.
							▲	++		(+)	+	+		Hearing ▼, Fractures	B.
		Infant ▼						+		+			▼	Cyclical neutropenia	B.H.
					▲			+		(+)					
Pedicles ▼	(▼)	(▼)		▼	Spur			+		(+)	Tib / Fib	+		Spinal stenosis	G.
								(+)			Tib / Fib	(+)			G.
											+	Disl. ulna ('Madelung')			G.
Pedicles ▼					▼			+			+	▼			
Pedicles ▼					▼							▼	▲ Hands		(G)
	Post cupping				▼	▼	++	++			+	▼	▼ (Hips)	(Gross joint laxity)	(G)
Pedicles (▼)				(▲)			+	+		(+)	Contracture	▼ 1st MC	▲ ▼	Cleft palate	R. (Cl.2) G.
	▼	▼		▼			(+)	Dumb-bell	▼		+		▼		(G)
Coronal Clefts	▼			▼	▼		(+)	▲				(+)	▲	Cleft palate; myopia; hearing	(G)
	Carinatum			Lace like			(+)	+					▼	(Mental retard:)	(G)
		▼ (improves later) ▼		(▼)	Spike					(+)	Fusion capit/ham Post-ax. poly.		(▲) Infant	Heart; hair ▼	(G)
		▼ (improves later) ▼		(▼)	Spike				(+)		(Post-ax. poly.)		(▲) Infant	(Nephritis)	(G)
		All May: — Med: ▲		▲	▼	▼	+	+	▲	(c. valga)	Hip dislocation contractures	Modelling ▼ MC 2-5 pointed bases		Mental retard:	B.G.
		Med: (▲)		▲	▼	▼	+	+	▲	(c. valga)	Contracture	As Hurler		Mental retard:	B.G.
											Contracture	Contracture			B.(G)
		Ant ▲		(▲)	(▼)	(▼)					Contracture			Mental retard:	B
		Post ▼		(▲)	(▼)	(▼)								Mental retard:	B.(G)
		Med: ▲		▲	▼	▼	+	+	▲	(c. valga)	Contracture	As Hurler			B.(G)
Carinatum		Med: ▲		▲	▼	▼	+	+		(c. valga)	G.valgum ++	As Hurler but well modelled	▲ Hip-early ▼ Hip-late	Joint laxity; Atlanto-axial instability	R. (Cl.2) B.(G)
		Med: (▲)		▲	▼	▼			+	(c. valga)		As Hurler		Periosteal cloaking	R.
							+	(+)			+		▼	Fractures	B.(G)
		▲ Dense				▲			▲	+	+	Modelling ▼		Fractures	B.
		'rosary'				(▲)		Cupped		(+)	+		▼ prem. fusion	Fractures	B.(G)
Pedicles ▼												MC 3, 4, 5 ▼		Hypocalcaemia	B.(G)
		(Beaded)		(Trefoil)			▲				+		▼	Fractures (Blue Sclerai) (Deafness)	(G)
													▼	Fractures	
	▼	Thin					(▲)				+	T.P. ▼	▼	Fractures	
Fusion delayed			▼	(Pubic symph: wide)								T.P. ▼	▼	(Pseudarthroses)	(G)
	(▲)	(▲)		Arcuate bands			▲					'Bone-in-Bone'		Fractures; Pancytopenia	(G)
Sandwich	(▲)	(▲)		Arcuate bands										(Fractures)	(B)
	+	▼			▼							T.P. ▼		Fractures	(G)
	(▲)	▲							▲	(early) ▲		Modelling ▼		Fractures	
		Med: ▲							▲			Modelling ▼			
	▼ Constrict;			Grooved ▼					▼		Wavy	Modelling ▼		Cosmetic only	
	▼ Constrict;			Grooved ▼	▲				▼	Constric:	Wavy	T.P. ▼			(G)
	(▲)	▲								▲				Pain; Muscle weakness	
	▲	▲								▲		Modelling ▼			
									Striations						

diagnosed over the age of 2 years; all are asymmetrical with shortening and/or malalignment confined to the affected part, with patchy sclerosis. Malignant change is rare, except in Maffucci.

Staging of puberty

See 'Centile charts for height, weight, and occipital-frontal circumference (OFC)' in this appendix. The staging below is taken from Tanner (1962).

Girls: pubertal stages (98th–2nd centiles)

Breast development

Stage 1   Pre-adolescent: elevation of papilla only.

Stage 2   Breast bud stage: elevation of breast and papilla as small mound. Enlargement of areola diameter (8.2–13.8 years).

Stage 3   Further enlargement and elevation of breast and areola, with no separation of their contours (9.7–14.3 years).

Stage 4   Projection of areola and papilla to form a secondary mound above the level of the breast (10.5–15.7 years).

Pubic hair

Stage 1   Pre-adolescent: the vellus over the pubes is not further developed than that over the abdominal wall, i.e. no pubic hair.

Stage 2   Sparse growth of long slightly pigmented downy hair, straight or slightly curled, chiefly along labia (9.4–14.4 years).

Stage 3   Considerably darker, coarser, and more curled. The hair spreads sparsely over the junction of the pubes (10.2–15.2 years).

Stage 4   Hair now adult in type, but the area covered is still considerably smaller than in the adult. No spread to the medial surface of the thighs (11.2–16 years).

Stage 5   Adult in quantity and type.

Menarche

11–15 years (98th–2nd centiles); 10.3–15.7 year (99.6th–0.4th centile).

Boys: pubertal stages (98th–2nd centiles)

Genital (penis) development

Stage 1   Pre-adolescent: testes, scrotum, and penis are of about the same size and proportion as in early childhood.

Stage 2   Enlargement of scrotum and testes. Skin of scrotum reddens and changes in texture. Little or no enlargement of the penis at this stage (9.8–14.2 years).

Stage 3   Enlargement of the penis, which occurs at first mainly in length; further growth of testes and scrotum (11.1–14.3 years).

Stage 4   Increased size of penis with growth and breadth and development of glans. Testes and scrotum larger; scrotal skin darkened (12.1–15.9 years).

Stage 5   Genitalia adult in size and shape.

Pubic hair

Stage 1   Pre-adolescent: The vellus over the pubes is not further developed than that over the abdominal wall, i.e. no pubic hair

Stage 2   Sparse growth of long slightly pigmented downy hair, straight or slightly curled, chiefly at the base of the penis (10.3–14.2 years).

Stage 3   Considerably darker, coarser, and more curled. The hair spreads sparsely over the junction of the pubes (11.1–14.9 years).

Stage 4   Hair now adult in type, but the area covered is still considerably smaller than in the adult. No spread to the medial surface of the thighs (12.1–15.9 years).

Stage 5   Adult in quantity and type.

References

Child Growth Foundation. *Boys four-in-one growth charts*. Harlow Printing Ltd, 1996.

Child Growth Foundation. *Girls four-in-one growth charts*. Harlow Printing Ltd, 1996.

Tanner JM. *Growth at adolescence*, 2nd edn. Blackwell Scientific, Oxford, 1962.

Index

N.B. 'f' following a page locator indicates a figure and 't' indicates a table.

A

3C (craniocerebellocardiac) syndrome (Ritscher–Schinzel syndrome) 67
22q11 deletion syndrome 76, 85, 175, 183, 366, 490–2, 521
  see also del (22q11), DiGeorge syndrome, Shprintzen or velocardiofacial syndrome (VCFS)
45, X/46, XY 544
46, XX/46, XY 544
47, XXX (Triple X syndrome) 494
47, XXY (Klinefelter syndrome) 496–7
47, XYY (XYY syndrome) 498–9
Aagenaes syndrome (cholestasis–lymphoedema syndrome) 198
Aarskog syndrome (faciogenital dysplasia) 57, 196–7, 224, 243
abdominal wall defects, anterior 566–7
abetalipoproteinaemia 53, 232, 233
acanthosis nigricans 211
achalasia–addisonianism–alacrima (AAA) syndrome (Allgrove syndrome) 264
achondrogenesis 631
achondroplasia 57, 136, 260–1, 631
achromatopsia 190, 406
acricephaly 212
acrocallosal syndrome (Schinzel syndrome) 215, 219, 249, 250
acrocephalopolysyndactyly type II (Carpenter syndrome) 219, 289
acrodysostosis 57
acrofacial dysostosis 229
  with limb defects 153
acromesomelic dysplasia (AMD) 57
Adams–Oliver syndrome 153, 236
Addison disease 264
adenosine deaminase deficiency 364
adoption 2–3
  genetic issues relating to 2–3
  genetic testing of children 29
ADPKD (adult polycystic kidney disease) 624, 625
adrenoleukodystrophy 97, 264
  see also X-linked adrenoleukodystrophy (X-ALD)
adrenomyeloneuropathy 264
adult cerebral adrenoleukodystrophy 264
AEG syndrome (anophthalmia–oesophageal–genital syndrome) 177, 201
aganglionic megacolon (Hirschsprung disease) 352–3
agenesis of the corpus callosum 248–9
agnathia–holoprosencephaly (agnathia–HPE) 131
Aicardi syndrome 83
Aicardi–Goutieres syndrome 107, 151
Alagille syndrome 86, 221
albinism 126–7, 190
albinoidism 126
Albright hereditary osteodystrophy (AHO) 57, 161, 193
alcohol, cancer risks 462
Alexander disease 97, 150, 163
Allgrove syndrome (achalasia–addisoninism–alacrima (AAA) syndrome) 264
alobar holoprosencephaly 130
alpha-1 antitrypsin deficiency 220–1, 266–7
Alport syndrome 268–9
Alstrom syndrome 61, 190, 194, 233

amblyopia 100, 224
amelogenesis imperfecta 257–8
amenorrhoea, female infertility and 586–7
amniocentesis 602
amniotic bands 153
amyoplasia 49
anaesthetic agents, sensitivity to 410–11
anal anomalies 42–4
anal atresias 42, 43
androgen insensitivity syndrome 270–1, 586
anencephaly 392, 395f
  recurrence risks 394f
aneuploidy 610
Angelman syndrome (del 15q11) 53, 127, 173, 272–3, 408, 521
angiofibromata 420
angiotensin-converting enzyme inhibitors (ACE inhibitors), in pregnancy 584
aniridia 46
anocerebrodigital syndrome (Pallister–Hall syndrome) 43, 131, 215
anomalies, minor congenital 180
anophthalmia 176–8
anophthalmia–oesophageal–genital syndrome (AEG syndrome) 171, 201
anterior segment eye malformations 46–7
  see also glaucoma
aortic root dimensions, normal range 684–6
APC (adenomatous polyposis coli) mutations 445
Apert syndrome 254–5, 289
aplasia cutis congenita 236–7
apple peel syndrome 202
arachnoid cysts 135, 249, 643
ARC syndrome 49, 222
Arnold–Chiari malformations 135
ARPKD (autosomal recessive polycystic kidney disease) 624, 625
arrhythmogenic right ventricular cardiomyopathy (ARVC) 361, 378–9
arrhythmogenic right ventricular dysplasia (ARVD) 361, 378–9
arthrogryposis (arthrogryposis multiplex congenita) 48–9, 123
arthrogryposis multiplex congenita–spinal muscular atrophy association 49
ARX (Aristaless related homeobox) gene abnormalities 165
Ashkenazi jews 444
  colorectal cancer in 436
Asperger syndrome 275
asphyxiating thoracic dystrophy (Jeune syndrome) 215
asplenia syndrome 148
assisted reproductive technology (ART) 568–70
association, definition 4
ataxia
  in adults 50–1
  in children 52–4
Ataxia telangiectasia 51, 304, 305
ataxic cerebral palsy 53, 70, 71
athetoid cerebral palsy 70, 71
ATR-16 syndrome (del 16p) 549
ATR-X syndrome (X-linked α-thalassaemia mental retardation syndrome) 165, 182, 272
atresia, oesophageal and intestinal 200–2
attenuated familial adenomatous polyposis (FAP) 444
autism 97, 166, 274–6
autism spectrum disorders 274–6

autoimmune polyendocrinopathy–candidiasis–ectodermal dystrophy (APECED) 620
autosomal dominant (AD) disorders 6–7, 50
autosomal dominant chondrodysplasia punctata 73
autosomal dominant Emery–Dreifuss muscular dystrophy 375
autosomal dominant HPE 131
autosomal dominant polycystic kidney disease 262–3
autosomal dominant retinitis pigmentosa 407
autosomal recessive (AR) inheritance 8–9
autosomal recessive disorders, carrier frequency and carrier testing 650–1
autosomal recessive hypercholesterolaemia (ARH) 358
autosomal recessive immunodeficiencies 367t
autosomal recessive polycystic kidney disease 262
autosomal recessive retinal dysplasia 230
autosomal reciprocal translocations
  background 500–2
  familial 504
  postnatal 506
  prenatal 508–9
Axenfeld–Rieger syndromes 46

B

bad news, breaking 10
Baller–Gerold syndrome 228
Bannayan–Riley–Ruvalcaba syndrome 211, 442
Bannayan–Riley–Ruvalcaba/Cowden syndrome 160, 162, 207
Bardet–Biedl syndrome 193, 215, 232, 625
Barth syndrome 61
Bartter syndrome 117
basal cell naevus syndrome (Gorlin syndrome) 162, 452–3
Batten disease 233
Baye's theorem 646–7
Beal syndrome (congenital contractural arachnodactyly) 380
Beare–Stevenson syndrome 289
Becker disease 389
Becker muscular dystrophy 302, 308–11, 323, 374
Beckwith–Wiedemann syndrome 61, 79, 128, 141, 206, 278, 487, 625
behavioural pattern profiles 648–9
Beighton scoring system 138
benign childhood epilepsy with centrotemporal spikes (BCECTS) 315
benign familial chorea 354
benign familial haematuria 269
benign familial neonatal–infantile seizures 315
benign joint hypermobility syndrome 138–9, 313
Bethlem myopathy 376
bilateral acoustic neurofibromatosis (neurofibromatosis type 2) 65, 160, 210, 397, 470–1
bilateral periventricular nodular heterotopia 166
biliary atresia 220
Binder syndrome 73, 182
biotinidase deficiency 188
bladder exstrophy 566
blepharophimosis 224

Blepharophimosis–ptosis–epicanthus inversus syndrome 225, 620
Blomstrand dysplasia 144
Bloom syndrome 304, 305, 487
blue cone monochromatism, X-linked 190
body wall complex (body stalk anomaly) 566
bone density, increased 144–5
bone marrow transplantation, HLA tissue typing for 569
BOR syndrome (branchiootorenal syndrome) 92, 109, 113, 262, 624
Börjeson–Forssman–Lehmann syndrome 165
Boston craniosynostosis 289
Bourneville disease (tuberous sclerosis) 208, 239, 262, 275, 420–3
bowed limbs 572–3
boys, pubertal stages 698
brachycephaly 212
brachydactyly 56–7
   type B 58
   type D 58
   type E 58
branchiooculofacial syndrome (Haemangiomatous branchial cleft syndrome) 83
branchio-otorenal syndrome 92, 109, 113, 262, 624
BRCA1 and *BRAC2* 426–9
BRCA1 and *BRCA2* mutations, likelihood of identifying 432t
breast cancer 426, 427, 428, 430–3
   criteria for evaluating a family history of 432t
   in men 430
breast MRI 434–5
breast surveillance 434–5
brittle bone disease (osteogenesis imperfecta) 122
broad thumbs 58–9
Bruck syndrome 123
Brugada syndrome 378–9
Bruton disease (X-linked agammaglobulinaemia) 365
butyrylcholinesterase deficiency 410

C

CADASIL 296
café au lait spots 210
campomelic dysplasia 39, 572
Camurati–Englemann syndrome 145
Canavan disease 97, 150, 163
cancer 425–88
   confirmation of diagnosis 440
   lifestyle factors 462
   patterns of 690–2
   surveillance methods 434–5
Cantu syndrome 79
carbamazepine, and fetal anticonvulsant syndrome 591
carbimazole, in pregnancy 584
carbimazole/methimazole embryopathy 183
carbohydrate-deficient glycoprotein syndrome 67, 180, 233
cardiac rhabdomyoma, isolated 421
cardiofaciocutaneous syndrome 61, 117, 163, 402
cardiomyopathy, dilated 302–3
Carey–Fineman–Ziter syndrome 254
Carmi syndrome 236
Carney complex 160, 467, 470
carnitine deficiency 61
Carpenter syndrome (acrocephalopoly-syndactyly type II) 219, 289
carrier status, testing for 28–9
cat-eye syndrome 43, 82, 109, 177, 552
cataracts 64–5
catecholaminergic polymorphic ventricular tachycardia 379
caudal regression 43
CD40 ligand deficiency (X-linked hyper-IgM syndrome) 365
cell division 510–13

Cenani–Lenz syndrome 255
centile charts for head circumference
   boys 0–18 years 660
   girls 0–18 years 661
centile charts for height, weight and head circumference 652–61
   boys 0–1 yr 653
   boys 0–20 yrs 655
   boys 1–5 yrs 654
   boys pre-term 652
   girls 0–1 yr 657
   girls 0–20 yrs 659
   girls 1–5 yrs 658
   girls pre-term 656
central neurofibromatosis (neurofibromatosis type 2) 65, 160, 210, 397, 470–1
central-core disease 410
cerebellar anomalies 66–8
cerebellar ataxia, autosomal dominant 191
cerebellar haemangioblastoma 485
cerebellar vermis aplasia 66
cerebello-oculo-renal syndromes 67
cerebral adrenoleukodystrophy
   adolescent 264
   childhood 264
cerebral palsy 70–1
cerebrooculofacioskeletal syndrome (COFS) 49, 65, 177, 304, 305
cerebrocostomandibular syndrome (Rib-gap syndrome) 175
Charcot–Marie–Tooth disease (hereditary motor and sensory neuropathy) 344–6, 349
CHARGE syndrome 82, 86, 109, 113, 177, 201
Charlevoix-Saguenay syndrome 53
Chediak–Higashi syndrome 127, 365
Chemotherapy 622
Chiari II malformation 66, 392
Chiari malformations 66
chickenpox (varicella) 640
CHILD syndrome 73
childhood ataxia with central hypomyelination 151
children
   with ataxia 52–4
   cardiomyopathy in under-10s 60–2
   developmental regression 96–8
   with dysmorphic features 102–4
   genetic testing for 29
   severe deafness in early childhood 90–3
choanal atresia 183
choledochal cysts 220
cholestasis–lymphoedema syndrome (Aagenaes syndrome) 198
cholesterol biosynthetic defects 188
chondrodysplasia punctata 65, 72–3
choriocarcinoma 556
chorion villus sampling, and placental biopsy 600
choroideraemia 233
chromosomal mosaicism 210
   postnatal 514–15
   prenatal 516–19
chromosomes 489–563
   haploid autosomal lengths 676
   ring 538–9
chronic granulomatous disease 365
chronic progressive external ophthalmoplegia (CPEO) 385
classical lissencephaly (type I lissencephaly) 156
cleft lip and palate 74–7
cleidocranial dysostosis 147
Clouston syndrome 257
clover leaf skull (Kleeblattschaedel) 212
club-foot (talipes) 574
coagulation disorders, inherited 338–40
cobblestone lissencephaly (type II lissencephaly) 156
cocaine, in pregnancy 584
cochlear implants 93
Cockayne syndrome 97, 233, 304, 305
Coffin–Lowry syndrome 79, 165
Coffin–Siris syndrome 79, 257

COFS (cerebrooculofacialskeletal syndrome) 49, 65, 177, 304, 305
Cohen syndrome 193, 233
coloboma 82–3
colobomatous microphthalmia 82
   and clefting 177
   non-syndromic 177
colonoscopy 434
colorectal adenomas 436, 444
colorectal cancer 436–8
   family history criteria for risk groups 437t
   odds ratio and lifetime risk of dying from 437t
   see also familial adenomatous polyposis; hereditary nonpolyposis colorectal cancer (HNPCC)
colour blindness 190
common variable immunodeficiency (CVID) 365
complete hydatidiform mole 556
conductive deafness 90
cone dystrophy 232
confidentiality, of genetic information 12
confined placental mosaicism 516
congenital absence of uterus and vagina (CAUV) 586
congenital adrenal hyperplasia (CAH) 39, 282–3, 586
congenital adrenal hypoplasia 282
congenital agranulocytosis (Kostmann syndrome) 365–6
congenital anomalies, minor 180
congenital bilateral absence of the vas deferens (CBAVD) 606
congenital contractural arachnodactyly (Beal syndrome) 380
congenital contractural archnodactyly 49
congenital cystic lung lesions 576
congenital diaphragmatic hernia 578–9
congenital fibrosis of the extraocular muscles 224
congenital heart disease 84–7
   maternal illness and the risk of 84t
   teratogens and the risk of 84t
congenital hydrocephalus 134–6
congenital idiopathic motor nystagmus 191
congenital insensitivity to pain with anhidrosis (CIPA) 252
congenital intestinal aganglionosis (Hirschsprung disease) 352–3
congenital leptin deficiency 194
congenital limb defects, classification 152
congenital magnesium malabsorption 188
congenital malformation, consultation with a child with 4–5
congenital myopathy 119
congenital myotonic dystrophy 119, 388
congenital rubella syndrome 628
congenital urethral obstruction 625
connexin 26 90
connexin 30 90
conotruncal anomaly face syndrome (22q11 deletion syndrome) 85, 175, 366, 490–2
Conradi–Hünermann syndrome (X-linked dominant chondrodysplasia punctata) 72
consanguinity 284–6
   developmental delay in the child with consanguineous parents 94–5
contiguous gene deletion involving *TSC2-ADPK1* 421
conversion charts, from English to metric units for height and weight 664–5
convulsions
   benign familial neonatal 315
   benign neonatal 188
corneal clouding 47, 88–9
corneal dystrophies 88
de Lange syndrome 154, 578, 631
corpus callosum, agenesis of the 248–9
Costello syndrome 61, 79, 117, 163, 207, 402–3
Cowden syndrome 442–3

craniodiaphyseal dysplasia 144
craniofrontonasal dysplasia 183, 196, 289
craniometaphyseal dysplasia 144, 145
craniosynostosis syndromes 113, 136, 213, 288–90
creatine kinase, levels in carriers of Duchenne muscular dystrophy 662
Cri du chat syndrome (del 5p) 548
Crigler–Najjar types 1 and 2 221
Cross syndrome 127
cross-linking agent repair 304
Crouzon syndrome 183, 289
cryptophthalmos 176, 224
Currarino syndrome 43, 576
cutis laxa 313
cyclic neutropenia 366
cystic fibrosis 202, 292–4
  male infertility and 293, 606
  pregnancy in women with 293–4
cystic hygroma 618
cystinosis 127
cytogenetic diagnoses, subtle rearrangements 602
cytomegalovirus (CMV) 580–1

D

Dandy–Walker malformation (DWM) 66, 582
dating ultrasound scanning, for prenatal diagnosis 598
de Grouchy syndrome (del 18q) 549
de Lange syndrome, mild 243
de Morsier's syndrome (septo-optic dysplasia) 204, 243, 249
deafness 268
  due to mutations in mitochondrial DNA 90
  severe deafness in early childhood 90–3
del (1p36) 548
del (1p44) 548
del (2p) 548
del (2q) 548
del (2q37) 57, 255
del (3p) 548
del (3q) 548
del (4p) (Wolf–Hirschhorn syndrome) 82, 173, 183, 548
del (4q) 548
del (5p) (cri du chat syndrome) 548
del (5q) 548
del (15q11–13) (Prader–Willi syndrome) 117, 119, 127, 192–3, 521
del (6p) 548
del (6q) 548
del (7p) 548
del (7q) 548
del (7q11.23) (Williams syndrome) 79, 85, 117, 402, 521
del (8p) 548
del (8q) 548
del (8q24) (Langer–Giedion syndrome) 161, 521
del (9p) 548
del (9q) 548
del (10p) 549
del (10q) 549
del (11p) 549
  del (11p13) WAGR 39, 143, 486, 521
del (12p) 549
del (13q) 549
del (14q) 549
del (15q) 549
del (15q11) (Angelman syndrome) 53, 127, 173, 272–3, 408, 521
del (16p) (ATR-16 syndrome) 549
del (16q) 549
del (17p11.2) Smith–Magenis syndrome 57, 79, 193, 521
del (17p13.3) (Miller–Dieker syndrome) 157, 158, 521, 549
del (17q) 549
del (18p) 549
del (18q) (de Grouchy syndrome) 549

del (19p) 549
del (19q) 549
del (20p) 549
del (20q) 549
del (21q) 549
del (22q11.2) DiGeorge syndrome 76, 85, 175, 183, 366, 490–2, 521
del (22q13.3) 207, 272, 549
del (Xp) 549
del (Xq) 549
del (11p13) WAGR 39, 143, 486, 521
deletions 520–2
  molecular diagnosis 602
Delleman syndrome (oculocerebrocutaneous syndrome) 113, 236
dementia 296–7
dental pits 420
dentatorubropallidoluysian atrophy (DRPLA) 50, 354
dentinogenesis imperfecta 258
Denver Developmental Screening Test 666
Denys–Drash syndrome 486
developmental delay
  in child with consanguineous parents 94–5
  consultation with a child with 4–5
  obesity with and without 192–4
  seizures with 238–40
developmental regression 96–8
diabetes, maturity-onset diabetes of the young 299
diabetes mellitus 298–300, 331
diabetes mellitus and diabetic embryopathy, maternal 612–13
diagnosis
  communicating a 10
  confirmation of 14
Diamond–Blackfan anaemia 219, 228
diastematomyelia 392
diastrophic dysplasia (dwarfism) 631
DiGeorge syndrome 366, 521
  see also 22q11 deletion syndrome, Shprintzen or Velocardiofacial syndrome (VCFS)
diploid mosaicism 514
diploid triploid mosaicism 255, 556
distal arthrogryposis type 1 49
distal spinal muscular atrophy 346, 412
dizygotic twins (non-identical twins) 636–7
DNA repair defects 65, 117, 172–3, 304–7, 366
dolicocephaly 212
dominant-negative mutation 19
Donnai–Barrow syndrome 578
Donohue syndrome (leprechaunism) 79, 117, 299
DOOR syndrome 219, 257
dopa-responsive dystonia (Segawa syndrome) 107, 349, 405
doublecortin 157
Down syndrome (trisomy 21) 524–5
Drash syndrome 39–40, 143
drugs, in pregnancy 584–5
Duane radial ray syndrome (Okihiro syndrome) 100, 153, 228
Duane retraction syndrome (Duane anomaly) 100
Dubowitz syndrome 117, 225
Duchenne muscular dystrophy 308–11
  creatine kinase levels in carriers 662
duplications 520–2
dysmorphic children 102–4
dysmorphism, consultation with a child with 4–5
dysmorphology
  definition 4
  examination checklist 670
dysosteosclerosis 145
dysplasia 4
dysraphism 392
dystonia 106–7
dystrophica myotonica (myotonic dystrophy) 65, 161, 224, 322, 388–90

E

ear anomalies 108–10
ear tags and pits 180
echogenic bowel (hyperechogenic bowel) 594
ectrodactyly, autosomal dominant 154
ectrodactyly–ectodermal dysplasia–clefting syndrome (EEC syndrome) 76, 154, 257
Edwards' syndrome (trisomy 18) 526–7
EEC syndrome (ectrodactyly–ectrodermal dysplasia–clefting syndrome) 76, 154, 257
Ehlers–Danlos syndrome 138–9, 312–13
  hypermobility type 380
  vascular type 380
Ellis–van Creveld syndrome 215
embryonic fetal development, overview 672–3
Emery–Dreifuss muscular dystrophy 302, 323, 375
EMG syndrome (Beckwith–Wiedemann syndrome) 61, 79, 128, 141, 206, 278, 487, 625
emphysema 266
encephalocele 392
encephalopathy, neonatal 186–9
enchondromatosis 161
endocrine abnormalities 141
endosteal hyperostosis 145
endrometrial surveillance 434
Englemann syndrome 145
epicanthic folds 180
epidermolysis bullosa dystrophica 237
epidermolysis bullosa-pyloric atresia 201, 236
epilepsy 238–40, 318–20
  classification 318t
  epileptic seizure classification 318t
  in infants and children 314–16
epiloia (tuberous sclerosis) 208, 239, 262, 275, 420–3
episodic ataxia 50
epispadias 142
espressivitiy 6
Evans myopathy 410
exercise, cancer risk reduction 462
exomphalos (omphalocele) 566
eyelid anomalies 224–6
eyes
  anterior segment eye malformations 46–7
  cataracts 64–5

F

Fabry disease 88, 361
facial asymmetry 112–14
facial features, coarse 78–80
facioauriculovertebral syndrome (Goldenhar syndrome, oculoauricularvertebral spectrum) 109, 112–13, 175, 177, 201
faciogenital dysplasia (Aarskog syndrome) 57, 196–7, 224, 243
facioscapulohumeral (facioscapuloperoneal) muscular dystrophy (FSHD) 322–3, 376
factor IX–haemophilia B 338
factor V Leiden, testing for 417t
factor VII deficiency 339
factor VIII deficiency 339
factor X deficiency 339
factor XI deficiency 339
Fahr disease 107
failure to thrive 116–17
Falconer's polygenic threshold model 24
familial adenomatous polyposis 160, 444–8, 450, 460
  see also colorectal cancer, hereditary nonpolyposis colorectal cancer
familial angiolipomatosis 160
familial brachial plexus neuropathy (hereditary neuralgic amyotrophy) 346
familial defective apoB-100 (FBD) 358
familial exudative vitreoretinopathy 230

familial hypercholesterolaemia 358
familial infiltrative fibromatosis 445
familial isolated hyperparathyroidism 467
familial macrocephaly 162
familial medullary thyroid cancer 352, 466
familial partial lipodystrophy (Dunnigan variety) 299
familial progressive intrahepatic cholestasis 221
familial Wilms tumour 486, 487
family tree sheet and symbols 674–5
Fanconi anaemia (FA) 219, 228, 304, 305–6, 487
Fanconi syndrome 631
fatty acid oxidation, and ketogenesis disorders 141
Feingold syndrome 201
female infertility and amenorrhoea 586–7
femur–fibula–ulna complex 154
fertility, pregnancy and 565–644
fetal akinesia sequence 49, 131
fetal alcohol syndrome 116–17, 177, 225, 243, 588–9
fetal anomaly scanning 598
fetal anticonvulsant syndrome 590–1
fetal echocardiography 598
fetal hydrocephalus 643
fetal hydrops 618
fetal magnetic resonance imaging 598–9
fetal sexing 598
fetomaternal alloimmunization 592–3
FG syndrome 43
fibrodysplasia ossificans progressiva 161
Filippi syndrome 255
FLAIR sequences 694
flexible sigmoidoscopy 434
Floating Harbor syndrome 183, 243
floppy infants 118–20, 139
fluconazole, in pregnancy 584
FMR1 (fragile X syndrome) 162, 163, 166, 275, 324–6
focal dermal hypoplasia (Goltz syndrome) 82, 177, 209, 236
focal dystonia 106
folinic acid-responsive seizures 188
fontanelle, large 146–7
forehead fibrous plaque 420
fostering 2–3
fractures, during childhood 122–4
fragile X pre-mutation carrier 620
fragile X pre-mutation tremor/ataxia syndrome 51
fragile X syndrome (FRAX) 162, 164, 166, 275, 324–6
Fraser syndrome 177, 225, 624
Frasier syndrome 40, 143, 486
Friedreich's ataxia (FRDA) 51, 53, 61, 346, 349, 361
frontometaphyseal dysplasia 145
frontonasal dysplasia 183, 196
frontotemporal dementia with parkinsonism, autosomal dominant 296
Fryns syndrome 88, 201, 230, 578
FSH receptor mutations 620
Fukayama congenital muscular dystrophy (FCMD) 157, 158

G

gain-of-function mutations (activating mutations) 19
galactokinase deficiency 65
galactosaemia 64, 221, 620
Gardner syndrome (familial adenomatous polyposis) 160, 444–8, 450, 460
gastric cancer 450–1
gastrointestinal surveillance 434
gastroschisis 566
geleophysic dysplasia 57
genetic code, and mutations 18–19
genetic information, confidentiality 12
genetic testing 3, 28–9

consent for 16–17
genetics consultation, communication skills 10
genitalia, ambiguous 38–41, 282
genomic imprinting 20–1
germline mosaicism 6, 32, 34
Gerstmann–Straussler disease 51
gestational trophoblastic tumour 556
Gilbert syndrome 221
Gillespie syndrome 47, 67
girls, pubertal stages 698
glaucoma 328–9, 382
    see also anterior segment eye malformations
glomus tumours, autosomal dominant 160
glucose-6-phosphate dehydrogenase deficiency 221
glutaric aciduria 252
glutaric aciduria type 1 162
glycogen storage disease 61
GM1 gangliosidosis 150, 198
GM2 gangliosidosis 150
Goldenhar syndrome (oculoauriculovertebral spectrum, facioauricolovertebral syndrome) 109, 112–13, 175, 177, 201,
Goltz syndrome (focal dermal hypoplasia) 82, 177, 209, 236
gonadal agenesis/dysgenesis 586
Gorlin syndrome 162, 452–3
Greig cephalopolysyndactyly 58, 196, 214–15, 219
Griscelli syndrome 127
Gryns 'anophthalmia plus' syndrome 177
gyrate atrophy of the choroid and retina 233

H

Haddad syndrome 352
HADHB deficiency 61
haemangiomatous branchial clefts (branchiooculofacial syndrome) 83
haemochromatosis 330–2
haemoglobin C β-thalassaemia 336–7
haemoglobin E β-thalassaemia 337
haemoglobinopathies 334–7
haemophilia 338–40
hair, unusual 256–8
Hallermann-Streiff syndrome 65, 177
hand–foot–genital syndrome 57, 143
haploid autosomal lengths 676
haploinsufficiency 19
Hardy–Weinberg equation 650
hearing aids 93
heart disease, congenital 84–7
hemiatrophy 128
hemifacial microsomia (oculoauriculovertebral spectrum) 109, 112–13,175, 177, 201
hemihyperplasia 113
hemihypertrophy
    isolated 128–9, 487
    and limb asymmetry 128–9
Hennekam syndrome 198
hereditary arthro-ophthalmopathy (Stickler syndrome) 65, 73, 76, 139, 175, 182, 380, 414–15
hereditary diffuse gastric cancer 450
hereditary haemorrhagic telangiectia (HHT) 342–3
hereditary motor and sensory neuropathy (HMSN) 344–6, 349
hereditary multiple exostoses 161
hereditary neuralgic amyotrophy (familial brachial plexus neuropathy) 346
hereditary neuropathy with liability to pressure palsies (HNPP) 346
hereditary nonpolyposis colorectal cancer, see also colorectal cancer, familial adenomatous polyposis
hereditary nonpolyposis colorectal cancer (HNPCC) 450, 454–8
    Amsterdam diagnosis criteria 456
    clinical definition 456t
    tumour risk 455t

hereditary persistence of fetal hemoglobin (HPFH) 334
hereditary spastic paraplegis (hereditary spastic paraparesis) 348–50
heredodegenerative dystonia 106
Hermansky–Pudlack syndrome 127
hernia, congenital diaphragmatic 578–9
heterotaxy 148
heterozygous β-thalassaemias 336
Hirschsprung disease 352–3
holoprosencephaly (HPE) 130–2, 642–3
holoprosencephaly polydactyly syndrome (Pseudotrisomy 13) 131
Holt–Oram syndrome 86, 153, 219, 229
homocystinuria 127, 328, 380, 417
homozygous α-thalassaemias 336
homozygous β-thalassaemias 335–6
Hoyerall–Hreidarsson syndrome (HHS) 67
HSCR (Hirschsprung disease) 352–3
Huntington disease (chorea) 50, 296, 354–6
    predictive testing 28
hyaline fibromatosis, juvenile 160
hydranencephaly 135, 643
hydrocephalus 134–6, 642, 643
hydrolethalus syndrome 214, 219, 631
hydrometacolpospolydactyly syndrome 215
hydrops 618
17β-hydroxysteroid dehydrogenase deficiency 40
hypercholesterolaemia 358
hyperechogenic bowel (hyperechoic bowel) 594
hyperechogenic (bright) kidneys 624
hyperglycinaemia, non-ketotic 187–8
hyperinsulinism, autosomal dominant 141
hyperlipidaemia 358–9
hypermobile joints 138–9
hyperostosis 144
hyperparathyroidism–jaw tumour syndrome 467, 487
hyperpyrexia 258, 410
hypertrophic (obstructive) cardiomyopathy 360–2, 378
hypochondroplasia 57, 243, 260
hypoglycaemia, in the neonate and infant 140–1
hypogonadotrophic hypogonadism 586, 607
hypohidrotic ectodermal dysplasia, X-linked 256
hypomelanosis of Ito 208, 210, 257, 514, 562
hypomelanotic macules 420
hypoparathyroidism, sensorineural deafness, renal dysplasia syndrome 92
hypophosphatasia 122, 147, 252
hypoplastic left heart syndrome 596
hypospadias 142–3
hypothalamic disorder 194
hypotonia 118, 119
hypoxic ischaemic encephalopathy 187

I

ichthyosis, X-linked 604
idic(15) (inverted duplicated chromosome 15 syndrome) 275, 552
idic(22) 552
idiopathic epilepsy 319
idiopathic hyperphosphatasia 145
idiopathic intrauterine growth retardation 116
idiopathic torsion dystonia, adult-onset 107
IFNγ receptor/interleukin 12 pathway defects 366
imaging in prenatal diagnosis 598–9
immunodeficiency and recurrent infections 364–8
immunoglobulin deficiencies, autosomal recessive 365
imprinting centres 21
in vitro fertilization (IVF) 568
incest 370
incontinentia pigmenti 209, 210, 231, 257
infantile hypophosphatasia 572, 631

infantile receptor dystrophies 406
infantile systemic hyalinosis 160
infections, immunodeficiency and recurrent 364–8
iniencephaly 392
interleukin 7 receptor alpha deficiency* 364–5
intestinal atresia, isolated 202
intracranial aneurysm 263
intracranial anomalies, structural 248–50
intracytoplasmic sperm injection (ICSI) 568
invasive techniques, and genetic tests in prenatal diagnosis 600–3
inversions 528–9
inverted duplicated chromosome 15 syndrome (idic (15)) 275, 552
inverted nipples 180
ISCN nomenclature 680–1
isolated cleft lip and palate 76
isolated tracheo-oesophageal fistula 202
isomerism 148
Ivemark syndrome 148

J

Janus-associated kinase 3 deficiency 365
jaundice, in neonates and infants 220–2
jejunal atresia (apple peel syndrome) 202
Jervell and Lange–Nielsen syndrome 378
Jeune syndrome (asphyxiating thoracic dystrophy) 215
Johanson–Blizzard syndrome 117, 183, 236
joint hypermobility 138–9
Joubert syndrome 66–7, 215, 233
juvenile haemochromatosis 330
juvenile Huntington disease 354
juvenile hyaline fibromatosis 160
juvenile myoclonic epilepsy 315
juvenile osteoporosis 122
juvenile Paget disease 145
juvenile parkinsonism, autosomal recessive 405
juvenile polyposis syndrome 460–1
juvenile X-linked retinoschisis 231

K

Kabuki syndrome 76, 82, 86, 225, 243
Kallmann syndrome 586, 607
Kartagener's syndrome 148
karyotypes 682–3
Kaufman–McKusick syndrome 215
Kearns–Sayre syndrome 233, 385
Kenny–Caffey syndrome 145
KID syndrome (Keratosis-icthyosis-deafness syndrome) 92
kidney disease 262–3, 624, 625
King–Denborough syndrome 410
kleeblattschaedel (clover leaf skull) 212
Klein–Waardenburg syndrome (WS3) 92
Klinefelter syndrome (47, XXY) 496–7, 606
Klippel–Feil anomaly (MURCS disorder) 100, 586, 624
Klippel–Trenaunay–Weber syndrome 128,198
Kniest dysplasia 414
Kostmann syndrome (congenital agranulocytosis) 365–6
Krabbe disease 107, 151
Kugelberg–Welander syndrome (SMA Type III) 412

L

Lacrimo-auriculo-dental-digital (LADD) syndrome 29, 58
lamotrigine, and fetal anticonvulsant syndrome 591
landfill sites, heritable diseases from residents living near 622

Landouzy–Dejerine muscular dystrophy (facioscapulohumeral muscular dystrophy) 322–3, 376
Langer–Giedion syndrome (del (8q24)) 161, 183, 257, 521
Laron syndrome 141
Larsen syndrome 139
laterality disorders 148–9
learning disability see mental retardation
Leber congenital amaurosis 67, 190, 406
Leber hereditary optic neuropathy 385
Leigh encephalopathy (subacute necrotizing encephalomyopathy) 372–3, 385
Leri–Weill dyschondrostosis (Leri–Weill syndrome) 243
lentigines 211
Lenz microphthalmia syndrome 177
Lenz–Majewski syndrome 144
LEOPARD syndrome 61, 211, 360, 402, 475
leprechaunism (Donohue syndrome) 79, 117, 299
leptin receptor deficiency 194
lethal multiple pterygium syndrome 579
leukocyte adhesion deficiency 365
leukodystrophy 150–1
leukoencephalopathy 150–1
Lewy body dementia 296, 404–5
Lhermitte–Duclos disease 442
Li–Fraumeni syndrome 464, 487
limbs
    hemihypertrophy and asymmetry 128–9
    limb girdle muscular dystrophies 322, 374–7
    limb reduction defects 152–4
    short 630–2
lipodystrophy syndromes 117, 299
lipomas, autosomal dominant 160
lissencephaly 119, 156–8, 239
    with cerebellar hypoplasia 67, 157, 158
lissencephaly sequence, isolated 157, 158
lithium, in pregnancy 584
lobar holoprosencephaly 130
Long QT syndrome 319, 378–9
loss-of-function mutation 19
Lowe oculo-cerebro-renal syndrome 65
lumps and bumps 160–1
lymphoedema–distichiasis syndrome 198
Lynch syndrome see hereditary nonpolyposis colorectal cancer

M

McCune–Albright syndrome 128, 210
macrocephaly 162–3
    see also overgrowth
macrocephaly–autism syndrome 163
macrocephaly–cutis marmorata telangiectatica congenital 207
macular degeneration (cone dystrophy) 232, 406
Maffucci syndrome 161
magnetic resonance imaging (MRI) 694
Majewski osteodysplastic primordial dwarfism II 183
male infertility, genetic aspects 606–8
malformation, definition 4
malignant hyperthermia 410
malignant peripheral nerve sheath tumours 399
malonyl-CoA decarboxylase deficiency 61
maple syrup urine disease 188
Marfan syndrome (MFS 1) 139, 380–3
    and ectopia lentis 328
    Ghent diagnostic criteria 381
    neonatal MFS 382
Marfan syndrome type II (MFS 2) 380
marfanoid habitus, with learning difficulties 382
Martin–Bell syndrome (fragile X syndrome) 162, 164, 166, 275, 324–6
Martinez–Frias syndrome 201
Marshall syndrome 414
maternal age, infertility and 610

maternal diabetes mellitus, and diabetic embryopathy 612–13
maternal phenylketonuria (PKU) 614–15
maternal serum oestriol 604
maternal uniparental disomy in chromosome 7, 243
maxillonasal dysplasia 182
Mayer–Rokitansky–Kuster–Hauser syndrome 586
Meacham syndrome 578
Meckel syndrome 177, 393
Meckel–Gruber syndrome 214, 625
MECP2 mutations 166
megalocornea 47
meiosis 510–11
    female 510–11
    male 511, 512f, 513f
melanocortin 4 receptor 194
MELAS syndrome 386
Melnick–Needles syndrome 144–5
Menkes syndrome 127, 252, 257
mental retardation 168–71
    with apparent X-linked inheritance 164–6
    offspring risks 170t
    recurrence risks for sibs 170t
    seizures with 238–40
MERRF syndrome 386
metabolic disorders
    investigation of lethal 678
    late-onset 296
metachromatic leukodystrophy 150
methylmalonic aciduria 61
MHC class 2 deficiency (bare lymphocyte syndrome) 365
microcephaly 172–3
microcephaly–lympoedema syndrome 198
microcornea 47
microdeletion chromosomal abnormalities 546–50
micrognathia 174–5
microlissencephaly 157
microphthalmia 176–8
    with linear skin defects 209, 236
Miller syndrome 109, 153
Miller–Dieker syndrome (MDS) 157, 158, 521, 549
Milroy primary congenital lymphoedema (Milroy disease) 198
minicore myopathy 410
minor congenital anomalies 180
miscarriages 610, 616–17
mismatch repair genes, recessive mutation 211
missense mutations 18–19
mitochondrial DNA diseases 384–7
mitochondrial inheritance 22–3
mitochondrial myopathy 323
mitochondrial respiratory chain disorders 221
mitosis 510f
MMIH syndrome 625
Moebius syndrome 100, 113, 153, 254, 389
Mohr-Majewski syndrome 215
molar-tooth sign 66
molecular karyotyping using arrays 547
moles 211
monosomy 1p36 194
monozygotic twins (identical twins) 637–8
mosaic tetrasomy 12p (Pallister–Killian syndrome) 79, 514, 518, 578
mosaic trisomy 2 516
mosaic trisomy 7 517
mosaic trisomy 8 514, 517, 530
mosaic trisomy 9 517
mosaic trisomy 13 517, 534
mosaic trisomy 15 517
mosaic trisomy 16 517, 532
mosaic trisomy 18 517, 526–7
mosaic trisomy 20 517–18
mosaic trisomy 21 518, 524–5
mosaic trisomy 22 514, 518
mosaic Turner syndrome 198, 620
mosaic variegated aneuploidy 487, 514–15

mosaicism
  postnatal chromosomal 514–15
  prenatal chromosomal 516–19
  sex chromosome 544–5
Mowat–Wilson syndrome 143, 173, 239, 249, 272, 352
MSX1 mutations and non-syndromic cleft lip and palate 76
Muenke syndrome 289
Muir–Torre syndrome 160, 454
Mulibrey-nanism syndrome 487
Müllerian aplasia 586
multicystic dysplastic kidney 624
multifactorial inheritance 24–5
multiple acyl-coA dehydrogenase deficiency 61
multiple carboxylase deficiency 188
multiple cutaneous and uterine leiomyomatosis 160
multiple endocrine neoplasia (MEN) 466–8
multiple endocrine neoplasia type 1 (MEN1) 466
multiple endocrine neoplasia type 2 (MEN2) 466
multiple endocrine neoplasia type 2A 352
multiple pregnancies, prenatal invasive techniques and genetic tests 602
multiple pterygium syndrome 224
multiple schwannomas (isolated familial schwannomatosis) 470
multisystem disease 444
MURCS disorder (Klippel–Feil anomaly) 100, 586, 624
muscle–eye–brain disease 67, 135, 157, 230, 643
muscular dystrophy 61
  congenital 119
  distribution of muscle weakness in different types of 668
mutation rates 6
mutations, genetic code and 18–19
MUTYH mutations 445
myasthenia gravis 224
myoclonic dystonia 107
myoclonic encephalopathy, early 188
myotonic dystrophy 65, 161, 224, 322, 388–90

N

naevoid basal cell carcinoma syndrome (Gorlin syndrome) 162, 452–3
naevus anaemicus 208
Nager acrofacial dysostosis (Nager syndrome) 109, 175, 229
nail patella syndrome 257, 328
nails, unusual 256–8
Nance–Horan syndrome 65
nanophthalmos (or simple microphthalmia) 176, 328
NARP (neuropathy–ataxia–retinitis pigmentosa) 386
nasal anomalies 182–4
Naxos disease 379
nemaline myopathy 322–3
neonatal alloimmune thrombocytopenia 592–3
neonatal diabetes 298
neonatal encephalopathy 186–9
neonatal haemochromatosis 221, 330
neonates, early infantile epileptic encephalopathy 188
nephroblastoma (Wilms tumour) 39, 143, 486–8
nephropathy 268
  non-syndromic 487
Neuhauser syndrome 47
neural tube defects 392–5
neuroacanthosis 355
neurofibromatosis type 1 (NF1) 128, 136, 160, 162, 163, 224, 396–400, 470
  café-au-lait spots 210
  diagnostic criteria 396t

frequency of complications 398t
  glaucoma 328
neurofibromatosis type 2 (NF2) 65, 160, 210, 397, 470–1
neuronal ceroid lipofuscinoses 97, 233
neuronal migration disorders 156–8
Nicolaides–Baraitser syndrome 79, 257
Niemann–Pick disease type A 222
night blindness, congenital stationary 190
Nijmegen breakage syndrome (NBS) 304, 306
nomograms 684
non-accidental injury 252–3
non-disjunction 535f
non-syndromic Wilms tumour 486–7
Noonan syndrome 60–1, 79, 85, 198, 224, 243, 360, 402–3
Norrie disease 230–1, 328
nuchal scanning 598
nuchal translucency 618
nucleotide excision repair 304
nystagmus 190–1

O

obesity
  cancer risks 462
  with and without developmental delay 192–4
ocular albinism, X-linked 190
ocular colobomata 82
ocular hypertelorism 196–7
oculoauriculovertebral spectrum (Goldenhar syndrome) 109, 112–13, 175, 177, 201
oculocerebrocutaneous (Delleman) syndrome 113, 236
oculocutaneous albinism 126–7, 190
oculodentodigital dysplasia 183, 255
oculopharyngeal myopathy 224
oedema 198–9, 618–19
OEIS complex 43, 201, 566
oesophageal atresia 201
oesophageal cancer 450
Ohdo syndrome 225
Ohtahara syndrome 188, 314, 315
Okihiro syndrome (Duane radial ray syndrome) 100, 153, 228
oligophrenin-1 166
Ollier disease 161
Ommen syndrome 364
Opitz FG syndrome 165
Opitz syndrome 43–4, 76, 143, 165, 183, 196, 201
optic nerve hypoplasia 190, 204
optic nerve pathway tumours 398–9
oral contraceptive pill, in pregnancy 584
oral-facial-digital syndromes 215, 255
  type 1 183, 262
  type 2 183
  type Mohr (II) and Varadi (VI) 67
organic acidaemias 188
oromandibular–limb–hypogenesis syndrome 153, 175, 254
OSMED (Weissenbacher–Zweymüller syndrome) 414
osteodysplastic dwarfisms 172, 183
osteogenesis imperfecta (brittle bone disease) 122, 123, 139, 252, 572, 631
osteopathia striata 145
osteopetrosis 144, 145
osteoporosis 122
osteoporosis–pseudoglioma syndrome 123, 230
otopalatodigital syndrome 145
  type 1 (Taybi syndrome) 58
  type 2 215
ovarian cancer 426, 427, 472–3
  chance of identifying a BRCA1/2 mutation 472t
  criteria for defining high-risk women 472t
ovarian surveillance 435

overgrowth 113, 206
  see also macrocephaly
oxycephaly 212

P

pachonychia congenita 257
pachytene diagram 500, 501f, 502f
Paget disease, juvenile 145
Pallister–Hall syndrome 43, 131, 215
Pallister–Killian syndrome (tetrasomy 12p) 79, 514, 518, 578
palmar creases, transverse 180
pantothenate kinase-associated neurodegeneration syndrome 107
papillorenal syndrome 83
paracentric inversions 528
paragangliomas 478
parathyroid cancer, sporadic 467
parietal foramina syndrome 147, 236
Parkinson disease 355, 404–5
partial androgen insensitivity syndrome (PAIS) 40, 270
partial hydatidiform mole 556
Patau syndrome (trisomy 13) 534–5
paternity testing 688
Pearson syndrome 386
PEHO syndrome 67, 97, 198, 239
Pelizaeus–Merzbacher disease 151, 165–6, 191
Pena–Shokeir syndrome 177
Pendred syndrome 92
penetrance 6
pericentric inversions 528
periventricular nodular heterotopia 158, 421
Perlman syndrome 207, 487
permanent neonatal diabetes 298
peroneal muscular atrophy (hereditary motor and sensory neuropathy) 344–6, 349
peroxisomal disorders 65, 188
persistent hyperinsulinaemic hypoglycaemia of infancy 141
persistent hyperplastic primary vitreous 230
Perthes disease 414
Peter anomaly 46
Peutz–Jeghers syndrome 211, 450, 460, 474–6
Pfeiffer syndrome 58, 219, 289
phaeochromocytoma 478
phenylketonuria (PKU) 127
  maternal 614–15
phytosterolaemia 358
piebaldism 208
Pierre-Robin sequence 74
pigmented naevi 211
plagiocephaly 212–13
poikiloderma 211
Poland anomaly 153
polycystic kidney disease 262–3
polymerase chain reaction-based analyses 602
polymicrogyria 157, 158
polymorphisms 547
polyposis syndrome, juvenile 460–1
polysplenia syndrome 148
porencephalic cysts 643
postaxial acrofacial dysostosis syndrome 153
postaxial polydactyly 214–16
Potter sequence 175
Prader–Willi syndrome (del 15q11–13) 117, 119, 127, 192–3, 521
pre-implantation genetic diagnosis (PGD) 26, 568–9
pre-implantation genetic screening (PGS) 569
preaxial polydactyly 218–19
predictive testing 28
pregnancy
  anticonvulsant therapy during 590–1
  drugs in 584–5
  and fertility 565–644
premature ageing 65
premature osteoporosis 122
premature ovarian failure 620–1
prenatal chromosomal mosaicism 516–19

prenatal diagnosis, invasive techniques and genetic tests 600–3
primary AR microcephaly 172
Pringle disease (tuberous sclerosis) 208, 239, 262, 275, 420–3
prion disease 296
pro-opiomelanocortin 194
progressive myoclonic epilepsy 97, 239
prophylactic laparoscopic salpingo-oophorectomy 473
prophylactic mastectomy 428
prophylactic salpingo-oophorectomy 427
Proteus syndrome 128, 160, 207, 397
  diagnostic criteria 129t
proximal 11p deletion syndrome 147
proximal myotonic myopathy 388–9
Prune-belly syndrome 625
pseudoachondroplasia 57, 261
pseudo-autosomal inheritance 32
pseudocholinesterase deficiency 410
pseudohermaphrodism 143
pseudohypoaldosteronism 282–3
pseudohypoparathyroidism 193, 243
pseudomosaicism 516
pseudoTORCH syndrome 135, 172, 643
pseudotrisomy 13 131
pseudo-warfarin embryopathy 73
PTEN hamartoma tumour syndrome (PHTS) 442
ptosis 224
puberty, staging of 698
purine nucleoside phosphorylase deficiency 364
pycnodysostosis 144, 147
pyelectasis, mild 625
Pyle dysplasia 145
pyridoxine-dependent seizures 188

R

Rabson–Mendenhall syndrome 299
radial ray defects, and thumb hypoplasia 228–9
radiation-induced heritable diseases 622
radiological investigations 694
Raine syndrome 144
recessive disorders, molecular diagnosis 602
5α-reductase deficiency 40
Refsum syndrome 233
renal agenesis 624
renal cell carcinoma 485
renal coloboma syndrome 83
renal cysts 485
  and diabetes 262
renal tract anomalies 624–6
Rendu–Osler–Weber syndrome (hereditary haemorrhagic telangiectia) 342–3
Renpenning syndrome 165
reproductive fitness 6
reproductive options, for future pregnancies 26
retinal angioma, solitary 484
retinal blindness, congenital 406
retinal dysplasia 230–1
retinal receptor dystrophies 232–4
retinitis pigmentosa 232, 406–7
retinoblastoma 480–2
  Knudson's hypothesis 480f
retinoids, in pregnancy 584
retinopathy of prematurity (ROP) 230
Rett syndrome 97, 272, 408–9
rhesus D 592
rhizomelic chondrodysplasia punctata 73
ring chromosomal abnormalities 211
ring chromosomes 538–9
Roberts syndrome 154, 228, 229
Robertsonian translocation (13q;14q) 534, 540–2
Robin sequence 74, 174–5
Robinow syndrome 57, 58, 197
  autosomal recessive 147
rod monochromatism (achromatopsia) 190, 406

Romano–Ward syndrome 378
Rothmund–Thomson syndrome 209, 306
Roussy–Levy syndrome 53
rubella 628–9
Rubinstein–Taybi syndrome (RTS) 59, 131, 173, 183, 243
Russell–Silver syndrome 116, 129, 243, 631

S

sacral pits and dimples 180
sacrococcygeal teratoma 576
Saethre–Chotzen syndrome 183, 224, 289
sagittal synostosis 289
Sanfilippo syndrome 97
scalp defects 236–7
scaphocephaly 212
Schimke immuno-osseous dysplasia 211
Schinzel syndrome (Acrocallosal syndrome) 215, 219, 249, 250
Schinzel–Giedion syndrome 144
schizencephaly 157, 158, 239
Schwachman–Diamond syndrome 117
Schwartz–Jampel syndrome 389
sclerocornea 47
sclerosis 144
sclerosteosis 145
Seckel syndrome 172
  and microcephalic primordial dwarfism 631
SEDC (spondyloepiphyseal dysplasia congenita) 414
Segawa syndrome (dopa-responsive dystonia) 107, 349, 405
segmental neurofibromatosis type 1 (NF1) 397
seizures
  with developmental delay/mental retardation 238–40
  in neonates 186–9
semilobar holoprosencephaly 130
sensorineural deafness 90
septo-optic dysplasia (de Morsier's syndrome) 204, 243, 249
sequence, definition 4
Setleis syndrome 236
severe combined immunodeficiencies (SCID) 364
sex chromosome aneuploidy, prenatal diagnosis 536
sex chromosome mosaicism 544–5
sex reversal 40
shagreen patches 420
Shah–Waardenburg syndrome, with Hirschsprung disease 92
shaken baby syndrome 252
short limbs 630–2
short rib-polydactyly syndromes 214, 631–2
short stature 242–4
SHORT syndrome 46
Shprintzen syndrome (velocardiofacial syndrome) 76, 85, 175, 183, 366, 490–2, 521
  see also del (22q11), DiGeorge syndrome
sickle cell anaemia 335
sickle cell β-thalassaemia 336
Silver–Russell syndrome 116, 129, 243, 631
Simpson–Golabi–Behmel syndrome 79, 162, 165, 206, 215, 487, 578
single hypopigmented macule 208
site-specific colorectal cancer see hereditary nonpolyposis colorectal cancer
sitosterolaemia 358
situs ambiguus 148
situs inversus 148
situs solitus 148
skeletal dysplasia 139, 246–7, 631, 632
  charts 696–7
  investigation of fetus and baby with 678
  undiagnosed 572, 632
skewed X-inactivation 32, 34
skin, unusual 256–8
skin lesions

patchy hypomelanotic 208–9
patchy pigmented 210
skin pigmentation, generalized disorders 126–7
skull shape, abnormalities 212–13
small bowel carcinomas 436
Smith–Lemli–Opitz syndrome 39, 67, 73, 76, 85, 222, 225
  holoprosencephaly 131
  hypospadias 142–3
  microcephaly 172
  postaxial polydactyly 215
  short limbs 631
Smith–Magenis syndrome (del 17p11.2) 57, 79, 193, 521
smoking, cancer risk of smokers 462
somatic mosaicism 6
Sotos syndrome 162, 206
spastic cerebral palsy 70, 71
spastic paraplegia 2, X-linked 165–6
spina bifida
  recurrence risks 394f
  schematic drawings of various types 392f
spina bifida cystica 392
spina bifida occulta 392
spinal muscular atrophy 119, 412–13
spinocerebellar ataxia 50, 53, 355, 405
splice-site mutations 19
steatocystoma multiplex 160
Steinert disease (myotonic dystrophy) 54, 161, 224, 322, 388–90
steroid sulphatase deficiency 604
Stickler syndrome 65, 73, 76, 139, 175, 182, 380, 414–15
Sturge–Weber syndrome 328
subacute necrotizing encephalomyelpathy (Leigh encephalopathy) 372–3, 385
subcortical band heterotopia 158
subdural haemorrhage 252
submicroscopic chromosomal abnormalities, and the chromosomal phenotype 546–50
subtelomeric deletions, clinical features 548
subtelomeric rearrangements 547
sulphite oxidase deficiency 188
supernumerary marker chromosomes
  postnatal 552–3
  prenatal 554–5
suxamethonium sensitivity 410
syndactyly 254
syndrome, definition 4
synpolydactyly 254

T

talipes calcaneovalgus 574
talipes equinovarus 574
TAR (thrombocytopenia–absent radius syndrome) 153, 228
tardive dyskinesia 355
tauopathies 404
Taybi syndrome (Otopalatodigital syndrome type 1) 58
Teebi syndrome(s) 197
teeth, unusual 256–8
Teunissen–Cremers syndrome 59
α-thalassaemias 336
β-thalassaemias 335
thanatophoric dysplasia 260, 572, 631
Thomsen disease 389
thrombocytopenia–absent radius syndrome (TAR synrome) 153, 228
thrombophilia 416–18
thryoid cancer 467
thumb hypoplasia, radial ray defects and 228–9
Timothy syndrome 378
tinea versicolor 208
toes, 2, 3 syndactyly 180
torsion dystonia, autosomal dominant early-onset 106
Townes–Brock syndrome 43, 109, 113, 219
toxoplasmosis 634

tracheo-oesophageal fistula 200, 201
transcription-coupled repair 304
transient neonatal diabetes 298
translocations
  autosomal reciprocal 500–2
  familial autosomal reciprocal 504
  postnatal autosomal reciprocal 506
  prenatal autosomal reciprocal 508–9
  Robertsonian 534, 540–2
Treacher Collins syndrome 76, 92, 109, 113, 175
tremors, benign essential 405
trichorinophalangeal syndrome (TRPS, Langer-Giedion syndrome) 161, 183, 257,521
trichothiodystrophy 304–5, 306
trigonocephaly 212
Triple X syndrome (47, XXX) 494
triplet repeat mutations 19
triploid mosaicism 514
triploidy 255, 393, 556–7
trisomies, and congenital heart disease 85
trisomy 13 (Patau syndrome) 231, 487, 578, 625
trisomy 18 (Edwards' syndrome) 487, 578
trisomy 21 (Down syndrome) 524–5
TrkB 194
truncating mutations 19
tuberous sclerosis (tuberous sclerosis complex) 208, 239, 262, 275, 420–3
Turcot syndrome 444, 454
Turner syndrome 85, 198, 558–60, 586, 620
  mild 243
turricephaly 212
twins, genetic testing for MZ 29
twins and twinning 636–8
tylosis 450

U

Ullrich congenital muscular dystrophy 119
ulnar–mammary syndrome 153–4, 215
ultrasound scanning
  for prenatal diagnosis 598
  three-dimensional 598
ungual fibromata 420
uniparental disomy 21, 116, 193
upper GI endoscopy 434
urea cycle disorders 188
urticaria pigmentosa 211
Usher syndrome 92, 232

V

VACTERL association 86, 153
valproate, and fetal anticonvulsant syndrome 591
Van Buchem disease 145
Van der Woude syndrome 76
vanishing white matter disease 151
varicella (chickenpox) 640

vascular Ehlers–Danlos syndrome (EDS) 312–13
vascular malformations 147
VATER/VACTERL association 43, 201, 229, 624
velocardiofacial syndrome (Shprintzen syndrome) 76, 85, 175, 183, 366, 490–2, 521
  see also 22q11 deletion syndrome, del (22q11),, DiGeorge syndrome
ventriculomegaly (prenatal) 642–4
vesico-ureteric reflux 625–6
Virchow–Robin spaces 162
visceral heterotaxy 148
vitamin K deficiency 73
vitiligo 126, 208
von Hippel–Lindau disease 262, 484–5
  complications and frequency 484t
von Recklinghausen disease see neurofibromatosis type 1
von Willebrand disease 339

W

Waardenburg syndrome 91, 208, 352
Wagner hereditary vitreoretinopathy/erosive retinopathy 414
WAGR (Wilms tumour–aniridia–genitourinary anomalies–mental retardation) 39, 143, 486, 521
Walker–Warburg syndrome 67, 135, 157, 158, 177, 230, 643
warfarin, in pregnancy 584
warfarin embryopathy 73, 182
Watson syndrome 397, 402
Weaver syndrome 206
Weissenbacher–Zweymüller syndrome (OSMED) 414
Werdnig–Hoffmann disease 412
Werner syndrome 306
West syndrome 315
Wiedemann–Beckwith syndrome (Beckwith–Wiedemann syndrome) 61, 79, 128, 141, 206, 278, 487, 625
Wiedemann–Rautenstrauch syndrome 65
Wildervank syndrome 100
Williams syndrome (del 7q11.23) 79, 85, 117, 402, 521
Wilms tumour 39, 143, 486–8
Wilson disease 355
Wiskott–Aldrich syndrome 365
Witkop syndrome 256–7
Wolf–Hirschhorn syndrome (4p-) 82, 173, 183, 548
Wolfram syndrome 299

X

X inactivation 562
X-autosome translocations 562–3

X-inactivation patterns 34
X-linked adrenoleukodystrophy 151, 264–5, 349
  see also adrenoleukodystrophy
X-linked agammaglobulinaemia (Bruton disease) 365
X-linked α-thalassaemia mental retardation syndrome (ATR-X) 165, 182, 272
X-linked Alport syndrome 268
X-linked autism 166
X-linked blue cone monochromatism 190
X-linked chondrodysplasia punctata 32, 73
X-linked cleft palate and ankyloglossia 76
X-linked dominant (XLD) inheritance 32–3
X-linked dystonia parkinsonism 107
X-linked Emery–Dreifuss muscular dystrophy 375
X-linked hydrocephalus 135, 643
X-linked hyper-IgM syndrome (CD40 ligand deficiency) 365
X-linked hypohidrotic ectodermal dysplasia 256
X-linked ichthyosis (steroid sulphatase (STS) deficiency) 604
X-linked immunodeficiencies 366t
X-linked isolated lissencephaly XLIS 166
X-linked laterality sequence 148
X-linked lissencephaly with abnormal genitalia (XLAG) 157
X-linked lymphoproliferative syndrome (Duncan syndrome) 365
X-linked mental retardation 164–6
X-linked ocular albinism 190
X-linked recessive (XLR) inheritance 34–5
X-linked retinitis pigmentosa (XLRP) 407
X-linked retinoschisis, juvenile 231
X-linked semi-dominant disorder 32
X-linked semi-dominant inheritance 34
X-linked severe combined immunodeficiencies (SCID) 364
X-linked spastic paraplegia 2, 165–6
xanthogranuloma, and chronic myelogenous leukaemia 399
xeroderma pigmentosum (XP) 305, 306
XYY syndrome (47, XYY) 498–9

Y

Y chromosome anomalies 606–7
Yunis–Varon syndrome 257

Z

Zellweger syndrome 73, 88, 119, 147, 221–2, 233, 625

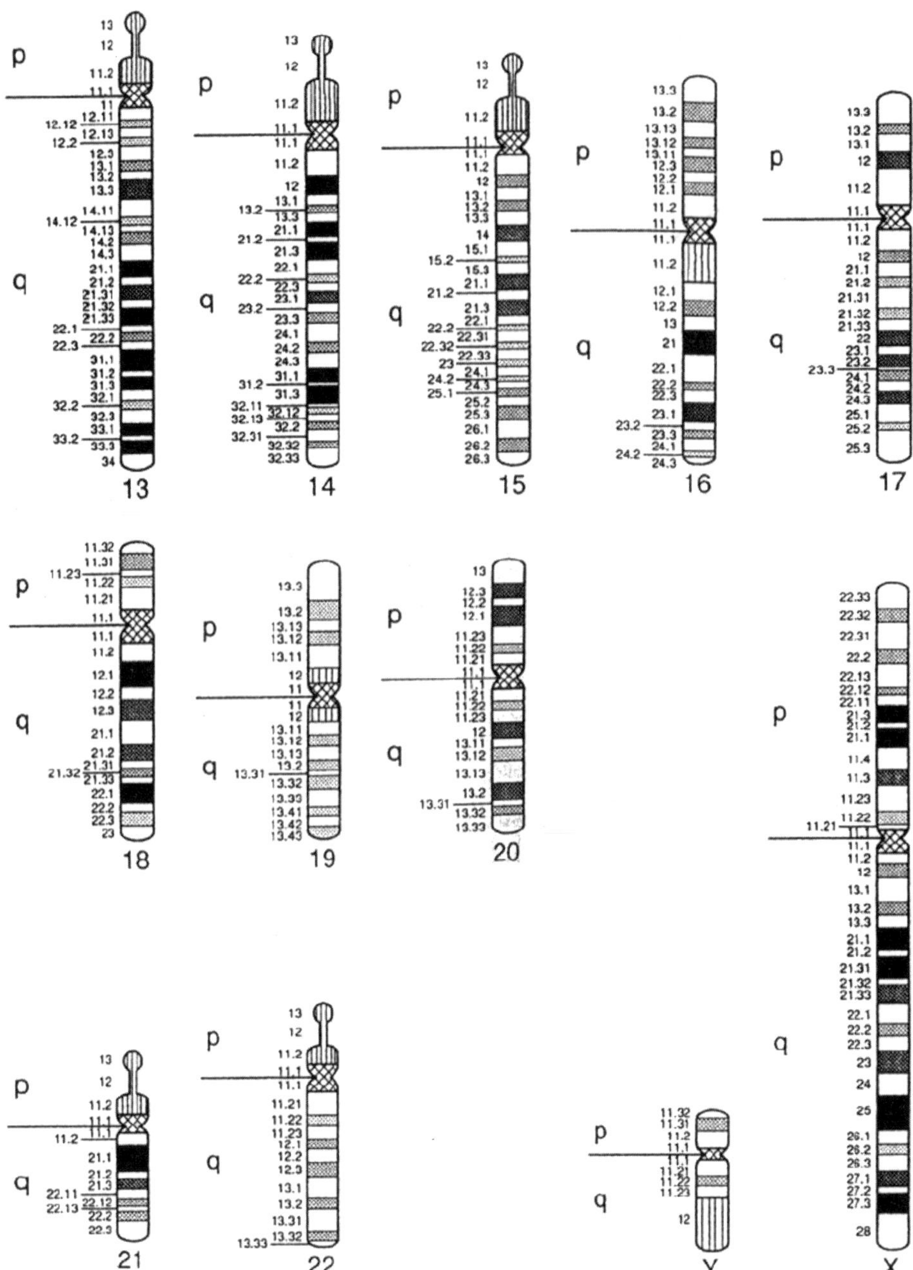

Figure *Continued*

Reference

Francke U. Digitized and differentially shaded human chromosome
  ideograms for genomic applications. *Cytogenet Cell Genet* 1994;
  65: 206–19.